AAOS

Comprehensive Orthopaedic Review

3

MW01056339

Wolters Kluwer

AAOS
American Academy of Orthopaedic Surgeons

AAOS Comprehensive Orthopaedic Review 3

Volume 2

EDITOR

Jay R. Lieberman, MD

Professor and Chairman
Department of Orthopaedic Surgery
Keck School of Medicine of USC
Los Angeles, California

Wolters Kluwer

AAOS
American Academy of Orthopaedic Surgeons

AAOS

AMERICAN ACADEMY OF ORTHOPAEDIC SURGEONS

Staff

American Academy of Orthopaedic Surgeons

Anna Salt Troise, MBA, *Chief Education Strategist*

Hans Koelsch, PhD, *Director, Publishing Partner Relationships*

Lisa Claxton Moore, *Senior Manager, Editorial*

Steven Kellert, *Senior Editor*

Wolters Kluwer Health

Brian Brown, *Director, Medical Practice*

Stacey Sebring, *Senior Development Editor*

Kerry McShane, *Senior Editorial Coordinator*

Jolene Carr, *Editorial Coordinator*

Erin Cantino, *Marketing Manager*

David Saltzberg, *Senior Production Project Manager*

Stephen Druding, *Design Coordinator*

Beth Welsh, *Senior Manufacturing Coordinator*

TNQ Technologies, *Prepress Vendor*

ISBN 978-1-9751-2717-6

Library of Congress Control Number: Cataloging in Publication data available on request from publisher.

Printed in China

Published 2020 by the
American Academy of Orthopaedic Surgeons
9400 West Higgins Road
Rosemont, IL 60018

Bone and Joint Initiative USA

RRS1909

Acknowledgments

Editorial Board, AAOS Comprehensive Orthopaedic Review, Third Edition

Kenneth Egol, MD *(Trauma)*
Joseph E. Milgram Professor of Orthopedic Surgery
Vice Chair for Education
Department of Orthopedic Surgery
NYU Langone Orthopedic Hospital
NYU School of Medicine
New York, New York

Geoffrey Marecek, MD *(Trauma)*
Assistant Professor of Clinical Orthopaedic Surgery
Department of Orthopaedic Surgery
Keck School of Medicine of USC
Los Angeles, California

Kurt Spindler, MD *(Sports Medicine)*
Orthopaedic Surgeon
Cleveland Clinic
Garfield Heights, Ohio

Seth Gamradt, MD *(Sports Medicine)*
Director of Orthopaedic Athletic Medicine
Associate Clinical Professor of Orthopaedic Surgery
Department of Orthopaedic Surgery
Keck School of Medicine of USC
Los Angeles, California

Jonathan G. Schoenecker, MD, PhD *(Pediatrics)*
Associate Professor of Orthopaedic Surgery
Jeffrey W. Mast Chair in Orthopaedics Trauma and Hip Surgery
Vanderbilt School of Medicine
Nashville, Tennessee

Rachel Y. Goldstein, MD, MPH *(Pediatrics)*
Assistant Professor, Pediatric Orthopaedics
Children's Hospital Los Angeles
Keck School of Medicine of USC
Los Angeles, California

Jeffrey E. Martus, MD, MS *(Pediatrics)*
Associate Professor, Orthopaedic Surgery
Vanderbilt University Medical Center
Nashville, Tennessee

Kristy L. Weber, MD *(Oncology)*
Chief of Orthopaedic Oncology
Department of Orthopaedic Surgery
University of Pennsylvania
Philadelphia, Pennsylvania

Peter S. Rose, MD *(Oncology)*
Professor of Orthopedic Surgery
Mayo Clinic
Rochester, Minnesota

Eric W. Tan, MD *(Foot and Ankle)*
Assistant Professor of Clinical Orthopaedic Surgery
Department of Orthopaedic Surgery
Keck School of Medicine of USC
Los Angeles, California

Jeremy J. McCormick, MD *(Foot and Ankle)*
Associate Professor, Orthopaedic Surgery
Director, Foot and Ankle Fellowship Program
Department of Orthopaedic Surgery
Washington University School of Medicine
St. Louis, Missouri

Contributors

Oussama Abousamra, MD
Assistant Professor
Department of Orthopaedic Surgery
Children's Hospital Los Angeles
Keck School of Medicine of USC
Los Angeles, California

Yousef Abu-Amer, PhD
Professor
Department of Orthopedic Surgery
Department of Cell Biology & Physiology
Washington University School of Medicine
St. Louis, Missouri

Samuel B. Adams, MD
Co-Chief, Division of Foot and Ankle Surgery
Director of Foot and Ankle Research
Assistant Professor
Department of Orthopaedic Surgery
Duke University Medical Center
Durham, North Carolina

Christopher S. Ahmad, MD
Professor of Orthopaedic Surgery
Department of Orthopaedic Surgery
Columbia University College of Physicians and Surgeons
New York, New York

Jay C. Albright, MD
Assistant Professor, CU Orthopedics
Surgical Director, Sports Medicine Center
Children's Hospital Colorado

Alexander W. Aleem, MD, MSc
Assistant Professor
Department of Orthopaedic Surgery
Washington University in St. Louis, School of Medicine
St. Louis, Missouri

Ram K. Alluri, MD
Resident Physician
Department of Orthopaedic Surgery
Keck School of Medicine of USC
Los Angeles, California

Annunziato Amendola, MD
Professor
Department of Orthopaedics
Duke University Hospitals
Durham, North Carolina

Steven M. Andelman, MD
Department of Orthopaedic Surgery
University of Connecticut
Farmington, Connecticut

John G. Anderson, MD
Orthopedic Associates of Michigan
Professor, Michigan State University College of Human Medicine
Professor, Michigan State University College of Osteopathic Medicine
Co-Director, Grand Rapids Orthopedic Foot and Ankle Fellowship Program
Assistant Program Director, Grand Rapids Spectrum Orthopedic Residency
Grand Rapids, Michigan

Paul A. Anderson, MD
Professor
Department of Orthopedics and Rehabilitation
University of Wisconsin-Madison
Madison, Wisconsin

Jack Andrish, MD
Retired Consultant
Department of Orthopaedic Surgery
Cleveland Clinic
Cleveland, Ohio

Shawn G. Anthony, MD, MBA
Assistant Professor
Department of Orthopedics
Mount Sinai Health System
New York, New York

Robert A. Arciero, MD
Professor
Department of Orthopaedic Surgery
University of Connecticut
Farmington, Connecticut

Elizabeth A. Arendt, MD
Professor and Vice Chair
Department of Orthopaedic Surgery
University of Minnesota
Minneapolis, Minnesota

George S. Athwal, MD, FRCSC
Professor
Department of Surgery
Western Ontario University
London, Ontario, Canada

Reed A. Ayers, MS, PhD
Research Assistant Professor
Department of Orthopedics
University of Colorado
Anschutz Medical Campus
Aurora, Colorado

Donald S. Bae, MD
Associate Professor
Department of Orthopaedic Surgery
Harvard Medical School
Boston Children's Hospital
Boston, Massachusetts

Hyun W. Bae, MD
Professor of Surgery
Department of Orthopaedic Surgery
Cedars-Sinai Medical Center
Director of Education
Cedars-Sinai Spine Center
Los Angeles, California

Keith Baldwin, MD, MSPT, MPH
Assistant Professor
Department of Orthopedic Surgery
Children's Hospital of Philadelphia
Philadelphia, Pennsylvania

Paul Beaulé, MD, FRCSC
Professor of Surgery
Division of Division of Orthopedics
Department of Surgery
University of Ottawa
Ottawa, Ontario, Canada

Kathleen S. Beebe, MD
Professor
Department of Orthopaedics
Rutgers New Jersey Medical School
Newark, New Jersey

John-Erik Bell, MD, MS
Associate Professor
Shoulder, Elbow, and Sports Medicine
Department of Orthopaedic Surgery
Dartmouth-Hitchcock Medical Center
Lebanon, New Hampshire

Gregory C. Berlet, MD
Orthopedic Foot and Ankle Center
Worthington, Ohio

Bruce Beynnon, PhD
Professor of Orthopedics and Director of Research
Department of Orthopedics and Rehabilitation
University of Vermont
Burlington, Vermont

Mohit Bhandari, MD, PhD, FRCSC
Professor and Academic Head
Department of Surgery
Division of Orthopaedic Surgery
McMaster University
Hamilton, Ontario, Canada

Jesse E. Bible, MD
Assistant Professor
Department of Orthopaedics
Penn State Health Medical Center
Hershey, Pennsylvania

Ryan T. Bicknell, MD, MSc, FRCS(C)
Associate Professor
Departments of Surgery and Mechanical and Materials Engineering
Queen's University
Kingston, Ontario, Canada

Allen T. Bishop, MD
Professor
Department of Orthopedic Surgery
Department of Neurosurgery
Mayo Clinic
Rochester, Minnesota

Philip E. Blazar, MD
Associate Professor
Department of Orthopaedic Surgery
Brigham and Women's Hospital
Harvard Medical School
Boston, Massachusetts

Andrew Bodrogi, MD, FRCSC
Department of Surgery
University of Ottawa
Ottawa, Ontario, Canada

Donald R. Bohay, MD, FACS
Co-Director, Grand Rapids Orthopaedic Foot and Ankle Fellowship
Orthopaedic Surgeon
Orthopaedic Associates of Michigan
Grand Rapids, Michigan

Frank C. Bohnenkamp, MD
OrthoIllinois
Algonquin, Illinois

Michael P. Bolognesi, MD
Professor
Department of Orthopaedic Surgery
Duke University Health System
Durham, North Carolina

Martin I. Boyer, MD, MSc, FRCS(C)
Carol B. and Jerome T. Loeb Professor of Orthopaedic Surgery
Co-Chief, Hand & Microsurgery Service
Department of Orthopaedic Surgery
Washington University School of Medicine
St. Louis, Missouri

Robert H. Brophy, MD
Professor
Department of Orthopaedic Surgery
Washington University School of Medicine
St. Louis, Missouri

Lance M. Brunton, MD
Excela Health Orthopaedics and Sports Medicine
Latrobe, Pennsylvania

William D. Bugbee, MD
Associate Professor
Director of Lower Extremity Reconstruction Fellowship
Department of Orthopaedic Surgery
Scripps Clinic
La Jolla, California

Zorica Buser, PhD
Assistant Professor of Research Orthopaedic Surgery and Neurological Surgery
Department of Orthopaedic Surgery
Keck School of Medicine of USC
Los Angeles, California

Sean V. Cahill, BA
Medical Research Associate
Department of Orthopaedics & Rehabilitation
Yale School of Medicine
New Haven, Connecticut

Kevin M. Casey, MD
Orthopaedic Surgeon
Kaiser Permanente Riverside Medical Center
Riverside, California

Thomas D. Cha, MD, MBA
Assistant Professor, Orthopedic Surgery
Harvard Medical School
Massachusetts General Hospital
Boston, Massachusetts

Peter N. Chalmers, MD
Assistant Professor
Department of Orthopaedic Surgery
University of Utah
Salt Lake City, Utah

Thomas J. Christensen, MD
Orthopaedic Surgeon
Reno Orthopaedic Clinic
Reno, Nevada

John C. Clohisy, MD
Professor
Department of Orthopedic Surgery
Washington University School of Medicine
St. Louis, Missouri

Peter A. Cole, MD
Division Medical Director for HealthPartners Orthopaedic Medical Group
Chair, Department of Orthopaedics, Regions Hospital
Professor, University of Minnesota Medical School
St. Paul, Minnesota

D. Nicole Deal, MD
Assistant Professor
Department of Orthopaedic Surgery
University of Virginia
Charlottesville, Virginia

Malcolm R. DeBaun, MD
Orthopaedic Surgery Resident
Department of Orthopaedic Surgery
Stanford University School of Medicine
Palo Alto, California

Niloofar Dehghan, MD, MSc, FRCS(C)
Assistant Professor
Department of Orthopaedic Surgery
University of Arizona College of Medicine – Phoenix
The CORE Institute
Phoenix, Arizona

Christopher Del Balso, BSc, MSc, MBBS, FRCSC
Lecturer/MD
Department of Surgery
Division of Orthopaedic Surgery
Western Ontario University
London, Ontario, Canada

Alejandro Gonzalez Della Valle, MD
Professor of Clinical Orthopaedic Surgery
Department of Orthopedic Surgery
Weill Cornell Medicine
Hospital for Special Surgery
New York, New York

Craig J. Della Valle, MD
Professor of Orthopaedic Surgery
Chief, Division of Adult Reconstructive Surgery
Rush University Medical Center
Chicago, Illinois

Gregory S. DiFelice, MD
Associate Professor
Department of Orthopedic Surgery
Weill Cornell Medicine
Hospital for Special Surgery
New York, New York

Benedict F. DiGiovanni, MD, FAOA
Professor
Department of Orthopaedics and Rehabilitation
University of Rochester School of Medicine and Dentistry
Rochester, New York

Jon Divine, MD, MS
Associate Professor of Orthopedics and Sports Medicine
Department of Orthopedics
University of Cincinnati Medical Center
Cincinnati, Ohio

Seth D. Dodds, MD
Associate Professor, Hand and Upper Extremity Surgery
Associate Program Director, Department of Orthopaedics
University of Miami, Miller School of Medicine
Miami, Florida

Warren R. Dunn, MD, MS
Professor
Department of Orthopaedic Surgery
University of Iowa
Iowa City, Iowa

Mark E. Easley, MD
Co-Chief, Division of Foot and Ankle Surgery
Assistant Professor
Department of Orthopaedic Surgery
Duke University Medical Center
Durham, North Carolina

Kenneth A. Egol, MD
Joseph E. Milgram Professor of Orthopedic Surgery
Vice Chair for Education
Department of Orthopaedic Surgery
NYU School of Medicine
New York, New York

Howard R. Epps, MD
Associate Professor
Department of Orthopaedic Surgery
Baylor College of Medicine
Texas Children's Hospital
Houston, Texas

Greg Erens, MD
Assistant Professor
Department of Orthopaedic Surgery
Emory University
Atlanta, Georgia

Blake A. Eyberg, MD
Resident Physician
Department of Orthopaedic Surgery
University of Arizona College of Medicine – Phoenix
Phoenix, Arizona

Robert Warne Fitch, MD
Assistant Professor
Vanderbilt Sports Medicine
Vanderbilt University Medical Center
Nashville, Tennessee

Valerie A. Fitzhugh, MD
Associate Professor, Pathology
Department of Pathology and Laboratory Medicine
Rutgers New Jersey Medical School
Newark, New Jersey

Jared R. H. Foran, MD
Director Total Joint Arthroplasty, OrthoColorado Hospital
Panorama Orthopaedics and Spine Center
Golden, Colorado

Frank J. Frassica, MD
Former Chairman
Department of Orthopedics
Johns Hopkins University
Baltimore, Maryland

Nathan L. Frost, MD
Pediatric Orthopaedic Surgeon
Mary Bridge Children's Hospital
Tacoma, Washington

Mark J. Gage, MD
Assistant Professor
Department of Orthopaedic Surgery
Division of Orthopaedic Trauma
Duke University
Durham, North Carolina

Alexia G. Gagliardi, BA
Research Assistant
Musculoskeletal Research Center
Children's Hospital Colorado
Aurora, Colorado

Braden Gammon, MD, MSc, FRCSC
Assistant Professor
Division of Orthopaedic Surgery
Department of Surgery
University of Ottawa
Ottawa, Ontario, Canada

Steven R. Gammon, MD
Orthopaedic Surgeon, Rocky Mountain Orthopaedic Associates
Director of Orthopaedic Trauma
St. Mary's Hospital Regional Medical Center
Grand Junction, Colorado

Joshua L. Gary, MD, FAOA
Associate Professor
Department of Orthopaedic Surgery
McGovern Medical School at UTHealth Houston
Houston, Texas

Charles L. Getz, MD
Associate Professor
The Rothman Institute
The Sidney Kimmel Medical College at Thomas Jefferson University
Philadelphia, Pennsylvania

Arash Ghaffari, MD
Clinical Instructor of Orthopaedic Surgery
Department of Orthopaedic Surgery
Keck School of Medicine of USC
Los Angeles, California

Joshua Allan Gillis, MD
Department of Plastic and Reconstructive Surgery
Maine General Medical Center
Augusta, Maine

Vijay K. Goel, PhD
Professor
Department of Bioengineering
University of Toledo
Toledo, Ohio

Charles A. Goldfarb, MD
Professor and Vice Chair
Department of Orthopedic Surgery
Washington University School of Medicine
St. Louis, Missouri

David Goss Jr, DO
Orthopedic Foot and Ankle Center
Worthington, Ohio

Gregory Gramstad, MD
Rebound Orthopedics
Portland, Oregon

Jonathan N. Grauer, MD
Professor
Department of Orthopaedics
Yale School of Medicine
New Haven, Connecticut

Amitava Gupta, MD, FRCS
Clinical Professor
Department of Orthopedic Surgery
University of Louisville
Louisville, Kentucky

Rajnish K. Gupta, MD
Associate Professor
Department of Anesthesiology
Vanderbilt University Medical Center
Nashville, Tennessee

Ranjan Gupta, MD
Professor of Orthopaedic Surgery, Anatomy & Neurobiology, and Biomedical Engineering
University of California, Irvine
Irvine, California

Raymond J. Hah, MD
Assistant Professor
Department of Orthopaedic Surgery
Keck School of Medicine of USC
Los Angeles, California

Andrea Halim, MD
Assistant Professor
Orthopedic Surgery
Yale School of Medicine
New Haven, Connecticut

David A. Halsey, MD
Associate Professor
Department of Orthopaedics and Rehabilitation
University of Vermont College of Medicine
Burlington, Vermont

Mark Halstead, MD
Assistant Professor
Department of Orthopedics and Pediatrics
Washington University
St. Louis, Missouri

Adam Halverson, DO
Orthopedic Foot and Ankle Center
Worthington, Ohio

Nady Hamid, MD
Shoulder & Elbow Center
OrthoCarolina
Charlotte, North Carolina

Erik N. Hansen, MD
Associate Professor
Department of Orthopaedic Surgery
University of California
San Francisco, California

Carl M. Harper, MD
Instructor
Department of Orthopaedic Surgery
Harvard Medical School
Boston, Massachusetts

Carolyn M. Hettrich, MD, MPH
Adjunct Professor
Department of Orthopedic Surgery
University of Kentucky
Lexington, Kentucky

Timothy E. Hewett, PhD
Director of Research
Department of Sports Health and Performance Instruction
The Ohio State University
Columbus, Ohio

Alan S. Hilibrand, MD
Joseph and Marie Field Professor of Spinal Surgery
The Rothman Institute
Jefferson Medical College
Philadelphia, Pennsylvania

Jason E. Hsu, MD
Assistant Professor
Department of Orthopaedics & Sports Medicine
University of Washington
Seattle, Washington

Clifford B. Jones, MD, FACS
Orthopaedic Traumatologist
Banner University Medical Center
Phoenix, Arizona

Morgan H. Jones, MD, MPH
Staff Physician
Department of Orthopaedic Surgery
Cleveland Clinic
Cleveland, Ohio

Christopher C. Kaeding, MD
Judson-Wilson Professor
Department of Orthopaedics
The Ohio State University Wexner Medical Center
Columbus, Ohio

Joseph B. Kahan, MD
Orthopaedic Surgery Resident, Yale-New Haven Hospital
Department of Orthopaedics & Rehabilitation
Yale University School of Medicine
New Haven, Connecticut

Sanjeev Kakar, MD, FAOA
Professor of Orthopaedic Surgery
Mayo Clinic
Rochester, Minnesota

Robin Kamal, MD
Assistant Professor
Chase Hand and Upper Limb Center
Department of Orthopaedic Surgery
Stanford University
Stanford, California

Linda E. A. Kanim, MA
Clinical and Translational Research
Spine Center
Cedars-Sinai Medical Center
Los Angeles, California

Robert M. Kay, MD
Vice Chief
Children's Orthopaedic Center
Children's Hospital Los Angeles
Los Angeles, California

Mary Ann Keenan, MD
Professor
Department of Orthopaedic Surgery
University of Pennsylvania
Philadelphia, Pennsylvania

Jay D. Keener, MD
Professor
Chief Shoulder and Elbow Service
Fellowship Director, Shoulder and Elbow Reconstruction
Department of Orthopaedic Surgery
Washington University School of Medicine
St. Louis, Missouri

James A. Keeney, MD
Chief, Adult Hip and Knee Reconstruction Service
Missouri Orthopaedic Institute
Associate Professor
University of Missouri School of Medicine
Columbia, Missouri

Brian A. Kelly, MD
Assistant Professor
Department of Orthopaedic Surgery
Washington University School of Medicine in St. Louis
St. Louis, Missouri

Michael Patrick Kelly, MD, MSc
Associate Professor of Orthopedic Surgery
Associate Professor of Neurological Surgery
Department of Orthopedic Surgery
Washington University, School of Medicine
St. Louis, Missouri

Safdar N. Khan, MD
The Benjamin R. and Helen Slack Wiltberger Endowed Chair in Orthopaedic Spine Surgery
Associate Professor and Chief of Division of Spine
Department of Orthopaedics
Adjunct Associate Professor, Department of Integrated Systems Engineering
Clinical Faculty, Spine Research Institute
The Ohio State University Wexner Medical Center
Columbus, Ohio

Vickas Khanna, MD, MHA, FRCSC
Assistant Professor, MacOrtho Program Director
Department of Surgery
McMaster University
Hamilton, Ontario, Canada

Michael L. Knudsen, MD
Assistant Professor of Orthopaedic Surgery
Department of Orthopaedic Surgery
University of Minnesota Medical School
Minneapolis, Minnesota

Jessica M. Kohring, MD
Northwest Orthopaedic Specialists
Spokane, Washington

Sanjit R. Konda, MD
Assistant Professor
Department of Orthopaedic Surgery
NYU School of Medicine
New York, New York

Marc S. Kowalsky, MD, MBA
Shoulder & Elbow Surgery
Orthopaedic & Neurosurgery Specialists
ONS Foundation for Clinical Research & Education
Greenwich, Connecticut

John E. Kuhn, MD, MS
Kenneth D. Schermerhorn Professor of Orthopaedic Surgery
Department of Orthopaedic Surgery
Vanderbilt University Medical Center
Nashville, Tennessee

Nikhil Kulkarni, MS
Research and Development Engineer
Department of Product Development
Medtronic Spine & Biologics
Memphis, Tennessee

Adam J. La Bore, MD
Associate Professor
Department of Orthopedic Surgery
Washington University in St. Louis
St. Louis, Missouri

Paul M. Lafferty, MD
Orthopedic Trauma and Adult Reconstruction
Twin Cities Orthopedics
North Memorial Medical Center
Robbinsdale, Minnesota

Mario Lamontagne, PhD
Emeritus Professor of Biomechanics
Faculty of Health Sciences
University of Ottawa
Ottawa, Ontario, Canada

Christian Lattermann, MD
Associate Professor
Director
Center for Cartilage Repair and Restoration
Department of Orthopaedic Surgery
University of Kentucky
Lexington, Kentucky

Melissa Leber, MD
Associate Professor
Departments of Orthopedics and Emergency Medicine
Mount Sinai Health System
New York, New York

Adam K. Lee, MD
Assistant Professor
Department of Orthopaedic Surgery
Keck School of Medicine of USC
Los Angeles, California

Daniel J. Lee, MD
Department of Orthopaedic Surgery
Washington University School of Medicine
St. Louis, Missouri

Francis Y. Lee, MD, PhD
Wayne O. Southwick Professor of Orthopaedics and Rehabilitation
Department of Orthopaedics & Rehabilitation
Yale School of Medicine
New Haven, Connecticut

Simon Lee, MD
Associate Professor
Department of Orthopedic Surgery
Rush University Medical Center
Chicago, Illinois

Yu-Po Lee, MD
Clinical Professor
Department of Orthopaedic Surgery
UC Irvine
Orange, California

James P. Leonard, MD
Orthopaedic Surgeon
Shoulder Reconstruction, Arthroscopy and Sports Medicine
Midwest Orthopaedic Consultants
Clinical Instructor, University of Illinois at Chicago
Chicago, Illinois

Philipp Leucht, MD
Associate Professor, Orthopaedic Surgery and Cell Biology
NYU School of Medicine
New York, New York

Fraser J. Leversedge, MD
Associate Professor
Department of Orthopaedic Surgery
Duke University
Durham, North Carolina

Bo Li, MD, PhD
Visiting Research Scientist
Department of Orthopaedics & Rehabilitation
Yale School of Medicine
New Haven, Connecticut

Jun Li, MD, PhD
Associate Professor
Department of Microbial Pathogenesis
Yale School of Medicine
New Haven, Connecticut

David G. Liddle, MD
Assistant Professor
Vanderbilt Sports Medicine
Vanderbilt University Medical Center
Nashville, Tennessee

Jay R. Lieberman, MD
Professor and Chairman
Department of Orthopaedic Surgery
Keck School of Medicine of USC
Los Angeles, California

Johnny Lin, MD
Assistant Professor
Department of Orthopedic Surgery
Rush University Medical Center
Chicago, Illinois

Dieter M. Lindskog, MD
Associate Professor
Department of Orthopaedics and Rehabilitation
Yale School of Medicine
New Haven, Connecticut

Frank A. Liporace, MD
Chairman and Vice President, Department of Orthopaedic Surgery
Chief, Division of Orthopaedic Trauma & Adult Reconstruction
Jersey City Medical Center - RWJBarnabas Health
Jersey City, New Jersey

Mario H. Lobao, MD
Fellow, Shoulder and Elbow Surgery
Department of Orthopaedic Surgery
MedStar Union Memorial Hospital
Baltimore, Maryland

David W. Lowenberg, MD
Clinical Professor
Department of Orthopaedic Surgery
Stanford University School of Medicine
Palo Alto, California

Scott J. Luhmann, MD
Professor
Department of Orthopedic Surgery
Washington University
St. Louis, Missouri

C. Benjamin Ma, MD
Professor
Vice Chair, Adult Clinical Operations
Chief, Sports Medicine and Shoulder Surgery
University of California, San Francisco
San Francisco, California

Robert A. Magnussen, MD
Assistant Professor
Department of Orthopaedic Surgery
The Ohio State University Medical Center
Columbus, Ohio

David R. Maish, MD
Chief, Adult Reconstruction (Central/South)
Geisinger Musculoskeletal Institute
Danville, Pennsylvania

Randall J. Malchow, MD
Associate Professor
Department of Anesthesiology
Vanderbilt University Medical Center
Nashville, Tennessee

Azeem Tariq Malik, MBBS
Spine Research Fellow
Division of Spine
Department of Orthopaedics
The Ohio State University Wexner Medical Center
Columbus, Ohio

Peter J. Mandell, MD
Assistant Clinical Professor
Department of Orthopaedic Surgery
University of California, San Francisco
San Francisco, California

P. Kaveh Mansuripur, MD
Department of Orthopedic Surgery
The Permanente Medical Group
Oakland, California

Geoffrey S. Marecek, MD
Assistant Professor of Clinical Orthopaedic Surgery
Keck School of Medicine of USC
Los Angeles, California

Robert G. Marx, MD, MSc, FRCSC
Professor
Department of Orthopedic Surgery
Weill Cornell Medicine
New York, New York

Bogdan A. Matache, MD, CM, FRCSC
Clinical Fellow
Department of Surgery
Western Ontario University
London, Ontario, Canada

Matthew J. Matava, MD
Professor
Department of Orthopedic Surgery
Washington University
St. Louis, Missouri

Travis H. Matheney, MD, MLA
Assistant Professor
Orthopaedic Surgery
Boston Children's Hospital
Harvard Medical School
Boston, Massachusetts

Stephanie W. Mayer, MD
Assistant Professor
Department of Orthopedic Surgery
University of Colorado
Denver, Colorado

Augustus D. Mazzocca, MS, MD
Professor
Department of Orthopaedic Surgery
University of Connecticut
Farmington, Connecticut

David R. McAllister, MD
Professor
Department of Orthopaedic Surgery
David Geffen School of Medicine at UCLA
Los Angeles, California

Christopher M. McAndrew, MD, MSc
Associate Professor
Department of Orthopaedic Surgery
Washington University in St. Louis
St. Louis, Missouri

Eric C. McCarty, MD
Chief, Sports Medicine
University of Colorado
Boulder, Colorado

Michael D. McKee, MD, FRCS(C)
Professor and Chairman, Department of Orthopaedic Surgery
University of Arizona College of Medicine – Phoenix
The CORE Institute
Phoenix, Arizona

Ross E. McKinney Jr, MD
Professor
Department of Pediatrics
Duke University School of Medicine
Durham, North Carolina

Michael J. Medvecky, MD
Section Chief of Sports Medicine
Associate Professor
Department of Orthopaedics & Rehabilitation
Yale School of Medicine
New Haven, Connecticut

Erin Meisel, MD
Attending Surgeon
Children's Orthopaedic Center
Children's Hospital Los Angeles
Los Angeles, California

Steve Melton, MD
Assistant Professor
Department of Anesthesiology
Duke University Medical Center
Durham, North Carolina

Gary A. Miller, MD
Associate Professor
Department of Orthopedic Surgery/VA
Washington University School of Medicine
St. Louis, Missouri

Timothy L. Miller, MD
Associate Professor
Department of Orthopaedics
The Ohio State University Wexner Medical Center
Columbus, Ohio

Nicole Montgomery, MD
Assistant Professor
Department of Orthopaedic Surgery
Baylor College of Medicine
Texas Children's Hospital
Houston, Texas

Richard E. Moon, MD, FRCPC, FACP, FCCP
Professor of Anesthesiology
Professor of Medicine
Duke University Medical Center
Durham, North Carolina

Steven L. Moran, MD
Professor of Orthopedic and Plastic Surgery
Department of Orthopedic Surgery
Mayo Clinic
Rochester, Minnesota

Steven J. Morgan, MD
Orthopaedic Traumatologist
Mountain Orthopaedic Trauma Surgeons
Swedish Medical Center
Englewood, Colorado

Thomas Edward Mroz, MD
Director, Center for Spine Health
Director, Spine Research Lab
Center for Spine Health
Departments of Orthopaedic and Neurological Surgery
Cleveland Clinic
Cleveland, Ohio

Raman Mundi, MD, MSc, PhD(c), FRCSC
Assistant Professor
Department of Surgery
University of Toronto
Toronto, Ontario, Canada

Margaret Siobhan Murphy-Zane, MD
Assistant Professor, Department of Orthopedic Surgery
University of Colorado School of Medicine
Children's Hospital Colorado
Denver, Colorado

Anand M. Murthi, MD
Chief, Shoulder and Elbow Surgery
Director, Shoulder and Elbow Research
Department of Orthopaedic Surgery
MedStar Union Memorial Hospital
Baltimore, Maryland

Denis Nam, MD, MSc
Associate Professor
Department of Orthopaedic Surgery
Rush University Medical Center
Chicago, Illinois

Surena Namdari, MD, MSc
Associate Professor of Orthopaedic Surgery
Director of Shoulder & Elbow Research
Rothman Orthopaedic Institute - Thomas Jefferson University
Philadelphia, Pennsylvania

Jeffrey J. Nepple, MD
Assistant Professor, Orthopaedic Surgery
Director, Young Athlete Center
Department of Orthopaedic Surgery
Washington University School of Medicine
St. Louis, Missouri

Wendy M. Novicoff, PhD
Assistant Professor
Department of Public Health Sciences
University of Virginia
Charlottesville, Virginia

Ryan M. Nunley, MD
Associate Professor and Fellowship Director
Joint Preservation, Resurfacing and Replacement Service
Washington University Orthopedics
Barnes Jewish Hospital
Chesterfield, Missouri

Reza Omid, MD
Associate Program Director
Associate Professor of Orthopedic Surgery
Shoulder & Elbow Surgery/Sports Medicine
Keck Medical Center of USC
Los Angeles, California

Christopher Ornelas, MD
Assistant Professor
Department of Orthopaedic Surgery
Keck School of Medicine of USC
Los Angeles, California

Peter J. Ostergaard, MD
Harvard Combined Orthopaedic Residency Program
Department of Orthopaedic Surgery
Massachusetts General Hospital
Boston, Massachusetts

Thomas Padanilam, MD
Toledo Orthopaedic Surgeons
Toledo, Ohio

Don Young Park, MD
Assistant Professor
Department of Orthopaedic Surgery
David Geffen School of Medicine at UCLA
Los Angeles, California

Richard D. Parker, MD
Professor
Department of Orthopedic Surgery
The Ohio State University College of Medicine
Cleveland, Ohio

Michael L. Parks, MD
Associate Professor of Clinical Orthopaedic Surgery
Department of Orthopedic Surgery
Weill Cornell Medicine
Hospital for Special Surgery
New York, New York

Javad Parvizi, MD, FRCS
Professor
Department of Orthopaedic Surgery
Rothman Institute at Thomas Jefferson University
Philadelphia, Pennsylvania

Rina P. Patel, MD
Assistant Professor
Department of Radiology
University of California, San Francisco
San Francisco, California

Brendan M. Patterson, MD, MPH
Assistant Professor
Department of Orthopedics and Rehabilitation
University of Iowa
Iowa City, Iowa

Tony Pedri, MD
Instructor, Orthopaedic Trauma Fellow
Department of Orthopaedics
Regions Hospital, University of Minnesota
St. Paul, Minnesota

Terrence Philbin, DO
Orthopedic Foot and Ankle Center
Worthington, Ohio

Gregory J. Pinkowsky, MD
Department of Orthopaedic Surgery
Summit Medical Group
West Orange, New Jersey

Kornelis Poelstra, MD, PhD
The Robotic Spine Institute of Silicon Valley
OrthoNorCal, Inc
Los Gatos, California

Gregory G. Polkowski, MD
Assistant Professor
Department of Orthopaedic Surgery
University of Connecticut Health Center
Farmington, Connecticut

Steven M. Raikin, MD
Professor
Department of Orthopaedic Surgery
Chief, Foot and Ankle Division
Rothman Institute at Thomas Jefferson University Hospital
Sydney Kimmel Medical School at Jefferson University
Philadelphia, Pennsylvania

Sean S. Rajaee, MD
Assistant Professor of Adult Reconstruction
Department of Orthopaedic Surgery
Cedars Sinai Medical Center
Los Angeles, California

David R. Richardson, MD
Associate Professor
Department of Orthopaedic Surgery
University of Tennessee-Campbell Clinic
Memphis, Tennessee

E. Greer Richardson, MD
Professor
Department of Orthopaedic Surgery
University of Tennessee-Campbell Clinic
Memphis, Tennessee

Michael D. Ries, MD
Arthroplasty Fellowship Director
Reno Orthopaedic Clinic
Reno, Nevada

K. Daniel Riew, MD
Professor, Orthopedic Surgery
Columbia University Medical Center
New York, New York

David C. Ring, MD, PhD
Associate Dean for Comprehensive Care
Department of Surgery and Perioperative Care
University of Texas at Austin Dell Medical School
Austin, Texas

Marco Rizzo, MD
Professor of Orthopedic Surgery
Department of Orthopedic Surgery
Mayo Clinic
Rochester, Minnesota

Scott B. Rosenfeld, MD
Associate Professor
Department of Orthopaedic Surgery
Baylor College of Medicine
Texas Children's Hospital
Houston, Texas

Tamara D. Rozental, MD
Chief, Hand and Upper Extremity Surgery
Professor of Orthopaedic Surgery
Department of Orthopaedic Surgery
Harvard Medical School
Beth Israel Deaconess Medical Center
Boston, Massachusetts

Khaled J. Saleh, MD, MSc, FRCSC, MHCM
Professor and Chairman
Division of Orthopaedic Surgery
Southern Illinois University School of Medicine
Springfield, Illinois

Vincent James Sammarco, MD
Orthopaedic Surgeon
OrthoCincy Orthopaedics & Sports Medicine
Cincinnati, Ohio

David W. Sanders, MD, MSc, FRCSC
Professor
Department of Surgery
Division of Orthopaedic Surgery
Western Ontario University
London, Ontario, Canada

Anthony A. Scaduto, MD
Professor and Executive Vice Chair
Department of Orthopaedic Surgery
University of California, Los Angeles
Orthopaedic Institute for Children
Los Angeles, California

Shadley C. Schiffern, MD
Shoulder & Elbow Center
OrthoCarolina
Charlotte, North Carolina

Perry L. Schoenecker, MD
Professor
Department of Orthopaedic Surgery
Washington University School of Medicine
St. Louis, Missouri

John A. Scolaro, MD, MA
Associate Professor
Department of Orthopaedic Surgery
University of California, Irvine
Orange, California

Jon K. Sekiya, MD
Professor Emeritus
Department of Orthopedic Surgery
University of Michigan
Ann Arbor, Michigan

Ritesh R. Shah, MD
Chief
Orthopedic Surgery
Advocate Illinois Masonic Medical Center
Illinois Bone and Joint Institute
Chicago, Illinois

Arya Nick Shamie, MD
Professor & Chief of Spine Surgery
Vice Chair of International Affairs
Department of Orthopaedic Surgery
David Geffen School of Medicine at UCLA
Los Angeles, California

Alexander Y. Shin, MD
Professor
Department of Orthopedic Surgery
Department of Neurosurgery
Mayo Clinic
Rochester, Minnesota

Allen K. Sills, MD, FACS
Chief Medical Officer, National Football League
Professor of Neurological Surgery
Department of Neurological Surgery
Vanderbilt University Medical Center
Nashville, Tennessee

Kern Singh, MD
Professor
Department of Orthopedic Surgery
Rush Medical College
Chicago, Illinois

David L. Skaggs, MD, MMM
Children's Hospital Endowed Chair of Pediatric Spinal Disorders
Chief of Orthopaedic Surgery
Children's Hospital Los Angeles
Professor of Orthopaedic Surgery
Keck School of Medicine of USC
Los Angeles, California

Matthew V. Smith, MD
Assistant Professor
Department of Sports Medicine
Department of Orthopedics
Washington University in St. Louis
St. Louis, Missouri

Michael D. Smith, MD
Department of Orthopaedic Surgery
Emory University
Atlanta, Georgia

Gary Solomon, PhD
Professor of Neurological Surgery (Retired)
Department of Neurological Surgery
Vanderbilt University Medical Center
Nashville, Tennessee

Nelson Fong Soohoo, MD
Associate Professor
Department of Orthopaedic Surgery
David Geffen School of Medicine at UCLA
Los Angeles, California

Samantha A. Spencer, MD
Immediate Past President, Massachusetts Orthopaedic Association
Assistant Professor of Orthopaedic Surgery
Department of Orthopaedic Surgery
Harvard Medical School
Staff Physician, Boston Children's Hospital
Boston, Massachusetts

Robert J. Spinner, MD
Professor
Department of Neurosurgery
Department of Orthopedic Surgery
Mayo Clinic
Rochester, Minnesota

Michael P. Steinmetz, MD
Chairman
Department of Neurological Surgery
Case Western Reserve University/MetroHealth Medical Center
Cleveland, Ohio

Daniel J. Stinner, MD, FACS
Assistant Professor
Department of Orthopaedic Surgery
Vanderbilt University Medical Center
Nashville, Tennessee

Karen M. Sutton, MD
Associate Attending
Department of Orthopedics
Hospital for Special Surgery
New York, New York

Robert Z. Tashjian, MD
Ezekiel R. Dumke, Jr. Presidential Endowed Professor
Department of Orthopedic Surgery
University of Utah School of Medicine
Salt Lake City, Utah

Ross Taylor, MD
Orthopaedic Surgeon
McLeod Orthopaedics Seacoast
Little River, South Carolina

Nirmal C. Tejwani, MD
Professor
Department of Orthopaedic Surgery
NYU School of Medicine
New York, New York

Stavros Thomopoulos, PhD
Robert E. Carroll and Jane Chace Carroll Professor
Professor of Biomechanics (in Orthopedic Surgery and Biomedical Engineering)
Director of Carroll Laboratories for Orthopedic Surgery
Vice Chair of Basic Research in Orthopedic Surgery
Columbia University
New York, New York

Vidyadhar V. Upasani, MD
Associate Professor
Department of Orthopedic Surgery
University of California San Diego
Rady Children's Hospital San Diego
San Diego, California

Gary F. Updegrove, MD
Assistant Professor
Penn State Bone and Joint Institute
Penn State Milton S. Hershey Medical Center
Hershey, Pennsylvania

Arya G. Varthi, MD
Assistant Professor
Department of Orthopaedics and Rehabilitation
Yale School of Medicine
New Haven, Connecticut

Kenneth M. Vaz, MD
Lower Extremity Reconstruction Fellow
Department of Orthopaedic Surgery
Scripps Clinic
San Diego, California

Armando F. Vidal, MD
Associate Clinical Professor
Department of Orthopaedics
The Steadman Clinic
Vail, Colorado

Jeffrey C. Wang, MD
Chief, Orthopaedic Spine Service
Co-Director USC Spine Center
Professor of Orthopaedic Surgery and Neurosurgery
USC Spine Center
Keck School of Medicine of USC
Los Angeles, California

Jeffry T. Watson, MD
Assistant Professor
Department of Orthopaedic Surgery
Vanderbilt University
Nashville, Tennessee

Kristy L. Weber, MD
Chief of Orthopaedic Oncology
Department of Orthopaedic Surgery
University of Pennsylvania
Philadelphia, Pennsylvania

David S. Wellman, MD
Assistant Professor
Department of Orthopedic Surgery
New York Medical College
Valhalla, New York

Samuel S. Wellman, MD
Associate Professor
Department of Orthopaedic Surgery
Duke University Health System
Durham, North Carolina

Peter G. Whang, MD, FACS
Associate Professor
Department of Orthopaedics and Rehabilitation
Yale School of Medicine
New Haven, Connecticut

Glenn N. Williams, PT, PhD, ATC
Associate Professor
Department of Physical Therapy and Rehabilitation Science
University of Iowa
Iowa City, Iowa

Seth K. Williams, MD
Associate Professor
Orthopedic Surgery
University of Wisconsin
Madison, Wisconsin

Brian R. Wolf, MD, MS
Professor
Department of Orthopaedic Surgery
University of Iowa
Iowa City, Iowa

Rick W. Wright, MD
Department Chair, Orthopaedic Surgery
Vanderbilt University Medical Center
Nashville, Tennessee

Raymond D. Wright Jr, MD
Associate Professor
Orthopaedic Traumatology
Orthopaedic Surgery and Sports Medicine
University of Kentucky College of Medicine
Lexington, Kentucky

Dane K. Wukich, MD
Professor and Chair
Department of Orthopaedic Surgery
University of Texas Southwestern Medical Center
Dallas, Texas

Jae Hyuk Yang, MD, PhD
Associate Professor
Department of Orthopaedic Surgery
Korea University Guro Hospital
Seoul, Korea

Richard S. Yoon, MD
Director, Orthopaedic Research
Division of Orthopaedic Trauma and Adult Reconstruction
Department of Orthopaedic Surgery
Jersey City Medical Center - RWJBarnabas Health
Jersey City, New Jersey

S. Tim Yoon, MD, PhD
Associate Professor
Department of Orthopaedic Surgery
Emory University
Atlanta, Georgia

Jim A. Youssef, MD
Orthopedic Spine Surgeon
Spine Colorado
Durango, Colorado

Elizabeth Yu, MD
Associate Professor
Division of Spine
Department of Orthopaedics
The Ohio State University Wexner Medical Center
Columbus, Ohio

Warren D. Yu, MD
Associate Professor and Chief of the Spine Section
Department of Orthopaedic Surgery
The George Washington University Hospital
Washington, DC

Preface

The third edition of *AAOS Comprehensive Orthopaedic Review* is both a significant step forward and a continuation of work done in previous editions. The first edition was published in 2009 and the second in 2014. This edition encompasses the fundamental knowledge of orthopaedic surgery, as well as a comprehensive review of the past 5 years of published literature and expanded coverage of topics that are becoming increasingly significant. With that in mind, seven completely new chapters have been added: Minimally Invasive Spine Surgery; Spinal Imaging; Biologics and Current Applications; Disorders of the Scapula; Geriatric Trauma; Compartment Syndrome; and Rib Cage Fractures and Flail Chest.

Like the second edition, the third edition is composed of 11 distinct sections, organized by subspecialty. The content is consistently structured in an outline format, allowing for rapid recall of material and streamlined readability. Each chapter concludes with 10 to 12 bibliographic entries and *Top Testing Facts,* which are designed as not only a "memory jogger" for the reader but also represent the information in the chapter that one would most likely be tested on.

All the chapters have been written by experts in each subject and rigorously reviewed. This text could not have been completed without the dedication and excellent work of the section editors: Matthew P. Abdel, MD; Paul A. Anderson, MD; Asheesh Bedi, MD; Kenneth Egol, MD; Brian Feeley, MD; Leesa M. Galatz, MD; Seth Gamradt, MD; Rachel Y. Goldstein, MD, MPH; Christopher Got, MD; Raymond Hah, MD; Jay D. Keener, MD; Geoffrey Marecek, MD; Jeffrey E. Martus, MD, MS; Jeremy J. McCormick, MD; Reza Omid, MD; Frank Petrigliano, MD; Peter S. Rose, MD; Jonathan G. Schoenecker, MD, PhD; Kurt Spindler, MD; Bryan Springer, MD; Eric W. Tan, MD; Kristy L. Weber, MD; and Jennifer Moriatis Wolf, MD. Many thanks and appreciation to the chapter authors who contributed their time to this important educational publication.

It is my hope that students, residents, and fellows preparing for board examinations and other tests will find that this edition is a comprehensive review text that provides a user-friendly way to enhance their orthopaedic knowledge. In addition, the text presents all orthopaedic surgeons with concise broad-based knowledge that they can use in their practices. Best of luck to everyone in their studies and careers.

Jay R. Lieberman, MD
Professor and Chairman
Department of Orthopaedic Surgery
Keck School of Medicine of USC
Los Angeles, California

Contents

VOLUME 2

Section 6 Shoulder and Elbow

Section 11 Oncology

Section 6

Shoulder and Elbow

Section Editors | JAY KEENER, MD
REZA OMID, MD

Chapter 69

Anatomy of the Shoulder, Arm, and Elbow

GREGORY GRAMSTAD, MD

I. SHOULDER

A. Osteology

1. Clavicle

   a. The clavicle is the first bone to ossify (fifth week of gestation); it is the only long bone to ossify by intramembranous ossification.

   b. The medial (sternal) epiphysis is the last ossification center to fuse, at age 20 to 25 years.

   c. The primary blood supply is periosteal; no nutrient artery is present.

2. Scapular body—The scapula has only one true diarthrodial articulation, the acromioclavicular (AC) joint.

   a. Normal shoulder motion is approximately two-thirds glenohumeral and one third scapulothoracic.

   b. Ossification of the scapular body begins at the eighth week of gestation.

   c. The scapular spine is an osseous ridge that separates the supraspinatus and infraspinatus fossae.

   d. The acromion has three ossification centers: the metacromion (base), the mesoacromion (middle), and the preacromion (tip). Failure of fusion results in os acromiale.

   e. The relationship between the acromial anatomy and rotator cuff disease remains controversial. The classification of acromial morphology (flat, curved, or hooked) is challenged by poor interobserver reliability.

3. Coracoid process

   a. The coracobrachialis muscle and the short head of the biceps tendon originate from the coracoid process.

   b. The pectoralis minor muscle inserts onto the medial coracoid process.

   c. The relationship between coracoid morphology and subscapularis tears is controversial.

4. Glenoid

   a. The subchondral bone of the glenoid is relatively flat; the articular concavity is augmented by cartilage and a circumferential labrum.

   b. The glenoid averages 5° of retroversion in relation to the axis of the scapular body.

5. Superior shoulder suspensory complex (SSSC)

   a. The SSSC provides a stable connection between the scapula and the axial skeleton.

   b. The SSSC is composed of the glenoid, the coracoid process, the coracoclavicular ligaments, the distal clavicle, the AC joint, and the acromion (**Figure 1**).

   c. The superior strut comprises the middle clavicle; the inferior strut comprises the lateral scapular border/spine of the scapula.

6. Proximal humerus

   a. The proximal humerus has three centers of ossification: the humeral head (4 to 6 months), the greater tuberosity (1 to 3 years), and the lesser tuberosity (3 to 5 years). They fuse to the shaft at age 17 to 20 years.

   b. The humeral head averages 19° of retroversion and 41° of inclination (neck-shaft angle).

   c. The greater and lesser tuberosities serve as attachment sites for the rotator cuff tendons.

Dr. Gramstad or an immediate family member is a member of a speakers' bureau or has made paid presentations on behalf of Acumed and serves as a paid consultant to or is an employee of Acumed.

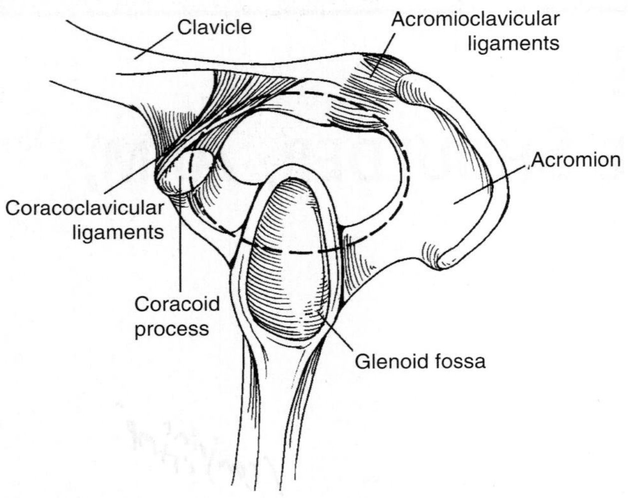

Figure 1 Illustration shows the bone–soft-tissue ring of the superior shoulder suspensory complex (dashed circle), lateral view. (Reproduced from Goss TP: Scapular fractures and dislocations: Diagnosis and treatment. *J Am Acad Orthop Surg* 1995;3[1]:22-33.)

d. The anterolateral ascending branch of the anterior humeral circumflex artery provides the primary blood supply to the humeral head. It travels proximally in the lateral aspect of the intertubercular groove. The terminal intraosseous portion of the artery enters at the proximal aspect of the intertubercular groove as the arcuate artery.

B. Joints and ligaments

1. Sternoclavicular (SC) joint
   a. The SC joint is the only true diarthrodial articulation between the upper appendicular and axial skeletons.
   b. The posterior SC joint capsule and ligaments are the primary stabilizers to anterior and posterior translation of the medial clavicle.
2. AC joint
   a. The AC joint is a small diarthrodial joint with an interposed fibrocartilaginous disk.
   b. The superior and posterior AC ligaments are the primary stabilizers to anterior and posterior (horizontal) translation of the clavicle.
   c. The coracoclavicular ligaments (conoid: medial; trapezoid: lateral) are the primary stabilizers to superior (vertical) translation of the distal clavicle.
3. Glenohumeral joint
   a. Dynamic stabilizers—The rotator cuff stabilizes the joint via joint compression. Positioning of the scapulothoracic joint also contributes to dynamic stability.
   b. Static stabilizers include articular congruity, the glenoid labrum, concavity-compression, negative intra-articular pressure, and the glenohumeral capsule and ligaments. The glenoid labrum provides concavity and up to 50% of marginal glenoid socket depth.
   c. The rotator interval is defined medially by the base of the coracoid, superiorly by the supraspinatus tendon, and inferiorly by the subscapularis tendon.
   d. The rotator interval contains the coracohumeral (CH) ligament, the superior glenohumeral ligament (SGHL), and the intra-articular portion of the long head of the biceps tendon. Laxity of the rotator interval results in inferior laxity (the sulcus sign), and contracture of the interval is seen with adhesive capsulitis.
   e. The CH ligament restricts external rotation in adduction, and it is a static restraint to inferior and posterior translation in adduction and external rotation.
   f. The SGHL is a primary static restraint against anterior translation with the arm at the side. With the CH ligament, the SGHL forms a pulley that provides restraint against medial subluxation of the long head of the biceps tendon.
   g. The middle glenohumeral ligament (MGHL) is a primary static restraint against anterior translation with the arm in external rotation and 45° of abduction.
   h. The anterior band of the inferior glenohumeral ligament (AB-IGHL) is a primary static restraint against anterior-inferior dislocation of the glenohumeral joint in 90° of abduction and external rotation (position of apprehension).
   i. The posterior band of the IGHL (PB-IGHL) is a primary static restraint against posterior-inferior translation in internal rotation and adduction.
4. Intrinsic scapular ligaments
   a. The superior transverse scapular ligament arises from the medial base of the coracoid overlying the suprascapular notch. The suprascapular artery runs superior to the ligament; the nerve runs deep to the ligament. Entrapment of the suprascapular nerve here causes denervation of both the supraspinatus and the infraspinatus.

6 | Shoulder and Elbow

TABLE 1

Musculature of the Shoulder Girdle

Muscle	Origin	Insertion	Innervation	Action
Trapezius	Spine	Scapular spine, acromion, clavicle	Cranial nerve XI	Scapular elevation
Latissimus dorsi	Spine	Humerus	Thoracodorsal	Extension, adduction, internal rotation
Serratus anterior	Ribs	Scapula	Long thoracic	Scapular stability
Pectoralis major	Anterior ribs, sternum, clavicle	Humerus	Medial/lateral pectoral	Adduction, internal rotation
Pectoralis minor	Anterior ribs	Coracoid	Medial pectoral	Scapular protraction
Deltoid	Scapular spine, acromion, clavicle	Humerus	Axillary	Abduction
Teres major	Scapula	Humerus	Lower subscapular	Extension, adduction, internal rotation
Subscapularis	Scapula	Lesser tuberosity	Upper/lower subscapular	Stability, internal rotation
Supraspinatus	Scapula	Greater tuberosity	Suprascapular	Stability, elevate, external rotation
Infraspinatus	Scapula	Greater tuberosity	Suprascapular	Stability, external rotation
Teres minor	Scapula	Greater tuberosity	Axillary	Stability, external rotation

b. The spinoglenoid ligament overlies the suprascapular nerve at the spinoglenoid notch. Entrapment, traction, or compression here causes denervation of the infraspinatus alone.

c. Coracoacromial ligament—This ligament originates from the lateral coracoid to insert on the anterior and lateral acromion.

C. Musculature of the shoulder girdle (**Table 1**)

D. Nerves

1. The brachial plexus is organized into roots, trunks, divisions, cords, and branches (**Figure 2**).

2. Axillary nerve (posterior cord)

a. The axillary nerve courses inferior to the glenohumeral joint, adjacent to the capsule, and is closest to the glenoid labrum at the 6 o'clock position on the glenoid, at an average of 12 mm.

b. The axillary nerve exits the axilla posteriorly, with the posterior humeral circumflex artery, through the quadrilateral space (medial: long head of triceps; lateral: humeral shaft; superior: teres minor; inferior: teres major) before dividing into anterior and posterior branches (**Figure 3**).

c. The posterior branch terminates into a muscular branch to the teres minor and a sensory branch to the skin overlying the lateral deltoid (superior lateral brachial cutaneous nerve). Loss of sensation over the lateral deltoid can signify palsy of the teres minor.

d. The muscular branch supplying the teres minor lies closest to the glenoid labrum and is most susceptible to injury during arthroscopic capsular procedures.

e. The anterior branch courses along the undersurface and innervates the deltoid muscle.

f. On average, the anterior branch to the deltoid is located 5 to 6 cm distal to the midlateral acromial margin, although it can be found as close as 3 cm. This distance is positively correlated to limb length; it is reduced by up to 30% with abduction of the arm to 90°.

3. Musculocutaneous nerve (lateral cord)

a. The main trunk penetrates the coracobrachialis muscle 3 to 8 cm distal to the tip of the coracoid.

b. It innervates the biceps brachii and the brachialis.

c. It terminates as the lateral antebrachial cutaneous nerve to the anterolateral forearm.

4. Suprascapular nerve (preclavicular branch)

a. This nerve transverses through the suprascapular notch (under the superior transverse scapular ligament), where it innervates the supraspinatus.

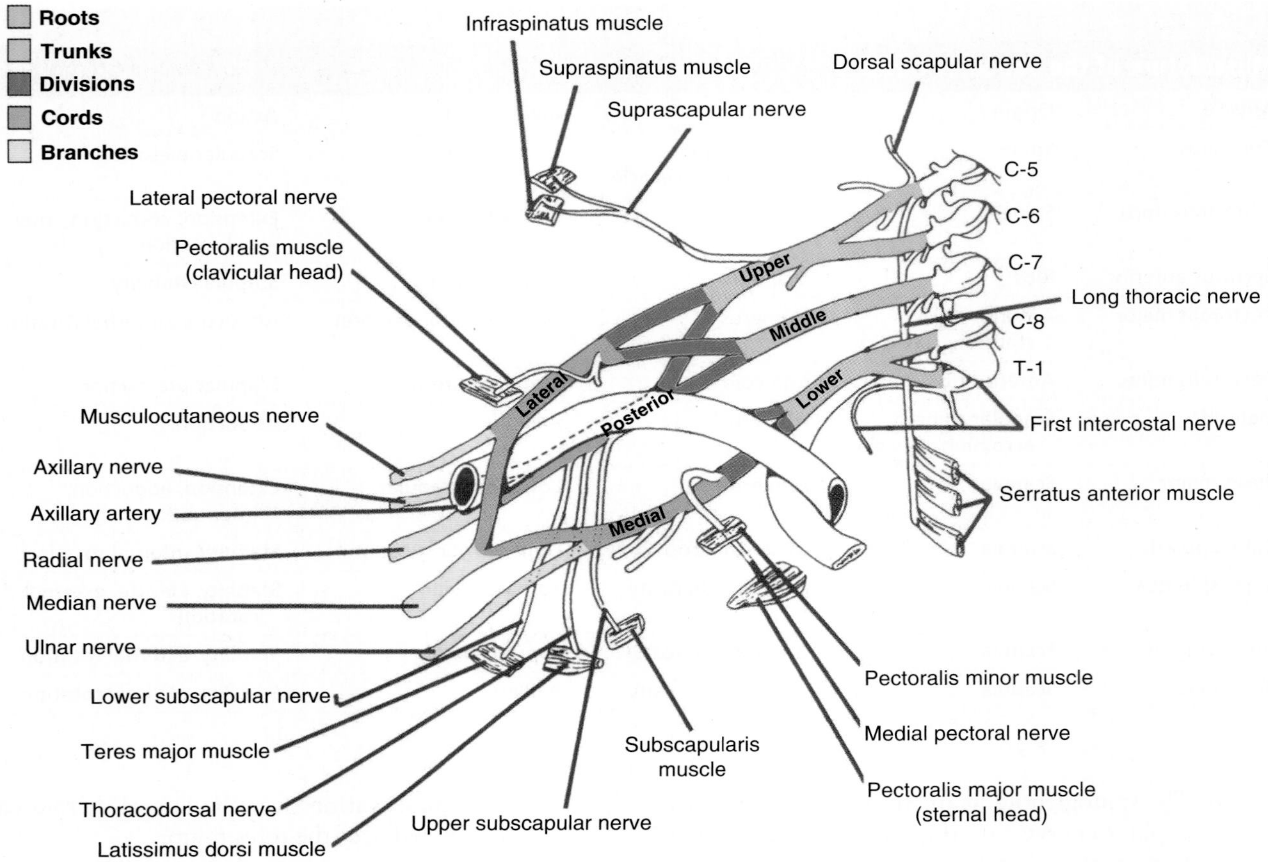

Figure 2 Illustration depicts the brachial plexus and its terminal branches. (Adapted from Thompson WO, Warren RF, Barnes RP, Hunt S: Shoulder injuries, in Schenck RC Jr, ed: *Athletic Training and Sports Medicine*, ed 3. Rosemont, IL, American Academy of Orthopaedic Surgeons, 1999, p 231.)

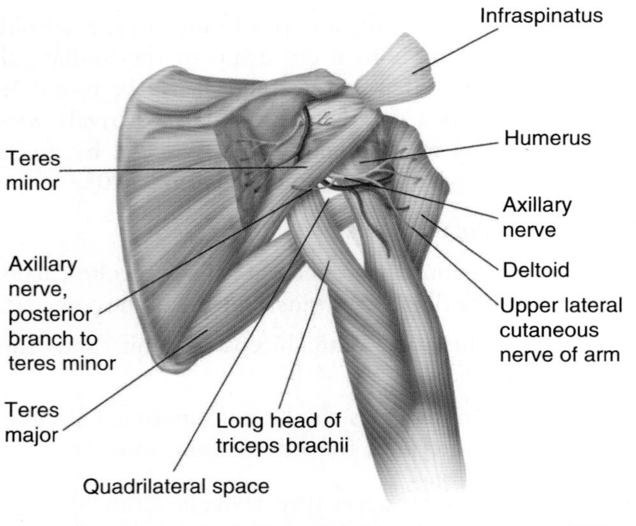

Figure 3 Illustration shows muscles and nerves of the posterior aspect of the shoulder.

b. Posteriorly, it traverses the spinoglenoid notch to innervate the infraspinatus.

c. It is found approximately 1.5 cm medial to the posterior rim of the glenoid and can be endangered in this location with transglenoid fixation techniques.

d. Suprascapular nerve compression at the suprascapular notch causes denervation of both the supraspinatus and the infraspinatus. Nerve compression at the spinoglenoid notch leads to selective denervation of the infraspinatus muscle.

e. Traction injury may occur from repetitive overhead activity or secondary to a retracted rotator cuff tear. Space-occupying lesions (eg, large perilabral cysts) can cause a direct compression injury, typically at the spinoglenoid notch.

5. Long thoracic nerve (preclavicular branch)—Injury (from axillary dissection or aggressive retraction of the middle scalene muscle) results in serratus anterior palsy and medial winging of the scapula (superior elevation of the scapula with medial translation and medial rotation of the inferior pole of the scapula).
6. Spinal accessory nerve (cranial nerve XI)—Injury (from cervical lymph node biopsy or radical neck dissection) results in trapezius palsy and lateral winging of the scapula (depression of the scapula with lateral translation and lateral rotation of the inferior pole of the scapula).

E. Arteries—The axillary artery is divided into three segments by the pectoralis minor muscle.

1. First part
    a. Found medial to the pectoralis minor muscle
    b. Has one branch: the superior thoracic artery
2. Second part
    a. Found deep to the pectoralis minor muscle
    b. Has two branches: the thoracoacromial trunk and the lateral thoracic artery
3. Third part
    a. Found lateral to the pectoralis minor muscle
    b. Has three branches: the subscapular artery (the circumflex scapular branch runs through the triangular space), the anterior humeral circumflex artery (the anterolateral ascending branch is the major blood supply to the humeral head), and the posterior humeral circumflex artery (accompanies the axillary nerve and exits posteriorly through the quadrilateral space) (**Figure 4**)

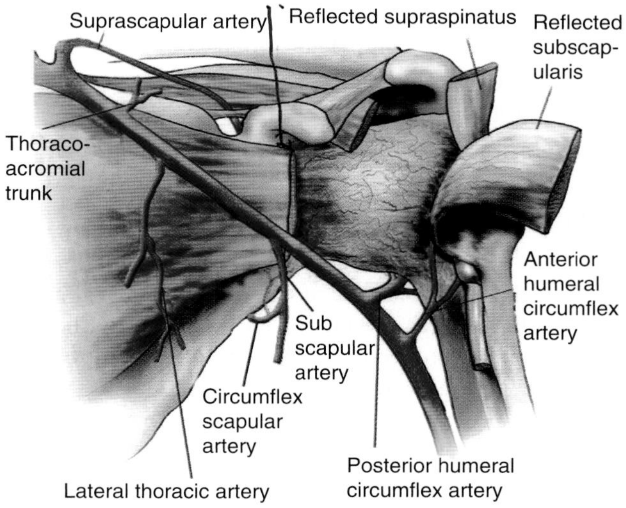

Figure 4 Illustration shows the vascularity of the anterior shoulder. (Adapted with permission from Andary JL, Petersen SA: The vascular anatomy of the glenohumeral capsule and ligaments: An anatomic study. *J Bone Joint Surg Am* 2002;84:2258-2265.)

F. Surgical approaches

1. Deltopectoral approach
    a. This is the workhorse approach to the shoulder.
    b. It uses the internervous plane between the deltoid (axillary nerve) and the pectoralis major (medial and lateral pectoral nerves) muscles.
    c. The cephalic vein is usually present in the interval.
    d. The clavipectoral fascia overlies the conjoined tendon (coracobrachialis and short head of the biceps) and the subscapularis.
    e. The musculocutaneous nerve is at risk for retraction injury medially.
    f. The axillary nerve (posterior cord of the brachial plexus) can be palpated on the anterior-inferior surface of the subscapularis, medial to the coracoid.
    g. The anterior circumflex humeral artery travels along the inferior subscapularis between the upper two-thirds and the inferior one-third (muscular portion).
2. Posterior approach
    a. The posterior approach is used most commonly for posterior capsular shift procedures and repair of glenoid fractures. Latissimus dorsi release (for transfer) can also be performed with this approach. The radial nerve lies anterior to the latissimus dorsi insertion on the humerus and is at risk of injury with tendon release.
    b. Identification of the quadrilateral space protects the axillary nerve and the posterior circumflex humeral artery.
    c. This approach uses the internervous plane between the teres minor (axillary nerve) inferiorly and the infraspinatus (suprascapular nerve) superiorly.
3. Lateral approach
    a. The lateral approach is commonly used for repair of the rotator cuff and greater tuberosity fractures.

b. A mini-open approach to the shoulder uses a deltoid split. The axillary nerve branch to the anterior deltoid is at risk of injury in this approach.

c. Alternatively, the deltoid is detached from the anterolateral acromion for wider exposure.

G. Arthroscopic anatomy of the shoulder

1. The long head of the biceps brachii exits the joint in the lateral aspect of the rotator interval and is stabilized against medial subluxation by the subscapularis (deep fibers) and a pulley composed of the CH ligament and the SGHL.

2. The superior biceps–labral anchor complex is anchored to the supraglenoid tubercle. A mobile and/or meniscoid superior glenoid labrum associated with an extension of articular cartilage over the superior glenoid rim can be a normal variant and must be differentiated from a traumatic disruption of the superior labrum (superior labral anterior to posterior [SLAP] tear) from bone.

3. The region of the anterosuperior labrum and MGHL origin has wide anatomic variability (**Figure 5**).

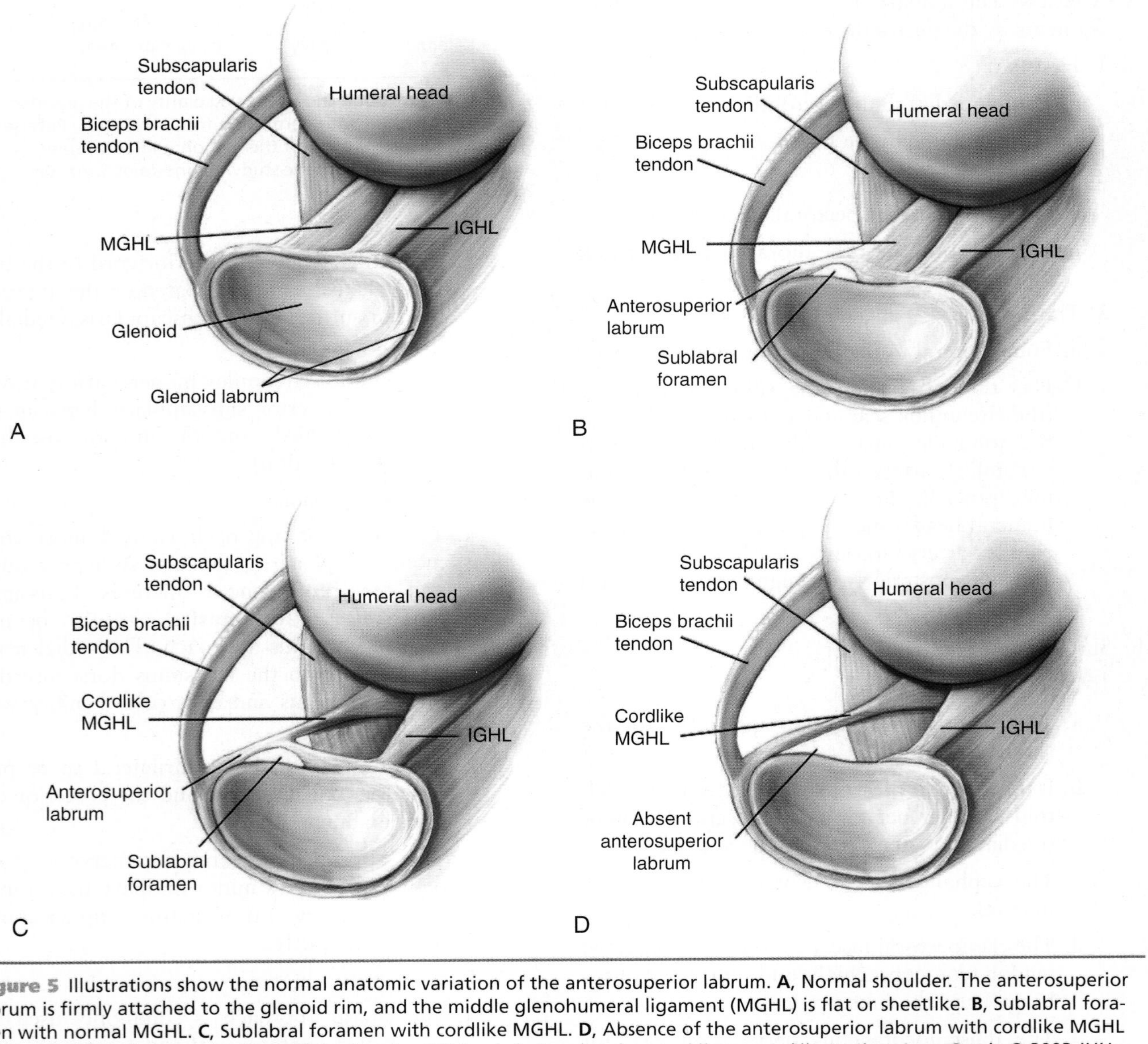

Figure 5 Illustrations show the normal anatomic variation of the anterosuperior labrum. **A**, Normal shoulder. The anterosuperior labrum is firmly attached to the glenoid rim, and the middle glenohumeral ligament (MGHL) is flat or sheetlike. **B**, Sublabral foramen with normal MGHL. **C**, Sublabral foramen with cordlike MGHL. **D**, Absence of the anterosuperior labrum with cordlike MGHL originating from the superior biceps–labral anchor. IGHL = inferior glenohumeral ligament. (Illustration: Juan Garcia © 2002 JHU AAM, Department of Art as Applied Medicine, The Johns Hopkins University School of Medicine.)

a. The most common anatomy is an attached labrum with a broad MGHL.

b. A sublabral foramen is often associated with a cordlike MGHL.

c. A cordlike MGHL with an absent anterosuperior labrum is a rare variant known as the Buford complex.

4. The glenoid chondrolabral junction does not define the margin of the osseous glenoid in its inferior half. The glenoid labrum overlies the osseous glenoid face from 2 to 7 mm in this region.

5. A central bare spot on the glenoid and a bare area on the posterior humeral head, adjacent to the infraspinatus insertion, normally are devoid of cartilage and are not representative of trauma or arthritis.

II. ARM AND ELBOW

A. Osteology

1. Humeral shaft

a. The deltoid inserts in a V shape at the deltoid tubercle.

b. The radial nerve lies within the spiral groove and lies directly posterior at the level of the deltoid tuberosity.

c. A supracondylar process, present in 1% to 3% of individuals, is located 5 to 7 cm proximal to the medial epicondyle and is a potential site of median nerve entrapment.

2. Distal humerus

a. The distal humerus is composed of an articular cylinder (spool) between the lateral and medial metaphyseal flares (columns) of the distal humerus.

b. The articular surface has approximately 30° of anterior tilt, 5° of internal rotation, and 6° of valgus.

c. The capitellum articulates with the radial head and is the site of idiopathic osteonecrosis (Panner disease) and osteochondritis dissecans lesions.

d. The trochlea has a high degree of articular congruency with the greater sigmoid notch of the olecranon.

e. The olecranon fossa receives the tip of the olecranon during terminal extension; the coronoid fossa receives the coronoid tip in flexion; and the radial fossa receives the radial head in flexion.

f. The lateral condyle serves as the origin for the lateral collateral ligaments.

g. The medial epicondyle serves as the origin for the medial collateral ligaments.

3. Proximal radius

a. The radial head functions as an important secondary stabilizer to valgus stress, particularly in medial collateral ligament–deficient elbows.

b. The radial head is elliptical and variably offset from the radial neck.

c. Cartilage encircles approximately 240° of the marginal radial head, with the lateral 120° ("safe zone") devoid of cartilage. This is an important consideration for the placement of internal fixation for radial head and neck fractures.

d. The proximal radial tuberosity provides the insertion site for the distal biceps tendon.

4. Proximal ulna—The ulnohumeral joint is the major osseous stabilizer of the elbow joint.

a. The coronoid acts as an anterior buttress to posterior dislocation.

b. The transverse sulcus at the midportion of the articular surface of the olecranon is normally devoid of cartilage.

c. The crista supinatoris (supinator crest) provides insertion of the lateral ulnar collateral ligament and the origin of the supinator muscle.

d. The sublime tubercle provides insertion for the anterior bundle of the medial collateral ligament.

B. Joint and ligaments

1. The elbow is a trochoginglymoid joint with three articulations: the ulnohumeral joint, the radiohumeral joint, and the proximal radioulnar joint.

a. The ulnohumeral joint is highly congruous and is nearly hingelike.

b. The radiohumeral and proximal radioulnar joints allow rotation.

2. Stability is provided by dynamic and static constraints.

a. Dynamic (muscular) stabilizers provide a variable degree of compression, with a net posterior vector. The common extensor origin at the lateral epicondyle provides restraint against varus and posterolateral rotatory forces.

b. Static stabilizers include bone, capsule, and ligaments.

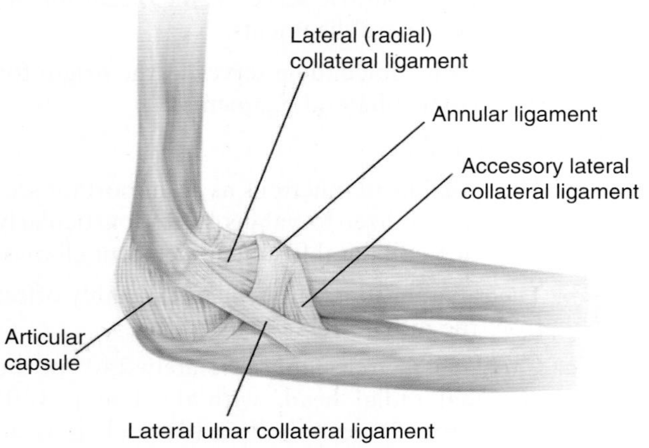

Figure 6 Illustration of the lateral aspect of the elbow depicts the lateral collateral ligament complex.

3. Ligaments (**Figure 6**)
   a. Annular ligament—stabilizes the proximal radioulnar joint.
   b. Lateral (radial) collateral ligament
   c. Lateral ulnar collateral ligament—acts as the primary stabilizer to posterolateral rotatory instability.
   d. Medial collateral ligament (**Figure 7**)
      - Anterior band: acts as the primary stabilizer to valgus stress
      - Posterior band: forms the floor of the cubital tunnel; limits flexion when contracted

C. Musculature—The origin, insertion, innervation, and action of the muscles of the elbow are given in **Table 2**.

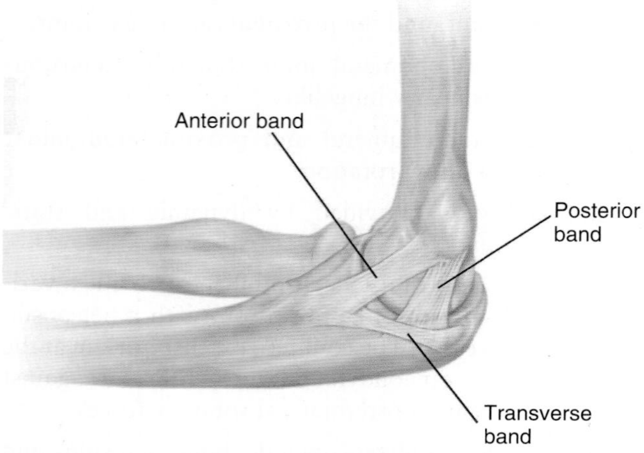

Figure 7 Illustration of the medial aspect of the elbow depicts the medial collateral ligament complex.

D. Nerves
1. Lateral antebrachial cutaneous nerve
   a. This nerve is the terminal branch of the musculocutaneous nerve (lateral cord).
   b. The musculocutaneous nerve runs between the biceps and the brachialis and emerges lateral to the distal tendon of the biceps brachii as the lateral antebrachial cutaneous nerve.
   c. The lateral antebrachial cutaneous nerve is at risk for injury during distal biceps repair (one-incision anterior approach).
2. Radial nerve (posterior cord)
   a. The radial nerve exits the triangular interval (teres major, medial humeral shaft, long head of the triceps).
   b. It travels with the profunda brachii artery, lateral to the deltoid insertion, into the spiral groove of the humerus. It lies directly posterior at the level of the deltoid tuberosity.
   c. It pierces the lateral intermuscular septum to enter the anterior compartment of the arm at approximately the junction of the middle and distal thirds of the humerus.
   d. It courses superficial to the elbow joint capsule, anterior to the midpoint of the radiocapitellar joint, where it is vulnerable to injury during arthroscopic or open anterior capsular release.
   e. Radial nerve palsy is most commonly associated with middle-third humeral fractures.
3. Ulnar nerve (medial cord)
   a. The ulnar nerve enters the posterior compartment of the brachium through the medial intermuscular septum at the arcade of Struthers.
   b. It passes through the cubital tunnel posterior to the medial epicondyle.
   c. The first motor branch to the flexor carpi ulnaris arises distal to the cubital tunnel.
4. Median nerve (lateral and medial cords)
   a. The median nerve courses distally medial to the brachial artery.
   b. It lies anterior to the brachialis muscle at the elbow joint.

E. Arteries
1. Brachial artery
   a. The brachial artery descends in the anterior compartment of the arm with the median nerve.

TABLE 2

Musculature of the Elbow

Muscle	Origin	Insertion	Innervation	Action
Biceps brachii	Long head—superior glenoid/labrum	Radial tuberosity	Musculocutaneous	Elbow flexion/supination
	Short head—coracoid			
Brachialis	Humerus, intermuscular septum	Coronoid	Musculocutaneous (medial), radial (lateral)	Elbow flexion
Brachioradialis	Humerus	Radial styloid	Radial	Elbow flexion
Triceps brachii	Medial head—humerus	Olecranon	Radial	Elbow extension
	Lateral head—humerus			
	Long head—inferior glenoid			
Anconeus	Lateral condyle	Ulna	Radial	Stability

b. Proximally, the nerve is medial to the artery.

c. Distally, the artery is medial to the nerve.

d. At the level of the elbow joint, the brachial artery branches into the radial and ulnar arteries.

2. The inferior ulnar collateral artery provides the only direct supply of oxygenated blood to the ulnar nerve proximal to the cubital tunnel.

3. The vascular supply to the lateral condyle is from the posterior aspect.

F. Surgical approaches—humeral shaft

1. Anterior/anterolateral approach

a. Proximally, the deltopectoral interval is used.

b. Distally, the superficial interval is between the biceps brachii (musculocutaneous nerve) and the brachialis (the musculocutaneous nerve medially and the radial nerve laterally).

c. The lateral antebrachial cutaneous nerve, located between the biceps and the brachialis, is retracted medially with the biceps.

d. The radial nerve is identified in the deep interval between the lateral brachialis (radial nerve) and the brachioradialis (radial nerve).

e. The brachialis is split (anterior approach) or subperiosteally reflected from the humerus and retracted medially and laterally (anterolateral approach).

2. Posterior approach

a. This approach allows exposure of the distal two-thirds of the humerus and the radial nerve.

b. The superficial interval is between the long and lateral heads of the triceps.

c. The radial nerve and the profunda brachii artery are identified in the spiral groove.

G. Surgical approaches—elbow

1. Lateral approaches are used for radiocapitellar surgery, capsular release/excision, and lateral collateral ligament repair/reconstruction.

a. The Kocher approach uses the plane between the anconeus (radial nerve) and the extensor carpi ulnaris (posterior interosseous nerve). Access to the joint anterior to the midplane of the radial head preserves the lateral ulnar collateral ligament.

b. The lateral column approach uses the plane along the lateral supracondylar ridge between the triceps posteriorly and the brachioradialis/extensor carpi radialis longus anteriorly.

2. Medial approach

a. The medial approach is used for medial capsular release/excision, coronoid fracture, and medial collateral ligament repair/reconstruction.

b. Identification and/or transposition of the ulnar nerve is often required.

c. The medial antebrachial cutaneous nerve is also identified and protected in the distal aspect of the incision.

3. Posterior approach

a. The posterior approach is a utilitarian extensile exposure for concomitant medial and lateral surgery, elbow arthroplasty, and distal humerus fractures.

b. Posterior exposure is obtained by split or reflection of the triceps or by osteotomy of the olecranon.

H. Biomechanical features of the elbow

1. Articular congruity contributes greatly to varus stability.
2. Valgus stability is divided equally among the medial collateral ligament, the anterior joint capsule, and the osseous articulation in elbow extension.
3. In 90° of flexion, the medial collateral ligament is the primary valgus stabilizer.
4. The carrying angle of the elbow is 11° of valgus.
5. Axial loading of the extended elbow is transmitted 40% through the ulnohumeral joint and 60% through the radiohumeral joint.
6. Most activities of daily living require elbow range of motion arcs comprising 100° (30° to 130°) of flexion/extension and 100° (50°/50°) of pronation/supination.
7. The center of rotation approximates a line through the isometric points on the lateral and medial epicondyles.

I. Arthroscopic anatomy of the elbow

1. The close proximity of neurovascular structures places them at risk of injury during arthroscopy (**Figure 8**).
   a. The proximal anterolateral portal is close to the radial nerve.
   b. The proximal anteromedial portal is close to the medial antebrachial cutaneous nerve.
2. The radial nerve lies close to the anterior capsule at the mid aspect of the radiocapitellar joint.
3. The ulnar nerve lies directly superficial to the joint capsule in the posteromedial gutter.
4. The most common neurologic complication after elbow arthroscopy is transient ulnar nerve palsy.

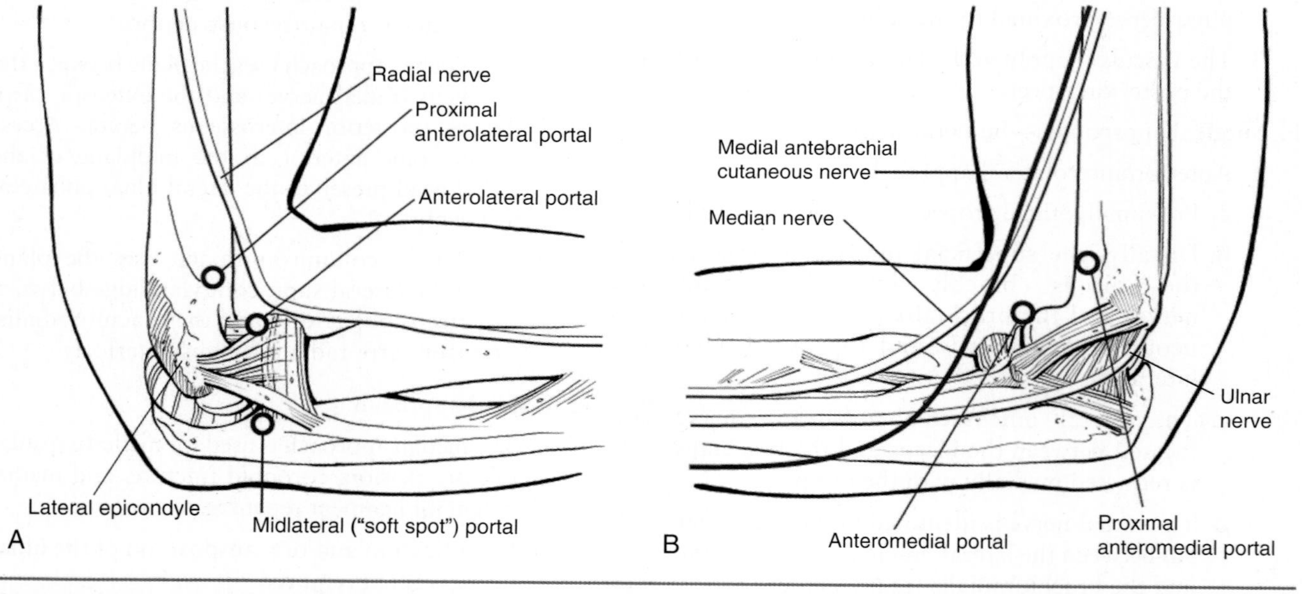

Figure 8 Illustrations demonstrate the location of the anterior portals used in arthroscopic surgery of the elbow. **A**, Lateral view of the elbow. The proximal anterolateral, anterolateral, and midlateral (soft spot) portals are shown in relation to the radial nerve. **B**, Medial view of the elbow. The anteromedial and proximal anteromedial portals are shown in relation to the median, ulnar, and medial antebrachial cutaneous nerves. (Reproduced from Yamaguchi K, Tashjian RZ: Set up and portals, in Yamaguchi K, King GJW, McKee MD, O'Driscoll SWM, eds: *Advanced Reconstruction: Elbow*. Rosemont, IL, American Academy of Orthopaedic Surgeons, 2007, pp 3-11.)

TOP TESTING FACTS

Anatomy of the Shoulder

1. The clavicle is the first bone to ossify, and the medial (sternal) epiphysis of the clavicle is the last ossification center to fuse, at age 20 to 25 years.
2. The deep insertion of the subscapularis and the biceps pulley (CH and SGHL ligaments) provide restraint against medial subluxation of the long head of the biceps tendon.
3. The anterior IGHL is a primary static restraint against anterior-inferior dislocation of the glenohumeral joint in 90° of abduction and external rotation (the position of apprehension).
4. Loss of sensation over the lateral shoulder indicates injury to the posterior branch of the axillary nerve and signifies possible teres minor palsy. The muscular branch to the teres minor lies closest to the glenoid and is most susceptible to injury during arthroscopic surgery involving the inferior capsule.
5. Suprascapular nerve compression at the suprascapular notch causes denervation of the supraspinatus and the infraspinatus. Nerve compression at the spinoglenoid notch leads to selective denervation of the infraspinatus muscle.
6. The lateral deltoid-splitting approach places the axillary nerve at risk of iatrogenic injury. The distance between the nerve and the lateral margin of the acromion is related to arm length and decreases with shoulder abduction.
7. Injury to the long thoracic nerve (serratus anterior) causes medial scapular winging, and injury to the spinal accessory nerve (trapezius) causes lateral scapular winging.

Anatomy of the Arm and Elbow

1. The lateral ulnar collateral ligament is the primary elbow stabilizer to posterolateral elbow rotatory instability. The anterior band of the medial collateral ligament is the primary valgus stabilizer in elbow flexion.
2. The radial nerve pierces the lateral intermuscular septum to enter the anterior compartment of the arm at the junction of the middle and distal thirds of the humerus. It courses superficial to the elbow joint capsule, anterior to the midpoint of the radiocapitellar joint, where it is vulnerable to injury during arthroscopic or open anterior capsular release.
3. Most activities of daily living require elbow range of motion arcs comprising 100° (30° to 130°) of flexion/extension and 100° (50°/50°) of pronation/supination.

Bibliography

Ball CM, Steger T, Galatz LM, Yamaguchi K: The posterior branch of the axillary nerve: An anatomic study. *J Bone Joint Surg Am* 2003;85(8):1497-1501.

Bauer GS, Blaine TA: Humeral shaft fractures: Surgical approaches, in Levine WN, Marra G, Bigliani LU, eds: *Fractures of the Shoulder Girdle*. New York, NY, Marcel Dekker, 2003, pp 221-247.

Burkhead WZ Jr, Scheinberg RR, Box G: Surgical anatomy of the axillary nerve. *J Shoulder Elbow Surg* 1992;1(1):31-36.

Fleming P, Lenehan B, Sankar R, Folan-Curran J, Curtin W: One-third, two-thirds: Relationship of the radial nerve to the lateral intermuscular septum in the arm. *Clin Anat* 2004;17(1):26-29.

Gleason PD, Beall DP, Sanders TG, et al: The transverse humeral ligament: A separate anatomical structure or a continuation of the osseous attachment of the rotator cuff? *Am J Sports Med* 2006;34(1):72-77.

Goss TP: Scapular fractures and dislocations: Diagnosis and treatment. *J Am Acad Orthop Surg* 1995;3(1):22-33.

Klimkiewicz JJ, Williams GR, Sher JS, Karduna A, Des Jar-dins J, Iannotti JP: The acromioclavicular capsule as a restraint to posterior translation of the clavicle: A biomechanical analysis. *J Shoulder Elbow Surg* 1999;8(2):119-124.

Morrey BF: Surgical exposures of the elbow, in Morrey BF, ed: *The Elbow and Its Disorders*, ed 3. Philadelphia, PA, Saunders, 2000, pp 109-134.

Morrey BF, An KN: Articular and ligamentous contributions to the stability of the elbow joint. *Am J Sports Med* 1983;11(5):315-319.

Morrey BF, Askew LJ, Chao EY: A biomechanical study of normal functional elbow motion. *J Bone Joint Surg Am* 1981;63(6):872-877.

O'Driscoll SW, Bell DF, Morrey BF: Posterolateral rotatory instability of the elbow. *J Bone Joint Surg Am* 1991;73(3):440-446.

Price MR, Tillett ED, Acland RD, Nettleton GS: Determining the relationship of the axillary nerve to the shoulder joint capsule from an arthroscopic perspective. *J Bone Joint Surg Am* 2004;86(10):2135-2142.

Rao AG, Kim TK, Chronopoulos E, McFarland EG: Anatomical variants in the anterosuperior aspect of the glenoid labrum: A statistical analysis of seventy-three cases. *J Bone Joint Surg Am* 2003;85(4):653-659.

Rispoli DM, Athwal GS, Sperling JW, Cofield RH: The macroscopic delineation of the edge of the glenoid labrum: An anatomic evaluation of an open and arthroscopic visual reference. *Arthroscopy* 2009;25(6):603-607.

Robertson DD, Yuan J, Bigliani LU, Flatow EL, Yamaguchi K: Three-dimensional analysis of the proximal part of the humerus: Relevance to arthroplasty. *J Bone Joint Surg Am* 2000;82(11):1594-1602.

Chapter 70
PHYSICAL EXAMINATION OF THE SHOULDER AND ELBOW

BOGDAN A. MATACHE, MD, CM, FRCSC
BRADEN GAMMON, MD, MSc, FRCSC
GEORGE S. ATHWAL, MD, FRCSC
RYAN T. BICKNELL, MD, MSc, FRCS(C)

I. SHOULDER

A. Draping/positioning—The patient should be draped appropriately to allow circumferential visualization of the sternoclavicular, acromioclavicular (AC), glenohumeral, scapulothoracic, and scapular surface anatomy bilaterally.

B. General inspection—The patient's general posture, any bone/soft-tissue deformity, incisions/scars, regions of swelling or erythema, muscle atrophy, and any asymmetry are noted. The scapulae are examined bilaterally for resting attitude and winging/dyskinesia with movement of the shoulder through its range of motion (ROM).

C. Palpation—The anatomic landmarks of the shoulder and elbow are palpated for evidence of swelling, warmth, tenderness, deformity, crepitus, or instability. Anteriorly, these include the sternoclavicular joint, clavicle, AC joint, coracoid process, and anterior glenohumeral joint. Posteriorly, the scapular margins, periscapular soft tissues, and posterior glenohumeral joint are assessed. Palpation of the supraspinatus and infraspinatus fossae can reveal small amounts of atrophy that may not be obvious on inspection. Laterally, on the proximal humerus, the lesser and greater tuberosities with their associated rotator cuff insertions are palpated, as are also the bicipital groove and subacromial space. Any crepitus with passive glenohumeral or scapulothoracic motion are noted. If palpation reveals pain, the examiner should clarify whether it reproduces the patient's typical symptoms.

D. Range of motion

1. The active ROM of the shoulder is initially assessed with the patient in the upright position. The following movements are observed: forward elevation, abduction, external rotation (with the arm adducted), and internal rotation behind the back. To isolate glenohumeral motion, horizontal adduction and both internal and external rotation in 90° of abduction are measured with the patient in the supine position.
2. Both shoulders are examined simultaneously, and differences in their rhythm and maximum ROM are noted. Associated scapulothoracic motion is also gauged, with the patient standing and with observation of elevation, depression, protraction, and retraction.

Dr. Athwal or an immediate family member has received royalties from CONMED Linvatec, Exactech, Inc., Imascap, Orthospace - Inspace, and Wright Medical Technology, Inc.; serves as a paid consultant to or is an employee of DePuy, A Johnson & Johnson Company and Stryker; has stock or stock options held in PrecisionOS and Wright Medical Technology, Inc.; has received research or institutional support from Smith & Nephew and Wright Medical Technology, Inc.; and serves as a board member, owner, officer, or committee member of the American Shoulder and Elbow Surgeons. Dr. Bicknell or an immediate family member is a member of a speakers' bureau or has made paid presentations on behalf of Biomet, CONMED Linvatec, DePuy, A Johnson & Johnson Company, and Zimmer; serves as a paid consultant to or is an employee of Biomet, DePuy, A Johnson & Johnson Company, and Zimmer; has received research or institutional support from CONMED Linvatec and DePuy, A Johnson & Johnson Company; and serves as a board member, owner, officer, or committee member of the American Academy of Orthopaedic Surgeons, the American Shoulder and Elbow Surgeons, and the Canadian Orthopaedic Association. Neither of the following authors nor any immediate family member has received anything of value from or has stock or stock options held in a commercial company or institution related directly or indirectly to the subject of this chapter: Dr. Matache and Dr. Gammon.

TABLE 1

Normal Glenohumeral Range of Motion

Parameter	Normal Values (°)
Forward elevation	170
Abduction	90
External rotation, arm adducted	70
Internal rotation, behind back	T7
Internal rotation in abduction	70
External rotation in abduction	100
Horizontal adduction	50

3. The passive ROM of the glenohumeral joint is observed and limitations or less commonly increased passive movements are noted. **Table 1** depicts normal values for each of these motions. These values can vary widely among patients, and comparing any shoulder motion with that of the normal contralateral shoulder is advantageous.

E. Rotator cuff strength—The patient is examined in the standing position, with the scapulae in a retracted and depressed position. Each muscle unit of the rotator cuff is isolated and tested in sequence. Power is graded with the Medical Research Council rating scale (**Table 2**).

1. The supraspinatus muscle is evaluated with the empty can and champagne toast tests.
   a. The empty can test is performed with the shoulder in 70° to 90° of abduction in the plane of the scapula and in internal rotation, with the forearm maximally pronated. Downward pressure is applied to the forearm, which the patient is asked to resist (**Figure 1**).
   b. The champagne toast test is performed with the shoulder in 30° of abduction in the plane of the scapula, 30° of forward elevation, and mild external rotation. The patient is asked to resist downward pressure applied to the upper arm (**Figure 2**). This position better isolates the abducting function of the supraspinatus from that of the deltoid.

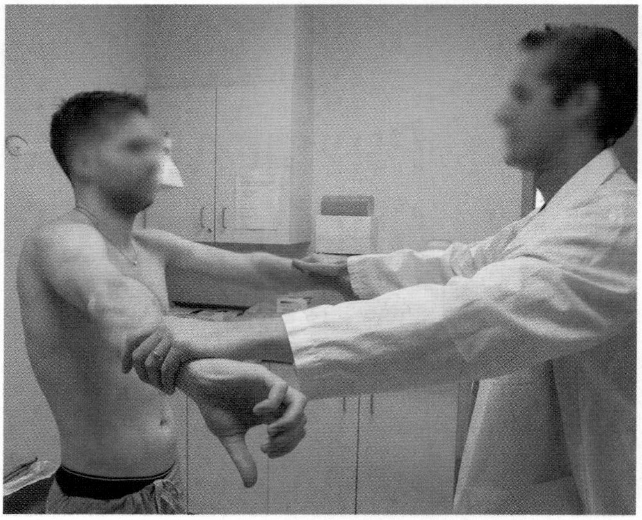

Figure 1 Photograph shows evaluation of supraspinatus muscle strength using the empty can test.

TABLE 2

Medical Research Council Grading Scale of Muscle Power

Grade	Findings
5	Normal
4	Weakness against resistance
3	Able to overcome gravity
2	Able to move with gravity eliminated
1	Flicker of movement
0	No muscle activation

2. The infraspinatus muscle is tested with the shoulder abducted 20° in the scapular plane and the elbow at 90° of flexion. The patient attempts to externally rotate the arm from 45° of internal rotation against the examiner's counterforce (**Figure 3**). If they are unable to do so, the examiner positions the arm in 5° less than maximal passive external rotation, to allow for capsular recoil, and asks the patient to hold the arm in this position as they release the wrist. If the patient's arm spontaneously falls back by more than 10° of internal rotation, the result is designated a positive external rotation "lag" or "dropping" sign, indicating insufficiency of the infraspinatus muscle.
3. The teres minor muscle is isolated with the elbow flexed to 90° and the arm in 90° of external rotation and 90° of abduction. Power is tested as the examiner tries to forcibly rotate the arm internally from its abducted and externally rotated position. If any weakness is perceived, the shoulder is passively placed in the above position and the patient is asked to maintain the arm as such against gravity. Inability to do so, defined by spontaneous internal rotation of the shoulder, is considered a positive "hornblower" sign, indicating teres minor insufficiency.

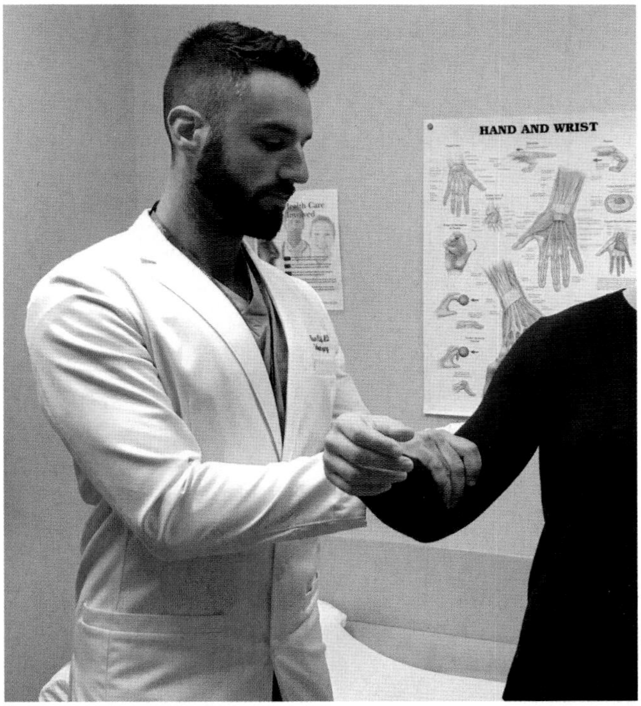

Figure 2 Photograph depicts the champagne toast test to evaluate supraspinatus muscle strength.

4. The subscapularis muscle can be tested with the belly-press, lift-off, and bear-hug tests.
    a. The belly-press maneuver is performed with the patient's hand pressing on the upper abdomen, with the elbow anterior to the wrist in the coronal plane. Both the power of the press and any tendency of the elbow to fall behind the wrist are noted.

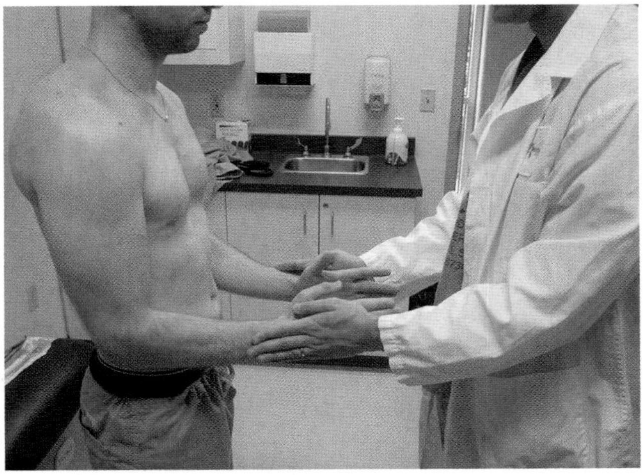

Figure 3 Photograph shows evaluation of infraspinatus muscle strength.

    b. The lift-off test is performed with the shoulder rotated internally and the dorsum of the patient's hand resting against the patient's ipsilateral sacroiliac joint. To ensure that the patient is not limited by internal joint stiffness, the examiner passively positions the back of the patient's hand away from the sacroiliac region and asks the patient to maintain that position. The patient's power in lifting the back of the hand against resistance from that position should be noted.
    c. The bear-hug test requires the patient to place the palm of the hand on the opposite shoulder, with the elbow anterior to the body. The patient maintains an internal rotation force in this position as the examiner attempts to externally rotate the patient's arm. Weakness of the arm compared with the arm on the contralateral side is considered a positive result, indicating a tear in the upper border of the subscapularis muscle or tendon (**Figure 4**).

F. Special tests
1. Glenohumeral internal rotation deficit (GIRD)/internal impingement in throwers—A pathology defined as the loss, in degrees, of internal rotation of the glenohumeral joint in the affected (throwing) shoulder compared with the nonaffected

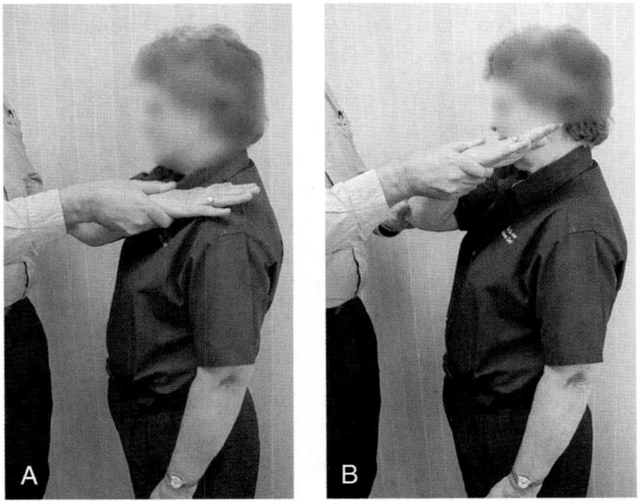

Figure 4 Photographs demonstrate the bear-hug test to examine for a tear in the upper border of the subscapularis muscle or tendon. **A**, A normal examination result. **B**, A positive test result, demonstrated by weakness. (Adapted with permission from Barth JR, Burkhart SS, De Beer JF: The bear-hug test: A new and sensitive test for diagnosing a subscapularis tear. *Arthroscopy* 2006;22[10]:1076-1084.)

shoulder. This loss is measured as the difference in internal rotation in abduction with the scapula stabilized.

a. The loss of internal rotation relates to a concomitant posterior capsular contracture, and external rotation is often increased with attenuation of the anterior capsule and glenohumeral ligaments. As the contracture evolves, the center of rotation of the humeral head shifts superiorly and posteriorly, which may result in impingement of the labrum and rotator cuff between the greater tuberosity and glenoid when the arm is abducted and externally hyperrotated.

b. This internal impingement may result in partial articular-side tears of the rotator cuff and superior labrum anterior to posterior (SLAP) lesions and should be evaluated in throwers with shoulder pain. Shoulders with a GIRD of more than 20° compared with the GIRD of the contralateral shoulder are considered at risk for injury.

2. Impingement—Neer test, Hawkins-Kennedy test

a. In the Neer impingement test, the patient's scapula is stabilized and the arm is passively taken through a full arc of forward elevation. In terminal forward elevation, pain is experienced at the anterior edge of the acromion and may indicate subacromial impingement syndrome or rotator cuff pathology. The diagnosis is confirmed when the pain is relieved by injecting 10 mL of 1% xylocaine beneath the anterior acromion (**Figure 5**).

b. In the Hawkins-Kennedy test, the examiner positions the patient's arm into internal rotation in 90° of abduction in the scapular plane. Pain in this position can indicate subacromial impingement syndrome or rotator cuff pathology, with the greater tuberosity pressed against the coracoacromial ligament and acromion (**Figure 6**).

3. AC joint—Instability, cross-arm test, Paxinos test

a. AC joint instability. In type 1 and 2 separations of the AC joint, there will be pain over the AC joint capsule and potentially a palpable gap compared with the contralateral AC joint. With higher grades of AC joint separation and disruption of the coracoclavicular ligaments, the distal clavicle will become progressively more unstable. Most commonly, the distal clavicle displaces superiorly and posteriorly.

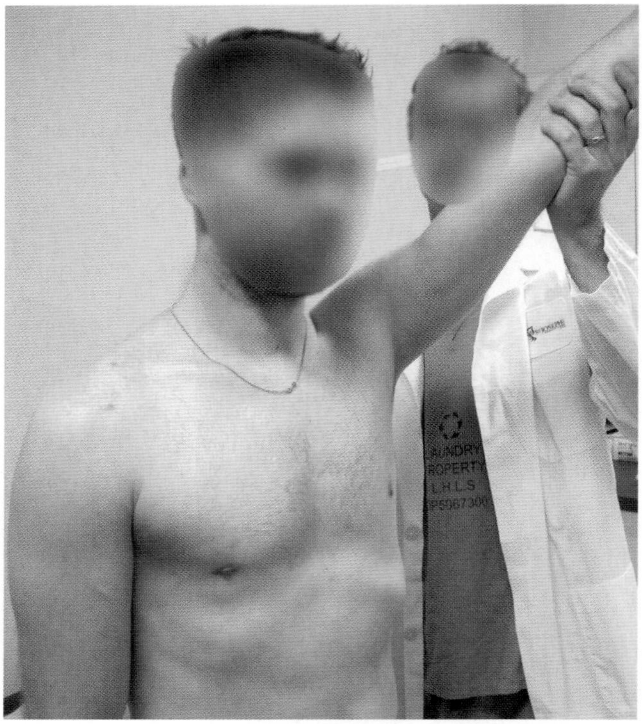

Figure 5 Photograph demonstrates the Neer impingement test for subacromial impingement syndrome.

b. In the cross-arm test, the patient's arm is brought into 90° of forward elevation and maximal adduction, producing axial compression across the AC joint. Pain at the AC joint can indicate degenerative pathology. When conducted with

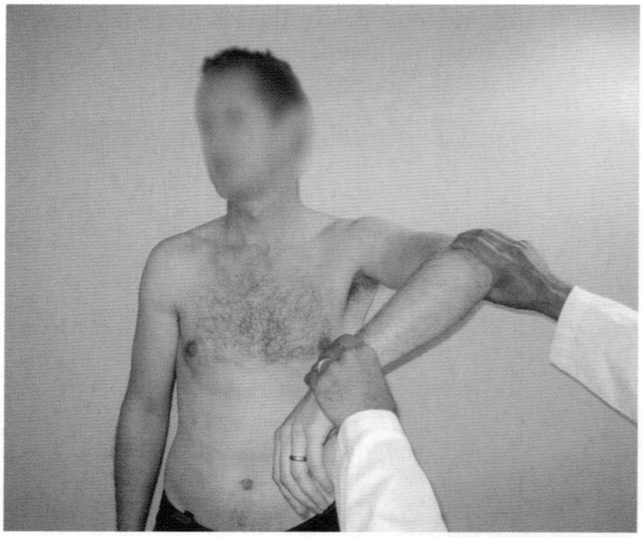

Figure 6 Photograph demonstrates the Hawkins-Kennedy test for subacromial impingement syndrome or rotator cuff pathology.

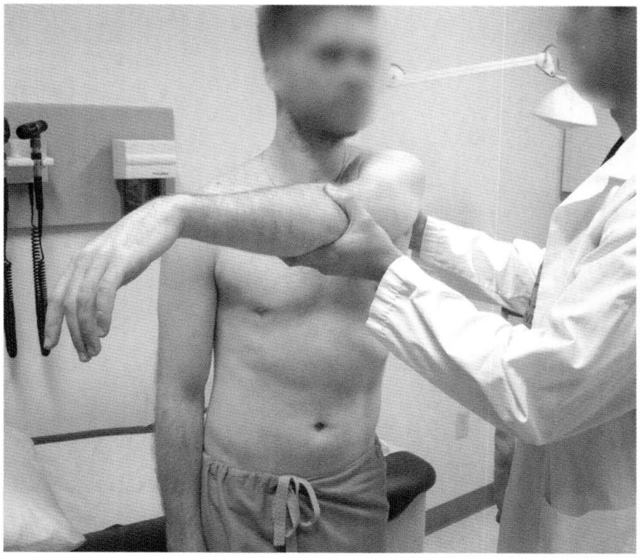

Figure 7 Photograph demonstrates the cross-arm test for degenerative pathology of the acromioclavicular joint.

the patient in the supine position and the scapula stabilized, this is also a test for posterior capsular tightness. Pain at the posterior aspect of the glenohumeral joint, with a diminished ROM compared with that on the contralateral side, indicates symptomatic contracture (**Figure 7**).

c. The Paxinos test is conducted with the patient's arm relaxed at the side of the body. The examiner then creates a shearing force across the AC joint by applying thumb pressure over the posterior acromion and counterpressure with the index finger over the distal clavicle. Pain at the AC joint can indicate degenerative changes in the joint.

4. SLAP tear—O'Brien test, crank test, biceps load test 2, anterior slide test

   a. The O'Brien test (also called the active compression test) is performed with the patient's arm in 90° of forward elevation, with the elbow in full extension, full internal rotation of the shoulder (thumb pointed down), and 10° to 15° of adduction. The examiner applies a downward force to the forearm that is resisted by the patient. Pain in the glenohumeral joint that is absent when the test is repeated with the shoulder in maximum external rotation (forearm supinated) indicates a SLAP tear (**Figure 8**).

   b. In the crank test, the patient is seated and the examiner positions the patient's arm at 160° of forward elevation in the scapular plane. The glenohumeral joint is axially loaded in this position along the axis of the humerus, with passive internal and external rotation of the humerus. Pain, particularly in external rotation of the humerus and with a catching sensation, indicates a SLAP tear (**Figure 9**).

   c. The biceps load test 2 is used to assess potentially isolated SLAP pathology, in contrast to the biceps load test 1, which is designed for patients with anterior shoulder instability and a SLAP tear. In the biceps load test 2, the patient is in

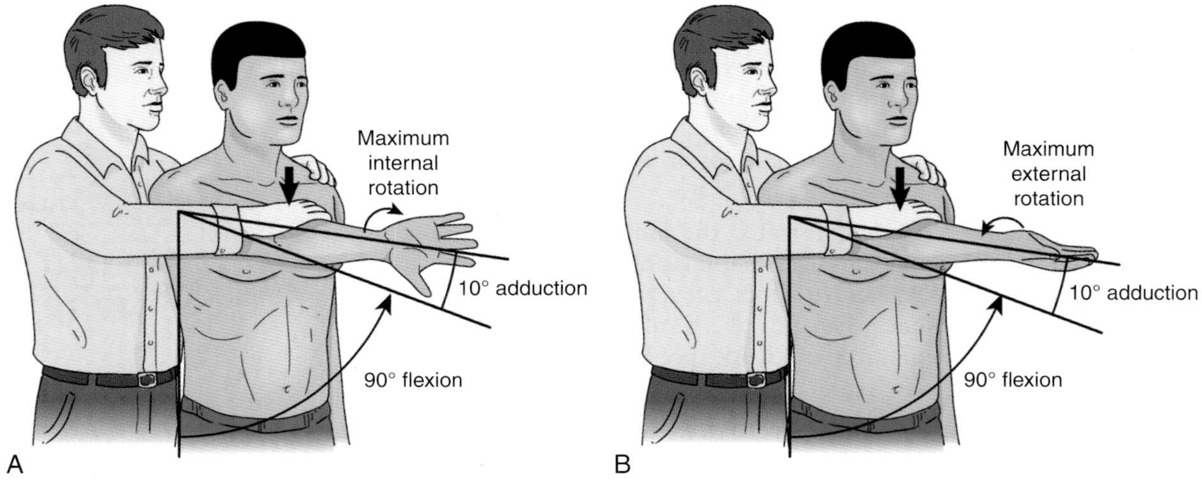

Figure 8 Illustration depicts the O'Brien test for a superior labrum anterior to posterior tear. **A,** The O'Brien test is performed with the patient's arm in 90° of forward elevation, with the elbow in full extension, full internal rotation of the shoulder (thumb pointed down), and 10° to 15° of adduction. The examiner applies a downward force to the forearm that is resisted by the patient. **B,** Pain in the glenohumeral joint that is absent when the test is repeated with the shoulder in maximum external rotation (forearm supinated) indicates a SLAP tear. (Adapted with permission from O'Brien SJ, Pagnani MJ, Fealy S, McGlynn SR, Wilson JB: The active compression test: A new and effective test for diagnosing labral tears and acromioclavicular joint abnormality. *Am J Sports Med* 1998;26[5]:610-613.)

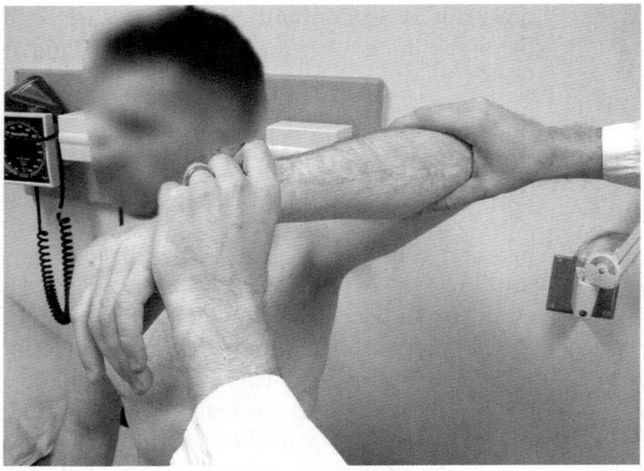

Figure 9 Photograph demonstrates the crank test for a superior labrum anterior to posterior tear.

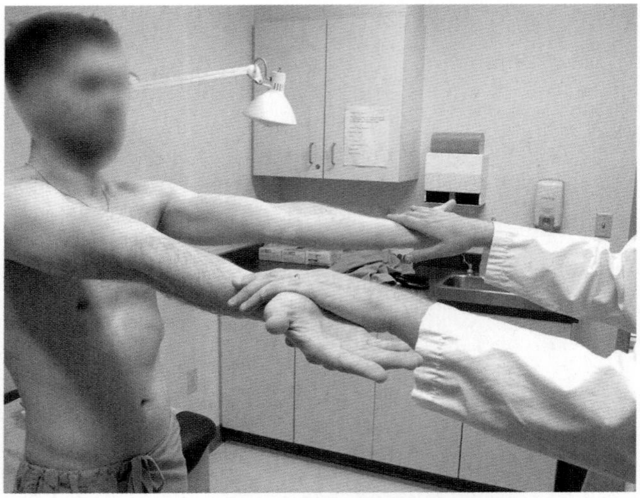

Figure 10 Photograph demonstrates the Speed test for pathology of the long head of the biceps tendon.

the supine position and the arm is placed into 120° of forward elevation and maximal external rotation. With the elbow in 90° of flexion, the forearm is supinated. The patient is asked to flex the elbow, with the examiner resisting this flexion. If this increases pain beyond its baseline severity, the test result is positive.

d. In the anterior slide test, the patient is examined in either the standing or sitting position with the hands on the hips and the thumbs pointed posteriorly. The examiner's hand cups the superior aspect of the patient's shoulder, with the tip of the examiner's index finger extending over the anterior aspect of the patient's acromion. The examiner's contralateral hand then applies a force to the patient's elbow, driving the humeral head anteriorly and superiorly. The patient is asked to resist this force. Pain and/or a click emanating from the front of the shoulder constitutes a positive test result.

e. Multiple studies have demonstrated the limited accuracy of various physical examination maneuvers for SLAP tears. A more accurate diagnosis can be made when positive results occur with a combination of SLAP-specific tests.

5. Pathology of the long head of the biceps (LHB)—Speed test, Yergason test, "3-Pack" test

   a. In the Speed test, the patient's arm is placed into 90° of forward elevation in the sagittal plane, with the elbow extended and the forearm supinated. A downward force is applied to the forearm, and pain in the anterior shoulder indicates pathology of the LHB tendon (**Figure 10**).

   b. In the Yergason test, the patient's arm is adducted, flexed to 90° at the elbow, and fully pronated. The examiner attempts to forcibly hold the forearm in pronation, and the patient counters with supination. Pain in the bicipital groove with resisted supination is a positive test result for pathology of the LHB tendon (**Figure 11**).

   c. The "3-Pack" test combines the O'Brien (active compression) test, throwing test, and bicipital tunnel palpation. The throwing test is performed with the elbow flexed 90° and the shoulder abducted 90° in the scapular plane and in maximal external rotation (late cocking position). The examiner provides resistance to

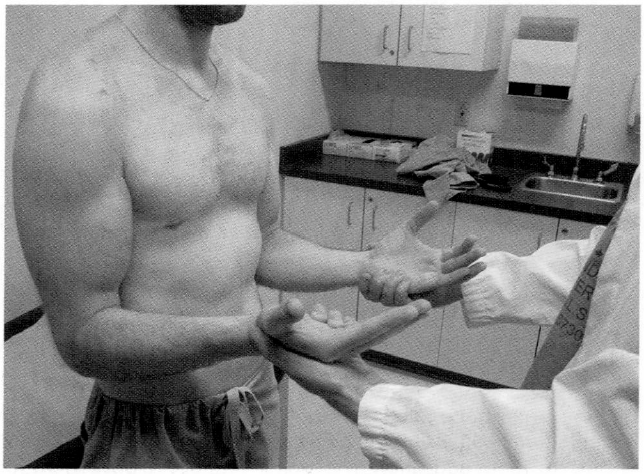

Figure 11 Photograph demonstrates the Yergason test for pathology of the long head of the biceps tendon.

the arm as the patient steps forward with the contralateral leg (early acceleration position). Pain with this maneuver indicates a positive result. Pain with each component of the "3-Pack" test is highly indicative of pathology of the LHB.

6. Glenohumeral joint instability
   a. It is important to assess for generalized ligamentous laxity. Signs of this may include hyperextension at the elbows and knees, the ability to place the palms of the hands on the floor with the knees extended, and the ability to bring the thumbs to the forearm. Excessive translation of the humeral head on the glenoid in this scenario may not be pathologic if it does not cause pain or diminish function.
      - In the load-and-shift test, the patient is placed in the supine position or is seated with the back against a chair to help stabilize the scapula. The examiner cups the patient's proximal humerus with one hand and uses the other hand to axially load the humerus while centering the humeral head in the glenoid fossa. The humeral head is then translated posteriorly and anteriorly, with observation of the degree of its translation and any accompanying symptoms. The modified Hawkins grading system can be used to determine the degree of translation (**Table 3**; **Figure 12**).
      - In the examination for the sulcus sign, the patient is seated and an axial traction force is applied to the arm. The examiner looks for an indentation or sulcus to form in the subacromial space as the humeral head subluxates inferiorly from the glenoid fossa. This can be a sign of generalized laxity or inferior instability of the shoulder. The examination should be repeated with the shoulder in both neutral rotation and maximum external rotation. The sign is considered especially indicative of inferior laxity if it is present in both neutral rotation and external rotation. Comparison should be made of the findings on examination of the contralateral shoulder (**Figure 13**).

TABLE 3

Grading of Translation With the Load-and-Shift Maneuver

Grade	Findings
0	Little or no translation (<25% of humeral head diameter)
1	Humeral head moves onto glenoid rim
2	Humeral head can be dislocated but spontaneously reduces
3	Humeral head does not relocate when pressure is removed

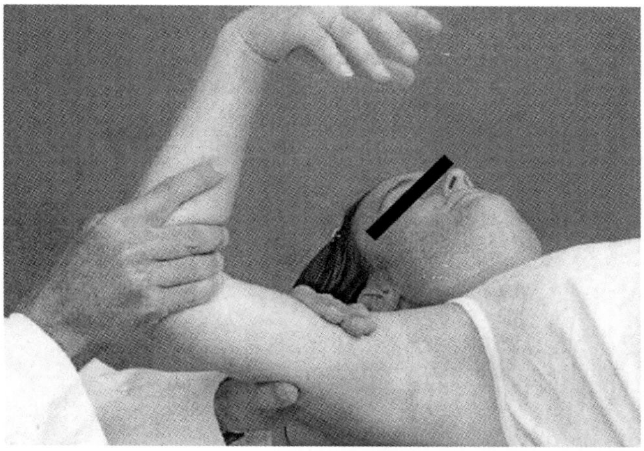

Figure 12 Photograph demonstrates the load-and-shift test for anterior and posterior instability of the shoulder. (Adapted with permission from Tzannes A, Paxinos A, Callanan M, Murrell GA: An assessment of the interexaminer reliability of tests for shoulder instability. *J Shoulder Elbow Surg* 2004;13:18-23.)

   b. Anterior instability—Anterior apprehension test, relocation test, and surprise test
      - In the anterior apprehension test, the patient is in the supine position with the patient's body at the edge of the examining table. The patient's arm is brought into 90° of abduction and full external rotation. Reproducing a sensation of instability constitutes a positive test result (**Figure 14**).
      - The relocation test is a continuation of the anterior apprehension test. This maneuver is performed when the anterior apprehension test elicits a patient report of a sensation of instability with the arm in abduction and external rotation. When this occurs, and with the arm in abduction and external rotation, a posteriorly directed force is applied to the humeral head, relocating it back into the glenoid fossa. Relief of the sensation of instability constitutes a positive test result (**Figure 15**).
      - The surprise test is the final component of this series of tests to assess anterior instability of the shoulder. A relocation maneuver is performed, with the patient's arm moved

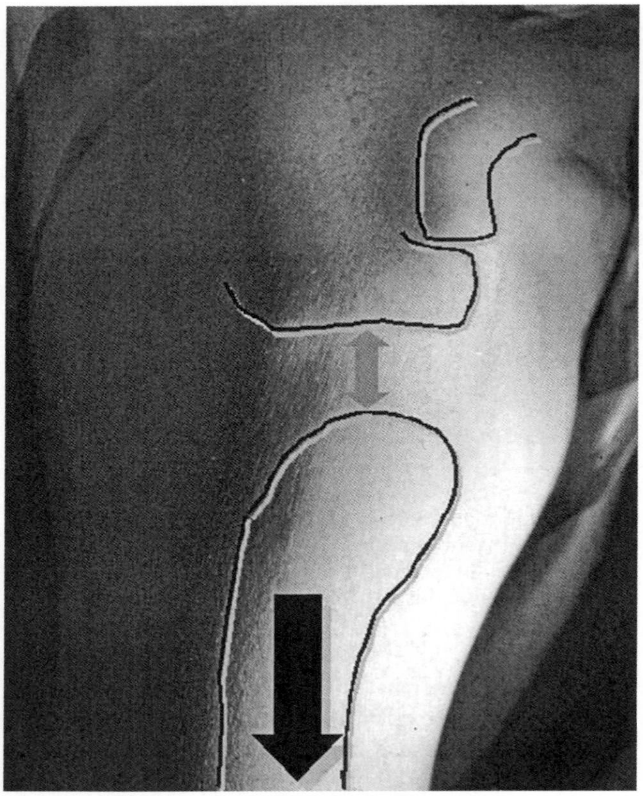

Figure 13 Photograph demonstrates the test for the sulcus sign, indicating generalized laxity or inferior instability of the shoulder. The arrow indicates the direction of force applied by the examiner. The double arrow depicts the sulcus formed between the humeral head and the acromion resulting from inferior subluxation. (Adapted with permission from Tzannes A, Paxinos A, Callanan M, Murrell GA: An assessment of the interexaminer reliability of tests for shoulder instability. *J Shoulder Elbow Surg* 2004;13:18-23.)

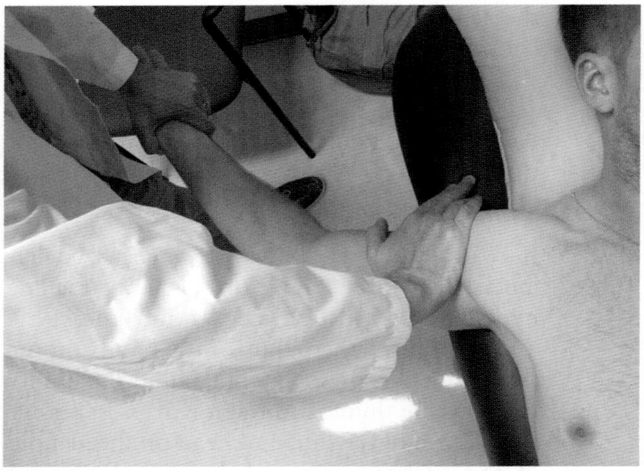

Figure 15 Photograph demonstrates the relocation test for anterior shoulder instability.

into further abduction and external rotation. A positive test result consists of reproducing a sensation of instability on release of the posteriorly directed relocation force on the shoulder (**Figure 16**).

c. Inferior instability—Gagey hyperabduction test. In this test, the patient's arm is brought into 90° of abduction. The scapula and acromion are stabilized and the ability to passively hyperabduct the arm through the glenohumeral joint is assessed. The ability to hyperabduct the arm by 20° or more compared with the contralateral arm is correlated with symptomatic instability of the shoulder (**Figure 17**). Also, pain or a reported sensation of instability may be elicited.

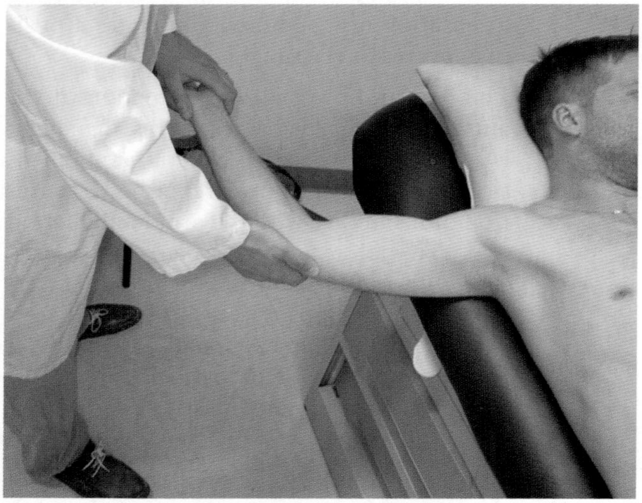

Figure 14 Photograph demonstrates the anterior apprehension test for anterior shoulder instability.

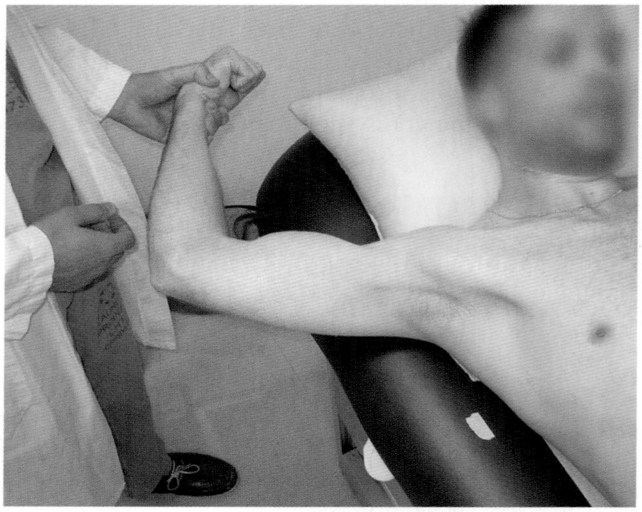

Figure 16 Photograph demonstrates the surprise test for anterior shoulder instability.

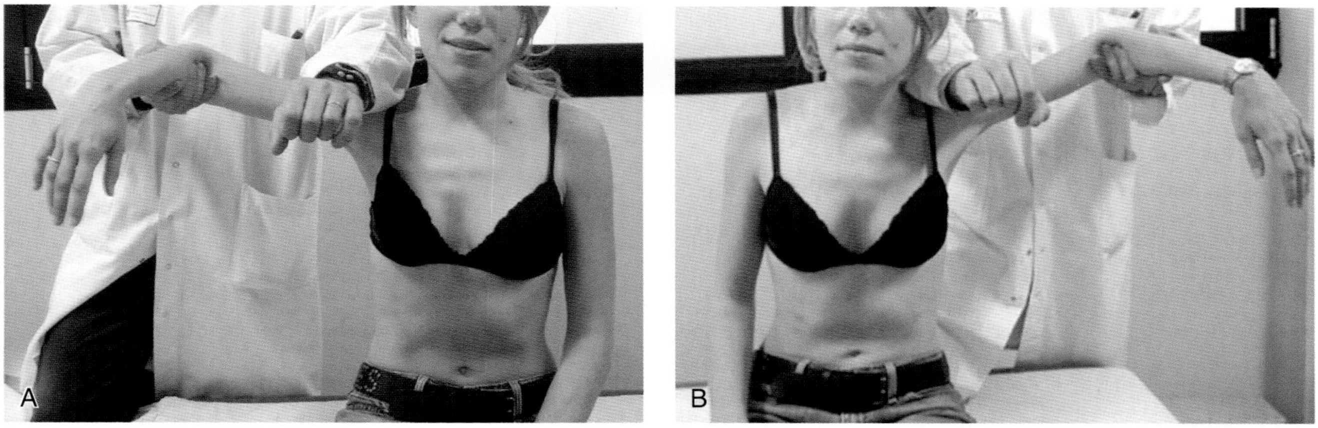

Figure 17 Photographs demonstrating that the comparative hyperabduction test is positive on the left shoulder (**B**) when it reproduces the patient's pain (deep pain recognized by the patient); it is asymmetrical compared with the contralateral side (**A**) (>20° of difference); and there is a soft end point (compared with the firm end point of the contralateral side). This test is considered to be the Lachman test of the shoulder. (Adapted with permission from Boileau P, Zumstein M, Balg F, Penington S, Bicknell RT: The unstable painful shoulder (UPS) as a cause of pain from unrecognized anteroinferior instability in the young athlete. *J Shoulder Elbow Surg* 2011;20:98-106.)

d. Posterior instability—Posterior jerk test. In this test, the patient is seated and the arm is brought to 90° of forward elevation and 90° of internal rotation. An axial load is applied to the humerus with a posteriorly directed force, moving the arm through an arc of motion in the axial plane. The examiner attempts to subluxate the patient's humeral head posteriorly and then extends the shoulder toward 90° of abduction. The sensation of instability or a clunk as the humeral head reduces on extension of the shoulder constitutes a positive test result.

G. Neurovascular examination—Detailed in **Table 4**

H. Cervical spine—A comprehensive examination of the shoulder should include an upper quarter screen, especially if a patient's symptoms of pain or paresthesias radiate to the medial scapula or below the elbow. The examination should include an assessment of the ROM of the cervical spine, Spurling manuever of the neck to assess for radicular pain, and assessments of myotomal strength, dermatomal sensation, and reflexes when indicated.

II. ELBOW

A. Draping/positioning—Circumferential visual access to the elbows, forearms, and hands bilaterally is necessary. The examination is generally performed with the patient in the sitting position. Some tests for lateral instability require supine positioning of the patient with the arm above the head.

B. General inspection—The presence of bony/soft-tissue deformities, including abnormalities of the carrying angle of the elbow, is noted. Cubitus valgus of 11° to 14° in men and 13° to 16° in women is normal (measured in full extension of the arm and supination of the forearm). The elbows on both sides of the body are compared.

1. The elbow is examined for incisions/scars, regions of swelling/erythema, muscle atrophy, or any asymmetry. Intra-articular elbow effusions may be appreciated by examining for loss of the normal lateral dimple in the anconeus triangle.
2. In situations in which the LHB has ruptured, a Popeye deformity may be present, and in the case of a retracted distal biceps tendon rupture, a reverse Popeye deformity may be present.

C. Palpation—The anatomic landmarks of the elbow are palpated for evidence of swelling, warmth, tenderness, deformity, and instability. If during palpation the examiner encounters a painful structure, clarification should always be made of whether it reproduces the patient's typical symptoms.

1. Laterally, the landmarks of the elbow include the lateral epicondyle, origin of the common extensor tendon, posterior interosseous nerve, radiocapitellar joint, radial head, and capitellum.
2. Medially, the examiner should assess the ulnotrochlear joint, medial epicondyle, cubital tunnel/ulnar nerve, and origin of the common flexor tendon.

TABLE 4

Neurovascular Examination of the Shoulder

Nerve	Muscle(s)	Actions
Spinal accessory (CN 11)	Trapezius	Elevation of shoulder, stabilization of scapula
Dorsal scapular	Rhomboids and levator scapulae	Rhomboids: Scapular retraction Levator scapulae: Scapular elevation
Long thoracic	Serratus anterior	Scapular protraction with forward arm elevation
Lateral pectoral	Pectoralis major (clavicular head)	Adduction of humerus
Medial pectoral	Pectoralis major (sternal head) and pectoralis minor	Pectoralis major: Adduction and internal rotation of humerus Pectoralis minor: Depression of scapula
Suprascapular	Supraspinatus and infraspinatus	Supraspinatus: Abduction of humerus, depression of humeral head Infraspinatus: External rotation of humerus
Subscapular	Subscapularis and teres major	Subscapularis: Internal rotation of humerus Teres major: Adduction and internal rotation of humerus
Axillary	Deltoid and teres minor	Deltoid: Abduction of humerus Teres minor: External rotation of humerus
Musculocutaneous	Biceps, brachialis, and coracobrachialis	Biceps: Flexion and supination of elbow Brachialis: Flexion of elbow Coracobrachialis: Flexion of elbow, flexion and adduction of humerus
Radial	Triceps (in upper arm)	Extension of elbow

3. Posteriorly, the olecranon and bursa, proximal radioulnar joint, and triceps tendon can be palpated.
4. The sublime tubercle and distal biceps tendon should be examined anteriorly.

D. Range of motion

1. Active ROM can be assessed with the patient sitting or standing. The following movements are observed: elbow flexion/extension and pronation/supination with the elbow at 90° of flexion. Passive ROM is subsequently assessed and limitations are noted.
2. Both elbows are examined simultaneously and differences are noted in rhythm and maximum achieved ROM. **Table 5** depicts normal values for flexion and pronation/supination of the elbow.
3. Crepitance on assessment of the elbow ROM should be noted.
4. The relationship of pain and ROM should be assessed. Midarc pain may signify acute joint inflammation, whereas end-arc pain is associated with joint contractures and osteoarthritis.

E. Strength—The patient is examined in the sitting or standing position with the elbow flexed to 90° and the forearm in neutral rotation. Each motion is isolated and tested in sequence. Strength is graded with the Medical Research Council rating scale. Resisted elbow flexion and extension are assessed; extension power generally is 70% of flexion power. Resisted pronation and supination are also tested; pronation power generally is 80% of supination power. Provocation of pain with resisted movements should be noted.

TABLE 5

Normal and Functional Elbow Ranges of Motion

Motion	Normal Range	Functional Range
Flexion	0° (extension) → 145° (full flexion)	30° → 130°
Pronation-supination	75° (pronation) → 85° (supination)	50° → 50°

F. Special tests

1. Instability:

   a. Varus/valgus—The patient is placed in a seated position with the shoulder fully externally rotated to stabilize movement through the glenohumeral joint. The elbow is flexed to 30° to disengage the olecranon from its fossa (which in full extension will lock the elbow and give a false sense of stability).

      - The lateral ligament complex, and specifically the lateral ulnar collateral ligament, is assessed with the application of a varus stress, with palpation for any gapping at the radiocapitellar interval. The forearm should be supinated during this maneuver to relax the lateral forearm extensors, which act as secondary stabilizers.
      - To test for instability on the medial side of the elbow, a valgus stress test is applied and the examiner palpates for any gapping at the ulnotrochlear joint. If present, this can indicate insufficiency of the medial collateral ligament (MCL). The forearm should be pronated during this maneuver to relax the medial forearm flexors, which act as secondary stabilizers (**Figure 18**).

   b. Moving valgus stress test—Described for athletes involved in throwing who have symptomatic attenuation of the MCL, this test involves abducting the shoulder to 90°. A valgus force is applied to the elbow and the elbow is then brought quickly through a complete arc from flexion to full extension. Pain experienced at 70° to 120° of this arc can indicate symptomatic insufficiency of the MCL (**Figure 19**).

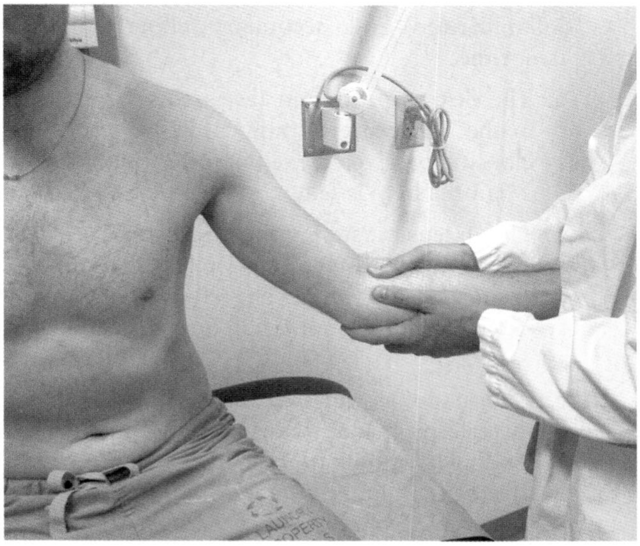

Figure 18 Photograph demonstrates the testing of varus and valgus elbow stability.

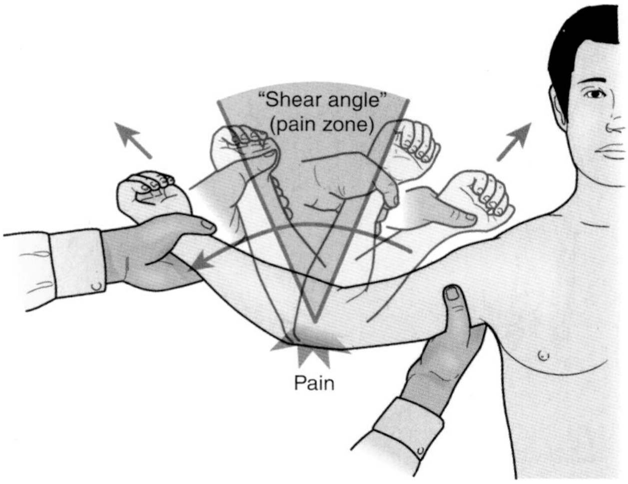

Figure 19 Illustration depicts the moving valgus stress test for insufficiency of the medial collateral ligament. (Adapted with permission from O'Driscoll SW, Lawton RL, Smith AM: The "moving valgus stress test" for medial collateral ligament tears of the elbow. *Am J Sports Med* 2005;33[2]:231-239.)

   c. Milking test—The patient positions the arm in adduction and external rotation at the shoulder, with the elbow flexed. The patient then reaches the contralateral arm underneath the elbow in question and, with the hand of the contralateral arm, applies traction to the thumb of the adducted and externally rotated arm, which creates a valgus moment across the elbow. The reproduction of pain across the medial aspect of the elbow constitutes a positive test result (**Figure 20**)

2. Posterolateral rotatory instability (PLRI): In posterolateral rotatory instability, the proximal radius and ulna remain as a unit, with a normal congruent articulation at the proximal radioulnar joint. Together, they rotate externally off the distal humerus in a spectrum of instability ranging from posterolateral subluxation of the radial head to full posterior ulnotrochlear dislocation. Generally, insufficiency of both the lateral ulnar collateral ligament and radial collateral ligament is required for PLRI. This differs from what occurs in proximal radioulnar joint instability as seen in Monteggia fractures.

   a. PLRI (lateral pivot shift) test—The patient is put in the supine position, and the affected arm is brought overhead. The humerus is stabilized, and the elbow is extended. With

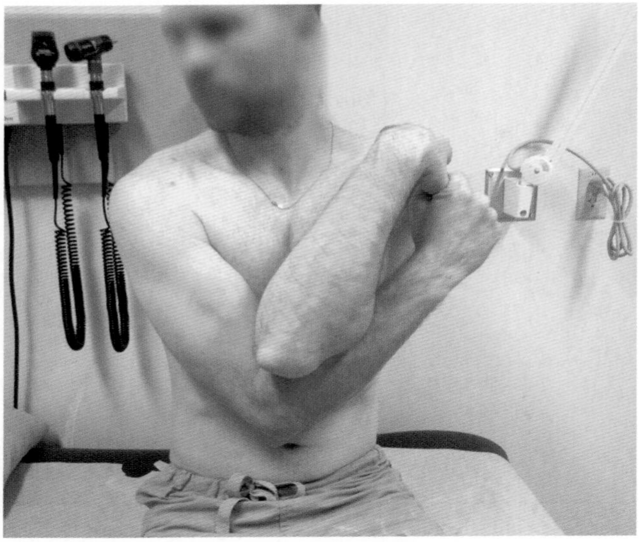

Figure 20 Photograph demonstrates the milking test for a tear of the ulnar collateral ligament.

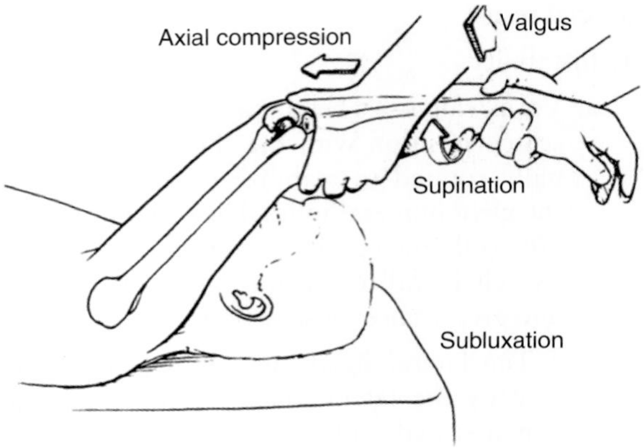

Figure 21 Illustration depicts the posterolateral rotatory instability test.

the elbow extended, the forearm is supinated and a valgus, axially directed load is applied to the elbow. In this position, the proximal ulna and radius are subluxated at the ulnotrochlear and radiocapitellar joints, respectively. The elbow is then progressively flexed, and a sense of apprehension accompanies its flexion. In the setting of PLRI, the unit consisting of the proximal ulna and radial head will reduce beyond 40° of flexion (the position of maximal displacement). Before this reduction occurs, a lateral skin dimple may be noted proximal to the radial head. Reduction is manifested by a palpable clunk as the radial head reduces. This test is challenging to perform in an awake patient, who often has difficulty relaxing sufficiently to properly perform the test (**Figure 21**).

b. Posterolateral drawer test—The elbow is flexed to 30°, and an AP force is applied to subluxate the ulna and radius off the distal humerus. The test is repeated at 90° of flexion, and a sensation of instability or palpable subluxation constitutes a positive test result. The posterolateral rotatory drawer test resembles this test, but instead, a hypersupination force is applied to the forearm, resulting in abnormal excessive posterolateral subluxation of the elbow.

c. Push-up and rising-from-chair tests—In the prone position, the patient attempts to push up from the floor with the forearms maximally supinated and the hands spaced wider than shoulder width. This applies a valgus, posteriorly directed load to the elbow. A positive test result consists of apprehension or instability as the elbow progresses from flexion to extension. The rising-from-chair test is a variation of this in which the patient pushes up and out of a chair, with the palms of the hands facing inward on the armrests and thus maximally supinating the forearm. As in the push-up test, the valgus, posteriorly directed forces across the elbow will aggravate symptoms of instability at approximately 40° of flexion. Relief of symptoms when the test is repeated with the forearm pronated (palms out) constitutes a positive test result.

3. Plica: Mechanical snapping with movement of the elbow through its ROM can be related to intra-articular plicae. Their presence can cause inflammation and secondary chondromalacia over time.

   a. The flexion-pronation test assesses for plicae in the anterolateral radiocapitellar joint. The elbow is passively flexed in full pronation, and a painful snap is felt.

   b. The extension-supination test can be used to assess for a posterolateral plica affecting the radiocapitellar joint. The elbow is passively extended in full supination and a painful snap is felt.

   c. Cubitus varus can alter the vector of pull for the triceps muscle, causing the distal triceps tendon to subluxate over the medial epicondyle of the humerus. When symptomatic, this is termed a snapping medial triceps. This condition also occurs in patients with hypertrophied triceps muscles, such as weight lifters.

4. Distal biceps tendon: Ruptures of the distal biceps tendon often manifest with pain and swelling in the antecubital fossa. Resisted flexion of the elbow and supination of the forearm can be painful. If the ruptured tendon is retracted, a reverse Popeye deformity may be present. The biceps crease interval can be determined by fully extending and supinating the elbow and measuring the distance between the main elbow flexion crease in the antecubital fossa and the distalmost aspect of the biceps muscle in its central axis. A biceps crease interval of >6 cm is predictive of a distal biceps tendon rupture. The belly of the biceps muscle should normally be seen to "rise and fall" with active flexion and extension of the elbow. The hook test can be used in the examination for a rupture of the distal biceps tendon. In this test, the patient flexes the elbow to 90° and fully supinates the forearm. The examiner's distal phalanx is inserted laterally beneath the distal biceps, hooking it and pulling the tendon forward. Inability to perform the test indicates a distal biceps tear (**Figure 22**).
5. Medial epicondylitis: Also termed golfer's elbow, medial epicondylitis is marked by degeneration and tendinosis of the common flexor origin at its attachment on the medial epicondyle. Direct palpation of this area will reproduce the pain experienced in golfer's elbow. Pain can also be reproduced with resisted flexion of the wrist and pronation of the forearm or passive wrist and elbow extension with supination. These tests stress the abnormal tissue and exacerbate symptoms, especially when coupled with direct palpation of the insertion of the common flexor tendon. Grip strength on the patient's affected side should also be compared with that on the opposite side.

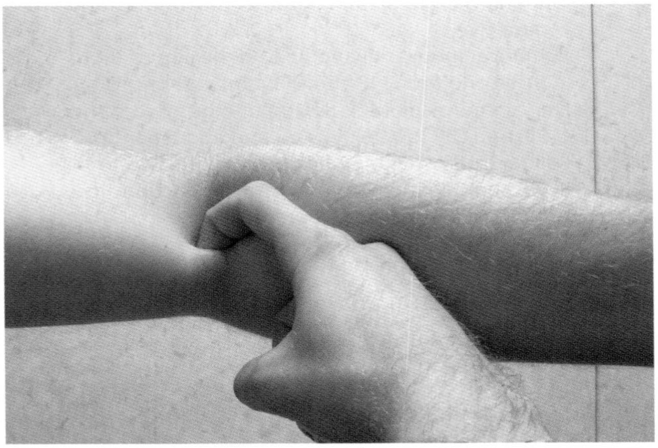

Figure 22 Photograph demonstrates the hook test for rupture of the distal biceps tendon.

6. Lateral epicondylitis: Also termed tennis elbow, lateral epicondylitis involves degeneration and tendinosis of the tendon of the extensor carpi radialis brevis muscle at its origin on the lateral epicondyle of the humerus. Direct palpation of this area will reproduce the pain of tennis elbow. Pain can also be reproduced with resisted wrist and long finger extension with the elbow in full extension (Maudsley test) or passive wrist and elbow flexion with pronation. Both of these maneuvers put tension on the abnormal tissue and will exacerbate symptoms, especially when coupled with direct palpation of the insertion of the extensor carpi radialis brevis tendon. Additionally, grip strength on the affected side will typically be diminished compared with that on the opposite side.
7. Ulnar nerve: Although it is important to examine all of the nerves in and around the elbow in patients with disorders of this joint, the ulnar nerve especially can be affected by many elbow disorders. Because of this, it should be evaluated closely for comorbid neuritis and compression.
   a. In examining the ulnar nerve, the examiner should palpate its course through a flexion-extension arc, assessing for evidence of subluxation over the medial epicondyle (which is particularly important if elbow arthroscopy is being considered because this is relatively contraindicated by ulnar nerve instability).
   b. The Tinel sign is identified by percussing the ulnar nerve along its length for signs of irritability. To exacerbate compression symptoms, the elbow is held in a hyperflexed position with the wrist extended for 1 minute, a procedure analogous to that in the Phalen test at the wrist. Any reproduction of numbness or paresthesia in the ulnar two digits of the hand is noted. The most common site of compression is at the cubital tunnel.
   c. The hand is evaluated for signs of severe ulnar neuropathy. These may include diminished two-point touch sensation, wasting of the interosseus muscles, clawing of the ulnar two digits, a positive Wartenberg sign (inability to adduct the little finger), and Froment sign (flexion of the thumb interphalangeal joint in pinching).
8. Neurovascular examination: The neurovascular examination of the elbow is detailed in **Table 6**.

TABLE 6

Neurovascular Examination of the Elbow

Nerve	Muscles	Actions
Radial	Brachioradialis, extensor carpi radialis longus	Brachioradialis: Flexion of elbow Extensor carpi radialis longus: Extension of wrist, deviation of radius
Posterior interosseous	Extensor carpi radialis brevis, supinator, extensor carpi ulnaris, extensor digitorum communis, abductor pollicis longus, extensor pollicis longus, extensor pollicis brevis, extensor indicis proprius	Supinator: Forearm supination Extensor carpi ulnaris: Wrist extension, ulnar deviation Extensor digitorum communis: MCP extension of digits two to five Extensor digiti quinti: MCP extension of digit five Abductor pollicis longus: Abduction of thumb in plane of palm Extensor pollicis longus and brevis: Extension of thumb Extensor indicis proprius: MCP extension of digit two
Median	Pronator teres, flexor carpi radialis, palmaris longus, flexor digitorum superficialis, lumbrical muscles, opponens pollicis, abductor pollicis brevis, flexor pollicis brevis	Pronator teres: Pronation of forearm Flexor carpi radialis: Flexion of wrist, deviation of radius Palmaris longus: Flexion of wrist Flexor digitorum superficialis: MCP and PIP flexion of digits two to five Lumbrical muscles I and II: MCP and PIP flexion of digits two and three, PIP and DIP extension Opponens pollicis: Flexion and opposition of thumb Abductor pollicis brevis: Abduction of thumb perpendicular to plane of palm Flexor pollicis brevis (superficial head): Thumb MCP joint flexion
Anterior interosseous	Flexor digitorum profundus (digits two and three), flexor pollicis longus, pronator quadratus	Flexor digitorum profundus flexion of digits two and three DIP flexion of digits two and three Flexor pollicis longus: Flexion of IP joint of thumb Pronator quadratus: Pronation of forearm
Ulnar	Flexor carpi ulnaris, flexor digitorum profundus (digits four and five), abductor digiti minimi, flexor digiti minimi, opponens digiti minimi, lumbrical muscles (digits three and four), interossei, adductor pollicis, palmaris brevis	Flexor carpi ulnaris: Flexion of wrist, deviation of ulna Flexor digitorum profundus (digits four and five): DIP joint flexion of digits four and five Abductor digiti minimi: Abduction of digit five Flexor digiti minimi: MCP flexion of digit five Opponens digiti minimi: Internal (palmar) rotation of digit five Lumbrical muscles III and IV: MCP flexion of digits three and four, PIP and DIP joint extension Dorsal interossei: MCP flexion of digits two to five, PIP and DIP joint extension and abduction Palmar interossei: MCP flexion of digits two to five, PIP and DIP joint extension and adduction Adductor pollicis: Adduction of thumb

DIP = distal interphalangeal; IP = interphalangeal; MCP = metacarpophalangeal; PIP = proximal interphalangeal

TOP TESTING FACTS

1. The external rotation lag or dropping sign indicates insufficiency of the infraspinatus muscle.
2. The belly-press and bear-hug tests assess for integrity and power of the subscapularis muscle.
3. GIRD is common in throwing athletes and may predispose to SLAP tears and partial articular supraspinatus tendon avulsion lesions.
4. The Paxinos test helps assess osteoarthritis of the AC joint.
5. Anterior shoulder instability should be assessed with a combination of the anterior apprehension, relocation, and surprise tests.
6. Partial tears of the MCL of the elbow manifest as pain with the moving valgus stress and milk tests.
7. During the posterolateral pivot shift test, the head of the radius will subluxate at 40° of flexion if PLRI (posterolateral rotatory instability) is present.
8. In the hook test, the examiners finger is inserted laterally beneath the distal biceps tendon.
9. The flexion-pronation test is used to identify plicae in the anterolateral radiocapitellar joint; the extension-supination test is used to identify posterolateral plicae in the radiocapitellar joint.
10. Signs of advanced ulnar neuropathy at the cubital tunnel include numbness, an ulnar clawhand with wasting of the interosseous muscles, Wartenberg sign, and Froment sign.

Bibliography

Barth JR, Burkhart SS, De Beer JF: The bear-hug test: A new and sensitive test for diagnosing a subscapularis tear. *Arthroscopy* 2006;22(10):1076-1084.

Chalmers PN, Cvetanovich GL, Kupfer N, et al: The champagne toast position isolates the supraspinatus better than the Jobe test: An electromyographic study of shoulder physical examination tests. *J Shoulder Elbow Surg* 2016;25:322-329.

Collin P, Treseder T, Denard PJ, Neyton L, Walch G, Lädermann A: What is the best clinical test for assessment of the teres minor in massive rotator cuff tears? *Clin Orthop Relat Res* 2015;473:2959-2966.

ElMaraghy A, Devereaux M, Tsoi K: The biceps crease interval for diagnosing complete distal biceps tendon ruptures. *Clin Orthop Relat Res* 2008;466:2255-2262.

Hawkins RJ, Kennedy JC: Impingement syndrome in athletes. *Am J Sports Med* 1980;8(3):151-158.

Kim SH, Ha KI, Ahn JH, Kim SH, Choi HJ: Biceps load test II: A clinical test for SLAP lesions of the shoulder. *Arthroscopy* 2001;17(2):160-164.

Lo IK, Nonweiler B, Woolfrey M, Litchfield R, Kirkley A: An evaluation of the apprehension, relocation, and surprise tests for anterior shoulder instability. *Am J Sports Med* 2004;32(2):301-307.

McFarland EG, Kim TK, Savino RM: Clinical assessment of three common tests for superior labral anterior-posterior lesions. *Am J Sports Med* 2002;30(6):810-815.

Neer CS II: Impingement lesions. *Clin Orthop Relat Res* 1983;173:70-77.

O'Brien SJ, Pagnani MJ, Fealy S, McGlynn SR, Wilson JB: The active compression test: A new and effective test for diagnosing labral tears and acromioclavicular joint abnormality. *Am J Sports Med* 1998;26(5):610-613.

O'Driscoll SW, Bell DF, Morrey BF: Posterolateral rotatory instability of the elbow. *J Bone Joint Surg Am* 1991;73(3):440-446.

O'Driscoll SW, Goncalves LB, Dietz P: The hook test for distal biceps tendon avulsion. *Am J Sports Med* 2007;35(11):1865-1869.

O'Driscoll SW, Lawton RL, Smith AM: The "moving valgus stress test" for medial collateral ligament tears of the elbow. *Am J Sports Med* 2005;33(2):231-239.

Parentis MA, Glousman RE, Mohr KS, Yocum LA: An evaluation of the provocative tests for superior labral anterior posterior lesions. *Am J Sports Med* 2006;34(2):265-268.

Snyder SJ, Karzel RP, Del Pizzo W, Ferkel RD, Friedman MJ: SLAP lesions of the shoulder. *Arthroscopy* 1990;6(4):274-279.

Taylor SA, Newman AM, Dawson C, et al: The "3-Pack" examination is critical for comprehensive evaluation of the biceps-labrum complex and bicipital tunnel: A prospective study. *Arthroscopy* 2017;33(1):28-38.

Walton J, Mahajan S, Paxinos A, et al: Diagnostic values of tests for acromioclavicular joint pain. *J Bone Joint Surg Am* 2004;86(4):807-812.

Chapter 71
IMAGING OF THE SHOULDER AND ELBOW

SHADLEY C. SCHIFFERN, MD
NADY HAMID, MD

I. SHOULDER

A. Radiographic evaluation of the shoulder

1. Indications—Conventional radiographs are appropriate for patients presenting with shoulder pain with any history of trauma, dislocation, night pain, or chronic shoulder pain.
2. Shoulder series—The standard shoulder series should include orthogonal views of the shoulder, including a true AP view in the scapular plane, an AP view, an axillary view, and a scapular Y view.
   a. True AP view in the scapular plane: Visualizes anterior greater tuberosity in profile. The x-ray beam is positioned perpendicular to the plane of the scapula, and the arm is held in neutral rotation with the shoulder in slight abduction (dynamic loading of cuff and deltoid), which can reveal proximal humeral migration.
   b. AP view: The arm is held in internal rotation. This view visualizes the posterior aspect of the greater tuberosity and the lesser tuberosity in profile. The x-ray beam is positioned perpendicular to the coronal plane of the body.
   c. Axillary view: Necessary view in evaluation of glenohumeral joint instability. This view enables to determine the humeral head position in the glenoid fossa. Often overlooked, this view may detect occult, locked posterior shoulder dislocation in a patient who exhibits a lack of passive external rotation. The axillary view is also helpful in evaluation of glenoid morphology in glenohumeral osteoarthritis and provides good visualization of the coracoid process, acromion, and distal clavicle.
   d. Scapular Y view: This view provides visualization of the coracoacromial arch and can reveal coracoacromial spurs, which have been closely associated with the presence of rotator cuff pathology. The scapula Y view is also a reliable alternative for evaluation of glenohumeral subluxation and dislocation. It can also show scapular body abnormalities (eg, osteochondroma, fracture) and acromial shape.
3. Special shoulder views—see **Table 1**.
4. Normal radiographic parameters
   a. The acromiohumeral distance is normally 7 to 14 mm. The width of the glenohumeral joint space should be symmetric superiorly and inferiorly.
   b. The coracoclavicular distance is normally 1.1 to 1.3 cm.
   c. Neer classified acromial morphology as follows: type I (flat), type II (curved), and type III (hooked). Type III acromial morphology has been shown to have a correlation with the presence of rotator cuff disease; however, no direct causal relationship has been demonstrated. The classification has shown relatively poor interobserver reliability.

B. CT

1. Indications
   a. Glenoid bone loss: CT with three-dimensional reconstructions is the advanced imaging study of choice for determining the extent of glenoid bone loss in the setting of shoulder instability (**Figure 1**).

Dr. Schiffern or an immediate family member serves as a paid consultant to or is an employee of Lima USA, Medacta, and Wright Medical Technology, Inc. Dr. Hamid or an immediate family member serves as a paid consultant to or is an employee of Biomet.

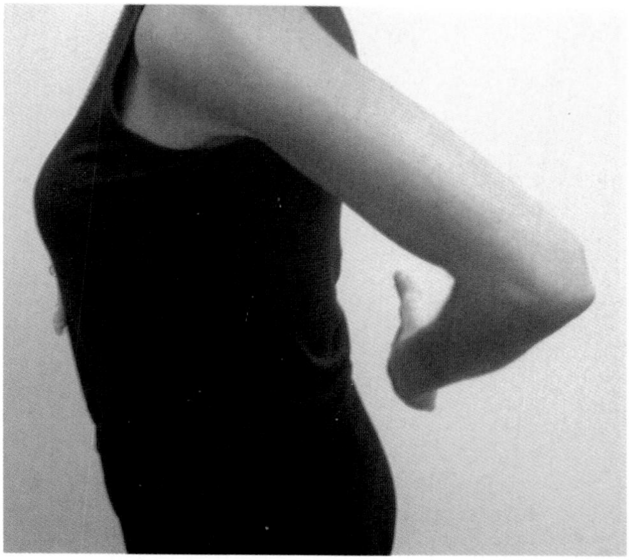

Figure 2 Photograph shows the modified lift-off test for subscapularis function. In this test, the patient places a hand behind the back, with the palm facing away from the body and then lifts the hand away from the back. A patient with a subscapularis tear will not be able to lift the hand off the back.

- AP view in external and internal rotation. Greater tuberosity excrescences pathognomonic for cuff disease.

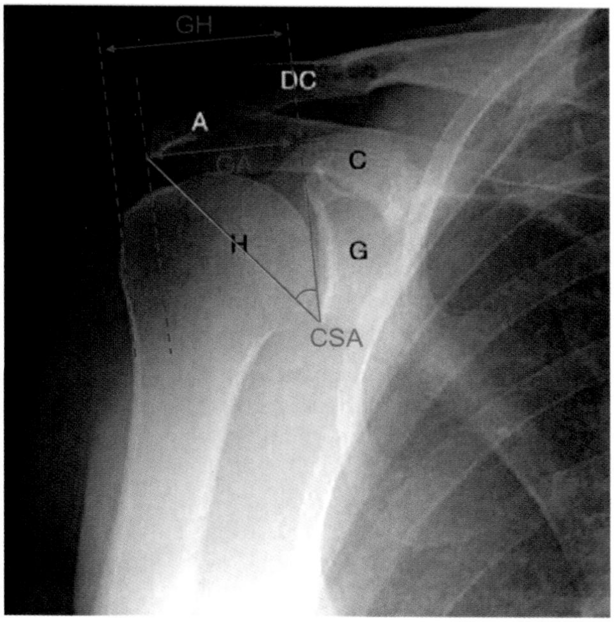

Figure 3 The glenohumeral joint space is evaluated on a true AP radiograph of a shoulder. A = acromion, C = coracoid, CSA = critical shoulder angle, DC = distal clavicle, G = glenoid, GA = glenoacromial distance, GH = glenohumeral distance, H = humerus. Acromion index (AI) = GA/GH

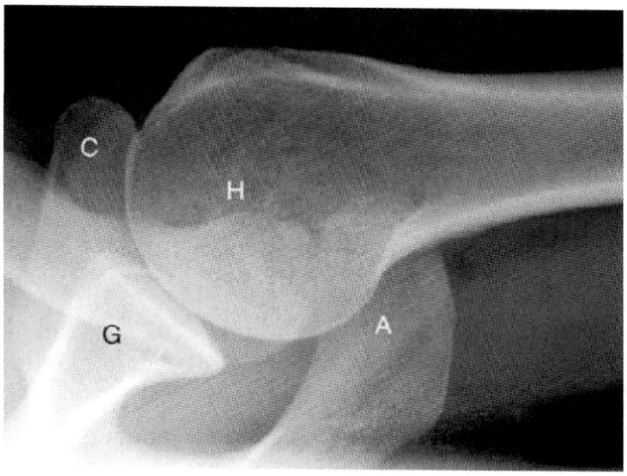

Figure 4 Axillary radiograph of a shoulder. A = acromion, C = coracoid, G = glenoid, H = humerus

- Supraspinatus outlet view: evaluate acromial morphology according to Bigliani (type 1 = flat; type 2 = curved; type 3 = hooked).
- Axillary view to assess glenohumeral joint morphology and joint space and rule out dislocations (**Figure 4**).

b. MRI

- MRI is the benchmark for diagnosing RCTs (94% sensitivity and 93% specificity).
- T2-weighted images best visualize RCTs (**Figure 5**).

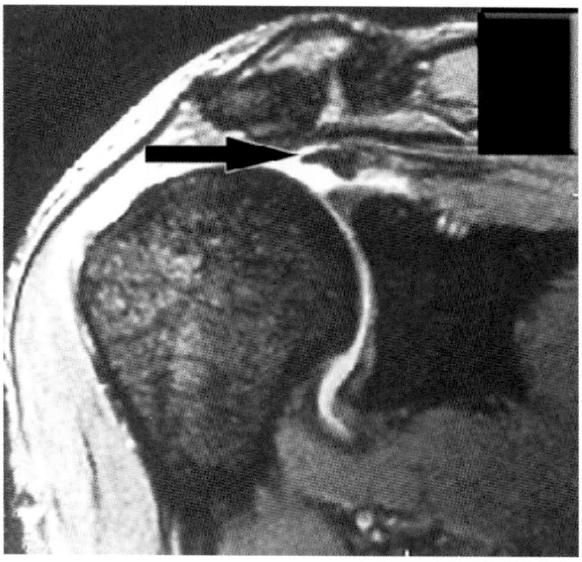

Figure 5 T2-weighted coronal oblique MRI demonstrates a supraspinatus tear (arrow).

- T1 sagittal oblique cuts reveal muscle/tendon retraction and muscle atrophy to determine chronicity, reparability, and outcome of surgical RCT repairs.
- Intra-articular contrast-enhanced magnetic resonance arthrography (MRA) is best for detecting partial-thickness RCTs (95% sensitivity and 95% specificity).

c. Ultrasonography
- Advantages: good accuracy (92% sensitivity and 93% specificity) and dynamic assessment of the cuff insertion.
- Disadvantages: operator dependent; limited assess of chondral lesions; poor sensitivity to diagnose partial-thickness RCTs.

d. CT arthrography
- Uncommon in the United States.
- Useful in postoperative assessment, retear evaluation in patients with retained metallic anchors causing artifact on MRI, and when MRI is contraindicated.

E. Classification
1. Time: acute versus chronic (>3 months from the onset of pain/injury).
2. Anatomic: supraspinatus, infraspinatus, teres minor, subscapularis, and combinations (1, 2, 3, or 4 tendons).
3. Thickness: Full-thickness (complete tears) or partial-thickness.
4. Size: small (0 to 1 cm), medium (1 to 3 cm), large (3 to 5 cm), and massive (>5 cm).
5. Shape: crescent (rotator cable preserved), U-shaped, L-shaped, and retracted-immobile.
6. Ellman classification for partial-thickness RCTs
   a. Location: articular side (PASTA lesions), bursal side, or intratendinous.
   b. Size/thickness: grade I <3 mm (<25%); grade II 3 to 6 mm (25% to 50%); grade III >6 mm (>50%).
7. Goutallier-Fuchs for fatty atrophy: T1 sagittal MRI cuts. Grade 0: normal muscle; grade 1: some fat streaks; grade 2: more muscle than fat; grade 3: fat evident on equivalent amount as muscle; grade 4: more fat than muscle.
8. Tangent sign corresponds with muscle atrophy and chronicity (**Figure 6**).

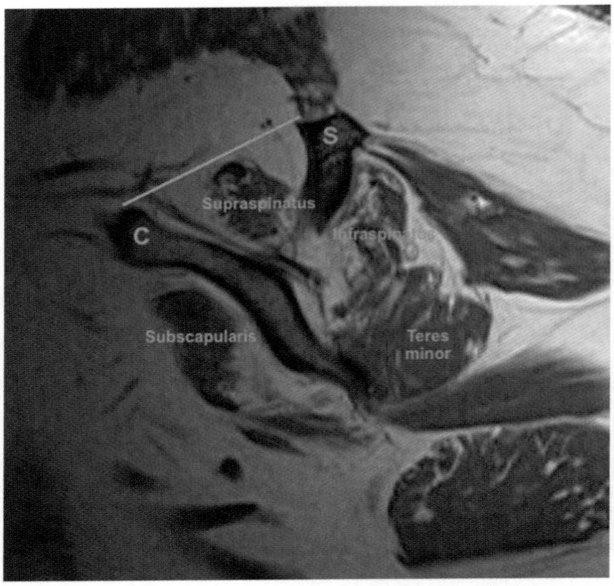

Figure 6 T1-weighted sagittal oblique MRI demonstrates a positive tangent sign. C = coracoid; S = scapular spine.

F. Treatment
1. Nonsurgical treatment: rest, ice, NSAIDs, physical therapy, corticosteroid injections.
   a. First-line treatment for most tears.
   b. Older, low demand, comorbidities.
   c. A recent UK meta-analysis demonstrated the natural history of RCTs is to improve over time, whether treated operatively or nonoperatively.
   d. Physical therapy (PT): stretching, cuff and periscapular stabilizers strengthening.
   e. Subacromial corticosteroid injections: improve pain and motion, facilitating PT; multiple injections are not recommended due to the risk of tendon degeneration and infection.
   f. Platelet-rich plasma: inconclusive evidence in literature to support its use for total or partial-thickness RCTs, neither as an adjuvant to repairs.
2. Surgical treatment
   a. Indications
      - Fail of nonsurgical treatment (>6 months).
      - Traumatic RCTs in active patients.
      - Acute full-thickness tears (<3 months)

- Older patients with chronic RCTs with good-quality muscle on MRI and low fatty-infiltration grades.
- Partial-thickness (PASTA) tear > 50%; if <50%, can treated with subacromial débridement alone.

b. Contraindications

- Infection.
- Advanced glenohumeral arthritis.
- Chronically retracted tendons and atrophic rotator cuff muscles.
- Fixed proximal migration of humeral head, with acromiohumeral interval <7 mm (rotator cuff arthropathy).
- Deltoid or axillary nerve dysfunction.

3. Surgical procedures

a. Arthroscopic: minimally invasive, equivalent results to open repair, and allows assessment and treatment of surrounding structures (biceps tenodesis, AC resection, cartilage débridement, labrum). Appropriate arthroscopic portals establishment is crucial.

- Posterior portal: 1 cm medial and 1 cm inferior to the posterolateral corner of the acromion.
- Rotator interval portal (used for intra-articular work): just lateral to the coracoid process.
- Anterolateral portal (used to access the subacromial space): 2 cm lateral/inferior to the lateral acromion.
- Posterolateral subacromial portals: 2 cm lateral/inferior to the posterolateral border of the acromion.

b. Mini-open cuff repair: lateral longitudinal incision and deltoid slitting.

- Avoid deltoid takedown, decreasing the risk of deltoid avulsion and postoperative weakness.
- Appropriate for small to medium tears and superior third subscapularis tears.
- Avoid splitting deltoid >5 cm distal from the anterolateral corner of the acromion to protect the axillary nerve

c. Open rotator cuff repair: transversal shoulder incision and deltoid detachment from acromion.

- Appropriate for repair RCT of all sizes, especially massive retracted RCTs.
- Subsequent repair of deltoid is important.

d. Rotator cuff repair constructs

- A large meta-analysis has indicated essentially equivalent results with single-row, double-row, or transosseous equivalent techniques.
- Single-row repair: single line of suture anchors based on top of the greater tuberosity, allowing simple sutures, mattress, or combined/cruciate for fixation.
- Double-row repair: medial anchors with sutures passed in a mattress fashion, and lateral anchors with simple sutures; lateral sutures are tied first.
- Transosseous equivalent: medial anchors with sutures passed in mattress fashion and sutures left long and captured by laterally based humeral anchors for a compression-type rotator cuff repair.
- Partial-thickness articular side tears (PASTA): >50% complete tear and repair; <50% débridement or in-situ repair is good tendon quality.
- Graft augmentation of RCTs: currently there is limited evidence supporting the use of allografts (human skin), xenografts (bovine dermal grafts), autograft (muscular fascia), or synthetic collagen grafts.
- Massive RCTs: partial repairs (subscapularis and infraspinatus) can be attempted to re-create both anterior and posterior force couples of the cuff, together with adjuvant procedures (AC resection, biceps tenodesis or tenotomy, suprascapular nerve decompression); the coracoacromial arch must be preserved to avoid iatrogenic anterosuperior escape of the humeral head.

e. Surgical options for massive irreparable RCTs in young patients

- Superior capsule reconstruction: equivocal results have been observed with dermal allograft or fascia lata autograft to reconstruct the superior capsule to restore shoulder stability and avoid superior escape, but randomized long-term outcomes are necessary to determine longevity and equivalence.

- Tendon transfers: require patient commitment to postoperative rehabilitation, and outcomes reported are very variable.
- Pectoralis major transfer for subscapularis: transferring the pectoralis underneath the conjoint tendon reproduces native force vectors of the subscapularis.
- Latissimus dorsi transfer for infraspinatus and/or supraspinatus: best results are on young laborers to restore external rotation and secondary gain of elevation; an intact subscapularis is mandatory; technically demanding procedure with risk of iatrogenic injuries to the radial and axillary nerves.
- Lower trapezius transfer to supraspinatus: superior biomechanics to restore elevation, but still lack clinical evidence. Requires allograft and can be performed open or combined arthroscopic and open with promising early results.

G. Complications

1. Infection (<1%): *Cutibacterium acnes* (most common), coagulase-negative *Staphylococcus*, *Peptostreptococcus*, and *Staphylococcus aureus*.
2. Deltoid dehiscence and weakness.
3. Recurrent tears: age >65 years, larger chronic tears, poor quality tendon, retraction, smoking, and uncontrolled diabetes.
4. Iatrogenic nerve injury: suprascapular and/or axillary.
5. Adhesive capsulitis: happens early after surgery, lasting from 6 months to 2 years to restore function; 5% evolve with permanent restriction of shoulder motion requiring arthroscopic release.
6. Persistent shoulder pain: look for associated pathologic conditions (biceps tendinosis, glenohumeral arthritis, instability, cervical radiculopathy, brachial plexitis, or Parsonage-Turner syndrome).

H. Pearls and pitfalls

1. Multiple corticosteroid injections should be avoided.
2. Open surgical procedures that involve deltoid detachment require meticulous deltoid repair to prevent dehiscence, which is a devastating complication.
3. Arthroscopy-specific complications include severe intraoperative edema, peripheral nerve neurapraxia, and failure of the rotator cuff repair due to technical difficulties intraoperatively.
4. Elderly patients often do well with nonsurgical treatments, including deltoid and periscapular muscles strengthening protocols.
5. Larger or massive rotator cuff repairs require tension-free repair, longer immobilization period and slower rehabilitation.

II. CUFF TEAR ARTHROPATHY

A. Epidemiology and overview

1. Cuff tear arthropathy (CTA) is the final stage of the shoulder impingement syndrome spectrum. It affects patients with long-term insufficient massive RCTs, superior migration of the humeral head toward the acromion, subchondral osteoporosis, humeral head collapse, and painful debilitating shoulder arthritis.
2. Initially known as Milwaukee shoulder syndrome due to the rapidly progressive destruction of cartilage and bone, noninflammatory joint effusion containing calcium hydroxyapatite crystals, synovial hyperplasia, and multiple loose bodies.
3. Affects women (3:1 female to male ratio), over 70 yo, more commonly on the dominant shoulder.
4. Risk factors: chronic RCT, hemorrhagic shoulder (oral anticoagulants and hematologic diseases), rheumatic disease, and crystal-induced arthropathy.

B. Pathogenesis

1. Neer suggested mechanical, nutritional, and crystal-induced arthropathy pathways (**Figure 7**), but no definitive pathogenesis has been identified.
2. Mechanical factors: insufficient cuff, superior migration of the humeral head, instability, eccentric wear of the glenoid, humeral head deformity, and decreased shoulder function.
3. Nutritional: hypomobility-induced cartilage atrophy, poor nutrition (decrease in glycosaminoglycans), dehydration, and subchondral osteoporosis
4. Crystalline-induced arthropathy: synovial-based matrix proteins degradation destroys rotator cuff tendons and cartilage; end-stage calcium-phosphate crystal deposition.

C. History and physical examination

1. Chronic shoulder pain, night pain, weakness, and stiffness.
2. Inspection: supraspinatus and infraspinatus atrophy, anterior prominence of humeral head with arm elevation (anterosuperior escape), and subcutaneous effusion.

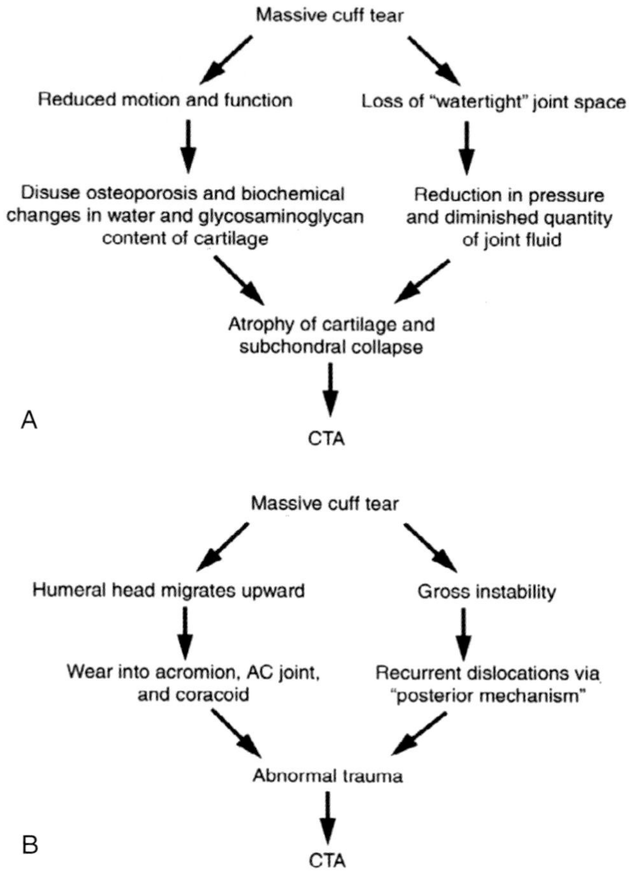

Figure 7 Illustrations depict the nutritional and mechanical pathways involved in cuff tear arthropathy (CTA). **A**, Nutritional factors include the loss of a so-called watertight joint space and a reduction in the pressure of the joint fluid that is required for the perfusion of nutrients to the articular cartilage. Both contribute to the atrophy of cartilage and disuse osteoporosis in the subchondral bone of the humeral head. **B**, Mechanical factors include upward, anterior, and posterior instability of the humeral head. Upward instability escalates wear into the anterior part of the acromion, the acromioclavicular (AC) joint, and the coracoid. (Adapted with permission from Neer CS II, Craig EV, Fukuda H: Cuff-tear arthropathy. *J Bone Joint Surg Am* 1983;65:1232-1244.)

3. Range of motion (ROM)
   a. Subacromial/glenohumeral crepitus with movement.
   b. Very limited ROM for elevation, external, and internal rotation.
   c. Pseudoparalysis: less than 60° elevation, lack of active external rotation, and incompetent subscapularis.
   d. Chronic long head of biceps rupture is usually present.
4. External rotation lag sign and hornblower sign (inability to keep external rotation when the shoulder is 90° flexed and 90° abducted, indicating teres minor insufficiency).

D. Imaging
1. Radiographs: AP, axillary, true AP.
   a. Acetabularization of the acromion and femoralization of the humeral head.
   b. Eccentric superior glenoid wear.
   c. Absence of typical peripheral osteophytes around the humeral head as seen on osteoarthritis.
   d. Osteopenia and subarticular sclerosis (snowcap sign).
   e. Loss of the coracoacromial arch, indicating anterosuperior escape.
2. MRI/CT scan: not routinely necessary, especially if radiographs show anterosuperior escape.
   a. Establishes the extent of RCT, retraction, and fatty infiltration.
   b. CT is helpful to quantify glenoid bone stock when reverse shoulder replacement is considered in cases of advanced arthropathy.

E. Classifications
1. Hamada—classification for rotator cuff arthropathy (**Figure 8**).
2. Favard—classification for rotator cuff arthropathy (**Figure 9**).
3. Sirveaux—classification for scapular notching after reverse shoulder replacements (**Figure 10**).

F. Treatment
1. Nonsurgical: rest, ice, NSAIDs, activity modification, physical therapy, subacromial corticosteroid injection, therapeutic ultrasonography, and laser therapy.
   a. If elevation >60°, deltoid-strengthening exercises protocol may improve function and pain relief.
   b. Pseudoparalytic shoulders usually do not improve with conservative measures.
2. Surgical treatment
   a. Indications: failed nonsurgical treatment, pseudoparalytic shoulder, and uncontrolled pain with conservative measures.
   b. Contraindications: deltoid dysfunction, noncompliant patients to postoperative rehabilitations, chronic infection, and poor glenohumeral bone stock.

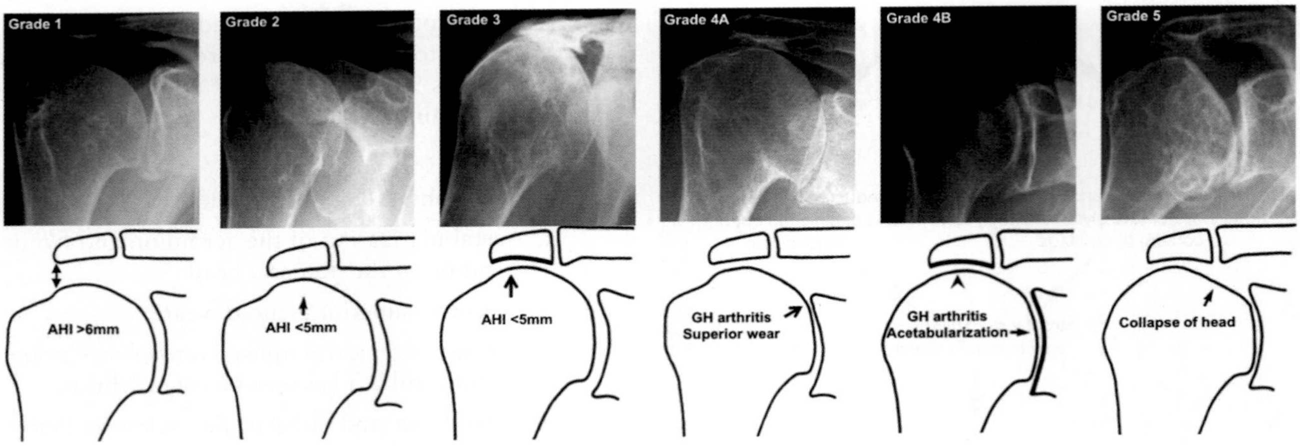

Figure 8 Radiographs and illustrations show the Hamada classification for rotator cuff arthropathy. (Adapted with permission from Hamada K, Yamanaka K, Uchiyama Y, Mikasa T, Mikasa M: A radiographic classification of massive rotator cuff tear arthritis. *Clin Orthop Relat Res* 2011;469[9]:2452-2460, Figures 1 through 5.)

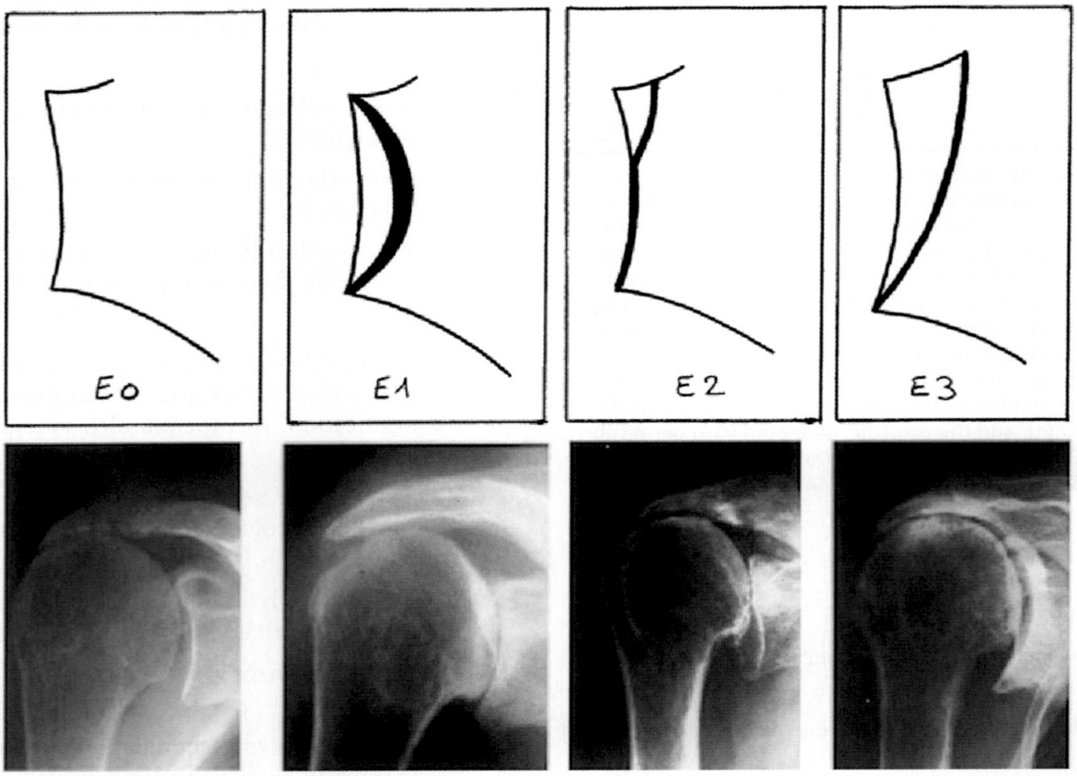

Figure 9 Illustrations and radiographs show the Favard classification for rotator cuff arthropathy. (Used with permission from Sirveaux F, Favard L, Oudet D, Huquet D, Walch G, Molé D: Grammont inverted total shoulder arthroplasty in the treatment of glenohumeral osteoarthritis with massive rupture of the cuff. *J Bone Joint Surg [Br]* 2004;86-B:388-395. [Figure 2, p 390].)

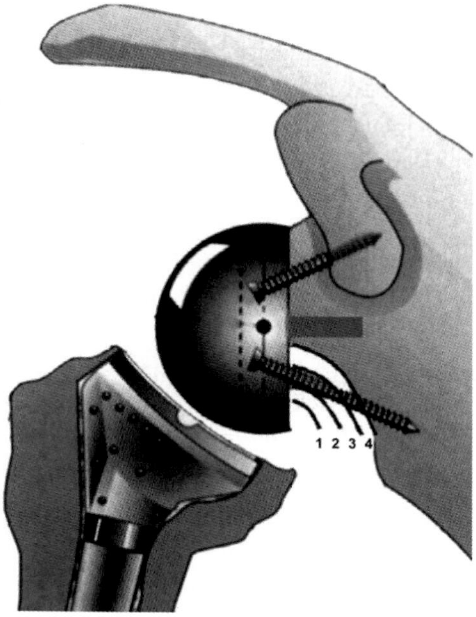

Figure 10 Illustration shows the Sirveaux classification for scapular notching. Numbers 1 to 4 represent the grade of notching according to the Sirveaux classification. Grade 1 notch is a defect contained within the inferior pillar of the scapular neck. Grade 2 notch is erosion of the scapular neck to the level of the inferior fixation screw of the baseplate. Grade 3 notch is extension of the bone loss over the lower fixation screw. Grade 4 notch is progression to the undersurface of the baseplate. (Used with permission from Sirveaux F, Favard L, Oudet D, Huquet D, Walch G, Molé D: Grammont inverted total shoulder arthroplasty in the treatment of glenohumeral osteoarthritis with massive rupture of the cuff. *J Bone Joint Surg* 2004;86:388-395. [Figure 3, p 391].)

3. Surgical procedures
   a. Arthroscopic débridement
      - Unpredictable outcomes.
      - Must preserve the coracoacromial arch (no CA ligament release or acromioplasty) to avoid anterosuperior escape.
      - Greater tuberosity "tuberoplasty" creates a smooth tuberosity-acromion interface.
      - Can be combined with adjuvant procedures: long head of biceps tenotomy or tenodesis and suprascapular nerve decompression.
   b. Hemiarthroplasty (humeral head replacement only)
      - Must have a functioning deltoid and preserved coracoacromial arch.
      - Indicated for young active patients.
      - The combination of concentric glenoid reaming and a humeral head component (CTA design) under the coracoacromial arch grant stability to prosthesis.

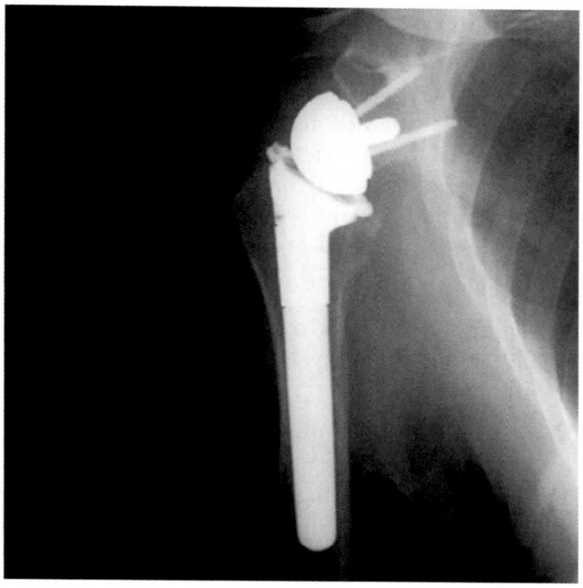

Figure 11 AP radiograph of a shoulder after reverse shoulder arthroplasty.

      - Outcomes are limited: pain relief only; no function improvement over 90° elevation can be promised to patients.
   c. Reverse shoulder arthroplasty (RSA; **Figure 11**)
      - Indications: pseudoparalytic shoulder; anterosuperior escape (insufficient coracoacromial arch); age >70 years (controversial).
      - Functioning deltoid and adequate glenoid bone stock are mandatory.
      - Grammont design prosthesis move the center of rotation inferiorly and medially to assist the deltoid fulcrum and improve active abduction.
      - Outcomes are good and reproducible, especially pain relief (greater than 30% improvement in Constant-Murley score) and improved elevation (over 100°); external or internal rotation may not improve due to infraspinatus/teres minor and subscapularis deficiency.
      - Good outcomes has extended the use of RSA to younger patients (>60 yo).
   d. Resection arthroplasty: salvage procedure indicated for very low-demand patients, multiple comorbidities, chronic osteomyelitis, deltoid insufficiency, alcoholism, multiple previous surgeries, and/or poor soft-tissue coverage.

6 | Shoulder and Elbow

e. Arthrodesis: indicated in salvage situations only; in general, it is poorly tolerated by older patients (other than 60 years).

f. Total shoulder arthroplasty (TSA) and resurfacing prosthesis are absolutely contraindicated for RCT arthropathy; they lead to early glenoid loosening via the "rocking horse" phenomenon and poor outcomes.

G. RSA rehabilitation

1. Sling is worn for 3 to 6 weeks, followed by gradual active and active-assisted range of motion in all planes.
2. Deltoid strengthening from supine to sitting is instituted at 6 to 8 weeks.
3. Many patients are taught a home exercise program and do not require formal physical therapy.

H. Complications

1. Prosthetic replacement (RSA and hemiarthroplasty): infection, perioperative hematoma, anterosuperior escape (hemiarthroplasty), instability, component wear, scapular notching, acromion stress fractures, and residual pain and dysfunction.
2. RSA has a relatively higher complication rate compared with hemiarthroplasty.
3. Scapular notching
   a. Unique complication of Grammont-style RSAs (neckless component design).
   b. Incidence: 44% to 96%, but the clinical relevance is still controversial in the literature.
   c. The medial and inferior center of rotation predispose to abutment of the humeral component with the inferior scapular neck.
   d. This is mitigated by more lateral offset designed prostheses.
   e. Sirveaux classified notching according to the glenoid neck erosion on AP radiographic images of the shoulder (**Figure 10**).

I. Pearls and pitfalls

1. Nonsurgical treatment should be maximized with physical therapy and NSAIDs.
2. Anterosuperior escape is an iatrogenic complication secondary to loss of the CA arch after aggressive acromioplasty in conjunction with rotator cuff insufficiency. To avoid anterosuperior escape, the CA arch should be preserved with arthroscopic débridement and arthroplasty.
3. Glenoid implantation, which leads to early glenoid failure (TSA), should be avoided.
4. Anterior deltoid strengthening may provide good function in elderly patients with massive RCTs.

TOP TESTING FACTS

Rotator Cuff Tears

1. Partial-thickness RCTs often progress in both size and symptoms.
2. To determine whether an RCT is chronic, MRI (especially in the sagittal oblique plane) should be used to measure muscle retraction and atrophy.
3. Older and less active patients may do well with nonsurgical treatment.
4. During repair of massive RCTs, the integrity of the CA ligament should be maintained to prevent iatrogenic anterosuperior escape.
5. An intact subscapularis tendon is required for latissimus dorsi tendon transfer.

Cuff Tear Arthropathy

1. Characteristics of CTA include a massive, chronic RCT; destruction of glenohumeral cartilage; osteoporosis of subchondral bone; and humeral head collapse.
2. Acetabularization of the acromion and femoralization of the humeral head are two radiographic features of CTA.
3. RSA is indicated if the patient has a pseudoparalytic CTA shoulder or is older than 70 years (controversial).
4. Anterosuperior escape is salvageable with RSA.
5. TSA is contraindicated in the treatment of CTA because it may lead to glenoid failure (the "rocking horse" phenomenon).
6. To avoid anterosuperior escape, the CA arch should be preserved with arthroscopic débridement and arthroplasty.

Bibliography

Chalmers PN, Granger E, Nelson R, Yoo M, Tashjian RZ: Factors affecting cost, outcomes and tendon healing after arthroscopic rotator cuff repair. *Arthroscopy* 2018;34(5):1393-1400. doi:10.1016/j.arthro.2017.11.015.

Codding JL, Keener JD: Natural history of degenerative rotator cuff tears. *Curr Rev Musculoskelet Med* 2018;11:77-85. doi:10.1007/s12178-018-9461-8.

Cuff DJ, Pupello DR: Prospective randomized study of arthroscopic rotator cuff repair using an early versus delayed postoperative physical therapy protocol. *J Shoulder Elbow Surg* 2012;21(11):1450-1455.

DeHaan AM, Axelrad TW, Kaye E, Silvestri L, Puskas B, Foster TE: Does double-row rotator cuff repair improve functional outcome of patients compared with single-row technique? A systematic review. *Am J Sports Med* 2012;40(5):1176-1185.

Guery J, Favard L, Sirveaux F, Oudet D, Mole D, Walch G: Reverse total shoulder arthroplasty: Survivorship analysis of eighty replacements followed for five to ten years. *J Bone Joint Surg Am* 2006;88(8):1742-1747.

Hamada K, Yamanaka K, Uchiyama Y, Mikasa T, Mikasa M: A radiographic classification of massive rotator cuff tear arthritis. *Clin Orthop Relat Res* 2011;469: 2452-2460. doi:10.1007/s11999-011-1896-9.

Hsu J, Keener JD: Natural history of rotator cuff disease and implications on management *Oper Tech Orthop* 2015;25(1):2-9. doi:10.1053/j.oto.2014.11.006.

Imam MA, Holton J, Horriat S, et al: A systemic review of the concept and clinical applications of bone marrow aspirate concentrate in tendon pathology. *SICOT J* 2017;3:58. doi:10.1051/sicotj/2017039.

Khatri C, Parsons H, Lawrence TM, et al: The natural history of full-thickness rotator cuff tears in randomized controlled trials: A systematic review and meta-analysis. *Am J Sports Med* 2019;47(7):1734-1743. doi:10.1177/0363546518780694.

Lenza M, Buchbinder R, Takwoingi Y, Johnston RV, Hanchard NCA, Faloppa F: Magnetic resonance imaging, magnetic resonance arthrography and ultrasonography for assessing rotator cuff tears in people with shoulder pain for whom surgery is being considered. *Cochrane Database Syst Rev* 2013;(9):CD009020. doi:10.1002/14651858.CD009020.pub2.

Li H, Chen Y, Chen J, Hua Y, Chen S: Large critical shoulder angle has higher risk of tendon retear after arthroscopic rotator cuff repair. *Am J Sports Med* 2018;46(8):1892-1900. doi:10.1177/0363546518767634.

Mall NA, Kim HM, Keener JD, et al: Symptomatic progression of asymptomatic rotator cuff tears: A prospective study of clinical and sonographic variables. *J Bone Joint Surg Am* 2010;92(16):2623-2633.

Nolan BM, Ankerson E, 'Mater JM: Reverse total shoulder arthroplasty improves function in cuff tear arthropathy. *Clin Orthop Relat Res* 2011;469(9):2476-2482.

Park HB, Yokota A, Gill HS, El Rassi G, MacFarland EG: Diagnostic accuracy of clinical tests for the different degrees of subacromial impingement syndrome. *J Bone Joint Surg Am* 2005;87(7):1446-1455. doi:10.2106/JBJS.D.02335.

Sirveaux F, Favard L, Oudet D, et al: Grammont inverted total shoulder arthroplasty in the treatment of glenohumeral osteoarthritis with massive rupture of the cuff. *J Bone Joint Surg Br* 2004;86-B:388-395. doi:10.1302/0301-620X.86B3.

Sobhy MH, Khater AH, Hassan MR, El Shazly O: Do functional outcomes and cuff integrity correlate after single-versus double-row rotator cuff repair? A systematic review and meta-analysis study. *Eur J Orthop Surg Traumatol* 2018;28(4):593-605. doi:10.1007/s00590-018-2145-7.

Yamaguchi K, Ditsios K, Middleton WD, Hildebolt CF, Galatz LM, Teefey SA: The demographic and morphological features of rotator cuff disease: A comparison of asymptomatic and symptomatic shoulders. *J Bone Joint Surg Am* 2006;88(8):1699-1704.

Chapter 73
THE UNSTABLE SHOULDER

STEVEN M. ANDELMAN, MD
AUGUSTUS D. MAZZOCCA, MS, MD
ROBERT A. ARCIERO, MD

I. OVERVIEW AND TERMINOLOGY

A. Laxity is a physiologic term that refers to the passive translation of the humeral head on the glenoid or over the glenoid rim. Laxity may be pathologic or physiologic.

B. Glenohumeral instability is a pathologic state in which glenohumeral laxity causes pain, subluxation, or dislocation.

II. CLASSIFICATION

A. Glenohumeral instability represents a spectrum of pathology based on the direction of laxity (anterior, posterior, or multidirectional) and the underlying cause (traumatic or atraumatic).

1. Traumatic anterior instability: a traumatic event causing an anteriorly directed force with the arm positioned in abduction and external rotation causing an anterior glenohumeral dislocation.
2. Traumatic posterior instability: a traumatic event causing a posteriorly directed force on an arm positioned in forward flexion and adduction causing a posterior glenohumeral dislocation.
3. Acquired/atraumatic instability: pathologic glenohumeral laxity due to repetitive trauma to the capsule and intraarticular structures of the shoulder (throwers).
4. Multidirectional instability: pathologic glenohumeral laxity with recurrent subluxation or dislocation in more than one direction.

III. ANATOMY

A. Glenohumeral stability depends on active and passive restraints.

1. Passive restraints: the primary passive restraint is the labrum, a cartilaginous ring that encircles the glenoid, deepening the glenoid fossa and serving as an attachment site for capsuloligamentous structures. The glenohumeral ligaments form a second important passive restraint and attach to the glenoid and labrum.
   a. The anterior band of the inferior glenohumeral ligament (IGHL) is the primary restraint to anterior translation of the humeral head with the arm in abduction and external rotation.
   b. The posterior band of the IGHL is the primary restraint to posterior translation of the humeral head with the arm in forward flexion and adduction.
   c. The superior glenohumeral ligament (SGHL), middle glenohumeral ligament (MGHL), and coracohumeral ligament also play important roles in glenohumeral stability.
2. Active restraints: the rotator cuff muscles and deltoid are the main active restrains to glenohumeral instability.

Dr. Mazzocca or an immediate family member serves as a paid consultant to or is an employee of Arthrex, Inc. and has received research or institutional support from Arthrex, Inc. Dr. Arciero or an immediate family member has stock or stock options held in Biorez; has received research or institutional support from Arthrex, Inc. and DJ Orthopaedics; and serves as a board member, owner, officer, or committee member of the American Orthopaedic Society for Sports Medicine and the American Shoulder and Elbow Surgeons. Neither Dr. Andelman nor any immediate family member has received anything of value from or has stock or stock options held in a commercial company or institution related directly or indirectly to the subject of this chapter.

This chapter is adapted from Spang JT, Mazzocca AD, Arciero R: The unstable shoulder, in Boyer MI, ed: *AAOS Comprehensive Orthopaedic Review*, ed 2. Rosemont, IL, American Academy of Orthopaedic Surgeons, 2014, pp 931-941.

IV. TRAUMATIC ANTERIOR INSTABILITY

A. Epidemiology and overview

1. Incidence: Traumatic anterior shoulder dislocation is the most common form of glenohumeral instability, representing 88% to 98% of all dislocations.
2. Recurrence rate: While age at the time of the initial dislocation has been considered the primary risk factor for redislocation, new reports have suggested a more complex picture identifying age at initial injury, sex, activity level, and the presence of bony lesions to the humeral head and glenoid as risk factors for recurrence.
    a. High recurrence rates (>80%) are seen in younger patients, males, and contact athletes and with the presence of a glenoid or humeral head bony defect.
    b. Lower recurrence rates (<10%) are seen in older patients and females and with the absence of glenoid or humeral head bony defects.

B. Pathoanatomy

1. Anterior glenohumeral dislocation typically occurs secondary to a traumatic event that leads to excessive abduction and external rotation causing anterior and inferior displacement of the humeral head over the glenoid.
2. A Bankart lesion (detachment of the anterior-inferior labrum and anterior band of the IGHL complex; **Figure 1**) is an important pathoanatomic finding that is present in 90% of all traumatic glenohumeral dislocations.

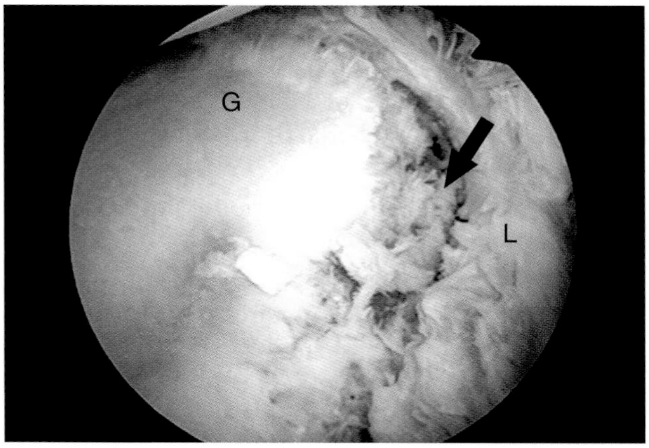

Figure 1 Arthroscopic view shows a Bankart lesion (arrow) of the inferior capsulolabral complex. G = glenoid, L = labrum

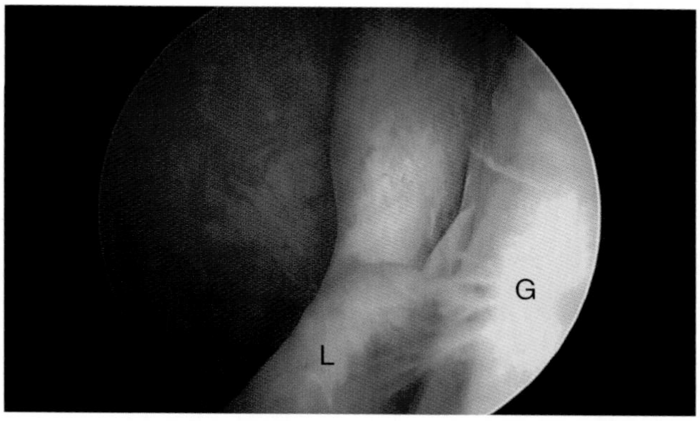

Figure 2 Arthroscopic view demonstrates an anterior labroligamentous periosteal sleeve avulsion (ALPSA) lesion. G = glenoid, L = labrum. (Adapted from Arciero RA, Spang JT: Complications in arthroscopic anterior shoulder stabilization: Pearls and pitfalls. *Instr Course Lect* 2008;57:113-124.)

3. A torn labrum may heal to the medial aspect of the glenoid neck (anterior labroligamentous periosteal sleeve avulsion [ALPSA]; **Figure 2**).
4. Associated injuries can include a humeral avulsion of the glenohumeral ligaments (HAGL) lesion (**Figure 3**) and a rotator cuff tear or greater tuberosity fracture.
5. Concomitant injury to the brachial plexus occurs in 13.5% of patients. The axillary nerve is the most common nerve injured followed by a mixed plexus injury.

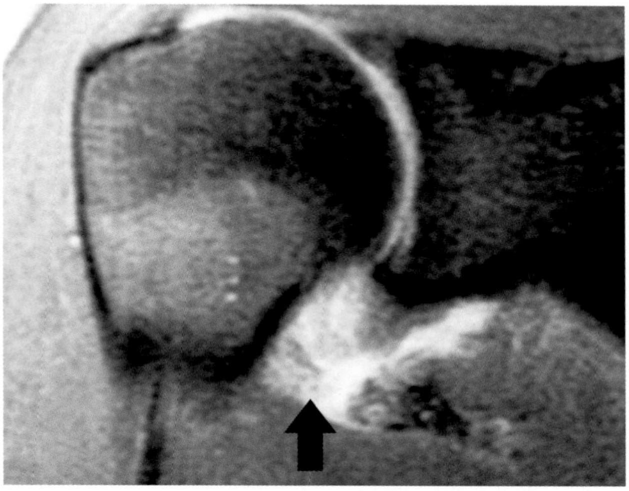

Figure 3 MRI shows a humeral avulsion of the glenohumeral ligaments (HAGL) lesion. The arrow indicates extravasated contrast material. (Adapted with permission from Bicos J, Mazzocca AD, Arciero RA: Anterior instability of the shoulder, in Schepsis AA, Busconi BD, eds: *Orthopaedic Surgery Essentials*. Philadelphia, PA, Lippincott Williams & Wilkins, 2006, p 221.)

6 | Shoulder and Elbow

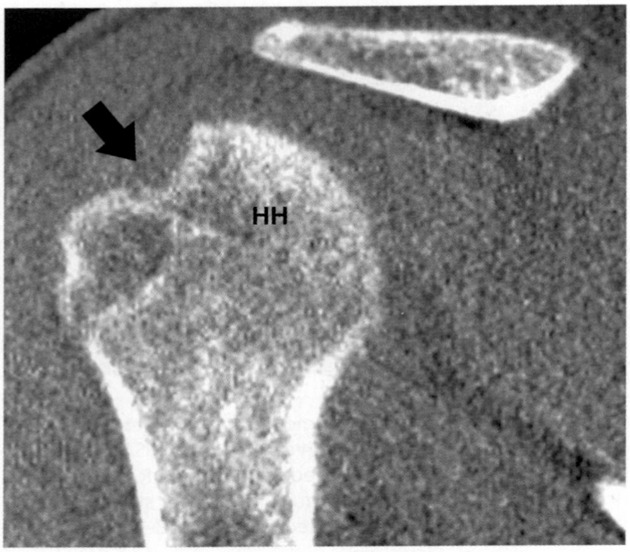

Figure 4 CT scan shows a Hill-Sachs lesion (arrow). HH = humeral head. (Adapted from Arciero RA, Spang JT: Complications in arthroscopic anterior shoulder stabilization: Pearls and pitfalls. *Instr Course Lect* 2008;57:113-124.)

6. The Hill-Sachs lesion (**Figure 4**) is a compression fracture of the posterosuperior humeral head caused by its impaction on the anterior-inferior glenoid rim after dislocation. The incidence of Hill-Sachs lesions is as high as 80% of all anterior dislocations.
7. A Bankart fracture is an anterior-inferior glenoid bony fracture which remains attached to the anterior-inferior labrum (**Figures** 5 and 6); in patients with recurrent anterior shoulder dislocations, the prevalence of anterior-inferior glenoid bone defects is 49%.

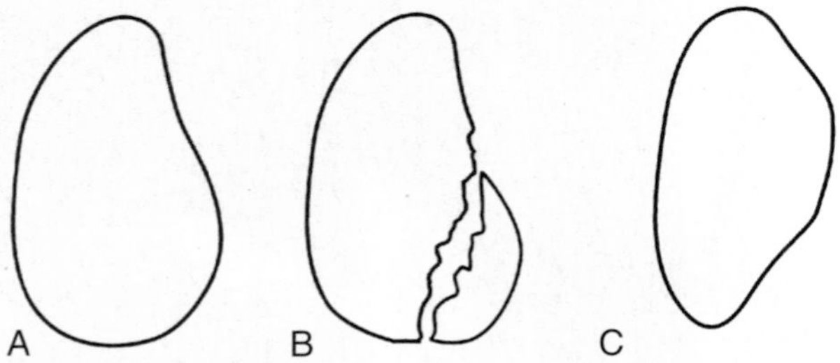

Figure 5 Illustrations depict normal and abnormal configurations of the glenoid. **A**, The normal shape of the glenoid is that of a pear, larger below than above. **B**, A bony Bankart lesion can create an inverted-pear configuration. **C**, A compression Bankart lesion also can create an inverted-pear configuration. (Reproduced from Burkhart SS: Recurrent anterior shoulder instability, in Norris TR, ed: *Orthopaedic Knowledge Update: Shoulder and Elbow*, ed 2. Rosemont, IL, American Academy of Orthopaedic Surgeons, 2002, pp 83-89.)

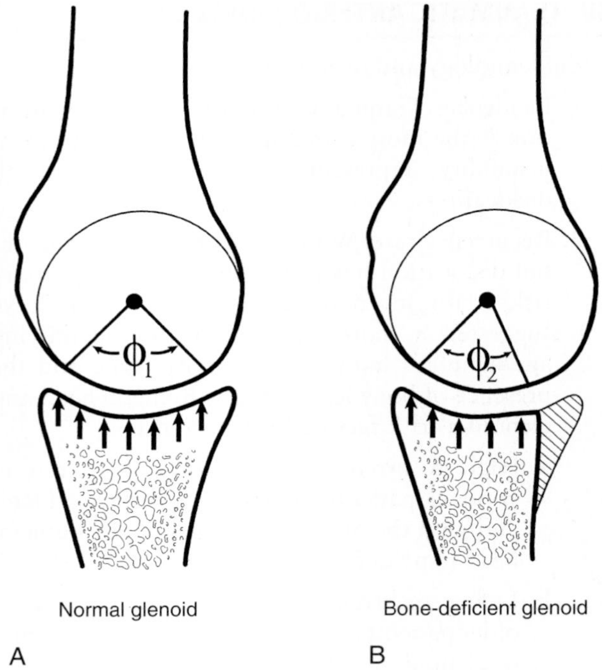

Figure 6 Illustrations show how glenoid bone loss shortens the "safe arc" through which the glenoid can resist axial forces. The safe arc represents the angle of contact between the glenoid and the humeral head. The normal glenoid (**A**) has a longer safe arc than the damaged glenoid (**B**). (Reproduced from Burkhart SS: Recurrent anterior shoulder instability, in Norris TR, ed: *Orthopaedic Knowledge Update: Shoulder and Elbow*, ed 2. Rosemont, IL, American Academy of Orthopaedic Surgeons, 2002, pp 83-89.)

C. Evaluation
   1. Patient history (**Table 1**).
   2. Physical examination
      a. Generalized hyperlaxity can be tested as part of the Beighton criteria.
      b. Load and shift test: anterior to posterior translation of the humerus
      c. Apprehension sign: in the supine position, the patient demonstrates apprehension to dislocation with abduction and external rotation.
      d. Relocation test: the patient demonstrates a decrease in apprehension with the application of posterior force on the shoulder in abduction and external rotation.

TABLE 1

Key Questions for Identifying Patients With Traumatic Anterior Shoulder Instability

Question	Value
What was the initial mechanism of injury?	Quantifies energy required for initial dislocation; greater energy suggests a greater likelihood of associated lesions (glenoid fracture, capsular tear).
What was the arm position at the time of injury?	Allows imaging and physical examination to be directed at locations of suspected pathology; abduction/external rotation would indicate a mechanism consistent with anterior instability.
Did the shoulder dislocate? Was a reduction required?	Need for reduction indicates a mechanism of injury sufficient to cause capsulolabral disruption.
Were radiographs taken at the time of the initial event?	Early radiographs may show bone fragments and can verify the direction of dislocation.
What was the length of disability following the event?	Delayed return to functional activities or persistent disability may indicate more extensive capsulolabral disruption.
How many episodes of disability have occurred since the index event? Were they dislocations? Subluxations? Were reductions required?	Multiple episodes increase concern for bony defects or concomitant damage and indicate the level of laxity.
Are there arm positions/activities that you avoid?	Allows assessment of current functional status; permits identification of direction of instability.
What activities would you like to resume?	Categorizes patient in terms of functional postoperative requirements.

Adapted from Arciero RA, Spang JT: Complications in arthroscopic anterior shoulder stabilization: Pearls and pitfalls. *Instr Course Lect* 2008;57:113-124.

3. Imaging
   a. Radiographs—Shoulder AP, scapular AP, and axillary views are standard images. Other helpful views include the West Point view (to visualize glenoid bone loss) and the Stryker notch view (to visualize Hill-Sachs lesions).
   b. CT is useful for detailed evaluation of bony injuries (**Figure 7**).
   c. MRI is useful for soft-tissue detail, labral lesions, HAGL lesions, and capsular tears; intra-articular contrast increases the sensitivity for soft-tissue injuries.

D. Treatment
1. Algorithms for the management are shown in **Figures 8** and **9**.
2. Nonsurgical treatment is a reasonable option for patients with a first-time anterior dislocation; however, they should be counseled as to the high rates of redislocation based on demographic criteria previously discussed. A brief 1 to 2 week period of immobilization is followed by range of motion (ROM) exercises.
3. Surgical indications
   a. Failure of nonsurgical management with recurrent instability.

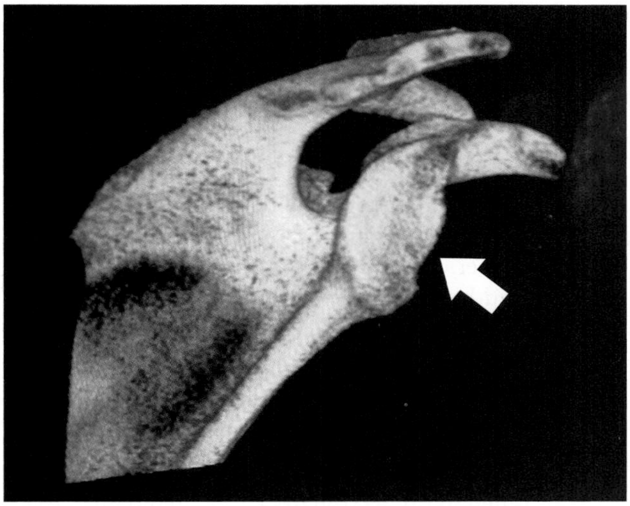

Figure 7 Three-dimensional CT scan shows bone loss in the anterior-inferior glenoid fossa (arrow). (Reproduced from Arciero RA, Spang JT: Complications in arthroscopic anterior shoulder stabilization: Pearls and pitfalls. *Instr Course Lect* 2008;57:113-124.)

   b. Patients younger than 25 years who engage in athletics or other high-demand activities may benefit from immediate surgical stabilization.

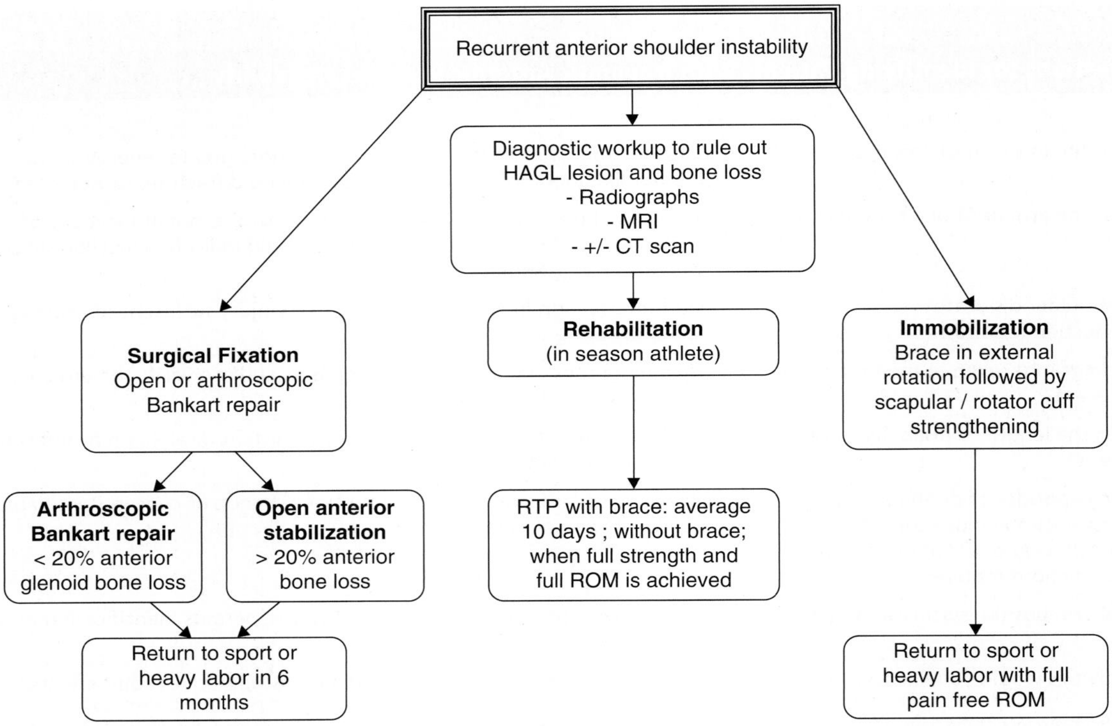

Figure 8 Algorithm demonstrates the management of recurrent anterior shoulder instability. HAGL = humeral avulsion of the glenohumeral ligaments, ROM = range of motion, RTP = return to play. (Adapted with permission from Bicos J, Mazzocca AD, Arciero RA: Anterior instability of the shoulder, in Schepsis AA, Busconi BD, eds: *Sports Medicine: Orthopaedic Surgery Essentials*. Philadelphia, PA, Lippincott Williams & Wilkins, 2006, p 221.)

c. Patients with significant bony injuries or rotator cuff tears require immediate surgical stabilization.

4. Surgical management: The goal of surgery is to anatomically repair the Bankart lesion, retension the anterior capsulolabral complex (**Figure 10**), and address all bony defects as necessary.
   a. Arthroscopic Bankart repair ± capsulorrhaphy: common option for first-time dislocators or recurrent instability without significant anterior glenoid bone loss with high rates of return to sport (97.5%)
   b. Open Bankart repair ± capsular shift: treatment of choice prior to the development of arthroscopic techniques. Large randomized studies show equivalent results with open and arthroscopic Bankart repair.
   c. Open bone-transfer procedures ± capsular shift: options include coracoid transfer (Bristow-Latarjet), iliac crest autograft, and distal tibial allograft. Classically indicated for "critical" anterior bone loss (>20%); however, recent studies have suggested that the presence of subcritical bone loss >13.5% is a risk factor for recurrent instability with soft-tissue repair alone.
   d. Management of engaging Hill-Sachs lesions: can be done in conjunction with any of the above procedures. Options include remplissage of the posterior rotator cuff, allograft reconstruction of the humeral surface, and resurfacing arthroplasty.
5. Surgical complications
   a. Recurrence of instability: large scale studies suggest near equivalent rates of recurrence between arthroscopic (4% to 15%) and open (5% to 10%) repair.
   b. Stiffness due to overtightening of the capsulolabral complex.
   c. Subscapularis failure with open surgical techniques.
6. Surgical pearls and pitfalls
   a. Failure to reconstruct and re-tension the anterior-inferior capsulolabral complex
   b. Failure to recognize and address glenoid or humeral bony defects.

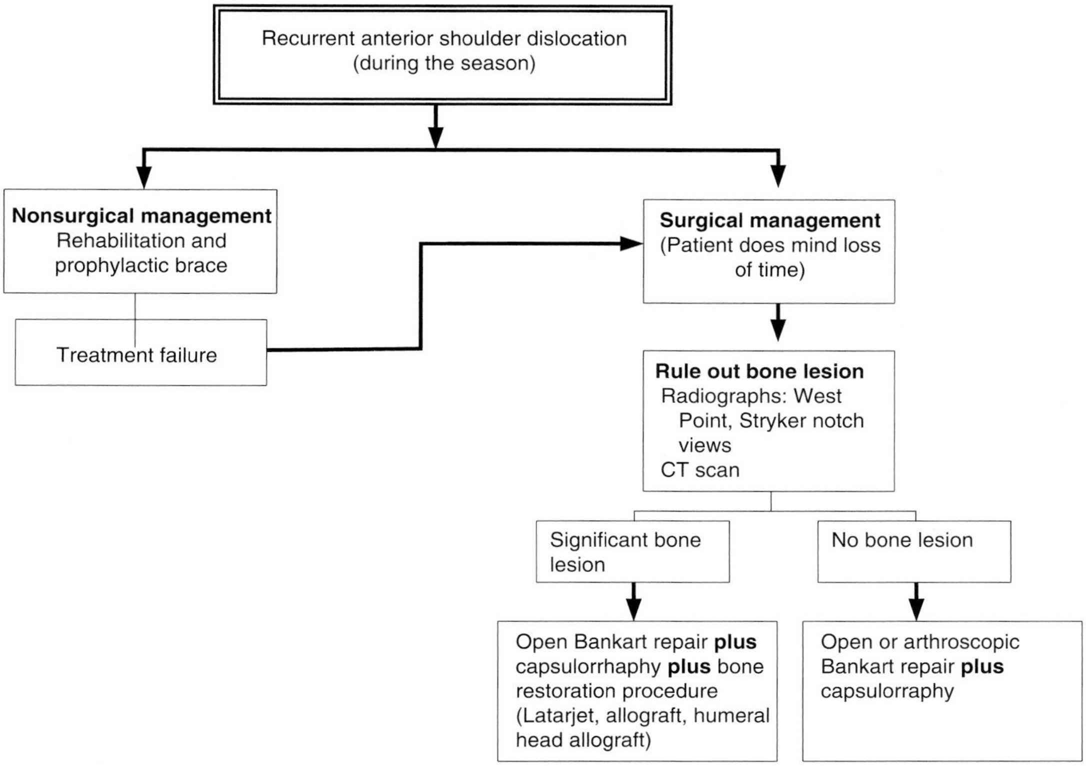

Figure 9 Algorithm demonstrates the management of anterior shoulder instability associated with recurrent anterior shoulder dislocation. (Adapted with permission from Bicos J, Mazzocca AD, Arciero RA: Anterior instability of the shoulder, in Schepsis AA, Busconi BD, eds: *Sports Medicine: Orthopaedic Surgery Essentials*. Philadelphia, PA, Lippincott Williams & Wilkins, 2006, p 221.)

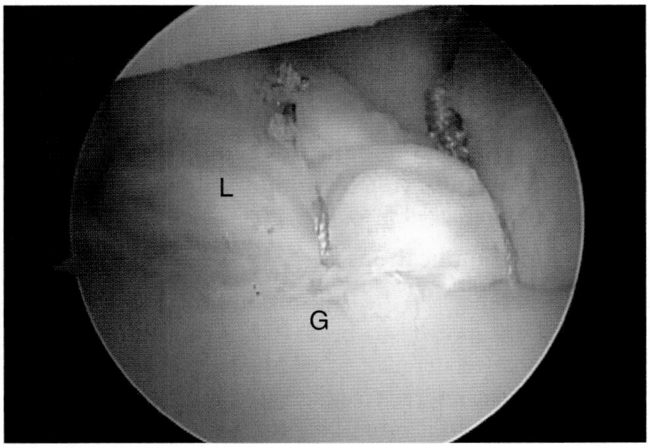

Figure 10 Arthroscopic view shows a completed arthroscopic Bankart repair, with restored labral bumper. G = glenoid, L = labrum. (Adapted from Arciero RA, Spang JT: Complications in arthroscopic anterior shoulder stabilization: Pearls and pitfalls. *Instr Course Lect* 2008;57:113-124.)

V. POSTERIOR INSTABILITY

A. Epidemiology and overview

1. Posterior glenohumeral instability is less common, accounting for 2% to 5% of all glenohumeral instability.
2. Up to 50% of traumatic posterior shoulder dislocations are undiagnosed upon presentation to hospital emergency departments.

B. Pathoanatomy

1. Traumatic posterior glenohumeral dislocation or recurrent instability can cause posterior labral tearing or disruption of the posterior IGHL.
2. A compression fracture of the anterosuperior portion of the humeral head (a reverse Hill-Sachs) may be present.

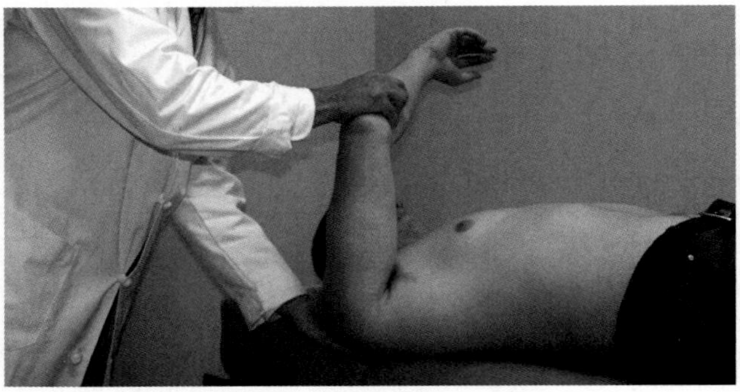

Figure 11 Photograph demonstrates the posterior stress test. A posterior force is applied through the humerus. The test is positive if palpable crepitus or subluxation is present. Pain is often elicited, but this finding is less specific for posterior shoulder instability. (Reproduced from Millett PJ, Clavert P, Hatch GF III, Warner JJ: Recurrent posterior shoulder instability. *J Am Acad Orthop Surg* 2006;14[8]:464-476.)

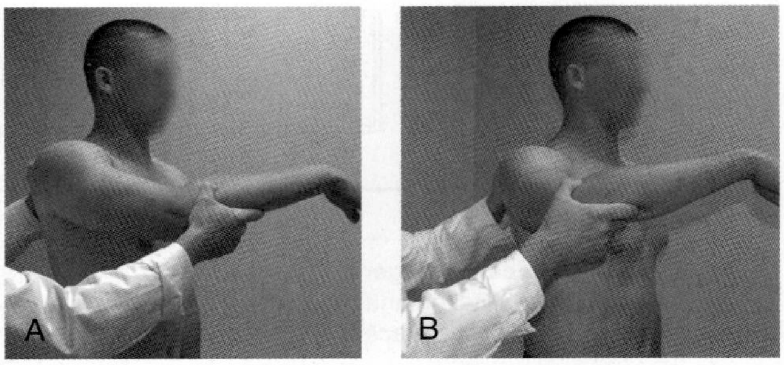

Figure 12 Photographs demonstrate the jerk test. **A**, A posterior force is applied along the axis of the humerus, with the arm in forward flexion and internal rotation. This will cause the humeral head to subluxate posteriorly out of the glenoid socket. **B**, As the arm is brought into extension, a clunk will be felt as the humerus reduces into the glenoid cavity. (Reproduced from Millett PJ, Clavert P, Hatch GF III, Warner JJ: Recurrent posterior shoulder instability. *J Am Acad Orthop Surg* 2006;14[8]:464-476.)

3. Posterior glenoid bone loss may be present in cases of recurrent instability.

C. Evaluation

1. History: A history of trauma with the arm locked in internal rotation.
   a. Volitional dislocation of the shoulder must be ruled out.
2. Physical examination
   a. An acute posterior dislocation will present with a prominent posterior shoulder and anterior coracoid and a limited ability to externally rotate the shoulder.
   b. Posterior instability can lead to compensatory scapular winging.
   c. Specialized tests to assess posterior stability include the posterior stress test (**Figure 11**) and jerk test (**Figure 12**).
3. Imaging: Same as for anterior shoulder instability discussed in Section IV.

D. Treatment

1. Nonsurgical: Nonsurgical treatment should always be attempted first. After a single traumatic injury, the arm should be immobilized in neutral rotation with the elbow in adduction. A 1 to 2 week period of immobilization is followed by therapy.
2. Surgical indications and contraindications
   a. Surgical intervention is indicated for patients that who have symptoms that interfere with activities or athletics and for failure of nonsurgical management.
   b. Surgery is contraindicated for voluntary dislocators.
3. Surgical management: The goal of surgery is to repair the posterior capsulolabral structures and to re-tension the posterior capsular to prevent recurrent instability.
   a. Soft-tissue procedures include open or arthroscopic labral repair and posterior capsular shift. Some authors recommend plication of the rotator interval (controversial).
   b. Options for an engaging reverse Hill-Sachs include structural bone graft to the humeral head, the McLaughlin or modified McLaughlin procedure (transfer of the lesser tuberosity or subscapularis into the defect), or resurfacing arthroplasty.
   c. Options for posterior glenoid bone loss include distal tibial allograft or autograft reconstruction (posterior acromion, iliac crest, distal clavicle).

E. Surgical complications

1. Recurrence is the most common complication and is reported to be 8.5% in the general population. Recurrence rates are highest in overhead athletes and recurrence rates increase with posterior glenoid bone loss >20%, which should be considered a contraindication to arthroscopic soft-tissue stabilization alone.
2. Shoulder stiffness or adhesive capsulitis—a concern with rotator interval plication
3. Overtightening of the posterior capsule can lead to anterior subluxation or coracoid impingement.

F. Surgical pearls and pitfalls

1. In arthroscopic labral repair, a high lateral portal provides better access than a standard posterior portal

G. Rehabilitation: Postoperatively, the shoulder should be placed in a rigid immobilizer with the arm abducted to 30° in neutral rotation. After a short period of immobilization, ROM exercises may begin. Strengthening should begin at 12 weeks. Patients may return to heavy labor or contact sports 6 months after surgery. Pooled published rate of return to any sport and to preinjury level of sport is 91% and 67%, respectively.

VI. MULTIDIRECTIONAL INSTABILITY

A. Epidemiology and overview: multidirectional instability (MDI) has variable presentations and is difficult to quantify. It is characterized by inferior laxity in addition to anterior and/or posterior laxity.

B. Pathoanatomy

1. There are two commonly associated anatomic lesions: A patulous inferior capsule which contains both the anterior and posterior bands of the IGHL (**Figure 13**) and functional deficiency of the rotator interval.
2. Labral tearing may occur with repeated subluxations or a traumatic event.

C. Evaluation

1. History: Symptoms include pain, weakness, ipsilateral paresthesias, popping or clicking of the shoulder, instability of the shoulder during sleep, difficulty with throwing, and pain when carrying heavy objects.
   a. Differential diagnoses include unidirectional shoulder instability, cervical disease, brachial plexitis, and thoracic outlet syndrome.
2. Physical examination
   a. Assess for generalized ligamentous laxity (Beighton criteria).
   b. A positive sulcus sign assesses the competency of the rotator interval. Tests described in Sections III and IV can be used to assess for anterior or posterior instability in the setting of MDI.
   c. Rotator cuff tendinitis in an individual <20 years should raise concern for MDI.

D. Treatment

1. Nonsurgical management: All patients with MDI should undergo extensive physical therapy (6 to 9 months) prior to consideration of surgical treatment.
2. Physical therapy should focus on rotator cuff strengthening, scapular kinematics, and proprioceptive training.
3. Surgical indications
   a. Surgery is appropriate for patients with pain and instability that interferes with normal or sport-related activity that have failed extensive nonsurgical treatment.
      - Approximately 20% of patients fail nonsurgical management.
4. Surgical contraindications
   a. Surgery is contraindicated for voluntary dislocators and patients who have not attempted physical therapy.
5. Surgical techniques
   a. Arthroscopic pancapsular plication ± rotator interval closure
      - If labral pathology is encountered, anterior or posterior labral repair is indicated.
      - To avoid asymmetric tightening, capsulorrhaphy should address the inferior redundancy in a balanced fashion.
   b. Open anterior-inferior capsular shift.

E. Complications: Recurrence of MDI (7% for both open arthroscopic techniques), axillary nerve injury, stiffness (rare), and subscapularis insufficiency (after open procedure).

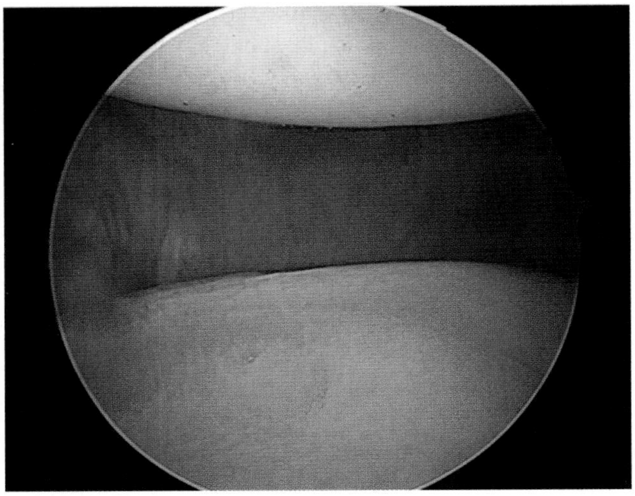

Figure 13 Arthroscopic view of a shoulder with a patulous capsule with an expanded inferior pouch. The glenoid is below, and the humeral head is above.

TOP TESTING FACTS

Anterior Instability

1. Age at time of initial dislocation is the most important predictor of recurrent anterior shoulder dislocation with patients <20 years having a much higher recurrence rate.
2. The main pathoanatomic components are anterior-inferior capsulolabral avulsion and bony defects of the glenoid and humeral head.
3. Open and arthroscopic management provide equivalent outcomes for primary stabilization.
4. Failure to recognize significant bone loss to the humeral head and glenoid can lead to failed surgical stabilization.

Posterior Instability

1. Trauma to a flexed, adducted arm can lead to posterior labral tearing and injury to the posterior glenoid and anterior humeral head.
2. Seizures, electrical shock, encephalitis, ethanol withdrawal, or electrolyte abnormalities may lead to traumatic posterior dislocation that is often missed on initial examination.
3. Tests to assess posterior shoulder stability are the posterior stress test and jerk test.

Multidirectional Instability

1. The pathoanatomic features of MDI are a patulous inferior capsule and functional deficiency of the rotator interval.
2. Presentation is variable and symptoms may include pain, weakness, paresthesias, clicking of the shoulder, instability during sleep, and difficulty with overhead activity.
3. A complete course of nonsurgical therapy focusing on rotator cuff strengthening and scapular kinematics should be attempted prior to consideration of surgical management.

Bibliography

Abdul-rassoul H, Galvin JW, Curry EJ, Simon J, Li X: Return to sport after surgical treatment for anterior shoulder instability: A systematic Review. *Am J Sports Med.* 2018:363546518780934.

Arciero RA, Wheeler JH, Ryan JB, McBride JT: Arthroscopic Bankart repair versus nonoperative treatment for acute, initial anterior shoulder dislocations. *Am J Sports Med* 1994;22(5):589-594.

Boileau P, Villalba M, Fiery JY, Balg F, Ahrens P, Neyton L: Risk factors for recurrence of shoulder instability after arthroscopic Bankart repair. *J Bone Joint Surg Am* 2006;88(8):1755-1763.

Castagna A, Delle Rose G, Borroni M, et al: Arthroscopic stabilization of the shoulder in adolescent athletes participating in overhead or contact sports. *Arthroscopy* 2012;28(3):309-315.

Dickens JF, Owens BD, Cameron KL, et al: The effect of subcritical bone loss and exposure on recurrent instability after arthroscopic Bankart repair in intercollegiate American football. *Am J Sports Med* 2017;45(8):1769-1775.

Dickens JF, Rue JP, Cameron KL, et al: Successful return to sport after arthroscopic shoulder stabilization versus nonoperative management in contact athletes with anterior shoulder instability: A prospective multicenter study. *Am J Sports Med* 2017;45(11):2540-2546.

Gaskill TR, Taylor DC, Millett PJ: Management of multidirectional instability of the shoulder. *J Am Acad Orthop Surg* 2011;19(12):758-767.

Longo UG, Rizzello G, Loppini M, et al: Multidirectional instability of the shoulder: A systematic Review. *Arthroscopy* 2015;31(12):2431-2443.

Nacca C, Gil JA, Badida R, Crisco JJ, Owens BD: Critical glenoid bone loss in posterior shoulder instability. *Am J Sports Med* 2018;46(5):1058-1063.

Piasecki DP, Verma NN, Romeo AA, Levine WN, Bach BR Jr, Provencher MT: Glenoid bone deficiency in recurrent anterior shoulder instability: Diagnosis and management. *J Am Acad Orthop Surg* 2009;17(8):482-493.

Shah A, Judge A, Delmestri A, et al: Incidence of shoulder dislocations in the UK, 1995–2015: A population-based cohort study. *BMJ Open.* 2017;7(11):e016112.

Wasserstein DN, Sheth U, Colbenson K, et al: The true recurrence rate and factors predicting recurrent instability after nonsurgical management of traumatic primary anterior shoulder dislocation: A systematic review. *Arthroscopy* 2016;32(12):2616-2625.

Watson L, Balster S, Lenssen R, Hoy G, Pizzari T: The effects of a conservative rehabilitation program for multidirectional instability of the shoulder. *J Shoulder Elbow Surg* 2018;27(1):104-111.

Chapter 74
ADHESIVE CAPSULITIS

JAY D. KEENER, MD

I. OVERVIEW/EPIDEMIOLOGY

A. Definition—Disorder of unknown etiology characterized by significant restriction of active and passive range of motion of the glenohumeral joint that occurs in the absence of a known intrinsic shoulder disorder.

B. Epidemiology—affects between 1% and 3% of the general population.

1. Women afflicted more commonly than men.
2. Typical age is between 40 and 60 years.

II. PATHOGENESIS

A. Exact etiology and pathogenesis is unknown.

B. Adhesive capsulitis felt to be an inflammatory-mediated fibrosis and contracture of the glenohumeral capsule.

C. Biopsy results:

1. Capsular tissue contains perivascular mononuclear cell infiltrates, absence of synovial lining, and extensive subsynovial fibrosis.
2. Increased cytokine levels are noted including transforming growth factor beta, platelet-derived growth factor, interleukin 1 beta, and tumor necrosis factor alpha.

D. Contracture of capsular tissue is noted.

1. Glenohumeral joint volume is reduced.
2. Obliteration of the axillary fold is noted.
3. Inflammation and thickening of the rotator interval capsule is seen along with characteristic contracture of the coracohumeral ligament (**Figure 1**).

Dr. Keener or an immediate family member serves as a paid consultant to or is an employee of Arthrex, Inc. and Wright Medical Technology, Inc.; has received research or institutional support from the National Institutes of Health (NIAMS & NICHD) and Zimmer; and serves as a board member, owner, officer, or committee member of the American Shoulder and Elbow Surgeons.

III. CLASSIFICATION OF ADHESIVE CAPSULITIS

A. Primary adhesive capsulitis occurs, by definition, in a joint with no intrinsic disease or damage.

B. Secondary adhesive capsulitis causes are typically related to previous trauma or prior surgery.

1. The pathogenesis of secondary adhesive capsulitis is likely not the same as the primary disease.
2. Previous trauma or surgery is more likely to result in adhesion formation within the humeroscapular interface (cuff/bursa to acromion/deltoid) in addition to glenohumeral joint capsular contracture.

IV. RISK FACTORS FOR PRIMARY ADHESIVE CAPSULITIS

A. The majority of cases are idiopathic in origin.

B. Greatest risk factor is previous diagnosis of adhesive capsulitis in the contralateral shoulder.

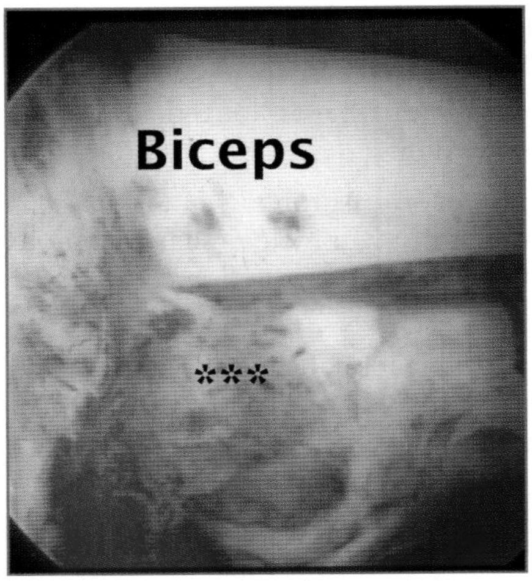

Figure 1 Intraoperative view (from posterior to anterior) of right shoulder with adhesive capsulitis. The rotator interval tissue (***) immediately inferior to the biceps is characteristically thickened and erythematous.

C. Hormonal causes include diabetes mellitus and hypothyroidism.

D. Cardiovascular disease.

E. Neurologic conditions that may predispose to frozen shoulder include cerebrovascular accident, Parkinson disease and Parsonage-Turner syndrome.

F. Other associated conditions include mastectomy/lumpectomy, prior chest wall surgery and Dupuytren disease.

V. NATURAL HISTORY

A. Onset of symptoms is often insidious but sometimes related to mild trauma or change in activity level.

B. Clinical stages are suggested but not definitive. There is considerable time overlap between proposed stages.

1. Stage 1—the "freezing" stage is associated with severe pain, including night pain. This stage is dominated by acute inflammatory pain with minimal capsular contracture. The duration is variable often ranging from 10 to 36 weeks.
2. Stage 2—the "frozen" stage is associated with profound capsular stiffness and limited range of motion. The severe inflammatory pain usually decreases, and pain is experienced when the limits of range of motion are reached. The duration is variable often ranging from 3 to 12 months.
3. Stage 3—the "thawing" stage is associated with a gradual spontaneous improvement in shoulder motion and function. The duration is variable often ranging from 1 to 3 years.

C. Gradual resolution of symptoms occurs spontaneously or with minimal intervention generally; however,

1. Recovery can be prolonged, especially without intervention.
2. Persistent measurable limitation in range of motion or low-grade pain has been noted in 50% to 60% of patients followed for more than 2 years.
3. Measurable loss of shoulder motion and function (greater than 1-year follow-up) frequently noted without intervention.

VI. CLINICAL EVALUATION

Adhesive capsulitis is primarily a clinical diagnosis.

A. Criteria for the diagnosis of idiopathic adhesive capsulitis are

1. Insidious onset of pain.
2. Global loss of active and passive glenohumeral joint motion.
   a. Passive elevation limited to 100°.
   b. 50% or greater loss of glenohumeral external rotation motion compared with the opposite shoulder.
   c. Capsular end feel at the limit of motion. This may not be present in the initial acute inflammatory stage of the disease.
3. Normal radiographs with the exception of disuse osteopenia.
4. Rotator cuff strength testing is usually normal and minimally painful.

B. Examination by stages of disease

1. Stage 1—Painful loss of range of motion where the onset of pain is noticed before the capsular limit of passive motion.
2. Stage 2—Painful loss of range of motion where the onset of pain occurs sequentially with the limits of passive motion.
3. Stage 3—Loss of movement where stiffness predominates and the patient can tolerate a capsular stretching with minimal pain.

C. Secondary adhesive capsulitis often has the same clinical examination findings as primary adhesive capsulitis, and there is a history of previous surgery or traumatic event such as a proximal humerus fracture.

D. Differential diagnosis includes glenohumeral arthritis, posterior glenohumeral joint fracture/dislocation, bicipital tenosynovitis, and rotator cuff disease, including calcific tendinitis of the rotator cuff and cervical radiculopathy.

VII. RADIOGRAPHIC EVALUATION

A. Adhesive capsulitis is primarily a clinical diagnosis.

B. Shoulder radiographs should be obtained to rule out other diagnoses including glenohumeral joint osteoarthritis, glenohumeral joint fracture/dislocation, boney neoplasm, and calcific tendinitis.

C. MRI/arthrography are not needed for diagnosis; however, specific findings are suggestive of adhesive capsulitis (**Figure 2**) and include

1. Obliteration of the axillary fold.
2. Thickening of the inferior capsule.
3. Thickening of the rotator interval tissue and coracohumeral ligament and reduced dimensions of the rotator interval.

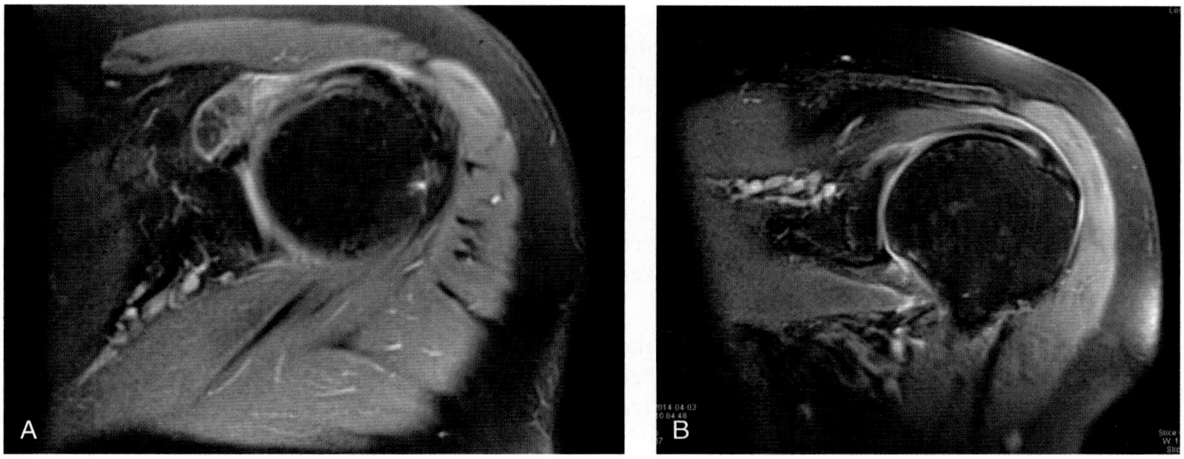

Figure 2 **A**, MRI axial image showing synovitis and thickening of the rotator interval tissue (*) in the anterior aspect of the shoulder. **B**, MRI coronal image showing thickening of the inferior capsule (*) and obliteration of the axillary recess.

VIII. MANAGEMENT

A. Conservative treatment: Recommended as initial treatment.

1. Exercise/physical therapy
   a. Both home-directed exercise and structured physical therapy are beneficial and represent the mainstay of treatment.
   b. Intense stretching can be poorly tolerated in the early and middle stages of adhesive capsulitis secondary to pain.
   c. Literature is inconclusive regarding advantages of modified rehabilitation techniques over standard stretching and joint mobilization exercises.
   d. The addition of static progressive splinting has shown benefit in addition to traditional rehabilitation in one randomized trial.
2. Nonsteroidal anti-inflammatory medications
   a. NSAIDs are often prescribed but have no proven benefit in treating adhesive capsulitis.
3. Oral corticosteroids
   a. Oral steroids have been shown to be beneficial for short-term pain relief and improvement in range of motion compared with placebo with no advantage after 6 weeks.
4. Corticosteroid injections
   a. Intra-articular injections of corticosteroids versus placebo injections have been proven to be beneficial for pain relief and improved clinical outcomes in multiple prospective randomized studies at short-term follow-up. Most studies show no long-term advantage when both groups also receive standard rehabilitation.
   b. Intra-articular injections have been shown to be as effective as physical therapy, manipulation, and hydrodilatation.
   c. Intra-articular steroid injections have been shown to be more beneficial for pain relief and improvement in motion than oral steroids or NSAIDs in prospective randomized trials at short-term follow-up, except one study showing an advantage to injections at 12 months follow-up.
   d. Similar benefits have been shown in with subacromial and intra-articular steroid injections in prospective randomized trials; however, early pain relief is generally better with glenohumeral injections.
5. Hydrodilatation aims to release capsular contracture by injection of large amounts of fluid (often including corticosteroids) into the glenohumeral joint often in a repeated manner.
   a. Hydrodilatation has not been shown to be more advantageous compared with conventional glenohumeral corticosteroid injections in two randomized trials.

B. Conservative treatment compared with surgical intervention.

1. There is insufficient evidence to suggest surgical intervention as the first-line treatment for adhesive capsulitis.

a. Better early return of motion was seen in a randomized trial comparing manipulation and arthroscopic release compared with glenohumeral corticosteroid injections; however, no differences were seen at 12 months follow-up.

b. There is no advantage to the addition of manipulation to a home exercise program compared with home exercises only in one randomized trial.

c. Similar results are seen comparing hydrodilatation and corticosteroid injection compared with manipulation in most randomized trials. However, one study showed better early motion when manipulation was combined with hydrodilatation compared with intra-articular injection with no difference between groups at 12 months.

C. Operative treatment

1. Indications for operative intervention include persistent pain and/or failure to shown improvements in range of motion after 3 to 6 months of conservative treatment.

2. Manipulation

a. Manipulation has been shown to be beneficial to safely improve range of motion and function in patients who have failed initial conservative treatment.

b. Manipulation offers no clear benefit over physical therapy, self-directed stretching, or steroid injections as an initial treatment modality for adhesive capsulitis.

c. Manipulation should not be performed as an isolated procedure for posttraumatic, postsurgical, and severe cases of adhesive capsulitis secondary to risk of humerus fracture.

3. Arthroscopic capsular release

a. Risk factors for need for surgical release include younger age, more severe restriction of range of motion, and failure to show improvement with initial conservative treatment.

b. Surgical technique should include release of the rotator interval tissue and anterior capsule with direct release of the inferior capsule or through manipulation.

- Additional release of the posterior capsule (pancapsular) is performed in cases in restricted internal rotation.
- Better early improvement in range of motion has been shown following pancapsular release compared with selective capsular release; however, differences are not maintained in the long term.
- Release of scapulohumeral adhesions within the subacromial and subdeltoid space should be performed prior to manipulation in posttraumatic and postsurgical adhesive capsulitis.

c. Multiple studies, often without control groups, have demonstrated safe and effective relief of pain and improvement in range of motion and function following arthroscopic release and manipulation.

d. Long-term outcomes (mean 7 years) demonstrate excellent return of function (similar motion to contralateral shoulder) following arthroscopic capsular release.

e. There is no clear advantage to arthroscopic release with manipulation compared with manipulation alone for the treatment of refractory adhesive capsulitis in one systematic review of existing literature.

f. Outcomes of release for postsurgical adhesive capsulitis results in less improvement in pain, satisfaction, and function compared with idiopathic and posttraumatic adhesive capsulitis.

4. Open capsular release

a. Open release is rarely performed today secondary to advances in arthroscopy.

b. Open releases may be indicated in cases where hardware may be removed and/or in cases of severe posttraumatic or postsurgical stiffness.

c. Open releases are often limited by the need to takedown the subscapularis tendon to adequately access the joint capsule.

TOP TESTING FACTS

1. Idiopathic adhesive capsulitis is primarily diagnosed by history and clinical examination rather than imaging studies.
2. The most common radiographic finding of patients with adhesive capsulitis are normal radiographs or mild osteopenia.
3. Given the existing literature, the most appropriate initial treatment for adhesive capsulitis is a combination of intra-articular corticosteroid injection and physical therapy.
4. One potential advantage of an image-guided glenohumeral intra-articular corticosteroid injection over a freehand subacromial injection is better early pain relief and tolerance to capsular stretching.
5. Regarding the treatment of refractory adhesive capsulitis of the shoulder, there is no clear advantage of manipulation alone over arthroscopic release and manipulation.
6. Postsurgical frozen shoulder will often resolve with time and continued rehabilitation and produces less consistent and poorer results following surgical release than idiopathic frozen shoulder.
7. Regarding physical therapy for idiopathic adhesive capsulitis, both home exercise programs and structured physical therapy have been shown to be effective treatments with no clear advantage of one over the other.
8. Adhesive capsulitis is commonly seen in middle-aged patients, often female and with an insidious onset of night pain.
9. The most common physical examination findings of a patient with adhesive capsulitis are limitation of overhead motion and severe pain and limited passive external rotation of the shoulder.
10. The natural history of untreated idiopathic adhesive capsulitis is predictable return of shoulder function and pain relief with some measurable loss of range of motion in most shoulders within 1 to 3 years.

Bibliography

Barnes CP, Lam PH, Murrell GA: Short-term outcomes after arthroscopic capsular release for adhesive capsulitis. *J Shoulder Elbow Surg* 2016;25(9):e256-e264.

Cho CH, Kim du H, Bae KC, et al: Proper site of corticosteroid injection for the treatment of idiopathic frozen shoulder: Results from a randomized trial. *Joint Bone Spine* 2016;83(3):324-329.

Grant JA, Schroeder N, Miller BS, Carpenter JE: Comparison of manipulation and arthroscopic capsular release for adhesive capsulitis: A systematic review. *J Shoulder Elbow Surg* 2013;22(8):1135-1145.

Jacobs LG, Smith MG, Khan SA, et al: Manipulation or intra-articular steroids in the management of adhesive capsulitis of the shoulder? A prospective randomized trial. *J Shoulder Elbow Surg* 2009;18(3):348-353.

Kivimaki J, Pohjolainen T, Malmivaara A, et al: Manipulation under anesthesia with home exercises versus home exercises alone in the treatment of frozen shoulder: A randomized, controlled trial with 125 patients. *J Shoulder Elbow Surg* 2007;16(6):722-726.

Le Lievre HM, Murrell GA: Long-term outcomes after arthroscopic capsular release for idiopathic adhesive capsulitis. *J Bone Joint Surg Am* 2012;94(13):1208-1216.

Lorbach O, Anagnostakos K, Scherf C, et al: Nonoperative management of adhesive capsulitis of the shoulder: Oral cortisone application versus intra-articular cortisone injections. *J Shoulder Elbow Surg* 2010;19(2):172-179.

Mun SW, Baek CH: Clinical efficacy of hydrodistention with joint manipulation under interscalene block compared with intra-articular corticosteroid injection for frozen shoulder: A prospective randomized controlled study. *J Shoulder Elbow Surg* 2016;25(12):1937-1943.

Reeves B: The natural history of the frozen shoulder syndrome. *Scand J Rheumatol* 1975;4(4):193-196.

Russell S, Jariwala A, Conlon R, et al: A blinded, randomized, controlled trial assessing conservative management strategies for frozen shoulder. *J Shoulder Elbow Surg* 2014;23(4):500-507.

Shaffer B, Tibone JE, Kerlan RK: Frozen shoulder. A long-term follow-up. *J Bone Joint Surg Am* 1992;74(5):738-746.

Zuckerman J, Cuomo F, Rokito A: Definition and classification of frozen shoulder: A consensus aprroach. *J Shoulder Elbow Surg* 1994;3(S72).

Chapter 75

Arthritis and Arthroplasty of the Shoulder

SURENA NAMDARI, MD, MSc

I. OSTEOARTHRITIS

A. Epidemiology and overview

1. Primary osteoarthritis (OA)—The cause is unknown but a genetic predisposition may be present.
2. The secondary cause of OA can be posttraumatic, postsurgical, or a result of persistent or recurrent shoulder instability.

B. Pathoanatomy—Primary OA of the shoulder

1. Posterior glenoid wear and posterior humeral head subluxation occur in up to 45% of shoulders affected by primary OA.
2. The anterior soft tissues, including the anterior capsule and the subscapularis, become contracted, limiting external rotation.
3. Joint space narrowing and periarticular osteophyte formation occur most commonly on the inferior aspects of the humeral head, and the result has been referred to as a "goat's beard."
4. Full-thickness rotator cuff tears rarely (5% to 10%) are associated with primary OA.

C. Evaluation

1. History
   a. Common symptoms include pain with activity, pain at night, decreased range of motion, and loss of function.
   b. A history of previous trauma, instability, or prior joint surgery should be sought for possible secondary causes of OA.
2. Physical examination
   a. Anterior soft-tissue flattening secondary to posterior subluxation may be seen. Because of inactivity, muscle atrophy also may be noted about the entire shoulder girdle, especially about the anterior deltoid.
   b. Common findings include crepitus, painful motion, and limited range of motion, especially external rotation.
   c. Rotator cuff strength usually is preserved.
3. Imaging
   a. Radiographs—AP, true glenohumeral AP, and axillary views should be obtained. Common findings include symmetric or asymmetric joint space narrowing, subchondral sclerosis, and osteophytes about the glenoid and humeral head (**Figure 1**). Posterior glenoid erosion (also known as a biconcave glenoid) with humeral head subluxation may be evident on axillary view radiographs (**Figure 2**).
   b. CT is the study of choice for evaluating bony changes about the joint.
      - Advanced software can be utilized for three-dimensional preoperative planning of glenoid reaming and implant placement (**Figure 3**).

Dr. Namdari or an immediate family member has received royalties from DJ Orthopaedics and Miami device solutions; is a member of a speakers' bureau or has made paid presentations on behalf of DJ Orthopaedics and Miami device solutions; serves as a paid consultant to or is an employee of DJ Orthopaedics, Flexion Therapeutics, Miami device solutions and Synthes; has stock or stock options held in Aevumed, Force Therapeutics, MD Live, MD Valuate, Orthophor, Parvizi Surgical Innovations and RubiconMD; has received research or institutional support from Arthrex, Inc., DJ Orthopaedics, Integra and Zimmer; and serves as a board member, owner, officer, or committee member of the Philadelphia Orthopaedic Society.

This chapter is adapted from Kwon Y, Mahoney A: Arthritis and arthroplasty of the shoulder, in Boyer MI, ed: *AAOS Comprehensive Orthopaedic Review*, ed 2. Rosemont, IL, American Academy of Orthopaedic Surgeons, 2014, pp 949-958.

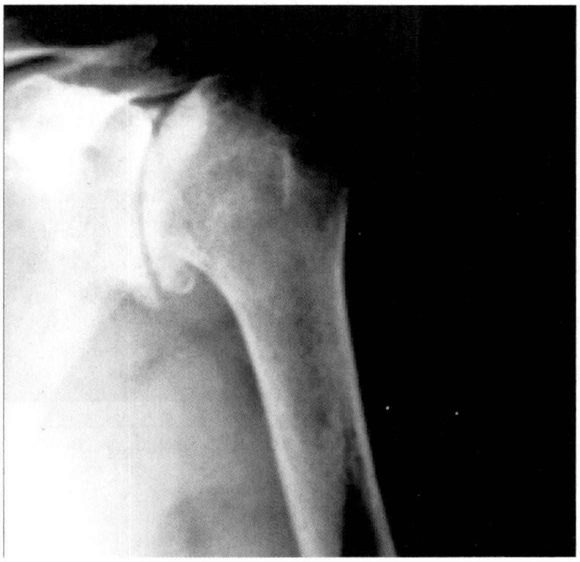

Figure 1 AP radiograph shows an osteoarthritic glenohumeral joint with subchondral sclerosis, cyst formation, humeral head flattening, and osteophyte formation. (Adapted from Chen AL, Joseph TM, Zuckerman JD: Rheumatoid arthritis of the shoulder. *J Am Acad Orthop Surg* 2003;11:12-24.)

- Planning software has been shown to influence surgical decision making and improve the accuracy of glenoid component positioning.
- The impact of three-dimensional virtual planning on functional outcomes and implant survival remains to be investigated.

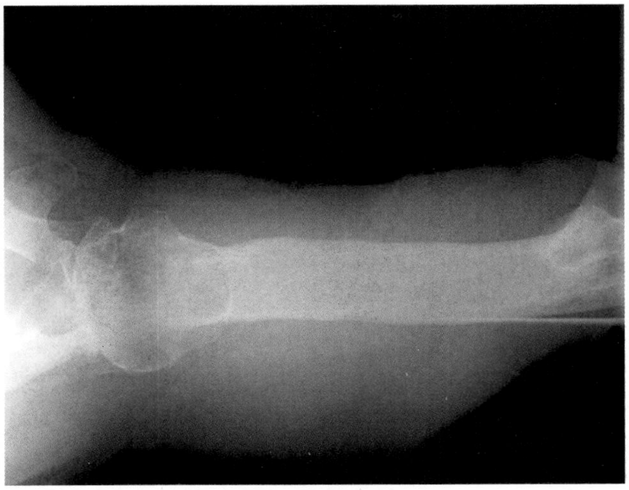

Figure 2 Axillary radiograph shows a shoulder with posterior glenoid erosion and posterior subluxation of the humeral head, which commonly are seen in osteoarthritis. (Courtesy of Leesa M. Galatz, MD, St Louis, MO.)

c. MRI is typically unnecessary for routine cases. It may provide additional information about the soft tissues, such as the rotator cuff, if clinical concerns exist, however.

D. Classification—Walch et al identified three types of glenoid morphology that are associated with primary glenohumeral OA based on erosion and bone loss which has subsequently been updated (**Figure 4**).

1. Type A—Concentric wear with no subluxation (59%)
   a. A1: Minor central erosion
   b. A2: Major central erosion
2. Type B—posterior humeral subluxation (32%)
   a. B1: Narrowing of the posterior joint space
   b. B2: Asymmetric loading of the posterior glenoid resulting in biconcave morphology
   c. B3: Monoconcave and posteriorly worn, with at least 15° of retroversion or at least 70% posterior humeral head subluxation
3. Type C—Glenoid retroversion greater than 25° from dysplasia (not acquired) (9%)
   a. C1: Monoconcave and without eccentric wear
   b. C2: Dysplastic glenoid with high pathologic retroversion, high premorbid version, and acquired posterior bone loss, giving it the appearance of a biconcave glenoid with posterior translation of the humeral head
4. Type D—Any level of glenoid anteversion or with humeral head subluxation of less than 40% (anterior subluxation)

E. Nonsurgical treatment

1. Medications such as NSAIDs and acetaminophen may provide symptomatic relief.
2. Intra-articular glenohumeral corticosteroid injection can provide substantial, but likely temporary, relief.
3. Physical therapy may provide some benefit if gentle stretching exercises are performed. Aggressive stretching and heavy weight training can exacerbate symptoms.
4. Several studies have demonstrated that viscosupplementation injections may provide some relief in patients with glenohumeral arthritis; however, these compounds have not yet produced sufficient evidence to warrant FDA approval, and any use about the shoulder is considered off-label.

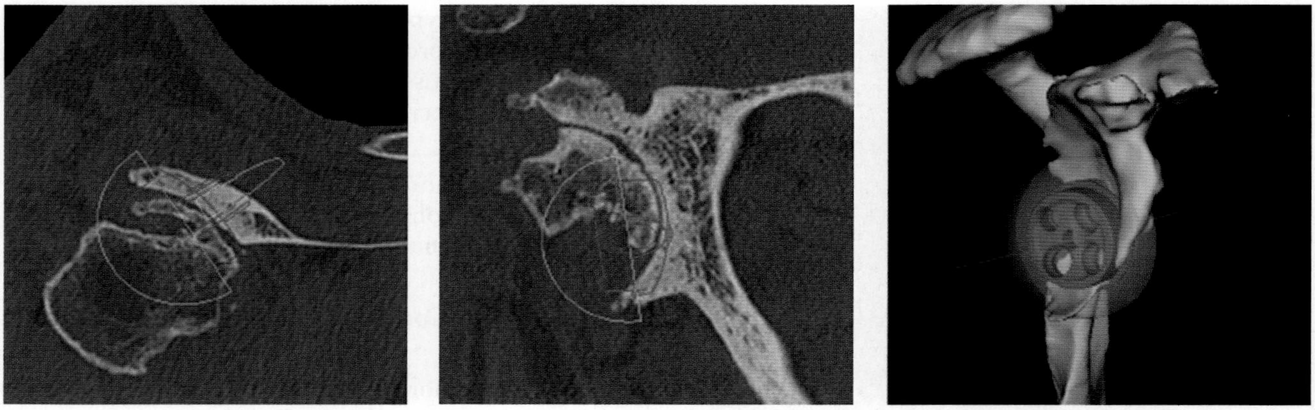

Figure 3 Example of virtual planning using a three-dimensional CT for a case of severe glenoid bone loss.

F. Surgical treatment

1. Indications—Persistent symptoms despite nonsurgical management; symptoms causing substantial disability and dysfunction that affect a patient's capacity to perform the activities of daily living
2. Arthroscopy
   a. Procedure may include removal of osteophytes, capsular release, loose body removal, chondroplasty, synovectomy, and/or axillary nerve neurolysis.
   b. Given the heterogeneity of procedures that can be performed arthroscopically, studies are difficult to interpret and variable in their support of the procedure.
   c. Poor candidates are those with advanced grades of arthritis, eccentric glenoid wear, and bipolar lesions.
   d. It is best suited for younger patients with a concentric glenoid and early radiographic arthritis.
3. Hemiarthroplasty
   a. Pain relief and range of motion are generally good but are less predictable than that following total shoulder arthroplasty (TSA). Pain relief with TSA is more predictable.
   b. Outcomes are suboptimal if the glenoid does not have a concentric surface to interact with the humeral head prosthesis.

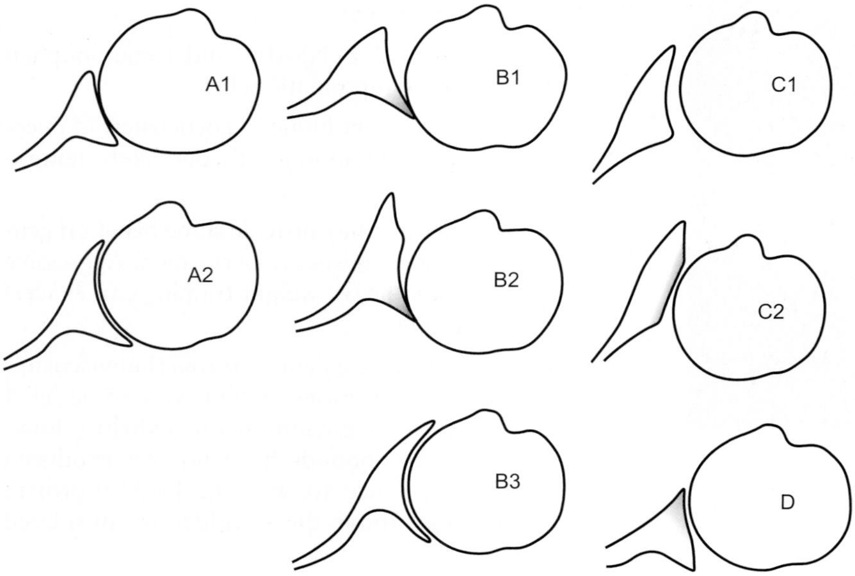

Figure 4 Illustrations depict the updated Walch classification of glenoid morphology associated with primary glenohumeral osteoarthritis. A1, Minor erosion. A2, Major erosion. B1, Narrowing of the posterior joint space, subchondral sclerosis, and osteophytes. B2, Posterior wear with a biconcave aspect to the glenoid. B3, Monoconcave and posteriorly worn (at least 15° of retroversion or at least 70% posterior humeral head subluxation). C1, Monoconcave glenoid with retroversion of more than 25° (dysplastic). C2, Biconcave glenoid with high premorbid retroversion (>25°), and acquired posterior bone loss. D, glenoid anteversion or with humeral head subluxation of less than 40% (anterior subluxation).

c. Hemiarthroplasty with biologic resurfacing of the glenoid (eg, meniscal allograft and Achilles allograft) has historical relevance for young patients. More recent studies have reported poor results, and this procedure has largely fallen out of favor.

d. Cuff tear arthroplasty of the humeral head is an option for patients with osteoarthritis, associated rotator cuff tears, and preserved overhead function. The prosthesis provides a larger area of lateral coverage to prevent the greater tuberosity from articulating against the undersurface of the acromion during abduction. Therefore, it may provide improved pain relief in patients with rotator cuff–deficient shoulders without pseudoparalysis.

4. Total shoulder arthroplasty

   a. TSA using a metallic humeral head and a cemented all-polyethylene glenoid prosthesis is the treatment of choice for elderly patients with OA.

   b. TSA provides reliable pain relief and range of motion.

   c. The 10-year survival rate is between 92% and 95%.

   d. Contraindications include active infection, a nonfunctioning deltoid, irreparable rotator cuff tears, brachial plexus palsy, and severe glenoid bone loss.

   e. The rocking horse phenomenon refers to the proposed mechanism of prosthesis failure in rotator cuff–deficient patients. The humeral head rocks superiorly and inferiorly like a rocking horse, causing premature glenoid loosening. This mechanism also may cause failure if subscapularis failure or anterior joint instability is present, allowing the humeral head to rock anteriorly and posteriorly.

5. Reverse TSA

   a. Reverse TSA is used to treat glenohumeral arthritis associated with large, irreparable rotator cuff tears.

   b. By reversing the relationship of the glenoid and the humeral head, the deltoid is placed at greater mechanical advantage to overcome the deficiency of the rotator cuff and elevate the shoulder. The fixed center of rotation of a reverse arthroplasty allows more efficient deltoid function without proximal humeral migration.

   c. Primarily used to treat elderly patients with irreparable cuff tears and pseudoparalysis; however, the indications continue to expand and evolve.

   d. Complication rates are substantially higher than those following TSA and include infection, dislocation, postoperative hematoma, acromion fracture, neurologic injury, intraoperative fracture, scapular notching, and deltoid pain.

   e. The 10-year survival rate is between 78% and 89%.

6. Arthrodesis

   a. Rarely indicated for OA; may be appropriate for patients with deltoid deficiency, young patients with high demands, or patients with persistent deep infection

   b. The optimal positioning for shoulder arthrodesis traditionally has been described to be 30° of abduction, 30° of forward flexion, and 30° of internal rotation. The actual position should be determined during the surgery to ensure that the ipsilateral hand can reach the mouth and the anterior waist line for improved functional capacity.

   c. Some patients report mild pain at the scapulothoracic joint caused by increased motion and fatigue.

G. Pearls and pitfalls

1. Generally, after shoulder arthroplasty, optimal results are obtained when the native anatomy of the shoulder is re-created.
2. Arthroplasty results are optimized when adequate soft-tissue releases and subscapularis mobilization are performed.
3. The retroversion of the humerus is highly variable, ranging from 10° to 45°, with a mean of 29°.
4. The mean native glenoid version is 1° of retroversion relative to the scapular body. This value can vary from 10° of retroversion to 10° of anteversion, however. Glenohumeral arthritis can result in excessive posterior glenoid wear.
5. Generally, 10° to 15° of glenoid retroversion can be corrected by eccentrically reaming the anterior glenoid rim.
6. Bone grafting, augmented glenoid components, or reverse arthroplasty may be necessary in the presence of severe glenoid bone loss that cannot be corrected with eccentric reaming alone.

7. Cement should not be used to compensate for glenoid bone loss because it can disintegrate over time.
8. The top of the humeral head should be approximately 5 to 8 mm superior to the top of the greater tuberosity.
9. Soft tissue must be balanced about the glenohumeral joint to obtain an optimal outcome.
10. In general, an anterior and inferior capsular release or removal is performed to optimize surgical exposure and to improve postoperative motion.
11. Rarely, posterior capsular imbrication may be needed to restore an appropriate soft-tissue balance.
12. Overstuffing the joint with an oversized humeral head should be avoided because this can cause increased joint reaction forces and tension on the rotator cuff.
13. Radiolucency around the glenoid component is a common finding; however, it does not always correlate with clinical failure.
14. Progressive radiolucency around the glenoid prosthesis is suggestive of glenoid loosening.
15. Debate over the optimal treatment of the subscapularis during TSA continues, and current options include tenotomy, peel, and lesser tuberosity osteotomy. Advocates of the osteotomy suggest that bone healing is more reliable than that seen following tendon-to-tendon healing. This has not been clinically demonstrated, however.
16. One of the more common complications of reverse TSA is inferior notching of the scapula. According to some studies, this may be associated with an inferior outcome. Placing the glenosphere on or below the inferior edge of the glenoid surface, inferior tilt, lateralization, and more vertical humeral component inclination angle may reduce the likelihood of this complication. Scapular notching may be related to the design of the implant.

II. INFLAMMATORY ARTHRITIS

A. Epidemiology and overview

1. Rheumatoid arthritis (RA) is the most prevalent form of inflammatory arthritis affecting the shoulder.
2. Of patients with RA for more than 5 years, 91% develop shoulder symptoms.
3. Other less common forms of inflammatory arthritis include spondyloarthropathies, disorders of connective tissue such as systemic lupus erythematosus, psoriatic arthritis, and crystalline deposition disorders.

B. Pathoanatomy

1. RA is a systemic autoimmune disorder that affects multiple joints.
2. Erosive pannus formation within the joint and the release of inflammatory cytokines result in cartilage damage, bone resorption, and soft-tissue degradation.
3. Up to 75% of patients with RA eventually develop rotator cuff pathology.
4. Between 25% and 30% of patients have full-thickness defects at the time of surgery.

C. Evaluation

1. History
   a. Most patients report generalized fatigue, pain in other joints, intermittent fever, and weight loss.
   b. Pain, swelling, progressive loss of motion, and weakness commonly are seen in the affected shoulder.
2. Physical examination
   a. Common findings during early stages of the disease include localized warmth and limited range of motion with pain. In a more chronic condition, crepitus and weakness also may be encountered.
   b. Periscapular atrophy may be noted if an associated rotator cuff tear is present.
   c. Sternoclavicular or acromioclavicular joint tenderness occurs in about one-third of patients with glenohumeral involvement.
3. Laboratory evaluation
   a. A complete blood cell count, erythrocyte sedimentation rate, C-reactive protein level, uric acid level, rheumatoid factor, serum complement, HLA-B27 screening, and antinuclear antibody titer are helpful in confirming the diagnosis.
   b. Arthrocentesis may be helpful in the setting of an acutely painful shoulder to rule out septic arthritis and crystalline arthropathies. Fluid tests include cell count, Gram stain, culture, and crystal analysis.
   c. Milwaukee shoulder (calcium hydroxyapatite crystalline arthropathy)—Aspirates contain blood-tinged fluid with debris, hydroxyapatite crystals, and inflammatory cells with a

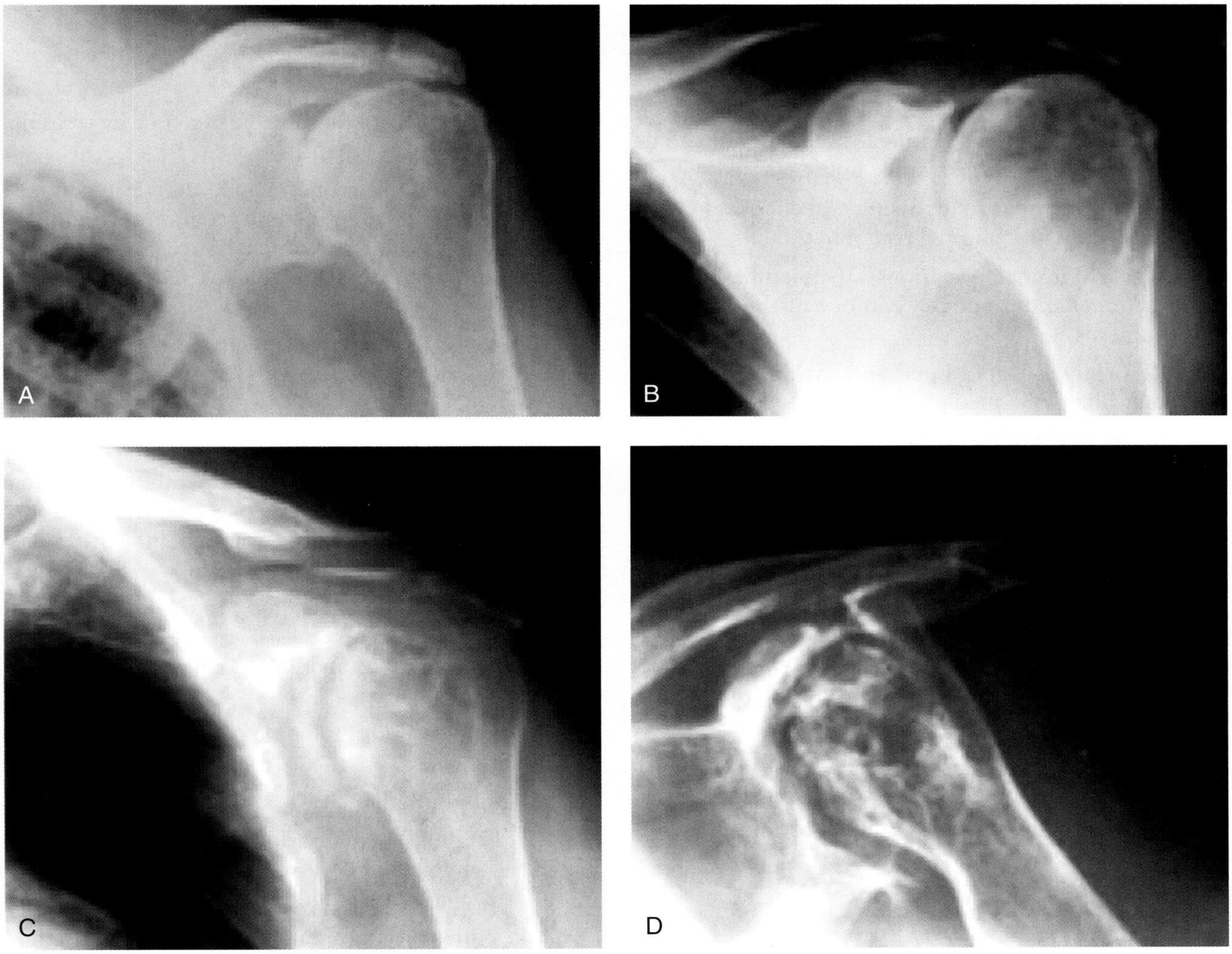

Figure 5 AP radiographs show changes associated with rheumatoid arthritis. **A**, Early changes of rheumatoid disease. Osteopenia (with minimal articular degenerative changes) and superior migration of the humeral head (consistent with rotator cuff compromise) are present. **B**, Intermediate changes of symmetric glenohumeral joint space loss and early cyst formation. **C**, As the disease progresses, more extensive erosion is evident around the humeral head and glenoid; progressive glenoid bone loss results in medialization of the humeral head. The superior migration of the humeral head indicates progressive rotator cuff deterioration. **D**, Extensive articular destruction, or arthritis mutilans, reflects end-stage changes with extensive erosions and bone loss. (Reproduced from Chen AL, Joseph TM, Zuckerman JD: Rheumatoid arthritis of the shoulder. *J Am Acad Orthop Surg* 2003;11:12-24.)

preponderance of monocytes. The diagnosis is confirmed by positive staining of the crystals with alizarin red.

d. Gout can be diagnosed by the characteristic negatively birefringent, needle-shaped deposition of sodium urate crystals.

e. Pseudogout joint fluid is characterized by positively birefringent, rhomboid-shaped calcium pyrophosphate dihydrate crystals.

4. Imaging

a. Radiography—Classic findings (**Figure 5**) for inflammatory arthritis of the shoulder include osteopenia, marginal erosions, and cyst formation. Advanced inflammatory arthritis is characterized by concentric joint space narrowing and medial glenoid wear. Large, irreparable rotator cuff tears may result in superior migration of the humeral head, "acetabularization" of the acromion, and rounding of the greater tuberosity.

b. CT should be performed when large bony defects or deformities are present.

c. MRI is useful for evaluating the integrity of the rotator cuff tendons and muscle quality.

6 | Shoulder and Elbow

d. A preoperative radiographic examination of the cervical spine is mandatory for patients with inflammatory arthritis to assess cervical spine stability before intubation.

D. Classification—Neer identified three types of shoulder RA based on radiographic findings.

1. Dry—Joint space narrowing, subchondral cysts, erosions with marginal osteophytes
2. Wet—Marginal erosions (sometimes quite extreme) and a pointed contour of the proximal humerus
3. Resorptive—Rapid bone and cartilage loss with centralization (medialization to the level of the coracoid process) of the glenohumeral joint

E. Nonsurgical treatment—The treatment of choice in modern inflammatory arthritis management

1. Medications
   a. Disease-modifying antirheumatic drugs have prevented many of the joint issues associated with inflammatory arthritis. These drugs work by disrupting the immune system, including the interleukin 1 antagonist and the tumor necrosis factor-α antagonist.
   b. NSAIDs also may be used to alleviate pain and inflammation.
2. Intra-articular corticosteroid injections may be used judiciously.
3. Physical therapy may help preserve motion.

F. Surgical treatment

1. Synovectomy
   a. May be appropriate for patients with active synovitis and mild articular involvement; this treatment is most beneficial during the early stages of the disease before joint destruction.
   b. The duration and efficacy of pain relief depend on the severity of the disease.
   c. Arthroscopic synovectomy is performed more commonly than open synovectomy.
   d. If the rotator cuff tendon is torn and cannot be repaired, the coracoacromial arch should be preserved to prevent anterosuperior escape of the humeral head.
2. Hemiarthroplasty—Historically, it has been indicated for advanced disease with massive irreparable rotator cuff tears; recently, however, reverse TSA has been used for this indication. Hemiarthroplasty still may be appropriate if the bone stock is inadequate to support a glenoid prosthesis and overhead active motion is maintained.
3. TSA
   a. TSA requires sufficient bone stock to support a glenoid prosthesis.
   b. The rotator cuff must be intact or have a small tear that is repairable.
   c. Contraindications include active infection, a nonfunctioning deltoid, a nonfunctioning or insufficient rotator cuff, irreparable rotator cuff tears, brachial plexus palsy, and severe glenoid bone loss.
   d. Overall outcome is good to excellent but slightly inferior compared with patients with OA.
4. Reverse TSA
   a. Ideally indicated for patients with rotator cuff arthropathy with pseudoparalysis; also may be indicated in elderly patients with inflammatory arthritis whose rotator cuff tissues have been severely compromised.
   b. The glenoid bone stock must be sufficient to support a prosthesis. In addition, patients must have a functional axillary nerve and deltoid muscle.
   c. The overall outcome is generally good to excellent.

G. Pearls and pitfalls

1. Substantial medialization of the joint may erode enough glenoid bone to preclude reaming and the insertion of a glenoid prosthesis.
2. In patients with inflammatory arthritis, osteopenia leads to a substantially higher risk for intraoperative iatrogenic fractures.
3. A long-stem humeral prosthesis should be avoided in patients with inflammatory arthritis because elbow arthroplasty may be necessary in the future.

III. OSTEONECROSIS

A. Epidemiology and overview

1. Posttraumatic osteonecrosis
   a. Four-part fracture-dislocations are associated with osteonecrosis in almost 100% of patients.
   b. Displaced four-part fractures are associated with osteonecrosis in 45% of patients.
   c. Valgus-impacted four-part fractures and three-part fractures have a much lower incidence of osteonecrosis (10% to 14%).
   d. Three-part fractures are associated with osteonecrosis in 14% of patients.

2. Atraumatic osteonecrosis
   a. The humeral head is the second most common site of atraumatic osteonecrosis; the femoral head is the most common.
   b. Systemic corticosteroid use is the most common cause of atraumatic osteonecrosis. The estimated incidence of atraumatic osteonecrosis after systemic corticosteroid use is 5% to 25%.
   c. Atraumatic osteonecrosis also is associated with alcohol abuse, sickle cell disease, Caisson disease, Gaucher disease, and systemic lupus erythematosus.

B. Pathoanatomy
1. Blood supply to the humeral head
   a. The main supply comes from the ascending branch of the anterior circumflex artery, which runs in the lateral bicipital groove and becomes intraosseous as the arcuate artery.
   b. A lesser contribution is made by the posterior humeral circumflex artery, which runs along the posteromedial aspect of the humeral neck to supply the humeral head.
   c. When the anterior circumflex artery has been compromised, the flow through the posterior humeral circumflex artery increases to maintain the blood supply to the humeral head.
2. The common final pathway of osteonecrosis is blood flow insufficiency, resulting in the death of cells within the bony matrix.
3. During subsequent bone resorption and remodeling, microfracture and subchondral bone collapse may result in joint incongruity and arthritic changes.

C. Evaluation
1. History
   a. Common symptoms include pain and weakness. In advanced disease, crepitus and loss of motion can be expected.
   b. The onset of symptoms is commonly insidious, which often causes the patient to delay seeking evaluation.
   c. A history of risk factors including prior surgery, fractures, alcohol abuse, corticosteroid use, and diving may be elicited.
2. Physical examination
   a. During the early stages of the disorder, the examination can be fairly normal, other than pain with motion.
   b. During the advanced stages, common findings include limited range of motion, crepitus, and weakness.
3. Imaging
   a. Radiographs—The most common site for osteonecrotic lesions is the superior middle portion of the humeral head, just deep to the articular cartilage. This area can be visualized best on an AP shoulder view with the arm in neutral external rotation (**Figure 6**).

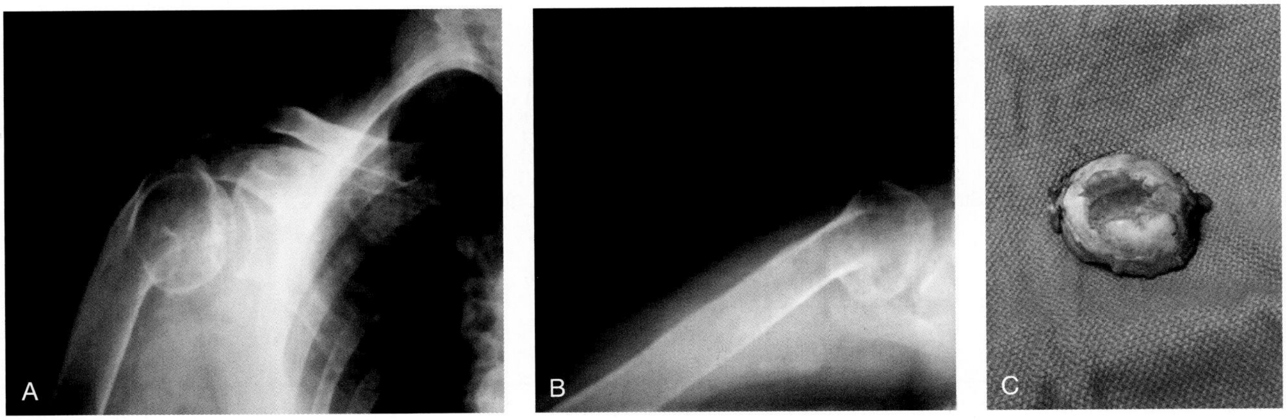

Figure 6 Images depict posttraumatic osteonecrosis. AP (**A**) and axillary (**B**) radiographic views. **C**, Photograph of a surgical specimen demonstrates subchondral collapse. (Adapted with permission from Sarris I, Weiser R, Sotereanos DG: Pathogenesis and treatment of osteonecrosis of the shoulder. *Orthop Clin North Am* 2004;35:397-404.)

b. MRI is the preferred imaging method, and its sensitivity in detecting early osteonecrotic lesions is nearly 100%.

c. When osteonecrosis of the humeral head is confirmed, radiographs of the hip must be obtained to rule out osteonecrosis of the femoral head. If hip radiographs are negative, MRI of the femoral head may be warranted in patients with hip pain.

D. Classification—The Cruess system (**Figure** 7)

E. Nonsurgical treatment

1. Medications may provide symptomatic pain relief. Associated synovitis of the joint also may be treated with NSAIDs.
2. Physical therapy can be useful for restoring or maintaining motion and strength.
3. Temporary activity modification, with restriction of overhead activities and strenuous use, may be helpful.

F. Surgical treatment

1. Core decompression

a. Indicated for early-stage disease without humeral head collapse; one study reported successful results in 94% of patients with stage I disease and 88% of those with stage II disease.

b. Clinical experience of core decompression in the humeral head is limited.

c. Core decompression can be performed after arthroscopy to confirm the integrity of the humeral head cartilage.

2. The role of vascularized bone grafting for osteonecrosis of the humeral head is unclear.
3. Hemiarthroplasty—Indicated for stage III or stage IV disease with humeral head collapse
4. For stage V disease, TSA must be considered.
5. Results after shoulder arthroplasty for osteonecrosis are generally inferior compared with those after shoulder arthroplasty for osteoarthritis.

G. Pearls and pitfalls

1. After subchondral collapse occurs in osteonecrosis, arthroplasty is the most reliable treatment option.
2. After a diagnosis of humeral head osteonecrosis has been established, other joints should be examined, especially the hip, because the femoral head is the most common site of osteonecrosis.

IV. COMPLICATIONS OF TOTAL SHOULDER ARTHROPLASTY

A. Glenoid loosening—The most common cause of TSA failure, accounting for approximately 30% of revisions in the setting of primary OA.

1. Humeral stem loosening—Generally uncommon after hemiarthroplasty or TSA; therefore, infection always must be considered when humeral head loosening is observed.

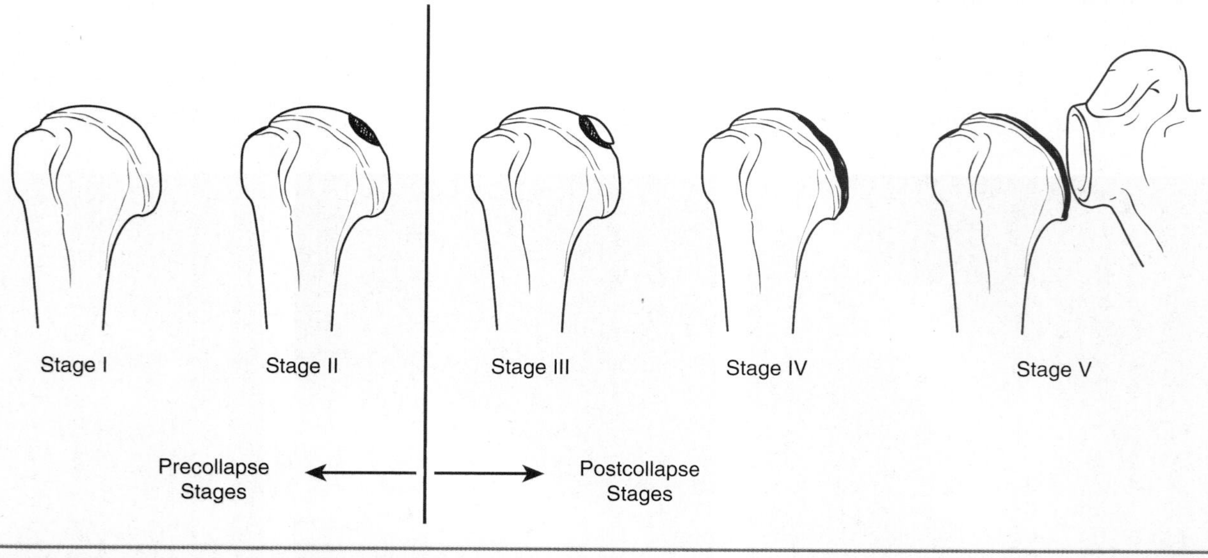

Figure 7 Illustrations demonstrate the Cruess classification system for osteonecrosis. The system includes five stages, based on radiographic appearance. In stage I, changes are not visible on plain radiographs but can be detected on MRIs. In stage II, sclerotic bone can be seen on plain radiographs. In stage III, a subchondral fracture (crescent sign) can be seen on radiographs. Stage IV is characterized by a collapse of the humeral head and joint incongruity that does not affect the glenoid. In stage V, arthritic changes are present in the glenoid.

2. Radiolucency around the glenoid prosthesis does not always correlate with clinical failure. Progressive radiolucency or component migration more reliably indicates component loosening.

B. Infection—General principles for infection control with shoulder arthroplasty are derived from the literature for treating infection following total hip and total knee arthroplasty. Early infection (<6 weeks after surgery) without evidence of prosthetic loosening may be treated with open irrigation and débridement. Late infections are best treated with implant removal, intravenous antibiotics, and single-stage or dual-stage reconstruction. A precontoured antibiotic-impregnated cement spacer may be useful in maintaining tissue tension during treatment with intravenous antibiotics during dual-stage revision. *Cutibacterium acnes* is a commonly recognized pathogen in TSA infections and usually is characterized as an indolent, low-virulence infection that can be difficult to diagnose.

C. Rotator cuff failure of subscapularis healing

1. Rotator cuff dysfunction often can result in premature glenoid loosening after TSA because of the rocking horse mechanism.
2. Subscapularis failure is a potential cause of shoulder pain after TSA. Treatment options include primary repair, pectoralis major tendon transfer, or revision reverse TSA.
3. Supraspinatus failure may occur after TSA or hemiarthroplasty, resulting in superior escape of the humerus. Treatment options include primary repair or revision to reverse TSA.

D. Postoperative stiffness is a complication that is best avoided with prevention. After adequate soft-tissue healing, aggressive physical therapy must be instituted to restore motion. In patients with severely restricted motion whose extensive therapy regimen is unsuccessful, arthroscopic release or infection workup may be required.

E. Neurologic injury is an uncommon complication. Most nerve complications involve the lateral cord and/or posterior cords of the brachial plexus are transient and resolve within 6 months The musculocutaneous nerve can be injured during the placement of retractors under the conjoint tendon. Manipulation of the humerus during shoulder arthroplasty (external rotation and extension) also can result in a general brachial plexus traction injury. Risk factors for neurologic injury include severe preoperative stiffness and revision surgery.

F. Intraoperative fracture—In patients with osteopenia (eg, inflammatory arthritis), a substantially higher risk for intraoperative iatrogenic fractures exists in both the glenoid and the humerus.

ACKNOWLEDGMENTS

The authors wish to recognize the work of Young W. Kwon, MD, PhD and Andrew P. Mahoney, MD who authored this chapter for the second edition of the *AAOS Comprehensive Orthopaedic Review*.

TOP TESTING FACTS

Osteoarthritis

1. Anterior capsule and subscapularis contractures are common in primary OA.
2. Rotator cuff tears rarely (5% to 10%) are associated with primary OA.
3. In primary OA of the shoulder, glenoid erosion typically occurs posteriorly with the associated humeral head posterior subluxation.
4. In TSA, rotator cuff insufficiency may result in a rocking horse phenomenon that results in premature loosening and failure of the glenoid component.
5. Compared with hemiarthroplasty, TSA is associated with more consistent pain relief.

Inflammatory Arthritis

1. Up to 75% of patients with inflammatory arthritis may have concomitant rotator cuff pathology, and 25% to 30% have full-thickness defects at the time of surgery.
2. Inflammatory arthritis is characterized by concentric joint space narrowing and medial glenoid wear.
3. Preoperative radiographic examination of the cervical spine is mandatory for patients with inflammatory arthritis to assess cervical stability.

4. Synovectomy, either arthroscopic or open, is most beneficial during the early stages of inflammatory arthritis, before articular joint destruction.
5. Substantial medialization of the joint may erode enough glenoid bone to preclude reaming and the insertion of a glenoid component.

Osteonecrosis

1. Osteonecrosis can have a posttraumatic or an atraumatic etiology.
2. The femoral head is the most common site of atraumatic osteonecrosis. The humeral head is the second most common.
3. Systemic corticosteroid use is the most common risk factor of atraumatic osteonecrosis; estimated incidence is 5% to 25%.
4. The most common initial site for osteonecrotic lesions is the superior middle portion of the humeral head, just deep to the articular cartilage. This area can be visualized best on an AP view of the shoulder with the arm in neutral external rotation.
5. MRI is the preferred imaging method because its sensitivity in detecting early osteonecrosis is nearly 100%.
6. Once osteonecrosis-related subchondral collapse occurs, arthroplasty is the most reliable treatment option.

Complications of Total Shoulder Arthroplasty

1. Glenoid loosening is the most common cause of TSA failure; it accounts for approximately 30% of revisions in the setting of primary OA.
2. *C acnes* is a low-virulent organism associated with shoulder arthroplasty infections and can be difficult to diagnose.
3. Rotator cuff tear is a common postoperative complication that may occur in the early or late postoperative period and result in pain, weakness, and decreased range of motion.

Bibliography

Boileau P, Watkinson D, Hatzidakis AM, Hovorka I: Neer Award 2005: The Grammont reverse shoulder prosthesis: results in cuff tear arthritis, fracture sequelae, and revision arthroplasty. *J Shoulder Elbow Surg* 2006;15(5):527-540.

Cofield RH: Total shoulder arthroplasty with the Neer prosthesis. *J Bone Joint Surg Am* 1984;66(6):899-906.

Ernstbrunner L, Andronic O, Grubhofer F, Camenzind RS, Wieser K, Gerber C: Long-term results of reverse total shoulder arthroplasty for rotator cuff dysfunction: a systematic review of longitudinal outcomes. *J Shoulder Elbow Surg* 2019;28(4):774-781.

Hovelius L, Saeboe M: Neer Award 2008: Arthropathy after primary anterior shoulder dislocation—223 shoulders prospectively followed up for twenty-five years. *J Shoulder Elbow Surg* 2009;18(3):339-347.

Iannotti J, Baker J, Rodriguez E, et al: Three-dimensional preoperative planning software and a novel information transfer technology improve glenoid component positioning. *J Bone Joint Surg Am* 2014;96(9):e71. doi:10.2106/JBJS.L.01346.

Iannotti JP, Jun BJ, Patterson TE, Ricchetti ET: Quantitative Measurement of Osseous pathology in advanced glenohumeral osteoarthritis. *J Bone Joint Surg Am* 2017;99(17):1460-1468. doi:10.2106/JBJS.16.00869.

Rugg CM, Gallo RA, Craig EV, Feeley BT: The pathogenesis and management of cuff tear arthropathy. *J Shoulder Elbow Surg* 2018;27(12):2271-2283.

Saltzman BM, Leroux TS, Verma NN, Romeo AA: Glenohumeral osteoarthritis in the young patient. *J Am Acad Orthop Surg* 2018;26(17):e361-e370.

Sperling JW, Cofield RH, Rowland CM: Minimum fifteen-year follow-up of Neer hemiarthroplasty and total shoulder arthroplasty in patients aged fifty years or younger. *J Shoulder Elbow Surg* 2004;13(6):604-613.

Chapter 76
DISORDERS OF THE ACROMIOCLAVICULAR JOINT

JAY D. KEENER, MD
BRENDAN M. PATTERSON, MD, MPH

I. ACROMIOCLAVICULAR JOINT ANATOMY AND BIOMECHANICS

A. Acromioclavicular (AC) joint anatomy

1. The AC joint is a synovial diarthrodial joint separated by a fibrocartilaginous disk that degenerates with age.
2. The angle of inclination of the distal clavicle and acromial facet articular surfaces is highly variable, ranging from near vertical to 50° angulation of the superolateral clavicle over the acromial facet.
3. The AC joint capsule surrounds the joint and is reinforced on all sides by the AC joint capsular ligaments. The AC joint capsular insertion on the acromion begins, on average, 2.8 mm (range, 2.3 to 3.3 mm) from the medial acromion and begins on the lateral clavicle a mean of 3.5 mm (range, 2.9 to 3.9 mm) from the distal clavicle.
4. The distal clavicle epiphysis fuses with the clavicle late, between the ages of 18 and 22 years.
5. The AC joint is innervated by branches of the lateral pectoral, suprascapular, and axillary nerves.

B. AC joint biomechanics

1. The clavicle rotates posteriorly 40° to 45° with full elevation of the shoulder; however, only 5° to 8° of rotation is seen at the AC joint because of the synchronous upward rotation of the scapula and sternoclavicular joint motion.
2. The horizontal stability of the clavicle is provided by the AC joint ligaments, especially the superior (50%) followed by the posterior (25%) ligaments.
3. The vertical stability of the clavicle is provided by the AC joint ligaments at physiologic loads and by the coracoclavicular (CC) ligaments at higher loads (**Figure 1**).
   a. The medially positioned conoid ligament is the strongest and most important vertical stabilizer of the AC joint at higher loads. The conoid ligament inserts into the conoid tubercle at the posteroinferior clavicle centered at a mean of 46 mm from the lateral end of the clavicle.

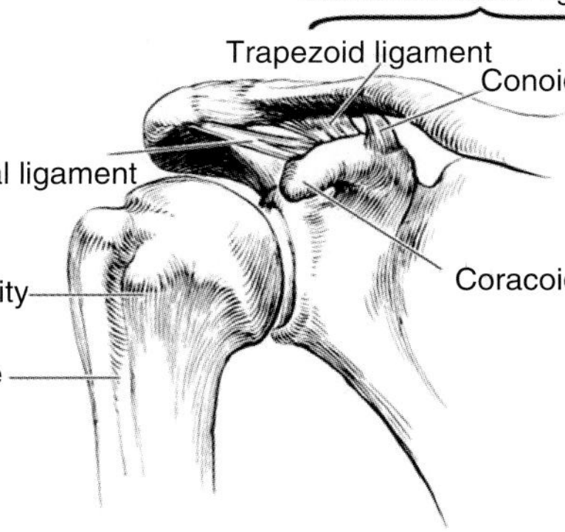

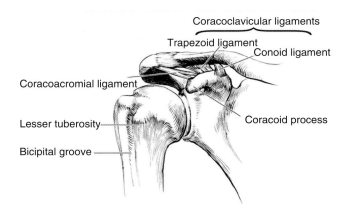

Figure 1 Illustration depicts the acromioclavicular (AC) joint. Static stabilizers include the AC capsule and the coracoclavicular ligaments, consisting of the trapezoid ligament laterally and the conoid ligament medially. (Reproduced from Simovich R, Sanders B, Ozbaydar M, Lavery K, Warner JJP: Acromioclavicular joint injuries: Diagnosis and management. *J Am Aced Orthop Surg* 2009;17[4]:207-219.)

Dr. Keener or an immediate family member has received royalties from Genesis, Shoulder Innovations and Wright Medical Technology, Inc.; serves as a paid consultant to or is an employee of Arthrex, Inc. and Wright Medical Technology, Inc.; has received research or institutional support from the National Institutes of Health (NIAMS & NICHD) and Zimmer; and serves as a board member, owner, officer, or committee member of the American Shoulder and Elbow Surgeons. Dr. Patterson or an immediate family member serves as a paid consultant to or is an employee of Disk-Criminator LLC.

b. The laterally positioned trapezoid ligament provides restraint against lateral translation of the clavicle in relation to the coracoid as well as vertical stability. The trapezoid ligament inserts at the undersurface of the clavicle centered at a mean of 25 mm from the lateral end of the clavicle.

4. The deltotrapezial fascia plays an important but unquantified role in AC joint stability.

5. Minimal (5- and 10-mm) resection of the distal clavicle increases the horizontal motion of the clavicle in cadaveric models, and further translation is seen when releasing the superior and posterior AC joint ligaments.

II. TRAUMATIC CONDITIONS OF THE AC JOINT

A. AC joint separation

1. Overview and epidemiology—Common injury; incidence is unknown

2. Pathoanatomy—Injury results in progressive disruption of the ligamentous support of the AC joint, beginning with the capsular ligaments and progressing to the CC ligaments.

3. Evaluation

a. History—The mechanism of injury is usually direct trauma resulting from a fall on the point of the shoulder. Indirect injuries are rare.

b. Physical examination of the AC joint

- Higher grade injuries result in prominence of the distal clavicle.
- Localized bruising, swelling, and tenderness are present in acute injuries.
- The sternoclavicular joint also should be evaluated for swelling, deformity, and tenderness.
- Range of motion (ROM) of rotator cuff strength typically is normal in chronic injuries but may be limited in acute injuries secondary to pain.
- The ability to reduce the deformity with manual pressure is important and, for higher grade injuries, can help differentiate nonsurgical versus surgical treatment.
- Horizontal plane translation of the distal clavicle should be assessed manually and compared with the opposite shoulder.
- A complete neurologic examination of the upper extremity should be performed to rule out brachial plexus injuries.
- Scapular motion should be carefully assessed as scapular dyskinesis can be seen with this type of injury.

c. Imaging—Plain radiographs include an AP view of the clavicle, a caudal tilt view, and an axillary view.

- The axillary view is needed to rule out posterior translation of the distal clavicle. The anterior aspect of the clavicle should lie in the same plane as the anterior aspect of the acromion.
- Normal coracoclavicular distance (between the superior aspect of the coracoid and the inferior clavicle) should be between 11 to 13 mm.
- Fracture of the base of the coracoid process should be ruled out. A coracoid fracture can result in superior displacement of the clavicle but an intact CC distance, creating a functionally equivalent AC joint separation.
- A Zanca view (a modified, underpenetrated AP view with a cephalic tilt of 10° to 15°) gives excellent detail of the distal clavicle.
- Weighted views include bilateral AP views with a weight tied to the wrists in relaxed standing. They help distinguish between type II and type III separations but rarely are indicated and often are not clinically helpful.

4. Rockwood classification (**Figure 2**)

a. Type I—AC ligament sprain, intact CC ligaments; radiographs show CC distance is normal.

b. Type II—AC ligament rupture, sprained but intact CC ligaments; radiographs show CC distance is normal.

c. Type III—Disruption of the AC and CC ligaments (**Figures 3** and **4**); characterized by increased CC distance; superior displacement of the clavicle of up to 100% of the clavicle width; the deformity is reducible.

- More recently a modification of type III injuries has been proposed consisting of type IIIA (horizontally stable) and type IIIB (horizontally unstable).

d. Type IV—Disruption of the AC and CC ligaments with posterior displacement of the clavicle; characterized by increased CC distance; distal clavicle is herniated into or through the deltotrapezial fascia; the deformity is not reducible.

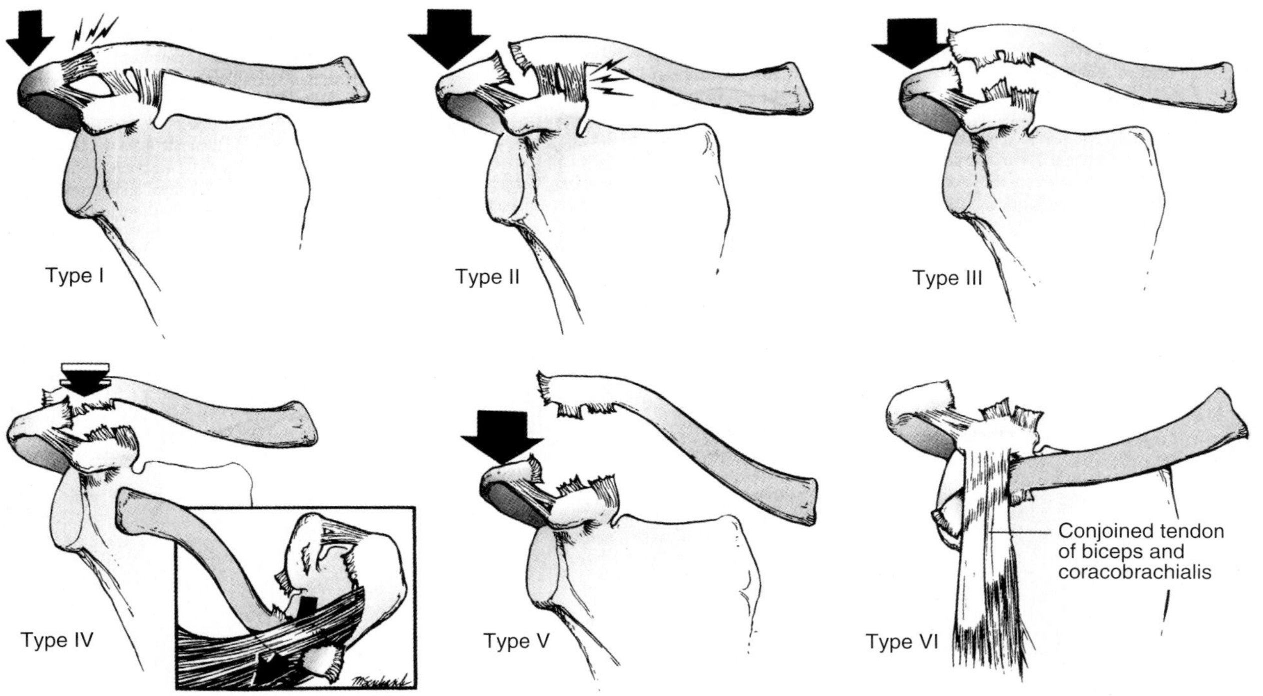

Figure 2 Illustrations show the Rockwood classification of acromioclavicular joint injuries. Arrows demonstrate the direction of displacement of the scapula or the clavicle. Inset for type IV demonstrates posterior herniation of the clavicle through the trapezial fascia.

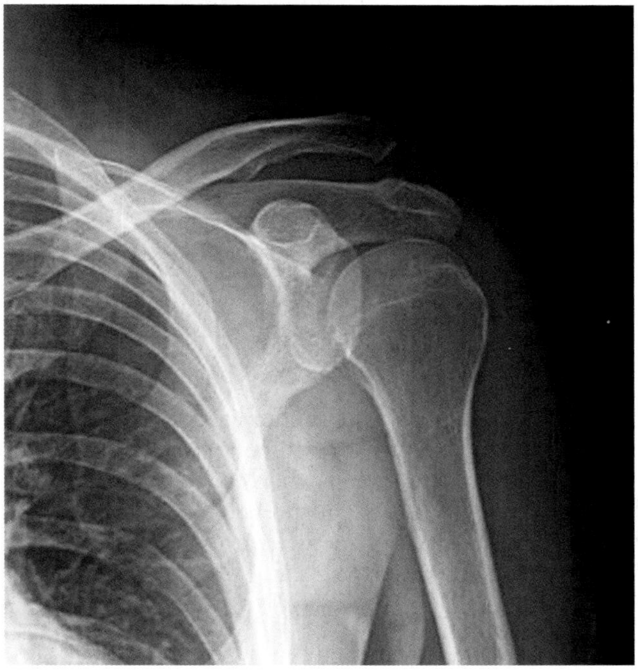

Figure 3 AP view of the left shoulder of a patient with type III acromioclavicular joint separation, with elevation of the clavicle relative to the acromion. Increased coracoclavicular distance is noted.

e. Type V—Disruption of the AC and CC ligaments with greater than 100% displacement of the clavicle superiorly; a markedly increased CC distance; deformity usually is not reducible because of herniation through the deltotrapezial fascia.

f. Type VI—Disruption of the AC and CC ligaments with inferior clavicle displacement; these rare injuries result in the distal clavicle lying under the acromion or coracoid process.

5. Nonsurgical treatment is recommended for type I and II injuries. Good functional outcomes can be expected.

a. Sling immobilization is followed by gradual active ROM exercises and stretching, then strengthening as tolerated.

b. Most patients regain full shoulder function within 4 to 6 weeks.

c. Patients are at increased risk for painful AC joint arthritis.

d. Between 30% and 50% of young, very active patients will have mild to moderate residual pain at the AC joint.

6 | Shoulder and Elbow

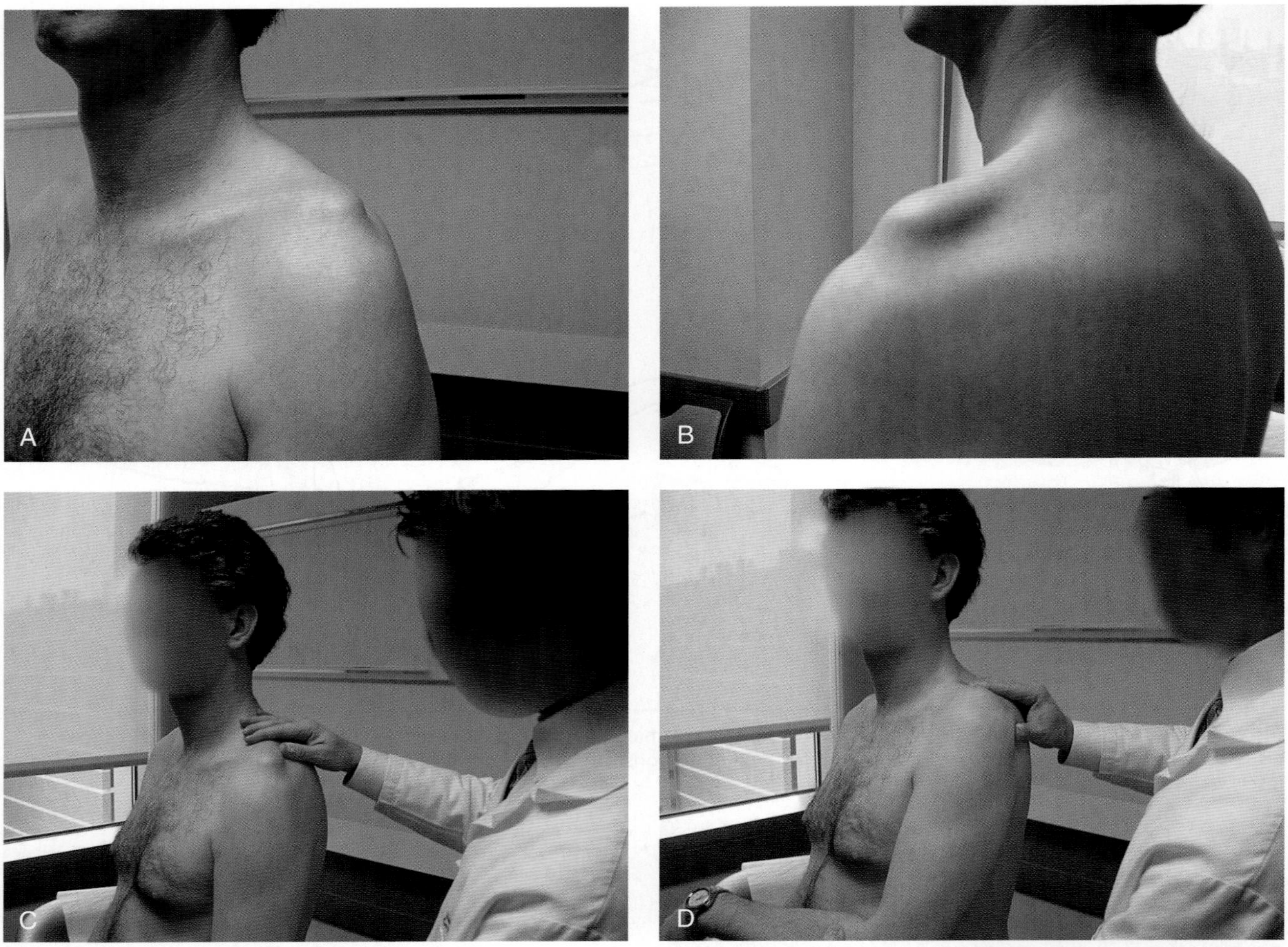

Figure 4 Photographs depict a type III acromioclavicular joint separation and disruption of the AC and coracoclavicular ligaments. **A**, Anterior view of the left shoulder of a chronic type III AC joint separation. Note the prominence of the distal clavicle. **B**, Posterolateral view of the same shoulder. **C**, Resting position of the distal clavicle before manual reduction. **D**, The examiner reduces the distal clavicle deformity by applying downward pressure to the clavicle and upward pressure through the elbow. The deformity is completely reducible, indicating the clavicle is not herniated through the deltotrapezial fascia.

6. The recommended treatment for type III injuries is controversial and depends on patient age and activity level.
   a. Multiple retrospective comparative studies have shown good clinical results and return to sport with nonsurgical treatment and no advantage from surgery. Criticisms of these studies primarily relate to the use of antiquated surgical techniques in the surgical groups.
   b. Meta-analysis and systematic reviews demonstrate similar outcomes for type III separations managed nonsurgically and surgically.
      - Nonsurgical treatment resulted in quicker recovery and return to work.
      - Surgical treatment resulted in an increase in complications.
   c. One prospective, randomized trial of type III and V injuries showed better results with nonsurgical treatment when clavicle displacement was less than 2 cm and better results with surgical management when the clavicle was displaced more than 2 cm.
7. Treatment for type IV, V, and VI injuries
   a. Nonsurgical treatment likely results in substantial residual pain and limited function; however, outcomes studies are limited.
   b. Surgical treatment is recommended for most patients.

8. Surgical indications
   a. Surgery is indicated for most acute type IV, V, and VI separations.
   b. Surgery can be performed acutely in selected type III separations in younger, physically active patients, manual laborers, patients with cosmetic concerns, or those with chronic injuries who have persistent symptoms.
   c. Surgery is also often recommended for patients with type IIIB (horizontally unstable) separations.
9. Acute surgery (less than 3 to 4 weeks following injury). Healing of the CC ligaments is reliable without the need for graft augmentation if adequate reduction and stabilization are achieved acutely.
   a. AC joint fixation—Implants spanning the acromion into the clavicle (Knowles pins) have high failure rates and implant-related complications and are not recommended. Hook plates provide reliable temporary fixation of acute injuries.
      - The hook plate must be removed because of acromial erosion.
      - Clinical results are good when using hook plates for acute injuries; however, they are not superior to other methods of fixation.
      - Hook plates are associated with various complications, including hook pullout, acromial erosion, and increased pain in some studies compared with other methods of fixation.
   b. CC interval fixation (acute)
      - Various acceptable fixation options exist, including suture loops, titanium button, coracoid suture anchors, and screw fixation.
      - Healing is predictable no matter which type of fixation is used; however, some laxity may develop, and hardware complications and fractures are seen.
      - Biomechanically, double-suture titanium button techniques approach the strength of the native CC ligaments.
      - Suture loops and suture anchor fixation provide better reduction strength than a Weaver-Dunn procedure without suture augmentation.
      - A recent study showed excellent clinical results in acute type III and V separations treated with an arthroscopic double-suture flip button technique despite radiographic signs of mild recurrent vertical and horizontal clavicle instability.
      - A potential benefit of arthroscopic treatment is the ability to both diagnose and address associated intra-articular pathology when present.
   c. Delayed surgical reconstruction
      - Reconstruction with tissue grafting is indicated when surgery is delayed more than 3 to 4 weeks following injury.
      - Anatomic reconstruction (**Figure 5**) of the conoid and trapezoid ligaments with tissue grafting provides better fixation strength and biomechanical stability than the Weaver-Dunn procedure, re-creating stability approaching the native state.
      - Improved functional outcomes and increased patient satisfaction have been reported at a minimum of 2 years follow-up for patients undergoing anatomic reconstruction.
      - Despite improved outcomes with surgical treatment, a review of the results of anatomic reconstruction reported an overall combined complication rate of up to 39%.
      - Potential complications of anatomic reconstruction include loss of reduction, clavicle and or coracoid fracture, symptomatic hardware, and infection.

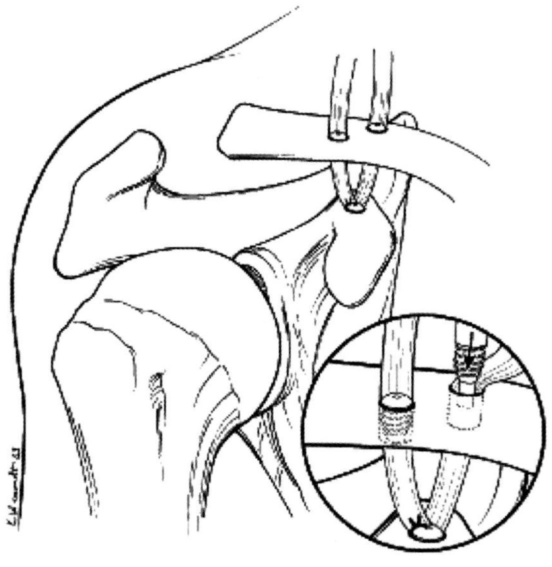

Figure 5 Illustration depicts an anatomic reconstruction of the coracoclavicular ligaments. Graft tissue is passed between the coracoid and the native insertions of the conoid and trapezoid ligaments on the undersurface of the clavicle. Alternatively, the graft can be passed under the coracoid process (not shown). (Reproduced with permission from Mazzocca AD, Santangelo SA, Johnson ST, Rios CG, Dumonski ML, Arciero RA: A biomechanical evaluation of an anatomical coracoclavicular ligament reconstruction. *Am J Sports Med* 2006;34[2]:236-246.)

6 | Shoulder and Elbow

- Recent clinical research has highlighted the importance of optimal tunnel position and preoperative templating to decrease the risk of loss of reduction.
- One prospective randomized trial showed better clinical results and maintenance of the reduction with anatomic reconstruction than with a Weaver-Dunn procedure.

d. Weaver-Dunn procedure (**Figure 6**)

- This procedure consists of the resection of the distal clavicle and transfer of the coracoacromial ligament into the distal clavicle with or without suture augmentation to the coracoid.
- Coracoacromial ligament transfer alone recreates only 20% of the native strength of the CC ligaments.
- Clinical results using the Weaver-Dunn procedure generally are good, especially when performed acutely. Incomplete loss of reduction can be seen in cases of chronic injury.

B. Physeal injuries of the distal clavicle—AC joint injuries in skeletally immature patients can result in a Salter-Harris physeal injury.

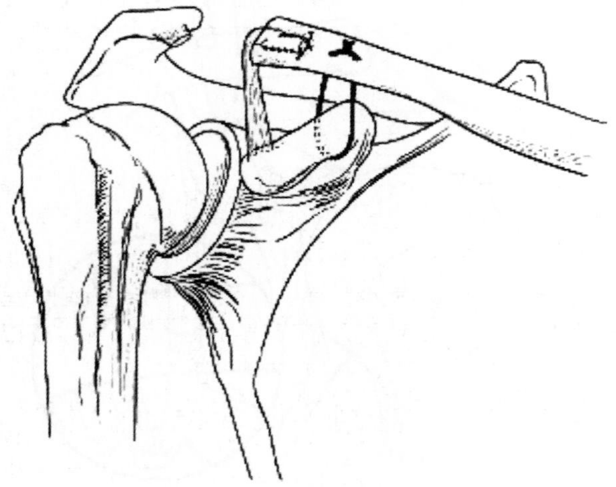

Figure 6 Illustration demonstrates the Weaver-Dunn acromioclavicular joint reconstruction. The coracoacromial ligament is released from the acromion and transferred to the endosteal canal of the lateral clavicle. Supplemental fixation is provided by a suture loop around the coracoid process and into the clavicle. (Reproduced with permission from Mazzocca AD, Santangelo SA, Johnson ST, Rios CG, Dumonski ML, Arciero RA: A biomechanical evaluation of an anatomical coracoclavicular ligament reconstruction. *Am J Sports Med* 2006;34[2]:236-246.)

III. ATRAUMATIC AND DEGENERATIVE CONDITIONS OF THE AC JOINT

A. Osteoarthritis

1. Epidemiology/pathoanatomy

a. More common with advanced age following degeneration of the intra-articular disk. Arthritic deterioration starts in early middle age.

b. More common in patients engaged in repetitive overhead or lifting activities.

c. Previous low-grade AC joint separations can result in painful arthritis.

d. The radiographic severity of arthritis does not always correlate with patient symptoms.

2. Evaluation

a. History

- Patients report activity-related pain.
- The pain is localized to the AC joint, with occasional radiation anteriorly or along the trapezius.
- Pain with heavy lifting or when sleeping on the affected side also is reported.

b. Physical examination

- Point tenderness is seen at the AC joint.
- Horizontal stability should be assessed.
- Pain at the AC joint with terminal elevation and cross-body motion often is seen.
- Selective injection of anesthetic into the AC joint can confirm the diagnosis.

c. Imaging

- Radiographs—An AP view and/or a Zanca view of the shoulder provides good visualization of the AC joint. Osteophyte formation, sclerotic reaction, and bone cysts are commonly seen.
- Bone and joint edema on MRI correlate with AC joint pain.

3. Nonsurgical treatment—Rest, ice, and NSAIDs are used initially; corticosteroid injections can also be used for diagnostic or therapeutic purposes.

4. Surgical treatment

a. Surgical indications include persistent pain and failure of nonsurgical treatment.

b. Relative contraindications include a previous low-grade separation with persistent horizontal plane instability.

c. Arthroscopic distal clavicle excision
   - Biomechanical evidence suggests a resection of 5 mm is needed to prevent contact between the clavicle and the acromion in the absence of instability.
   - Care should be taken to preserve the posterior and superior AC ligaments.
   - Pain relief is reliable (in >90% of patients) in the absence of instability.
   - Previous traumatic instability is associated with persistent pain in 30% to 40% of cases following distal clavicle excision.
   - One systematic review showed slightly better results with arthroscopic excision than with open distal clavicle excision.
   - Direct comparison studies have shown similar or better results with arthroscopic excision than with open techniques.

d. Open distal clavicle resection (Mumford procedure)
   - Between 5 and 10 mm of the distal clavicle should be resected.
   - Meticulous repair of the deltotrapezial fascia is important.

5. Rehabilitation
   a. Acute—zero to 7 days postoperative; sling, ice, and pendulum exercises
   b. Subacute—1 to 6 weeks postoperative
      - Gradually increase in shoulder ROM; gentle passive stretching and ROM as tolerated.
      - Reduce sling use as pain permits.
      - Avoid heavy lifting or strengthening exercises.
   c. Late recovery—more than 6 weeks
      - Full shoulder ROM and stretching
      - Initiate rotator cuff, scapular stabilizer, and deltoid strengthening.
      - Heavy weight lifting and return to full activities as tolerated. Residual pain/soreness can persist for 3 to 4 months and can be aggravated by heavy lifting. Therefore, activity progression should be modified according to symptoms.

B. Distal clavicle osteolysis
   1. Pathology—Localized hyperemia of the distal clavicle, resulting in inflammation, bone resorption, microfractures, and secondary arthritis of the AC joint
   2. Epidemiology
      a. More common in males
      b. Seen in younger patients
      c. Associated with heavy lifting (weight lifters) or repetitive motions
   3. Examination findings include localized pain, swelling, and tenderness similar to those seen in symptomatic AC joint arthritis.
   4. Nonsurgical treatment includes rest, NSAIDs, ice, activity modification, and corticosteroid injections.
   5. Surgical treatment
      a. Indications are persistent pain despite nonsurgical treatment.
      b. Options include arthroscopic or open distal clavicle excision.
      c. Surgery is successful in more than 90% of patients.

TOP TESTING FACTS

1. The horizontal plane stability of the clavicle is provided by the AC ligaments, specifically the posterior and superior portions.
2. The normal CC distance on an AP radiograph should be less than 11 to 13 mm.
3. The treatment of type I and II AC joint separations should be nonsurgical. Good functional outcomes can be expected.
4. The surgical indications for type III separations are controversial, and current literature does not provide a high level of evidence favoring nonsurgical or surgical management.
5. The treatment of type IV, V, and VI separations should be surgical in medically fit patients.
6. Acute fixation (within 3 to 4 weeks of injury) of high-grade AC joint separations can be successfully performed with various fixation options and without the use of tendon graft.

7. Delayed reconstruction of AC joint separations requires biologic augmentation, either ligament transfer or tendon grafting, in addition to CC stabilization.
8. Anatomic AC joint reconstructions are biomechanically superior to nonanatomic techniques, such as the Weaver-Dunn procedure.
9. Distal clavicle excision for the management of painful AC joint arthritis has a higher failure rate in patients with a history of previous low-grade AC joint separations.
10. Resection of the distal clavicle for AC joint arthritis should be limited to 5 to 10 mm of bone.

Bibliography

Bannister GC, Wallace WA, Stableforth PG, Hutson MA: The management of acute acromioclavicular dislocation: A randomised prospective controlled trial. *J Bone Joint Surg Br* 1989;71(5):848-850.

Beitzel K, Sablan N, Chowaniec DM, et al: Sequential resection of the distal clavicle and its effects on horizontal acromioclavicular joint translation. *Am J Sports Med* 2012;40(3):681-685.

Beitzel K, Mazzocca AD, Bak K, et al: ISAKOS upper extremity committee consensus statement on the need for diversification of the Rockwood classification for acromioclavicular joint injuries. *Arthroscopy* 2014;30(2):271-278.

Cook JB, Shaha JS, Douglas RJ, et al: Clavicular bone tunnel malposition leads to early failures in coracoclavicular ligament reconstructions. *Am J Sports Med* 2013;41(1):142-148.

Deshmukh AV, Wilson DR, Zilberfarb JL, Perlmutter GS: Stability of acromioclavicular joint reconstruction: Biomechanical testing of various surgical techniques in a cadaveric model. *Am J Sports Med* 2004;32(6):1492-1498.

Korsten K, Gunning AC, Leenen LP: Operative or conservative treatment in patients with Rockwood type III acromioclavicular dislocation: A systematic review and update of current literature. *Int Orthopaedics* 2014;38:831-838.

Martetsclager F, Horan MP, Warth RJ, Millett PJ: Complications after anatomic fixation and reconstruction of the coracoclavicular ligaments. *Am J Sports Med* 2013;41(12):2896-2903.

Millett PJ, Horan MP, Warth RJ: Two-year outcomes after primary anatomic coracoclavicular ligament reconstruction. *Arthroscopy* 2015;31(10):1962-1973.

Mazzocca AD, Santangelo SA, Johnson ST, Rios CG, Dumonski ML, Arciero RA: A biomechanical evaluation of an anatomical coracoclavicular ligament reconstruction. *Am J Sports Med* 2006;34(2):236-246.

Pensak M, Grumet RC, Slabaugh MA, Bach BR Jr: Open versus arthroscopic distal clavicle resection. *Arthroscopy* 2010;26(5):697-704.

Rios CG, Arciero RA, Mazzocca AD: Anatomy of the clavicle and coracoid process for reconstruction of the coracoclavicular ligaments. *Am J Sports Med* 2007;35(5):811-817.

Robertson WJ, Griffith MH, Carroll K, O'Donnell T, Gill TJ: Arthroscopic versus open distal clavicle excision: A comparative assessment at intermediate-term follow-up. *Am J Sports Med* 2011;39(11):2415-2420.

Rockwood CA, Williams GR, Young DC: Disorders of the acromioclavicular joint, in Rockwood CA, Matsen FA, eds: *The Shoulder*. Philadelphia, PA, WB Saunders, 1998, pp 483-553.

Salzmann GM, Paul J, Sandmann GH, Imhoff AB, Schöttle PB: The coracoidal insertion of the coracoclavicular ligaments: An anatomic study. *Am J Sports Med* 2008;36(12):2392-2397.

Scheibel M, Droschel S, Gerhardt C, Kraus N: Arthroscopically assisted stabilization of acute high-grade acromioclavicular joint separations. *Am J Sports Med* 2011;39(7):1507-1516.

Schlegel TF, Burks RT, Marcus RL, Dunn HK: A prospective evaluation of untreated acute grade III acromioclavicular separations. *Am J Sports Med* 2001;29(6):699-703.

Stine IA, Vangsness CT: Analysis of the capsule and ligament insertions about the acromioclavicular joint: A cadaveric study. *Arthroscopy* 2009;25(9):968-974.

Taft TN, Wilson FC, Oglesby JW: Dislocation of the acromioclavicular joint: An end-result study. *J Bone Joint Surg Am* 1987;69(7):1045-1051.

Tauber M, Gordon K, Koller H, Fox M, Resch H: Semitendinosus tendon graft versus a modified Weaver-Dunn procedure for acromioclavicular joint reconstruction in chronic cases: A prospective comparative study. *Am J Sports Med* 2009;37(1):181-190.

Walz L, Salzmann GM, Fabbro T, Eichhorn S, Imhoff AB: The anatomic reconstruction of acromioclavicular joint dislocations using 2 TightRope devices: A biomechanical study. *Am J Sports Med* 2008;36(12):2398-2406.

Weinstein DM, McCann PD, McIlveen SJ, Flatow EL, Bigliani LU: Surgical treatment of complete acromioclavicular dislocations. *Am J Sports Med* 1995;23(3):324-331.

Chapter 77
Disorders of the Sternoclavicular Joint

JASON E. HSU, MD
JAY D. KEENER, MD

I. STERNOCLAVICULAR JOINT ANATOMY AND BIOMECHANICS

A. Sternoclavicular (SC) joint anatomy

1. The SC joint is a synovial saddle-type articulation between the medial edge of the clavicle and the manubrium of the sternum.
2. The joint lacks bony stability and primarily depends on ligamentous restraints for stability (**Figure 1, A**).
3. Anterior and posterior SC ligaments are critical to the stability of the SC joint.
   a. The posterior SC ligament is stronger than and twice as thick as the anterior ligament.
   b. The posterior SC ligament is the primary restraint to anterior and posterior translation.
   c. The anterior SC ligament is a secondary stabilizer to anterior translation.
4. The costoclavicular (rhomboid) ligament is lateral to the joint and is the largest ligament of the sternoclavicular joint, originates at the medial edge of superior first rib, and inserts onto the costoclavicular tubercle on the medial end of the clavicle.
   a. Originates at the superomedial edge of the first rib.
   b. Inserts onto the costoclavicular tubercle on the medial end of the clavicle.

Dr. Hsu or an immediate family member has received royalties from DJ Orthopaedics and serves as a paid consultant to or is an employee of DJ Orthopaedics and Miami Device Solutions. Dr. Keener or an immediate family member has received royalties from Genesis, Shoulder Innovations and Wright Medical Technology, Inc.; serves as a paid consultant to or is an employee of Arthrex, Inc. and Wright Medical Technology, Inc.; has received research or institutional support from the National Institutes of Health (NIAMS & NICHD) and Zimmer; and serves as a board member, owner, officer, or committee member of the American Shoulder and Elbow Surgeons.

5. The intra-articular disk ligament runs from the synchondrosis of the first rib to the sternum and passes through the SC joint.
   a. Divides the SC joint into two spaces and attaches to the anterior and posterior capsular ligaments.
   b. Acts as a checkrein to medial displacement of the medial clavicle.
6. The interclavicular ligament connects the medial aspect of each clavicle to the SC joint capsule and the upper portion of the sternum.
7. The subclavius muscle originates just lateral to the costoclavicular ligament on the first rib and has an insertion on the inferior surface of the clavicle; it provides stability to the SC joint by preventing upward displacement of the clavicle.
8. The SC joint is bounded by muscular layers anteriorly and posteriorly.
   a. A musculoaponeurotic layer anterior to the SC joint is composed of the superficial portion of the clavicular insertion of the sternocleidomastoid and the clavicular portion of the pectoralis major.
   b. The sternohyoid, sternothyroid, and scalene muscles lie posterior to the SC joint along the inner third of the clavicle.
9. The vascular supply to the SC joint is provided by branches from the internal thoracic and suprascapular arteries.
10. The SC joint is innervated by branches from the medial supraclavicular nerve and the nerve to the subclavius.
11. Vital neurovascular and thoracic structures—the innominate vessels, internal jugular vein, vagus nerve, phrenic nerve, trachea, and

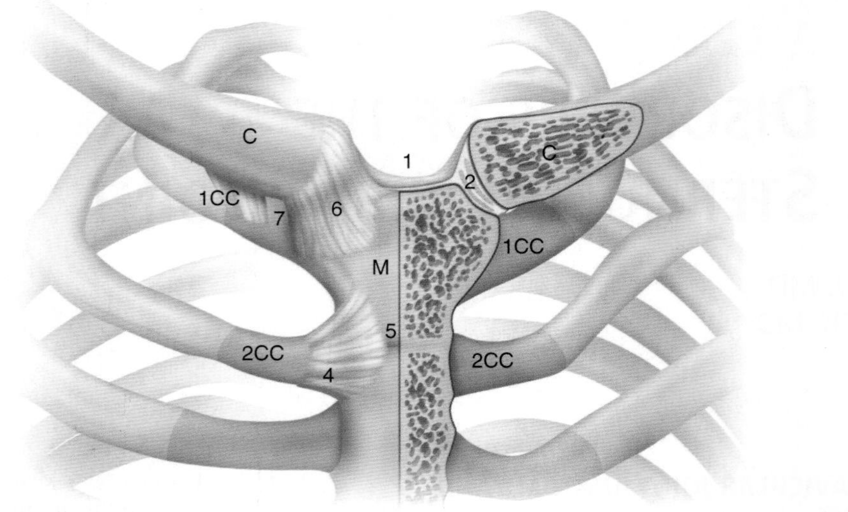

A

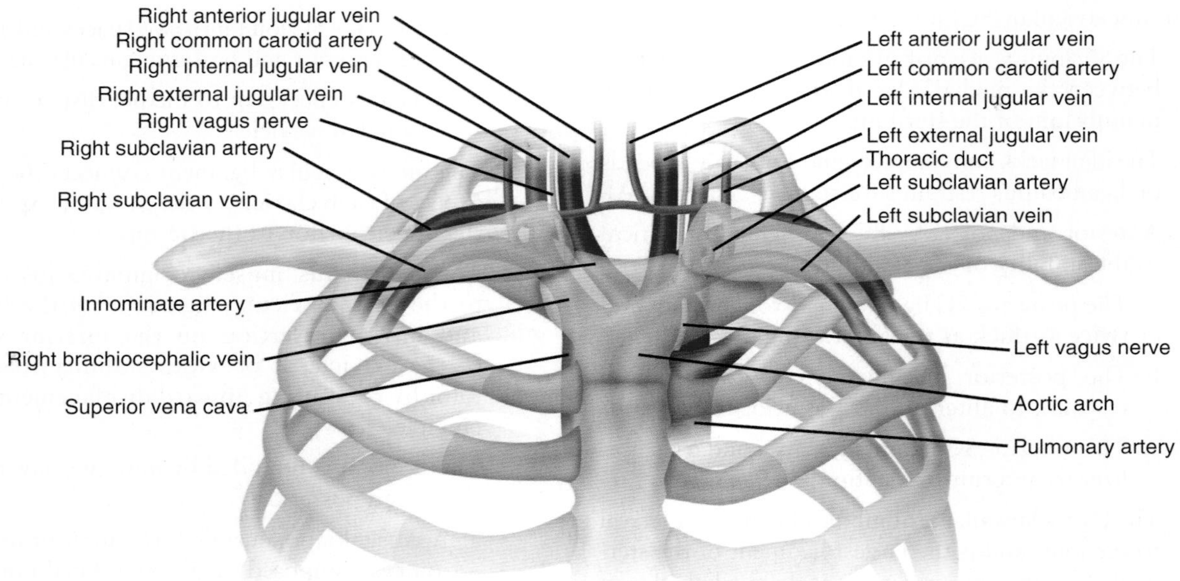

B

Figure 1 Illustrations depict the sternoclavicular (SC) joints. **A**, The anatomy of the SC joints is shown, viewed from the anterior aspect, with the left joint intact and the right joint in coronal section. 1 = interclavicular ligament, 2 = SC joint disk, 4 = costochondral capsule, 5 = sternum, 6 = SC joint capsule, 7 = costoclavicular ligament, C = clavicle, CC = costochondral cartilage, M = manubrium. **B**, Major vessels posterior to the SC joint are shown.

esophagus—lie posterior to the SC joint and are at risk with posterior dislocations and during surgery (**Figure 1, B**).

12. The medial clavicular epiphysis is the last epiphysis to ossify (at approximately 18 years) and the last to close (at approximately 25 years).

B. SC joint biomechanics
   1. The clavicle elevates approximately 35° in the coronal plane with shoulder abduction.
      a. The clavicle elevates 4° for each 10° of arm elevation, up to 90°.
      b. Negligible motion of the clavicle occurs after 90° of arm elevation.
   2. The clavicle rotates 45° around its longitudinal axis.

II. TRAUMATIC CONDITIONS OF THE STERNOCLAVICULAR JOINT

A. Overview and epidemiology

1. Traumatic dislocations of the SC joint comprise only 1% of all joint dislocations and 3% of all upper extremity dislocations.
2. The most common causes of traumatic SC joint dislocations are motor vehicle accidents, athletic accidents, and falls from a height.
3. Anterior dislocations are more common than posterior dislocations.
4. Posterior dislocations can be associated with mediastinal compromise in up to 25% of patients.

B. Pathoanatomy

1. Substantial force to the shoulder girdle or the medial clavicle is required to disrupt the strong ligamentous complex surrounding the SC joint.
2. A direct force to the anteromedial clavicle results in a posterior SC dislocation.
3. An indirect force to the posterolateral shoulder, which causes the shoulder to roll forward, results in a posterior SC dislocation (**Figure 2, A**).
4. An indirect force to the anterolateral shoulder, which causes the shoulder to roll backward, results in an anterior SC dislocation (**Figure 2, B**).
5. Injuries in patients with an open physis often result in physeal disruption rather than ligamentous injury.
6. Trauma to the SC joint can result in an intra-articular disk injury without ligamentous instability, causing localized pain, swelling, and early arthritis.

C. Evaluation

1. History
   a. The mechanism of injury helps distinguish the direction of subluxation or dislocation.
   b. Patients typically report pain and swelling after trauma to the shoulder girdle or the chest.
   c. Patients with a posterior dislocation show higher levels of pain and may report shortness of breath, difficulty swallowing, or a sensation of choking.
2. Physical examination
   a. In mild sprains with intact ligaments, tenderness and swelling of the SC joint and pain with movement of the upper extremity occur but no instability with palpation.

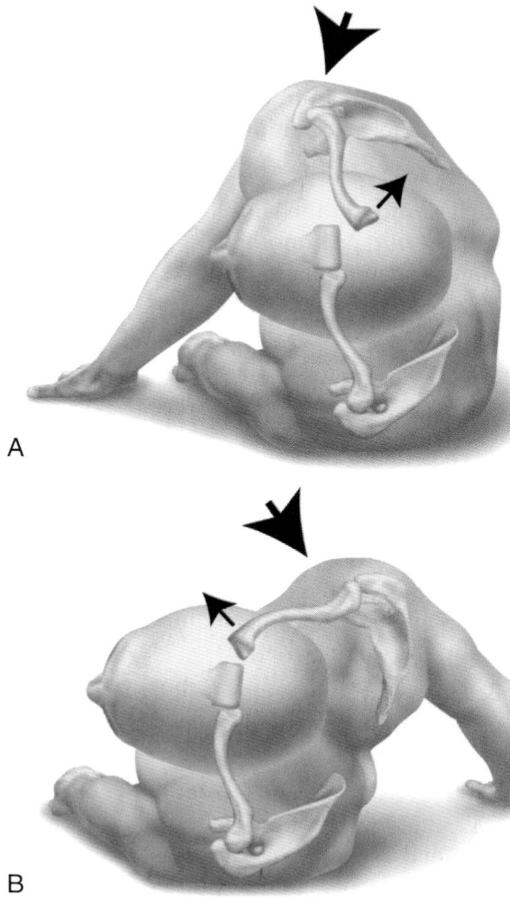

Figure 2 Illustrations show the mechanisms that produce anterior or posterior dislocations of the sternoclavicular joint when a patient is lying on the ground. **A**, A compression force is applied to the posterolateral aspect of the shoulder; the medial end of the clavicle will be displaced posteriorly. **B**, If a lateral compression force is directed from the anterior position, the medial end of the clavicle is dislocated anteriorly.

   b. In more severe sprains with partial disruption of the ligaments, subluxation of the SC joint may be substantial.
   c. An anterior dislocation presents with prominence of the medial clavicle.
   d. The corner of the sternum may be palpable in a posterior dislocation.
   e. Soft-tissue swelling may make the diagnosis more difficult.
   f. Compression of the mediastinal structures may present with venous congestion of the face or the ipsilateral arm, stridor, cough, dysphagia, and diminished breath sounds caused by pneumothorax. Deep vein thrombosis in the upper extremity vessels has been reported with chronic posterior SC dislocations.

g. Full examination of the shoulder girdle and the thorax should be performed to rule out other fractures, a concomitant injury to the acromioclavicular joint, or other upper extremity and thoracic wall injuries.

3. Imaging
   a. A chest radiograph should be obtained acutely to rule out pneumothorax, pneumomediastinum, or hemopneumothorax.
   b. Standard AP radiographs can be supplemented by additional views.
      - The serendipity view is obtained by tilting the beam 40° cephalad (**Figure 3**).
      - The Heinig view is an oblique view obtained by directing the beam perpendicular to the joint.
   c. Radiographs may be difficult to interpret because of bony overlap; cross-sectional CT axial imaging may be required for definitive diagnosis (**Figure 4**).
   d. Because of the late closure of the medial clavicular epiphysis, MRI may help distinguish physeal separations from frank dislocations in patients younger than 25 years.
   e. CT angiograms and venograms should be obtained if the presentation is cause for concern for vascular abnormalities.

D. Treatment

1. Nonsurgical
   a. Patients with SC joint sprains and subluxations can be treated with ice, analgesia, and a short period of sling immobilization.
   b. Patients should avoid contact activities for 6 weeks or until symptoms resolve.
   c. Chronic recurrent anterior instability is difficult to manage nonsurgically; observation and activity modification are appropriate if minimally symptomatic.
2. Closed reduction
   a. Acute dislocations can be treated with attempted closed reduction under conscious sedation or general anesthesia.
   b. Posterior dislocations should be reduced urgently, particularly if any signs of mediastinal compromise are present.
   c. The patient is positioned supine with a bolster between the scapulae.
   d. For anterior dislocations, traction is applied to the abducted arm, and reduction can be obtained with direct pressure over the medial clavicle (**Figure 5, A**).
   e. For posterior dislocations, the arm also is placed in 90° of abduction with traction to the arm. An extension force applied to the shoulder may release the medial clavicle from behind the manubrium (**Figure 5, B**).
   f. An alternative reduction technique for posterior dislocations is to provide traction in adduction, with a downward force to the shoulders.
   g. If reduction is unsuccessful by manipulation, percutaneous reduction with towel clips (**Figure 5, C**) or open reduction with or without ligament reconstruction under general anesthesia is performed.
   h. After reduction, the arm is immobilized for 6 weeks in a figure-of-8 brace or sling; strenuous or contact activities are avoided for 3 months.
   i. Posterior dislocations are more likely to remain reduced than are anterior dislocations.
3. Open reduction
   a. Open reduction is considered for acute posterior dislocations that have not responded to closed management.
   b. A cardiothoracic surgeon should be available to assist in case any intrathoracic structural damage is found.
4. Surgical reconstructive techniques
   a. Ligament reconstruction can be considered for chronic symptomatic instability that has failed appropriate nonsurgical management.
   b. Most often, chronic posterior SC joint instability is fixed and requires surgical reconstruction. Anterior instability may be recurrent or fixed, and nonsurgical treatment should be maximized.
   c. The anterior and posterior SC ligaments can be reconstructed with semitendinosus tendon passed in a figure-of-8 fashion through drill holes in the medial clavicle and the manubrium (**Figure 6**).
   d. The subclavius tendon can be routed through a drill hole in the medial clavicle and sutured to itself to reconstruct the costoclavicular ligament.
   e. The intra-articular disk ligament can be inserted into the medullary canal of the medial clavicle, similar to a Weaver-Dunn procedure for the lateral clavicle.

Sewell MD, Al-Hadithy N, Le Leu A, Lambert SM: Instability of the sternoclavicular joint: Current concepts in classification, treatment and outcomes. *Bone Joint J* 2013;95-B(6):721-731.

Spencer EE, Kuhn JE, Huston LJ, Carpenter JE, Hughes RE: Ligamentous restraints to anterior and posterior translation of the sternoclavicular joint. *J Shoulder Elbow Surg* 2002;11(1):43-47.

Spencer EE Jr, Kuhn JE: Biomechanical analysis of reconstructions for sternoclavicular joint instability. *J Bone Joint Surg Am* 2004;86(1):98-105.

Chapter 78
Superior Labrum Anterior to Posterior Tears and Lesions of the Proximal Biceps Tendon

MARC S. KOWALSKY, MD, MBA

I. INTRODUCTION

A. A superior labrum anterior to posterior (SLAP) lesion is the detachment of the superior portion of the glenoid labrum, including the anterior and posterior aspects.

B. The long head of the biceps brachii tendon at its insertion may or may not be involved.

C. Typically occurs in patients who perform repetitive overhead activities, such as the overhead athlete, but also may occur in acute trauma.

II. ANATOMY

A. The glenoid labrum consists of parallel collagen fibers that course around the circumference of the glenoid.

   1. The superior labrum inserts on the superior glenoid rim, medial to the articular cartilage margin, through a transitional zone of fibrocartilage.
   2. A normal synovial recess exists between the meniscoid or triangular superior labrum and the articular cartilage extension over the superior glenoid rim.

B. Vascularity to the glenoid labrum originates from the scapular, circumflex scapular, and posterior circumflex humeral arteries via capsular or periosteal vessels (**Figure 1**).

C. Of the biceps tendon, 40% to 60% attaches to the supraglenoid tubercle 5 mm medial to the superior glenoid rim; the remainder attaches directly to the superior glenoid labrum.

   1. The biceps tendon typically attaches entirely (type I) or predominantly posterior (type II) on the superior labrum. Alternatively, the labral attachment of the biceps tendon may have equal anterior and posterior contributions (type III) or, less commonly, predominantly anterior (type IV).
   2. The biceps tendon is an intra-articular but extrasynovial structure within the glenohumeral joint.
   3. Vascularity of the biceps tendon is provided primarily by the ascending branch of the anterior humeral circumflex artery, which travels within the bicipital groove. An avascular zone exists at its proximal portion, close to the superior glenoid.
   4. The biceps tendon passes through the bicipital groove, or intertubercular groove, between the greater and lesser tuberosities. Stability of the biceps within this region is afforded by the biceps sling, or pulley, consisting of fibers from the following:
      a. Subscapularis tendon
      b. Supraspinatus tendon
      c. Coracohumeral ligament
      d. Superior glenohumeral ligament

III. PATHOPHYSIOLOGY

A. The glenoid labrum enhances glenohumeral joint stability by increasing the surface area of the glenoid and by serving as an attachment site for the glenohumeral ligaments.

B. The superior labrum/biceps anchor complex serves as a secondary restraint to anterior translation in abduction and external rotation.

Neither Dr. Kowalsky nor any immediate family member has received anything of value from or has stock or stock options held in a commercial company or institution related directly or indirectly to the subject of this chapter.

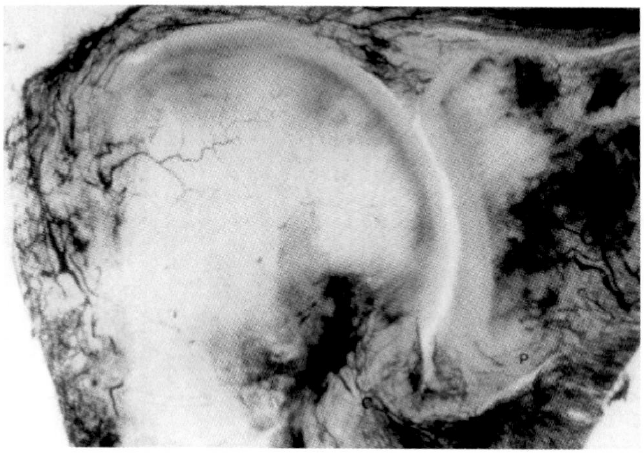

Figure 1 Histologic coronal section of the glenohumeral joint, demonstrates the capsular and periosteal contributions to the vascularity of the labrum as well as the meniscoid superior labrum and synovial recess created by the articular cartilage extension beyond the superior glenoid rim. C = capsular contributions, P = periosteal contributions. (Reproduced with permission from Cooper DE, Arnoczky SP, O'Brien S, et al: Anatomy, histology, and vascularity of the glenoid labrum: An anatomic study. *J Bone Joint Surg Am* 1992;74:46-52.)

C. The long head of the biceps brachii has been described as a static humeral head depressor and a secondary stabilizer to anterior and posterior translation, but it has not been shown to serve an important dynamic role in glenohumeral joint kinematics or stability.

D. Various mechanisms have been described in the pathogenesis of superior labral tears, including

1. Direct traction to the biceps tendon,
2. Internal impingement, and
3. Peel-back—May be the primary mechanism in throwers. With the shoulder in abduction and external rotation, the orientation and pull of the biceps pull the labrum off the posterosuperior glenoid. May be exacerbated by posterior capsular contracture.

E. Unique aspects of glenohumeral joint kinematics in the throwing athlete are relevant to the etiology of superior labral tears.

1. Contracture of the posterior band of the inferior glenohumeral ligament exerts a posterior force on the ligament, which tethers the humeral head and shifts the glenohumeral contact point posterosuperiorly in composite abduction and external rotation.
2. This posterosuperior shift allows hyperexternal rotation at the glenohumeral joint by avoiding abutment of the greater tuberosity against the posterosuperior glenoid and by increasing the redundancy of the anterior-inferior capsule.

TABLE 1

Classification of Superior Labrum Anterior to Posterior Tears

Type	Description
I	Degenerative fraying
II	Unstable biceps anchor
III	Bucket-handle tear, intact biceps anchor
IV	Bucket-handle tear, unstable biceps anchor
V	Type II + anterior-inferior extension (Bankart lesion)
VI	Type II + unstable flap
VII	Type II + middle glenohumeral ligament extension
VIII	Type II + posterior extension
IX	Circumferential
X	Type II + posteroinferior extension (reverse Bankart lesion)

Adapted from Maffet MW, Gartsman GM, Moseley B: Superior labrum-biceps tendon complex lesions of the shoulder. *Am J Sports Med* 1995;23(1):93–98; Powell SE, Nord KD, Ryu RKN: The diagnosis, classification, and treatment of slap lesions. *Oper Tech Sports Med* 2004;12:99–110; and Snyder SJ, Karzel RP, Del Pizzo W, Ferkel RD, Friedman MJ: SLAP lesions of the shoulder. *Arthroscopy* 1990;6(4):274–279.

3. This posterosuperior shift in the humeral head with resultant hyperexternal rotation accounts for the exacerbation of internal impingement of the rotator cuff on the posterosuperior labrum and the peel-back mechanism of superior labral tears.

IV. CLASSIFICATION

A. SLAP tears are classified into 10 types (**Table 1**).

B. The original classification of SLAP tears consisted of four types.

1. Type I: degenerative fraying with an intact biceps anchor (**Figure 2, A**)
2. Type II: unstable biceps anchor detached from the underlying glenoid (**Figure 2, B**)
   a. Type IIa: anterosuperior
   b. Type IIb: posterosuperior
   c. Type IIc: combined anterior and posterior
3. Type III: bucket-handle tear with an intact biceps anchor (**Figure 2, C**)
4. Type IV: bucket-handle tear with extension into the biceps tendon (**Figure 2, D**)

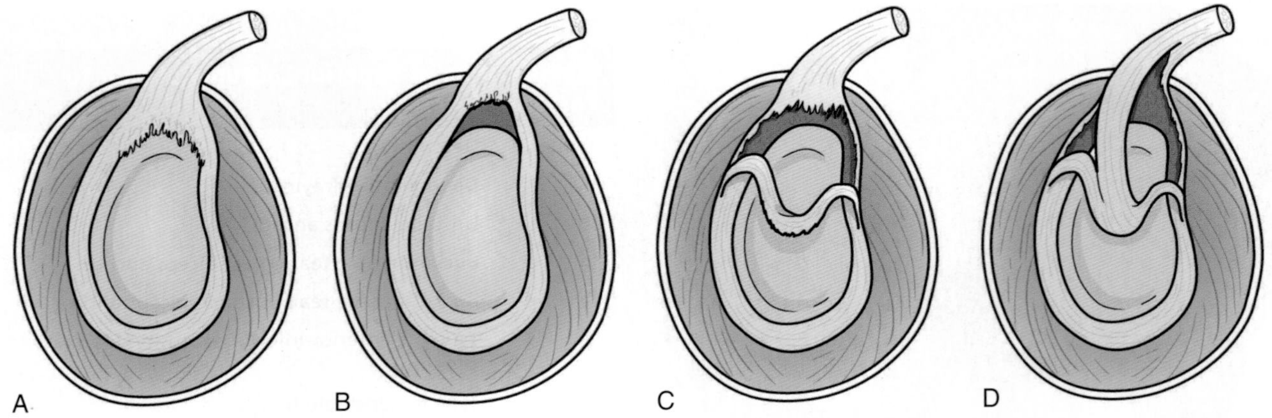

Figure 2 Drawings depict the four types of superior labrum anterior to posterior (SLAP) tears. **A**, Type I SLAP tear: Degenerative fraying with an intact biceps anchor. **B**, Type II SLAP tear: Unstable biceps anchor is detached from the underlying glenoid. **C**, Type III SLAP tear: Bucket-handle tear with an intact biceps anchor. **D**, Type IV SLAP tear: Bucket-handle tear with extension into the biceps tendon. (Adapted with permission from Powell SE, Nord KD, Ryu RKN: The diagnosis, classification, and treatment of SLAP lesions. *Oper Tech Sports Med* 2004;12:99-110.)

C. The classification was later expanded to include types V through X.

D. It is critical to recognize normal anatomic variants of the anterosuperior labrum on diagnostic imaging and arthroscopy, which are not pathologic and should not be repaired, including

1. Anterior sublabral foramen
2. Anterior sublabral foramen with cordlike middle glenohumeral ligament
3. Absent anterosuperior labrum with cordlike middle glenohumeral ligament

E. Classification of biceps tendon pathology is typically descriptive.

1. Tear versus synovitis
2. Extent of tear based on percentage of the entire tendon
3. Location of pathology
4. Presence of subluxation or dislocation of the biceps from the bicipital groove

V. DIAGNOSIS

A. A history of acute trauma, consisting of sudden traction or compression to the affected extremity, may be present.

B. SLAP tears can be associated with a previous subluxation or dislocation event.

C. Insidious onset of symptoms associated with SLAP tears is most common in overhead throwing athletes.

D. Pain caused by a SLAP tear often is localized deep within the glenohumeral joint and can be associated with mechanical symptoms, fatigue or a "dead arm" sensation of the extremity during overhead activities, or frank weakness of the rotator cuff in a concomitant paralabral cyst.

E. Various provocative tests have been described for SLAP tears and biceps pathology, but none have sufficient accuracy to confirm the diagnosis.

1. O'Brien active compression test: The affected extremity is positioned in 90° of forward elevation, slight adduction, and maximum internal rotation; the patient performs resisted forward elevation; the test is repeated in maximum external rotation. The test is positive if pain occurs deep within the shoulder in maximum internal rotation, then improves with maximum external rotation.
2. Crank test: The affected extremity is elevated to 160° in the scapular plane; axial force is applied to the extremity while the humerus is passively rotated. The test is positive if pain, clicking, or catching is reproduced.
3. Biceps load I and II test: The affected extremity is abducted to 90° to 120° and maximally externally rotated; the forearm is maximally supinated; and the elbow is flexed against resistance. The tests are positive if pain or apprehension worsens with resisted elbow flexion.
4. Anterior slide test: The hand of the affected extremity is placed on the hip with the thumb posterior; one hand of the examiner is placed on the elbow of the affected extremity, exerting a slight anterior and axial force to the extremity; the patient is asked to resist this force to the

elbow. The test is positive if pain, a pop, or a click is reproduced.

5. Speed test: The affected extremity is elevated to 90° in full supination with the elbow extended; the patient resists downward pressure on the extremity by the examiner. The test is positive if pain is experienced in the anterior shoulder or glenohumeral joint.
6. Dynamic labral shear test: The affected arm is externally rotated and progressively abducted while horizontally extended. A positive test is characterized by reproducible painful click deep in the shoulder in the mid-arc of abduction.
7. Yergason test: The affected extremity is adducted against the side with the elbow flexed to 90° in full pronation; the patient then supinates against resistance. The test is positive if pain is experienced in the bicipital groove or glenohumeral joint.

F. Speed and Yergason tests demonstrate poor sensitivity, moderate specificity, and poor accuracy. Diagnostic injection of local anesthetic with or without corticosteroid into the glenohumeral joint or bicipital groove may aid in confirming the diagnosis.

G. Including two sensitive tests (active compression and crank tests) and a specific test (Speed test) increases the overall accuracy.

H. Physical examination should include assessment of rotator cuff strength and infraspinatus atrophy to identify patients who may have suprascapular nerve compression from a paralabral ganglion cyst.

I. An instability examination should be performed.

J. Assessment of throwing athletes includes the total arc of rotation to identify those with a glenohumeral internal rotation deficit.

K. MRI is the imaging modality of choice.

1. Diagnostic accuracy of MRI may be improved by positioning the arm in abduction and external rotation. Recent systematic review and meta-analysis confirm that magnetic resonance (MR) arthrography does improve the diagnostic performance of an MRI for the detection of a SLAP tear.
2. Diagnostic accuracy of MRI ranges widely in the literature. Overdiagnosis of SLAP tears is common as normal anatomy can be misconstrued as pathologic. Accurate diagnosis is predicated on clinical examination and concordant MRI findings and cannot be confirmed until the time of surgery.

L. Ultrasonography can be useful in the dynamic assessment of the biceps tendon.

VI. TREATMENT

A. Nonsurgical

1. Injection of local anesthetic with corticosteroid into the glenohumeral joint or bicipital groove is diagnostic and potentially therapeutic.
2. Aspiration of the spinoglenoid notch cyst can be done to treat suprascapular nerve compression.
3. Physical therapy for superior labral tears consists of rotator cuff strengthening, periscapular muscular strengthening, and posteroinferior capsular stretching.
4. In the general population, predictive factors for failure of nonsurgical management include history of trauma, positive compression-rotation test, and participation in overhead sports. In baseball players, advanced age, prolonged symptoms, pitching, presence of exostosis of the posterior band of the inferior glenohumeral ligament (Bennett lesion), and presence of partial articular rotator cuff tear have been associated with failure of conservative management.

B. Surgical—Indicated for patients who experience symptoms despite months of nonsurgical management.

1. Treatment based on classification
   a. Type I degenerative tears typically demonstrate fraying, with an intact biceps anchor. Débridement alone is sufficient.
   b. Type II tears are unstable due to the involvement of the biceps anchor. Reattachment of the labrum to the superior glenoid rim is indicated.
      - In patients older than 40 years, biceps tenodesis may be preferred over SLAP repair secondary to concerns for complications such as retear and excessive stiffness.
   c. Type III tears are managed by débriding the unstable bucket-handle labral tear.
   d. Type IV tears are managed given the status of the torn biceps tendon.
      - If less than 25% to 50% of the biceps tendon is involved, the tear and its extension into the tendon are débrided.
      - If 25% to 50% or more of the biceps tendon is involved, biceps tenodesis or tenotomy with labral débridement or repair is indicated.
2. Technique
   a. Portals
      - Viewing: The standard posterior viewing portal typically is used.

6 | Shoulder and Elbow

- Working: Anterosuperior and anterior-inferior portals. Alternatively, the portal of Neviaser can be used to pass the shuttling device beneath the labral tissue (1 cm medial to the acromion at its junction with the scapular spine and posterior border of the distal clavicle).
- Anchor placement: Anterosuperior rotator interval portal. An accessory transrotator cuff posterolateral portal can be used for anchors placed posterior to the biceps tendon. The portal of Wilmington also has been described for this purpose (pierce cuff at myotendinous junction).
- The transrotator cuff portal has been used in a cannulated manner for anchor placement and suture shuttling.

b. Fixation

- Various techniques exist for anchor placement and suture configuration during superior labral repair. Overconstraining of the biceps anchor should be avoided.
- Ideal anchor placement depends on the anatomy of the patient's biceps insertion on the superior labrum and the anatomy of the labral tear.
- Knotless implants eliminate the need for arthroscopic knot tying and, with a horizontal mattress suture configuration, decrease the potential adverse effects of bulky intra-articular suture material.

c. Concomitant pathology

- Paralabral ganglion cysts: Often accompany SLAP tears and should be recognized on preoperative MRI; can cause suprascapular nerve compression and resultant rotator cuff weakness; can be decompressed using aspiration at the time of surgery.
- Subacromial bursitis: Subacromial procedures performed in conjunction with a superior labral repair should be done with caution because they may increase the risk of postoperative stiffness.
- Rotator cuff tear: In a patient with concomitant rotator cuff and superior labral tears, it is imperative to determine whether the SLAP tear is an incidental finding or if both lesions contribute to the patient's symptoms. It is generally preferable to perform a biceps procedure, rather than a SLAP repair, when a concomitant rotator cuff repair is performed.

- Biceps tendon pathology
  - Indications for surgery include a symptomatic SLAP tear with biceps involvement, tearing of the tendon of 25% to 50% or more of the tendon, tendon subluxation or dislocation due to disruption of the biceps pulley, or intraoperative findings consistent with tenosynovitis or tendinosis, with concordant preoperative examination and imaging.
  - Alternative treatment primarily includes tenotomy or tenodesis. In biceps tendon instability, acceptable outcomes have not been achieved with pulley repair or reconstruction.
  - Biceps tenotomy: Benefits include the technical ease of the procedure and of the postoperative rehabilitation, and advantages in elderly, less active patients, who, along with patients with large arms, are less likely to be negatively affected by cosmetic deformity, cramping, or fatigue of the biceps muscle.
  - Biceps tenodesis: Removal of the intra-articular portion of the tendon (a pain generator), with more distal reinsertion of the tendon to maintain the length-tension relationship of the biceps muscle. Concern exists that proximal tenodesis may be associated with a higher incidence of persistent pain due to the preservation of a potentially pathologic tendon and tenosynovium within the bicipital groove. Distal tenodesis, below the groove in a suprapectoral or subpectoral region, removes the biceps tendon from the joint and bicipital groove, thus mitigating the risk of persistent postoperative pain.
    - Soft-tissue fixation: The biceps tendon can be reinserted with a variety of implants. The simplest technique relies on interference of the bulky tendon against the entrance of the biceps pulley or on fixation to the overlying rotator interval using suture.
    - Osseous fixation: Arthroscopic or open tenodesis can be performed with more rigid fixation of the tendon to bone, including suture anchors, cortical buttons, or interference screws. In a prospective, randomized comparison, interference screw fixation demonstrated slightly higher risk of tenodesis rupture compared with suture anchor fixation.

- Tenotomy has been associated with cosmetic deformity, cramping, fatigue, and reduced supination strength. No evidence of the overall superiority of tenodesis exists in the literature.

3. Rehabilitation
   a. Postoperatively, the surgical extremity typically is protected in a sling for about 4 weeks.
   b. A gradual, progressive range of motion protocol is begun immediately. Full range of motion should be achieved within the first 6 weeks.
   c. Strengthening, beginning with the periscapular musculature and advancing to the rotator cuff, typically begins at approximately 4 weeks. Dynamic functional activities are introduced at 3 months, with return to sports deferred for 4 to 6 months.
   d. Rehabilitation should be modified to account for the concomitant treatment of associated pathology.
4. Outcomes
   a. Modern techniques and implants have been associated with favorable results after SLAP repair in both pain and return to function. The ability to return to sports is unpredictable, however.
   b. In managing SLAP tears, some evidence exist that biceps tenodesis has more favorable results and lower complication rates than SLAP repair and should be considered in less active patients or those older than 40 years. Recent systematic review and meta-analysis suggest an advantage of biceps tenodesis with respect to patient satisfaction and return to sport.
   c. A recent double-blind, randomized, controlled trial demonstrated a lack of difference in outcomes among sham surgery, SLAP repair, and biceps tenodesis.
5. Complications
   a. SLAP repair: Retear, stiffness, persistent pain, rotator cuff tear from the transrotator cuff portal
   b. Biceps tenodesis: Biceps tendon rupture at the site, bicipital groove pain with proximal tenodesis, biceps pain particularly from overtensioning of the tendon, humeral fracture
   c. Biceps tenotomy: Cramping, fatigue or weakness of flexion, supination, cosmetic deformity

TOP TESTING FACTS

1. A normal synovial recess exists between the superior labrum and the articular cartilage extension over the superior glenoid rim; it should not be confused for a labral tear.
2. SLAP tears can occur from direct trauma, internal impingement of the labrum on the posterosuperior rotator cuff, or torsional force on the biceps anchor during throwing, causing a peel-back of the labrum from the superior glenoid rim.
3. The sublabral foramen and cordlike middle glenohumeral ligament are normal anatomic variants of the anterosuperior labrum. Errant repair can restrict external rotation.
4. No single provocative test is sufficient to confirm the diagnosis of a superior labral tear or biceps lesion. A combination of sensitive and specific tests increases the accuracy of the physical examination.
5. Nonsurgical treatment can resolve pain effectively and restore function in patients with SLAP tears or biceps lesions.
6. The surgical treatment of SLAP tears depends on the status of the biceps anchor. Degenerative or flap tears without involvement of the anchor can be débrided. Labral tears with an unstable biceps anchor require reattachment to the superior glenoid rim or biceps tenodesis.
7. Superior labral tears can be associated with paralabral ganglion cysts. Spinoglenoid notch cysts cause isolated infraspinatus weakness. Cysts that involve the suprascapular notch cause supraspinatus and infraspinatus weakness.
8. SLAP repair with subacromial procedures should be performed with caution because of the risk of stiffness. Associated pathology should be addressed when clinically indicated. In a concomitant SLAP and rotator cuff tear, no advantage exists to SLAP repair compared with biceps tenotomy.
9. Biceps tendon subluxation or dislocation should be treated with biceps tenotomy or tenodesis.
10. Biceps tenotomy has been associated with cosmetic deformity, cramping, and fatigue, but no substantial difference in overall outcomes has been demonstrated between tenotomy and tenodesis.

Bibliography

Arirachakaran A, Boonard M, Chaijenkij K, Pituckanotai K, Prommahachai A, Kongtharvonskul J: A systematic review and meta-analysis of diagnostic test of MRA versus MRI for detection superior labrum anterior to posterior lesions type II-VII. *Skeletal Radiol* 2017;46(2):149-160.

Beyzadeoglu T, Circi E: Superior labrum anterior posterior lesions and associated injuries: Return to play in elite athletes. *Orthop J Sports Med* 2015;3(4):2325967115577359.

Burkhart SS, Morgan CD: The peel-back mechanism: Its role in producing and extending posterior type II SLAP lesions and its effect on SLAP repair rehabilitation. *Arthroscopy* 1998;14(6):637-640.

Grossman MG, Tibone JE, McGarry MH, Schneider DJ, Veneziani S, Lee TQ: A cadaveric model of the throwing shoulder: A possible etiology of superior labrum anterior-to-posterior lesions. *J Bone Joint Surg Am* 2005;87(4):824-831.

Hsu AR, Ghodadra NS, Provencher MT, Lewis PB, Bach BR: Biceps tenotomy versus tenodesis: A review of clinical outcomes and biomechanical results. *J Shoulder Elbow Surg* 2011;20(2):326-332.

Hurley ET, Fat DL, Duigenan CM, Miller JC, Mullett H, Moran CJ: Biceps tenodesis versus labral repair for superior labrum anterior-to-posterior tears: A systematic review and meta-analysis. *J Shoulder Elbow Surg* 2018;27(10):1913-1919.

Jang SH, Seo JG, Jang HS, Jung JE, Kim JG: Predictive factors associated with failure of nonoperative treatment of superior labrum anterior-posterior tears. *J Shoulder Elbow Surg* 2016;25(3):428-434.

Kuhn JE, Lindholm SR, Huston LJ, Soslowsky LJ, Blasier RB: Failure of the biceps superior labral complex: A cadaveric biomechanical investigation comparing the late cocking and early deceleration positions of throwing. *Arthroscopy* 2003;19(4):373-379.

Maffet MW, Gartsman GM, Moseley B: Superior labrum-biceps tendon complex lesions of the shoulder. *Am J Sports Med* 1995;23(1):93-98.

Meserve BB, Cleland JA, Boucher TR: A meta-analysis examining clinical test utility for assessing superior labral anterior posterior lesions. *Am J Sports Med* 2009;37(11):2252-2258.

Pagnani MJ, Deng XH, Warren RF, Torzilli PA, Altchek DW: Effect of lesions of the superior portion of the glenoid labrum on glenohumeral translation. *J Bone Joint Surg Am* 1995;77(7):1003-1010.

Powell SE, Nord KD, Ryu RKN: The diagnosis, classification, and treatment of SLAP lesions. *Oper Tech Sports Med* 2004;12:99-110.

Schroder CP, Skare O, Reikeras O, Mowinckel P, Brox JI: Sham surgery versus labral repair or biceps tenodesis for type II SLAP lesions of the shoulder: A three-armed randomised clinical trial. *Br J Sports Med* 2017;51(24):1759-1766.

Snyder SJ, Karzel RP, Del Pizzo W, Ferkel RD, Friedman MJ: SLAP lesions of the shoulder. *Arthroscopy* 1990;6(4):274-279.

3. Medial epicondylitis is most commonly seen in the fourth and fifth decades of life.
4. It affects men and women equally.
5. The dominant arm is affected in 75% of patients.
6. The primary etiology is repetitive stress, although medial epicondylitis can also be caused by trauma.
7. It is seen in athletes (baseball pitchers, javelin throwers, golfers, bowlers, weight lifters, and racket sport players) and also in laborers (eg, carpenters, construction workers).

B. Anatomy and pathoanatomy

1. Anatomy
    a. Medial epicondylitis most commonly affects the origins of the pronator teres and flexor carpi radialis muscles.
    b. The mechanism of injury is thought to be repetitive stress/overuse that causes microtrauma to the origin of the flexor-pronator muscles.
    c. Ulnar nerve irritation is often seen because of local inflammation.
    d. In athletes, medial epicondylitis occurs with repeated substantial valgus force on the elbow, which is absorbed by the flexor-pronator group, thereby reducing forces on the anterior band of the ulnar collateral ligament.
    e. The anterior band of the ulnar collateral ligament is deep to the pronator teres and flexor carpi radialis and is the primary valgus stabilizer of the elbow.
2. Histology
    a. The histopathology of angiofibroblastic hyperplasia Nirschl described for lateral epicondylitis is also seen in medial epicondylitis.
    b. As with lateral epicondylitis, inflammation is not typically seen.

C. Evaluation

1. History
    a. Repetitive use of the elbow, repetitive valgus stress, and repetitive gripping are reported.
    b. Pain that worsens with gripping activities is localized to the medial epicondyle.
    c. A history of numbness or tingling in the ulnar digits suggests ulnar neuritis.
    d. A history of trauma to the elbow should be documented.
2. Differential diagnosis
    a. Ulnar collateral ligament injury and resulting instability
    b. Cubital tunnel syndrome
    c. Occult fracture
    d. Cervical radiculopathy
    e. Triceps tendinitis
3. Physical examination
    a. Tenderness to palpation is noted slightly anterior and distal to the medial epicondyle, over the origins of the pronator teres and flexor carpi radialis.
    b. Resisted wrist flexion and forearm pronation exacerbate symptoms at the elbow.
    c. Local inflammation may manifest by swelling and warmth.
    d. A flexion contracture is sometimes seen in chronic cases.
    e. Examination for ulnar collateral ligament injury:
        - Pain is deeper and is reproduced with moving valgus stress test and milking maneuver, rather than with resisted wrist flexion.
        - History of throwing sports or injury is the norm.
    f. Examination for cubital tunnel syndrome:
        - Tinel test at the cubital tunnel
        - Elbow-flexion compression test
        - Assessment of ulnar nerve stability with elbow flexion should be performed.
4. Imaging
    a. Radiography
        - Plain radiographs are typically normal.
        - Stress radiographs may be useful in cases of suspected ulnar collateral ligament injury.
        - Posteromedial osteophytes and joint space narrowing may signal valgus extension overload syndrome.
    b. Magnetic resonance imaging
        - MRI may detect ulnar collateral ligament injury.
        - It may identify loose bodies in the elbow or posteromedial arthritic change.
        - It also may show rupture of the flexor-pronator origin from the epicondyle.

- MRI is not diagnostic of medial epicondylitis, but it may signal change in the flexor-pronator origin.

c. Electromyography/nerve conduction velocity studies are useful if ulnar nerve dysfunction is found on history and physical examination.

D. Treatment

1. Nonsurgical treatment for medial epicondylitis is similar to that for lateral epicondylitis. Nonsurgical treatment should always be tried first for isolated medial epicondylitis.

a. Activity modification

b. NSAIDs

c. Physical therapy (flexor-pronator stretching and strengthening)

d. Injections—The medication should ideally be delivered into the space deep to the flexor-pronator origin. Avoid posterior placement to avoid ulnar nerve damage.

e. Acupuncture

f. Bracing treatment (counterforce, wrist)

g. Iontophoresis, phonophoresis

2. Surgical treatment

a. Indications

- Lack of response to 6 to 12 months of nonsurgical treatment
- Clear diagnosis (distracting diagnoses ruled out)

b. Contraindications

- Inadequate trial of nonsurgical treatment
- Patient noncompliance with nonsurgical treatment

c. Surgical technique

- The incision is centered just anterior and distal to the medial epicondyle, with protection of the medial antebrachial cutaneous nerve.
- The ulnar nerve should be identified and protected posterior to the medial epicondyle. If substantial ulnar nerve symptoms exist preoperatively, decompression or transposition should be considered as part of the surgical procedure.
- The interval between the pronator teres and flexor carpi radialis is identified and incised.
- Pathologic tendon tissue is excised.
- The epicondyle is decorticated.
- The anterior band of the ulnar collateral ligament deep to the flexor-pronator is evaluated.
- Postoperative management consists of brief immobilization followed by early range of motion. Strengthening does not begin until week 6.
- Results are inferior when ulnar nerve symptoms are present preoperatively. Overall data on surgical treatment of medial epicondylitis are sparse.

E. Complications

1. Ulnar nerve injury from traction or surgical trauma
2. Medial antebrachial cutaneous neuropathy
3. Infection

F. Pearls and pitfalls

1. Correct diagnosis is critical. An understanding of the appropriate physical examination and appropriate use of imaging allows differentiation between ulnar collateral ligament injury and medial epicondylitis.
2. Proper surgical indications are paramount because patients with concomitant ulnar nerve symptoms have less favorable outcomes.
3. Identification and protection of the ulnar nerve and the medial antebrachial cutaneous nerve branches helps avoid injury.

TOP TESTING FACTS

Lateral Epicondylitis

1. The lesion of lateral epicondylitis is typically found in the origin of the ECRB.
2. Nirschl termed the histologic lesion "angiofibroblastic hyperplasia."
3. Differential diagnosis of lateral epicondylitis includes radial tunnel syndrome and radiocapitellar plica.
4. PA and lateral radiographs are usually normal.
5. Nonsurgical treatment is attempted initially and is usually effective.

6. Surgical injury of the lateral ulnar collateral ligament results in iatrogenic PLRI of the elbow.
7. The lesion of medial epicondylitis is typically found in the pronator teres and flexor carpi radialis.
8. Medial epicondylitis must be distinguished from ulnar collateral ligament injury and valgus elbow instability.
9. Surgical treatment of medial epicondylitis is less successful when ulnar neuropathy is present preoperatively.
10. Injury to the medial antebrachial cutaneous nerve during surgery for medial epicondylitis can cause a painful neuroma.

Bibliography

Aben A, De Wilde L, Hollevoet N, et al: Tennis elbow: Associated psychological factors. *J Shoulder Elbow Surg* 2018;27(3):387-392.

Clark T, McRae S, Leiter J, Zhang Y, Dubberly J, McDonald P: Arthroscopic versus open lateral release for the treatment of lateral epicondylitis: A prospective randomized clinical trial. *Arthroscopy* 2018:34(12):3177-3184.

Coombes BK, Bisset L, Brooks P, Khan A, Vicenzino B: Effect of corticosteroid injection, physiotherapy, or both on clinical outcomes in patients with unilateral lateral epicondylalgia: A randomized controlled trial. *JAMA* 2013;309(5):461-469.

Degen RM, Cancienne JM, Camp CL, Altchek DW, Dines JS, Werner BC: Three or more preoperative injections is the most significant risk factor for revision surgery after operative treatment of lateral epicondylitis: An analysis of 3863 patients. *J Shoulder Elbow Surg* 2017;26(4):704-709.

Krogh TP, Fredberg U, Stengaard-Pedersen K, Christensen R, Jensen P, Ellingsen T: Treatment of lateral epicondylitis with platelet-rich plasma, glucocorticoid, or saline: A randomized, double-blind, placebo-controlled trial. *Am J Sports Med* 2013;41(3):625-635.

Kroslak M, Pirapakaran K, Murrell GAC: Counterforce bracing of lateral epicondylitis: A prospective, randomized, double-blinded, placebo-controlled clinical trial. *J Shoulder Elbow Surg* 2019;28(2):288-295.

Kroslak M, Murrell GAC: Surgical treatment of lateral epicondylitis: A prospective, randomized, double-blinded, placebo-controlled clinical trial. *Am J Sports Med* 2018;46(5):1106-1113.

Lian J, Mohamadi A, Chan JJ, et al: Comparative efficacy and safety of nonsurgical treatment options for enthesopathy of the extensor carpi radialis brevis: A systematic review and meta-analysis of randomized placebo-controlled trials. *Am J Sports Med* 2018:363546518801914. [Epub ahead of print].

Regan W, Wold LE, Coonrad R, Morrey BF: Microscopic histopathology of chronic refractory lateral epicondylitis. *Am J Sports Med* 1992;20(6):746-749.

Shim JW, Yoo SH, Park MJ: Surgical management of lateral epicondylitis combined with ligament insufficiency. *J Shoulder Elbow Surg* 2018;27(10):1907-1912.

Chapter 80
ELBOW STIFFNESS

ALEXANDER W. ALEEM, MD, MSc

I. OVERVIEW

A. Most activities of daily living (ADLs) require elbow range-of-motion (ROM) arcs comprising 100° (30° to 130°) of flexion/extension and 100° (50°/50°) of pronation/supination.

1. More contemporary tasks (eg, cell phone and mouse/computer work) require more flexion and pronation than other ADLs.

B. Flexion and supination loss generally causes more disability than extension and pronation loss.

II. EPIDEMIOLOGY

A. Elbow stiffness is often associated with arthritis or trauma (dislocations and/or fractures).

B. Other causes

1. Congenital: arthrogryposis, radial head dislocation
2. Cerebral palsy
3. Head injury: risk of heterotopic ossification
4. A burn that results in contracted skin eschar or heterotopic ossification.

III. PATHOANATOMY

A. Intrinsic pathologic conditions—These include intra-articular fractures and malunions, joint incongruity, intra-articular loose bodies and adhesions, inflammatory arthropathy, osteochondritis dissecans, post-traumatic arthritis, osteoarthritis, and osteonecrosis.

B. Extrinsic pathologic conditions—These include heterotopic ossification, skin conditions such as eschar after a burn, muscle conditions such as myositis ossificans, capsular fibrosis/adhesions, and postoperative hardware impingement.

IV. EVALUATION

A. History

1. Duration of the elbow contracture
2. Initial injury
3. Previous surgical procedures
4. Trials of splinting, therapy, or injections
5. Complications of surgery
6. The patient's work, life demands, and goals

B. Physical examination

1. Function of the upper extremity (shoulder, wrist, and hand) should be assessed.
2. The soft tissue surrounding the elbow should be examined for previous skin incisions/grafts, eschar, or infection.
3. ROM should be assessed.
   a. Active and passive flexion, extension, supination, and pronation should be evaluated. (The contralateral elbow should be examined for comparison.) A goniometer should be used for accurate measurement.
   b. If the elbow has less than 90° to 100° of flexion, the posterior bundle of the medial collateral ligament (MCL) is contracted and must be released to restore flexion.
   c. Pain should be assessed for during the mid arc or at the terminal ends of motion. Mid arc ROM pain is more common with intrinsic disease and may not improve with contracture release alone.

Neither Dr. Aleem nor any immediate family member has received anything of value from or has stock or stock options held in a commercial company or institution related directly or indirectly to the subject of this chapter.

This chapter is adapted from Murthi AM: Elbow stiffness, in Boyer MI, ed: *AAOS Comprehensive Orthopaedic Review* 2. Rosemont, IL, American Academy of Orthopaedic Surgeons, 2014, pp 993-997.

4. Neurovascular examination
   a. The ulnar nerve is of utmost importance because of its anatomic proximity to the elbow. The posterior bundle of the MCL forms the floor of the cubital tunnel, along the course of the ulnar nerve.
   b. Electromyography/nerve conduction velocity studies should be performed if any question about neurologic dysfunction exists.
   c. An assessment for ulnar nerve subluxation should be performed. Subluxation of the nerve is a relative contraindication for an arthroscopic procedure secondary to possible iatrogenic nerve injury.
   d. Verify if ulnar nerve has been transposed if history of prior surgical procedures.

C. Imaging
1. Radiographs should always be obtained.
   a. AP, lateral, and oblique radiographs are standard, with serial radiography as follow-up when heterotopic ossification is present.
   b. The primary bony landmarks include the ulnohumeral joint, coronoid process, radial head, capitellum, radiocapitellar joint, olecranon tip, coronoid/olecranon fossae, and trochlear ridge.
2. CT is helpful when assessing for malunion architecture and the location and pattern of osteophytes and/or loose bodies. Three-dimensional CT is used to check for heterotopic ossification. CT is not necessary when the stiffness is entirely soft-tissue related. If any joint incongruity or abnormal bony anatomy is present, however, CT is beneficial.
3. MRI can be used to evaluate ligaments and tendons, but it is rarely indicated.

V. CLASSIFICATION

A. Contractures can be classified as intrinsic, extrinsic, or mixed-type.

B. Intrinsic contracture—The primary cause of stiffness is related to intra-articular pathology. Common causes include intra-articular fracture malunion, joint incongruity (acquired or congenital), inflammatory arthropathy, osteochondritis dissecans, and posttraumatic arthritis or osteoarthritis, in which intrinsic disease leads to the loss of articular cartilage and the formation of marginal osteophytes (at the coronoid and olecranon tips and fossae) that can limit motion.

C. Extrinsic contracture—The primary cause of stiffness is outside the elbow joint. Common causes are heterotopic ossification, skin conditions such as eschar after a burn, muscle conditions such as myositis ossificans, and capsular contracture, which commonly complicates both simple and complex elbow injuries.

D. Mixed-type contracture
1. This is the most common type; it includes osteoarthritis and posttraumatic contractures.
2. Late sequelae of an intrinsic pathologic condition can lead to extrinsic stiffness.

VI. TREATMENT

A. Nonsurgical treatment
1. Nonsurgical treatment may be attempted in virtually all patients with elbow stiffness in whom the treatment described below will not worsen the condition.
2. Nonsurgical treatment includes the following:
   a. Physical therapy (active and passive ROM) and NSAIDs for 6 to 12 weeks
   b. Intra-articular corticosteroid injections
   c. Splinting/ROM regimen
      - Dynamic splinting
      - Progressive static stretch
      - Turnbuckle orthosis (adjustable static type)

B. Surgical treatment
1. Indications
   a. Extrinsic contractures—Surgical release is ideally indicated for extrinsic contractures when the joint surface is congruous and normal joint architecture is maintained.
   b. Intrinsic contractures—Surgical release can be helpful for some contractures of intrinsic origin, such as osteoarthritis; once the joint surface is altered or incongruous, however, the results are much less predictable, especially if patient reports of mid arc pain.
   c. A patient in whom a course of nonsurgical treatment has failed
   d. A patient who will be compliant with postoperative therapy
   e. Heterotopic ossification—This can be resected once it is mature, as evidenced by well-corticalized margins of the new bone and a lack of changes on serial radiographs.

2. Contraindications
   a. Intra-articular ankylosed elbow
   b. A neurologic elbow disorder
   c. Charcot elbow
   d. A deficient skin envelope (may need a rotational flap)
   e. Posttraumatic arthritis
   f. Surgical release rarely is indicated for mild contractures (<40°) or for cases with severe articular incongruity.
3. Anesthesia—Surgery can be performed with general with regional, regional alone, or general alone.

C. Surgical approaches and procedures
1. Arthroscopic capsular release/osteocapsular arthroplasty
   a. Indications—This procedure is indicated for patients with osteoarthritis or extrinsic capsular contractures.
   b. Procedure—Arthroscopic capsular release is a technically demanding procedure because of the small joint space and the close proximity of neurovascular structures.
      - Posterior compartment—Olecranon tip/fossa osteophytes and loose bodies are débrided; posterior capsular release is performed. Débridement/suction is avoided medially to protect the ulnar nerve. A mini-open incision may be used to release the posterior bundle of the MCL to help gain flexion and protect the ulnar nerve.
      - Anterior compartment—Coronoid tip/fossa osteophytes and radial fossa osteophytes are débrided and loose bodies are removed; anterior capsulotomy/capsulectomy is performed.
      - To improve visualization and protect neurovascular structures, accessory portals and retractors should be used judiciously.
      - The neurovascular structures must be protected. The radial nerve is at greatest risk, followed by the ulnar and median nerves. Strategies to protect the neurovascular structures include insufflating the joint before establishing the portals, using proximally positioned medial and lateral portals in the anterior compartment, keeping the elbow flexed when establishing anterior portals, using retractors during débridement and capsulotomy, releasing the anterior capsule proximally, and avoiding cautery and shavers in the posterior medial gutter (ulnar nerve).

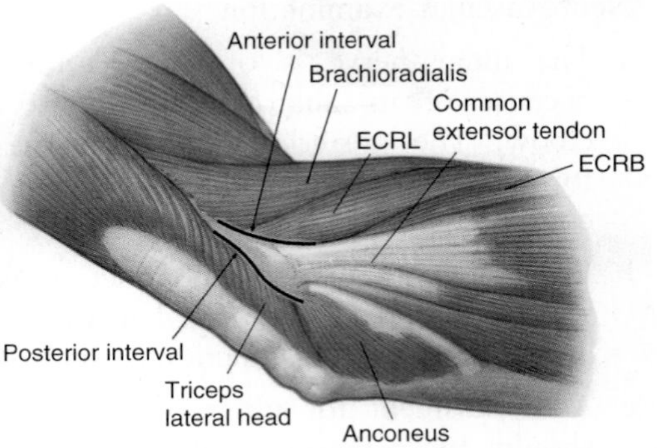

Figure 1 Illustration shows the lateral column approach for treating stiffness of the elbow. This approach is used to address the anterior and posterior aspects of the joint by exposing the capsule through the anterior interval, which consists of the distal fibers of the brachioradialis and the extensor carpi radialis longus (ECRL). The posterior interval simply consists of elevating the lateral margin of the triceps from the posterior aspect of the lateral column. ECRB = extensor carpi radialis brevis. (Reproduced with permission from the Mayo Foundation for Medical Education and Research, Rochester, MN. All rights reserved.)

2. Open lateral column (Morrey) approach (**Figure 1**)
   a. Indications—Extrinsic and/or intrinsic contracture that has failed nonsurgical treatment. Must be combined with a medial release when severe loss of flexion is noted.
   b. Procedure
      - The lateral column approach can be performed through a posterior or lateral skin incision.
      - The extensor carpi radialis longus/brachioradialis muscles are elevated anteriorly and the triceps muscle is elevated posteriorly.
      - The brachialis muscle is mobilized off the anterior capsule.
      - The anterior capsule is released and excised.
      - The coronoid tip/fossae are débrided.
      - The olecranon tip/fossae are decompressed.
      - The radiocapitellar joint is débrided.
      - The posterior capsule is released/excised.
3. Open medial "over the top" (Hotchkiss) approach (**Figure 2**)
   a. Indications—This approach is indicated for patients with extrinsic contractures, associated medial side heterotopic ossification, ulnar neuropathy, and/or preoperative flexion limited to 90° to 100°.

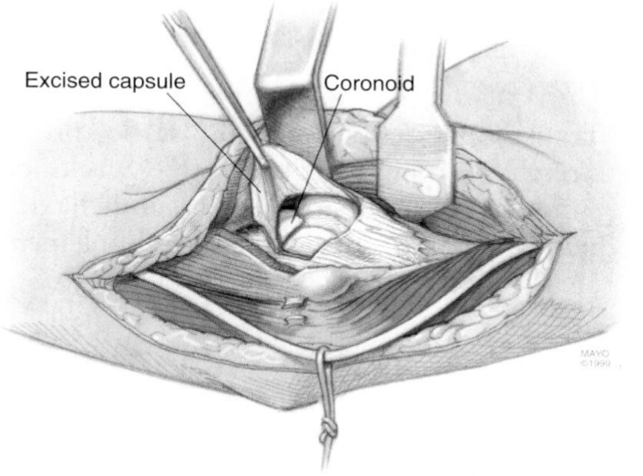

Figure 2 Illustration depicts the open medial approach. The capsule is exposed by reflecting the pronator teres from the anterior aspect of the capsule. The ulnar nerve is identified and protected. (Reproduced with permission from the Mayo Foundation for Medical Education and Research, Rochester, MN. All rights reserved.)

b. Procedure
- The ulnar nerve is decompressed or transposed.
- The posterior band of the MCL and/or the capsule is released to increase flexion.
- The surgeon should work anterior to the flexor/pronator mass and may need to release proximally to assess the anterior capsule.
- The anterior capsule is excised.
- The coronoid tip/fossae are débrided.

4. Combined approach

a. Indications
- Cases of significant elbow stiffness in which a unilateral approach is inadequate for complete elbow release
- Cases in which previous hardware removal is necessary
- Select cases with medial and lateral heterotopic ossification

b. Procedure
- A posterior skin incision, with medial and lateral skin flaps, is made.
    - Can also consider using a dual incision approach medially and laterally.
- If the elbow has less than 90° to 100° of flexion, the posteromedial band of the MCL and the posterior capsule are released to restore flexion; ulnar nerve decompression or transposition should be considered.

5. Interposition arthroplasty—Interposition arthroplasty is a procedure in which the distal humerus is resurfaced with biologic material. An external fixator often is used to distract the joint and provide stability in the immediate postoperative period.

a. Indications—The procedure is considered for intrinsic contractures in young patients (20 to 50 years) with articular cartilage destruction in whom the anatomic architecture of the distal humerus and proximal ulna are relatively preserved.

b. Procedure
- A hinged external fixator is used for distraction and to maintain stability.
- Interposition—Interpositional arthroplasty grafts may include autologous fascia, dermis, allograft Achilles tendon, dermal allografts, and xenografts
- The collaterals are reconstructed if necessary.

6. Total elbow arthroplasty

a. Indications—Total elbow arthroplasty is indicated only for older, low-demand individuals with intrinsic disease and joint contracture.

b. The procedure has a high failure rate in young, active individuals with posttraumatic arthritis.

c. Following total elbow arthroplasty, patients have a permanent 5-lb lifting restriction.

D. Complications

1. Postoperative heterotopic ossification—Prophylactic treatment with indomethacin or low-dose radiation therapy should be considered for both arthroscopic or open releases.
2. Neurovascular compromise—The ulnar nerve is at greatest risk and usually is transposed anteriorly.
3. Ulnar neurapraxia is often associated with an acute increase in flexion when preoperative flexion is limited to 90° to 100° and the ulnar nerve has not been decompressed.
4. Superficial infections
5. Prolonged drainage/seroma is common with open releases.
6. Recurrent contracture
7. Skin/wound healing problems

E. Rehabilitation

1. Continuous passive motion (CPM) through full ROM, under regional anesthesia. The efficacy of CPM is debated, however. To be used for 3 to 6 weeks if maintaining or improving ROM.

6 | Shoulder and Elbow

2. Active and active-assisted ROM therapy. To be used for 3 to 6 months to maintain and increase ROM.
3. Compressive elbow stockings to "pump out" edema. To be used for 3 to 6 weeks to decrease postoperative swelling.
4. Compressive cooling elbow wraps. To be used for 3 to 6 weeks to decrease postoperative swelling and inflammation.
5. Nighttime extension splinting. To be used for a minimum of 6 weeks to maintain elbow extension.
6. Transition to dynamic or static progressive stretch splinting. Instituted at 6 weeks postoperatively to increase ROM in both flexion and extension. Can consider earlier implementation in more severe cases of contracture.

TOP TESTING FACTS

1. Most activities of daily living require elbow ROM arcs comprising 100° (30° to 130°) of flexion/extension and 100° (50°/50°) of pronation/supination.
2. CT scans are helpful to understand the anatomy of intrinsic elbow contractures with changes in the bony architecture.
3. Surgical release is ideally indicated for extrinsic contractures when the joint surface is congruous and normal joint architecture is maintained.
4. Arthroscopic procedures require careful portal placement to minimize the risk of nerve injury. The radial nerve is at greatest risk, followed by the ulnar and median nerves.
5. Open surgical approaches include the lateral column and the medial "over the top" approaches. Either approach or a combined approach can be performed through a single posterior incision.
6. The medial approach is indicated for patients with extrinsic contractures, associated MCL calcification, and ulnar neuropathy.
7. If the elbow has less than 90° to 100° of flexion, the posteromedial band of the MCL and the posterior capsule should be released to restore flexion; ulnar nerve decompression or transposition should be considered.
8. To prevent postoperative heterotopic ossification, prophylactic treatment with indomethacin or low-dose radiation therapy should be considered.
9. Progressive static stretch or dynamic splinting should be considered at 6 weeks after surgery for residual stiffness.
10. Continuous passive motion may help improve ROM in extreme cases of contracture.

Bibliography

Attum B, Obremskey W: Posttraumatic elbow stiffness: A critical analysis review. *JBJS Rev* 2016;4(9).

Evans PJ, Nandi S, Maschke S, Hoyen HA, Lawton JN: Prevention and treatment of elbow stiffness. *J Hand Surg Am* 2009;34(4):769-778.

Keener JD, Galatz LM: Arthroscopic management of the stiff elbow. *J Am Acad Orthop Surg* 2011;19(5):265-274.

Kodde IF, van Rijn J, van den Bekerom MP, Eygendaal D: Surgical treatment of post-traumatic elbow stiffness: A systematic review. *J Shoulder Elbow Surg* 2013;22(4):574-580.

Lindenhovius AL, Doornberg JN, Brouwer KM, Jupiter JB, Mudgal CS, Ring D: A prospective randomized controlled trial of dynamic versus static progressive elbow splinting for posttraumatic elbow stiffness. *J Bone Joint Surg Am* 2012;94(8):694-700.

Mansat P, Morrey BF: The column procedure: A limited lateral approach for extrinsic contracture of the elbow. *J Bone Joint Surg Am* 1998;80(11):1603-1615.

Morrey BF: The posttraumatic stiff elbow. *Clin Orthop Relat Res* 2005;431:26-35.

Morrey BF: Surgical treatment of extraarticular elbow contracture. *Clin Orthop Relat Res* 2000;370:57-64.

Nguyen D, Proper SI, MacDermid JC, King GJ, Faber KJ: Functional outcomes of arthroscopic capsular release of the elbow. *Arthroscopy* 2006;22(8):842-849.

Park MJ, Chang MJ, Lee YB, Kang HJ: Surgical release for posttraumatic loss of elbow flexion. *J Bone Joint Surg Am* 2010;92(16):2692-2699.

Sardelli M, Tashjian RZ, MacWilliams BA: Functional elbow range of motion for contemporary tasks. *J Bone Joint Surg Am* 2011;93(5):471-477. doi:10.2106/JBJS.I.01633.

Sodhi N, Khlopas A, Vaughn MD, et al: Manufactured brace modalities for elbow stiffness. *Orthopedics* 2018;41(1):e127-e135.

Stans AA, Maritz NG, O'Driscoll SW, Morrey BF: Operative treatment of elbow contracture in patients twenty-one years of age or younger. *J Bone Joint Surg Am* 2002;84(3):382-387.

Zheng W, Liu J, Song J, Fan C: Risk factors for development of severe post-traumatic elbow stiffness. *Int Orthop* 2018;42(3):595-600.

Chapter 81
ACUTE AND RECURRENT ELBOW INSTABILITY

GARY F. UPDEGROVE, MD
CHARLES L. GETZ, MD

I. OVERVIEW/EPIDEMIOLOGY

A. The elbow is the second most commonly dislocated joint in adults and the most commonly dislocated joint in children.

B. Dislocations represent 10% to 25% of all elbow injuries.

C. The highest incidence of elbow dislocation is in patients of age 10 to 20 years.

D. Recurrent instability occurs as a result of ligamentous, bony, or combined injuries.

II. PATHOANATOMY

A. The stability of the elbow joint is provided by static and dynamic constraints (**Figure 1**).

1. Primary static constraints
   a. Ulnohumeral articulation
   b. Anterior bundle of the medial collateral ligament (MCL)
   c. Lateral collateral ligament (LCL) complex, including the lateral ulnar collateral ligament (LUCL)

2. Secondary static constraints
   a. Capsule (most stabilizing effect with elbow extended)
   b. Radiocapitellar articulation (important secondary valgus stabilizer)
   c. Common flexor and extensor tendon origins

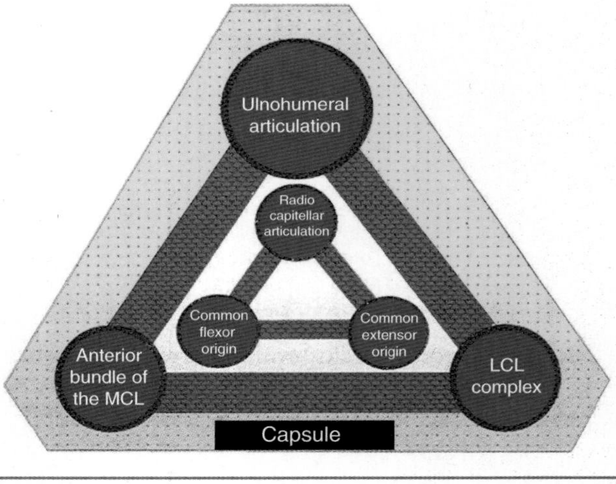

Figure 1 Illustration demonstrates how the static constraints in the elbow are analogous to the defenses of a fortress. The primary static constraints to elbow instability are the ulnohumeral articulation, the anterior bundle of the medial collateral ligament (MCL), and the lateral collateral ligament (LCL) complex, including the lateral ulnar collateral ligament. The secondary constraints include the capsule, the radiocapitellar articulation, and the common flexor and extensor tendon origins. (Adapted with permission from the Mayo Foundation for Medical Education and Research, Rochester, MN. All rights reserved.)

Dr. Getz or an immediate family member has received royalties from Zimmer; is a member of a speakers' bureau or has made paid presentations on behalf of Mitek and Zimmer; serves as an unpaid consultant to Zimmer; has stock or stock options held in OBERD; and has received research or institutional support from Zimmer. Neither Dr. Updegrove nor any immediate family member has received anything of value from or has stock or stock options held in a commercial company or institution related directly or indirectly to the subject of this chapter.

This chapter is adapted from Armstrong AD, Getz CL: Simple elbow dislocations and recurrent elbow instability, in Boyer MI, ed: *AAOS Comprehensive Orthopaedic Review*, ed 2. Rosemont, IL, American Academy of Orthopaedic Surgeons, 2014, pp 999-1004, 1005-1009.

3. Dynamic constraints
    a. Dynamic constraint is provided by the muscles that cross the elbow joint (the anconeus, triceps, and brachialis).
    b. These muscles apply compressive force.
4. The MCL becomes the primary constraint to valgus instability when the radial head is resected. Injuries to the MCL in isolation are typically well tolerated, except in overhead throwers.
5. The coronoid blocks rotational instability and posterior subluxation of the ulna from the posterior pull of the triceps or when weight bearing on the hand.
    a. 50% of the coronoid height is needed to provide substantial stability.
    b. Sagittal plane fractures of the coronoid may disrupt the MCL insertion or cause substantial articular deformity.
6. The lateral collateral ligaments—the lateral ulnar collateral ligament (LUCL) and the radial collateral ligament (RCL)—prevent rotational subluxation of the forearm away from the humerus. Both the LUCL and RCL must be compromised for the lateral ligaments to become insufficient.
    a. The radial head plays a minor role in posterolateral rotatory stability by tensioning the LUCL.

B. Mechanisms of injury for posterolateral dislocations
1. The classic mechanism is thought to be a combination of axial load, external rotation of the forearm (supination), and valgus force (valgus posterolateral). A progressive circular disruption of the soft tissues occurs beginning on the lateral side of the elbow (**Table 1**).
2. Posterolateral elbow dislocation may also occur with a combination of axial load, external rotation of the forearm, and varus force.
3. The lateral collateral ligament complex is disrupted with all elbow dislocations. Some authors believe that the MCL is always disrupted with elbow dislocation, but this is controversial.

III. ACUTE DISLOCATION

A. Physical examination
1. Neurovascular status should be documented (both before and after elbow reduction).
2. Open injuries and compartment syndrome, which require immediate surgical treatment, should be ruled out.

B. Imaging
1. Plain AP and lateral radiographs of the elbow are necessary to document congruent reduction.
2. Oblique views may be useful to identify periarticular fractures.
3. CT is useful to identify associated osseous injury.
4. With an incongruous reduction, CT or MRI should be considered to identify potential incarcerated osteocartilaginous fragments.

C. Classification
1. Elbow dislocations are classified according to whether they are simple or complex and the direction of displacement.
2. Simple versus complex dislocation
    a. Simple—Dislocation without osseous injury

TABLE 1

Stages of Soft-Tissue Disruption

Stage	Description
1	Disruption of the LUCL
2	Disruption of the other lateral ligamentous structures and the anterior and posterior capsule
3	Disruption of the MCL
3A	Partial disruption of the MCL
3B	Complete disruption of the MCL
3C	Distal humerus stripped of soft tissues; severe instability results in dislocation or subluxation

Adapted from O'Driscoll SW: Acute, recurrent, and chronic elbow instabilities, in Norris TR, ed: *Orthopaedic Knowledge Update: Shoulder and Elbow*, ed 2. Rosemont, IL, American Academy of Orthopaedic Surgeons, 2002, pp 313-323.
LUCL = lateral ulnar collateral ligament; MCL = medial collateral ligament

b. Complex—Dislocation with osseous injury
   - "Terrible triad"—Characterized by an elbow dislocation with an LCL complex tear, a radial head fracture, and a coronoid fracture.
   - Varus posteromedial rotatory instability—Characterized by an LCL tear with a fracture of the medial facet of the coronoid or a comminuted coronoid fracture.

3. Direction of displacement (position of the distal fragment relative to the proximal fragment)
   a. Posterior dislocations are most common. They can be
      - Posterior
      - Posterolateral
      - Posteromedial (**Figure 2**)

   b. Anterior, medial, lateral, and divergent dislocations also occur.

D. Treatment

1. An algorithm for nonsurgical and surgical treatment of simple elbow dislocations is shown in (**Figure 3**).

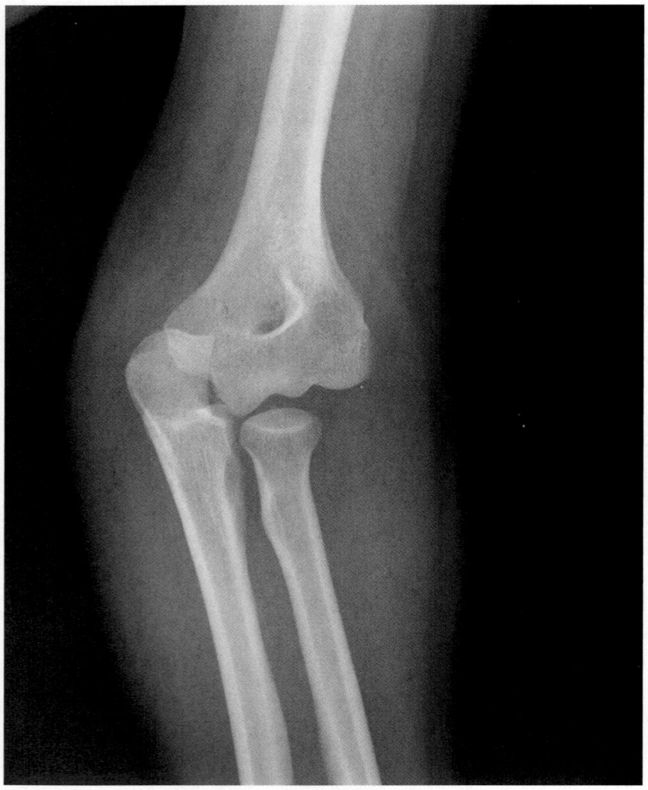

Figure 2 AP radiograph demonstrates a posteromedial dislocation of the elbow.

2. Nonsurgical treatment
   a. Reduction of the joint under adequate analgesia is performed first. Reduction maneuver for posterior dislocations: A controlled reduction is done by applying inline traction, progressive elbow flexion, and anterior directed force to the olecranon.
   b. Postreduction stability is assessed. In posterior dislocations, the elbow is typically more unstable in extension. Therefore, the elbow should be immobilized at 90° of flexion.

3. If the LCL is disrupted and the MCL is intact, the elbow will be more stable with the forearm in pronation.

4. If the LCL and the MCL are disrupted, the forearm should be immobilized in neutral (**Figure 4**).

5. A posterior splint is applied. Typically, the forearm is placed in a splint for 5 to 7 days, with the elbow positioned at 90° and with appropriate forearm rotation.

6. Postreduction radiographic assessment (AP and lateral views with the elbow at 90° and appropriate forearm rotation) is performed to confirm concentric reduction. Attention is directed to ensuring a concentric ulnohumeral reduction and alignment of the radial head with the capitellum. Once reduction is confirmed, the arm is immobilized for 5 to 7 days. Depending on stability, the splint can be removed to allow early active range of motion exercises using a brace with or without an extension block.

E. Surgical indications and contraindications

1. Indications
   a. Stability of the elbow cannot be achieved with reduction and immobilization.
   b. Osteochondral fragment or soft-tissue entrapment prevents concentric reduction.
   c. Complex dislocation–associated fractures are present.
   d. Open injuries are present.
   e. Neurovascular injuries requiring surgical care are present.

2. Relative indication—Reducible joint that is unstable (dislocates) when the elbow is extended between 90° and 60°.

3. Contraindications—Patients with severe medical comorbidities.

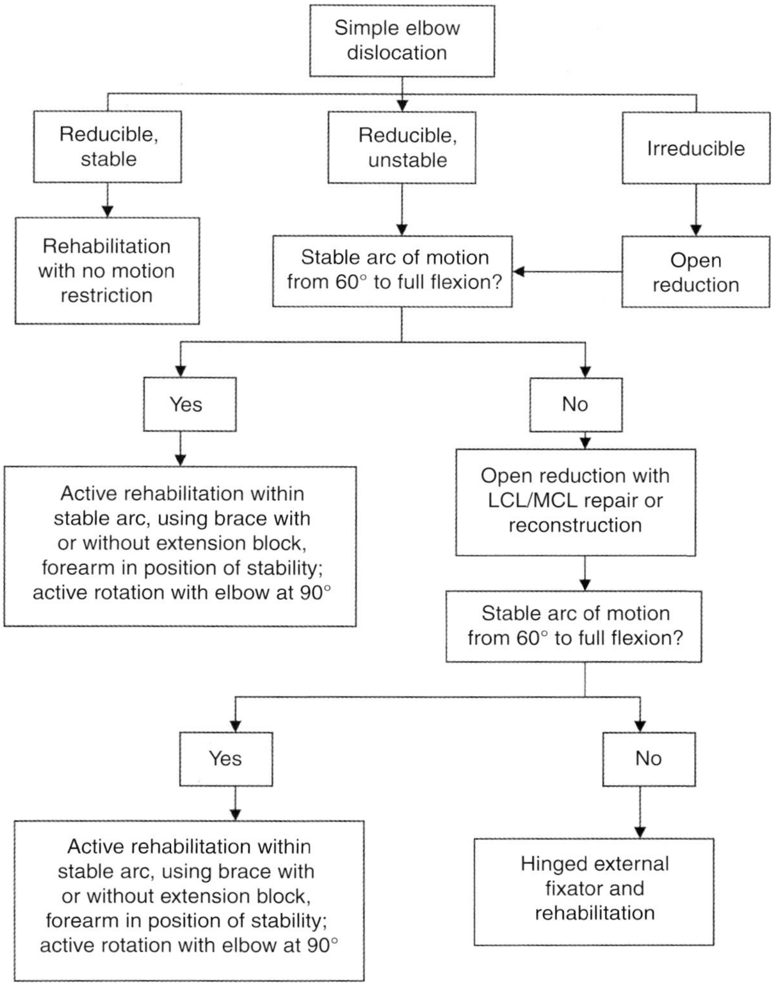

Figure 3 Algorithm for nonsurgical and surgical treatment of simple elbow dislocation. LCL = lateral collateral ligament; MCL = medial collateral ligament. (Adapted from Armstrong AD: Acute, recurrent, and chronic elbow instability, in Galatz LM, ed: *Orthopaedic Knowledge Update: Shoulder and Elbow*, ed 3. Rosemont, IL, American Academy of Orthopaedic Surgeons, 2008, pp 461-476.)

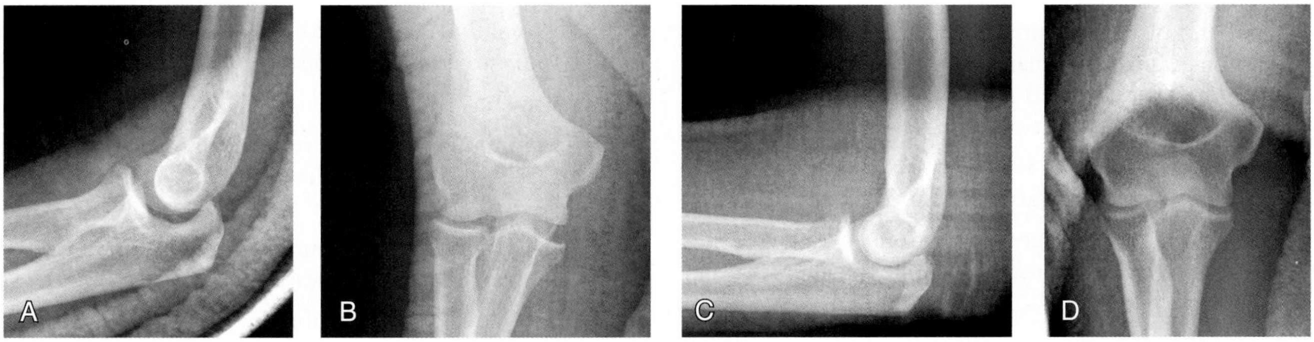

Figure 4 Postreduction lateral (**A**) and AP (**B**) elbow radiographs of a patient who sustained a direct lateral elbow dislocation. The forearm was positioned in pronation. Note the incongruency of the ulnohumeral joint on the lateral view and the medial gapping on the AP view. The splint was changed, and the forearm was repositioned in neutral, allowing for a congruent reduction of the elbow joint, as seen on the lateral (**C**) and AP (**D**) views. The forearm position in pronation accentuated a medial-side injury, whereas neutral forearm rotation allowed a concentric reduction by off-loading the medial- and lateral-side soft-tissue injuries.

F. Surgical procedures

1. The incision can be made in the posterior midline or on the lateral elbow over the Kocher interval (extensor carpi ulnaris and anconeus) with or without a medial approach.
2. Open reduction of the elbow with repair (or reconstruction) of the LCL complex is performed; then stability is assessed.
3. If the elbow is still unstable, the MCL is repaired (or reconstructed); then stability is assessed again.
4. Hinged or static external fixation is required only if the elbow is unstable after other surgical procedures (listed above) have failed to maintain a concentric, stable reduction.

G. Complications

1. Loss of extension (most common)
   a. Early active range of motion exercises can help prevent or minimize occurrence.
   b. Static, progressive splinting may be initiated when the elbow is less inflamed (typically, 6 to 8 weeks after injury).
2. Neurovascular injuries
3. Compartment syndrome
4. Articular surface injuries
5. Chronic or recurrent elbow instability. Residual laxity is common with stress radiographs; however, recurrent instability is seen in less than 10% to 20% of cases.
6. Late osteoarthritis
7. Heterotopic ossification

H. Pearls and pitfalls

1. The most common pitfall is failure to attain and maintain a concentric reduction after surgical or nonsurgical treatment. The joint must be reduced concentrically, and treatment does not stop until satisfactory reduction is achieved.
2. Forearm rotation is used to its fullest advantage to attain or maintain concentric reduction.
3. Early active range of motion through a stable arc with the use of splints can help prevent contracture.
4. If open reduction is required, a stepwise surgical approach should be followed.

I. Rehabilitation—Depending on the postoperative stability of the elbow, active range of motion exercises may begin using a brace with or without an extension block. The extension block may be decreased gradually or removed at approximately 2 to 3 weeks for a goal of full active extension approximately 6 to 8 weeks after injury. Active range of motion exercises are performed through the stable arc, maintaining the most stable position of the forearm through the arc of motion. Active pronation and supination with the elbow at 90° is initiated as soon as the splint is removed (5 to 7 days after injury), to prevent rotational contracture.

IV. VALGUS INSTABILITY

A. Mechanism and pattern of injury—acute valgus instability in nonthrowers

1. Valgus instability also can occur after a fall on an outstretched hand and a direct valgus load.
2. Injury to the anterior band of the MCL is the essential lesion.

B. Physical examination

1. Findings associated with acute valgus instability include tenderness to palpation along the MCL and medial elbow bruising and swelling.
2. Ulnar nerve irritation at the cubital tunnel can result from stretching of the nerve during throwing in the unstable elbow.
3. Rupture of the flexor-pronator group can occur from traumatic valgus load to the elbow.

C. Imaging

1. Radiographs are typically normal with valgus instability. In skeletally immature patients, injury to the medial epicondyle physis may be seen.
2. MRI is not necessary but can confirm diagnosis and assess the integrity of the flexor/pronator muscle/tendon.
3. CT may be obtained in cases of medial fracture, especially if there is concern for displacement or an incarcerated fragment.

D. Treatment

1. Traumatic ruptures are typically managed with a period of immobilization and early physical therapy.
   a. During the early mobilization period, valgus stress must be avoided.
   b. Only a small number of patients with traumatic valgus instability will experience recurrent instability.
   c. Surgical indications
      - Medial physeal fracture—the presence of an incarcerated fragment or displacement of the fragment more than 5 mm (relative indication).

- Skeletally mature—high-demand athlete or severe displacement of flexor/pronator tendon (relative indications).

V. POSTEROLATERAL ROTATORY INSTABILITY

A. Overview

1. Posterolateral rotatory instability (PLRI) may occur after elbow dislocation, iatrogenically, or in a delayed fashion after varus malunion of the distal humerus.
2. Insufficiency of the LUCL is the essential lesion.
3. Deficiencies in the coronoid, radial head, and MCLs can further destabilize the elbow in a rotational manner.

B. Mechanism of injury

1. A fall onto an outstretched hand that supinates the forearm with a valgus thrust and axially loads the forearm leads to PLRI.
    a. PLRI is primarily an instability pattern of the ulnohumeral articulation, with secondary involvement of the radiocapitellar joint.
    b. The radioulnar articulation remains stable.
2. The elbow dislocates as a result of progressive failure of the lateral collateral ligaments (RCL and LUCL), the anterior capsule, and possibly the MCL (**Figure 5**). In many cases, the common extensor origin is avulsed proximally from the lateral epicondyle.
3. In only a small number of patients with an elbow dislocation lead to recurrent PLRI of the elbow. Most patients are successfully treated by brief immobilization and early protected range of motion.
4. Tardy posterolateral elbow instability is a potential late complication of a varus supracondylar humerus malunion.
    a. In tardy posterolateral elbow instability, the abnormal lateral thrust across the joint line caused by the malunion slowly stretches the LUCL over time.

C. Physical examination

1. The physical examination tests attempt to recreate the mechanism of injury of forearm supination and axial load.
2. The most common physical examination tests that are performed to detect PLRI are the PLRI stress test, the posterior drawer test, the table top relocation test, the push-up test, and the chair-rise test.

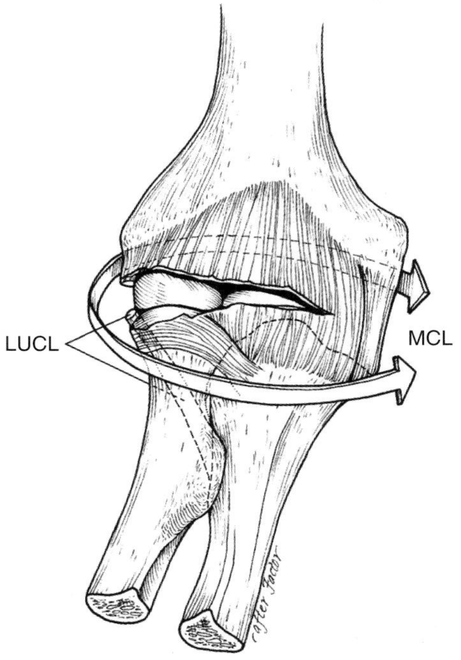

Figure 5 Illustration demonstrates how excessive rotation of the forearm leads to progressive disruption of the lateral ulnar collateral ligament (LUCL) that may propagate to include the anterior capsule and even the medial collateral ligament (MCL).

D. Imaging

1. In purely ligamentous PLRI, radiographs will be normal; however, associated lesions of the radial head, capitellum, coronoid, and articular surface may be seen.
2. CT is helpful to evaluate for associated bone injury.
3. MRI is unreliable to assess the integrity of the LUCL because of the oblique course of the ligament. Cartilaginous injury can be appreciated on magnetic resonance arthrogram, however.

E. Treatment

1. Avoiding provocative positions, bracing treatment, and strengthening of the extensors can decrease symptoms in milder cases.
2. For grossly unstable elbows and elbows in which nonsurgical treatment fails, LUCL reconstruction with a graft is indicated.
3. Graft material may be autograft or allograft. Palmaris longus, plantaris, gracilis, lateral triceps fascia, or other common tendon graft material may be used.

6 | Shoulder and Elbow

VI. VARUS POSTEROMEDIAL INSTABILITY

A. Mechanism and pattern of injury

1. Varus posteromedial instability (VPMI) may occur after a fall on an outstretched hand that applies a varus thrust to the elbow.
2. A combined sagittal coronoid fracture and LUCL injury are the essential lesions.
3. The instability occurs as the distal humerus subluxates into the proximal ulnar lesion. When this occurs, the proximal ulna rotates in a posterior and varus direction producing incongruency.
4. On the lateral aspect of the elbow, traction tears the lateral ligaments occur, usually without bony injury.

B. Physical examination—Decreased range of motion, painful arc of motion, and, sometimes, crepitus are noted on examination.

C. Imaging

1. With VPMI, AP radiographs will show a loss of articular congruency of the medial joint line and/or a sagittal coronoid fracture. Opening of the radiocapitellar articulation is common indicating injury to the lateral ligaments.
2. Radial head fractures are not seen with this injury pattern. This distinguishes VPMI from a terrible triad injury.
3. CT is the best study to define the orientation and size of the coronoid fracture (**Figure 6**).

D. Treatment

1. Early recognition of the instability pattern and treatment is needed to avoid rapid onset of posttraumatic arthritis.

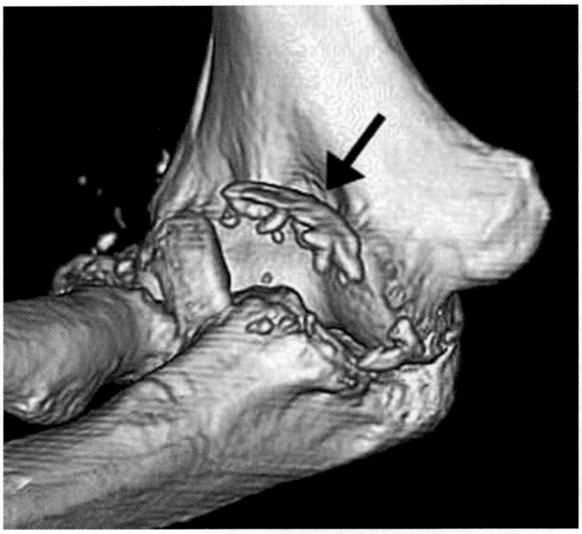

Figure 6 Three-dimensional CT scan demonstrates an anteromedial coronoid fracture. The arrow indicates the fracture fragment. (Reproduced from Steinmann SP: Coronoid process fractures. *J Am Acad Orthop Surg* 2008;16:519-529.)

2. Treatment of VPMI consists of repair of the lateral collateral ligament and restoration of the proximal ulnar joint surface and/or open reduction and internal fixation of the coronoid fracture.
3. Anteromedial coronoid fractures that are small, minimally displaced, and demonstrate no evidence of elbow subluxation may be treated nonoperatively.
4. Outcomes are improved with anatomic reduction and secure coronoid fixation. Varus malalignment of the anteromedial facet or varus subluxation of the elbow lead to arthritic changes and poor functional results.

6 | Shoulder and Elbow

TOP TESTING FACTS

1. The three primary static constraints of the elbow are the ulnohumeral bony articulation, the anterior bundle of the MCL, and the LCL complex (including the LUCL).
2. The three secondary static constraints of the elbow are the capsule, the radial head, and the common flexor and extensor tendon origins.
3. The dynamic constraints are the muscles that cross the elbow joint (the anconeus, triceps, and brachialis); these muscles apply compressive force.
4. In posterolateral dislocations, the classic mechanism of injury is thought to be a combination of axial load, external rotation of the forearm (supination), and valgus force (valgus posterolateral). A progressive circular disruption of the soft tissues occurs.
5. Most elbow dislocations are successfully treated by brief immobilization followed by early protected range of motion therapy.

6. The joint must be reduced concentrically, and treatment should not stop until satisfactory reduction is achieved.
7. In posterior dislocations, the elbow is typically more unstable in extension. Therefore, the elbow should be immobilized in at least 90° of flexion. If the LCL is disrupted and the MCL is intact, the elbow will be more stable with the forearm in pronation. If the LCL and the MCL are disrupted, pronation of the forearm may draw attention to the medial injury, and the forearm should be positioned in neutral to off-load the lateral- and medial-side injuries.
8. Loss of extension is the most common complication following the treatment of simple elbow dislocations.
9. PLRI is primarily an ulnohumeral instability problem. Chronic PLRI is best treated by reconstructing the LUCL.
10. VPMI is characterized by anteromedial facet fracture (sagittal plane fracture with MCL insertion) and LUCL tear. VPMI is treated surgically by repairing the anteromedial facet of the coronoid and, usually, repairing the LUCL.

Bibliography

Boretto JG, Rodriguez Sammartino M, Gallucci G, De Carli P, Ring D: Comparative study of simple and complex open elbow dislocations. *Clin Orthop Relat Res* 2014;472(7):2037-2043.

Chan K, Faber KJ, King GJW, Athwal GS: Selected anteromedial coronoid fractures can be treated nonoperatively. *J Shoulder Elbow Surg* 2016;25(8):1251-1257.

Hwang J-T, Shields MN, Berglund LJ, Hooke AW, Fitzsimmons JS, O'Driscoll SW: The role of the posterior bundle of the medial collateral ligament in posteromedial rotatory instability of the elbow. *Bone Joint J* 2018;100-B(8):1060-1065.

Murthi AM, Keener JD, Armstrong AD, Getz CL: The recurrent unstable elbow: Diagnosis and treatment. *J Bone Joint Surg Am* 2010;92(8):1794-1804.

Pollock JW, Brownhill J, Ferreira L, McDonald CP, Johnson J, King G: The effect of anteromedial facet fractures of the coronoid and lateral collateral ligament injury on elbow stability and kinematics. *J Bone Joint Surg Am* 2009;91(6):1448-1458.

Ramirez MA, Stein JA, Murthi AM: Varus posteromedial instability. *Hand Clin* 2015;31(4):557-563.

Richard MJ, Aldridge JM III, Wiesler ER, Ruch DS: Traumatic valgus instability of the elbow: Pathoanatomy and results of direct repair. *J Bone Joint Surg Am* 2008;90(11):2416-2422.

Chapter 82
ARTHRITIS AND ARTHROPLASTY OF THE ELBOW

PETER N. CHALMERS, MD

I. OSTEOARTHRITIS

A. Epidemiology and overview
   1. Symptomatic primary osteoarthritis of the elbow is relatively rare, affecting 2% of the population.
   2. The average age of presentation is 50 years (range, 20 to 70 years).
   3. Men are affected more often than women (4:1 ratio).
   4. Hand dominance and strenuous manual labor are associated with primary osteoarthritis of the elbow.
   5. Secondary causes include trauma, osteochondritis dissecans, and synovial osteochondromatosis.

B. Pathoanatomy
   1. Osteoarthritis of the elbow is characterized by osteophyte formation, capsular contracture, and loose bodies, often with relative preservation of the joint space.
   2. Periarticular hypertrophic osteophytes act as a mechanical block at the end ranges of flexion and extension.
   3. Rarely, advanced disease presents with joint space narrowing.
   4. Osteoarthritis typically involves the radiocapitellar joint articular cartilage preferentially, with relative preservation of the ulnohumeral articular surfaces.

Dr. Chalmers or an immediate family member serves as a paid consultant to or is an employee of Arthrex, Inc. and Mitek.

C. Evaluation
   1. History
      a. Patients typically present with loss of terminal extension and flexion and painful catching/clicking or locking of the elbow.
      b. Pain is typically noted at the end ranges of motion and not through the midrange.
      c. Night pain is not typical; if present, an inflammatory cause of the arthritis should be considered.
      d. The degree of disability caused by osteoarthritis, which depends on the patient's vocation and physical disability, should be determined.
   2. Physical examination
      a. Inspection—Check for prior surgical incisions and joint effusion at the lateral soft spot.
      b. Assess range of motion—Pain is usually felt at the end ranges of flexion and extension rather than throughout the arc.
      c. Forearm rotation is relatively preserved until later in the disease process.
      d. Ulnar neuropathy is present in up to 50% of patients.
   3. Imaging
      a. Radiographs—Standard AP and lateral radiographs should be obtained (**Figure 1**). Radiographs typically show osteophyte formation at the coronoid process (anterior and medial), coronoid fossa, radial fossa, radial head, olecranon tip, and olecranon fossa. Joint spaces at the ulnohumeral joint usually

This chapter is adapted from Armstrong AD: Arthritis and arthroplasty of the elbow, in Boyer MI, ed: *AAOS Comprehensive Orthopaedic Review*, ed 2. Rosemont, IL, American Academy of Orthopaedic Surgeons, 2014, pp 1011-1017.

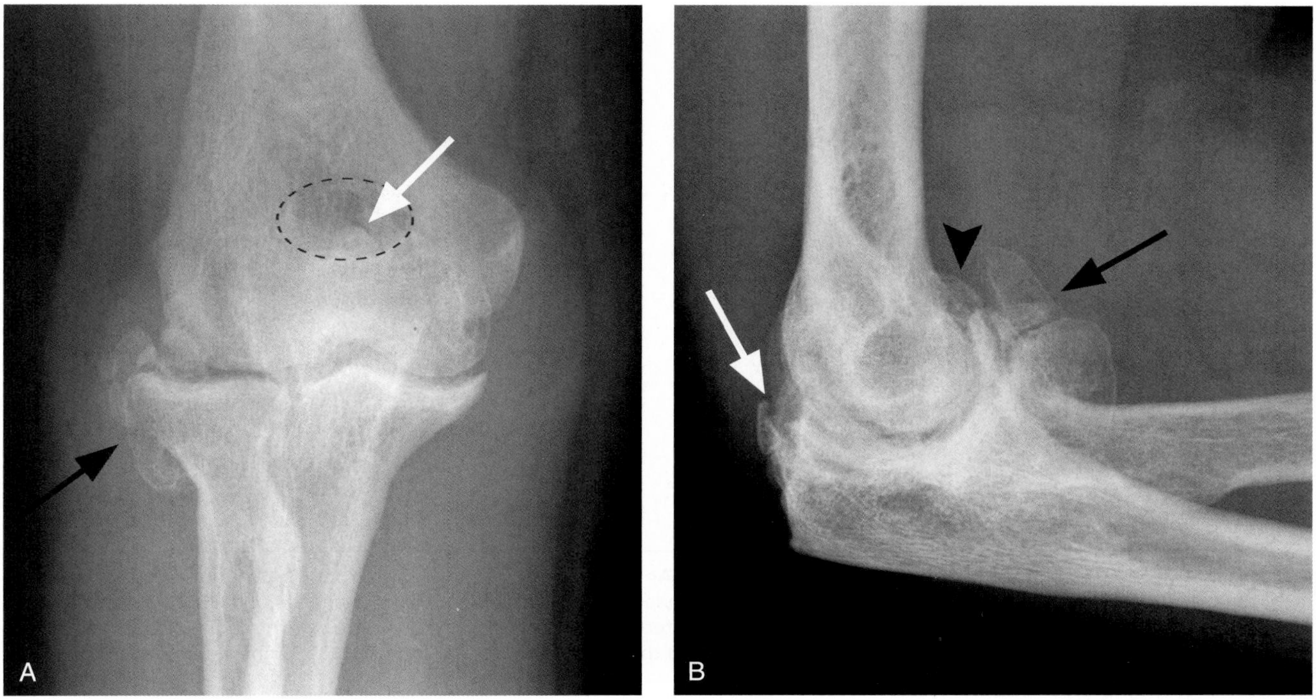

Figure 1 Radiographs of an osteoarthritic elbow. AP view (**A**) shows peripheral osteophytes around the radial head (black arrow) and the tip of the olecranon (white arrow) with a loss of normal contour of the olecranon fossa (broken line). Lateral view (**B**) shows osteophytes at the tip of the coronoid (black arrow), at the tip of the olecranon (white arrow), and at the radial and coronoid fossae (black arrowhead).

are preserved, and those at the radiocapitellar joint are mildly narrowed. Loose bodies may be evident, and radiographs typically underestimate the number present.

b. CT—May be useful for surgical planning; it allows a detailed assessment of osteophytes and the presence of loose bodies.

D. Treatment

1. Nonsurgical treatment—Rest, NSAIDs, corticosteroid injections, and activity modification are the mainstays of treatment.

2. Surgical indications

a. Failure to respond to nonsurgical interventions

b. Loss of motion that interferes with activities of daily living

c. Painful locking or catching of the elbow

3. Surgical procedures

a. Joint-sparing procedures such as débridement, excision of osteophytes, capsular release, and removal of loose bodies are preferred. These procedures can be performed arthroscopically.

b. Total elbow arthroplasty is rarely indicated, and it is not indicated for patients younger than 65 years or physically active patients because of concerns about implant longevity.

c. Open procedures

- Outerbridge-Kashiwagi arthroplasty is the classic open procedure. In this procedure, the olecranon fossa is trephinated and osteophytes are removed.
- Limitations of the Outerbridge-Kashiwagi procedure are incomplete anterior release and incomplete osteophyte removal anteriorly.
- Either a medial or lateral column approach can be used for open débridement, loose body removal, osteophyte resection, and capsulectomy depending upon the location of the pathology and concomitant procedures to be performed.

d. Arthroscopic procedures (**Figure 2**).

- Contraindications include severe contracture and periarticular heterotopic ossification. Relative contraindications: prior ulnar nerve transposition and prior extensive open procedures.
- Osteocapsular arthroplasty refers to the arthroscopic technique for elbow joint

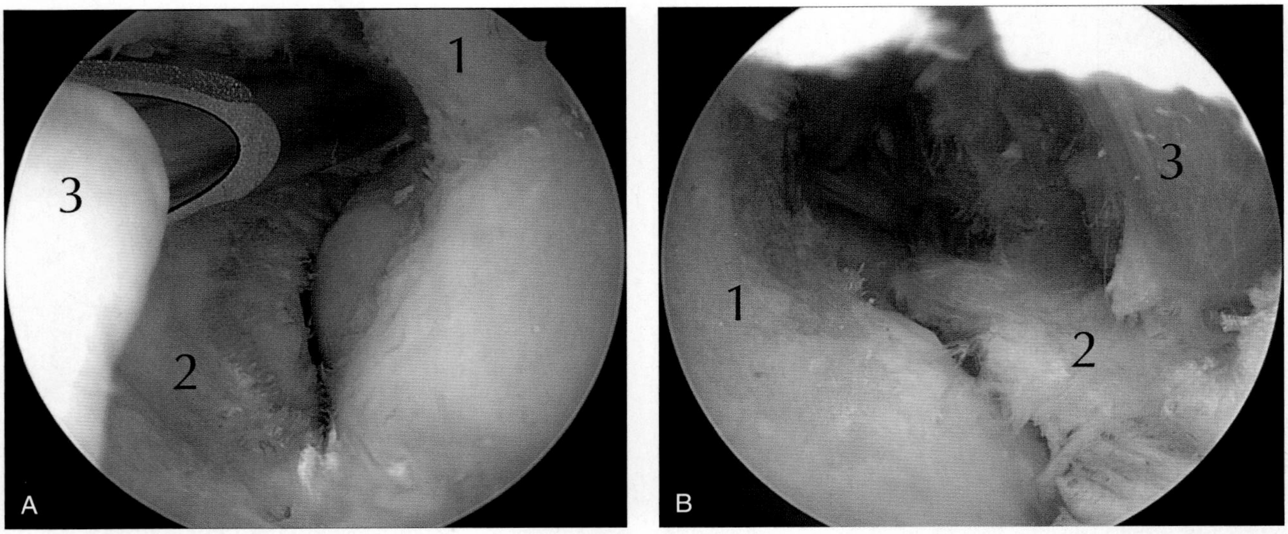

Figure 2 Arthroscopic images from osteocapsular arthroplasty. **A**, This predebridement image from the anterior compartment demonstrates (1) osteophytes, (2) a thickened and inflamed capsule with calcific deposits, and (3) a loose body. **B**, This postdebridement image from the anterior compartment demonstrates (1) osteophyte resection with restoration of the radial and coronoid fossa and (2) capsulotomy where the cut edge of the capsule and the underlying brachialis muscle (3) can be seen.

débridement; it involves capsular release, loose body removal, and excision of osteophytes.

e. Regardless of the type of procedure used, ulnar nerve transposition and release of the posterior bundle of the medial collateral ligament (MCL) should be considered for patients who have less than 90° to 100° of elbow flexion.

E. Complications

1. Infection—Can manifest as superficial (minor wound complications) or deep. Deep infections in the elbow are more common than other joints treated arthroscopically (0.8% to 2.2%). Infection related to intraoperative corticosteroid injections.
2. Stiffness (heterotopic ossification)
3. Hematoma formation
4. Transient nerve palsies—Complicate 1% to 3% of cases. Radial and ulnar most common.
5. Synovial ganglion formation

F. Pearls and pitfalls

1. During arthroscopic surgery, joint distention moves the capsule away from bone, but the distance between the neurovascular structures and the capsule remain unchanged; therefore, the nerves remain at risk with capsular work.
2. Neurovascular structures at risk during portal placement, débridement, and capsular release include median nerve (anteromedial), the ulnar nerve (posteromedial), and the radial nerve (lies adjacent to the anterolateral capsule).
3. The brachialis muscle protects the median nerve and brachial artery during capsular procedures.
4. The olecranon fossa is an oval structure that is wider in the medial to lateral dimension.
5. The olecranon osteophytosis extends medially and laterally and not just at the tip. Resection needs to be extended along the medial and lateral aspects of the olecranon to allow maximal extension and prevent impingement along the medial and lateral posterior columns.
6. Coronoid osteophytosis extends medially and not just at the tip. Resection should be extended medially if necessary to maximize the restoration of flexion range of motion. Restoring the normal radial fossa anatomy, in addition to the coronoid fossa, is also necessary to improve flexion.

G. Rehabilitation

1. Early active range of motion or continuous passive motion is critical.
2. Nighttime extension splinting.
3. Pharmacologic prophylaxis for heterotopic ossification is not typically prescribed, but it may be used at the discretion of the surgeon.
4. A static, progressive splinting program may be implemented at approximately 6 to 8 weeks, when the elbow is less swollen.

II. INFLAMMATORY ARTHRITIS

A. Epidemiology and overview

1. Rheumatoid arthritis is the most common inflammatory disease in adults.
2. In 20% to 50% of patients with rheumatoid arthritis, the elbow is affected.
3. Other less common inflammatory conditions include psoriasis, systemic lupus erythematosus, and pigmented villonodular synovitis.

B. Pathoanatomy

1. Rheumatoid arthritis typically presents initially as an intense synovitis that distends the joint and causes pain and loss of motion.
2. If synovitis persists, secondary changes develop.
   a. Fixed flexion contracture
   b. Attenuation of the soft tissues and instability
   c. Instability of the radial head, through laxity of the annular ligament
   d. Ulnar neuropathy
   e. Radial neuropathy has also been reported
3. As rheumatoid arthritis progresses, the articular cartilage becomes involved, with destruction and periarticular erosion and cyst formation. The end result is a severely deformed joint with loss of bone, loss of joint space, and progressive joint instability.
4. Loss of motion
5. Pain throughout range of motion
6. Ulnar neuropathy

C. Evaluation

1. Physical examination
   a. Range of motion is assessed.
   b. Varus and valgus stability are evaluated. Rheumatoid arthritis often results in soft-tissue attenuation, which can lead to joint instability.
   c. A thorough examination of the cervical spine is essential; many patients with rheumatoid arthritis have concomitant cervical spine abnormalities.
   d. Ulnar neuropathy may or may not be present.
2. Imaging
   a. AP and lateral plain radiographs should be obtained.
   b. Patients scheduled for surgical procedures should have plain preoperative radiographs of the cervical spine.

TABLE 1

Larsen Grading System for Rheumatoid Arthritis

Stage	Description
1	Involves the soft tissues and has near-normal radiographs.
2	Presents with periarticular erosions and mild cartilage loss; there may be evidence of soft-tissue swelling and osteopenia on radiographs.
3	Radiographs show marked joint space narrowing.
4	Progresses to advanced erosions penetrating the subchondral bone plate.
5	Radiographs show advanced joint damage and loss of articular contour.

Data from Trail IA: Arthroplasty in synovial-based arthritis of the elbow, in Williams GR Jr, Yamaguchi K, Ramsey ML, Galatz LM, eds: *Shoulder and Elbow Arthroplasty*. Philadelphia, PA, Lippincott Williams & Wilkins, 2005, pp 381-339.

D. Classification

1. Rheumatoid arthritis is classified according to the Larsen grading system (**Table 1**) or the Mayo Clinic classification system (**Table 2**).
2. The Larsen grading system is based on radiographic appearance (**Table 1**).

TABLE 2

Mayo Clinic Classification of the Rheumatoid Elbow

Grade	Description
I	No radiographic abnormalities except periarticular osteopenia with accompanying soft-tissue swelling. Mild to moderate synovitis is generally present.
II	Mild to moderate joint space reduction with minimal or no architectural distortion. Recalcitrant synovitis that cannot be managed with nonsteroidal anti-inflammatory medications alone.
III	Variable reduction in joint space with or without cyst formation. Architectural alteration, such as thinning of the olecranon or resorption of the trochlea or capitellum. Synovitis is variable and may be quiescent.
IV	Extensive articular damage with loss of subchondral bone and subluxation or ankylosis of the joint. Synovitis may be minimal.

Data obtained from Morrey BF, Adams RA: Semiconstrained arthroplasty for the treatment of rheumatoid arthritis. *J Bone Joint Surg Am* 1992;74:479-490.

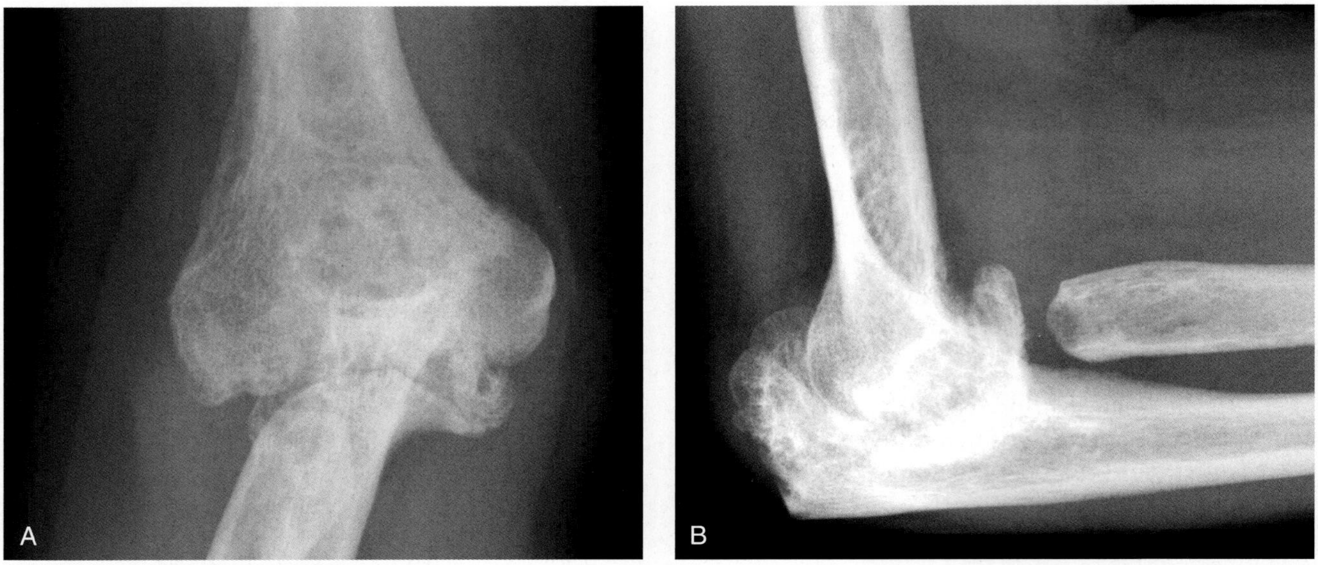

Figure 3 AP (**A**) and lateral (**B**) radiographs show an elbow with Larsen stage 5 rheumatoid arthritis.

E. Treatment

1. Nonsurgical

   a. The medical management of the systemic and joint pathology with disease-modifying antirheumatic medications should be optimized. This requires collaborative effort with a rheumatologist.

   b. Resting splints during the day and/or night may be useful.

   c. Intra-articular steroid injections also may be useful for temporary pain relief.

2. Surgical indications

   a. Patients with Larsen stage 1 or 2 radiographs (Mayo grade I or II) are candidates for a synovectomy with or without radial head resection if the pain cannot be controlled with medical management.

   b. In Larsen stages 3 through 5 in elderly individuals, surgical consideration should be geared toward total elbow arthroplasty (**Figure 3** and **4**).

   c. Historically, rheumatoid arthritis was the primary indication for total elbow arthroplasty, but its use has decreased with improved medical treatment.

3. Elbow implants—The bearing surfaces of elbow arthroplasty implants are highly variable. Most implants are semiconstrained to allow some buffering of forces across the articulation. The two basic types of elbow implants are linked and unlinked prostheses.

   a. Linked implants are joined by a “sloppy hinge” to allow for some varus and valgus laxity during range of motion of the elbow; early prosthetic loosening is a concern with these implants, especially in active patients.

   b. In unlinked implants, the humeral and ulnar components are not joined, and stability is provided by the surrounding soft tissues; instability is the main concern with this implant construct.

   c. In patients with inflammatory arthritis, the soft tissues often are attenuated, and the threshold for using a linked prosthesis is lower.

4. Contraindications for total elbow arthroplasty

   a. Active infection or Charcot joint disease is an absolute contraindication.

   b. Relative contraindications include active patients, patients younger than 65 years old, and patients without full neurologic control of the extremity.

5. Surgical procedures

   a. Radial head excision is controversial.

   b. Total elbow arthroplasty is indicated when loss of joint space and/or loss of normal joint architecture is present. A midline posterior elbow incision typically is used. Options for posterior elbow approaches include triceps splitting; triceps elevation, either medial

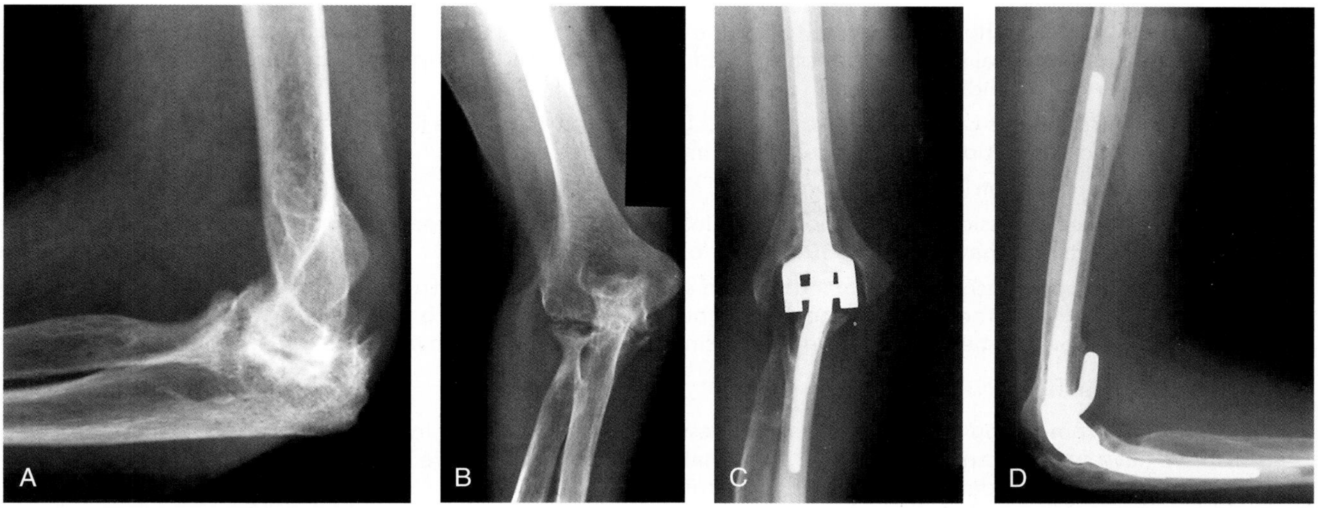

Figure 4 Lateral (**A**) and AP (**B**) preoperative radiographs depict an elbow with Larsen stage 5 rheumatoid arthritis. AP (**C**) and lateral (**D**) views obtained 6 years postoperatively show a satisfactory result following total elbow replacement. (Adapted from Morrey BF, O'Driscoll SW: Elbow arthritis, in Norris TR, ed: *Orthopaedic Knowledge Update: Shoulder and Elbow*. Rosemont, IL, American Academy of Orthopaedic Surgeons, 1997, pp 379-386.)

(classic Bryan and Morrey approach) or lateral; or the lateral paraolecranon triceps-on approach. The latter can prevent postoperative triceps rupture. Implant survival is less for total elbow arthroplasty than for hip or knee arthroplasty, with 20 year survival rates of 61% to 68%.

F. Complications

1. Complication rates as high as 43% have been reported for total elbow arthroplasty.
2. Arthroplasty complications include infection, instability, loosening, wound healing problems, ulnar neuropathy, and triceps insufficiency.
   a. Risk factors for infection include previous surgery involving the elbow, a previous infection of the elbow, psychiatric illness, severe RA, male sex, wound drainage, or a revision surgery on the elbow for any cause.
   b. Patients with postoperative *Staphylococcus epidermidis* infections are at high risk for recurrent infections.
   c. In acute infections consideration can be given to irrigation and débridement with component retention, although this has only a 50% success rate. A two-stage revision is recommended when treating chronically infected total elbow arthroplasties but has only a 50% rate of implantation of new components free of infection at final follow-up.
3. Instability is a complication of unlinked implants.
4. Loosening is a complication of linked implants.
5. Wound healing is an issue because the skin is typically of poor quality and atrophic as a result of long-term corticosteroid use.
6. Triceps insufficiency can cause pain and weakness.

TOP TESTING FACTS

Osteoarthritis

1. Symptomatic primary osteoarthritis of the elbow is relatively rare; men are affected more often than women (4:1 ratio).
2. Hand dominance and strenuous manual labor are associated with primary osteoarthritis of the elbow.
3. Patients typically present with loss of terminal flexion and extension and painful catching/clicking or locking of the elbow.

4. Radiographs typically show osteophyte formation at the coronoid process (anterior and medial), coronoid fossa, radial fossa, radial head, olecranon tip, and olecranon fossa. Joint spaces at the ulnohumeral joint is usually preserved or mildly narrowed.
5. Nonsurgical treatments can be effective for reducing symptoms but have limited effectiveness for improving range of motion limitations and pain related to impinging osteophytes.
6. Joint-sparing surgical procedures are preferred.
7. Ulnar nerve decompression/transposition and release of the posterior bundle of the MCL should be considered for patients who have less than 90° to 100° of elbow flexion.
8. Elbow arthroscopy is technically demanding, and several neurovascular structures that are at risk during the procedure include the radial, ulnar, and median nerves. However, unlike other joints, arthroscopic débridement in the elbow can be very effective at reducing symptoms and improving range of motion.

Inflammatory Arthritis

1. A thorough examination of the cervical spine is essential for all patients; many patients with rheumatoid arthritis have concomitant cervical spine abnormalities. Plain preoperative radiographs of the cervical spine should be obtained in patients scheduled for surgical procedures.
2. Patients with Larsen stage 1 or 2 radiographs (Mayo grade I or II) are candidates for a synovectomy with or without radial head resection if the pain cannot be controlled with medical management.
3. Total elbow arthroplasty is indicated primarily for patients with rheumatoid arthritis who are low demand and have Larsen stage 3 to 5 lesions.
4. Instability is a complication of unlinked implants.
5. Loosening is a complication of linked implants.
6. Complication rates for total elbow arthroplasty are high, and survival rates are lower than hip or knee arthroplasty, but many appropriately selected patients will experience substantial benefit from elbow arthroplasty.

Bibliography

Adams JE, King GJ, Steinmann SP, Cohen MS: Elbow arthroscopy: Indications, techniques, outcomes, and complications. *J Am Acad Orthop Surg* 2014;22(12):810-818.

Antuña SA, Morrey BF, Adams RA, O'Driscoll SW: Ulnohumeral arthroplasty for primary degenerative arthritis of the elbow: Long-term outcome and complications. *J Bone Joint Surg Am* 2002;84(12):2168-2173.

Frostick SP, Elsheikh AA, Mohammed AA, Wood A: Results of cementless total elbow arthroplasty using the discovery elbow system at a mean follow-up of 61.8 months. *J Shoulder Elbow Surg* 2017;26(8):1348-1354.

Kelly EW, Morrey BE, O'Driscoll SW: Complications of elbow arthroscopy. *J Bone Joint Surg* 2001;83:25-34.

Kim SJ, Kim JW, Lee SH, Choi JW: Retrospective comparative analysis of elbow arthroscopy used to treat primary osteoarthritis with and without release of the posterior band of the medial collateral ligament. *Arthroscopy* 2017;33(8):1506-1511.

Krukhaug Y, Hallan G, Dybvik E, Lie SA, Furnes ON: A survivorship study of 838 total elbow replacements: A report from the Norwegian Arthroplasty Register 1994–2016. *J Shoulder Elbow Surg* 2018;27(2):260-269.

Kwak JM, Kholinne E, Sun Y, Lim S, Koh KH, Jeon IH: Clinical outcome of osteocapsular arthroplasty for primary osteoarthritis of the elbow: Comparison of arthroscopic and open procedure. *Arthroscopy* 2019;35(4):1083-1089. pii:S0749-8063(18)31143-5. doi:10.1016/j.arthro.2018.11.057.

Nelson GN, Wu T, Galatz LM, Yamaguchi K, Keener JD: Elbow arthroscopy: Early complications and associated risk factors. *J Shoulder Elbow Surg* 2014;23:273-278.

Nishida K, Hashizume K, Nasu Y, et al: Mid-term results of alumina ceramic unlinked total elbow arthroplasty with cement fixation for patients with rheumatoid arthritis. *Bone Joint J* 2018;100-B(8):1066-1073.

Pham TT, Delclaux S, Huguet S, Wargny M, Bonnevaille N, Mansat P: Coonrad-Morrey total elbow arthroplasty for patients with rheumatoid arthritis: 54 prostheses reviewed at 7 years average follow-up (maximum, 16 years). *J Shoulder Elbow Surg* 2018;27(3):398-403.

Sanchez-Sotelo J, Baghdadi YMK, Morrey BF: Primary linked semiconstrained total elbow arthroplasty for rheumatoid arthritis: A single-institution experience with 461 elbows over three decades. *J Bone Joint Surg Am* 2016;98(20):1741-1748.

Zmistowski B, Pourjafari A, Padegimas EM, et al: Treatment of periprosthetic joint infection of the elbow: 15-year experience at a single institution. *J Shoulder Elbow Surg* 2018;27(9):1636-1641. doi:10.1016/j.jse.2018.05.035.

Chapter 83

Distal Biceps & Triceps Tendon Injuries

REZA OMID, MD

I. ANATOMY

A. Bicipital (radial) tuberosity—Lies on the opposite side of the radius in relation to the radial styloid; it has a mean length of 22 to 26 mm and a mean width of approximately 10.4 to 13.6 mm (**Figure 1**). The bicipital tuberosity has a protuberance just anterior to the biceps insertion that acts as a supination CAM. Maintenance of this tuberosity height may be important for supination strength.

B. Distal biceps tendon

1. The biceps tendon inserts on the posterior and ulnar margin of the radial tuberosity.
2. The long head of the distal tendon inserts on the proximal (and slightly more posterior) aspect of the footprint; the short head of the distal tendon inserts on the distal aspect of the tuberosity (**Figure 2**).
3. The average length of the biceps tendon insertion on the tuberosity is 15 to 21 mm, and the average width is approximately 3.5 mm, indicating that the tendon insertion does not occupy the entire bicipital tuberosity.
4. The distal insertion of the short head allows it to act as a more powerful flexor of the elbow (15% greater than the long head), and the slightly more posterior insertion of the long head on the tuberosity provides a greater lever arm for supination.
5. The tendon fibers of the distal biceps rotate predictably in the coronal plane (**Figure 3**). The short head is medial to the long head at the myotendinous junction. The distal biceps tendon then externally rotates 90° as it descends to the tuberosity. This rotation positions the short head distal to the long head on the footprint.

Dr. Omid or an immediate family member has received royalties from Integra and Medacta and serves as a paid consultant to or is an employee of Integra and Medacta.

C. The lacertus fibrosus usually originates from the distal short head of the biceps tendon and blends ulnarly with the fascia of the forearm. With forearm contraction, the lacertus fibrosus pulls the biceps tendon medially. An intact lacertus can prevent severe retraction of a torn distal biceps tendon.

II. EPIDEMIOLOGY

A. Rupture occurs most often in the dominant extremity of men between the ages of 40 and 60 years, but these injuries have been reported in women as well.

B. The mechanism of injury is typically an eccentric load applied to the biceps. Usually, an unexpected extension force is applied to the elbow in 90° of flexion.

C. Smokers have a risk of injury that is 7.5 times greater than nonsmokers.

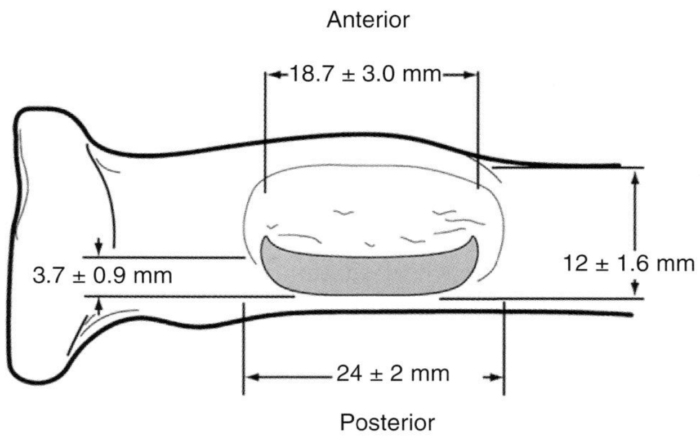

Figure 1 Illustration depicts the footprint of the distal biceps tendon on the bicipital tuberosity. Note that most of the tuberosity is uncovered. (Reproduced from Hutchinson HL, Gloystein D, Gillespie M: Distal biceps tendon insertion: An anatomic study. *J Shoulder Elbow Surg* 2008;17:342-346.)

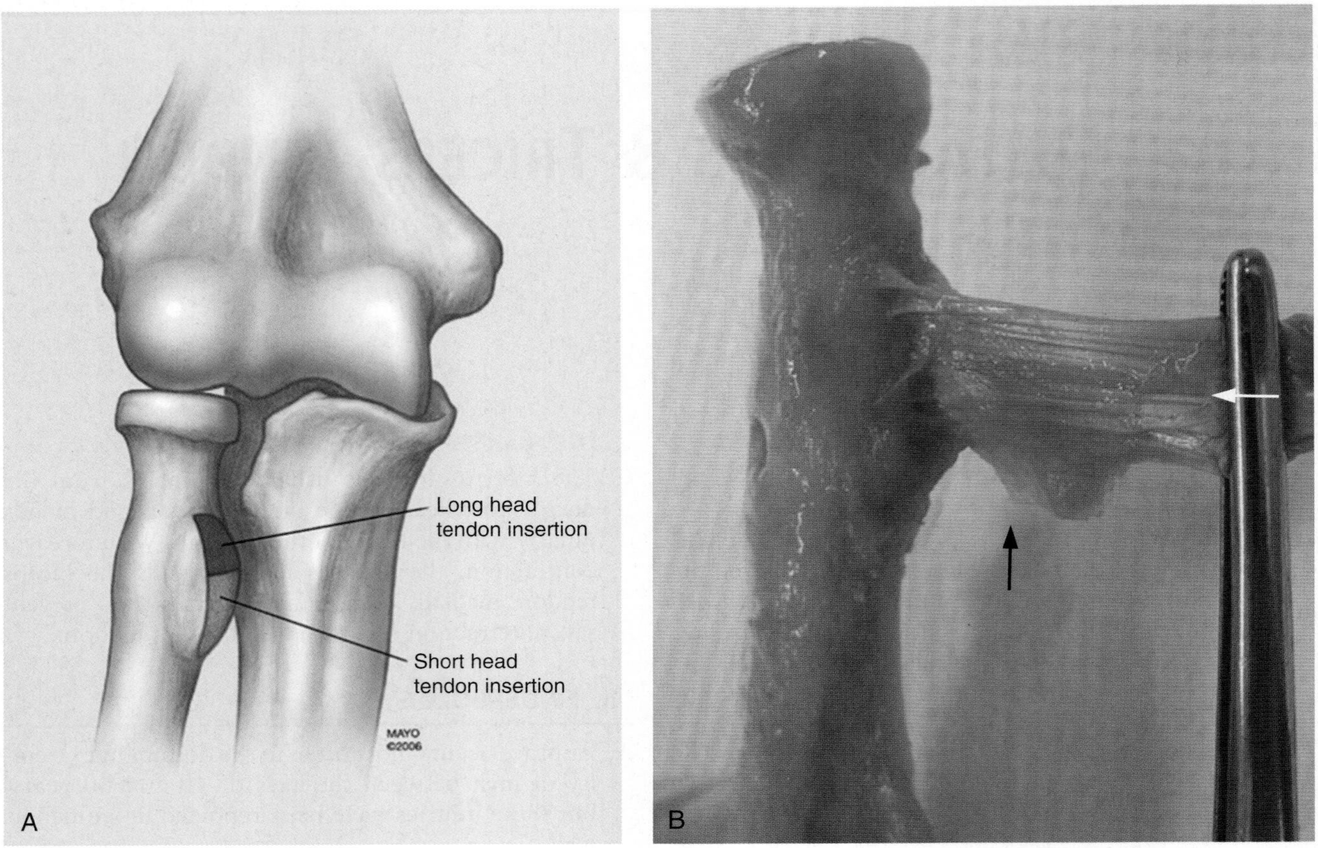

Figure 2 **A**, Illustration shows the insertion points of the distal biceps tendon on the bicipital tuberosity. The short head inserts more distal on the tuberosity than does the long head. **B**, In this photograph of cadaver specimen, the short head is detached and a demarcation can be seen between the long head and the short head of the tendon. Black arrow identifies the detached short head and the white arrow identifies the demarcation. (Reproduced from Athwal GS, Steinmann SP, Rispoli DM: The distal biceps tendon: Footprint and relevant clinical anatomy. *J Hand Surg Am* 2007;32:1225-1229.)

III. PATHOANATOMY

A. The tendon of the distal biceps muscle most commonly avulses off the radial tuberosity with a small amount of remnant tendon, but injury can also occur at the musculotendinous junction or midtendon.

B. Complete avulsions of the distal biceps tendon are thought to be more common than partial tears, but the exact incidence of partial tears is unknown.

C. Proposed mechanisms for rupture of the tendon include the hypovascularity of the tendon (**Figure 4**), mechanical impingement between the radial tuberosity and the ulna, inflammation of the bursa surrounding the tendon, and intrinsic degeneration.

D. The distance between the lateral border of the ulna and the radial tuberosity is 48% less with the forearm fully pronated than it is in full supination, supporting a mechanical etiology.

E. A commonly associated factor for tendon rupture is the use of anabolic steroids with a risk for a first tendon rupture is nine times higher.

F. Partial tears can occur on the undersurface of the tendon (radial surface), where spurring occurs. Isolated ruptures of the short head of the bifurcated biceps tendon have been described. Degenerative intratendinous ganglion formation is seen in approximately 30% of partial tears.

IV. EVALUATION

A. History

1. Patients report a sudden, sharp, tearing pain, often followed by ecchymosis and deformity within the muscle (reverse Popeye sign).

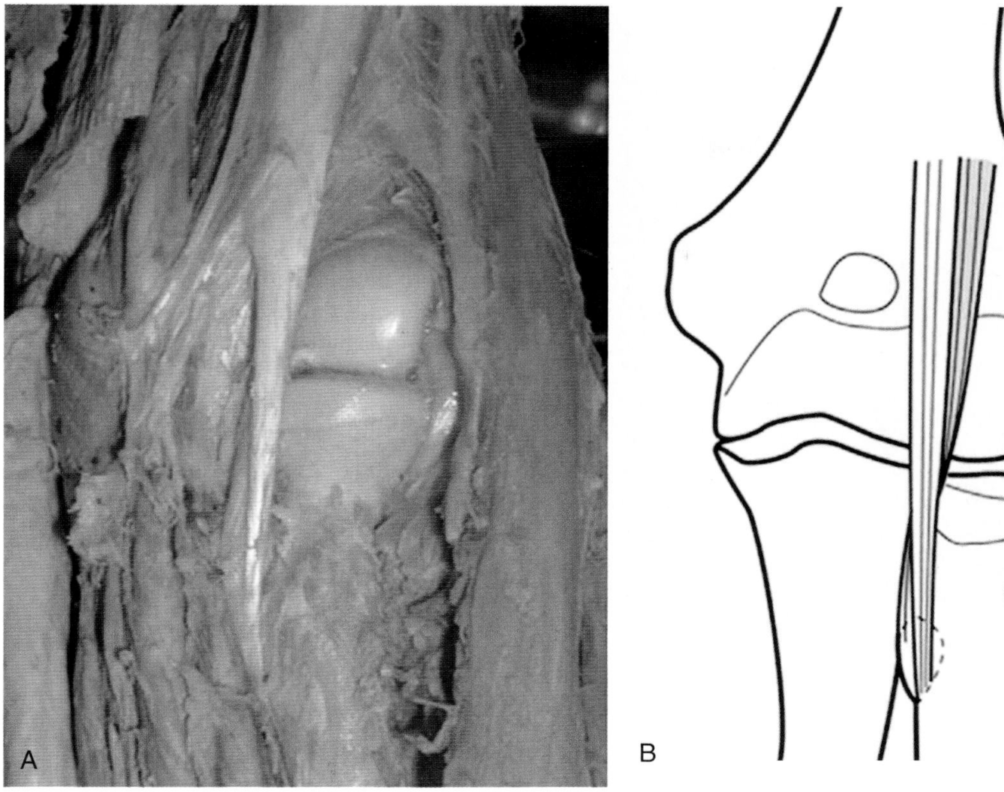

Figure 3 Photograph of cadaver specimen (**A**) and illustration (**B**) show the predictable external rotation of the distal biceps tendon. (Reproduced from Kulshreshtha R, Singh R, Sinha J, Hall S: Anatomy of the distal biceps brachii tendon and its clinical relevance. *Clin Orthop Relat Res* 2007;456:117-120.)

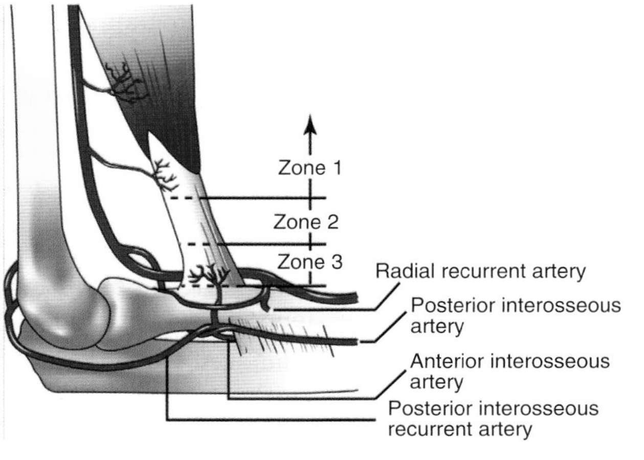

Figure 4 Illustration depicts the vascularity of the distal biceps tendon. Zone 1, a watershed zone, is where ruptures typically occur, Zone 2 is avascular, and Zone 3 is vascularized. (Reproduced from Miyamoto RG, Elser F, Millett PJ: Distal biceps tendon injuries. *J Bone Joint Surg Am* 2010:92:2128-2138.)

2. Supination weakness may be significant initially; however, it can improve with time. Flexion weakness is reported less commonly because of the intact brachialis, which is the predominant flexor of the arm. The patient should be asked about supination-specific activities.
3. Patients with partial tears may not describe an acute event but may instead report an insidious onset of anterior elbow pain.

B. Physical examination
1. Antecubital ecchymosis and tenderness may be present.
2. Proximal retraction of the biceps muscle is usually evident.
3. The hook test is performed by using the index finger to "hook" the tendon from the lateral side of the elbow.
4. The biceps squeeze test is similar to the Thompson test for Achilles tendon rupture. Squeezing the biceps should elicit supination with an intact tendon.

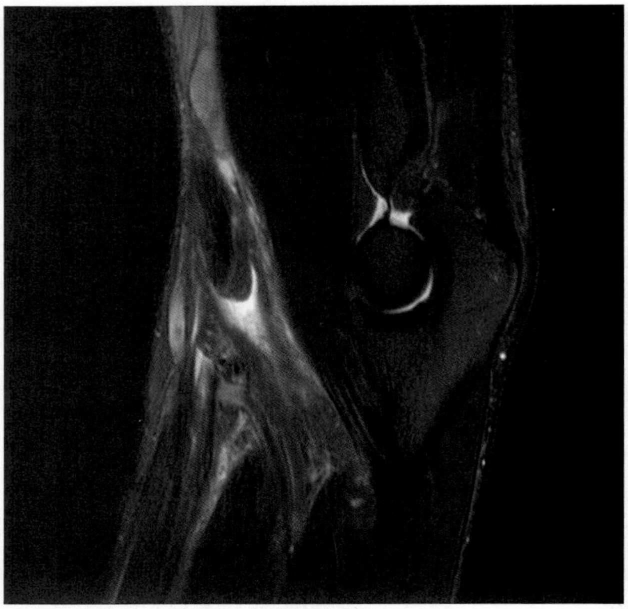

Figure 5 Sagittal T2-weighted fat-saturated MRI demonstrates a rupture of the distal biceps tendon anterior to the brachialis muscle, with edema tracking along the path of injury. (Courtesy of the University of Southern California Department of Radiology.)

5. The strength of elbow flexion and supination should be evaluated. In complete disruptions, supination is usually weak. With partial ruptures, supination strength is maintained but is often painful. Terminal supination is preferentially affected because the supinator muscle's moment arm decreases between neutral and terminal supination. A terminal supination lag sign may also be helpful.

C. Imaging

1. Plain radiographs are usually normal; however, hypertrophic changes at the radial tuberosity can be suggestive of a chronic tendon enthesopathy.
2. MRI is helpful in confirming the diagnosis (**Figure 5**), especially when the lacertus fibrosus is still intact. The flexed abducted supinated (FABS) position can be used to better visualize the biceps tendon on MRI. MRI may also be helpful in diagnosing a musculotendinous junction rupture.
3. Ultrasonography can be useful but is operator dependent.

V. TREATMENT

A. Nonsurgical

1. Nonsurgical treatment of distal biceps tendon ruptures can be recommended for very low-demand patients or those not medically fit for surgery. Nonsurgical treatment can yield acceptable outcomes, with modestly reduced strength and endurance and little or no pain.
2. Biomechanical studies has shown that supination strength will decrease up to 40%, and flexion strength will decrease up to 30% with loss of biceps function.
3. Fatigue or lack of endurance with supination and loss of terminal supination are the most common functional deficits noticed by patients treated nonsurgically.

B. Surgical

1. Most complete ruptures are treated surgically.
2. Indications
   a. The primary indication for repair is a complete rupture of the distal biceps tendon. Repair aims to prevent chronic pain and weakness in young, active patients with heavy occupational or recreational demands.
   b. Another surgical indication is a partial tear of the distal biceps that has failed to respond to nonsurgical measures. This is typically seen if the tear involves >50% of the tendon fibers.
3. Relative contraindications
   a. Repair of a distal biceps rupture may not be indicated in medically unfit patients with low functional demands.
   b. Primary repair should be cautiously attempted in chronic tears that have significant retraction and scarring. In these situations, consideration should be given to autograft/allograft reconstruction.
   c. Musculotendinous ruptures should generally be treated nonsurgically.

C. Surgical procedures

1. General considerations
   a. Anatomic repair to the biceps tuberosity is preferred over nonanatomic repair to the brachialis, to restore supination strength.
   b. Modern fixation techniques with transosseous tunnels, suture anchors, cortical buttons, and interference screws all provide adequate fixation to allow early range of motion. Biomechanical studies have shown cortical buttons to be mechanically superior to suture anchors and interference screws; however, clinical studies has failed to show a difference in rerupture rates.

c. A delay (>6 to 8 weeks) in surgical management of retracted tears may require tendon grafting because of fixed contracture of the biceps muscle, but the precise definition of chronic tears as well as the requirements for grafting have not been clearly defined.

2. Partial tears

a. Most partial tears with less than 50% involvement of the tendon seen on MRI can be treated nonsurgically.

b. If symptoms persist, the tear can be completed, débrided, and repaired back to the tuberosity.

3. Single-incision repair

a. Historically, distal biceps ruptures were repaired through a single extensile anterior incision. A high incidence of neurovascular injuries as well as loss of supination strength resulting from nonanatomic repairs led to the development of two-incision techniques.

b. More recently, less invasive single-incision techniques have regained popularity due to the use of modern tendon fixation techniques.

c. Tendon to bone fixation can be accomplished with suture anchors, a cortical button, and/or interference screws but clinical studies have failed to show a difference in rerupture rates.

4. Two-incision repair

a. The original two-incision technique was complicated by heterotopic ossification and radioulnar synostosis, so a modified muscle-splitting two-incision technique (**Figure 6**) was proposed, which reduced the incidence of synostosis. Instead of elevating the anconeus and possibly violating the ulnar periosteum, the modified two-incision technique splits the muscle fibers of the extensor carpi ulnaris (ECU) or extensor digitorum communis (EDC) as well as the supinator. However, splitting the supinator muscle can lead to postoperative fatty infiltration of the supinator muscle (seen on MRI), which has been associated with loss of supination strength postoperatively.

b. Tendon fixation with double-incision repairs usually is accomplished creating a bone trough and heavy sutures placed in transosseous bone tunnels. Maintenance of the tuberosity height during repairs was found to be associated with improved supination strength (due to maintenance of the anterior protuberance which acts like a supination CAM).

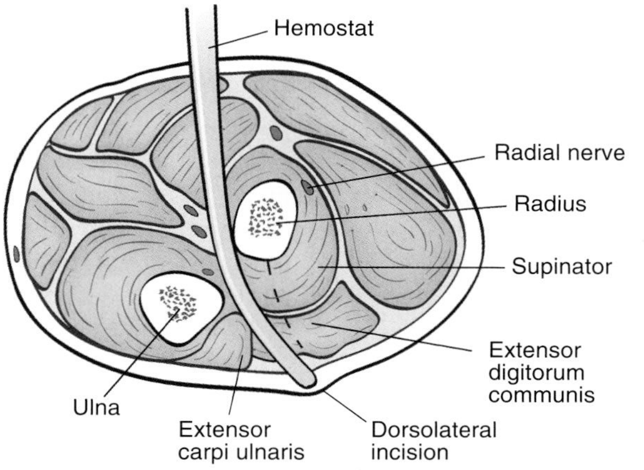

Figure 6 Illustration depicts the muscle-splitting two-incision approach. Notice that the tips of the hemostat are turned away from the ulna to prevent contact with the periosteum. This technique is used instead of the subperiosteal technique to prevent the formation of heterotopic ossification and subsequent radioulnar synostosis. (Reproduced from Kelly EW, Morrey BF, O'Driscoll SW: Complications of repair of the distal biceps tendon with the modified two-incision technique. *J Bone Joint Surg Am* 2000;82:1575-1581.)

Therefore, the classic bone trough used for anatomic two-incision repairs has been called into question recently.

c. Two-incision repairs may allow a better recreation of the anatomic location of tendon attachment on the posterior aspect of the radial tuberosity.

5. Chronic tears

a. Anatomic direct repair can generally be attempted up to 6 to 8 weeks after injury; however, this time frame is poorly defined.

b. Reconstruction of chronic retracted tears have been performed using semitendinosus autograft/allograft, acellular dermal allograft, and Achilles allograft.

c. Nonanatomic repair of the distal biceps tendon to the brachialis muscle was historically recommended but will fail to restore supination strength and generally should not be performed.

6. Outcomes

a. Both single-incision and two-incision techniques are effective at restoring elbow flexion and supination strength, with no significant difference in outcomes.

b. Biomechanical studies have demonstrated the importance of proper anatomic restoration of the tuberosity footprint.

c. Most studies demonstrate a restoration of strength and endurance to within 90% of normal compared with the opposite limb.

d. A randomized prospective study comparing single- and two-incision distal biceps repair showed slightly greater (10%) final flexion strength with two-incision repair and a higher rate (40% vs 7%) of transient lateral antebrachial cutaneous nerve injuries with single-incision repair.

e. Factors associated with loss of supination strength after distal biceps repair include

- Nonanatomic anterior site of the tendon
- Decreased height of the radial tuberosity
- Supinator muscle fatty infiltration

7. Complications

a. Tendon reruptures are uncommon (0%-5%) and typically occur within the first 2 to 3 weeks and are rare after 6 weeks.

b. The two most common complications are transient nerve injuries (most commonly the lateral antebrachial cutaneous nerve) and the formation of heterotopic bone, which may or may not limit forearm rotation.

c. Injury to the lateral antebrachial cutaneous nerve can occur with either technique but is more common with the single-incision technique, due to deep retraction on the radial side of the wound.

d. The incidence of posterior interosseous nerve (PIN) palsy after single-incision distal biceps repairs was 3.2% in one study and typically resolved by 3 months post-op. A recent study looking at 784 repairs found that PIN palsy was more common with the two-incision technique. A cadaveric study demonstrated that the use of a cortical button in combination with a two-incision technique jeopardizes the PIN due to the trajectory of the exiting drill holes in relation to the nerve.

e. Radioulnar synostosis and heterotopic ossification have been reported with the single-incision technique as well but studies consistently show higher rates with the two-incision technique.

f. The use of indomethacin (75 mg) for up to 6 weeks postoperatively was found to significantly reduce (37% vs 1%) the incidence of radioulnar synostosis after distal biceps repair without any adverse events.

VI. REHABILITATION

A. Contemporary fixation techniques provide sufficient fixation strength to allow early motion of the elbow and forearm.

B. Generally, a brief period of immobilization is followed by progressive range of motion exercises. Strengthening is usually delayed until 2 to 3 months postoperatively.

VII. DISTAL TRICEPS TENDON INJURIES

Distal Triceps Tendon Ruptures

Anatomy

A. The triceps brachii muscle is the primary extensor of the elbow joint.

B. The mean length of the superficial triceps tendon is 15.2 cm (range, 13.3 to 17.1 cm) measured from the tip of the olecranon to the most proximal extent of the tendon medially.

C. The distal aspect of the extensor tendon is more expansive laterally, where fibers of the triceps fascia blend with the brachioradialis and common wrist extensors. This lateral triceps expansion is continuous with the superficial fascia of the anconeus muscle and antebrachial fascia inserting into the radial aspect of the proximal ulna distally.

D. The medial triceps tendon inserts directly into the medial aspect of the olecranon process without expansion (**Figure 7**).

E. The medial aspect of the tendon is thicker than the lateral aspect and consistently shows a distinct, thickened, rolled tendon edge medially.

F. The mean medial to lateral width of the tendon insertional footprint is 20.9 mm (or 78% maximal width of the olecranon).

G. The mean proximal to distal maximum length of the tendon footprint is 13.4 mm.

H. The mean length from the tip of the olecranon process to the most proximal aspect of the tendon insertion near the curved apex of the olecranon is 14.8 mm.

Pathophysiology

A. Most common mechanism of injury is a sudden eccentric load to a contracting triceps muscle, such as a fall onto an outstretched arm.

B. Ruptures most commonly occur at the tendon-bone insertion, but muscle belly ruptures and tears at the musculotendinous junction also occur.

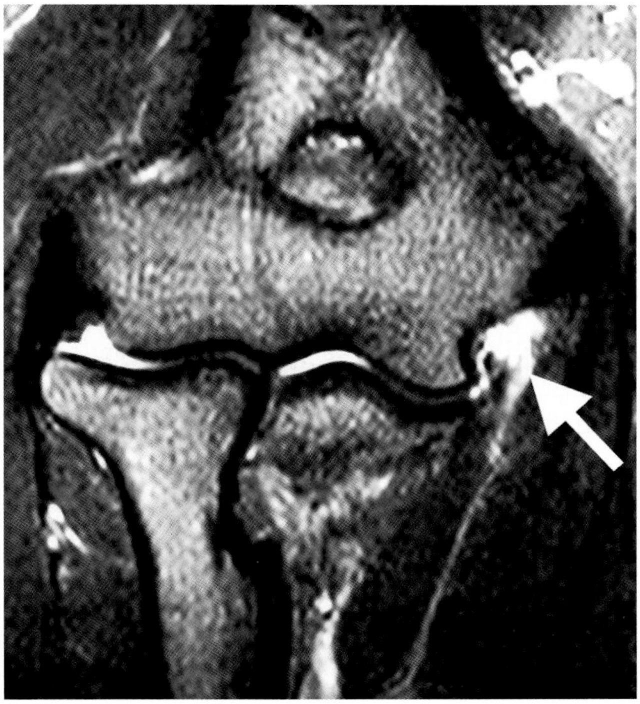

Figure 2 MRI of the elbow demonstrates a medial collateral ligament tear (arrow). (Reproduced with permission from Ahmad CS, ElAttrache NS: MUCL reconstruction in the overhead athlete. *Techniques in Orthopaedics* 2006;21(4):290-298.)

c. Magnetic resonance arthrography enhanced with intra-articular gadolinium improves the diagnosis of partial undersurface tears.

d. Dynamic ultrasonography can help detect increased laxity with valgus stress; however, the diagnostic quality of the results is operator dependent.

C. Treatment

1. Nonsurgical treatment includes a period of rest from throwing. Flexor-pronator strengthening and optimization of throwing mechanics is followed by a progressive throwing program or reduced throwing demands.

2. Surgical

a. Indications—Failure of nonsurgical treatment; patients must be willing to undergo the extensive postoperative rehabilitation program.

- Although controversial, MCL repair may be considered in amateur overhead athletes when MRI imaging demonstrates an avulsion of the ligament from either the sublime tubercle or medial epicondyle with good to normal ligament tissue quality.

b. Contraindications—Asymptomatic athletes with low valgus demands on the elbow (often minimally symptomatic) and patients who cannot or are unwilling to undergo the extensive postoperative rehabilitation program.

3. Surgical procedures

a. Surgical techniques currently used for MCL reconstruction include the modified Jobe technique (**Figure 3**, A), the docking technique (**Figure 3**, B), and the hybrid interference screw technique (**Figure 3**, C).

b. A muscle-splitting approach is preferred, to limit morbidity to the flexor-pronator mass.

c. Ulnar nerve transposition is reserved for patients with subluxating nerves or motor weakness.

d. MCL repair with or without internal brace augmentation has shown to provide encouraging results with less invasive surgery and faster rehabilitation. However, current research is limited and further studies with longer-term follow-up are needed.

D. Complications include ulnar nerve or medial antebrachial cutaneous nerve injury, ulnar or epicondylar fracture, elbow stiffness, and failure to achieve the preinjury level of throwing ability.

E. Pearls and pitfalls

1. Ulnar nerve complications can occur.

2. The medial antebrachial cutaneous nerve lies at the distal aspect of the incision.

F. Rehabilitation

1. Active wrist, elbow, and shoulder ROM exercises are initiated early in the postoperative period.

2. Strengthening exercises begin 4 to 6 weeks postoperatively, but valgus stress is avoided until 4 months after surgery.

3. A progressive throwing program is initiated 4 months postoperatively.

4. A return to competitive throwing is permitted 1 year after surgery if the shoulder, elbow, and forearm are pain free and full ROM has returned.

G. Surgical outcomes

1. Surgical outcomes are generally good with an overall return to sport rate for MCL reconstruction of 86% with a 10.4% complication rate (transient ulnar neuritis is the most frequent complication).

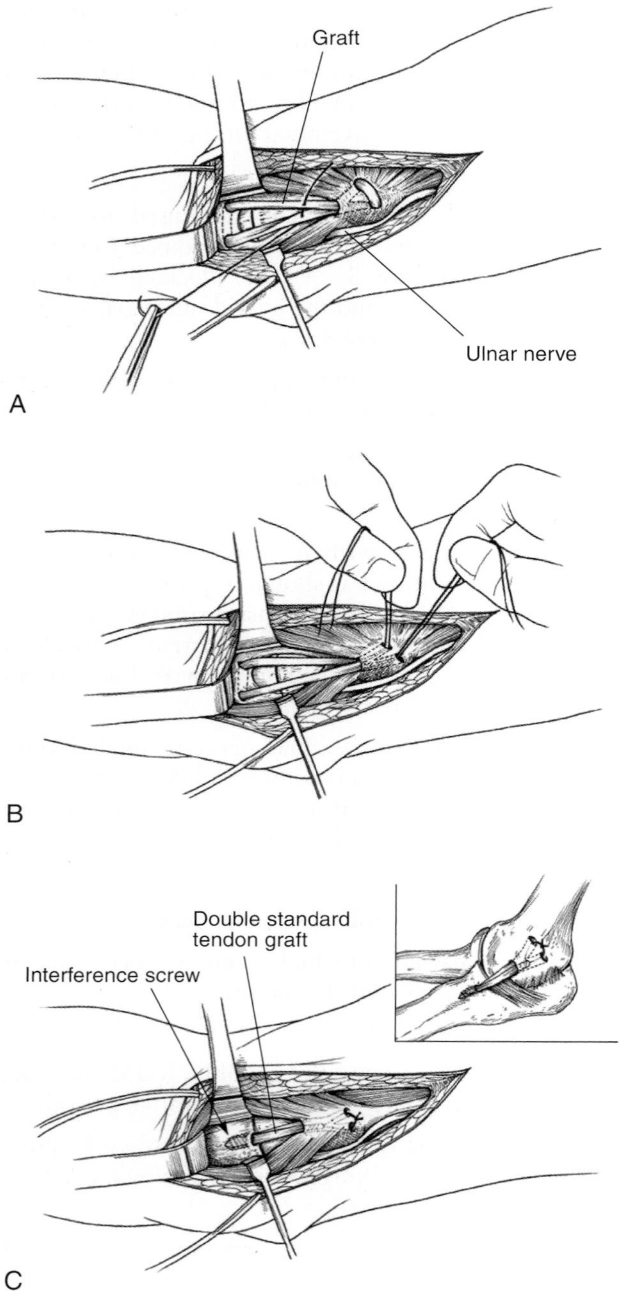

Figure 3 Drawings show the surgical techniques for medial collateral ligament reconstruction. **A**, Modified Jobe technique with muscle-splitting approach, figure-of-8 reconstruction, and ulnar nerve in situ. **B**, Docking technique with graft limbs tensioned into the humeral docking tunnel. **C**, Hybrid reconstruction technique with interference screw fixation on the ulna and docking fixation on the humerus. (Panel **A** adapted with permission from Kvitne RS, Jobe FW: Ligamentous and posterior compartment injuries, in Jobe FW, ed: *Operative Techniques in Upper Extremity Sports Injuries*. St. Louis, MO, Mosby, 1996, pp 411-430. Panels **B** and **C** reproduced from Ahmad CS, ElAttrache NS: Elbow valgus instability in the throwing athlete. *J Am Acad Orthop Surg* 2006;14:693-700.)

6 | Shoulder and Elbow

2. Concomitant flexor-pronator mass tear, ulnohumeral chondromalacia, and native MCL ligament calcification are all associated with inferior outcomes and lower return to sport rates following MCL reconstruction.
3. MCL repair with internal brace augmentation has recently shown to provide early promising results (92% return to play at a mean of 6.7 months) in carefully selected throwers.

III. VALGUS EXTENSION OVERLOAD SYNDROME AND POSTERIOR IMPINGEMENT

A. Epidemiology and overview
   1. During throwing, the olecranon is repeatedly and forcefully driven into the olecranon fossa, exerting shear forces on the medial aspect of the olecranon tip and the olecranon fossa. This process may cause cartilage injury and the development of osteophytes.
   2. Medial ligamentous laxity commonly exacerbates the condition.
   3. This constellation of injuries is called valgus extension overload syndrome.

B. Pathoanatomy
   1. The pathoanatomy of valgus extension overload syndrome includes chondrosis, osteophyte development on the posteromedial olecranon and humerus, and loose bodies.
   2. The ulnohumeral articulation contributes to elbow stability. Olecranon resection increases valgus angulation and MCL strain during valgus stress.

C. Evaluation
   1. History
      a. Patients report posteromedial elbow pain that occurs during the deceleration phase of throwing as the elbow reaches terminal extension. Pain may also occur during acceleration.
      b. Loss of terminal elbow extension may occur.
   2. Physical examination
      a. Crepitus and tenderness over the posteromedial olecranon may be noted.
      b. Pain is reproduced when the elbow is forced into extension.
      c. Elbow flexion contracture may be seen.
   3. Imaging
      a. AP, lateral, oblique, and axillary views of the elbow may reveal posteromedial olecranon osteophytes and/or loose bodies.

b. CT with two-dimensional reconstruction and three-dimensional surface rendering best visualizes the pathology.

c. MRI may be most helpful in evaluating associated injuries including partial or complete tears of the MCL.

D. Treatment

1. Nonsurgical

a. Activity modification with a period of rest from throwing, intra-articular corticosteroid injections, NSAIDs, and course of dedicated flexor-pronator muscle strengthening.

b. Pitching instruction should be started to correct flaws in pitching technique that may contribute to the injury.

2. Surgical

a. Indications—Patients who continue to have symptoms in spite of nonsurgical treatment.

b. Contraindications—MCL insufficiency is a relative contraindication for isolated olecranon débridement.

3. Surgical procedures

a. Diagnostic elbow arthroscopy, removal of osteophytes on the posteromedial aspect of the olecranon, removal of loose bodies, and débridement of chondromalacia.

b. To prevent increased strain on the MCL, it is important to remove only the osteophyte and not the normal olecranon.

4. Complications—Overaggressive olecranon resection may result in valgus instability of the elbow.

E. Surgical outcomes

1. Surgical outcomes are generally good with a cited return to sport rate for arthroscopic posteromedial decompression between 68% and 85%.

2. Careful evaluation of possible concomitant MCL injury is required, as treating the secondary effects of MCL insufficiency without treating the underlying MCL pathology will lead to unsatisfactory results and an increased revision surgery rate.

TOP TESTING FACTS

1. OCD must be differentiated from Panner disease. OCD is more common in skeletally immature athletes who engage in repetitive activities, such as throwing or gymnastics.
2. Physical examination findings in capitellum OCD include lateral elbow tenderness, crepitus, and often a 15° to 20° flexion contracture.
3. Initial treatment of stable OCD lesions includes activity modification, avoidance of throwing or related sports, NSAIDs, and, occasionally, a short period of immobilization for acute symptoms.
4. Unstable OCD lesions with gross mechanical symptoms require surgical repair.
5. The anterior oblique ligament of the MCL complex is the strongest and is the primary stabilizer to valgus stress. The ligament originates on the anterior-inferior edge of the medial epicondyle and inserts on the sublime tubercle of the ulna.
6. Valgus torque generated at the elbow during throwing maneuvers is highest in the late cocking and early acceleration phases of throwing.
7. Patients with MCL injuries report medial elbow pain during the acceleration phase of throwing; pain may occur only when throwing at more than 50% to 75% of maximal effort.
8. Surgical techniques currently used for MCL reconstruction include the modified Jobe technique, the docking technique, and the hybrid interference screw technique. A muscle-splitting approach is preferred, to limit morbidity to the flexor-pronator mass.
9. Ulnar nerve transposition is reserved for patients with subluxating nerves or motor weakness.
10. Patients with valgus extension overload report posteromedial elbow pain that occurs during the deceleration phase of throwing as the elbow reaches terminal extension. Pain during acceleration also may occur.

Bibliography

Ahmad CS, Park MC, Elattrache NS: Elbow medial ulnar collateral ligament insufficiency alters posteromedial olecranon contact. *Am J Sports Med* 2004;32(7):1607-1612.

Baumgarten TE, Andrews JR, Satterwhite YE: The arthroscopic classification and treatment of osteochondritis dissecans of the capitellum. *Am J Sports Med* 1998;26(4):520-523.

Bruce JR, Andrews JR: Ulnar collateral ligament injuries in the throwing athlete. *J Am Acad Orthop Surg* 2014;22(5):315-325.

Clain JB, Vitale MA, Ahmad CS, Ruchelsman DE: Ulnar nerve complications after ulnar collateral ligament reconstruction of the elbow: A systematic review. *Am J Sports Med* 2019;47(5):1263-1269.

Churchill RW, Munoz J, Ahmad CS: Osteochondritis dissecans of the elbow. *Curr Rev Musculoskelet Med* 2016;9(2):232-239.

Dugas JR, Looze CA, Capogna B, et al: Ulnar collateral ligament repair with collagen-dipped fibertape augmentation in overhead-throwing athletes. *Am J Sports Med* 2019;47(5):1996-1102.

Erickson BJ, Chalmers PN, Bush-Joseph CA, Verma NN, Romeo AA: Ulnar collateral ligament reconstruction of the elbow: A systematic review of the literature. *Orthop J Sports Med* 2015;3(12):1-7.

Park JY, Yoo HY, Chung SW, et al: Valgus extension overload syndrome in adolescent baseball players: Clinical characteristics and surgical outcomes. *J Shoulder Elbow Surg* 2016;25(12):2048-2056.

Paulino FE, Villacis DC, Ahmad CS: Valgus extension overload in baseball players. *Am J Orthop (Belle Mead NJ)* 2016;45(3):144-151.

Thompson WH, Jobe FW, Yocum LA, Pink MM: Ulnar collateral ligament reconstruction in athletes: Muscle-splitting approach without transposition of the ulnar nerve. *J Shoulder Elbow Surg* 2001;10(2):152-157.

Westermann RW, Hancock KJ, Buckwalter JA, Kopp B, Glass N, Wolf BR: Return to sport after operative management of osteochondritis dissecans of the capitellum: A systematic review and meta-analysis. *Orthop J Sports Med.* 2016;4(6):1-8.

Chapter 85
DISORDERS OF THE SCAPULA

REZA OMID, MD

I. ANATOMY

A. The scapulothoracic articulation consists of muscles and bursae that lie between the scapula and thoracic cage to allow for smooth shoulder motion.

B. The scapula typically spans the second to seventh ribs and has three borders (medial, lateral, and inferior).

C. Approximately 6% of scapulae have a hooked shape prominence known as *Luschka tubercle* at the superomedial angle.

D. The suprascapular notch is located at the lateral portion of the superior scapular border near the base of the coracoid process. The transverse scapular ligament extends across the notch, with the suprascapular artery lying above the ligament and the suprascapular nerve running below the ligament. The spinoglenoid notch lies below the lateral border of the scapular spine with the suprascapular artery and nerve passing through it. Variability of the spinoglenoid ligament (inferior transverse scapular ligament) exists.

E. Movement at the scapulothoracic articulation is dictated by the coordinated effort between several muscles as there is no direct bony attachment to the chest wall beyond the clavicle through the acromioclavicular and sternoclavicular joints. While a total of 17 muscles are known to attach to the scapula, several are directly involved at the scapulothoracic articulation.

F. Three muscle layers have been described: superficial, intermediate, and deep (**Figure 1**).

   1. Superficial layer:
      a. Trapezius: inserts on the scapular spine and acromion and helps laterally rotate the scapula to elevate the acromion for shoulder elevation
      b. Latissimus dorsi: some have aberrant attachments to the inferior angle of the scapula

   2. Intermediate layer:
      a. Levator scapulae: inserts on the superomedial angle of the scapula elevates and anteriorly tilts the scapula
      b. Rhomboid major: inserts on the medial border of the scapula from the level of the scapular spine and below. Medially rotates the scapula.
      c. Rhomboid minor: insert on the medial border of the scapula above the rhomboid major. Medially rotates the scapula.

   3. Deep layer: provides a cushion between the scapula and the thoracic wall
      a. Serratus anterior: originates from the upper 8-9 ribs and inserts on the entire medial border of the scapula. Very important scapular stabilizer, which fixes the position of the scapula to the chest wall, allowing for a stable fulcrum during arm elevation.
      b. Subscapularis: originates from the medial scapular body anteriorly and inserts on the lesser tuberosity of the humerus, medial to the bicipital groove

G. Two anatomic (major) and four adventitial (minor) bursae at the scapulothoracic articulation have been described (**Figure 2**). The two anatomic (major) bursae include the infraserratus (scapulothoracic) bursa and the supraserratus (subscapularis) bursa.

H. The *spinal accessory nerve* runs in the posterior triangle of the neck between the posterior border of the sternocleidomastoid and the anterior border of the upper trapezius. It then travels with the superficial branch of the transverse cervical artery along the central aspect of the levator scapulae and deep to the trapezius.

I. The *dorsal scapular nerve* and artery lie deep to the levator scapulae and rhomboid minor and major and courses approximately 2 to 3 cm medial to the vertebral border of the scapula.

J. The *long thoracic nerve* courses along the anterior margin of the serratus anterior.

Dr. Omid or an immediate family member has received royalties from Integra and Medacta and serves as a paid consultant to or is an employee of Integra and Medacta.

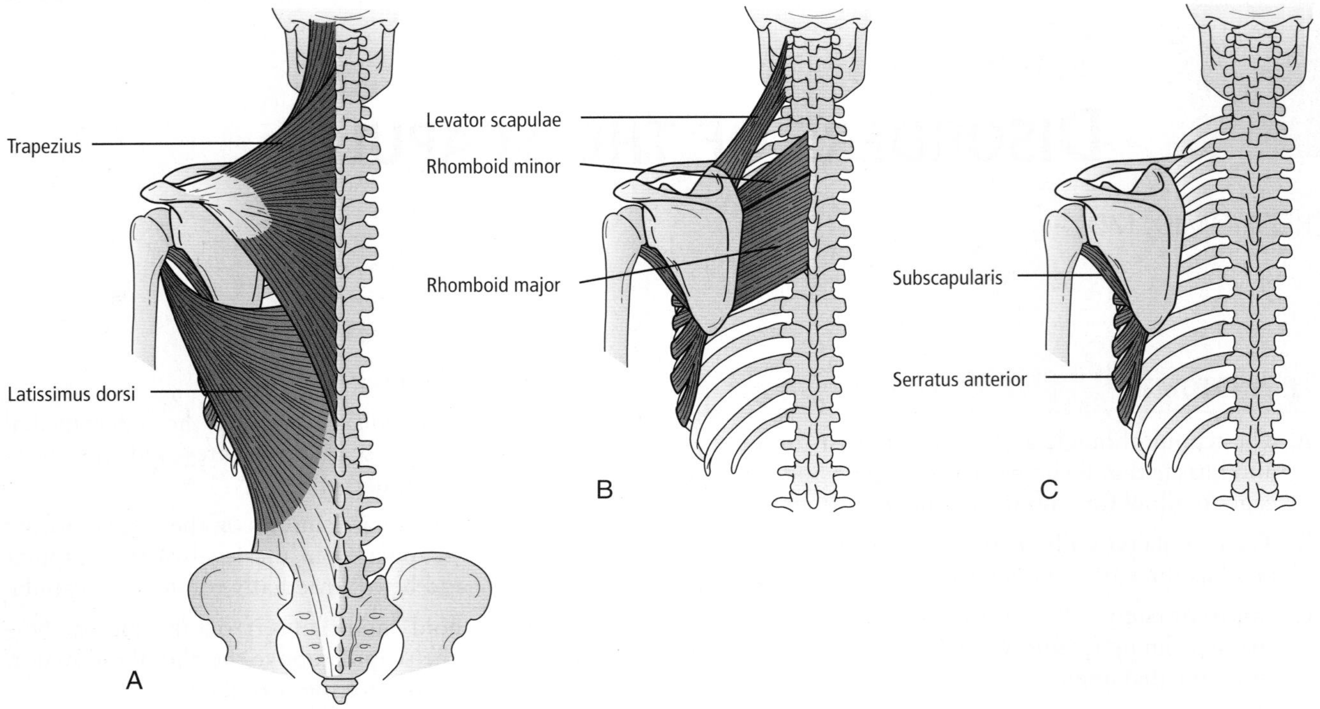

Figure 1 Illustrations showing the three muscle layers that have been described surrounding the scapula—**(A)** superficial: trapezius and latissimus dorsi; **(B)** intermediate: levatore scapulae, rhomboid major, and rhomboid minor; **(C)** deep: subscapularis and serratus anterior.

K. The *suprascapular nerve* (C5/6) originates from the superior trunk of the brachial plexus and courses toward the suprascapular notch with the suprascapular artery.

1. There are three scapular motions (retraction/protraction, lateral/medial rotation, anterior/posterior tilt) (**Figure 3**).
2. The ratio of glenohumeral to scapulothoracic motion during shoulder abduction is 2:1.
3. As the arm elevates, the center of rotation of the scapula moves superiorly and medially with lateral displacement of the inferior angle (lateral rotation) (**Figure 4**).

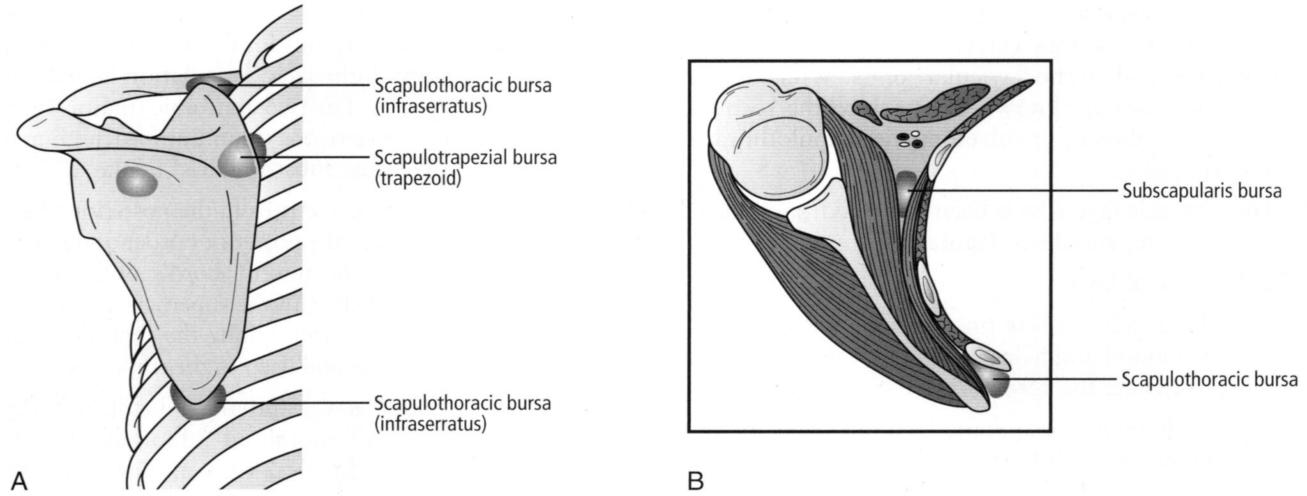

Figure 2 Illustrations showing the six bursae that have been described surrounding the scapula; two major bursae and four adventitial bursae. **(A)** Posterior view of the scapula; **(B)** axial view of the scapula showing the two major bursae of the scapula. The scapulothoracic bursae are involved in snapping scapula syndrome.

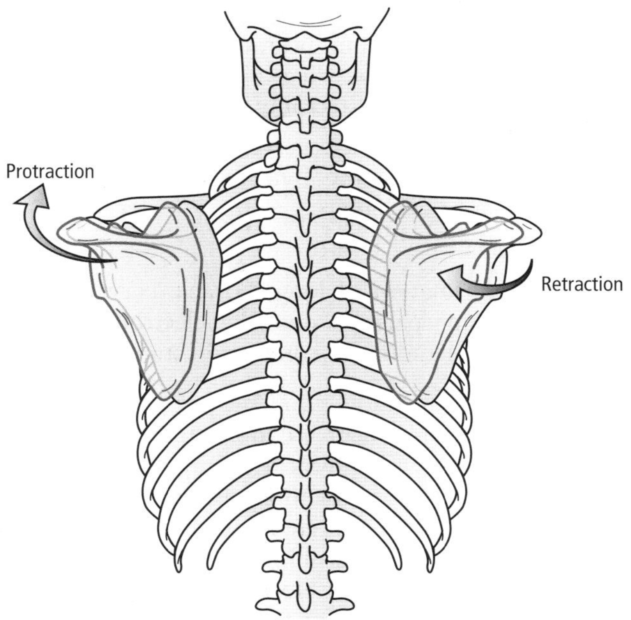

Figure 3 Two scapular motions (protraction and retraction) are illustrated here.

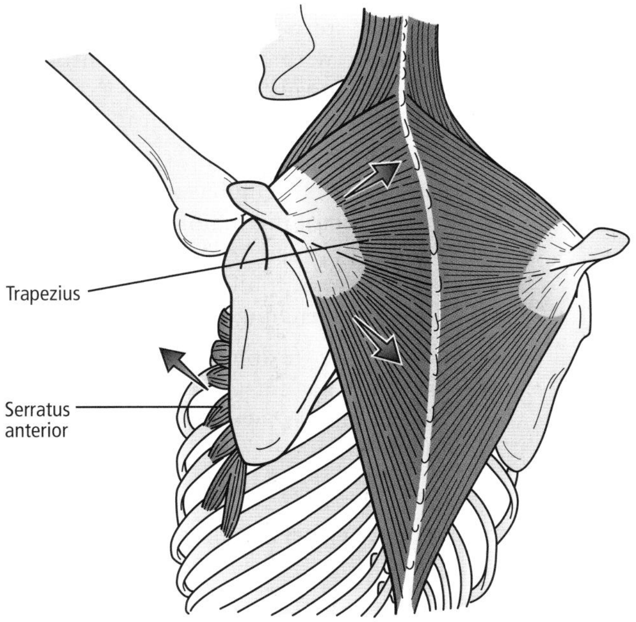

Figure 4 Illustrations showing the major scapular stabilizers (trapezius and serratus anterior) controlling scapular motion. The trapezius (especially the lower trapezius) laterally rotates the scapula on the chest wall allowing for acromial elevation and greater glenohumeral abduction. The serratus anterior stabilizes the medial border of the scapula against the chest wall to provide a stable fulcrum for glenohumeral motion. Arrows show the muscle line of pull.

4. Anterior tilt (cranial elevation) of the scapula is accomplished by the upper trapezius and pectoralis minor and countered by gravity and the latissimus dorsi (the primary scapular depressor). The serratus anterior and lower trapezius also act to posteriorly tilt and laterally rotate the scapula.
5. Medial rotators of the scapula include the rhomboid major/minor and levator scapulae. Lateral rotators of the scapula include the lower and middle trapezius as well as the serratus anterior and lower trapezius.
6. Protractors of the scapula include the serratus anterior and pectoralis major/minor.
7. Retractors of the scapula include the middle trapezius and rhomboid major/minor.

II. SCAPULAR WINGING

Scapular winging can be primary, secondary (from glenohumeral or subacromial pathology), or volitional (in setting of psychological disorders).

A. Causes of Scapular Winging
   1. primary scapular winging can be divided into three categories
      a. Neurologic
         - Long thoracic nerve (serratus anterior)
         - Spinal accessory nerve (trapezius)
         - Dorsal scapular nerve (rhomboids and levator scapulae)
      b. Osseous
         - Osteochondromas
         - Fracture malunion
      c. Soft tissue
         - Contracture
         - Muscle avulsion or agenesis
         - Scapulothoracic bursitis
   2. Secondary scapular winging can be due to
      a. Glenohumeral pathology (posterior shoulder instability)
      b. Subacromial pathology

B. Serratus Anterior Winging (Medial Winging)

   Due to long thoracic nerve palsy.
   1. Presentation
      a. Pain due to fatigability secondary to the other periscapular muscles compensating. More severe pain can be indicative of brachial plexus neuritis (Parsonage-Turner syndrome).

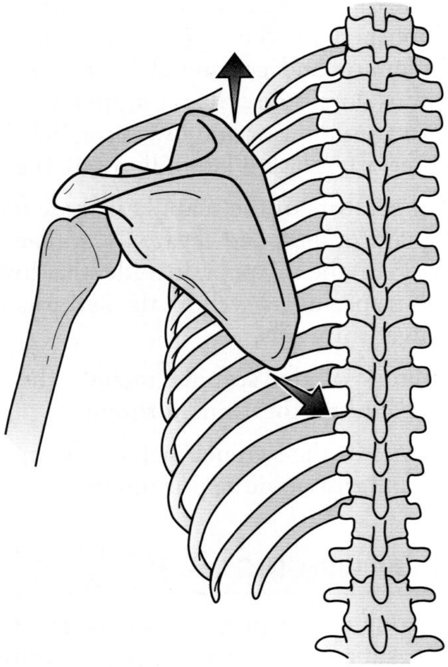

Figure 5 Illustration demonstrating that serratus anterior palsy results in medial rotation of the scapula and winging of the medial border of the scapula due to loss of the stabilizing effect of the serratus anterior holding the scapula against the chest wall. This leads to premature subacromial impingement and loss of shoulder elevation. Arrows depict the direction of deformity. (Reproduced from Srikumaran U, Wells JH, Freehill MT, Tan EW, Higgins LD, Warner JJP: Scapular winging: A great masquerader of shoulder disorders. *J Bone Joint Surg Am* 2014;96:e122(1-13).)

b. On examination, the scapula is elevated superiorly (anterior tilt), a prominent medial border and medial rotation of the inferior pole (**Figure 5**).

c. Shoulder elevation not possible above 110° to 120°, which may lead to the development of external (subacromial) impingement due to poor acromial elevation.

d. This winging is most pronounced by forward elevation but can also be exacerbated with resisted forward elevation (seen while attempting wall push ups).

e. Resolution/improvement seen with "scapular compression test" (manual compression of the scapula against the chest wall).

2. Incidence/Etiology

a. Damage (blunt trauma or stretching in athletes) to the long thoracic nerve (C5-7 nerve roots) is the most common neurologic cause of scapular winging.

b. Injury can also occur from a number of nontraumatic etiologies such as viral illness, drug reaction, Parsonage-Turner syndrome, iatrogenically from positioning in the operating room or wearing a heavy backpack, and postradical mastectomy.

c. The long thoracic nerve has a substantial C7 component so C7 nerve root compression must be excluded.

3. Diagnosis

a. Confirmation of long thoracic nerve/serratus anterior palsy is done by electromyography (EMG) and nerve conduction studies (NCS).

4. Treatment

a. Initial treatment is nonsurgical for most patients with physical therapy for strengthening of the periscapular muscles and passive stretching of the glenohumeral joint to prevent adhesive capsulitis. Most patients recover spontaneously within one year, but may take up to two years for full recovery. Up to 25% of patients will require surgery.

b. If nerve salvage is not possible, dynamic stabilization by muscle transfers and scapulothoracic fusion are potential surgical options.

- Dynamic stabilization is the most common treatment used. The classic transfer included the sternocostal head of the pectoralis major with a fascia lata autograft (or semitendinosus autograft) extension inserted into the inferior-lateral aspect of the scapula.
- "Direct transfers" emphasized direct contact of the pectoralis major tendon on the scapula (as opposed to "indirect" attachment with autograft/allograft extension) to prevent graft stretching.
- Scapulothoracic fusion is less commonly used because patients can lose up to 1/3 total elevation as well as up to 50% pseudarthrosis.

C. Trapezius Winging (Lateral Winging)

Due to spinal accessory nerve palsy.

1. Presentation

a. Pain due to overcompensation from the levator scapulae, rhomboid major, and rhomboid minor.

b. On examination, patient may have an asymmetric neckline with the affected shoulder depressed (angel-wing deformity).

c. The inferior angle of the scapula will displace and wing laterally (**Figure 6**).

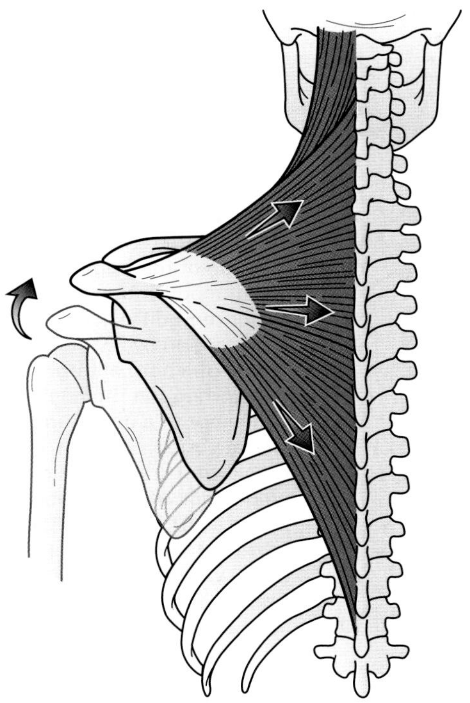

Figure 6 Illustration showing that normal trapezius function is broken down into three components: the upper trapezius elevates and laterally rotates the scapula, the middle trapezius retracts the scapula, and the lower trapezius lateral retracts the scapula. Because the trapezius is the only muscle to insert on the acromion, trapezius paralysis results in significant shoulder depression. (Waiter MJ, Bigliani LU: Spinal accessory nerve injury. *Clin Ortho Relat Res* 1999;368:5-16.)

d. Winging is worsened with abduction and resisted external rotation; may improve with forward elevation.

e. Active-elevation lag sign and triangle sign have been described.

2. Incidence/Etiology

   a. Damage to the spinal accessory nerve may occur during procedures in the posterior triangle of the neck (cervical node biopsy, post-carotid endarterectomy).

3. Diagnosis

   a. Diagnosis of trapezius palsy is confirmed by EMG/NCS.

4. Treatment

   a. Initial treatment is nonsurgical with physical therapy. Patients who have greater than one year of symptoms are unlikely to benefit from nonsurgical management.

   b. Surgical treatment: If nerve salvage is not possible, dynamic stabilization by muscle transfers and scapulothoracic fusion are potential surgical options.

      - **Eden-Lange procedure:** Transfer of the levator scapulae and rhomboid insertions laterally to effectively position the scapula medially and thus improve the mechanical advantage of these periscapular muscles and eliminate winging. The levator scapulae substitutes for the upper third of the trapezius, the rhomboid major for the middle third and the rhomboid minor for the lower third. Results are variable at best with excellent outcomes reported in only 57% to 75% of patients.
      - The **"T3 transfer"** alters the original Eden-Lange surgery by changing the line of pull on the scapula. This theoretically provides a more anatomic reconstruction of the trapezius for improved lateral rotation (**Figure 7**).

D. Rhomboid Winging (Lateral Winging)

Less common cause of primary neurologic scapular winging.

1. Presentation

   a. Patients mostly complain of pain along the medial border of the scapula, very similar to trapezius winging.

   b. Scapula is slightly depressed and translated with the inferior angle rotated laterally. Rhomboid winging is typically not as severe as other forms of winging and may be less symptomatic.

2. Incidence/Etiology

   a. Damage to the dorsal scapular nerve, which arises from the C5 nerve root (C5 radiculopathy must be assessed as a potential etiology).

3. Diagnosis

   a. Diagnosis of a rhomboid palsy is confirmed by EMG/NCS.

4. Treatment

   a. Initial treatment is nonsurgical with physical therapy for trapezius strengthening. Unlike other forms of neurapraxic scapular winging, rhomboid winging is not likely to improve spontaneously.

   b. Surgical treatment is rarely indicated and involves a fascial sling procedure in which two grafts are utilized to connect the lower vertebral border of the scapula to the spinal muscles and inferior angle of the scapula to the fibers of the latissimus dorsi. The teres major is

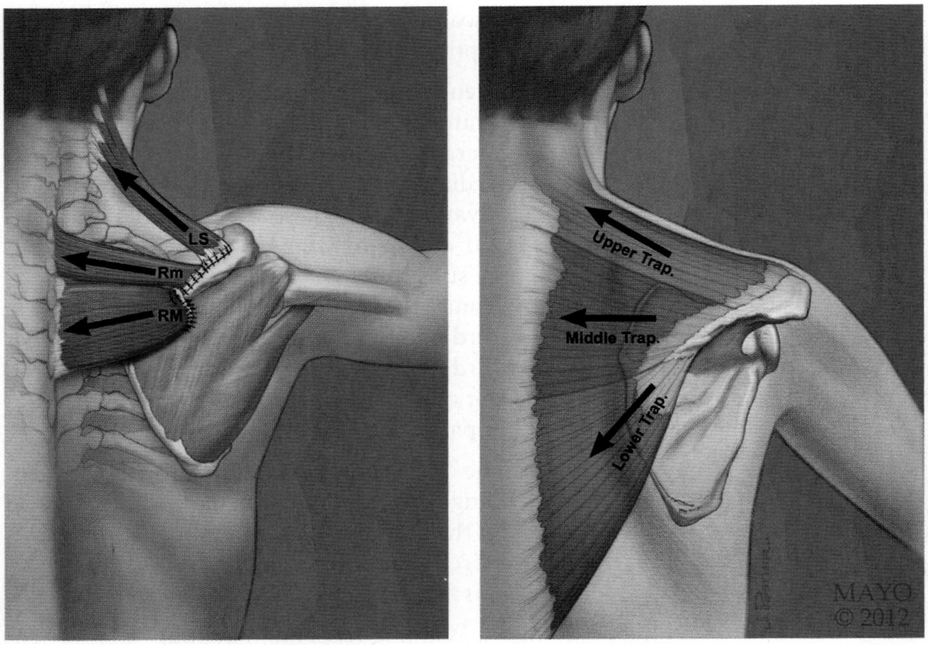

Figure 7 Illustration demonstrating that the traditional Eden-Lange procedure results in medial rotation of the scapula on the chest wall which is different that the normal function of the trapezius. The recent modification attempts to better reproduce normal trapezius function by restoring the line of pull of a normal trapezius by transferring the rhomboid major and minor to a more superior and lateral position on the scapula. LS = levator scapulae; Rm = rhomboid minor; RM = rhomboid major. (Elhassan BT, Wagner ER: Outcomes of triple-tendon transfer, an Eden-Lange variant, to reconstruct trapezius paralysis. *J Shoulder Elbow Surg* 2015;24:1307-1313.)

transferred from its insertion on the humerus to a spinous process.

E. Primary Scapular Winging Secondary to Muscle Disorders

1. Traumatic ruptures of periscapular muscles can lead to winging, the presentation of which depends on the specific injury.
2. Congenital absence of the serratus anterior and trapezius muscles has been reported and are tolerated well without significant scapular dysfunction.

a. Sprengel Deformity

- Congenital anomaly of scapular development in which the scapula remains small and undescended secondary to an interruption of the embryonic subclavian blood supply. This leads to scapular hypoplasia and winging with limited scapulothoracic motion. Patients typically have deficiencies in both forward elevation and abduction.
- May require surgical correction for severe functional deformities with surgery ideally being performed between the ages of 3 and 8 years (patients older than 8 years have an increased risk of nerve injury). Advanced imaging should be performed to assess for presence of an omovertebral bar connecting the superomedial border of the scapulae to one of the lower cervical vertebrae.
  - Woodward procedure: This procedure includes resection of any omovertebral bar division of the vertebral attachments of the trapezius, rhomboids, and levator scapulae with correction of scapular rotation and reattachment of these muscular origins to more caudal vertebrae. This may be combined with clavicular osteotomy to prevent compression of the brachial plexus.
  - Green procedure: Resection of the prominent superior border of the scapula, subperiosteal division of the medial scapular muscle attachments, displacement of the scapula inferiorly, and reattachment after appropriate translation.

b. Facioscapulohumeral Dystrophy

- Genetic neuromuscular dystrophy presenting in the second decade of life with shoulder girdle weakness, scapulothoracic instability, and limitations in flexion and abduction. The deltoid is typically spared and disease progression is slow.
- Given the involvement of multiple periscapular muscles, dynamic muscle transfers are not as effective as scapulothoracic fusion. If stability of the scapulothoracic articulation is achieved, the deltoid is typically sufficiently functional for elevation and improved function.

F. Primary Scapular Winging Secondary to Osseous Abnormalities

1. Scapular winging can occur secondary to osteochondromas of the scapula (the most common scapular bony tumor) or malunion of a prior scapula fracture.

G. Secondary Scapular Winging

1. Normal EMG/NCS findings are suggestive of secondary winging.
2. A common cause of secondary medial winging is posterior glenohumeral instability. As the shoulder subluxates out posteriorly, the scapula attempts to capture the humeral head by winging medially.
3. Contractual winging is an example of when soft tissue contracture can produce secondary scapular winging. Contractual winging can also occur in the setting of fibrosis of the deltoid in which cases winging decreases with arm elevation and increases with lowering of the arm.
4. Glenohumeral motion is reflexively limited in the setting of a painful shoulder, thus leading to increased work of the periscapular muscles. As the periscapular muscles fatigue with this increased workload, secondary winging occurs.
5. The treatment for secondary scapular winging is to address the primary pathology

III. SNAPPING SCAPULA

A. Presentation

1. Snapping scapula is also known as scapulothoracic bursitis. This phenomenon is characterized by a tactile-acoustic sensation occurring with anomalous tissue between the chest wall and the scapula. This is typically a painless presentation though some patients report pain that correlates with this phenomenon. This may occur following trauma (either a single episode or repetitive motion of the scapulothoracic joint) and is believed to be caused by abnormal motion between the anterior (ventral) surface of the scapula and the chest wall.
2. Patients should be evaluated for any scoliosis as this may alter scapular motion by changing the contour of the chest wall.
3. Approximately 6% of scapulae have a hooked shape prominence known as Luschka tubercle at the superomedial angle.
4. Osteochondromas are a common cause of snapping scapula syndrome and can be excised if symptomatic. However, chondrosarcoma must be considered in the differential diagnosis when evaluating lesions in the scapulothoracic articulation.
5. Elastofibroma dorsi are a result of friction between the chest wall and the scapula that can present with snapping scapula. These are circumscribed, but not encapsulated, benign lesions formed of collagen, adipose, and elastin.
6. Scapulothoracic bursitis may also be a result of abnormal scapular motion in the setting of muscle overuse, muscle imbalance, or glenohumeral pathology. Baseball pitchers may exhibit similar symptoms in the setting of overuse fatigue leading to SICK scapula.

B. Diagnosis

1. Standard radiographs which include an AP view, a true AP, a scapular Y view, and an axillary view. Routine CT scan is not indicated, and MRI is useful if suspicious for a soft-tissue lesion.

C. Treatment

1. Most patients with scapulothoracic crepitus/bursitis can be managed nonsurgically with physical therapy, anti-inflammatories, and corticosteroid injections with local anesthetics.
2. Surgical intervention is usually reserved for those with a clearly identifiable osseous or soft-tissue lesion and can be done arthroscopically or open to remove inflamed bursae as well as resection of prominent portions of the superomedial scapula.

IV. SICK SCAPULA SYNDROME

A. SICK (Scapular malposition, Inferior medial border prominence, Coracoid pain and malposition, and dysKinesis of scapular movement) scapula syndrome is an extreme form of scapular dyskinesis is an overuse muscular fatigue syndrome, which causes anterior shoulder pain in the throwing athlete who presents with "dead arm" complaints. The hallmark feature of this syndrome is the appearance of the involved shoulder to be lower than the other (due to scapular protraction).

B. Altered kinematics of the scapula upon dynamic use falls into three clinically recognizable patterns of scapular dyskinesis:

1. Type 1: associated with labral pathology; inferior medial scapular prominence
2. Type 2: associated with labral pathology; medial scapular prominence
3. Type 3: associated with external (subacromial) impingement and rotator cuff pathology rather

than labral pathology; superomedial border scapular prominence

C. The scapula initially protracts, rotating about a horizontal axis, with the upper scapula rotating anteroinferiorly. Protraction of the scapula makes the shoulder appear to be lower than the opposite side. The pectoralis minor tightens as the coracoid tilts inferiorly and shifts laterally away from the midline, and its insertion at the coracoid becomes very tender.

V. SUPRASCAPULAR NEUROPATHY

A. Suprascapular neuropathy (SSN) is an uncommon cause of shoulder pain resulting from an injury to the suprascapular nerve due to compression or traction.

B. The most common presenting symptom in patients with SSN is deep, posterior shoulder pain.

C. Etiologies for SSN may include repetitive overhead activities (tightening of the spinoglenoid ligament with internal rotation of the glenohumeral joint), traction from a rotator cuff tear (>3 cm retraction), and compression from a space-occupying lesion (paralabral cysts) at the suprascapular or spinoglenoid notch.

D. On examination, atrophy of the supraspinatus and/or infraspinatus fossa can be seen. Tenderness to palpation posterior to the clavicle in the region between the clavicle and the scapular spine (deep to the trapezius); weakness with resisted abduction and external rotation of the shoulder.

E. EMG/NCS are helpful in the diagnosis but false-negative results are possible.

F. Initial treatment of isolated SSN is typically nonsurgical, consisting of physical therapy, nonsteroidal anti-inflammatory drugs, and activity modification; however, surgical treatment (open or arthroscopic) is indicated when there is extrinsic nerve compression or progressive pain and/or weakness, unresponsive to conservative measures.

TOP TESTING FACTS

1. Serratus anterior winging medial winging due to long thoracic nerve palsy where the scapula is elevated superiorly (anterior tilt), a prominent medial border and medial rotation of the inferior pole.
2. The long thoracic nerve has a substantial C7 component so C7 nerve root compression must be excluded with serratus winging.
3. Muscle transfer of the sternocostal head of the pectoralis major with a fascia lata (or semitendinosus) autograft augmentation inserted into the inferior-lateral aspect of the scapula is the most common treatment used for serratus palsy.
4. Trapezius lateral winging due to spinal accessory nerve palsy where the scapula is displaced inferiorly and laterally.
5. Damage to the spinal accessory nerve may occur during procedures in the posterior triangle of the neck (cervical node biopsy, post-carotid endarterectomy).
6. Dynamic muscle transfers (Eden-Lange procedure) are used for trapezius palsy and involves transfer of the levator scapulae and rhomboid insertions laterally on the scapula.
7. Rhomboid winging (lateral winging) is a much less common cause of primary neurologic scapular winging and presents very similar to trapezius winging and typically treated nonsurgically.
8. Damage to the dorsal scapular nerve, which arises from the C5 nerve root, can be due to C5 radiculopathy and must be assessed as a potential etiology in rhomboid winging.
9. Sprengel deformity is a congenital anomaly of scapular development in which the scapula remains small and undescended secondary to an interruption of the embryonic subclavian blood supply.
10. Snapping scapula (scapulothoracic bursitis) is characterized by a tactile-acoustic sensation occurring with anomalous tissue between the chest wall and the scapula. Osteochondromas, elastofibromas, and scapulothoracic bursal inflammation are the most common causes.
11. SICK (Scapular malposition, Inferior medial border prominence, Coracoid pain and malposition, and dysKinesis of scapular movement) scapula syndrome is an extreme form of scapular dyskinesis and an overuse muscular fatigue syndrome, which causes anterior shoulder pain in the throwing athlete who presents with "dead arm" complaints.
12. Suprascapular neuropathy (SSN) is an uncommon cause of deep posterior shoulder pain resulting from an injury to the suprascapular nerve due to compression or traction.

Bibliography

Bigliani LU, Compito CA, Duralde XA, Wolfe IN: Transfer of the levator scapulae, rhomboid major, and rhomboid minor for paralysis of the trapezius. *J Bone Joint Surg Am* 1996;78:1534-1540.

Boykin RE, Friedman DJ, Higgins LD, Warner JJ: Suprascapular neuropathy. *J Bone Joint Surg Am* 2010;92(13):2348-2364.

Chalmers PN, Saltzman BM, Feldheim TF, et al: A comprehensive analysis of pectoralis major transfer for long thoracic nerve palsy. *J Shoulder Elbow Surg* 2015;24:1028-1035.

Connor PM, Yamaguchi K, Manifold SG, Pollock, Flatow EL, Bigliani LU: Split pectoralis major transfer for serratus anterior palsy. *Clin Ortho Relat Res* 1997;341:134-142.

Elhassan BT, Wagner ER: Outcomes of triple-tendon transfer, an Eden-Lange variant, to reconstruct trapezius paralysis. *J Shoulder Elbow Surg* 2015;24:1307-1313.

Galano GJ, Bigliani LU, Ahmad CS, Levine WN: Surgical treatment of winges scapula. *Clin Ortho Relat Res* 2008;466:652-660.

Povacz P, Resch H: Dynamic stabilization of winging scapula by direct split pectoralis major transfer: A technical note. *J Shoulder Elbow Surg* 2000;9:76-78.

Roren A, Fayad F, Poiraudeau S, et al: Specific Scapular kinematic patterns to differentiate two forms of dynamic scapular winging. *Clin Biomech* 2013;28:941-947.

Seror P, Lenglet T, Nguyen C, Ouakenine M, Lefevre-Colau MM: Unilateral winged scapula: Clinical and electrodiagnostic experience with 128 cases, with special attention to long thoracic. Nerve palsy. *Muscle & Nerve* 2018;57:913-920.

Seror P, Stojkovic T, Lefevre-Colau MM, Lenglet T: Diagnoses of unilateral trapezius muscle palsy: 54 cases. *Muscle & Nerve* 2017;56:215-223.

Steinmann SP, Wood MB: Pectoralis major transfer for serratus paralysis. *J Shoulder Elbow Surg* 2003;12:555-560.

Streit JJ, Lenarz CJ, Shishani Y, et al: Pectoralis major tendon transfer for the treatment of scapular winging due to long thoracic nerve palsy. *J Shoulder Elbow Surg* 2012;21:685-690.

Srikumaran U, Wells JH, Freehill MT, Tan EW, Higgins LD, Warner JJP: Scapular winging: A great masquerader of shoulder disorders. *J Bone Joint Surg Am* 2014;96:e122(1-13).

Section 7

Trauma

Section Editors | KENNETH A. EGOL, MD
GEOFFREY MARECEK, MD

Chapter 86

EVALUATION OF THE TRAUMA PATIENT

JOSHUA L. GARY, MD, FAOA

I. DEFINITION AND EPIDEMIOLOGY

A. Definition—A trauma patient has sustained injury owing to traumatic mechanism. A polytrauma patient is defined by an injury severity score (ISS) ≥16.

B. Epidemiology

1. Injury is the leading cause of death for Americans aged 45 and younger and is the leading cause for years of life lost. It is the fourth leading cause of death for Americans of any age. In 2014, almost 150,000 trauma deaths were reported in the United States, with 20% (approximately 30,000) preventable with optimal trauma care.
2. In 2013, estimated cost in the United States for injuries and work-loss was $671 billion.
3. 14,000 people die every day as a result of injury, or one life is lost every 6 seconds owing to trauma. 90% of traumatic deaths occur in countries classified as low- and middle-income.
4. From 2000 to 2010, the largest increase in American trauma mortality was for patients in their 40s and 50s, and with the aging baby boomers, this is expected to continue to progress toward older patients.
5. Fatal injuries
   a. Major mechanisms of injury for traumatic injury and deaths in 2012 are listed in **Table 1**.
   b. Unintentional death accounts for 62.3% of trauma-related mortality with suicide accounting for 35.0% and homicide 2.7% as of 2010.

Dr. Gary or an immediate family member is a member of a speakers' bureau or has made paid presentations on behalf of Smith & Nephew and Stryker; has stock or stock options held in Summitt Medventures; and serves as a board member, owner, officer, or committee member of the AO North America and the Orthopaedic Trauma Association.

II. MORTALITY AND THE GOLDEN HOUR

A. Three peak times of death after trauma

1. About 50% occur within minutes, from a neurologic injury or massive hemorrhage.
2. Another 30% occur within the first few days after injury, most commonly from a neurologic injury.
3. The final 20% occur days to weeks after injury as a result of infection and/or multiple organ failure.

B. The "Golden Hour"

1. Popularized by R Adams Cowley as the 60 minutes immediately after life-threatening injury to provide a sense of urgency for proper trauma care
2. Traumatic brain injury and uncontrolled hemorrhage are the major causes of mortality within the first hour after trauma.
3. Following a U.S. Secretary of Defense mandate to evacuate all critically injured soldiers in Operation Enduring Freedom and Operation Iraqi Freedom within 60 minutes, mortality dropped from 16.0% premandate to 9.9% postmandate.

TABLE 1

Mechanisms of Injury Deaths Worldwide

Mechanism of Injury[a]	Percentage of Deaths
Road traffic injuries	24%
Other unintentional injuries	18%
Suicide	16%
Falls	14%
Homicide	10%

[a]Data are from 2012.

7 | Trauma

4. Median time to death for patients with shock is 2 hours and for patients with traumatic brain injury is 29 hours. For those with combined shock and traumatic brain injury, the median time to death is 4 hours.
5. Sepsis and multiorgan dysfunction only cause 2% of deaths in trauma patients.

III. PREHOSPITAL CARE AND FIELD TRIAGE

A. General principles
   1. Rapid assessment to identify life-threatening injuries
   2. Appropriate interventions to address life-threatening conditions (airway, breathing, circulation, external hemorrhage control). The goal of prehospital care is to minimize preventable deaths.
   3. Rapid transport to appropriate facility based upon patients injuries

B. Components of field assessment
   1. Goals
      a. Should be quick and systematic
      b. Patients with potentially life-threatening injuries must be transported quickly to the closest appropriate hospital. Definitive care for internal hemorrhage cannot be provided at the scene.
   2. Mechanisms of injury that may result in major injuries include:
      a. Falls of more than 15 feet
      b. Motor vehicle collisions in which a fatality has occurred, a passenger has been ejected, extrication has taken longer than 20 minutes
      c. Motor pedestrian collision
      d. Motorcycle collisions in which the vehicle was traveling faster than 20 mph
      e. Penetrating injury
   3. Primary survey (ABCDE—Airway, Breathing, Circulation, Disability, Exposure)
      a. Performed just as in Advanced Trauma Life Support (ATLS) to establish priorities for management and continued during transport until arrival at hospital of definitive care.
      b. Treatment is initiated as problems are identified (same as ATLS).
   4. Indications for field intubation
      a. Glasgow Coma Scale total score less than 8 (inability to maintain an airway)
      b. Need for ventilation
      c. Potentially threatened airway (eg, inhalation injuries or expanding neck hematoma)
      d. Ventilation is required if respiration rate is less than 10 breaths per minute.
   5. External bleeding is controlled with direct pressure.
   6. Transport should not be delayed just to start fluids. Prehospital blood product transfusions have not been shown to decrease mortality rates compared with patients receiving prehospital non–blood product volume replacement.
   7. Secondary survey
      a. Performed according to ATLS, perhaps during transport
      b. AMPLE history (Allergies to medications, Medications the patient is taking, Pertinent medical history, Last time eaten, Events leading to the injury)
   8. Extremity trauma
      a. Bleeding associated with fractures can be life-threatening.
      b. Circumferential pelvic compression with pelvic binders or sheets is now recommended for patients with suspected pelvic ring disruptions and shock.
      c. External hemorrhage is controlled with direct pressure. Extremity tourniquets for severe bleeding associated with open fractures decrease mortality.
      d. Immobilization of the extremity helps control internal bleeding. Gross correction of obvious deformities also helps improve tissue perfusion and lessens ongoing soft-tissue compromise.
      e. A traction splint can be used for suspected femur fractures because it stabilizes the fracture and controls pain. It is contraindicated in patients with obvious knee injuries or deformities.
   9. Amputations
      a. Tourniquets are used to control bleeding until arrival to hospital.
      b. The amputated parts are cleaned by rinsing them with lactated Ringer solution.
      c. The parts are covered with sterile gauze moistened with lactated Ringer solution and placed in a plastic bag.

d. The bag is labeled and placed in another container filled with ice.

e. The part must not be allowed to freeze or be immersed directly in an aqueous medium.

f. The part is transported with the patient.

IV. TRAUMA SCORING SYSTEMS

A. Components of present scoring systems include physiologic data, anatomic data, a combination of the two, and specialized data.

B. Although no single scoring system has been universally adapted, each has advantages and disadvantages.

C. Glasgow Coma Scale

1. Attempts to score the function (level of consciousness) of the central nervous system. The sum of the scores for the eye opening, verbal response, and motor response is the score (**Table 2**).

2. The verbal score is eliminated for intubated patients and the score is modified with a "T" after the numerical score.

D. Abbreviated Injury Scale (AIS)

1. Developed to accurately rate and compare injuries sustained in motor vehicle accidents

2. Injuries are scored from 1 (minor injuries) to 6 (fatal within 24 hours).

3. A total of 73 different injuries can be scored, but it includes no mechanism to combine the individual injury scores into one score.

TABLE 2

Glasgow Coma Scale

	Parameter		
Score	**Eye Opening**	**Verbal Response**	**Motor Response**
6			Obeys command
5		Oriented	Localized pain
4	Spontaneous	Confused	Withdraws from pain
3	To voice	Inappropriate	Flexion to pain
2	To pain	Incomprehensible	Extension to pain
1	None	None	None

E. Injury Severity Score (ISS)

1. The sum of the squares of the three highest AIS scores of six regions provides an overall severity score (includes head and neck, face, thorax, abdomen, pelvis, extremities).

2. Each region is scored on a scale from 1 (minor injury) to 6 (almost always fatal).

3. Any region with an AIS score of 6 is automatically assigned an ISS value of 75, which represents a nonsurvivable injury.

4. A score of 16 or higher frequently is used as the definition of major trauma and correlates well with mortality.

5. Because ISS scores only one injury per body region, it does not reflect patient morbidity associated with multiple lower extremity fractures.

F. New ISS

1. This modification of the ISS sums the squares of the AIS scores of the three most substantial injuries, even if they occur in the same anatomic area.

2. Better predictor of survival than the ISS

3. One study looking at orthopaedic blunt trauma patients found the New ISS to be superior to the ISS.

G. Trauma and Injury Severity Score (trISS)

1. Predicts mortality based on postinjury anatomic and physiologic abnormalities

2. Uses age, the Revised Trauma Score (calculated in the emergency department), the ISS (calculated using discharge diagnosis), and whether the injury mechanism was blunt or penetrating

3. The data from any institution can then be compared with the mortality data from the Major Trauma Outcomes Study conducted by the American College of Surgeons in 1990.

V. INITIAL HOSPITAL WORKUP AND RESUSCITATION

A. Goals

1. Diagnosis and treatment of life-threatening injuries takes priority over a sequential, detailed, definitive workup.

2. ATLS, which provides a systematic method to evaluate trauma patients, was developed to teach this concept and ultimately improve patient survival.

B. Components of ATLS

1. Primary survey

   a. A systematic effort to identify life-threatening injuries immediately

   b. Treatment and resuscitation are performed simultaneously as problems are identified.

   c. Consists of evaluation of ABCDEs, which may need to be repeated because patient reevaluation constantly occurs during this step

   d. Chest and AP pelvic radiographs should be performed in all blunt trauma patients to identify potential life-threatening sources of bleeding.

   e. Placement of tourniquets for hemorrhage control with uncontrolled extremity bleeding and circumferential pelvic compression with a pelvic sheet or binder for volume expanding pelvic ring disruptions are treatments related to evaluation of circulation.

2. Secondary survey

   a. Performed after primary survey when immediate life-threatening injuries have been addressed.

   b. Consists of a head-to-toe physical examination and detailed medical history (if available). Intended to diagnose and treat injuries that are not an immediate threat to life.

   c. Intravenous antibiotics should be given to patients with open fractures as early as possible. Early antibiotics have been shown to be the most important factor in limiting infection rates after open fractures. Cefazolin is the drug of choice for all open fractures unless contraindicated. The addition of an aminoglycoside, even for type III open fractures, is controversial.

   d. Advanced imaging

      - CT usually performed as part of the secondary survey.
      - CT scans of the entire chest, abdomen, pelvis, and extremities may now be rapidly performed with newer scanners and protocols.
      - Patient should be stabilized hemodynamically to tolerate the scan with minimal risk.
      - CT scans have largely replaced a lateral cervical spine (C-Spine) radiograph. C-spine precautions with a cervical collar should be maintained for blunt trauma patients until proper radiologic and physical examinations are performed.
      - Failure to obtain an AP pelvis radiograph before CT may result in delayed diagnosis of hip dislocations and volume expanding pelvic ring disruptions and unnecessary repeat CT scans and radiation exposure to the patient.
      - Focused Assessment for the Sonographic Evaluation of the Trauma Patient (FAST) may be used for patients with shock. As with radiographic evaluation, FAST is obtained quickly and can be performed in the trauma bay. FAST is accurate for the detection of free intraperitoneal fluid and visualizing blood in the pericardial sac and dependent regions of the abdomen, including the right and left upper quadrants and pelvis, but it cannot detect isolated bowel injuries and does not reliably detect retroperitoneal injuries.
      - MRI is rarely indicated early in the management of trauma patients. Patients with cervical spine dislocations without progressive neurologic deficit may benefit from MRI before closed reduction attempts to identify interbody disk herniation within the spinal canal that may cause neurologic impairment with closed reduction.

3. Tertiary survey

   a. Performed when patients are awake, alert, and responsive and involves a detailed physical examination and review of all imaging modalities of the entire body to identify injuries not previously identified.

   b. Injuries to the hands and feet are the most commonly missed injuries in trauma patients.

C. Shock

1. Results in decreased end-organ perfusion. Hypovolemic shock is the most common type in trauma patients. Multiple forms of shock may also be present in a single patient.

2. Signs, symptoms, and laboratory findings

   a. Hypovolemic shock (**Table 3**)

      - Decreased peripheral or central pulses; peripheral vasoconstriction is an early compensatory mechanism for shock.
      - Pale and/or cool, clammy extremities
      - Tachycardia
      - Hypotension is a sign of severe shock and may be a late finding, especially in younger patients with better physiological compensatory abilities.

7 | Trauma

TABLE 3

Symptoms of Hypovolemic Shock by Hemorrhage Class

Hemorrhage Class	Blood Volume Loss (%)	Blood Loss	Symptoms
I	15	750 mL	Minimal
II	15-30	750-1,500 mL	Tachycardia, tachypnea, mild mental status Changes, decreased pulse pressure
III	30-40	1,500-2,000 mL	Decreased systolic blood pressure
IV	>40	>2 L	Severe mental status changes

- Altered level of consciousness may indicate a brain injury, hypovolemic shock, or both.
- Decreased urine output
- Acidosis, elevated base deficit, elevated lactate, elevated IL-6, anemia, elevated PT/INR/PTT, hypocoagulability on thrombelastography (TEG), elevated IL-6

b. Cardiogenic shock
- Hypotension and lack of tachycardia
- Abnormal electrocardiogram findings
- Elevated troponins and CK-MB

c. Neurogenic shock
- Altered neurologic examination
- Hypotension and bradycardia

D. Shock resuscitation
1. Systolic blood pressure <90 mm Hg on arrival is a risk factor for mortality.
2. Two large bore intravenous lines should be obtained on arrival. Intraosseous access may also be obtained for resuscitation.
3. Early transfusion with whole blood (1 unit packed red blood cells: 1 unit fresh frozen plasma: 1 unit platelets) decreases mortality
4. Rapid TEG (r-TEG) curves can be used to guide components of blood product resuscitation.
5. Urine output is also used to monitor the adequacy of resuscitation.
6. "Stop the bleed." Circumferential pelvic compression should be used for pelvic ring disruptions associated with shock, and tourniquets should be placed for open extremity injuries with uncontrolled hemorrhage to limit mortality.

VI. ASSOCIATED INJURIES

A. Neck injuries
1. Cervical spine injuries are assumed in trauma patients until ruled out with appropriate imaging and physical examination in an awake and alert patient.
2. The neck is immobilized until it has been proven that no injury exists.

B. Pelvic (retroperitoneal) versus intra-abdominal bleeding
1. These two injuries may coexist.
2. If diagnostic peritoneal lavage is performed in the presence of a pelvis fracture, it should be supra-umbilical and performed early, before the pelvic hematoma can track anteriorly. CT can also be used.
3. Circumferential pelvic compression with a sheet or binder should be used early and *should not be removed* until the patient is adequately resuscitated.
   a. If a sheet is used, holes may be cut in the sheet for groin access or placement of external fixator pins or resuscitation iliosacral screws.
   b. If a binder is used and centered on the greater trochanters, a second binder can be placed just caudal before releasing a binder centered over the greater trochanters for groin and abdominal access (**Figure 1**).
4. Hemodynamically unstable patients that do not respond to circumferential compression and resuscitation should be considered for pelvic angiography, if rapidly available (<45 minutes).

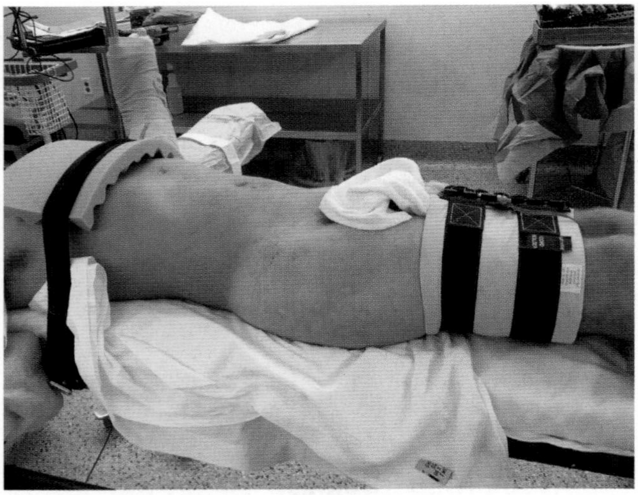

Figure 1 Clinical photograph of a second binder placed caudal to allow for groin and abdominal access in a damage control situation. This was placed before releasing the first binder that had been centered over the greater trochanters.

5. Pelvic packing is an alternative strategy if angiography is not readily available, the pelvic ring should be provisionally stabilized with circumferential compression, external fixation, c-clamp type devices, or combinations of these devices before packing. It remains controversial among trauma surgeons.

C. Head injuries
  1. Autoregulation of cerebral blood flow is altered after a head injury, and blood flow may become dependent on the mean arterial blood pressure.
  2. Secondary brain injury may develop if hypoperfusion or hypoxia occurs after the initial insult.
  3. Whether early definitive fracture surgery has an adverse effect on neurologic outcome remains subject to debate. At least one study that used neuropsychologic testing showed that this is not the case. Maintenance of cerebral perfusion and oxygenation remain the important goals during surgery.
  4. Early surgery that results in high volume blood loss and increases resuscitation may require invasive monitoring to ensure that adequate cerebral blood flow is maintained during surgery. Detailed multidisciplinary discussion with general surgery, neurosurgery, and orthopaedic surgery often helps chart the proper course while minimizing risk to the patient.

VII. DECISION TO OPERATE: SURGICAL TIMING

A. Determining the extent of resuscitation
  1. Indications for damage control:
     a. Systolic blood pressure ≤ 90 mm Hg
     b. Abnormal TEG values associated with hypocoagulability
     c. Elevated lactate (>2.0)
     d. Base deficit ≥ 4
     e. Worsening trend for lactate and base deficit are better indications for damage control orthopaedics than absolute values.
     f. Hypothermia is defined as core body temperature <35°C and should be corrected before definitive fixation.
     g. Soft tissues not appropriate for definitive fixation in a resuscitated patient
  2. Early appropriate care
     a. Single-center prospective data
     b. Recommends definitive fixation of pelvic ring, acetabulum, femur, and/or spine within 36 hours when:
        - Lactate <4.0 mmol/L
        - pH ≥7.25
        - Base deficit ≤5.5 mmol/L
     c. Decreased hospital and ICU length of stay and complications including infection, sepsis, venous thromboembolic disease, multiorgan dysfunction and failure, pneumonia, and adult respiratory distress syndrome (ARDS) were seen in appropriately resuscitated patients definitively fixed with 36 hours of presentation.

B. Damage control operations
  1. External fixation lower extremity fractures and dislocations
     a. Femoral shaft fractures
        - Should be stabilized within 24 hours with external fixation if the patient's condition does not allow for intramedullary nail
        - Patients with thoracic injury with increased peak airway pressures or abnormal chest radiograph should be strongly considered for external fixation, even if hemodynamically appropriate for intramedullary nailing.
        - Femoral reaming may increase risk for pulmonary complications, including ARDS

- External fixation of femoral shaft fractures allows for mobilization with physical therapy
- Conversion to intramedullary nail can take place up to 3 weeks after external fixation without apparent increased risk for infection

b. Tibial shaft fractures
- Usually only needed in association with open fractures, compartment syndrome, and/or vascular injuries to allow for revascularization or soft-tissue care.
- External fixation or provisional plating with mini-fragment (2.4 or 2.7 mm) plates may be used to temporize in certain fracture patterns in open injuries.
- Mobilization with physical therapy can take place with long or short leg splints before definitive stabilization.

c. Tibial plateau fractures and knee dislocations
- Indicated for injuries with associated vascular injuries. Should be performed *before revascularization* to avoid repair or bypass with a shortened extremity and graft tension with delayed restoration of length.
- Usually indicated for tibial plateau fractures that are length unstable to allow for soft-tissue healing before definitive fixation

d. Ankle and foot injuries
- Indicated for open rotational ankle fractures unable to undergo definitive stabilization because of patient condition or soft-tissue swelling
- Closed, length unstable pilon fractures are provisionally brought to length and reduced with external fixation to allow for soft-tissue injury to resolve before definitive fixation.
- Foot fractures and dislocations with soft tissues at risk may be provisionally stabilized with external fixation and/or provisional pinning with Kirschner wires.

2. External fixation ± resuscitation iliosacral screws for hemodynamically unstable pelvic ring disruptions
   a. Indicated for persistent hemodynamic instability after circumferential compression and blood product resuscitation and angiography
   b. Indicated for open injuries with perineal wound for soft-tissue management
3. Débridement and irrigation of open fractures
4. Fasciotomies

TOP TESTING FACTS

1. Injury is the leading cause of death in Americans ≤45 years of age.
2. Mortality significantly decreased in the Iraq and Afghanistan wars after a mandate to evacuate critically injured soldiers to field hospitals within 60 minutes of injury.
3. The goal of prehospital care is to limit preventable deaths.
4. Tourniquets for extremity injuries with uncontrolled hemorrhage decrease mortality.
5. The ISS is the sum of the squares of the three highest AIS scores.
6. Polytrauma is defined as ISS ≥16.
7. Trauma patients should be evaluated and managed per ATLS protocol with initial imaging including chest and AP pelvis radiographs.
8. Systolic blood pressure ≤90 on arrival to the hospital is associated with increase mortality.
9. Hemodynamically unstable patients with volume expanding pelvic ring disruptions should have circumferential pelvic compression that should not be removed until the patient has been resuscitated or mechanically stabilized for the bony injuries.
10. The base deficit or lactate level on admission is predictive of complication rates and mortality.

Bibliography

Florence C, Haegerich T, Simon T, Zhou C, Luo F: Estimated lifetime medical and work-loss costs of emergency department–treated nonfatal injuries—United States, 2013. *MMWR Morb Mortal Wkly Rep* 2015;64(38):1078-1082.

Holcomb JB, Tilley BC, Baraniuk S, et al: Transfusion of plasma, platelets, and red blood cells in a 1: 1: 1 vs a 1: 1: 2 ratio and mortality in patients with severe trauma: The PROPPR randomized clinical trial. *JAMA* 2015;313(5):471-482.

Holcomb JB, Swartz MD, DeSantis SM, et al: Multicenter observational prehospital resuscitation on helicopter study (PROHS). *J Trauma Acute Care Surg* 2017;83(1 suppl 1):S83.

Kotwal RS, Howard JT, Orman JA, et al: The effect of a golden hour policy on the morbidity and mortality of combat casualties. *JAMA Surg* 2016;151(1):15-24.

Lack WD, Karunakar MA, Angerame MR, et al: Type III open tibia fractures: Immediate antibiotic prophylaxis minimizes infection. *J Orthopaedic Trauma* 2015;29(1):1-6.

National Academies of Sciences, Engineering, and Medicine: 2016. *A National Trauma Care System: Integrating Military and Civilian Trauma Systems to Achieve Zero Preventable Deaths After Injury*. Washington, DC: The National Academies Press. doi:10.17226/23511.

Rhee P, Joseph B, Pandit V, et al: Increasing trauma deaths in the United States. *Ann Surg* 2014;260(1):13-21.

Tisherman SA, Schmicker RH, Brasel KJ, et al: Detailed description of all deaths in both the shock and traumatic brain injury hypertonic saline trials of the Resuscitation Outcomes Consortium. *Ann Surg* 2015;261(3):586.

Vallier HA, Moore TA, Como JJ, et al: Complications are reduced with a protocol to standardize timing of fixation based on response to resuscitation. *J Orthopaedic Surg Res* 2015;10(1):155.

World Health Organization: *Injuries and Violence: The Facts*. 2014. Available at: http://www.who.int/violence_injury_prevention/media/news/2015/Injury_violence_facts_2014/en/. Accessed October 1, 2018.

Chapter 87
Gunshot Wounds and Open Fractures

DANIEL J. STINNER, MD, FACS

I. GUNSHOT WOUNDS

A. Epidemiology

1. Firearm-related deaths in the United States totaled 39,773 in 2017, up from 31,224 in 2007.
2. Approximately half of patients with gunshot wounds (GSWs) have positive alcohol and/or drug screens; and one-quarter test positive for two or more drugs.
3. The extremities are the most common location for a nonfatal GSW.

B. Ballistics

1. Velocity is only one of several factors that determine the extent of damage caused by a bullet. Other factors include the shape, weight, diameter, jacketing, and tumbling characteristics of the bullet, as well as characteristics of the target.
2. Low-velocity bullets are defined as those traveling <2,000 ft/s (eg, from handguns).
3. High-velocity bullets are defined as those traveling >2,000 ft/s (eg, from M16 military rifles, most hunting rifles).
4. Shotguns deliver ammunition at a low velocity (typically between 1,000 to 1,400 ft/s) but can cause a high degree of destruction at close range.
   a. Shotgun blasts can inflict either high-energy injuries or low-energy injuries.
   b. Damage caused by shotgun blasts is determined by three factors: distance from the target, load (mass of the individual pellets), and chote (shot pattern).
5. When a bullet strikes tissue, the following three things occur:
   a. Mechanical crushing of tissue, forming the permanent cavity
   b. Elastic stretching of the tissue at the periphery of the permanent cavity by the dissipation of imparted kinetic energy, causing a temporary cavity
   c. A shock wave, which may cause tissue damage at a distance from the immediate bullet contact area
6. With higher velocity injuries, the temporary cavity is larger and fills with water vapor at a low atmospheric pressure, causing a momentary vacuum to form, which may attract contaminating foreign material.

C. Energy

1. The kinetic energy (KE) of a bullet is proportional to its mass (m) and its velocity squared (v^2). This is represented by the equation $KE = \frac{1}{2}(mv^2)$. For example, an M16 and a 0.22-caliber handgun fire a round of approximately the same size; however, the velocity of the M16 bullet is three times greater, thereby generating almost 10 times the kinetic energy.
2. Factors affecting the efficiency of energy transfer to the surrounding tissue
   a. The KE at the time of impact
   b. Stability and entrance profile of the bullet

Dr. Stinner or an immediate family member serves as a board member, owner, officer, or committee member of the American Academy of Orthopaedic Surgeons, the Orthopaedic Trauma Association, and the Society of Military Orthopaedic Surgeons.

This chapter is adapted from Riehl JT, Haidukewych GJ, Koval KJ: Gunshot wounds and open fractures, in Boyer MI, ed: *AAOS Comprehensive Orthopaedic Review* 2. Rosemont, IL, American Academy of Orthopaedic Surgeons, 2014, pp 265-273.

c. Caliber, construction, and configuration of the bullet, eg, mushrooming, tumbling, fragmentation. Tumbling (bullet flipping end over end) causes a greater amount of tissue displacement, than do other behaviors, and more of the kinetic energy of the bullet is imparted to the tissue.

d. Distance and path within the body (retained or exiting)

e. Characteristics of the tissue (Bone is not very elastic, capillaries are prone to rupture, arteries are typically resistant unless direct impact, and large nerves in the surrounding soft tissues may sustain a neurapraxia unless direct impact.)

D. Bullet entrance and exit

1. Secondary missiles can be created when a bullet contacts a dense object, such as a belt buckle or button, or tissue, such as bone or teeth. Secondary missiles may cause significant damage and additional permanent cavities.

2. An abrasion ring is produced at the entrance wound when the skin is damaged by clothing scraping the skin as the bullet penetrates it. The ring is stellate in the palm and sole.

3. Four categories of entrance wounds exist:

a. Contact—The muzzle of the gun is against the target at the time the gun is fired, causing blackened, seared margins.

b. Near-contact—The muzzle is a short distance away, causing powder soot deposit.

c. Intermediate—Gunpowder tattooing is present.

d. Distant—The muzzle is distant from the target.

4. Exit wounds are typically larger than entrance wounds, with a more irregular shape. When no exit wound is present, all of the kinetic energy of the bullet has been dissipated into the tissue.

E. Tissue parameters

1. The extent of injury to the tissue is related to the dissipation of kinetic energy for the crush or stretch of tissue, the production of secondary missiles, and cavitation.

2. Retained intra-articular bullet fragments can result in lead toxicity secondary to synovial fluid breakdown of the lead component of the bullet and absorption into the bloodstream.

3. Bullets are not sterilized by firing, and they introduce additional contaminants from clothing, the skin, and the bowel as they pass into sterile tissues.

F. Clinical evaluation

1. Initial assessment begins with Advanced Trauma Life Support (ATLS) protocols.

2. A thorough history should be obtained, including the type of firearm, its distance from the target, and the direction.

3. All clothing should be removed, and the skin should be examined for entrance and exit wounds.

4. Extremities should be evaluated for swelling, deformity, ecchymosis, and crepitus.

5. A thorough neurovascular examination should be performed on the injured extremity. Nerve injury can occur at a site remote from the immediate path of the bullet.

6. Biplanar radiographs of the injured limb should be obtained, including the joints above and below the injury.

7. A GSW near a major joint should raise strong suspicion of penetration into that joint.

G. Treatment

1. Treatment depends on wound size, contamination, and the amount of devitalized tissue.

2. Tetanus immunization status should be updated if necessary. Antibiotics are administered in the emergency department.

3. Low-velocity wounds

a. Outpatient treatment can be considered for stable fractures that exhibit minimal soft-tissue injury and are without neurovascular compromise. Superficial wound cleansing and skin-edge débridement can be performed in the emergency department. Upon discharge, patients are placed on oral antibiotics (eg, first-generation cephalosporin) for 7 to 10 days.

b. Indications for surgical treatment include retained bullet fragments in the subarachnoid or joint space; vascular injury; gross contamination; a prominent missile in the palm or sole; and severe tissue damage, including compartment syndrome and an unstable fracture requiring fixation.

4. High-velocity wounds

a. Surgical débridement—Evaluate muscle tissue for color, consistency, contractility, and capacity to bleed.

b. Stabilization of fracture (**Figure 1**)

c. Delayed wound closure, graft/flap planning as necessary

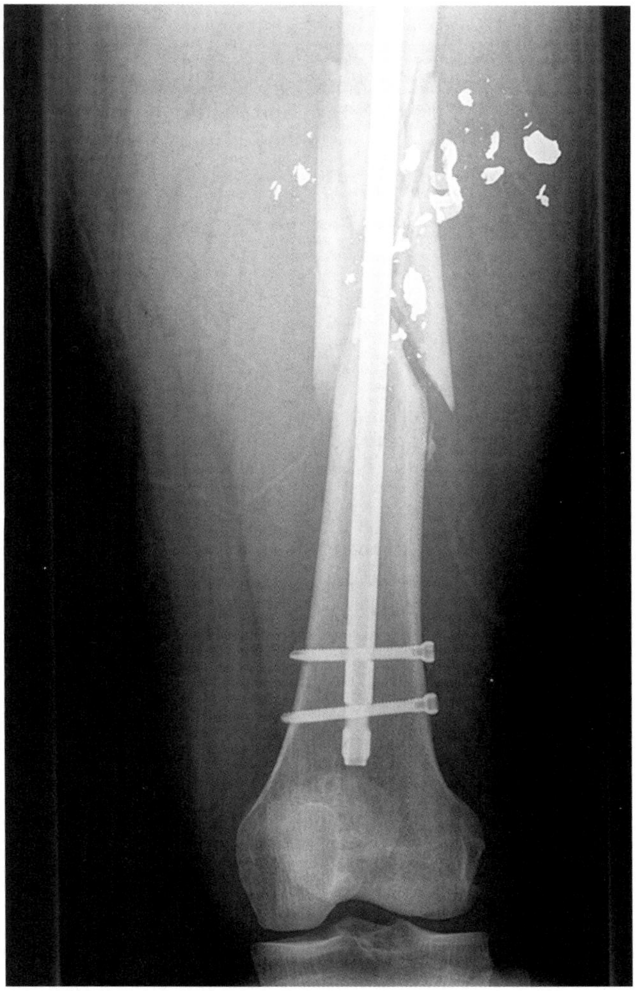

Figure 1 AP radiograph shows intramedullary nailing of a gunshot femoral shaft fracture. (Reproduced from Dougherty PJ, Najibi S: Gunshot fractures of the femoral shaft, in Dougherty PF, ed: *Gunshot Wounds*. Rosemont, IL, American Academy of Orthopaedic Surgeons, 2011, p 109.)

5. Transabdominal GSWs to the hip and pelvis
   a. Intra-articular contamination should be managed with urgent débridement and irrigation with fixation if required
   b. Although data are limited, transabdominal GSWs that result in extra-articular fractures with stable fracture patterns can be managed nonoperatively with broad-spectrum antibiotics for a minimum of 24 hours at the surgeon's discretion.

H. Complications
1. Infection—Occurs in 1.5% to 5% of patients; severity of injury is a contributing factor, and antibiotics help prevent infection after GSW.
2. Foreign bodies
   a. Historically, retained missile fragments have been presumed to be well tolerated.
   b. If symptoms develop late or with superficial or intra-articular location, surgical intervention is indicated.
   c. Clothing may be drawn into the wound at the time of injury and should be removed if present.
   d. In close-range shotgun injuries (<4 ft), shotgun wadding may be present within the wound and should be removed.
3. Neurovascular damage
   a. Greater in high-velocity injuries
   b. Temporary cavitation may result in traction or avulsion injuries to neurovascular structures outside the immediate path of the missile.
   c. Though controversial, observation is warranted for most neurologic deficits
4. Lead toxicity
   a. Synovial or cerebrospinal fluid is caustic to lead components of bullet missiles, resulting in lead breakdown products that may produce severe synovitis and low-grade lead poisoning.
   b. Lead also may be introduced into the bloodstream through phagocytosis by macrophages. Rarely, this mechanism leads to lead toxicity.

II. OPEN FRACTURES

A. Definition—An open fracture is a soft-tissue injury that includes a fracture. Communication is present between the fracture site and an overlying break in the skin (**Figure 2**).

B. Clinical evaluation
1. Initial assessment begins with an evaluation of airway, breathing, circulation, disability, and exposure (ABCDE).
   a. Roughly one-third of patients with open fractures have associated injuries; therefore, life-threatening injuries must be assessed, and treatment must begin immediately. The treating physician must take care not to allow the presence of an open fracture to distract from associated injuries to the head, chest, abdomen, pelvis, and spine.

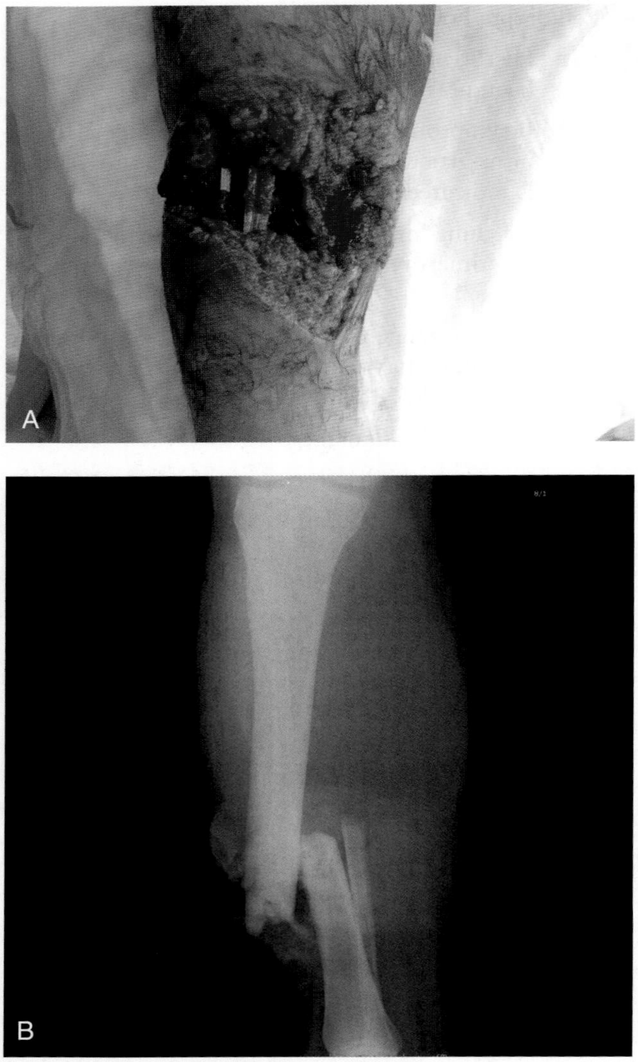

Figure 2 Clinical photograph (**A**) and AP radiograph (**B**) of a Gustilo-Anderson type IIIB open tibial shaft fracture.

b. All four extremities must be assessed for injury and, when possible, a detailed neurovascular examination must be undertaken. A complete soft-tissue assessment, palpation for tenderness, and observation of any deformity also are included in the initial evaluation.

2. Emergency department care

a. Tetanus prophylaxis should be given when appropriate (**Table 1**), and antibiotic treatment should begin immediately.

b. Bleeding should be controlled by direct pressure rather than by limb tourniquets or blind clamping.

TABLE 1

Requirements for Tetanus Prophylaxis

	For Clean, Minor Wound		For All Other Wounds	
Immunization History	**dT**	**TIG**	**dT**	**TIG**
Incomplete (<3 doses) or not known	+	–	+	+
Complete but >10 yr since last dose	+	–	+	–
Complete and <10 yr since last dose	–	–	–*	–

dT = diphtheria and tetanus toxoids, TIG = tetanus immune globulin, + = prophylaxis required, – = prophylaxis not required, * = required if >5 yr since last dose

c. Manual exploration of the wound in the emergency department is not indicated if formal surgical intervention is planned. Exploration in the emergency department risks further contamination and hemorrhage as well as neurovascular injury.

d. The open wound can be covered with saline-moistened gauze, and the extremity can be splinted.

3. Compartment syndrome must be considered a possibility in all extremity fractures.

C. Radiographic evaluation

1. In any case of suspected open fracture, AP and lateral radiographs of the affected area should be obtained, in addition to radiographs that include the joints above and below. These radiographs should be obtained as soon as possible to allow preoperative planning to begin.

2. CT is ordered as clinically indicated. In cases of periarticular fractures when temporary spanning external fixation is planned, CT often is best delayed until after the joint has been spanned so as to provide the most information possible.

3. Angiography is obtained based on the clinical suspicion of vascular injury, the type of injury, and the following indications:

a. Knee dislocation (or equivalent; eg, medial tibial plateau fracture) with asymmetric pulses

b. A cool, pale foot with poor distal capillary refill

c. High-energy injury in an area of compromise (eg, trifurcation of the popliteal artery)

d. Any lower extremity injury with documented ankle brachial index <0.9

TOP TESTING FACTS

Gunshot Wounds

1. Missile velocity is arbitrarily categorized into two groups: low-velocity (<2,000 ft/s) and high-velocity (>2,000 ft/s).
2. Shotgun blasts can inflict either high-energy injuries or low-energy injuries.
3. The permanent cavity is caused by mechanical crushing of soft tissues. The temporary cavity results from tissue that has been elastically stretched. The shock wave can cause tissue damage at a site distant from the path of the bullet.
4. Nerve injury can occur at a site remote from the immediate path of the bullet.
5. The energy imparted to human tissue by a bullet depends on the energy of the bullet on impact, the energy upon exit, and the behavior of the bullet while within the target.
6. Outpatient treatment may be appropriate in certain low-velocity GSWs.
7. A GSW that passes through the abdomen before passing through the hip joint requires débridement of the joint. If the GSW passes through the abdomen and creates a stable, extra-articular fracture, it can be managed with observation and broad-spectrum antibiotics.

Open Fractures

1. One-third of patients with open fractures will have associated injuries.
2. Antibiotics should be given as soon as possible in the treatment of open fractures.
3. In open fractures, fracture stabilization provides protection from further soft-tissue injury.
4. For mangled extremities, the indications for limb salvage versus amputation are controversial.
5. The number of medical comorbidities is a significant predictor of infection in patients with open fractures.

Bibliography

Agel J, Evans AR, Marsh JL, et al: The OTA open fracture classification. *J Orthop Trauma* 2013;27(7):379-384. doi:10.1097/BOT.0b013e3182820d31.

D'Alleyrand J-CG, Manson TT, Dancy L, et al: Is time to flap coverage of open tibial fractures an independent predictor of flap-related complications? *J Orthop Trauma* 2014;28(5):288-293.

FLOW Investigators: A trial of wound irrigation in the initial management of open fracture wounds. *N Engl J Med* 2015; 373(27):2629-2641.

Gustilo RB, Anderson JT: Prevention of infection in the treatment of one thousand and twenty-five open fractures of long bones: Retrospective and prospective analyses. *J Bone Joint Surg Am* 1976;58(4):453-458.

Gustilo RB, Mendoza RM, Williams DN: Problems in the management of type III (severe) open fractures: A new classification of type III open fractures. *J Trauma* 1984;24(8):742-746.

Johnson JP, Karam M, Schisel J, Agel J: An evaluation of the OTA-OFC system in clinical practice : A multicenter study with 90 days outcomes. *J Orthop Trauma* 2016;30(11):579-583.

Lack WD, Karunakar MA, Angerame MR, et al: Type III open tibia fractures : immediate antibiotic prophylaxis minimizes infect. *J Orthop Trauma* 2015;29(1):1-6.

Marsh JL, Hao J, Cuellar DO, et al: Does the OTA open fracture classification predict the need for limb amputation? A retrospective observational cohort study on 512 patients. *J Orthop Trauma* 2016;30(4):194-198.

Miller AN, Carroll EA, Pilson HT-P: Transabdominal gunshot wounds of the hip and pelvis. *J Amer Acad Orthop Surg* 2013;21:286-292.

National Center for Injury Prevention & Control: Centers for Disease Control & Prevention: *Web-Based Injury Statistics Query & Reporting System (WISQARS) Injury Mortality Reports, 1981-2017*. Available at http://www.cdc.gov/injury/wisqars/index.html. Accessed January 21, 2019.

Sathiyakumar V, Thakore RV, Stinner DJ, Obremskey WT, Ficke JR, Sethi MK: Gunshot-induced fractures of the extremities: A review of antibiotic and debridement practices. *Curr Rev Musculoskelet Med* 2015;8(3):276-289.

Streubel PN, Stinner DJ, Obremskey WT: Use of negative-pressure wound therapy in orthopaedic trauma. *J Am Acad Orthop Surg* 2012;20(9):564-574.

Tosti R, Rehman S: Surgical management principles of gunshot-related fractures. *Orthop Clin North Am* 2013;44(4):529-540.

Weber D, Dulai SK, Bergman J, Buckley R, Beaupre LA: Time to initial operative treatment following open fracture does not impact development of deep infection: A prospective cohort study of 736 subjects. *J Orthop Trauma* 2014;28(11):613-619.

Chapter 88
Nonunions, Malunions, and Osteomyelitis

GEOFFREY S. MARECEK, MD

I. NONUNION

A. Definitions

1. Delayed union—a fracture that is progressing more slowly toward healing than would normally be expected; however, achieving union remains possible.
2. Nonunion—a fracture in which all reparative processes have ceased without bony healing. All progress toward union has ceased; union cannot be achieved without further intervention.

B. Etiology

1. Risk factors—nonunions are often multifactorial in nature; broadly, nonunions can be attributed to factors related to the patient, the injury, and the treatment (**Table 1**).
2. Infection—Infection alone does not preclude fracture healing; however, it can contribute to the failure of a fracture to progress to union. The presence of infection should be suspected in all nonunions.

C. Evaluation

1. History
   a. A thorough history is imperative; understanding the mechanism of injury, prior surgical and nonsurgical interventions, and identifying factors that may have contributed to a nonunion are critical first steps.

Dr. Marecek or an immediate family member serves as a paid consultant to or is an employee of Globus Medical, Nuvasive, Stryker, Synthes, and Zimmer; has received research or institutional support from BoneSupport AB; and serves as a board member, owner, officer, or committee member of the Orthopaedic Trauma Association and the Western Orthopaedic Association.

   b. Any history of infection or use of antibiotics outside the perioperative period should be recorded.
2. Physical examination
   a. A detailed evaluation of distal pulses and patency of vessels is essential.
   b. Motor and sensory function in the limb must be assessed.
   c. The status of the soft-tissue envelope, prior incisions, flaps, areas of compromised skin, etc, is critical
   d. An assessment of the stability or stiffness of the nonunion provides useful information for treatment.
   e. The limb should be evaluated for deformity, including rotational deformity and any resultant limb-length discrepancy.
   f. All nonunions should be evaluated for signs of infection.
3. Imaging studies
   a. High-quality orthogonal radiographs are necessary.
   b. If limb-length discrepancy or deformity of the lower extremity is a potential issue, a full-length, weight-bearing view of both lower extremities is required.
   c. Comparison views of the contralateral limb help with preoperative planning.
   d. A CT scan may provide additional detail regarding union and articular injury or malreduction, but quality may be limited by the presence of metal implants.

This chapter is adapted from Lowenberg D: Nonunions, malunions, and osteomyelitis, in Boyer MI, ed: *AAOS Comprehensive Orthopaedic Review 2*. Rosemont, IL, American Academy of Orthopaedic Surgeons, 2014, pp 275-284.

a. This matrix is avascular, making it difficult for antibiotics to penetrate.

b. Depending on the microbe, the biofilm layer usually forms between 8 and 14 days following planktonic colonization of the bone.

3. Biofilm represents the "first-line response" of bacterial colonization, in which the initial colony invasion "falls on the sword" to create a bacteria-friendly environment for the rest of the colony to inhabit. It consists of a dead bacterial sludge milieu.

4. A mature biofilm complex represents the greatest barrier to treatment and effective eradication of musculoskeletal infections, especially if the infection involves bone or is implant related. This is due to the fact that the microbes enter into a sessile phase with markedly reduced metabolic rate, as well as the fact that the biofilm itself impairs efficacy because it represents a barrier to diffusion.

D. Evaluation

1. Clinical presentation

a. A draining sinus tract with abscess formation is the classic presentation of osteomyelitis. Often, the sinus tracts are multifocal in nature.

b. In acute osteomyelitis secondary to trauma, the clinical manifestation is exposed bone or a nonhealing, soupy, soft-tissue envelope over the bone.

c. Indolent infections might present with only chronic swelling and induration, occasionally accompanied by recurrent bouts of cellulitis.

2. Imaging

a. Radiographic evaluation of the affected limb segment is performed.

b. Osteomyelitis can present radiographically as areas of osteolysis acutely, then chronically as areas of dense sclerotic bone because of the avascular, necrotic nature of osteomyelitic bone.

c. When a necrotic segment of free, devascularized, infected bone is left in a limb over time, it becomes radiodense on radiographs and is called a sequestrum (**Figure 4**). Occasionally, it will be engulfed and surrounded or walled off by healthy bone; it is then called an involucrum.

3. Laboratory studies

a. Hematologic profiles are routine in the evaluation of osteomyelitis.

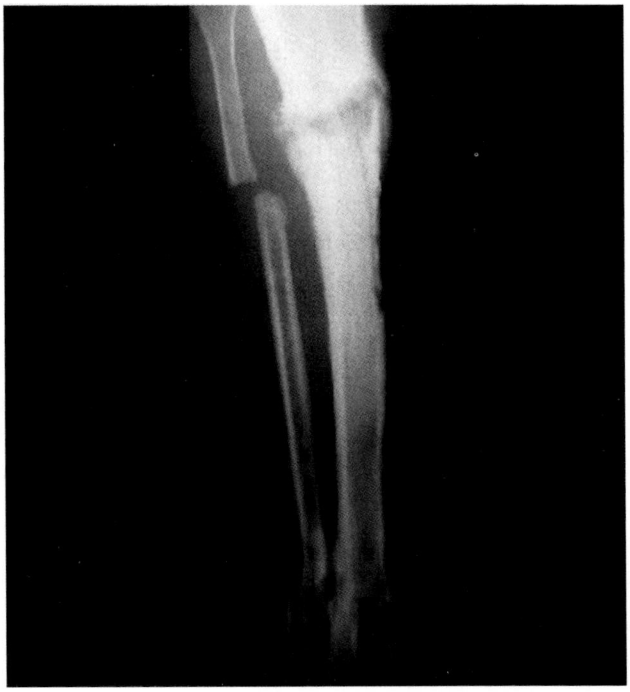

Figure 4 AP radiograph from a 24-year-old man 2 years after an open tibia fracture. The dense, necrotic cortical bone at the medial border of the tibia represents a sequestrum.

- Blood tests that should be ordered include CBC with differential, ESR, and CRP.

b. In acute osteomyelitis, elevated white blood cell (WBC) count, platelet count, ESR, and CRP level may be present; neutrophilia of the differential often is present.

c. In chronic osteomyelitis, the WBC and platelet counts usually are normal. Often, the ESR is normal as well; occasionally, the CRP level also is normal.

d. Surgery or trauma also can elevate the platelet count, ESR, and CRP level. The platelet count generally returns to normal once the hemoglobin level has stabilized to a more normal range. The CRP value usually normalizes within 2 to 4 weeks, and the ESR returns to normal within 4 to 8 weeks.

4. Tissue culture

a. The diagnosis of osteomyelitis depends on obtaining appropriate culture specimens.

b. The benchmark for proper diagnosis is obtaining good tissue samples for culture. If an abscess cavity exists, this can sometimes be performed adequately with needle aspiration.

c. Appropriate bacterial and fungal plating of the specimen is important.

d. In chronic osteomyelitis, the culture specimens sometimes fail to grow. This does not mean that infection is absent, but rather that the offending organisms cannot be grown successfully. Often, patients with chronic osteomyelitis have received multiple courses of antibiotic therapy, making it hard to grow the organisms in a laboratory setting.

e. Much new interest has focused on using polymerase chain reaction (PCR) analysis of specimens to determine whether microbial DNA is present as a way of diagnosing microbial infection.

E. Classification

1. The most widely accepted clinical staging system for osteomyelitis is the Cierny-Mader system (**Table 2**).

a. This system considers the anatomy of the bone involvement (**Figure 5**), then subclassifies the disease according to the physiologic status of the host (**Table 3**).

b. This staging method helps define the lesion and the ability of the host to deal with the process.

c. Prognosis has been well correlated with the physiologic host subclassification.

F. General treatment principles

1. Once the osteomyelitis has been staged and the condition of the host has been defined and optimized, a treatment plan individualized to the patient's condition and goals can be determined.

2. Ideally, the goal of treatment is complete eradication of the osteomyelitis with a preserved soft-tissue envelope, a healed bone segment, and preserved limb length and function.

3. Because of the extreme variation in the way osteomyelitis presents and manifests itself in different people, there is a paucity of good evidence-based data to aid in making treatment guidelines.

G. Surgical treatment

1. Surgical débridement

a. Surgical débridement is the cornerstone of osteomyelitis treatment.

- Adequate débridement is achieved when all infected and devitalized bone and tissue have been excised.

b. Débridement of any dense fibrotic scar is also necessary because it is often quite avascular and represents a poor soft-tissue bed for healing.

c. Atrophic skin that has become adherent to the bone (eg, the medial border of the tibia) also requires débridement because of its impaired blood supply and compliance.

d. It may not be possible to preserve enough bone or tissue for a functional limb; in these cases, amputation may be required or preferred.

2. Skeletal stabilization

a. Skeletal stabilization of the affected limb is necessary when mechanical instability results from débridement.

- This includes all type IV lesions and some type III lesions where a large amount of bone has been removed.

TABLE 2

Cierny-Mader Staging System for Osteomyelitis

Stage	Anatomic Type	Typical Etiology	Treatment
1	Medullary	Infected intramedullary nail	Removal of the infected implant and isolated intramedullary débridement
2	Superficial; no full-thickness involvement of cortex	Chronic wound, leading to colonization and focal involvement of a superficial area of bone under the wound	Remove layers of infected bone until viable bone is identified
3	Full-thickness involvement of a cortical segment of bone; endosteum is involved, implying intramedullary spread	Direct trauma with resultant devascularization and seeding of the bone	Noninvolved bone is present at same axial level, so the osteomyelitic portion can be excised without compromising skeletal stability
4	Infection is permeative, involving a segmental portion of the bone	Major devascularization with colonization of the bone	Resection leads to a segmental or near-segmental defect, resulting in loss of limb stability

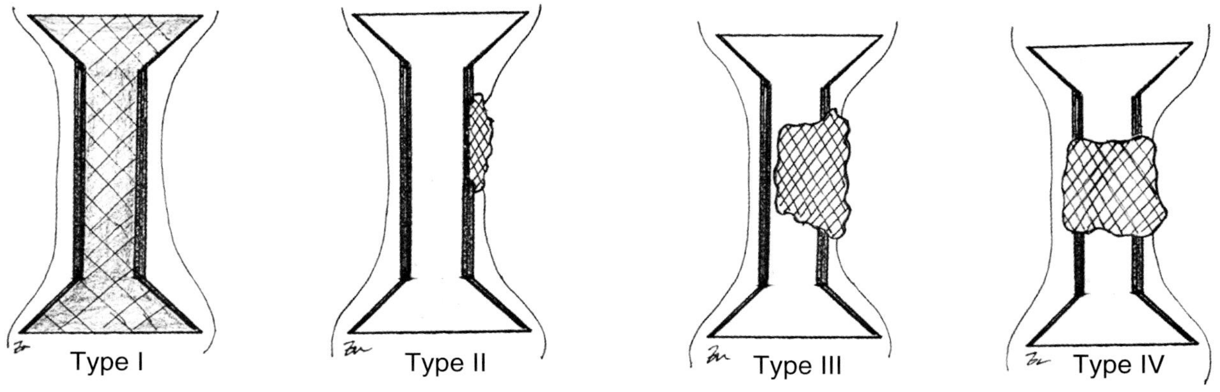

Figure 5 Illustrations show the Cierny-Mader anatomic classification of osteomyelitis. Type I is intramedullary osteomyelitis; type II is superficial osteomyelitis with no intramedullary involvement; type III is invasive localized osteomyelitis with intramedullary extension, but with a maintained, stable, uninvolved segment of bone at the same axial level; and type IV is invasive diffuse osteomyelitis, with involvement of an entire axial segment of bone such that excision of the involved segment leaves a segmental defect of the limb. (Reproduced from Ziran BH, Rao N: Infections, in Baumgaertener MR, Tornetta P III, eds: *Orthopaedic Knowledge Update: Trauma*, ed 3. Rosemont, IL, American Academy of Orthopaedic Surgeons, 2005, p 132.)

- If a segmental defect is created with the débridement, then proper planning in skeletal stabilization must occur from the start, with a clear and comprehensive plan established to gain bony stability of the limb.

b. Stabilization is accomplished most often with external fixation. It also can be accomplished with antibiotic-impregnated cement-coated medullary nails or plates.

c. For small defects (<2 cm), acute shortening remains a reasonable option for treatment, especially in the upper extremity.

- Delayed bone grafting or osteomyocutaneous free tissue transfer is also possible after infection eradication.

d. For some large osseous defects, the best option remains bone transport using distraction osteogenesis.

TABLE 3

Physiologic Host Classification Used With the Cierny-Mader Osteomyelitis Classification System

Type	Infection Status	Factors Perpetuating Osteomyelitis	Treatment
A	Normal physiologic responses to infection	Little or no systemic or local compromise; minor trauma or surgery to affected part	No contraindications to surgical treatment
B (local)	Locally active impairment of normal physiologic responses to infection	Cellulitis, prior trauma (such as open fracture, compartment syndrome, and free flap), or surgery to area; chronic sinus; free flap	Consider healing potential of soft tissues and bone, and anticipate the need for free tissue transfer and hyperbaric oxygen
B (systemic)	Systemically active impairment of normal physiologic responses to infection	Diabetes, immunosuppression, vascular disease, protein deficiency, or metabolic disease	Consider healing potential of soft tissues and treat correctable metabolic or nutritional abnormalities
C	Severe infection	Severe systemic compromise and stressors	Because treatment of condition is worse than the condition itself, suppressive treatment or amputation is recommended

Reproduced from Ziran BH, Rao N: Infections, in Baumgaertener MR, Tornetta P III, eds: *Orthopaedic Knowledge Update: Trauma*, ed 3. Rosemont, IL, American Academy of Orthopaedic Surgeons, 2005, p 133.

3. Dead-space management
   a. Débridement creates a dead space; this space requires appropriate management while the infection is being eradicated.
      - The dead space can be filled by means of local muscle mobilization, a rotational muscle flap, a free muscle flap, a free fasciocutaneous flap, or a rotational perforator-based flap.
   b. The VAC sponge is a useful short-term adjunct to assist in dead-space management until definitive soft-tissue coverage is achieved.
      - If placed directly over cortical bone for an extended period, it can result in dessication and death of the cortical bone beneath.
   c. Antibiotic-impregnated PMMA beads are a time-honored method for managing dead space; they also provide an effective means of local, high-dose antibiotic delivery.
      - Most surgeons make their own beads by mixing PMMA with tobramycin and vancomycin powder.
      - Other antibiotics used include gentamycin, erythromycin, tetracycline, and colistin. In general, heat-stable antibiotics can be used.
      - Resorbable materials, including calcium sulfate, calcium phosphate, and hydroxyapatite ceramic beads with antibiotic impregnation, have recently been introduced, but their clinical efficacy has not yet been well established.
   d. Antibiotic-impregnated PMMA beads can be used effectively with or without a closed soft-tissue envelope.
      - With an open soft-tissue envelope, the beads can be placed and then the limb and wound wrapped with an adhesive-coated plastic film laminate. This provides a biologic barrier with high-dose local antibiotic delivery and usually does well for 4 to 6 days before requiring changing because of leakage.
      - With a closed soft-tissue envelope, the beads can be left in for an extended period to further ensure that infection has been controlled.
4. Soft-tissue coverage
   a. A close working relationship with a microsurgeon experienced in soft-tissue mobilization and free tissue transfer is imperative in managing osteomyelitis with soft-tissue void or an impaired soft-tissue envelope.
   b. Rotational flaps are a good adjuvant for certain soft-tissue defects or when a microsurgeon is not available.
   c. Flap coverage combined with bone transport to fill large bone and soft-tissue defects is safe and effective and has good long-term results.
5. Antibiotic coverage
   a. Parenteral antibiotics are administered after débridement has been performed.
   b. Treatment protocols frequently involve a 6-week intravenous antibiotic regimen.
   c. With the sharp increase in organisms developing antibiotic resistance (such as methicillin-resistant *Staphylococcus aureus* and vancomycin-resistant *Enterococcus*), an appropriate antibiotic regimen may need to include daptomycin.
   d. In certain instances (C hosts), long-term antibiotic suppression can be the treatment of choice.

H. Distraction osteogenesis
1. Due to the frequency of segmental defects in osteomyelitis treatment, bone transport using distraction osteogenesis is often required.
2. Distraction osteogenesis is the process of creating new bone or "regenerate" by gradual distraction at a corticotomy site.
   a. A corticotomy is a low-energy periosteum-sparing osteotomy.
3. Distraction osteogenesis requires a latency phase followed by distraction at the proper rate and rhythm. A typical latency period is 5 to 10 days depending on the bone and healing potential at the corticotomy.
   a. The standard rate and rhythm is 1 mm distraction per day divided into 0.25-mm increments (ie, four times daily).
   b. Slower distraction or smaller increments may be necessary in other long bones (ie, not the femur).
4. The consolidation phase typically lasts twice as long as the distraction phase.

TOP TESTING FACTS

Nonunions

1. Stable fixation is paramount for successful treatment of nonunions.
2. A biologically viable environment at the nonunion site is also essential. The bone ends may have excellent biologic capacity, or a biologic stimulus may be required.
3. Infection and endocrinological abnormalities are two contributing factors to nonunions that should be addressed concomitantly with surgical treatment.
4. A healthy, well-vascularized soft-tissue envelope is necessary for the healing of tenuously vascularized diaphyseal bone ends. Use of free or rotational muscle or skin flaps enhances the healing environment.

Malunions

1. Accurate assessment of a malunion using physical examination and radiologic evaluation is critical for successful treatment.
2. A variety of treatment options exist and must be individualized to the patient, deformity location and severity, and surrounding soft-tissue envelope.

Osteomyelitis

1. Radical débridement of all nonviable bone, soft tissue, and inert material is the critical step in the treatment of osteomyelitis.
2. Proper dead-space management and soft-tissue coverage are similarly important.
3. The host and the bone involvement should be staged properly at the beginning of treatment so that an appropriate treatment plan can be established.
4. Biofilm currently represents the major limiting factor in eradicating microbes with antibiotics in the care of infection, especially implant-related and bone infections.
5. Local and parenteral antibiotic treatment is the standard of care.

Bibliography

Barger J, Fragomen A, Rozbruch R: Antibiotic-coated interlocking intramedullary nail for the treatment of long bone osteomyelitis. *J Bone Joint Surg Rev* 2017;5(7):e5.

Bishop JA, Palanca AA, Bellino MJ, et al: Assessment of compromised fracture healing. *J Am Acad Orthop Surg* 2012;20(5):273-282.

Brinker MR, O'Connor DP, Monla YT, et al: Metabolic and endocrine abnormalities in patients with nonunions. *J Orthop Trauma* 2007;21(9):634-642.

Hernigou P, Poignard A, Beaujean F, et al: Percutaneous autologous bone marrow grafting for nonunions: Influence of the number and concentration of progenitor cells. *J Bone Joint Surg* 2005; 87(7): 1430-1437.

Stucken C, Olszewski DC, Creevy WR, et al: Postoperative diagnosis of infection in patients with nonunions. *J Bone Joint Surg* 2013;95(15):1409-1412.

Swanson EA, Garrard ED, Bernstein DT, et al: Results of a systematic approach to exchange nailing for the treatment of aseptic femoral nonunions. *J Orthop Trauma* 2015;29(1):21-27.

Swanson EA, Garrard ED, O'Connor DP, et al: Results of a systematic approach to exchange nailing for the treatment of aseptic tibial nonunions. *J Orthop Trauma* 2015;29(1):28-35.

Watson JT: Distraction osteogenesis. *J Am Acad Orthop Surg* 2006;14(10 Spec No.):5168-5174.

Zura R, Xiong Z, Einhorn T, et al: Epidemiology of fracture nonunion in 18 human bones. *JAMA Surg* 2016;151(11):e162775.

Chapter 89
Fractures of the Clavicle, Scapula, and Glenoid

PETER A. COLE, MD
STEVEN R. GAMMON, MD
TONY PEDRI, MD

I. CLAVICULAR FRACTURES

A. Anatomy and biomechanics

1. Clavicle osteology
   a. The clavicle is the only long bone to ossify by intramembranous ossification.
   b. It serves as the primary stabilizer between the axial skeleton (via the sternoclavicular [SC] joint) and the appendicular skeleton (via the acromioclavicular [AC] joint).
2. Coracoclavicular (CC) ligaments
   a. Conoid—medial; trapezoid—lateral.
   b. The CC ligaments are the primary stabilizers to superior (vertical) translation of the distal clavicle.
3. Superior shoulder suspensory complex (SSSC)
   a. The SSSC is a bone–soft-tissue ring that provides a stable connection of the glenoid and scapula to the clavicle.
   b. The SSSC is composed of four bony landmarks—distal clavicle, acromion, coracoid process, and glenoid neck—and the supporting ligamentous complexes of the AC joint and the CC ligaments (**Figure 1**).
4. Blood supply
   a. The primary blood supply to the clavicle is periosteal; there is no nutrient blood supply.
   b. The clavicle is subcutaneous, and its muscular envelope includes the platysma, pectoralis major, deltoid, and some of the strap muscles of the neck.
5. Radiographic appearance
   a. The clavicle forms a unique S-shaped curve on the axial view.
   b. The distal clavicle is flat in the AP plane.

B. Overview and epidemiology

1. Clavicular fractures account for 3.8% of all fractures and 35.0% to 45.0% of all shoulder girdle injuries.
2. Approximately 15% of clavicular fractures are distal third, 80% are middle third, and 5% are medial third.
3. Medialization of a clavicular fracture more than 20 mm is associated with a measurable decrease in functional outcome.

C. Evaluation

1. History
   a. Injury—Most clavicular fractures are related to a lateral blow to the shoulder from a fall (most common) or a direct blow to the clavicle.
   b. A small percentage of clavicular fractures are associated with more severe injuries, including scapulothoracic dissociation, scapular fractures, rib fractures, pneumothorax, and neurovascular compromise.
2. Physical examination
   a. The typical deformity of middle-third fractures is caused by a medial fragment pulled superiorly by the sternocleidomastoid muscle, with the weight of gravity pulling downward on the lateral fragment.

Dr. Cole or an immediate family member has stock or stock options held in BoneFoams Inc. and LLC and has received research or institutional support from Stryker and Synthes. Neither of the following authors nor any immediate family member has received anything of value from or has stock or stock options held in a commercial company or institution related directly or indirectly to the subject of this chapter: Dr. Pedri and Dr. Gammon.

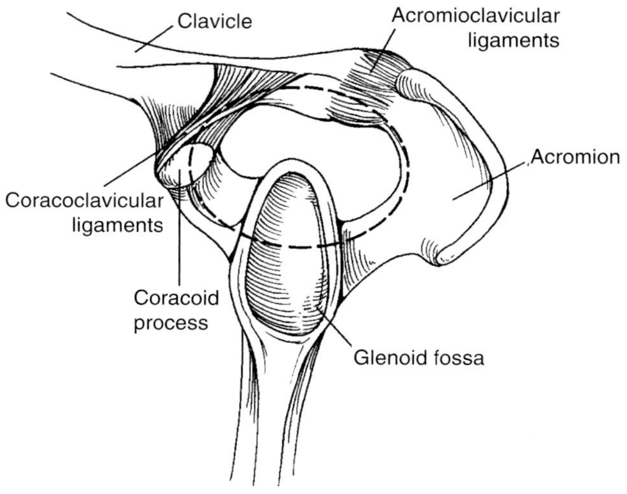

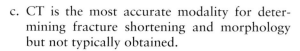

Figure 1 Illustration shows a lateral view of the bone–soft-tissue ring of the superior shoulder suspensory complex. (Reproduced from Goss TP: Scapular fractures and dislocations: Diagnosis and treatment. *J Am Aced Orthop Surg* 1995;3:22-23.)

b. A distal neurovascular examination is important because of the proximity of the brachial plexus and the subclavian vessels to the zone of injury.

c. Tenting of the skin should be evaluated carefully because it can be a sign of impending open fracture.

3. Imaging

a. Upright and supine radiographs, including an AP view of the clavicle and a 15° cephalad tilt view, should be obtained to define displacement when the patient is upright (**Figure 2**).

b. A bilateral panoramic view of both shoulders should be obtained to measure clavicular shortening.

c. CT is the most accurate modality for determining fracture shortening and morphology but not typically obtained.

D. Classification

1. The Allman classification defines fractures of the proximal (medial), middle (midshaft), and distal (lateral) thirds of the clavicle (**Figure 3**).

2. Neer classified lateral-third fractures based on the integrity of the CC ligament complex and the involvement of the AC joint (**Figure 4**).

3. Medial third fractures are classified according to the displacement and involvement of the SC joint.

E. Treatment

1. Lateral-third clavicular fractures

a. Nonsurgical treatment is reserved for all nondisplaced or minimally displaced fractures. Type II and type V fractures (especially type IIB) have a higher incidence of nonunion because of deforming forces.

b. Surgical treatment is considered for type II fractures because of the high incidence of nonunion.

c. Surgical fixation options include Kirschner wire fixation, tension band constructs, locking plates, and "Hook Plates.".

- Similar results have been shown with and without coracoclavicular ligament reconstruction or augmentation.
- Results of Hook Plate fixation have demonstrated favorable radiographic and clinical outcomes though they must be removed requiring a second surgery.

d. Complications include AC joint arthritis in intra-articular variants, nonunion, and loss of fixation.

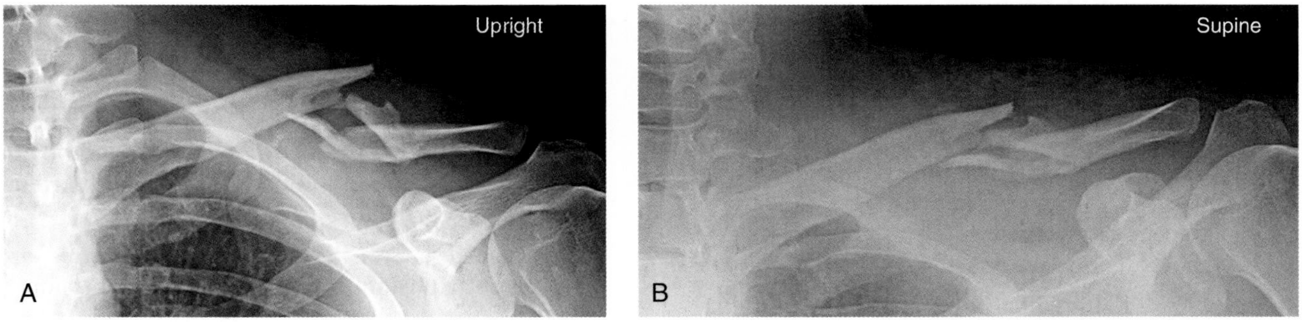

Figure 2 AP radiographs of a patient with a midshaft clavicle fracture show increased displacement when the patient is upright (**A**) compared with supine (**B**).

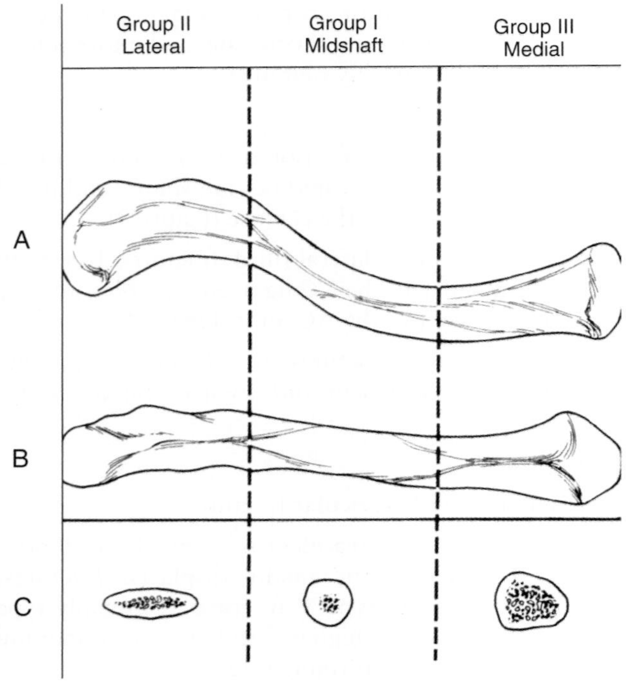

Figure 3 Diagram demonstrates the Allman classification system of clavicle fractures, which divides the clavicle into thirds. Group I (middle third) constitutes 69%-85% of fractures; group II (distal [lateral] third) makes up 12%-28%; and group III (medial third) represents 3%-6%.

2. Middle-third clavicular fractures
   a. Nonsurgical treatment is appropriate for nondisplaced or minimally displaced middle-third fractures. Treatment includes initial immobilization and the use of a sling is sufficient. Better clinical results and improved patient satisfaction with the use of sling compared with figure of eight bracing treatment have been shown.
   b. Surgical indications include open fractures or fractures with concomitant injuries to subclavian neurovascular structures, 100% displacement, more than 20 mm of shortening, highly comminuted fractures, and multiple upper or lower extremity fractures (polytrauma).
   c. Implant choices include intramedullary screw or elastic nail fixation, superior plate fixation, anterior-inferior plate fixation, and dual plating techniques. Both superior and anterior-inferior plating techniques have advantages. Recent biomechanical literature has reported that superior plating may be better for axial compression and anterior-inferior plating better for cantilever bending. Randomized controlled trials have found no difference in time to union or rates of hardware removal.
   d. Surgical complications include iatrogenic neurovascular injury, subclavian thrombosis, pneumothorax, injury to the supraclavicular nerves, hardware prominence, infection, nonunion, and even death.
3. Medial third clavicular fractures
   a. Nonsurgical treatment is appropriate for most medial third clavicular fractures that are nondisplaced or minimally displaced.
   b. Surgical intervention is reserved for fractures with significant displacement or posterior displacement into the mediastinum.
   c. Surgical procedures—Open reduction and internal fixation (ORIF) with plate and screws is used, with SC joint augmentation or reconstruction if the fracture is very medial and has little or no fixation to the medial clavicle.
   d. Complications are similar to those seen in posterior SC dislocation.
      - Retrosternal and mediastinal injuries are seen, including vascular, pulmonary, esophageal, cardiac, and neurologic injuries. Thoracic surgeon backup is important.
      - Hardware migration into the mediastinum has also been reported, causing late intrathoracic or vascular injury when Kirschner wires are used.

F. Rehabilitation
1. Nonsurgically treated clavicular fractures require a short period of immobilization (2 to 4 weeks), with simple Codman exercises followed by full active-assisted and passive range of motion. Strengthening generally begins by 6 to 10 weeks.
2. Surgically treated clavicular fracture rehabilitation typically begins immediately with full active-assisted and passive range of motion. Strengthening is begun 4 to 6 weeks postoperatively.

G. Pearls and pitfalls
1. Scapulothoracic dissociation should be considered in the presence of severe displacement when substantial distraction of the clavicle fragments or forequarter is evident on chest radiographs or when neurovascular injury to the upper extremity has occurred.
2. Displaced lateral-third clavicular fractures are inherently unstable and are prone to nonunion.
3. Completely displaced middle-third clavicular fractures treated nonsurgically have a nonunion rate of 15% to 20%.

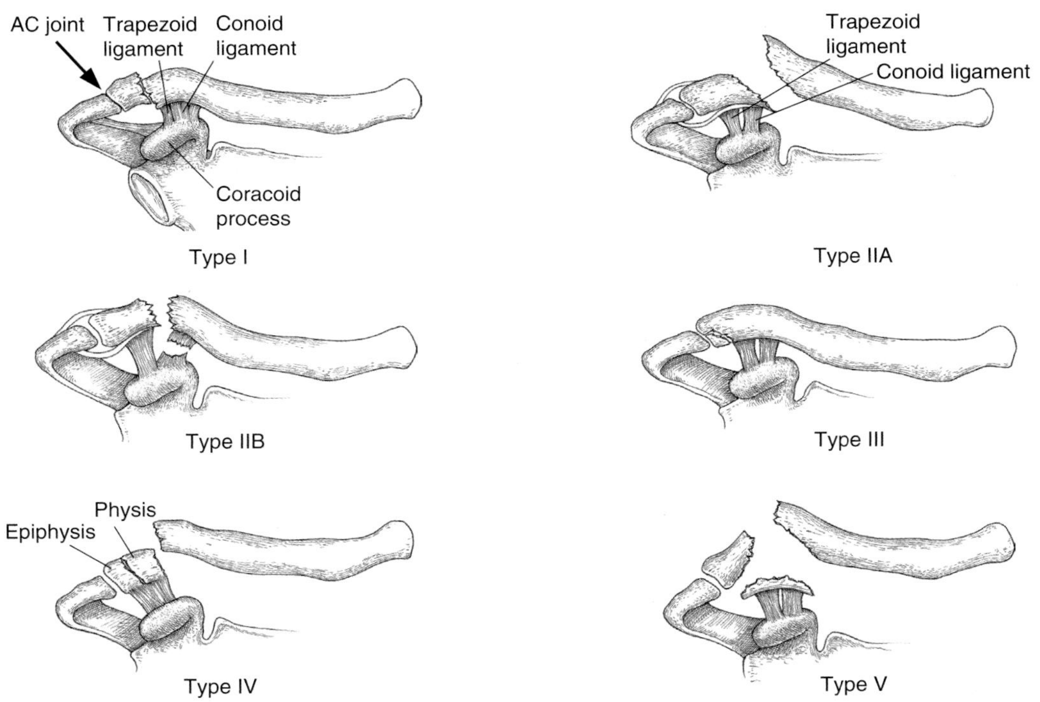

Figure 4 Illustration shows the Neer classification of distal clavicular fractures. Type I fractures occur lateral to the coracoclavicular (CC) ligaments but do not extend into the acromioclavicular (AC) joint. Type II fractures are subdivided into type IIA or type IIB, based on the fracture pattern relative to the CC ligaments. Type IIA fractures occur just medial to the CC ligaments, resulting in greater displacement, and type IIB fractures occur between the conoid and the trapezoid ligaments. Type III fractures involve intra-articular extension into the AC joint without ligamentous disruption. Type IV fractures occur in skeletally immature individuals and mimic an AC joint dislocation. Type V fractures represent an avulsion of the CC ligaments from the clavicle with an associated distal clavicular fracture. (Reproduced from Banerjee R: Management of distal clavicle fractures. *J Am Acad Orthop Surg* 2011;19:392-401.)

4. Additional risk factors for nonunion after clavicular fractures include advanced age, distal-fifth fractures, displaced transverse fractures, female sex, and comminuted displaced middle-third fractures.
5. Nonsurgical management of completely displaced clavicular fractures is associated with slower functional return, more muscle fatigability, patient perception of poorer cosmesis, more symptomatic malunions, and a greater percentage of nonunions than such fractures managed surgically.

II. SCAPULAR AND GLENOID FRACTURES

A. Anatomy and biomechanics

1. Glenoid
   a. The labrum deepens the pear-shaped glenoid fossa by up to 50%.
   b. Glenoid version is 2° of anteversion relative to the scapular body.
2. Body of the scapula
   a. Ossification begins at the eighth week of gestation.
   b. Two-thirds of shoulder motion is glenohumeral, and one-third is scapulothoracic.
   c. The scapula is the origin or insertion for 18 muscles.
3. Spine
   a. The spine of the scapula is an osseous bridge that separates the supraspinatus from the infraspinatus origin.
   b. The spinoglenoid notch is a potential site of suprascapular nerve tethering or compression.
4. Acromion—Has three ossification centers: the meta-acromion (base), the mesoacromion (mid), and the preacromion (tip).
5. Coracoid process
   a. Site of muscular attachments for the coracobrachialis, the short head of the biceps, and the pectoralis minor
   b. Site of ligament attachments for the CC ligaments

6. Superior shoulder suspensory complex (**Figure 1**)
    a. Composed of the distal clavicle, acromion, coracoid process, glenoid, and ligamentous structures of the AC joint and CC ligaments
    b. Plays important role in shoulder stability and biomechanics

B. Overview and epidemiology
1. Scapula fractures account for only 3% to 5% of shoulder girdle injuries and less than 1% of all fractures.
2. Scapula fractures tend to result from high-energy events such as motor vehicle or motorcycle accidents, which account for approximately 90% of all fractures; however, a bimodal age distribution is beginning to develop with an increase in fragility fractures of the elderly.
3. Scapular fractures are associated with hemothorax or pneumothorax in 80% of cases, with ipsilateral extremity injury in 50%, head injury in 15%, cervical injury in 15%, and neurovascular injury in 10%.
4. Scapular fractures are missed or the diagnosis is delayed in up to 15% of multiply injured patients.

C. Pathoanatomy
1. Mechanism of injury
    a. Direct, blunt, lateral to medial force trauma causes scapular body, neck, and glenoid fractures.
    b. An axial load on an outstretched extremity can cause scapular neck and glenoid fractures.
    c. Glenohumeral dislocation can cause anterior (bony Bankart) or posterior (reverse bony Bankart) glenoid fractures.
2. Scapulothoracic dissociation is a lateral displacement of the scapula associated with severe soft-tissue injury and brachial and vascular injury of the extremity.

D. Evaluation
1. History—Patients typically present with a history of high-energy blunt trauma to the shoulder. A history that includes baseline level of function and the patient's occupation, recreation, and handedness should be obtained.
2. Physical examination
    a. The incidence of injuries associated with scapular and glenoid fractures is high (90%). Identifying the mechanism of injury is helpful in determining other injuries.
    b. A thorough neurovascular examination of the affected extremity should be performed.
    c. The skin should be examined for abrasions or open wounds that should delay surgical intervention.
3. Imaging
    a. A true AP (Grashey), transscapular (Y), and axillary view should be obtained.
        - Obtaining quality radiographs is often difficult secondary to patient discomfort and a lack of radiographic protocols.
        - Radiographic parameters include intra-articular step-off, lateral border offset (medialization), glenopolar angle (angle on the true AP view of the glenoid surface relative to the inferior wing), and angulation seen on the transscapular view.
    b. CT scan with three-dimensional reconstruction is the benchmark for measuring radiographic parameters and visualizing the full picture of the scapula. If the scapular fracture is displaced more than 1 cm, CT should be obtained for accurate measurements (**Figure 5**).

E. Classification—Classification is based on the fracture's location on the scapula.
1. The Ogawa classification of coracoid fractures is shown in **Table 1**.
2. The Kuhn classification of acromial fractures is shown in **Table 2**. It is important not to mistake an os acromiale for an acute fracture.
3. The AO-OTA classification of scapular fractures is based on involvement of the processes, the neck, body, and glenoid (**Figure 6**).
4. The Ideberg classification of glenoid fractures has been modified by Mayo to make a more practical classification by adding fracture patterns that also involve the body, acromion, and/or coracoid process (**Figure 7**).
5. Disruption of the SSSC can be classified as a single, double, triple, or quadruple lesion.
6. Scapulothoracic dissociation can be classified by the presence or absence of a brachial plexus injury.

F. Nonsurgical indications—Most scapular fractures are minimally to moderately displaced and can be treated nonsurgically.

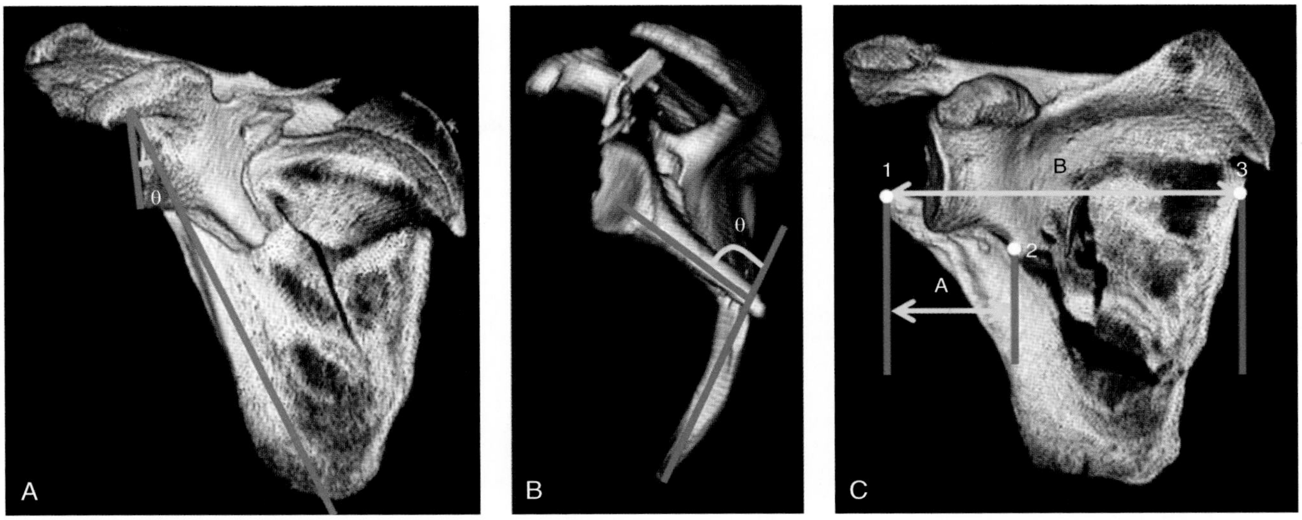

Figure 5 Three-dimensional CT reconstructions of the scapula demonstrate the accurate measurements of displacement and deformity for surgical decision making. **A**, Measurement of the glenopolar angle (GPA) represents the relationship of the glenoid surface on the AP view relative to the inferior wing. Normal GPA is 35°-45°. **B**, Scapular Y view demonstrates the angulation of the scapular body. Translation can also be well visualized on this view. **C**, Measurement of the medialization of the glenoid relative to the scapular body on the AP view. 1 = lateral-most point of the distal fragment, 2 = lateral-most point of the proximal fragment, 3 = medial-most point on the scapula at the level of the fracture, line A = medial/lateral displacement, line B = width of the scapula at the level of the fracture. (Reproduced from Cole PA, Gauger EM, Schroder LK: Management of scapular fractures. *J Am Acad Orthop Surg* 2012;20[3]:130-141.)

TABLE 1

Ogawa Classification of Coracoid Fractures

Type of Fracture	Characteristics
1	Fracture occurs proximal to the coracoclavicular ligaments and is associated with other injuries to the superior shoulder suspensory complex, which results in double disruptions.
2	Fracture occurs toward the tip of the coracoid.

TABLE 2

Kuhn Classification of Acromial Fractures

Type of Fracture	Characteristics
I	Nondisplaced or minimally displaced
II	Displaced but does not compromise the subacromial space
III	Displaced and compromises the subacromial space

G. Surgical indications

1. Coracoid and acromion fractures—Surgical indications include painful nonunion, at least 1 cm of displacement, multiple disruption of the SSSC, or a concomitant ipsilateral scapular fracture requiring surgical intervention.
2. Glenoid fractures—Surgery is indicated when an intra-articular gap or step-off of greater than 4 mm or glenohumeral instability is present after dislocation. Usually at least 20% of the joint must be involved to be indicated.
3. Scapular body fractures
   a. Surgery may be indicated when any of the following is present.
      - Lateral border offset (medialization) of at least 20 mm
      - Glenopolar angle of 22° or less
      - Angulation as seen on the transscapular view of at least 45°
      - Completely displaced double disruptions of the SSSC

Scapula

Bone: Scapula 14

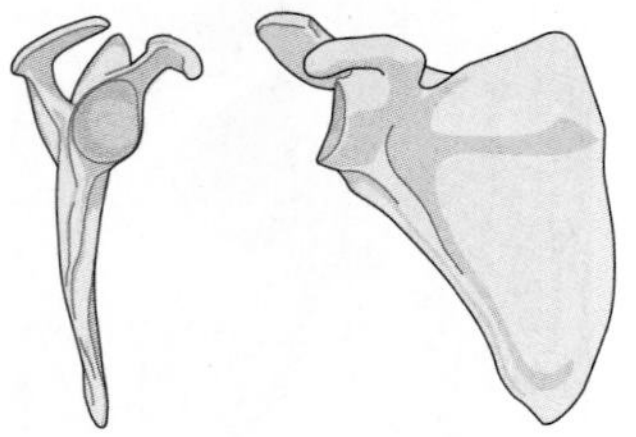

14

Locations:

Scapula, **process**
14A

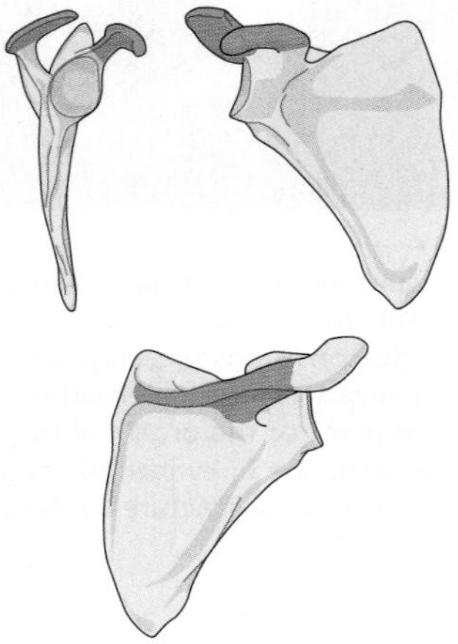

Scapula, **body**
14B*

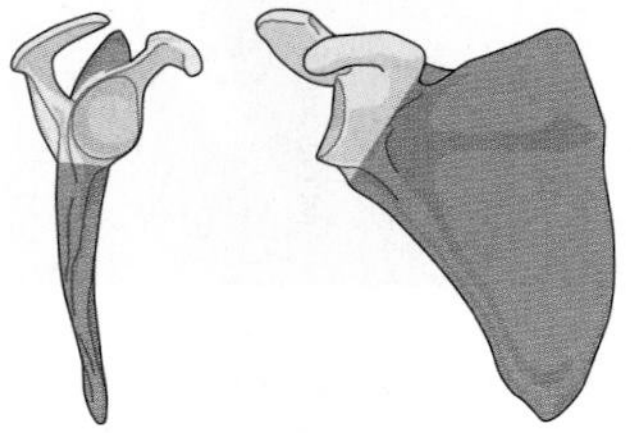

Scapula, **glenoid fossa**
14F*

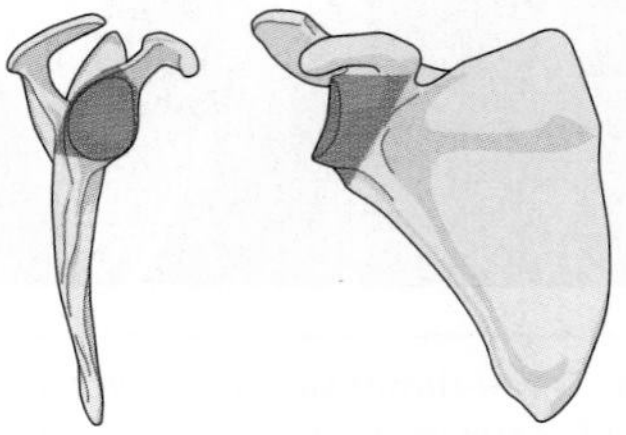

* Qualifications for process fractures:
x Coracoid P1
y Acromion P2
z Both processes P3
(These qualifications may be added to any fracture coded as type B or type F)

14A

Location: Scapula, **process** 14A

Types:

Scapula, process, **coracoid fracture**
14A1

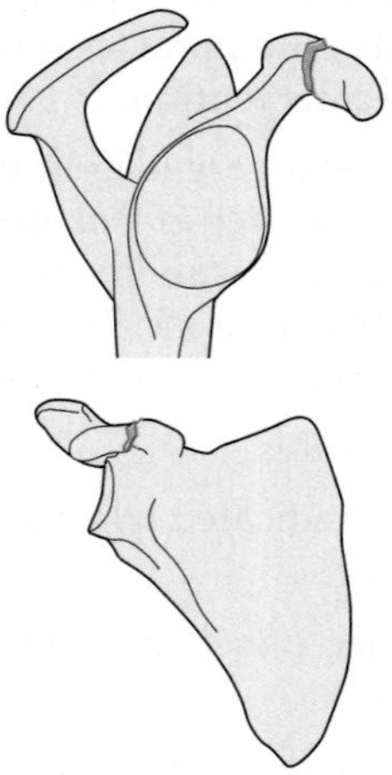

Scapula, process, **acromion fracture**
14A2

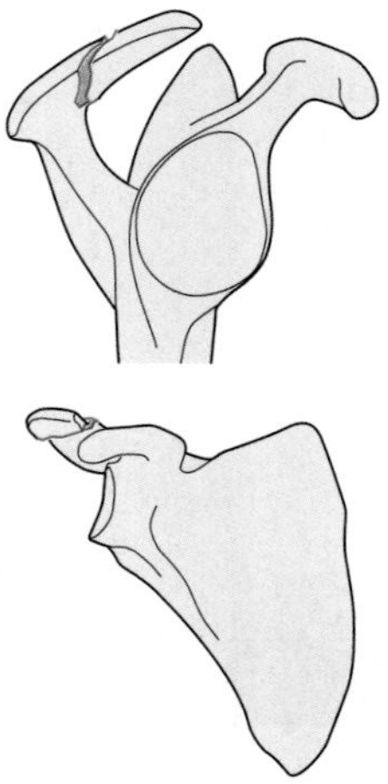

Scapula, process, **spine fracture**
14A3

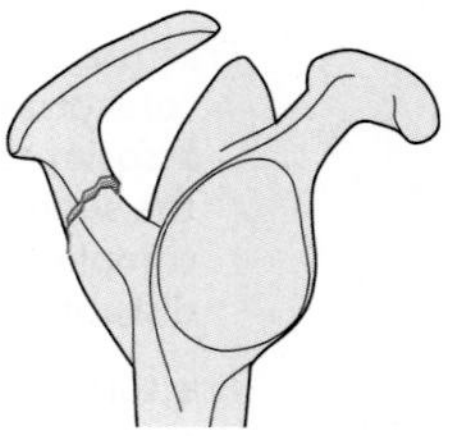

Qualifications *are optional and applied to the fracture code where the asterisk is located as a lower-case letter within rounded brackets. More than one qualification can be applied for a given fracture classification, separated by a comma. For a more detailed explanation, see the compendium introduction.*

Figure 6 The 2018 AO/OTA or OTA/AO Fracture and Dislocation Classification Compendium. (*J Orthop Trauma* 2018;32(Suppl 1), reprinted with permissions.)

14B

Location: Scapula, **body** 14B

Types:

Scapula, body, **fracture exits the body at 2 or less points**
14B1*

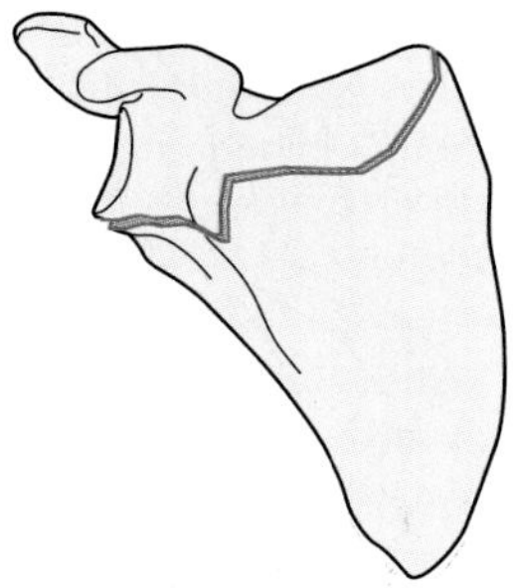

Scapula, body, **fracture exits the body at 3 or more points**
14B2*

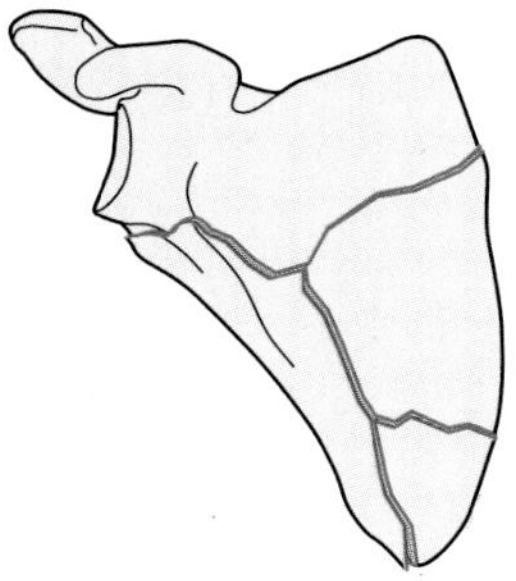

Qualifications:
l Lateral border fracture exit
m Medial border fracture exit
s Superior border fracture exit
g Area immediately lateral to base of coracoid (glenoid side exit)

14F

Location: Scapula, **glenoid fossa** 14F

Type:
Scapula, glenoid fossa, **through the extraarticular subchondral bone of the glenoid fossa (glenoid neck)** 14F0

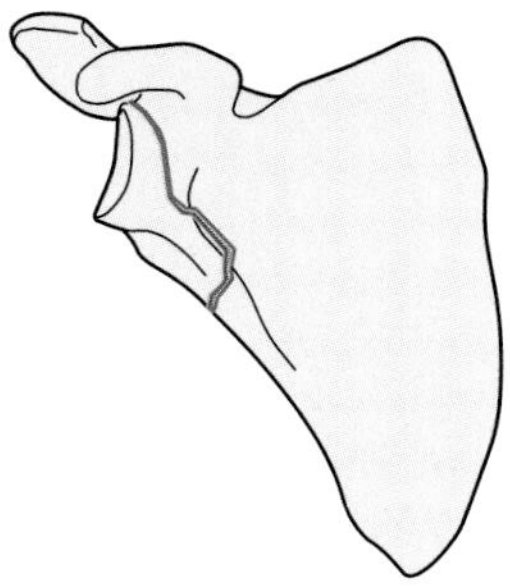

Figure 6 Cont'd

Type: Scapula, glenoid fossa, **simple fracture** 14F1

Groups:

Scapula, glenoid fossa, simple,
anterior rim fracture
14F1.1*

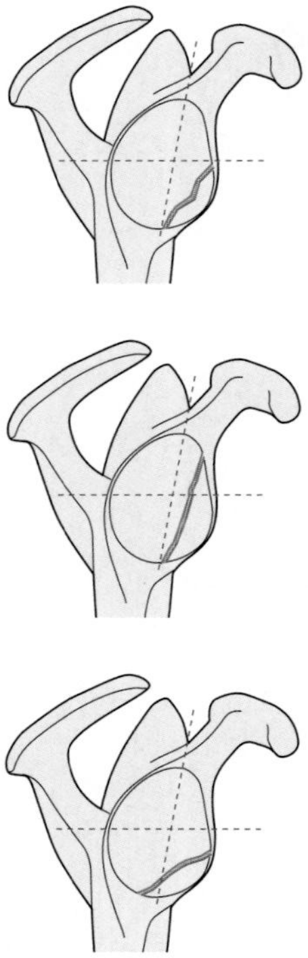

Scapula, glenoid fossa, simple,
posterior rim fracture
14F1.2*

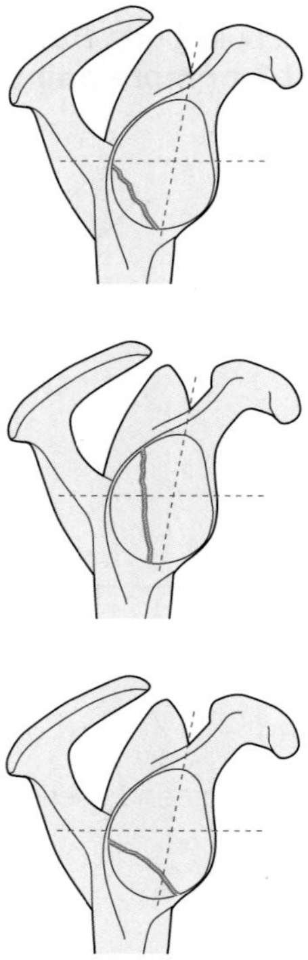

Scapula, glenoid fossa, simple,
transverse or short oblique fracture
14F1.3*

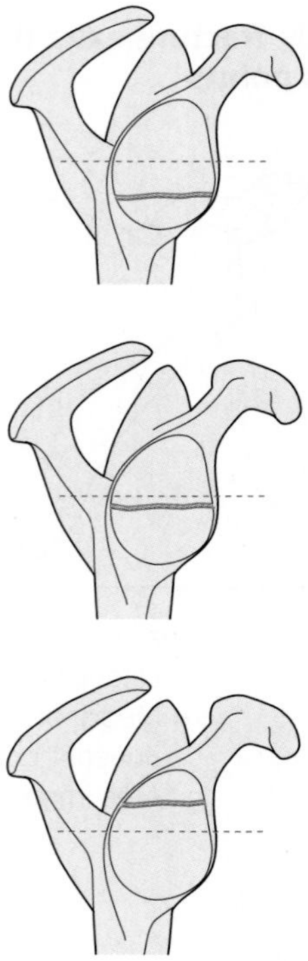

*Qualifications:
- f Infraequatorial rim fracture located in lower quadrant
- r Rim fracture anterior or posterior to maximum glenoid meridian with exits superior and inferior to the glenoid equatorial line
- t Fracture is located in two infraequatorial anterior and posterior quadrants with side of fracture defined by the center of fracture line

*Qualifications:
- i Infraequatorial
- e Equatorial
- p Supraequatorial

→ For more information about the four glenoid fossa quadrants, please refer to the Appendix.

Type: Scapula, glenoid fossa, **multifragmentary (three or more fracture lines)** 14F2

Groups:

Scapula, glenoid fossa, multifragmentary (3 or more articular fragments), **glenoid fossa fracture**
14F2.1

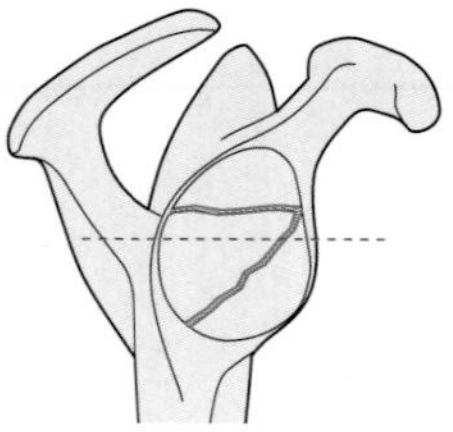

Scapula, glenoid fossa, multifragmentary (3 or more articular fragments with rim exits), **central fracture dislocation**
14F2.2

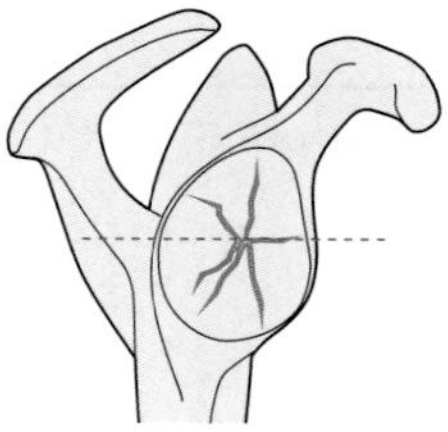

NOTE: Glenoid fractures with extension into the body are classified as a glenoid fracture, with the body fracture code added to the end of the code in square brackets [ ].

Figure 6 Cont'd

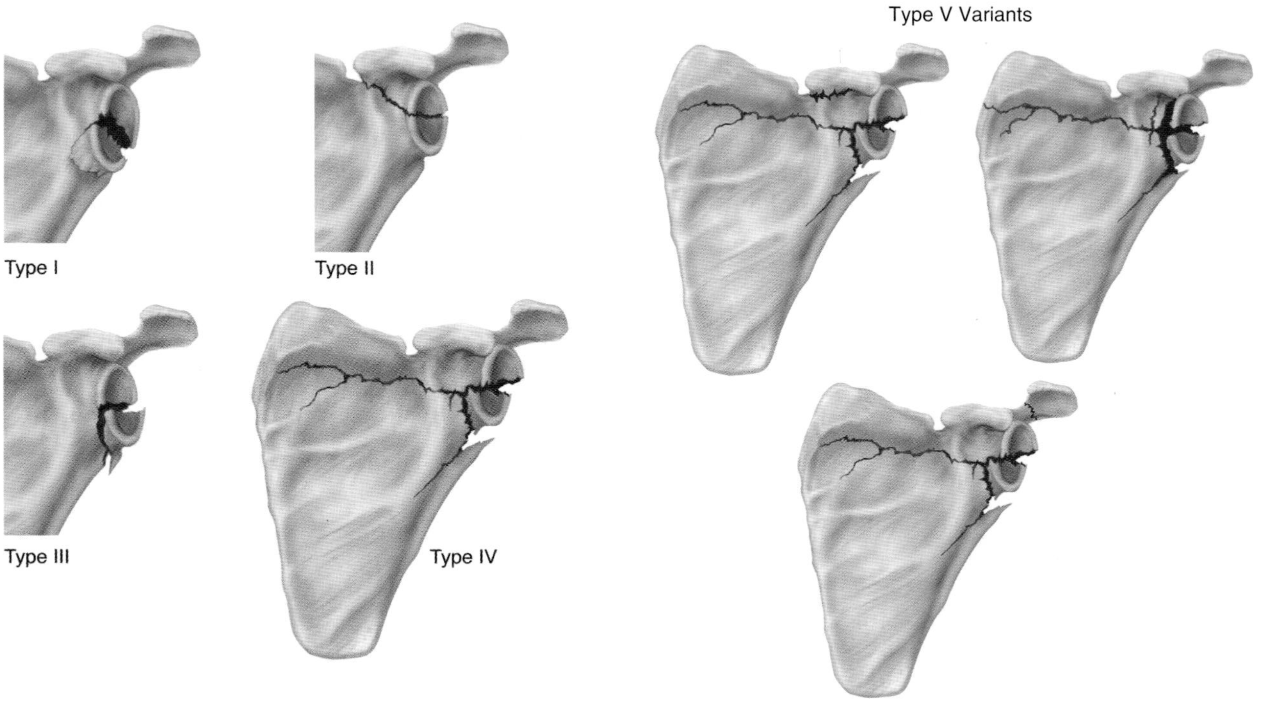

Figure 7 Illustrations depict the Mayo modification of the Ideberg classification of glenoid fractures. Type I injuries represent isolated involvement of the anterior-inferior joint surface (bony Bankart) and may be associated with shoulder dislocation. Type II injuries consist of a displaced articular segment involving the superior third to one half of the articular surface in continuity with the coracoid. Type III fractures encompass the inferior or inferoposterior portion of the fossa in continuity with a variable portion of the lateral border. Type IV patterns involve the inferior articular surface, with extension into the body, frequently with a stellate pattern that at times can involve the spine. The displaced articular segment may be free or contiguous with the lateral border of the body. Type V fractures represent a type IV pattern plus an additional coracoid, acromial, or free superior articular component.

b. If the fracture does not meet surgical criteria, weekly follow-up radiographs should be obtained for the first 2 to 3 weeks to ensure that no progressive displacement of an unstable fracture is present.

4. Double disruptions ("floating shoulder") as well as triple and quadruple disruptions of the SSSC can lead to discontinuity or malposition of the glenohumeral joint relative to the scapular body.

H. Surgical approach

1. The deltopectoral approach is used for anterior and superior glenoid fractures as well as coracoid fractures.
2. The transaxillary approach is sometimes beneficial for anterior-inferior glenoid fractures that extend into the scapular neck.
3. Posterior approaches
   a. A straight posterior approach is used for fractures isolated to the posterior glenoid, scapular neck, and/or the lateral border of scapula.
   b. The Judet approach is the most commonly used approach for scapular fractures. The incision begins at the acromion, courses along the spine of the scapula, and angles down along the vertebral border of the scapula. The surgeon can elevate the entire teres minor, infraspinatus, and posterior deltoid off the medial border of the scapula or can work in the interval between the infraspinatus and the teres minor while elevating the deltoid or splitting the muscle in line with its fibers.
   c. Other modifications have been described to minimize surgical dissection in posterior approaches including the deltoid sparing modified Judet approach.

I. Complications

1. Complications of scapular fractures are related primarily to the severity of the traumatic injury and associated injuries.
2. Axillary nerve injury is associated with fractures related to shoulder dislocation or traction.

J. Pearls and pitfalls
   1. Suprascapular nerve injury is associated with scapular neck fractures that involve the spinoglenoid and suprascapular notches. Preoperative electromyography (EMG) is recommended if the fracture involves the spinoglenoid notch and more than 2 weeks have elapsed since injury.
   2. Deformity and dysfunction are related.
   3. Length, alignment, rotation, and articular congruity are treatment principles, as for any bone.

K. Rehabilitation
   1. Nonsurgically treated scapular and glenoid fractures typically are immobilized in a sling or shoulder immobilizer with gentle Codman exercises for 2 weeks and then advanced to full active and passive range of motion after 3 weeks, beginning with resistive activities at 6 weeks post-injury.
   2. For surgically treated scapular and glenoid fractures, immediate full active and passive range of motion typically is prescribed for the first 4 weeks; then, a gradual strengthening program is initiated.
   3. Anterior approaches that involve subscapularis takedown require limitations in passive shoulder external rotation for 6 weeks.

TOP TESTING FACTS

1. The nonunion rate for displaced clavicular fractures treated nonsurgically is approximately 15%.
2. Risk factors for nonunion after clavicular fractures include advanced age, clavicular fractures of the distal fifth, displaced transverse fractures, female sex, and comminuted displaced middle-third fractures.
3. Nonsurgical management of completely displaced clavicular fractures is associated with slower functional return, more muscle fatigability, patient perception of poorer cosmesis, more symptomatic malunions, and a greater percentage of nonunions than such fractures managed surgically.
4. Surgical indications include open fractures or fractures with concomitant injuries to subclavian neurovascular structures, 100% displacement, more than 20 mm of shortening, highly comminuted fractures, and multiple upper or lower extremity fractures (polytrauma).
5. There is no difference in union or hardware removal with superior versus anterior-inferior clavicle plating.
6. Scapulothoracic dissociation should be suspected if vascular or neurological injury is present.
7. The acromion has three ossification centers; the meta-acromion (base), the mesoacromion (mid), and the preacromion (tip).
8. Scapular fractures are associated with hemothorax or pneumothorax in 80% of cases, ipsilateral extremity injury in 50%, head injury in 15%, cervical injury in 15%, and neurovascular injury in 10%.
9. The benchmark diagnostic test to measure angular deformities and displacement in scapular fractures with the greatest accuracy and reproducibility is the three-dimensional CT scan.
10. Surgical indications for scapular fractures include displaced intra-articular glenoid fractures, displaced double lesions of the SSSC, angulated scapular neck and body fractures greater than 45°, glenopolar angle of <20°, and lateral border offset (medialization) greater than 20 mm in active patients who demand optimal shoulder function.

Bibliography

Ahrens PM, Garlick NI, Barber J, Tims EM: The clavicle trial: A multicenter randomized controlled trial comparing operative with nonoperative treatment of displaced midshaft clavicle fractures. *J Bone Joint Surg Am* 2017;99(16):1345-1354.

Anavian J, Gauger EM, Schroder LK, Wijdicks CA, Cole PA: Surgical and functional outcomes after operative management of complex and displaced intra-articular glenoid fractures. *J Bone Joint Surg Am* 2012;94(7):645-653.

Banerjee R, Waterman B, Padalecki J, Robertson W: Management of distal clavicle fractures. *J Am Acad Orthop Surg* 2011;19(7):392-401.

Canadian Orthopaedic Trauma Society: Nonoperative treatment compared with plate fixation of displaced midshaft clavicular fractures: A multicenter, randomized clinical trial. *J Bone Joint Surg Am* 2007;89(1):1-10.

Choo AM, Schottel PC, Burgess AR: Scapulothoracic dissociation: Evaluation and management. *J Am Acad Orthop Surg* 2017;25(5):339-347.

Cole PA, Gauger EM, Schroder LK: Management of scapular fractures. *J Am Acad Orthop Surg* 2012;20(3):130-141.

Ersen A, Atalar AC, Birisik F, Saglam Y, Demirhan M: Comparison of simple arm sling and figure of eight clavicular bandage for midshaft clavicular fractures A RANDOMISED CONTROLLED STUDY. *Bone Joint J* 2015;97B(11):1562-1565.

Goudie EB, Clement ND, Murray IR, et al: The influence of shortening on clinical outcome in healed displaced midshaft clavicular fractures after nonoperative treatment. *J Bone Joint Surg Am* 2017;99(14):1166-1172.

Hill BW, Anavian J, Jacobson AR, Cole PA: Surgical management of isolated acromion fractures: Technical tricks and clinical experience. *J Orthop Trauma* 2014;28(5):e107-113.

Hill BW, Jacobson AR, Anavian J, Cole PA: Surgical management of coracoid fractures: Technical tricks and clinical experience. *J Orthop Trauma* 2014;28(5):e114-122.

Ideberg R, Grevsten S, Larsson S: Epidemiology of scapular fractures: Incidence and classification of 338 fractures. *Acta Orthop Scand* 1995;66(5):395-397.

Konigshausen M, Coulibaly MO, Nicolas V, Schildhauer TA, Seybold D: Results of non-operative treatment of fractures of the glenoid fossa. *Bone Joint J*. 2016;98-b(8):1074-1079.

Lee W, Choi CH, Choi YR, Lim KH, Chun YM: Clavicle Hook Plate fixation for distal-third clavicle fracture (neer type II): Comparison of clinical and radiologic outcomes between neer types IIA and IIB. *J Shoulder Elbow Surg*. 2017;26(7):1210-1215.

Mayo KA, Benirschke SK, Mast JW: Displaced fractures of the glenoid fossa: Results of open reduction and internal fixation. *Clin Orthop Relat Res* 1998;347:122-130.

Mulawka B, Jacobson AR, Schroder LK, Cole PA: Triple and quadruple disruptions of the superior shoulder suspensory complex. *J Orthop Trauma* 2015;29(6):264-270.

Nourian A, Dhaliwal S, Vangala S, Vezeridis PS: Midshaft fractures of the clavicle: A meta-analysis comparing surgical fixation using anteroinferior plating versus superior plating. *J Orthop Trauma* 2017;31(9):461-467.

Obremskey WT, Lyman JR: A modified Judet approach to the scapula. *J Orthopaedic Trauma* 2004;18(10):696-699.

Qvist AH, Vaesel MT, Jensen CM, Jensen SL: plate fixation compared with nonoperative treatment of displaced midshaft clavicular fractures: A randomized clinical trial. *Bone Joint J* 2018;100-b(10):1385-1391.

Schroder LK, Gauger EM, Gilbertson JA, Cole PA: Functional outcomes after operative management of extra-articular glenoid neck and scapular body fractures. *J Bone Joint Surg Am* 2016;98(19):1623-1630.

Tatro JM, Schroder LK, Molitor BA, Parker ED, Cole PA: Injury mechanism, epidemiology and hospital trends of scapula fractures: A 10-year retrospective study of the National Trauma Data Bank. *Injury*. January 2019.

Chapter 90
PROXIMAL HUMERAL FRACTURES

CLIFFORD B. JONES, MD, FACS
BLAKE A. EYBERG, MD

I. EPIDEMIOLOGY

A. Frequency—4% to 5% of all adult fractures (common)

B. Age and sex—bimodal distribution

1. High energy—younger men and boys
2. Low energy—older women
3. Patterns can be similar based on the extent of the osteoporosis, however.

II. PATHOANATOMY

A. Osseous

1. The proximal humerus is composed of four parts: the head, greater tuberosity, lesser tuberosity, and diaphysis.
2. The head is divided from the diaphysis via the surgical neck (distal to the tuberosities) and anatomic neck (proximal to the tuberosities).
3. Fractures extending into the surgical neck versus the anatomic neck affect the surgical options based on the fixation techniques and the vascular supply (see Section II.B).
4. The greater tuberosity has the supraspinatus, infraspinatus, and teres minor insertions. The lesser tuberosity has the subscapularis insertion.
5. Deforming forces about the proximal humerus include pectoralis major, pulling the shaft anterior and medial, subscapularis bringing the lesser tuberosity and articular surface into internal rotation, and supraspinatus, infraspinatus, and teres minor externally rotating the greater tuberosity.

B. Vascular (**Figure 1**)

1. The axillary artery courses medially to the humerus and supplies the proximal humerus via the anterior and posterior humeral circumflex arteries.
2. The anterior humeral circumflex branches into the arcuate artery of Liang, which courses the bicipital groove and terminates as a major blood supply to the greater tuberosity and the humeral head (36%).
3. The posterior humeral circumflex artery is another major blood supply (64%) and traverses the posterior head via the capsule, terminating in the greater tuberosity and the posterior humeral head.
4. Fracture patterns via the tuberosity and neck detachment disrupt the vascular supply to the humeral head and affect articular/head viability.
5. The vascular viability of the humeral head is optimized with 8 mm or more of the intact medial calcar.

C. Neural

1. The axillary nerve courses from anterior to posterior in close proximity to the inferior glenoid neck, anterior-inferior capsular pouch, and humeral heck; therefore, it is the site of the most common peripheral nerve injury.
2. Fracture-dislocations are associated with the highest risk of axillary nerve injury, which can occur in 20% to 50% of all fracture-dislocations (based on electromyographic analysis). This risk increases with glenohumeral dislocation and age.

Dr. Jones or an immediate family member has received royalties from Lippincott and OsteoConcentric; is a member of a speakers' bureau or has made paid presentations on behalf of Stryker; serves as a paid consultant to or is an employee of OsteConcentric and Stryker; and serves as a board member, owner, officer, or committee member of the Arizona Orthopaedic Society, the Banner University Medical Center – Phoenix, the Center Chief Orthopaedic Spine Institute, and the Orthopaedic Trauma Association. Neither Dr. Eyberg nor any immediate family member has received anything of value from or has stock or stock options held in a commercial company or institution related directly or indirectly to the subject of this chapter.

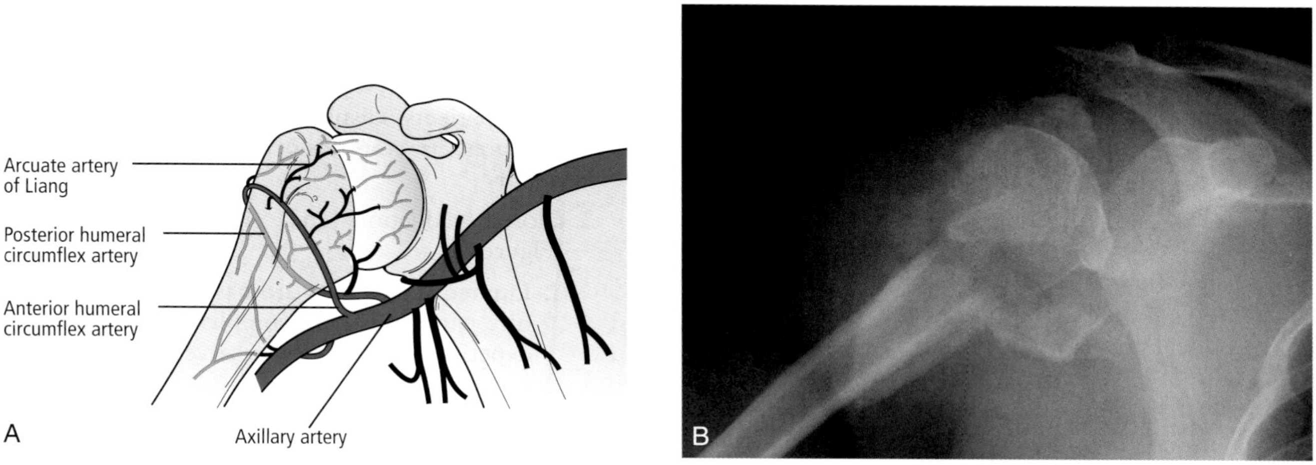

Figure 1 The illustration **(A)** and radiograph **(B)** demonstrate the proximal humeral vascularity: axillary artery, anterior humeral circumflex artery, arcuate artery of Liang, and posterior humeral circumflex artery.

III. EVALUATION

A. History

1. The preinjury functioning and comorbidities as well as the level of patient compliance should be determined. Patient and surgeon expectations should be determined.
2. The mechanism of injury should be determined.
    a. Low energy—The osseous quality should be confirmed.
    b. High energy—Associated injuries, nerve function, and vascular integrity should be evaluated.
    c. Glenohumeral integrity (dislocation, labrum, rotator cuff) should be discerned.

B. Physical examination

1. The entire shoulder, neck, and thorax (pulmonary) are examined for associated injuries.
2. Neural examination is confirmed to best of ability (pain limits motor function).

C. Imaging (**Figure 2**)

1. Injury radiographs (shoulder trauma series), including true AP (Grashey), axillary (to ensure head reduction but may falsely exaggerate

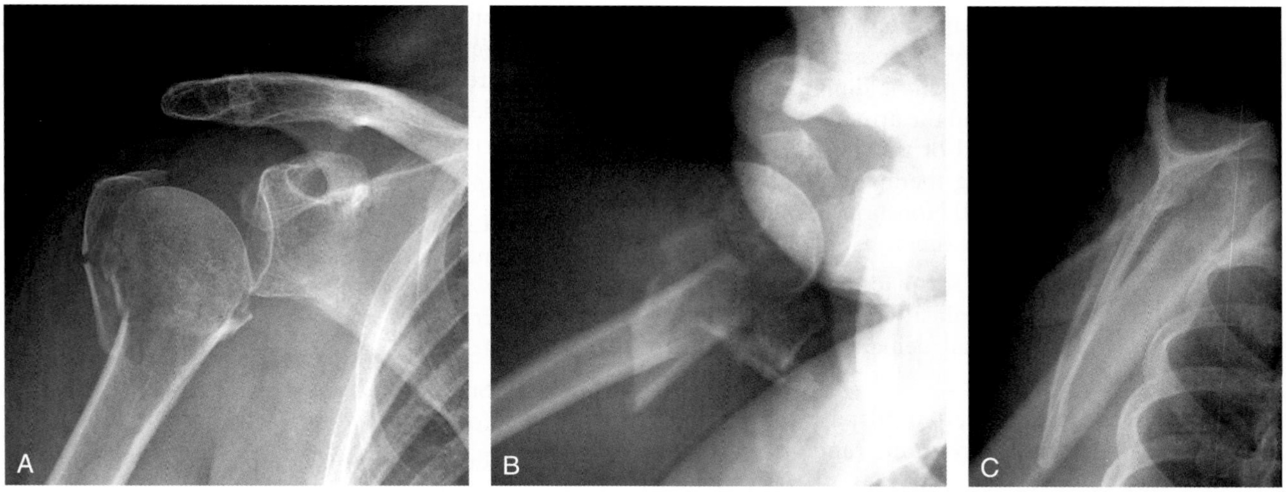

Figure 2 **A**, True AP (Grashey), **B**, axillary, and **C**, scapular Y shoulder radiographs demonstrating a complex comminuted proximal humeral fracture.

fracture angulation), and scapular Y views, are indicated in all fractures.

2. CT with reconstruction with three-dimensional averaging facilitates imaging of head-split fractures (marginal impaction, percentage of head involvement), fracture-dislocations, associated glenoid lesions (determine approaches), and extensive comminution with difficulty evaluating fracture patterns on plain radiography.
3. MRI has limited indications, including associated dislocation (labrum, anterior capsule, superior labrum anterior to posterior lesion, rotator cuff integrity).

IV. CLASSIFICATION

A. Based on fracture pattern and, therefore, vascular viability, healing, and outcomes

B. Codman classification—Fracture lines along physeal scars; therefore, four segments (head, greater tuberosity, lesser tuberosity, diaphysis)

C. Neer classification—Displaced with 1 cm or greater and 45° (**Figure 3**); has poor interobserver reliability

D. Orthopaedic Trauma Association/AO Foundation classification—Comprehensive long-bone classification based on location, stability, comminution, and dislocation (**Figure 4**)

V. TREATMENT

A. Nonsurgical

1. Nonsurgical treatment is not simply "benign neglect." Frequent follow-up examination and imaging are required. Fracture realignment is facilitated with sitting erect imaging, which allows the weight of the arm to offset muscle forces about the shoulder. After the pain is diminished, callus formation is present, and the arm moves as a functional unit, self-directed or therapy-assisted exercises can begin. Starting therapy too early or too late may be detrimental. Nonsurgical intervention is successful most of the time.
2. Indications—Minimal displacement, impacted displaced fractures, medical comorbidities, osteoporosis, low functional demand, and low outcome expectations.
3. Includes a sling and rest until pain diminishes; then a rotator cuff program, range of motion (ROM) activities, and activities of daily living (ADLs) are initiated until the patient becomes skilled at a daily home program.

B. Surgical

1. Indications—Young, high-demand patients, elderly patients with high expectations, cooperative patients, displaced unstable nonimpacted fractures, fracture-dislocations, adequate bone quality
2. Closed reduction and percutaneous pinning (**Figure 5**)
   a. Limited indications are based on simple fracture pattern, patient compliance, and surgeon experience, primarily reserved for pediatric population.
   b. Contraindications—Should not be used in dislocations (need for early ROM), metaphyseal comminution/diaphyseal extension (problems achieving a stable anchor point), severe osteoporosis (relative), or head-split fracture (unable to achieve early ROM and stable fixation).
   c. Pins are inserted initially under power and then advanced by hand terminally to avoid head penetration; two to four lateral-to-proximal and two greater tubercle pins (90-90 fixation) are inserted divergently and cut under the skin to avoid infection.
   d. Pins are removed at 6 weeks in the office or surgical suite; then unlimited ROM and strengthening are initiated.
3. Open reduction and internal fixation (ORIF) (**Figure 6**)
   a. Indications—All types of fractures, including head split, diaphyseal extension, and comminution
   b. Contraindications—Unreconstructable fracture patterns, fracture-dislocation may be a relative contraindication to ORIF in the elderly patient as half of these may undergo revision surgery for failure.
   c. Implants
      - Limited fixation—Combination of pin, cannulated screw, suture, and tension band wiring; best reserved for isolated tuberosity fractures and impacted (not comminuted) fractures.
      - Standard plate/screw implants—Reserved for very good quality bone
      - Locked plating implants—Used in compromised bone, comminution, and short-segment fixation. This has become the most

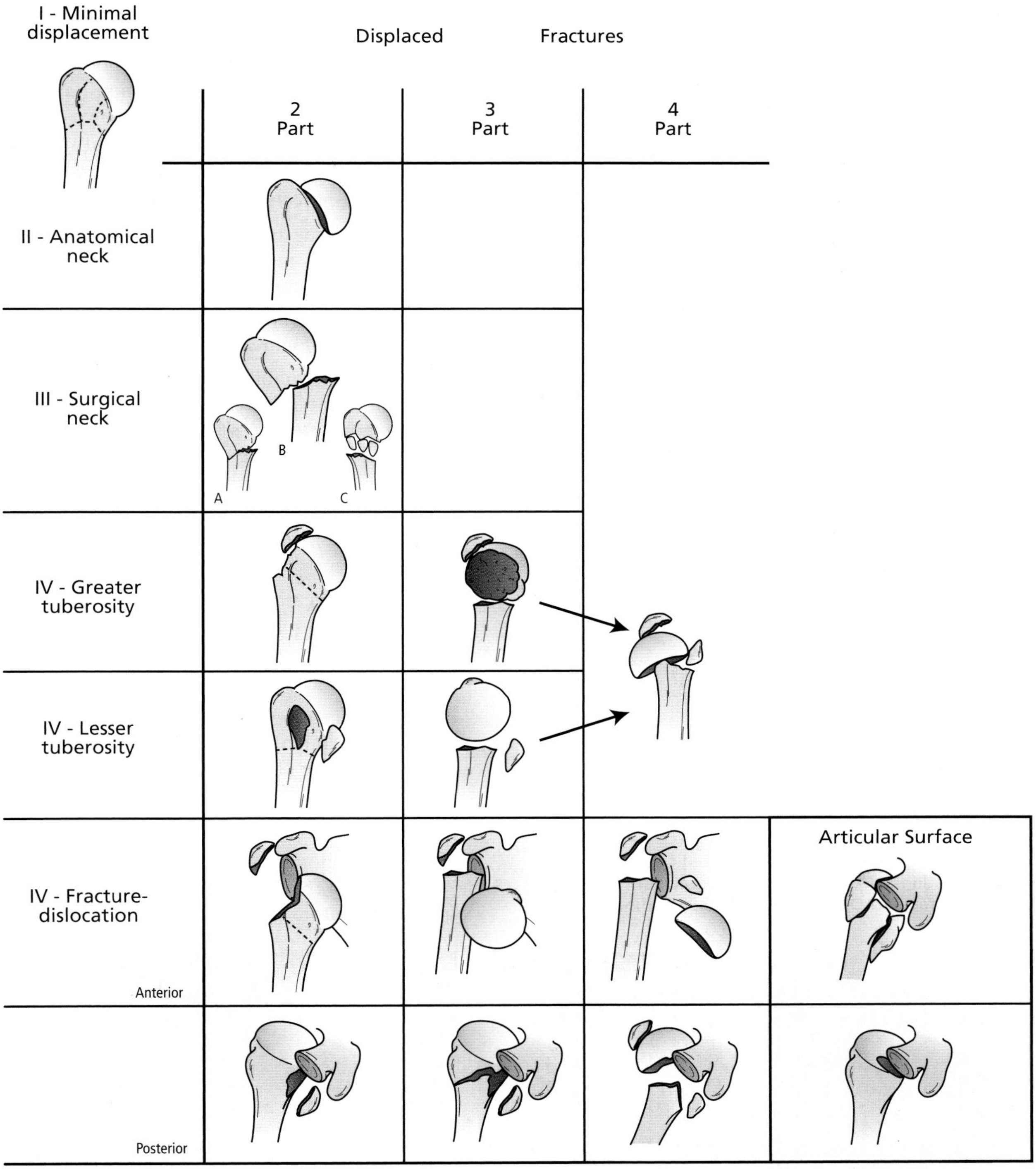

Figure 3 Chart demonstrates the Neer proximal humeral classification.

common implant of choice for proximal humerus fixation based on the poor track record of other fixation methods. Despite this, failures are all too common based on many factors.

d. Approaches

- Deltopectoral—Workhorse, most common; can fix or replace through this approach; may be problematic with displaced greater tuberosity fractures.

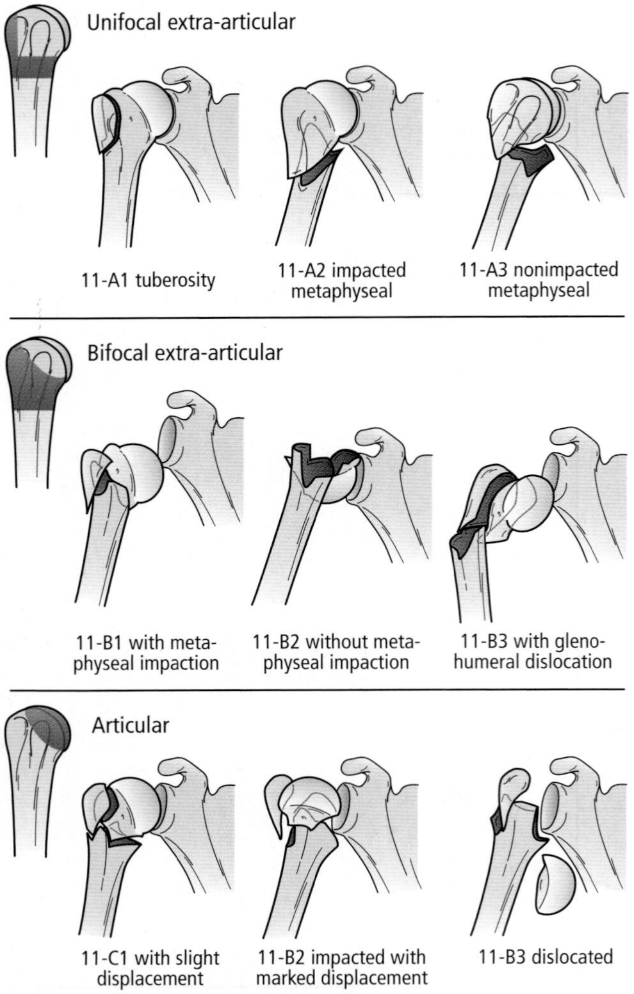

Figure 4 Chart demonstrates the Orthopaedic Trauma Association (OTA)/Arbeitesgemeinschaft fur Osteosynthesefragen (AO) proximal humeral classification.

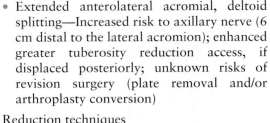

- Extended anterolateral acromial, deltoid splitting—Increased risk to axillary nerve (6 cm distal to the lateral acromion); enhanced greater tuberosity reduction access, if displaced posteriorly; unknown risks of revision surgery (plate removal and/or arthroplasty conversion)

e. Reduction techniques
- Soft-tissue integrity should be maintained, especially medially along the calcar.
- Rotator cuff attachments are used for tuberosity mobilization and stabilization with sutures (**Figure 7**).
- Joystick mobilization of head, tuberosity, and shaft with provisional 2.5 mm Schantz pin insertion. Also, an aid for reduction as a unit for fracture-dislocations.
- With comminution and limited calcar stability, medially inserted fibular strut graft insertion and mechanics (endosteal substitution) may be considered.

f. Plate application
- Lateral to the bicipital groove to enhance symmetrical screw insertion and diminish head penetration
- Distal to the rotator cuff insertion to avoid subacromial impingement and enhance calcar screw ("kickstand" screw) insertion
- Usually involves elevation of the deltoid insertion
- Care should be taken to avoid dissection or plate application distal and/or posterior to the deltoid (radial nerve).

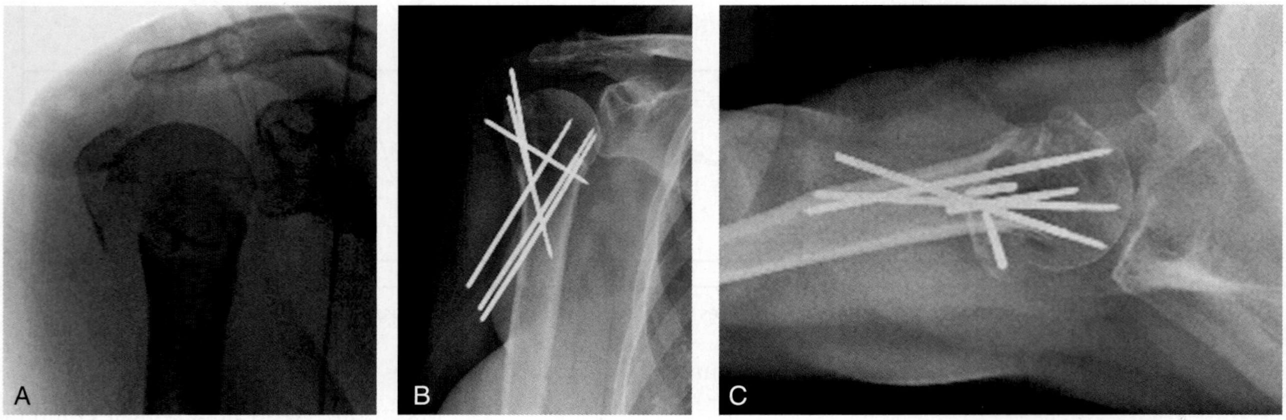

Figure 5 **A**, Radiograph of a four-part valgus impacted proximal humeral fracture with displaced greater tuberosity fracture. **B** and **C**, Postoperative radiographs of closed reduction percutaneous pinning utilizing 2.5 mm terminally threaded Schantz pins manually inserted, symmetrically and divergently deep into the subchondral bone but not through, and two pins inserted under power into the greater tuberosity, ending in the medial proximal diaphysis.

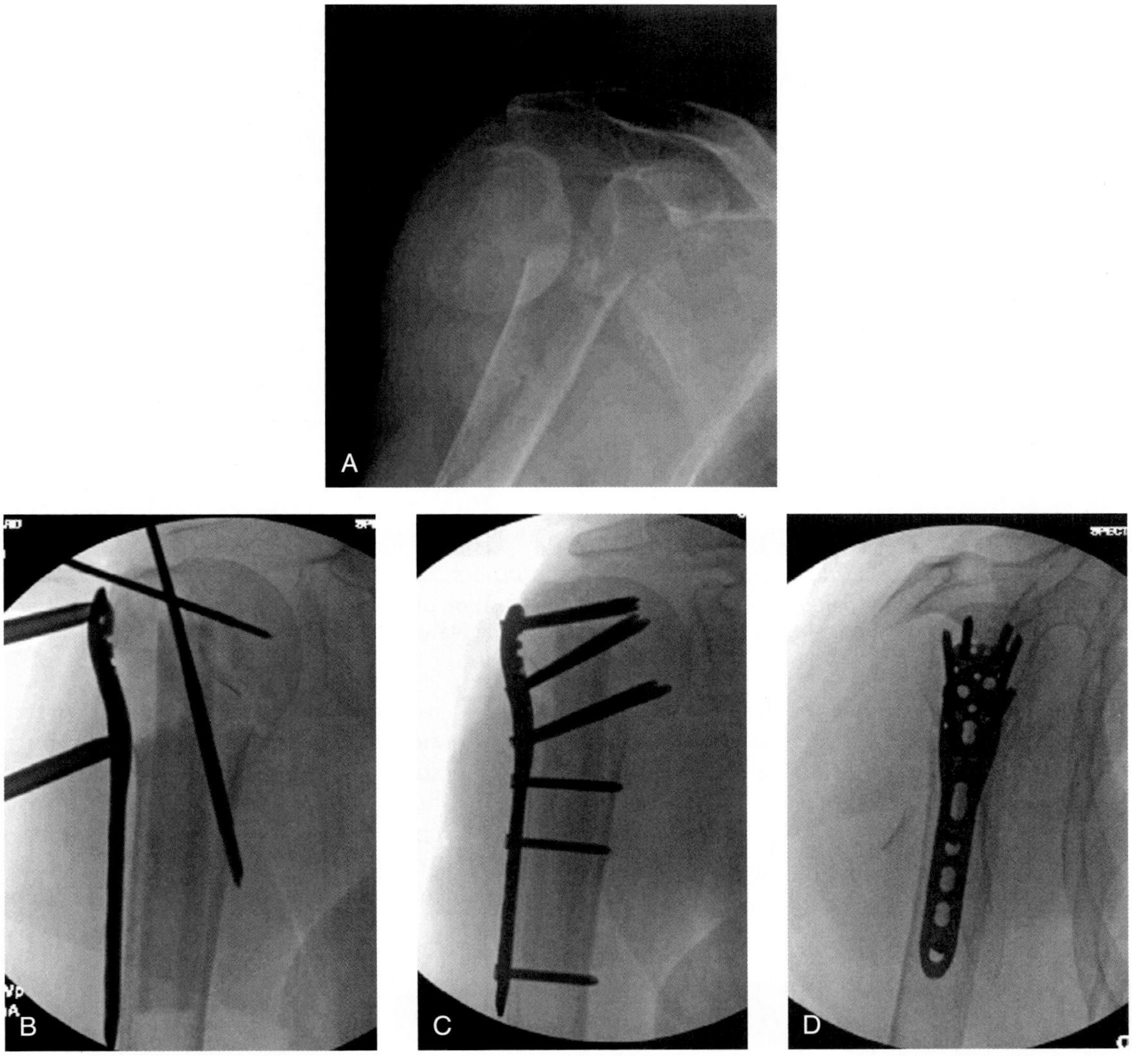

Figure 6 Radiographs (**A**) demonstrate a displaced unstable two-part proximal humeral fracture. Intraoperative imaging (**B**) demonstrates intramedullary fibular strut and preliminary 2.5 mm terminally threaded Schantz pin as joystick reduction and preliminary fixation. Final imaging demonstrates AP (**C**) and scapular Y (**D**) radiographs of locked plate fixation with symmetrical screw spread within the head, no intra-articular screws, and inferior "kickstand" screws along the calcar.

4. Intramedullary nailing (IMN) (**Figure 8**)
    a. Indications—All fracture types, especially diaphyseal extension, segmental, and comminution
    b. Contraindications—Head-split fractures, osteoporosis (relative)
    c. Rotator cuff approach
    d. Intra-articular insertion (through the articular surface and medial to the greater tuberosity)
    e. Joysticks should be used for reduction of the proximal segment out of varus and to expose the insertion site in relation to the diaphysis.
5. Arthroplasty
    a. Indications—Older population, unstable three- and four-part fractures, articular comminution, fracture-dislocations, osteoporosis, patterns that cannot be reconstructed, compromised head vascularity.
    b. Contraindications—Young patients.
    c. Hemiarthroplasty (**Figure 9**)
        - Indications—Intact or repairable cuff, no evidence of glenohumeral arthritis
        - Relative indication—Young patient with nonreconstructable articular head fragment
        - Expected pain control with variable function

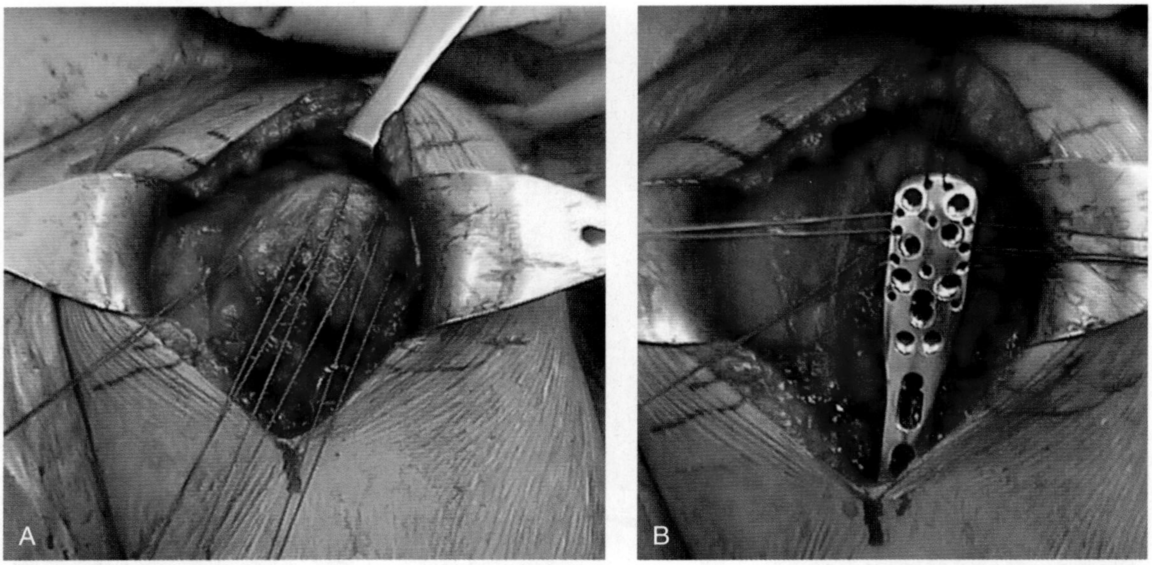

Figure 7 Intraoperative picture (**A**) demonstrates #2 Ethibond suture fixation of the rotator cuff insertion sites. Intraoperative picture of final plate application demonstrates (**B**) suture fixation through the plate holes to counteract rotator cuff deforming forces.

d. Total shoulder arthroplasty—Hemiarthroplasty indications (rare) with a relatively younger patient, intact cuff, preexisting glenohumeral arthrosis, skilled surgeon

e. Reverse shoulder arthroplasty (**Figure 10**)—Hemiarthroplasty indications with tuberosity that cannot be reconstructed; preexisting cuff dysfunction/irreparable tear; surgeon experienced in the technique. Current evidence supports that in the setting of proximal humerus fracture where arthroplasty is the chosen method of repair, reverse shoulder arthroplasty likely leads to more consistent and reproducible outcomes compared

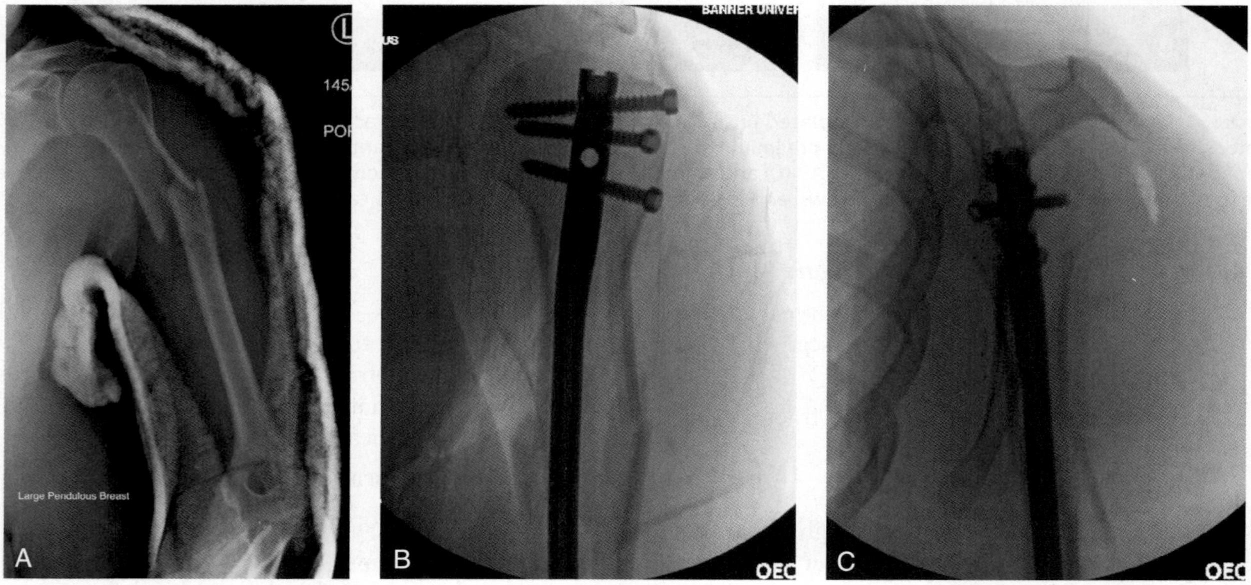

Figure 8 Radiograph demonstrates (**A**) injury of a minimally displaced proximal humeral fracture with diaphyseal extension in a 67-year-old, obese, active female who opted for operative fixation. Final intraoperative AP (**B**) and lateral (**C**) images demonstrate proximal humeral intramedullary nail fixation with anatomical alignment and fixation of tuberosities, no intra-articular screws, and realignment with the diaphyseal fracture.

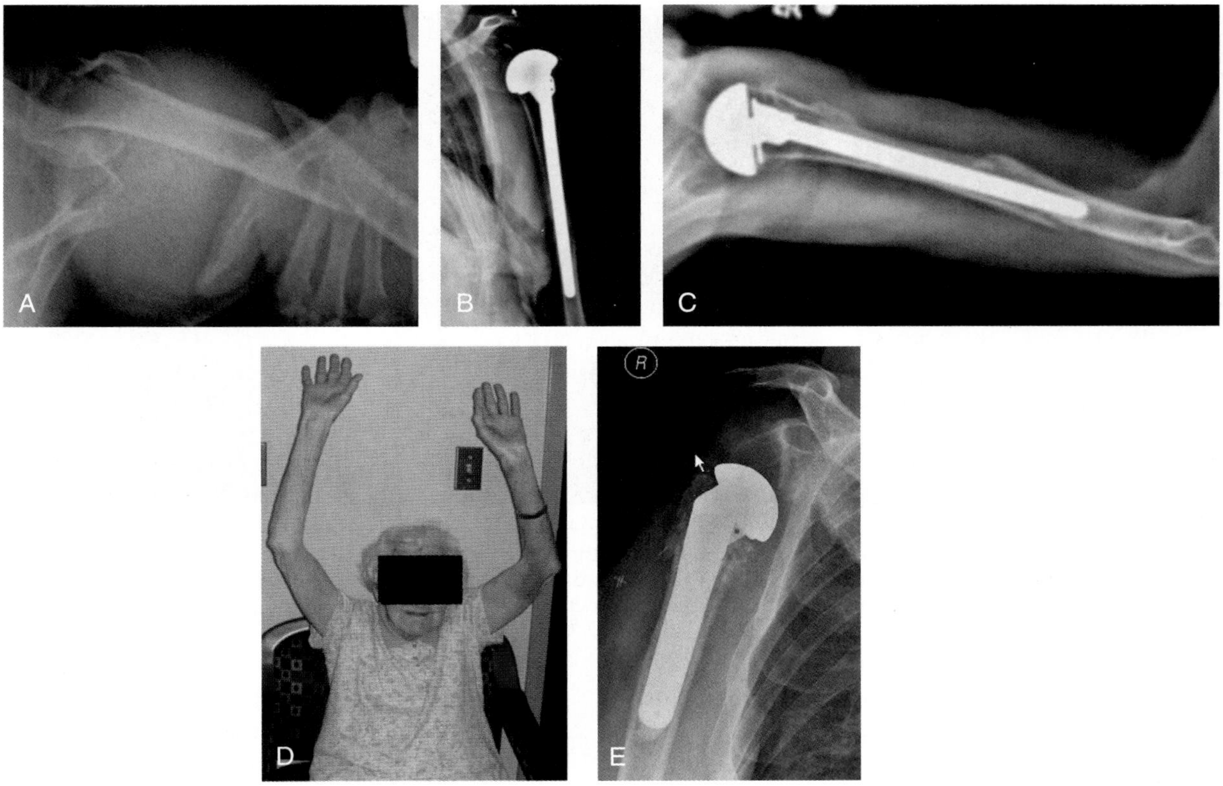

Figure 9 Radiograph (**A**) of complex proximal humeral head fracture-dislocation with ipsilateral shaft in an elderly frail 84-year-old female with osteoporosis. Final radiographs AP (**B**) and lateral (**C**) demonstrate final long-stem hemiarthroplasty of the shoulder with successful repair and union of the tuberosities, concentric humeral head position, and realignment and healing of the shaft fracture. Final clinical picture (**D**) demonstrates near full functional return. In contradistinction, AP (**E**) radiograph demonstrates resorption of the tuberosities and pseudosubluxation of the humeral head.

with hemiarthroplasty and/or total shoulder arthroplasty.

f. Arthroplasty, particularly reverse shoulder arthroplasty, is a viable salvage for failed ORIF or IMN of proximal humerus fractures in the elderly.

VI. COMPLICATIONS

A. Malunion (**Figure 11**)

1. Variable association with function and outcome
2. Posterior/cephalad greater tuberosity common and complex to revise

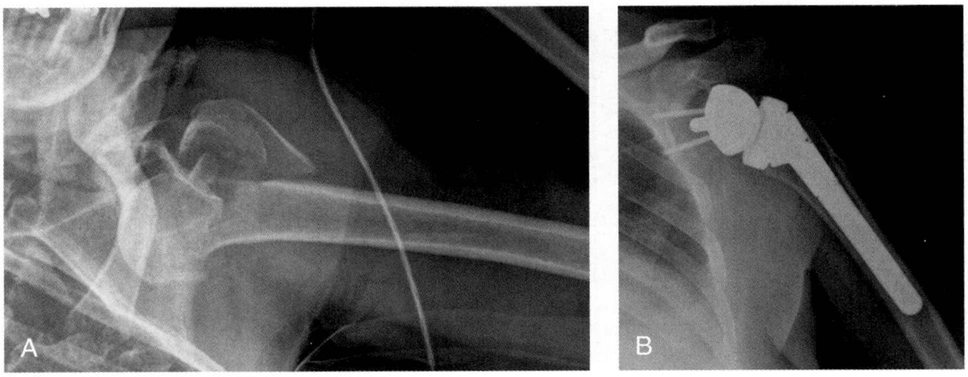

Figure 10 Radiostereometric analysis (RSA) radiograph demonstrates (**A**) complex proximal humeral four-part proximal humeral fracture-dislocation in an elderly 75-year-old male with osteoporosis. Radiograph demonstrates (**B**) a well-inserted reverse shoulder arthroplasty with appropriate glenosphere position, uncemented humeral stem, and suture repair of the great tuberosity.

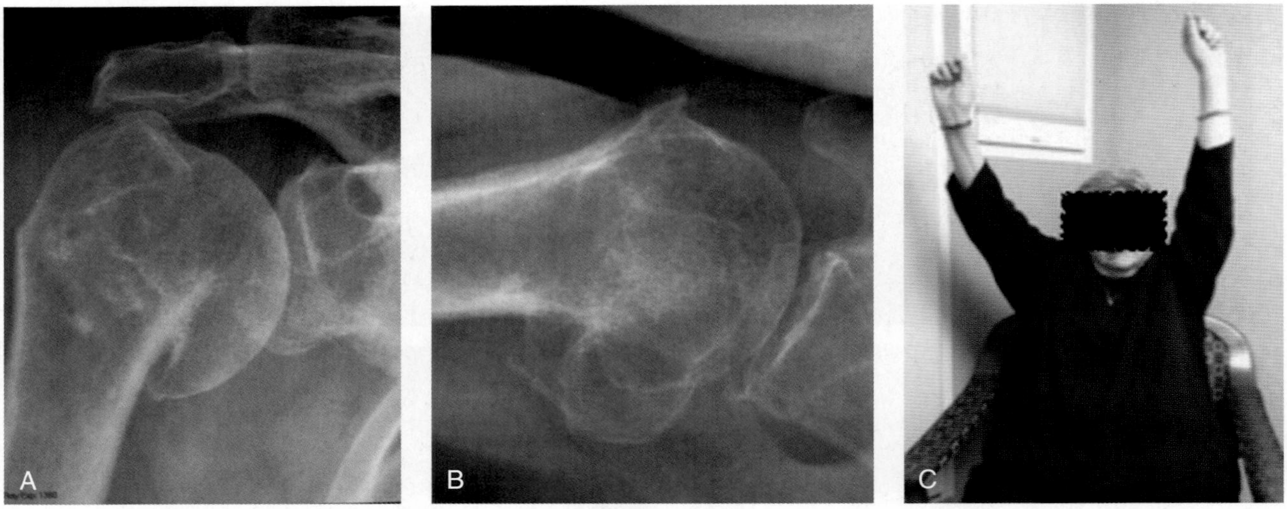

Figure 11 Final AP (**A**) and axillary (**B**) radiographs demonstrate a three-part healed proximal humeral malunion with typical varus, tuberosity impingement, and posterior-superior displacement of the greater tuberosity. Photograph demonstrates that despite this elderly female's malunion, she has compensated and functional activities of daily living (**C**).

3. Usual varus and apex anterior
   a. More common with nonsurgical techniques
   b. Diminished with full intraoperative imaging
   c. Results in increased implant failure
4. Options—Nonsurgical, osteotomy, arthroplasty

B. Nonunion (**Figure 12**)
1. Usually accompanies neck fractures
2. Usually atrophic and unstable
3. Difficult to reconstruct secondary to blood supply, osteoporosis (existing and disuse), scarring, and rotator cuff contracture
4. Options—ORIF with locked plating, grafting, and compression; arthroplasty (difficult with shortened and osteoporotic tubercles); and reverse shoulder arthroplasty (complex procedure, skilled/experienced surgeon, and possibly better for cuff dysfunction and tuberosity nonunion/resorption)

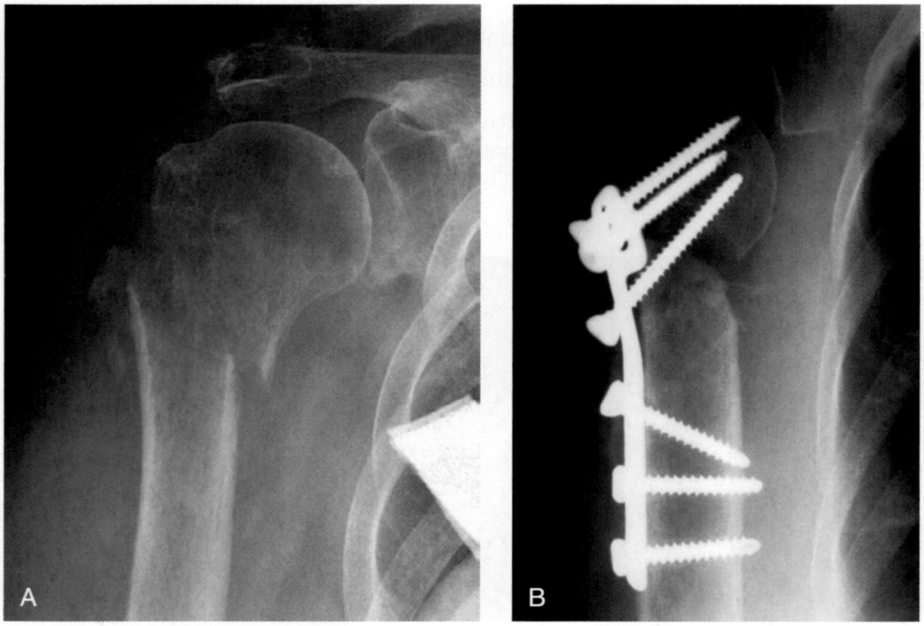

Figure 12 Radiograph (**A**) demonstrates a two-part proximal humeral fracture that was treated nonoperatively in a 45-year-old female resulting in an oligotrophic proximal humeral nonunion. Radiograph (**B**) demonstrates a two-part proximal humeral fracture that was treated with nonlocked antiquated proximal humeral plating in a 68-year-old osteoporotic, smoking, female.

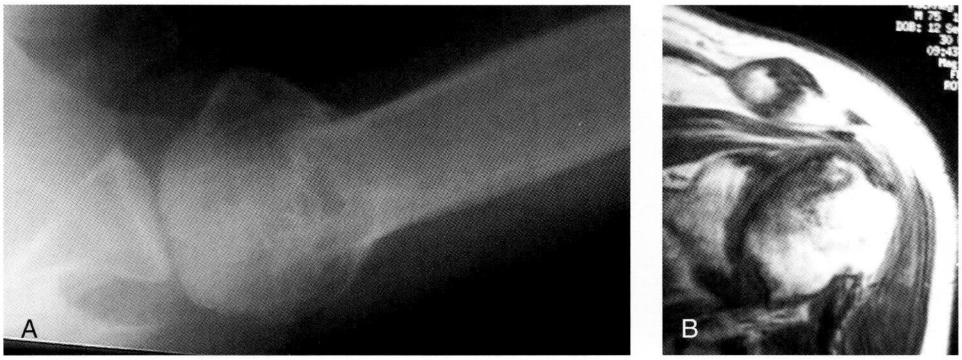

Figure 13 Two-year status post closed reduction percutaneous pinning (CRPP) of a complex three-part proximal humeral fracture of an 85-year-old farmer, who presented with stiffness, achiness, and some activity-related pain, with an axillary radiograph (**A**) and MRI (**B**) images of osteonecrosis.

C. **Posttraumatic** osteonecrosis (**Figure 13**)
   1. Increased incidence with four-part fractures, small calcar (<8 mm), and dislocations
   2. Rates are lower than historic reports
   3. Can be limited or extensive

D. Infection
   1. Open fracture increases incidence
   2. Complex problem to eradicate
   3. Usually results in chondrolysis and head resorption

E. Prominent and migrating implants (**Figure 14**)
   1. Proximal plate insertion can result in subacromial impingement.

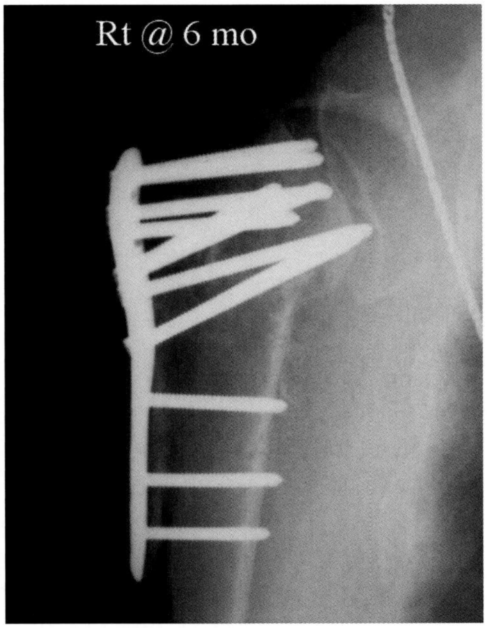

Figure 14 Radiograph demonstrates a three-part proximal humeral fracture that was treated with locked open reduction and internal fixation resulting in osteonecrosis, prominent intra-articular screws, and glenoid erosion.

   2. Intra-articular screw penetration more common with locked screws, diminished with calcium phosphate cement as bone void filler
   3. Screw loosening occurs with comminution and/or osteoporosis.
   4. Avascular head collapse with locked screws can result in glenoid erosion.
   5. Pin migration can occur when these implants are used in poor-quality bone.

F. Shoulder dyskinesia (**Figure 15**)
   1. Variable association based on ADLs
   2. Occurs with or without malunion
   3. Difficult problem to determine etiology and reverse
   4. Many elderly or low-demand patients tolerate or accommodate for limitations

VII. REHABILITATION

A. Nonsurgical treatment
   1. Sling and rest until pain dissipates; passive motion should be started within 2 weeks.
   2. Gradual return to ADLs and rotator cuff program.
   3. Caution should be used with greater tuberosity fractures; to avoid further displacement, active motion should not begin for 6 weeks after fracture consolidation.

B. Surgical treatment
   1. Fixation should be stable enough to begin immediate passive ROM (forward flexion, abduction) but with limited external rotation to neutral.
   2. When fracture consolidated is attained (usually 6 weeks), unlimited ROM, rotator cuff rehabilitation, and strengthening with an emphasis on ADLs should be initiated.
   3. Transition to daily home program at 10 to 12 weeks

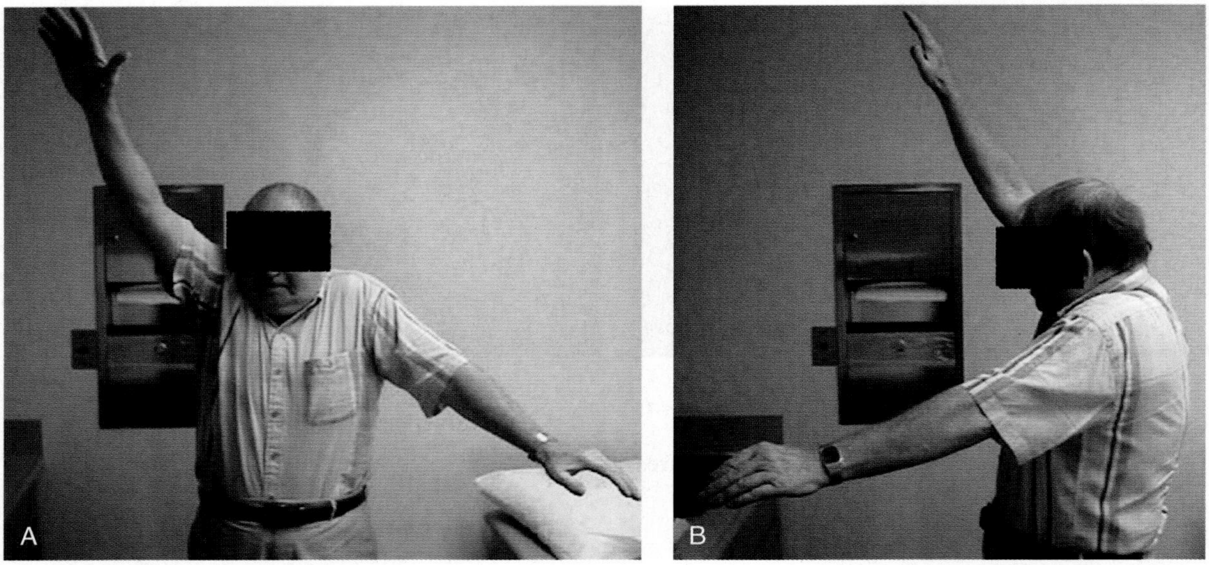

Figure 15 Clinical images (**A** and **B**) demonstrate unsuccessful treatment of this 80-year-old male's proximal humeral fracture with shoulder dyskinesia, pseudoparalysis of the shoulder, no external rotation, and compensated scapulothoracic motion.

VIII. OUTCOMES

A. Variable, based on preexisting function, rotator cuff integrity, the extent of injury, reduction quality, patient expectations, and ADLs.

B. Continued improvement can be expected for up to 1 year.

C. Optimal results usually require a compliant patient and extensive rehabilitation.

ACKNOWLEDGMENTS

The author wishes to recognize the work of Andrew Green, MD, for his contribution to *AAOS Comprehensive Orthopaedic Review* and this chapter.

TOP TESTING FACTS

1. The main or dominant arterial blood supply to the humeral head is the posterior humeral circumflex artery.
2. Head-split fractures have a high rate of osteonecrosis.
3. Minimally displaced fractures are best treated nonsurgically.
4. The axillary nerve is affected most commonly at the time of injury.
5. An axillary radiograph is key to ensure glenohumeral reduction.
6. Proximal humeral fractures are classified based on the number of parts and pattern.
7. Locking plate fixation has become the implant of choice for most proximal humerus fractures.
8. The deltopectoral approach is the approach most often utilized for fractures about the proximal humerus.
9. Arthroplasty is reserved for fractures and dislocations in poor bone that cannot be reconstructed.
10. Screw penetration is the most common complication following ORIF with locked plates and screws.

Bibliography

Agel J, Jones CB, Sanzone AG, Camuso M, Henley MB: Treatment of proximal humeral fractures with Polarus nail fixation. *J Shoulder Elbow Surg* 2004;13(2):191-195.

Athwal GS, Sperling JW, Rispoli DM, Cofield RH: Acute deep infection after surgical fixation of proximal humeral fractures. *J Shoulder Elbow Surg* 2007;16(4):408-412.

Bengard MJ, Gardner MJ: Screw depth sounding in proximal humerus fractures to avoid iatrogenic intra-articular penetration. *J Orthop Trauma* 2011;25(10):630-633.

Court-Brown CM, Garg A, McQueen MM: The epidemiology of proximal humeral fractures. *Acta Orthop Scand* 2001;72(4):365-371.

Duparc F, Muller JM, Fréger P: Arterial blood supply of the proximal humeral epiphysis. *Surg Radiol Anat* 2001;23(3):185-190.

Egol KA, Ong CC, Walsh M, Jazrawi LM, Tejwani NC, Zuckerman JD: Early complications in proximal humerus fractures (OTA types 11) treated with locked plates. *J Orthop Trauma* 2008;22(3):159-164.

Egol KA, Sugi MT, Ong CC, Montero N, Davidovitch R, Zuckerman JD: Fracture site augmentation with calcium phosphate cement reduces screw penetration after open reduction-internal fixation of proximal humeral fractures. *J Shoulder Elbow Surg* 2012;21(6):741-748.

Gardner MJ, Boraiah S, Helfet DL, Lorich DG: The anterolateral acromial approach for fractures of the proximal humerus. *J Orthop Trauma* 2008;22(2):132-137.

Gardner MJ, Voos JE, Wanich T, Helfet DL, Lorich DG: Vascular implications of minimally invasive plating of proximal humerus fractures. *J Orthop Trauma* 2006;20(9):602-607.

Gardner MJ, Weil Y, Barker JU, Kelly BT, Helfet DL, Lorich DG: The importance of medial support in locked plating of proximal humerus fractures. *J Orthop Trauma* 2007;21(3):185-191.

Georgousis M, Kontogeorgakos V, Kourkouvelas S, Badras S, Georgaklis V, Badras L: Internal fixation of proximal humerus fractures with the polarus intramedullary nail. *Acta Orthop Belg* 2010;76(4):462-467.

Gerber C, Schneeberger AG, Vinh TS: The arterial vascularization of the humeral head: An anatomical study. *J Bone Joint Surg Am* 1990;72(10):1486-1494.

Harrison AK, Gruson KI, Zmistowski B, et al: Intermediate outcomes following percutaneous fixation of proximal humeral fractures. *J Bone Joint Surg Am* 2012;94(13):1223-1228.

Hertel R, Hempfing A, Stiehler M, Leunig M: Predictors of humeral head ischemia after intracapsular fracture of the proximal humerus. *J Shoulder Elbow Surg* 2004;13(4):427-433.

Hettrich CM, Boraiah S, Dyke JP, Nevaiser A, Helfet DL, Lorich DG: Quantitative assessment of the vascularity of the proximal part of the humerus. *J Bone Joint Surg Am* 2010;92:934-938.

Jones CB, Sietsema DL, Williams DK: Locked plating of proximal humeral fractures: Is function affected by age, time, and fracture patterns? *Clin Orthop Relat Res* 2011;469(12):3307-3316.

Keener JD, Parsons BO, Flatow EL, Rogers K, Williams GR, Galatz LM: Outcomes after percutaneous reduction and fixation of proximal humeral fractures. *J Shoulder Elbow Surg* 2007;16(3):330-338.

Levy JC, Badman B: Reverse shoulder prosthesis for acute four-part fracture: Tuberosity fixation using a horseshoe graft. *J Orthop Trauma* 2011;25(5):318-324.

Marsh JL, Slongo TF, Agel J, et al: Fracture and dislocation classification compendium – 2007: Orthopaedic Trauma Association classification, database and outcomes committee. *J Orthop Trauma* 2007;21(10, suppl):S1-S133.

Martinez AA, Bejarano C, Carbonel I, Iglesias D, GilAlbarova J, Herrera A: The treatment of proximal humerus nonunions in older patients with reverse shoulder arthroplasty. *Injury* 2012;43(suppl 2):S3-S56.

Neer CS II: Displaced proximal humeral fractures: I. Classification and evaluation. *J Bone Joint Surg Am* 1970;52(6):1077-1089.

Prasarn ML, Achor T, Paul O, Lorich DG, Helfet DL: Management of nonunions of the proximal humeral diaphysis. *Injury* 2010;41(12):1244-1248.

Emil Schemitsch M: *Open Reduction and Internal Fixation Versus Acute Arthroplasty for the Management of Common Extremity Injuries: Evidence-Based Decision Making*. In: Aaron Nauth M, Michael D, McKee M, Hans J, Kreder M, Andrew H, Schmidt M, eds. AAOS Instructional Course Lectures, 2018, vol 67.

Sebastiá-Forcada E, Cebrián-Gómez R, Lizaur-Utrilla A, Gil-Guillén V: Reverse shoulder arthroplasty versus hemiarthroplasty for acute proximal humeral fractures. A blinded, randomized, controlled, prospective study. *J Shoulder Elbow Surg* 2014;23(10):1419-1426.

Sebastia-Forcada E, Lizaur-Utrilla A, Cebrian-Gomez R, Miralles-Muñoz FA, Lopez-Prats FA: Outcomes of reverse total shoulder arthroplasty for proximal humeral fractures: Primary arthroplasty versus secondary arthroplasty after failed proximal humeral locking plate fixation. *J Orthop Trauma* 2017;31(8):e236-e240.

Solberg BD, Moon CN, Franco DP, Paiement GD: Surgical treatment of three and four-part proximal humeral fractures. *J Bone Joint Surg Am* 2009;91(7):1689-1697.

Südkamp NP, Audige L, Lambert S, Hertel R, Konrad G: Path analysis of factors for functional outcome at one year in 463 proximal humeral fractures. *J Shoulder Elbow Surg* 2011;20(8):1207-1216.

Tejwani NC, Liporace F, Walsh M, France MA, Zuckerman JD, Egol KA: Functional outcome following one-part proximal humeral fractures: A prospective study. *J Shoulder Elbow Surg* 2008;17(2):216-219.

Voos JE, Dines JS, Dines DM: Arthroplasty for fractures of the proximal part of the humerus. *Instr Course Lect* 2011;60:105-112.

Voos JE, Dines JS, Dines DM: Arthroplasty for fractures of the proximal part of the humerus. *J Bone Joint Surg Am* 2010;92(6):1560-1567.

Willis M, Min W, Brooks JP, et al: Proximal humeral malunion treated with reverse shoulder arthroplasty. *J Shoulder Elbow Surg* 2012;21(4):507-513.

Chapter 91

FRACTURES OF THE HUMERAL SHAFT AND THE DISTAL HUMERUS

RICHARD S. YOON, MD
FRANK A. LIPORACE, MD

I. FRACTURES OF THE HUMERAL SHAFT

A. Epidemiology

1. Humerus fractures account for 3% of all fractures and most commonly occur in the middle third of the bone.
2. They exhibit a bimodal age distribution, with peak incidence in the third decade of life for males and the seventh decade for females.
3. In the younger age group, high-energy trauma is more frequently the cause. Lower energy mechanisms are more common in older patients.

B. Anatomy

1. The anatomy of the humerus varies throughout its length (**Figure 1**).
   a. The shaft is generally cylindrical and provides origin and insertion points for the pectoralis, deltoid, biceps, coracobrachialis, brachialis, and triceps muscles.
   b. These origins and insertions determine the displacement of the major fracture fragments.
   c. Distally, the humerus becomes triangular, and its intramedullary (IM) canal terminates approximately 2 to 3 cm proximal to the olecranon fossa.
   d. Medial and lateral septae delineate the posterior and anterior compartments of the arm.
2. The main neurovascular structures of the arm and forearm traverse the soft tissues overlying the humerus. Posteriorly, the spiral groove houses the radial nerve. Its location is approximately 14

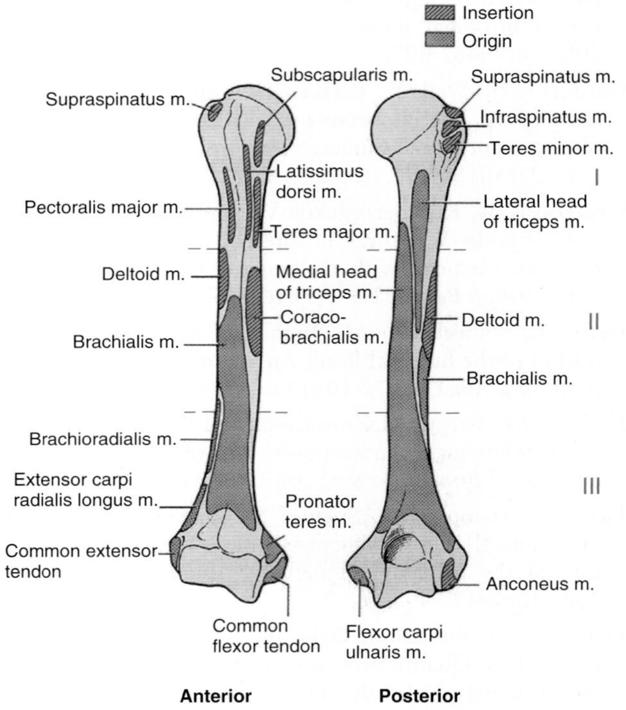

Figure 1 Illustrations show the shaft of the humerus, including the division into three surfaces (I, II, and III). m = muscle. (Adapted with permission from Browner BD, Jupiter JB, Levine AM, Trafton PG, eds: *Skeletal Trauma*, ed 2. Philadelphia, PA, WB Saunders, 2002, p 1524.)

Dr. Yoon or an immediate family member is a member of a speakers' bureau or has made paid presentations on behalf of Surgical Care Affiliates (SCA); serves as a paid consultant to or is an employee of Arthrex, Inc., DePuy, A Johnson & Johnson Company, LIfeNet Health, Orthobullets, ORTHOXEL, Synthes, and Use-Lab; serves as an unpaid consultant to BuiltLean; has stock or stock options held in Taithera Inc.; and has received research or institutional support from Biomet, Coventus, Synthes, and Wright Medical Technology, Inc. Dr. Liporace or an immediate family member has received royalties from Biomet; is a member of a speakers' bureau or has made paid presentations on behalf of Biomet, Stryker, and Synthes; serves as a paid consultant to or is an employee of Biomet, Medtronic, Stryker, and Synthes; and serves as an unpaid consultant to AO.

cm proximal to the lateral-distal articular surface and 20 cm proximal to the medial-distal articular surface. It lies directly posterior to the deltoid tuberosity.

C. Surgical approaches

1. Anterolateral approach—May be extensile but usually is considered for proximal third to middle third humeral shaft fractures.

    a. The radial nerve can be identified distally between the brachialis and brachioradialis muscles and traced proximally as it pierces the intermuscular septum.

    b. The brachialis (innervated by the radial and musculocutaneous nerves) is split to spare its dual innervation and protect the radial nerve during retraction.

2. Posterior approach—Most effective for the distal two-thirds of the shaft from the deltoid insertion and distally. The deltoid muscle prevents extension of this approach proximally to the shoulder.

    a. The radial nerve can be identified in the spiral groove in this approach. The interval between the lateral and long heads of the triceps is used, with elevation of the medial (deep) head off the posterior aspect of the shaft.

    b. The ulnar nerve emerges medially from deep to the medial head of the triceps. It courses distally through the cubital tunnel. It can be palpated along the medial aspect of the triceps along the distal third of the humerus.

    c. The radial nerve can be identified approximately 4 cm proximal to the point of confluence through the posterior approach.

3. Other approaches—The percutaneous, anterior, anteromedial, and direct lateral approaches have been described and may be used based on wound considerations, other injuries (eg, need for associated vascular repair), or the need for other approaches based on concomitant injuries.

D. Mechanism of injury and associated injuries

1. Distal humerus shaft fractures may be caused by high-energy or low-energy trauma. In patients with osteoporosis or osteopenia, bone mineral density is decreased, so less force is required for injury (eg, a fall from a standing position).

2. Torsional, bending, axial, or a combination of these forces can result in humeral fractures. Direct impact or blast injury (eg, gunshot wounds) also can cause these fractures.

3. With any long bone injury, associated proximal or distal articular fractures or dislocations may be present, necessitating a complete radiographic examination of the bone, including the joint above and joint below.

4. In high-energy injuries, forearm and wrist radiographs are warranted to rule out associated forearm fractures (such as floating elbow).

E. Clinical evaluation

1. Patients typically present with pain, swelling, and deformity about the arm (most frequently shortening and varus).

2. The fracture pattern is related to the mechanism of injury and bone quality. Therefore, a careful history is important to rule out pathologic processes that would require further workup.

3. Careful neurovascular examination is important because radial nerve (distal shaft) and ulnar nerve (articular) injuries are not uncommon associated findings.

F. Radiographic studies

1. A standard radiographic series of AP and lateral views should be acquired.

2. When obtaining the transthoracic lateral view, rotating the patient prevents rotation of the distal fragment and avoids the risk of further soft-tissue or nerve injury.

3. Radiographic series should include the shoulder and elbow ("joint above and joint below") to rule out associated injuries.

4. Traction views for intra-articular fractures may aid in preoperative planning for severely comminuted fractures that meet surgical indications.

5. Advanced imaging studies need to be considered only when a concomitant intra-articular injury is present or a pathologic process is suspected based on the history and initial radiographic evaluation.

G. Classification—Several different systems have been used to classify humeral shaft fractures.

1. The AO/Orthopaedic Trauma Association (OTA) classification system uses a combination of numbers and letters to describe the fracture: bone number (humerus = 1); location (diaphysis = 2); fracture pattern (simple = A, wedge = B, complex = C); and severity (1 through 3) (**Figure 2**).

2. The descriptive classification system is based on the location relative to the pectoralis and the deltoid. It provides information about the relative direction and displacement of the main fracture fragments.

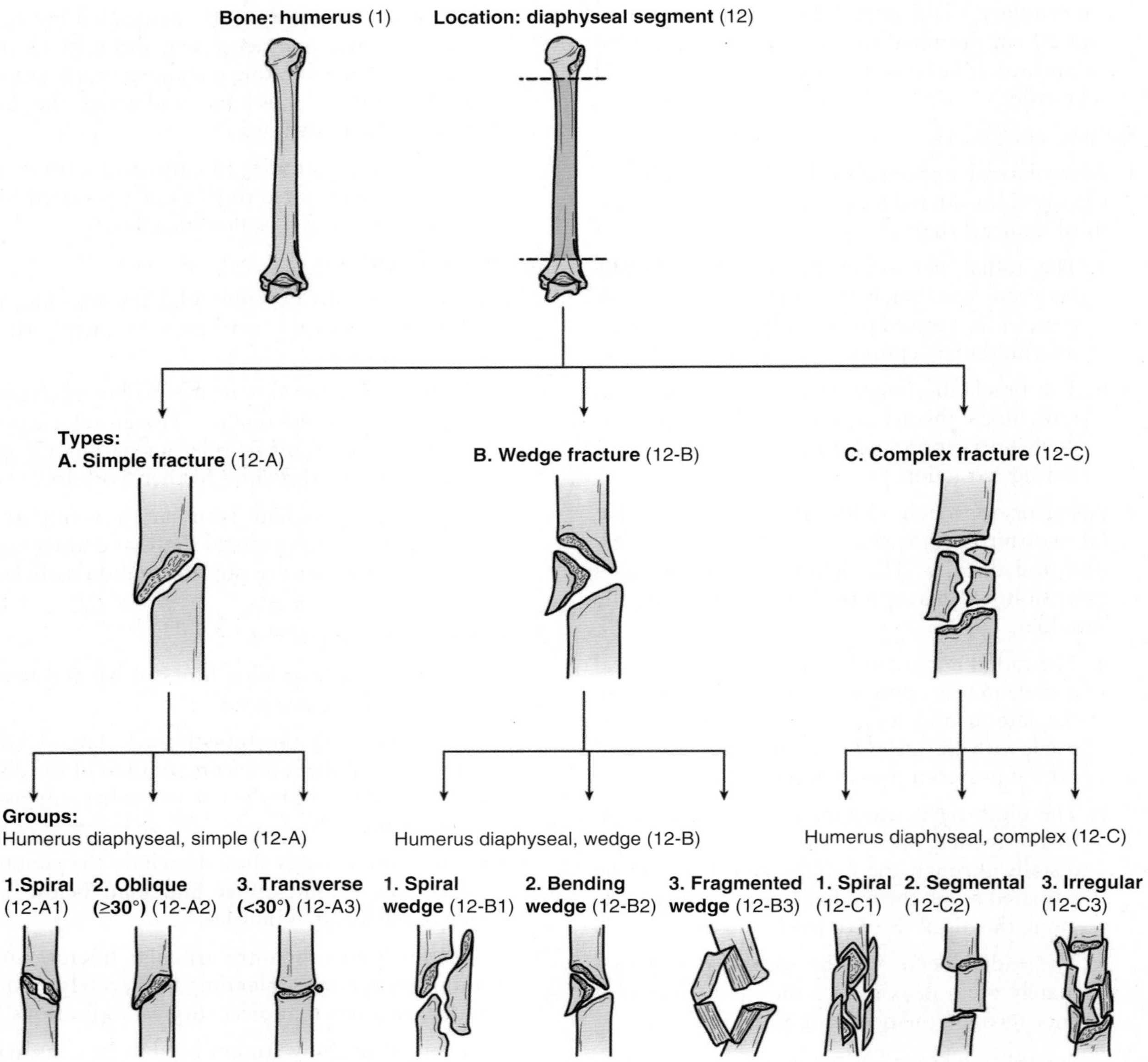

Figure 2 Algorithm depicts the Orthopaedic Trauma Association (OTA) classification of humeral shaft fractures.

3. A classification system based on fracture characteristics (transverse, oblique, spiral, segmental, comminuted) can aid in determining treatment (**Figure 3**).

H. Nonsurgical treatment

1. This is the treatment of choice for most humeral shaft fractures. Historical literature has reported good results with these techniques.
2. Closed treatment may involve initial coaptation splinting followed by a functional brace or a hanging arm cast.

a. The coaptation splint is used for 7 to 10 days, followed by application of a fracture brace in the office.

b. Weekly radiographs are have been called into question.

c. Immediately on fracture brace application, the patient is encouraged to do pendulum exercises for shoulder mobility. Isometric biceps, triceps, and deltoid muscle exercises, as well as active wrist and hand exercises also are encouraged.

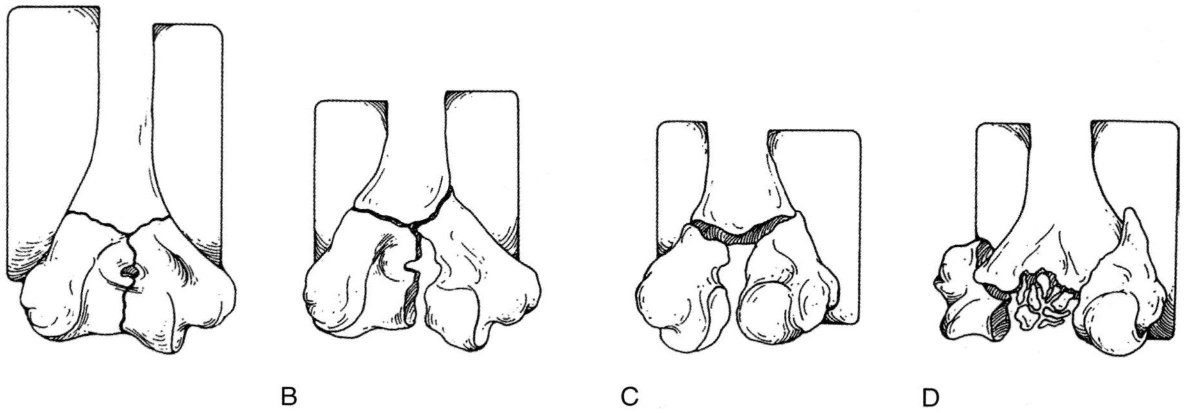

Figure 3 Illustrations depict the types of intercondylar fractures. **A**, Type I nondisplaced condylar fracture of the elbow. **B**, Type II displaced but not rotated T-condylar fracture. **C**, Type III displaced and rotated T-condylar fracture. **D**, Type IV displaced, rotated, and comminuted condylar fracture. (Reproduced with permission from the Mayo Foundation for Medical Education and Research, Rochester, MN. All rights reserved.)

d. The patient is instructed to adjust the tension of the fracture brace as needed and to sleep in a semi-erect position until 4 to 6 weeks after injury.

e. The fracture brace is worn for 10 to 12 weeks, until no pain or mobility is present with palpation at the fracture site, more than 90° of shoulder and elbow motion is painless, and bridging callus is seen radiographically on three of four cortices.

3. Hanging arm casts may be considered for shortened oblique, spiral, and transverse fractures. The cast should extend from 2 cm proximal to the fracture, across the 90° flexed elbow, and to the wrist; the forearm should be in neutral rotation. Suspension straps are attached to loops on the forearm aspect of the cast to aid in alignment.

4. No consensus exists on acceptable alignment, but it has been proposed that 20° apex anterior or posterior angulation and 30° varus/valgus angulation, 15° malrotation, and 3 cm of shortening are acceptable.

5. A recent meta-analysis review yielded no currently published studies that included randomized controlled trials to ascertain whether surgical intervention of humeral shaft fractures gives a better or worse outcome than nonsurgical management.

I. Surgical treatment

1. The absolute and relative indications for surgical treatment are listed in **Table 1**.

2. Outcomes—Open fractures have been shown to have a 12.0% infection rate without fixation and a 10.8% infection rate with fixation.

TABLE 1

Indications for Surgical Treatment of Humeral Shaft Fractures

Absolute Indications	Relative Indications
Concomitant vascular injury	Multiply injured patient
Severe soft-tissue injury	Concomitant head injury
Open fractures Floating elbow	Inability to maintain an acceptable reduction closed
Concomitant displaced humeral articular injuries	Segmental fractures
Pathologic fractures	Transverse or short oblique fractures in a young athlete

3. Surgical procedures

a. Open reduction and plate fixation

- Fixation with plate-and-screw constructs have union rates up to 94%, with low infection rates (0% to 6%) and low incidence of iatrogenic nerve injury (0% to 5%); they also allow the multiply injured patient to bear weight through the injured extremity.
- Conventional plating is usually performed with a broad 4.5-mm plate and three or four screws per side for axial and torsional stability.
- To improve resistance to bending when using a long plate, screw placement should include "near-near" and "far-far" relative to the site of the fracture.

7 | Trauma

- In osteoporotic bone, locked plating has been shown to improve stability and resistance to torsional stresses.
- Minimally invasive plating (MIPO) technique has been described but not yet demonstrated clinical advantages over traditional ORIF.

b. IM nailing

- Advocated by some as an alternative to plate fixation.
- Originally, nonlocking flexible nails were used and inserted in an antegrade or retrograde fashion, but newer interlocking nails have become more common and allow better rotational control.
- IM nails can be useful in segmental fractures, in the multiply injured patient to limit positioning changes, and in pathologic fractures.
- IM nails have been shown to withstand higher axial and bending loads than plates, although plated humerus fractures have been shown clinically to allow full weight bearing and have not shown a higher incidence of malunion or nonunion.
- IM nailing of humerus fractures has been shown to result in a higher incidence of shoulder pain and a potential risk to neurovascular structures when locking long nails distally.
- Comparison of plating with nailing for humerus shaft fractures has shown that plating results in less need for revision, a lower nonunion rate, and fewer shoulder problems.
- When using locked IM nails, a greater mismatch of nail diameter and shape occurred with retrograde nailing than antegrade nailing and necessitated substantially more reaming, which could increase bone weakness and the risk of a supracondylar fracture.

c. External fixation

- Indications—Staged external fixation is indicated for severe soft-tissue injury, bone defects, vascular injury with acute repair, the medically unstable patient, and infected nonunions.
- When applying external fixation, care must be taken to avoid neurovascular structures.
    - Typically, the elbow joint is spanned with two lateral pins placed proximal to the fracture in the humeral diaphysis and two pins in the ulna or radius, depending on whether a forearm injury is present.
    - The ulna is the preferred location for pin placement, when possible, because of its subcutaneous location, the limited risk to neurovascular structures, and the ability to maintain pronation-supination mobility during the period of external fixation.
    - An open approach is recommended for the humeral pins because of the variability of nerve courses in the region. An open approach also should be used if the distal pins are placed in the radius.

4. Surgical pearls

a. To minimize shoulder pain, a medial starting point for antegrade IM nailing has been suggested.

- The interval between the anterior and middle thirds of the deltoid is split, and an inline-splitting incision of the rotator cuff is made. This allows a direct path to the IM canal and an easier side-to-side tendon closure.
- The surgeon must be aware that the humeral canal ends 2 to 3 cm proximal to the olecranon fossa and narrows distally, which can result in a risk for fracture distraction when impacting the nail.

b. When plating from a posterior approach, the radial nerve must be identified.

- The radial nerve can be located by bluntly dissecting deep to bone at a point approximately 4 cm superior to the proximal aspect of the triceps fascia.

J. Rehabilitation

1. Humeral shaft fractures treated nonsurgically should undergo rehabilitation as described previously.
2. Surgically treated fractures can be splinted for 3 to 7 days to rest the soft tissues. Subsequently, active and passive range of motion (ROM) of the shoulder, elbow, wrist, and hand can progress.
3. Resistance strengthening exercises may begin postoperatively or, if nonsurgical treatment has been done, when callus with no motion or pain at the fracture sight is evident.

K. Complications

1. Radial nerve palsy

a. Humerus fractures often are associated with radial nerve palsies, whether from the time of injury, from attempted closed reduction, or during surgical intervention.

b. A recent meta-analysis of 4,517 fractures found an overall 11.8% incidence of concomitant radial nerve palsies in transverse and spiral fractures, with the middle and distal third of the humeral shaft most frequently involved.
   - Almost all recover.
   - Substantially different rates of recovery were reported for complete (77.6%) versus incomplete (98.2%) palsies and closed (97.1%) versus open (85.7%) injuries.
   - Barring open injury, vascular injury, a segmental fracture, or floating elbow, no difference in recovery between early and late exploration could be deduced.

c. For a concomitant nerve injury in patients who do not require surgical treatment of the fracture, electromyography and/or nerve conduction velocity studies should be obtained 6 weeks post injury. In patients who require surgical treatment, exploration is done at the time of surgery.

d. For secondary palsies that occur during fracture reduction, it has not been clearly established that surgery improves the ultimate recovery rate when compared with the results of nonsurgical management. Delayed surgical exploration should be done after 3 to 4 months if no evidence of recovery is apparent using electromyography or nerve conduction velocity studies.

2. Vascular injury is rare and may be the result of a penetrating injury (eg, industrial accident, gunshot wound). Revascularization should be attempted within 6 hours.

3. Interlocking with humeral nails can place the axillary nerve at risk proximally and the lateral antebrachial cutaneous nerve, the median nerve, or the brachial artery at risk distally. These risks can be minimized by using a limited open approach, with careful blunt dissection to bone when applying interlocking screws.

4. When passing the reamer through an area of comminution, consider turning off the reamer and pushing it through the area manually to avoid damage to the radial nerve.

5. When radial nerve dysfunction is present preoperatively and IM nailing is chosen, a limited open approach should be considered to ensure that the fracture site is clear of neurovascular structures before nail placement.

6. Nonunions—Although union rates are relatively high with humeral shaft fractures, nonunions do occur.
   a. Motion, avascularity, gap, and infection are all potential causes of nonunion.
   b. In osteopenia and osteoporosis, stability can be achieved with locked plates.

7. Infected nonunions
   a. Eradication of the infection is important to help achieve union.
   b. In select cases of severe infection, temporary or definitive external fixation along with resection of affected tissue and antibiotic treatment may be required.
   c. Whether required by atrophic nonunion or infection, resection and shortening of up to 4 cm can be tolerated.

8. Nerve conduction velocity studies can be considered after 6 weeks to help determine a baseline for the prognosis and severity of the nerve injury.

9. Ultrasonography also has been suggested as a modality for nerve evaluation but depends on the quality of the technician, the radiologist, and the ultrasonography machine.

II. DISTAL HUMERUS FRACTURES

A. Epidemiology
   1. Intercondylar fractures are the most common distal humerus fracture pattern.
   2. Fractures of the capitellum constitute approximately 1% of all elbow injuries.
   3. Fractures of a single condyle (lateral is more common than medial) account for 5% of all distal humerus fractures.

B. Anatomy (**Figure 4**)
   1. The elbow is a constrained, hinged joint. The ulna rotates around the axis of the trochlea, which is positioned in relative valgus and external rotation.
   2. The capitellum articulates with the proximal radius and is involved with forearm rotation, not elbow flexion/extension. Posteriorly, the capitellum is nonarticular and allows for distal posterior hardware placement.
   3. Medially, the medial collateral ligament originates on the distal surface of the medial epicondyle. The ulnar nerve resides in the cubital tunnel in a subcutaneous location.

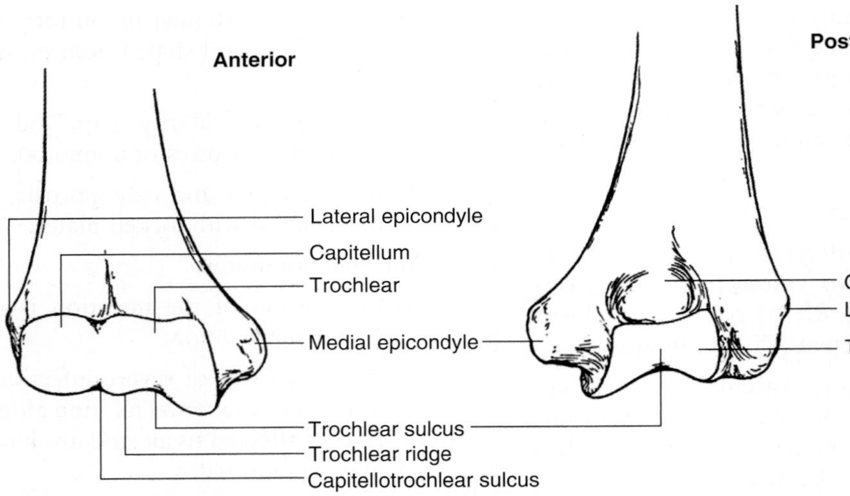

Figure 4 Illustrations demonstrate the anterior and posterior views of the anatomy of the distal articular surface of the humerus. The capitellotrochlear sulcus divides the capitellar and trochlear articular surfaces. The lateral trochlear ridge is the key to analyzing humeral condyle fractures. In type I fractures, the lateral trochlear ridge remains with the intact condyle, providing medial-to-lateral elbow stability. In type II fractures, the lateral trochlear ridge is a part of the fractured condyle, which may allow the radius and ulna to translocate in a medial-to-lateral direction in relation to the long axis of the humerus. (Reproduced with permission from Koval KJ, Zuckerman JD, eds: *Handbook of Fractures*, ed 2. Philadelphia, PA, Lippincott Williams and Wilkins, 2002, p 98.)

4. Laterally, the lateral collateral ligament originates on the lateral epicondyle, deep to the common extensor tendon.

C. Classification

1. Classifications of fractures of the distal humerus traditionally were descriptive and based on the number of columns involved and the location of the fracture (supracondylar, transcondylar, condylar, and bicondylar; **Table 2**).
2. The AO/OTA classification system divides these fractures into type A (extra-articular), type B (partial articular), and type C (complete articular).
   a. Each category is subclassified based on the degree and location of fracture comminution.
   b. It has been shown that the AO/OTA classification has substantial stand-alone agreement for interobserver reliability in fracture type (A, B, and C) but is less reliable for subtype.

TABLE 2

Descriptive and Anatomic Classifications of Distal Humerus Fractures

Intra-articular Fractures	Extra-articular/ Intracapsular Fractures	Extracapsular Fractures
Single-column fractures Medial (high/low) Lateral (high/low) Divergent	High transcolumnar fractures Extension Flexion Abduction Adduction	Medial epicondyle
Two-column fractures T pattern (high/low) Y pattern H pattern λ pattern (medial/lateral)	Low transcolumnar fractures Extension Flexion	Lateral epicondyle
Capitellar fractures		
Trochlear fractures		

D. Surgical approaches

1. Extra-articular and partial articular fractures typically are approached through a posterior triceps-splitting or triceps-sparing approach.
   a. For a triceps-splitting approach, a posterior incision is made and carried deep to the triceps, which is subsequently split between the long and lateral heads and distally at its ulnar insertion.
   b. The triceps-sparing approach involves mobilization of the ulnar nerve and subsequent elevation of the entire extensor mechanism in continuity, progressing from medial to lateral.
   c. An alternative approach is the posterior triceps-preserving approach. It involves mobilization of the triceps off the posterior humerus from

the medial and lateral aspects of the intermuscular septum. The ulnar nerve (medially) and the radial nerve (laterally and proximally) are identified and preserved.

d. For the extensor mechanism approach, a recent study yielded mean elbow ROM arcs exceeding 100° and reported 90% of triceps extension strength maintained.

2. Simple fractures often can be stabilized using one of these approaches with lag screws alone or screws and an antiglide plate.

3. For an isolated lateral column or capitellar fracture, a lateral (Kocher or Kaplan) approach may be considered.

4. Complete articular fractures can be repaired using one of the aforementioned approaches if adequate articular reduction and fixation can be achieved. Complex articular injury may require direct visualization through a transolecranon osteotomy.

   a. It is necessary to find and free the ulnar nerve before performing an olecranon osteotomy. A chevron-style osteotomy pointing distally is made at the level of the "bare area" of the olecranon.

   b. Some surgeons drill and tap the proximal ulna for larger screw insertion before osteotomizing the olecranon to facilitate later fixation.

   c. After the osteotomy is complete, the entire extensor mechanism can be reflected proximally to allow visualization of the entire distal humerus.

   d. Osteotomy repair can be performed using Kirschner wires and a tension band, a long large-fragment IM screw fixation with a tension band, a plate and screws.

   e. The olecranon osteotomy has potential complications, including nonunion and hardware discomfort.

5. Patients with open distal humerus injuries have been shown to have worse functional and ROM scores than those with closed fractures.

6. Regardless of the fixation approach used, the goals of fixation are anatomic articular reduction, stable internal fixation, and early range of elbow motion.

   a. In patients with unreconstructible or missing segments of the articular surface, care must be taken to avoid decreasing the dimensions of the trochlea and limiting the ability for flexion and extension.

   b. After articular reduction is accomplished, stable fixation of the distal end to the metadiaphyseal component with restoration of the mechanical axis is performed.

E. Mechanism of injury

1. Distal humerus fractures can result from low-energy falls (common in the elderly) or high-energy trauma with extensive comminution and intra-articular involvement (eg, gunshot wounds, motor vehicle accidents, falls from a height).

2. The amount of elbow flexion at the time of impact can affect the fracture pattern.

   a. A transcolumnar fracture results from an axial load directed through the forearm with the elbow flexed 90°.

   b. With the elbow in a similar position but with direct impact on the olecranon, an olecranon fracture with or without a distal humerus fracture may result.

   c. With the elbow in more than 90° of flexion, an intercondylar fracture may result.

   d. Clinically may have similar presentation to a terrible triad injury (which involves fractures of the medial collateral ligament, the coronoid, and the radial head/neck).

F. Clinical evaluation

1. Patients typically present with elbow pain and swelling. Crepitus or gross instability with attempted elbow ROM is often observed.

2. Excessive motion testing should not be performed because of the risk of further neurovascular injury.

3. A careful neurovascular examination should be performed because all neurovascular structures to the forearm and hand cross the area of injury, and sharp bone fragments can cause damage, especially to the radial nerve, the ulnar nerve, and the brachial artery.

4. Serial compartment examinations may be required because of extreme cubital fossa swelling or in the obtunded patient to avoid missing a volar forearm compartment syndrome with resultant Volkmann contracture.

G. Radiographic evaluation

1. AP and lateral views of the humerus and elbow are required.

2. When concomitant elbow injuries are present, forearm and wrist radiographs may be needed.

3. To aid in preoperative planning, traction radiographs, oblique radiographs, and CT scans may be of value.

4. Three-dimensional CT scans improve the intraobserver and interobserver reliability of two commonly used classification systems.

H. Supracondylar fractures are AO/OTA type A fractures that are distal metaphyseal and extra-articular.

1. Nonsurgical treatment is reserved for nondisplaced or minimally displaced fractures or for comminuted fractures in older, low-demand patients.
   a. A splint is applied for 1 to 2 weeks before initiating ROM exercises.
   b. At 6 weeks, with progressive evidence of healing, immobilization may be discontinued completely.
   c. Up to 20° of loss of condylar shaft angle may be acceptable.
2. Surgical treatment is indicated for most displaced fractures and for those associated with an open injury or a vascular injury.
   a. Open reduction and internal fixation (ORIF) typically is performed, with plates placed on the medial and lateral columns.
   b. Biomechanical analysis demonstrates that both 90-90 locked plating (medial and posterolateral) and bicolumnar (parallel) locked plating (medial and lateral) constructs are effective in supplying adequate stability (although parallel locked plating is biomechanically stronger than 90-90, both exhibit characteristics well above what is necessary for stable fixation).
3. ROM exercises may be initiated when the soft tissues allow.

I. Transcondylar fractures

1. Epidemiology—Transcondylar fractures traverse both columns, reside within the joint capsule, and typically are seen in elderly patients.
2. Mechanism of injury—These fractures occur with a flexed elbow or a fall on an outstretched hand with the arm in abduction or adduction.
3. Clinical evaluation—The examiner must be wary of a Posadas fracture, which is a transcondylar fracture with anterior displacement of the distal fragment and concomitant dislocation of the radial head and proximal ulna from the fragment.
4. Treatment
   a. Nonsurgical and surgical management follow recommendations and principles similar to those for supracondylar fractures.
   b. Total elbow arthroplasty may be considered in elderly patients with very distal fractures and poor bone quality.

J. Intercondylar fractures (**Figure 3**)

1. Epidemiology—Intercondylar fractures are the most common distal humerus fracture; frequently they are comminuted.
2. Classification
   a. According to the OTA classification, they are type C fractures.
   b. **Table 3** lists the descriptive types.
3. Pathoanatomy—The medial flexor mass and lateral extensor mass are responsible for rotation and proximal migration of the articular surface.
4. Treatment
   a. Treatment is primarily surgical, using medial and lateral plate fixation according to the principles and fixation types described previously.

TABLE 3

Two-Column Intercondylar Distal Humerus Fractures

Type	Description
High T fracture	A transverse fracture line divides both columns at or proximal to the olecranon fossa
Low T fracture	Similar to the high T fracture except the transverse component is through the olecranon fossa, making treatment and fixation more difficult
Y fracture	Oblique fracture lines cross each column and join in the olecranon fossa, extending vertically to the joint surface
H fracture	The trochlea is a free fragment and at risk for osteonecrosis. The medial column is fractured above and below the medial epicondyle, whereas the lateral column is fractured in a T or Y configuration
Medial λ fracture	The most proximal fracture line exits medially. Laterally, the fracture line is distal to the lateral epicondyle, rendering a very small fragment left for fixation on the lateral side.
Lateral λ fracture	The most proximal fracture line exits laterally. Medially, the fracture line is distal to the medial epicondyle, rendering a very small fragment left for fixation on the medial side
Multiplane fracture	This represents a T fracture with concomitant coronal fracture lines

Chapter 92

FRACTURES OF THE ELBOW

NILOOFAR DEHGHAN, MD, MSc, FRCS(C)
MICHAEL D. MCKEE, MD, FRCS(C)

I. RADIAL HEAD FRACTURES

A. Epidemiology and overview

1. Approximately 20% of all elbow fractures involve the radial head.
2. Radial head fractures can occur in isolation; however, they often are associated with more complex injuries, such as associated elbow fractures, dislocations, and soft-tissue injuries.
3. The radial head plays an important role as a secondary valgus stabilizer of the elbow.

B. Pathoanatomy

1. Radial head fractures typically result from a fall on an outstretched hand with the forearm in pronation, which results in an axial load on the elbow.
2. Of patients with radial head fractures, 30% have other soft-tissue and skeletal injuries, including carpal fractures, distal radioulnar joint (DRUJ), and interosseous membrane disruption, coronoid fractures, Monteggia fracture-dislocations, capitellar fractures, and medial and lateral collateral ligament injuries.

C. Classification—The Mason classification of radial head fractures is shown in **Table 1**

D. Evaluation

1. History
   a. Fractures of the radial head typically occur following a fall on an outstretched hand.

Dr. Dehghan or an immediate family member has received royalties from ITS; serves as a paid consultant to or is an employee of Acumed, LLC, bioventus and Zimmer; and serves as a board member, owner, officer, or committee member of the Orthopaedic Trauma Association. Dr. McKee or an immediate family member has received royalties from Elsevier Inc., ITS, Springer, Stryker, and Wolters- Kluwer publishing; serves as a paid consultant to or is an employee of Acumed, LLC, Bioventus, ITS, Nexsens, and Stryker; and serves as a board member, owner, officer, or committee member of the Canadian Orthopaedic Association and the Orthopaedic Trauma Association.

TABLE 1

Mason Classification of Radial Head Fractures

Fracture Type	Characteristic(s)
I	Fracture is minimally displaced
II	Fracture is displaced
III	Fracture is comminuted and displaced
IV[a]	Fracture of the radial head with dislocation of the ulnohumeral joint

[a]Type IV added by Johnston.

   b. The patient should be questioned carefully about concomitant wrist, forearm, or shoulder pain.
2. Physical examination
   a. Pain with palpation over the radial head.
   b. The surgeon should examine elbow range of motion (ROM) and assess for a block to pronation/supination or flexion/extension.
   c. The surgeon should examine the forearm, wrist, and elbow for tenderness along the course of the interosseous membrane (Essex-Lopresti lesion), instability of the DRUJ, pain at the medial side of the elbow (medial collateral ligament [MCL]), and pain at the lateral side of the elbow (lateral collateral ligament [LCL]).
   d. Lateral elbow pain and tenderness or limitation in elbow or forearm motion should alert the examiner to the possibility of a radial head fracture.
3. Imaging
   a. AP and lateral radiographs of the elbow are routinely obtained.
   b. Nondisplaced fractures of the radial head may not be visible; however, they may be diagnosed by elevation of the anterior and posterior fat pads (the sail sign) by an intra-articular hemarthrosis.

c. The radiocapitellar view is accomplished by positioning the patient as for a lateral view but angling the tube 45° toward the shoulder.

d. For comminuted fractures, CT can delineate the location, number, and size of the fragments and is rapidly emerging as a standard imaging method for more complicated radial head fractures.

4. Joint aspiration—Aspiration of the intra-articular hematoma and injection of a local anesthetic can be helpful when assessing mechanical blocks to motion.

E. Treatment

1. Nonsurgical—Most minimally displaced (<3 mm) radial head fractures can be treated nonsurgically if no block to ROM is present, with a brief period of immobilization (7-10 days maximum) in a sling or posterior splint for pain relief followed by early ROM exercises.

2. Surgical—Radial head fractures that are significantly displaced, block motion (especially rotation) or are part of more complicated injury patterns are candidates for surgical repair.

3. Surgical procedures

a. Open reduction and internal fixation (ORIF) options

- Screws—Mini fragment screws (2.7 or 2.0 mm) or headless screws with differential pitch (eg, Herbert screw, headless compression screw) should be countersunk to prevent screw prominence.
- Plates and screws—Plates should be placed in the "safe zone," the part of the radial head that does not articulate with the proximal ulna, which is the arc between the lines drawn through the radial styloid and the Lister tubercle (**Figure 1**).

b. Radial head replacement for comminuted fractures

- This is a good treatment option in cases with more than three fracture fragments, which have a higher rate of failure with surgical fixation (**Figure 2**).
- Radial head fracture fixation has a higher failure rate if there is associated elbow instability.
- The most commonly used radial head replacement prosthesis is a modular, metallic, smooth stem noncemented prosthesis.
- The ideal method of fixation of radial head prostheses remains elusive, but there is evidence that press-fit prostheses with a rough surface that do not obtain ingrowth or loosen can cause extensive osteolysis.

c. Radial head excision—The radial head is an important secondary stabilizer of the elbow; therefore, radial head excision alone is contraindicated in clinical settings in which extensive damage to the primary stabilizers (MCL: valgus instability; coronoid: posterior instability; interosseous membrane: longitudinal instability; LCL: posterolateral rotatory instability) is present.

F. Pearls and pitfalls

1. Isolated fractures heal best with early mobilization after 7 to 10 days.
2. Hardware should be applied to the safe zone.
3. Radial head fractures with three or more fragments have a higher incidence of unsatisfactory results with fixation. The surgeon should consider replacement, rather than fixation, for such fractures.
4. Radial head excision alone is contraindicated in the presence of other destabilizing injuries.

G. Rehabilitation

1. For nondisplaced radial head fractures: immobilization in a sling for 7 to 10 days followed by early ROM exercises.
2. For other nonsurgically treated stable fractures and for surgically treated fractures: immobilization in a posterior splint for 7 to 10 days, followed by early ROM exercises.

H. Complications of radial head fractures

1. Stiffness (especially forearm rotation)
2. Replacement of the radial head with a prosthesis that is too large (overstuffing the joint)
3. Fracture displacement (occurs in <5% of cases)
4. Radiocapitellar arthritis
5. Infection
6. Loss of fixation

II. OLECRANON FRACTURES

A. Epidemiology and overview

1. Olecranon fractures can result from several different mechanisms, including a direct blow, a fall on an outstretched hand with the elbow in

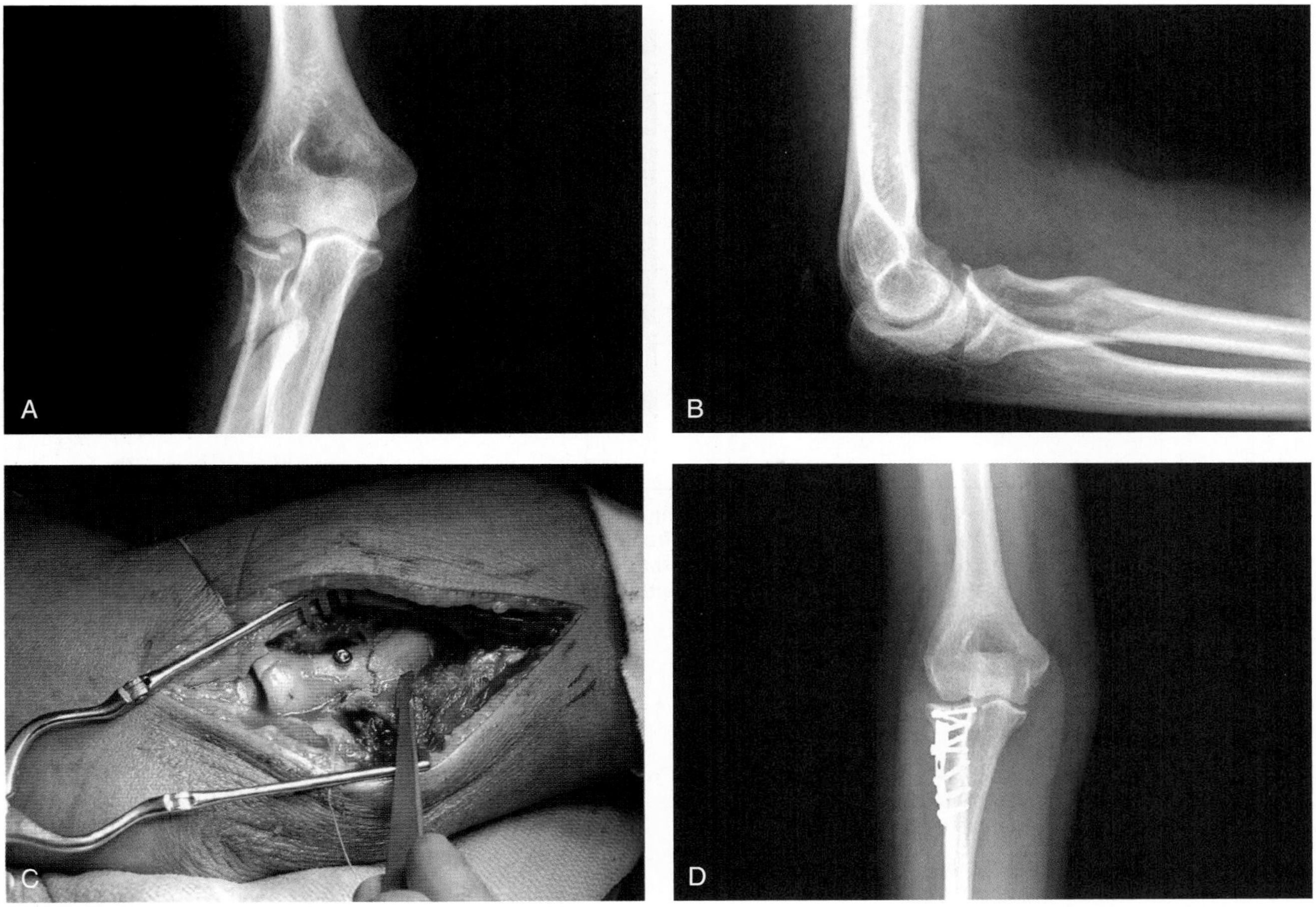

Figure 1 An active 32-year-old woman sustained a comminuted, displaced, intra-articular radial head and neck fracture. The patient had minimal, painful forearm rotation preoperatively. Preoperative AP (**A**) and lateral (**B**) radiographs demonstrate the fracture. **C**, Intraoperative photograph shows countersunk screw fixation of the head fracture and initial lag screw fixation of the neck fracture. The fixation was placed in the "safe zone," the nonarticular portion of the neck, in an arc subtended by lines through the radial styloid and the Lister tubercle. A mini fragment plate was subsequently applied. **D**, Postoperative AP radiograph shows the completed procedure.

flexion, or high-energy trauma that is associated with radial head fractures or elbow dislocation.

2. Sudden and violent triceps muscle contraction can produce an avulsion fracture of varying size of the olecranon tip.
3. A bimodal distribution of olecranon fractures is seen in young patients with high-energy trauma and elderly patients with low-energy trauma such as a fall from standing.

B. Pathoanatomy

1. The olecranon and the coronoid process form the greater sigmoid notch, which articulates with the trochlea of the distal humerus. The intrinsic anatomy of this articulation allows flexion/extension movement of the elbow joint and provides stability for the elbow.
2. The olecranon also serves as the insertion for the triceps tendon, which blends with the periosteum of the proximal ulna.
3. The exposed position of the olecranon renders it vulnerable to direct trauma and violent muscular contractions (from the triceps).

C. Classification—The Colton classification of olecranon fractures is shown in **Table 2**. This classification system can aid in decision making regarding treatment options, as outlined below.

D. Evaluation

1. History
    a. The history may help distinguish a triceps avulsion from an actual direct blow to the elbow.
    b. Pain usually is localized to the posterior part of the elbow.

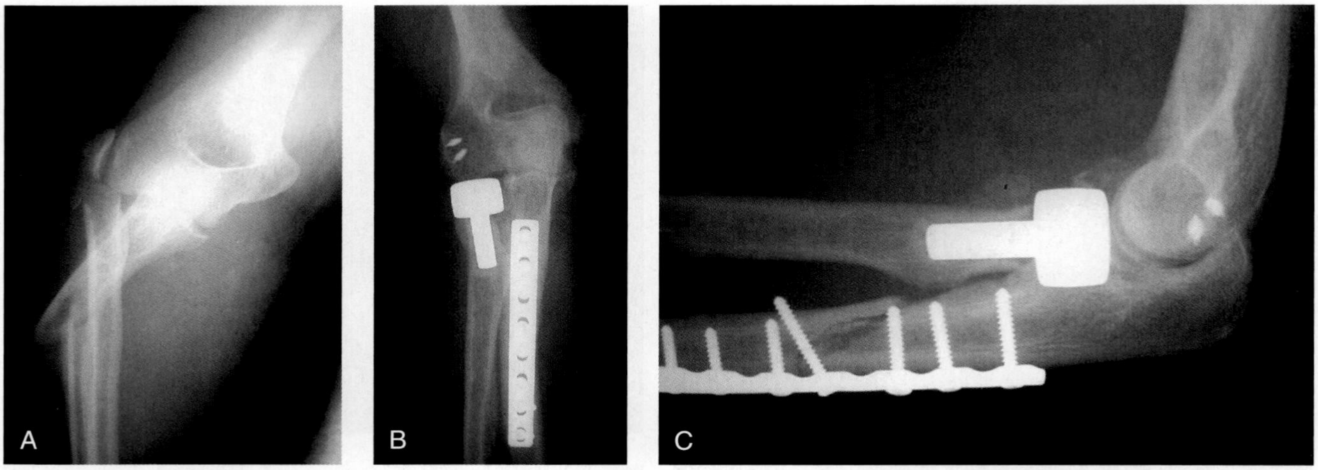

Figure 2 A 37-year-old patient sustained a Monteggia variant injury in a fall. **A**, Preoperative AP radiograph shows an angulated fracture of the proximal ulna with a comminuted posterolateral fracture-dislocation of the radial head. AP (**B**) and lateral (**C**) radiographs show the elbow following open reduction and internal fixation of the ulnar shaft; radial head replacement with a modular, metallic prosthesis; and repair of the lateral collateral ligament with suture anchors in the lateral column.

TABLE 2

Colton Classification of Olecranon Fractures

Fracture Type	Characteristics
I	Fracture is nondisplaced and stable, with <2 mm of separation; the extensor mechanism is intact and the patient is able to extend the elbow against gravity with flexion to 90°
II	Fracture is displaced Type IIA—Avulsion Type IIB—Oblique and transverse Type IIC—Comminuted Type IID—Fracture-dislocation

2. Physical examination
   a. Given the subcutaneous location of the olecranon, the fracture itself may be palpable.
   b. Extensive posterior swelling is typical.
   c. A careful examination of the integrity of the extensor mechanism (with gravity eliminated) can aid surgical decision making.
   d. If present, open wounds are typically posterior and result from the direct impact of the posterior surface of the elbow against an unyielding structure.
3. Imaging
   a. Plain radiographs are usually sufficient for isolated fractures of the olecranon.
   b. A true lateral radiograph is necessary to accurately identify the plane of the fracture and the number of fracture fragments. The examiner also should assess for fracture comminution and impaction.
   c. In more complex cases, CT may help delineate the comminution or impaction better; however, this is not routinely required.

E. Treatment
1. Goals—The goals of olecranon fracture management include articular restoration, preservation of the extensor mechanism, elbow stability, avoidance of stiffness, and minimization of complications.
2. Nonsurgical
   a. Nondisplaced fractures (Colton type I) or minimally displaced fractures can be treated effectively by immobilizing the limb in a long arm splint or cast with the elbow flexed at 30° to 90° for 2 to 4 weeks.
   b. There is recent evidence that displaced olecranon fractures in the setting of elderly patients (>75 years of age) or those with extensive comorbidities can be treated nonoperatively, which may result in lower complications compared with surgical fixation. Age as well as patient's activities and functional demands should be taken into account for decision making.

3. Surgical
    a. Displaced fractures (Colton type II and its subtypes) require surgical fixation in healthy, active patients to preserve the strength of the extensor mechanism and maintain intra-articular congruity.
    b. Contraindications include active infection and severe medical comorbidities.
4. Surgical procedures
    a. Tension band wiring technique over two Kirschner wires (K-wires)
        - Indications—Isolated, transverse fractures that are proximal to the coronoid, without significant comminution, and not associated with ligamentous instability.
        - This technique does not resist angular forces or stabilize complex fracture patterns.
        - Contraindications—Significantly comminuted fractures of the proximal ulna (**Figure 3**), especially those with associated elbow instability.
        - Insertion of K-wires into the anterior cortex of the ulna distal to the fracture line enhances fixation strength and may help prevent backing out. The surgeon must be aware of overpenetration of the anterior cortex, however, which may result in a decrease in ROM and risk injury to the anterior interosseous nerve.
    b. Dorsal plate application to the posterior aspect of the proximal ulna (**Figure 4**)

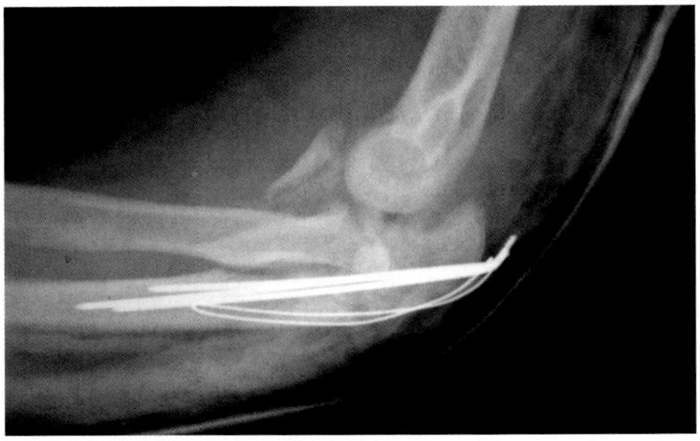

Figure 3 Lateral radiograph of the elbow of a 42-year-old man who sustained an early, recurrent posterior subluxation of the elbow following attempted fixation of a proximal ulnar fracture using a tension band technique demonstrates that the coronoid fragment has not been stabilized and the associated fracture of the radial head has not been addressed.

        - Dorsal plate application is the preferred fixation method if comminution or associated ligamentous injury with instability is present.
        - The terminal aspect of the triceps insertion can be elevated and then repaired following plate application to minimize prominence.
    c. Fragment excision and triceps reattachment for osteoporotic, comminuted fragments composing less than 50% of the olecranon.
        - May be beneficial for elderly (>70 years of age), low-demand patients whose bones are osteoporotic enough to compromise fixation (although nonoperative treatment of such patients should now be considered a superior option).
        - This procedure cannot be performed if associated ligamentous instability is present.
5. Pearls and pitfalls
    a. The tension band technique should be used only for fractures that are proximal to the base of the coronoid and that occur secondary to eccentric loads.
    b. In factures that are amendable to tension band fixation technique as well as plate fixation, the use of a plate may decrease subsequent hardware removal.
    c. Dorsal contoured plate application is the preferred fixation method in fractures secondary to bending mechanisms (including those distal to the coronoid), fractures with comminution, fracture-dislocations, or associated ligamentous injury with instability.
6. Rehabilitation
    a. Nonsurgically managed fractures that are minimally displaced with an intact extensor mechanism can be immobilized in a long arm splint with radiographic monitoring and mobilized at 4 weeks.
    b. Surgically managed fractures are splinted for up to 1 week for pain control and to allow swelling to subside.
        - Active and gentle passive motion is then initiated, but resisted extension is specifically restricted until clinical and radiographic evidence of fracture healing is apparent, usually at 6 weeks postoperatively.
        - Older patients who typically use forceful elbow extension to rise from a chair or a toilet should be advised to avoid this activity until fracture union occurs.

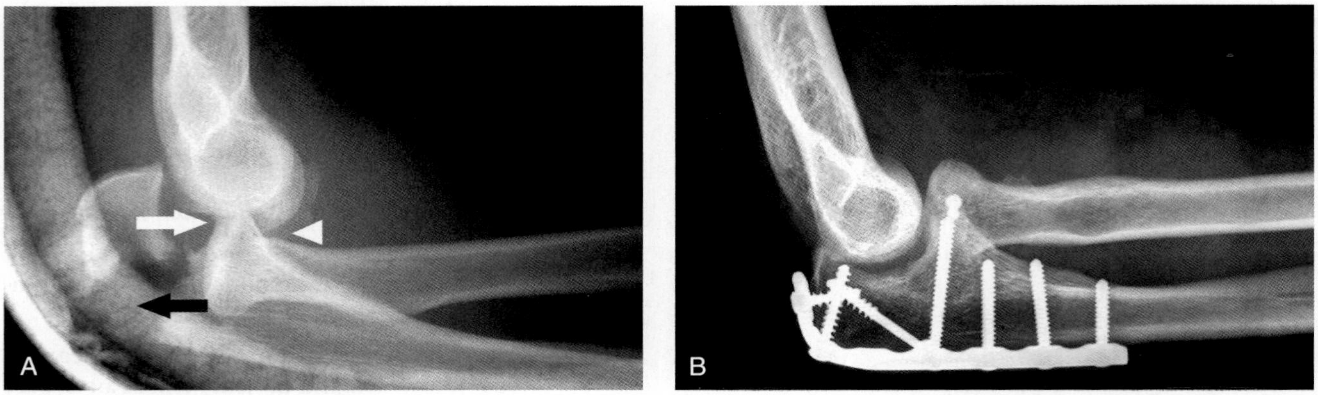

Figure 4 Lateral radiographs from a 17-year-old boy who sustained an elbow dislocation. **A**, Preoperative radiograph demonstrates the dislocation and associated olecranon (black arrow), coronoid (white arrowhead), and radial head (white arrow) fractures. **B**, Postoperative lateral radiograph shows the elbow following open reduction and internal fixation of the radial head fragment with a single countersunk Herbert screw, plate fixation of the ulna, and repair of the lateral collateral ligament through drill holes in the lateral column. A concentric reduction of the radiocapitellar and ulnohumeral joints was achieved, with sufficient stability to initiate immediate motion, enhancing the functional result.

7. Complications
    a. Stiffness (typically with terminal extension).
    b. Loss of reduction is rare if the proper principles of fixation are followed. As described previously, tension band wiring of fractures associated with comminution or elbow instability can lead to failure of the construct and loss of reduction and should be treated with plate fixation instead.
    c. Nonunion is rare, but malunion (especially of unreduced, impacted articular fragments) may result in posttraumatic arthritic change and stiffness.
    d. Hardware prominence and the need for hardware removal after fracture healing are common because of the subcutaneous nature of the olecranon. There is evidence that compared with tension band fixation the use of precontoured olecranon plates may decrease hardware prominence and hardware removal rates.
    e. Overpenetration of the anterior cortex with K-wires can result in a decrease in pronation/supination and puts the anterior interosseous nerve at risk for injury.

III. PROXIMAL ULNAR FRACTURES

A. Epidemiology and overview
1. Although they may seem complex, proximal ulnar fractures tend to fall into one of the three basic injury patterns.
    a. Simple olecranon fractures—No associated elbow instability or dislocation present
    b. Transolecranon fracture-dislocations—Fracture of the olecranon with associated elbow instability or dislocation
    c. Monteggia fractures and variants—Fracture of the proximal third ulna with associated radial head dislocation (specifically from the proximal radioulnar joint) or proximal radius fracture
2. Most of these injuries require surgical intervention.
3. Posterior fracture-dislocations of the proximal ulna are associated with a high incidence of radial head fractures and LCL injuries.

B. Pathoanatomy
1. A fall directly on the elbow can produce a transolecranon fracture-dislocation because the distal humerus acts as a pile driver and drives through the trochlear notch of the ulna.
2. A fall on an outstretched hand results in a posteriorly directed force vector to the elbow and can produce a posterior fracture-dislocation or a (posterior) Monteggia fracture.

C. Classification—The Bado classification defines four types of Monteggia fractures according to the direction of displacement of the radial head and other characteristics (**Table 3**). A Bado type II injury, which is associated with a posterior radial head dislocation, is the most common type of injury pattern in adults. This subtype is associated with the highest complication rate.

TABLE 3

Bado Classification of Monteggia Fractures

Fracture Type	Description		Direction of Displacement of the Radial Head	Characteristic(s)
I	Fracture of the middle or proximal third of the ulna	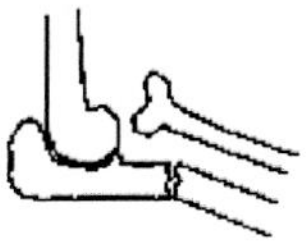	Anterior	More common in children and young adults
II	Fracture of the middle or proximal third of the ulna	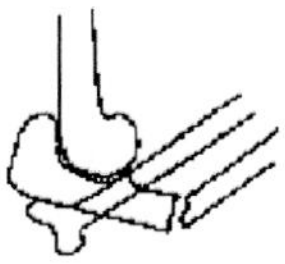	Posterior	Comprise most (70%-80%) Monteggia fractures in adults
III	Fracture of the ulna distal to the coronoid process	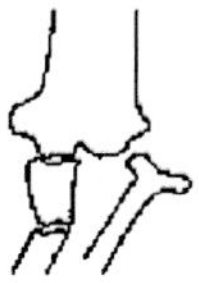	Lateral	More common in children
IV	Fracture of the middle or proximal third of the ulna and fracture of the proximal third of the radius	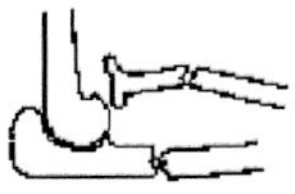	Any direction	Least common

Adapted from Turner RG, King GAW: Proximal ulnar fractures and fracture dislocations, in Galatz LM, ed: *Orthopaedic Knowledge Update: Shoulder and Elbow*, ed 3. Rosemont, IL, American Academy of Orthopaedic Surgeons, 2008, pp 517-529.

D. Evaluation

1. History

   a. The history should include a clarification of the exact mechanism of injury, any sensation of dislocation with spontaneous reduction, and any associated upper extremity pain or discomfort.

   b. Any reports of wrist and/or forearm pain should alert the treating surgeon to the possibility of a more complex injury pattern.

2. Physical examination

   a. The elbow is typically swollen, especially posteriorly.

   b. If present, open wounds are usually posterior or posterolateral.

   c. Neurologic examination, especially of the posterior interosseous nerve, should be performed.

   d. The wrist should be examined for any evidence of a distal radioulnar injury (a bipolar forearm injury).

3. Imaging

   a. Radiographs

   - Plain radiographs are the mainstay of imaging; they usually show the general injury pattern.
   - On normal AP and lateral radiographs, a line drawn through the center of the proximal radial shaft and the center of the radial head should bisect the capitellum. If the radial head does not line up with the capitellum, concern should arise about subluxation or dislocation of the radial head (**Figure 5**).
   - Repeat radiographs obtained after a gentle reduction and splinting can provide more detailed information. It is important to look for associated bony injuries in this situation; radial head fractures, coronoid fragments, and collateral ligament avulsions are common.
   - The proximal ulna has a slight dorsal bend averaging 6°, called the proximal ulna dorsal angle (PUDA). Radiographic imaging of

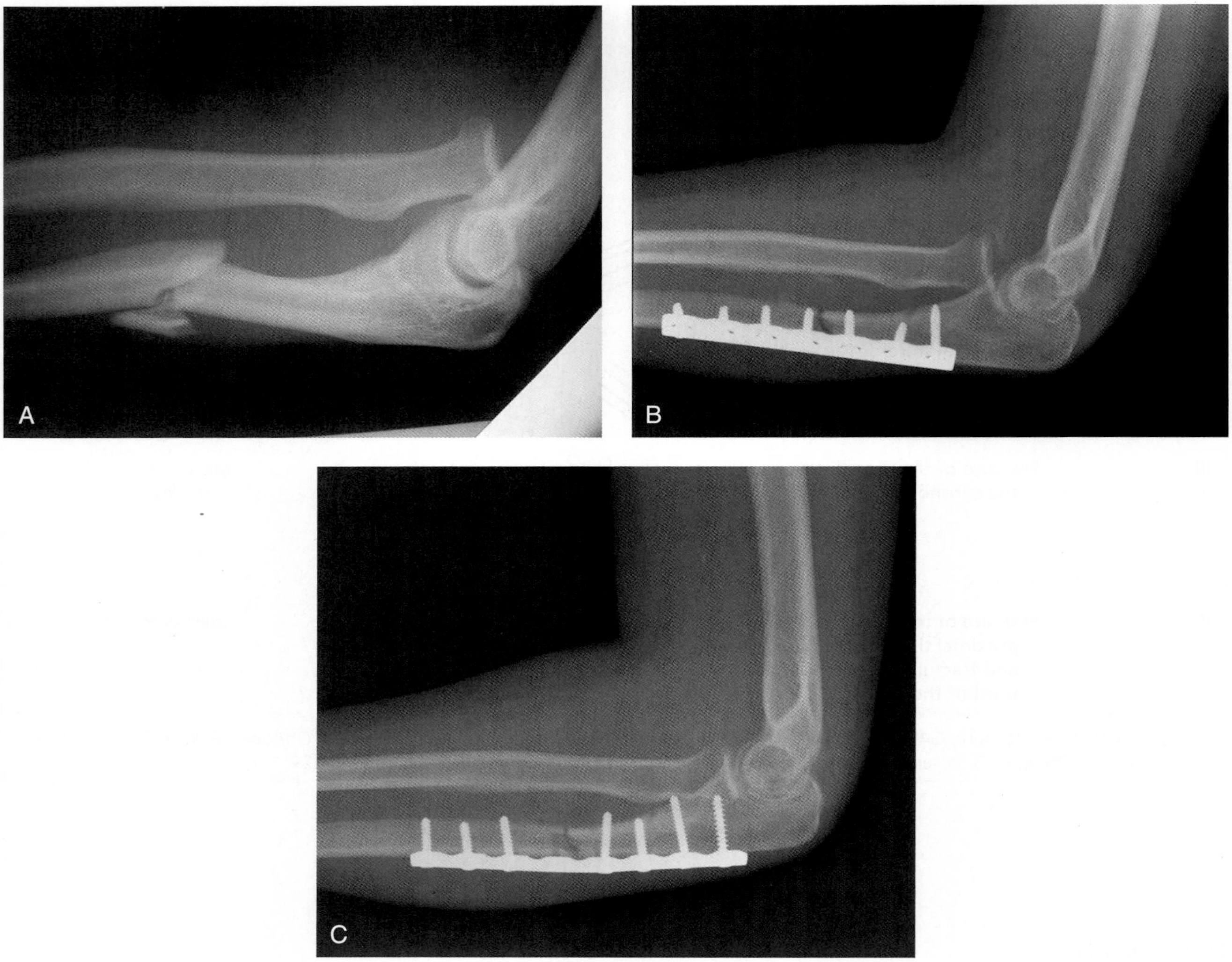

Figure 5 **A**, Preoperative lateral radiograph of the elbow shows a Monteggia fracture, with fracture of the proximal ulnar shaft and an associated anterior radial head displacement. **B**, Postoperative lateral radiograph obtained after attempted fixation that resulted in malreduction of the proximal ulnar shaft, due to placement of a strait plate without a dorsal bend to accommodate the proximal ulna dorsal angle (PUDA). This malreduction has caused anterior subluxation of the radial head. **C**, Postoperative lateral radiograph obtained after revision surgical fixation of the proximal ulna with a plate that has a slight dorsal bend, to fit the patient's natural PUDA. Notice the radial head has appropriately reduced after anatomic reduction of the proximal ulna.

the contralateral elbow can help determine the patients' natural PUDA.

b. CT may help define the size and location of fracture fragments and in confirming associated injuries.

E. Treatment

1. Nonsurgical—Stable, noncomminuted fractures of the proximal ulna that are not associated with other injuries about the elbow can be treated nonsurgically. This injury pattern is relatively rare, however; most require surgical intervention.

2. Surgical

a. Complex proximal ulnar fractures often contain a substantial coronoid fragment, which is typically triangular and involves 50% to 100% of the coronoid process. This fragment is important for re-creating the anterior buttress of the greater sigmoid notch of the proximal ulna.

b. Coronoid reduction and fixation is a critical component of elbow stability.

c. Once the main proximal-distal fragment fracture line of the ulna is reduced, visualization and repair of the coronoid become difficult. Thus, it is important to fix the coronoid fragment (usually with lag screws) to the distal ulnar fragment before reducing the primary ulnar fracture line.

d. Fixation of the proximal ulnar fracture should be performed with a small fragment compression plate contoured to project proximally around the tip of the olecranon.

e. A similar approach is used for Monteggia fracture patterns: ORIF of the ulna with a 3.5-mm compression plate through a posterior approach.

f. Ulnar fracture malreduction is the usual cause of any residual subluxation or dislocation of the radiocapitellar joint (**Figure 5**).

F. Pearls and pitfalls

1. Failure to recognize associated radial head and LCL injuries can lead to recurrent instability.
2. Loss of fixation from inadequate plate selection, length, or placement is exacerbated by the osteoporotic bone of older individuals.
3. Extensive soft-tissue damage, the use of surgical approaches that expose radial and ulnar fracture sites together (often necessary), prolonged immobilization, or concomitant radial head injury can lead to radioulnar stiffness or even synostosis.
4. Ulnar fracture malreduction is the most common cause of residual radial head malalignment in a Monteggia fracture-dislocation.
5. When utilizing straight/noncontoured plates to fix proximal ulna fractures, it is important to place a slight dorsal bend to match the natural PUDA. Failure to do this will lead to malreduction of the proximal ulna and persistent dislocation of the radial head in the setting of Monteggia fractures (**Figure 5**).

G. Rehabilitation

1. Postsurgical rehabilitation depends largely on the fracture/ligament fixation obtained intraoperatively and on the results of stability testing at the conclusion of the procedure.
2. Typically, a well-padded posterior splint is applied with the elbow at 90° and the forearm in pronation to protect a lateral-side ligament repair.
3. If adequate stability has been achieved, early motion with active and gentle passive exercises is instituted within 1 week after surgery, and the patient is weaned from the splint.
4. Strengthening is instituted at 6 to 8 weeks. Even in marginally repaired fractures, active muscle contraction of the dynamic stabilizers, such as the flexor-pronator mass and the common extensor origin, may improve the concentric stability of the ulnohumeral joint, analogous to active deltoid exercises in a shoulder with inferior subluxation after trauma.

H. Complications

1. The reported complication rate for fractures of the proximal ulna is high.
2. Simple fractures tend to heal well, but management of complex fractures has been hampered by a poor understanding of injury patterns and deforming forces, inadequate fixation, and prolonged immobilization of tenuously repaired fractures (**Figure 3**).
3. The risk of proximal radioulnar synostosis is increased by multiple surgeries, extensive soft-tissue damage or dissection, exposure of the radius and ulna together, and concomitant radial head injuries.

IV. CORONOID FRACTURES

A. Epidemiology and overview

1. The coronoid acts as the anterior buttress of the greater sigmoid notch of the olecranon, and it is the primary resistor of posterior elbow subluxation or dislocation.
2. A coronoid fracture, identified in as many as 10% to 15% of elbow injuries, is pathognomonic of an episode of elbow instability.
3. Fractures at the base of the coronoid can exacerbate elbow instability because the sublime tubercle is the attachment site for the anterior bundle of the MCL, and the tip of the coronoid is the attachment site for the middle part of the anterior capsule.
4. Associated injuries are common, including fracture of the radial head or olecranon, injury to the LCL or MCL, or associated elbow dislocation.

B. Pathoanatomy

1. An intact coronoid resists posterior elbow displacement.
2. The coronoid typically is fractured as the distal humerus is driven against it during an episode of posterior subluxation or severe varus stress.
3. Previously, type I and even some type II coronoid fractures (see Classification below) were

considered avulsion fractures produced by the anterior capsule; however, this does not describe the mechanism of injury, which is primarily a shearing force.

4. The medial facet is important for varus stability, and the sublime tubercle just distal to it provides insertion for the MCL.
5. Anteromedial facet fractures occur from a primarily varus force, are often associated with an LCL injury, and represent a distinct subtype of injury.
6. Posteromedial rotatory instability results from anteromedial coronoid fracture and disruption of the LCL.
7. Posterolateral rotatory instability is associated with injury to the LCL; it is often associated with radial head fracture and coronoid tip fracture.

C. Classification

1. The Regan and Morrey classification is shown in **Table 4**.
2. O'Driscoll classification—O'Driscoll has proposed a more comprehensive classification scheme that subdivides the coronoid injury based on the location and the number of coronoid fragments. This scheme is important because it recognizes fractures of the anteromedial facet caused by a varus posteromedial rotatory force (**Figure 6**).
3. Anteromedial facet fractures are a different entity from the usual coronoid fractures. They may involve the rim, the tip, or the sublime tubercle and result in varus and posteromedial rotatory instability. These fractures result from a varus injury mechanism, commonly require surgical fixation with a buttress plate used medially, and usually are associated with LCL avulsions.

TABLE 4

Regan and Morrey Classification of Coronoid Fractures

Fracture Type	Characteristics
I	Fracture of the tip of the coronoid process
II	Fracture involves ≤50% of the coronoid process
III	Fracture involves >50% of the coronoid process

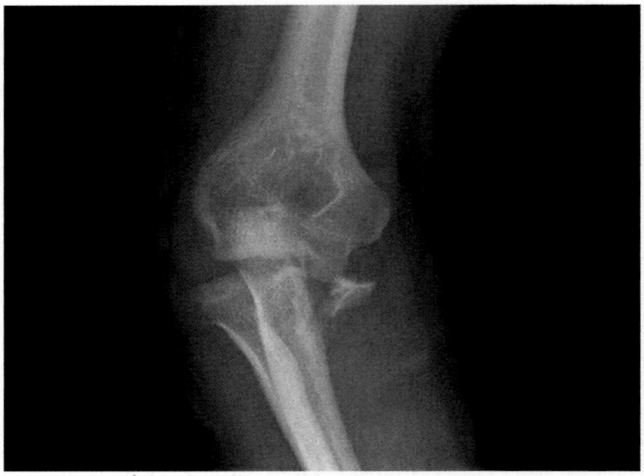

Figure 6 AP radiograph of the elbow of a young man demonstrates a posteromedial rotatory elbow injury from a varus deforming force. The varus position of the joint, with an avulsion of the lateral collateral ligament and a compression fracture of the anteromedial facet of the coronoid, is seen clearly. This injury pattern requires buttress plate fixation of the coronoid fracture and lateral ligament repair for an optimal outcome.

D. Evaluation

1. History
   a. A history of dislocation with spontaneous reduction may be elicited.
   b. Pain in the forearm or wrist may be a sign of associated injuries that require further evaluation and imaging.
2. Physical examination
   a. Examination for instability is difficult but important for an accurate diagnosis.
   b. A varus attitude of the elbow and pain on varus stress indicate a posteromedial rotatory injury (**Figure 6**).
3. Imaging
   a. Standard AP and lateral radiographs should be obtained; however, the amorphous structure of the coronoid and the overlap of adjacent structures can make interpretation difficult.
   b. CT can be useful in this setting, especially for higher grades of comminuted coronoid fractures.

E. Treatment

1. Nonsurgical
   a. The decision to treat a coronoid fracture surgically or nonsurgically is based on the associated injuries (radial head fracture, collateral

ligament tears) and the evaluation of elbow joint stability.

b. A minimally displaced type I or II fracture with no associated injuries and a stable elbow on examination is rare but may be treated with a brief period of immobilization for pain control followed by early ROM exercises. Most elbow dislocations are more stable with the forearm in pronation.

2. Surgical

a. Most coronoid fractures require surgical fixation because of elbow instability and are associated with other fractures or ligamentous injuries.

b. Concurrent injuries (radial head fracture, ligament tears) also must be addressed.

c. Surgical approach

- Lateral—This is ideal in cases associated with fracture of the radial head when the radial head will be replaced. The Kocher, Kaplan, or Hotchkiss approach may be used, depending on the presence of other injuries requiring fixation. After the radial head is removed, the coronoid can be visualized easily and repaired. The LCL complex also can be repaired at the end of the case.
- Medial—This is ideal for coronoid fractures that cannot be accessed from the lateral side because of the presence of the radial head or in situations with anteromedial facet fractures, which are visualized better from the medial side. Intervals include working between the two heads of the flexor carpi ulnaris or splitting the flexor-pronator mass more anteriorly as described by Hotchkiss. This approach is preferred for those anteromedial facet fractures that result from a varus force and require buttress plating. The MCL may be repaired at the end of the case.

d. Types of fixation

- Small type I or II coronoid fractures can be repaired with suture fixation by passing sutures through drill holes in the proximal aspect of the ulna and capturing the coronoid fragment and anterior elbow capsule for fixation.
- Larger type II or III coronoid fractures may require retrograde screws or plate insertion.
- Fractures involving the medial facet can be repaired with a buttress plate for rigid fixation.
- Hinged external fixation may be used to help maintain stability in difficult or revision cases.

F. Pearls and pitfalls

1. In the setting of a complex proximal ulnar fracture, the coronoid fragment is an important bulwark against recurrent posterior subluxation.
2. Larger coronoid fragments frequently include the insertion of the MCL.
3. In the setting of a complex proximal ulnar fracture, the coronoid fragment should be repaired before the main ulnar fracture is reduced.
4. Fixation of the coronoid fragment can be performed with cannulated screws from the posterior surface of the ulna.
5. Anteromedial facet fractures are best treated with a buttress plate via a medial approach.

G. Rehabilitation

1. Rehabilitation depends on an intraoperative examination at the conclusion of the procedure.
2. A thermoplastic resting splint is applied with the elbow at 90° and the forearm in the neutral position.
3. The terminal 30° of extension is restricted for the first 2 to 4 weeks.
4. Shoulder abduction, which places a varus moment on the arm, is avoided for the first 4 to 6 weeks in fractures/fracture-dislocations with varus instability.
5. Increasing evidence shows that some residual ulnohumeral "sagging" or gapping after the surgical repair of elbow injuries may rapidly improve under the influence of the dynamic muscle contraction that early active motion provides.

H. Complications

1. Complication and repeat surgery rates are high.
2. Complications include stiffness of the elbow, recurrent instability of the elbow, posttraumatic arthritic degeneration, and heterotopic ossification.
3. Failure to appreciate—and surgically repair—the underlying associated elbow instability results in early failure of fixation (**Figures 3** and **6**).

TOP TESTING FACTS

Radial Head Fractures

1. The forearm and wrist should be examined carefully in all cases of radial head fracture.
2. Most radial head fractures can be treated nonsurgically.
3. Isolated radial head fractures do best with early mobilization, not prolonged casting. The patient should not be immobilized for more than 7 to 10 days.
4. Radial head fractures that block motion or are significantly displaced can be treated with ORIF.
5. If a plate is used for radial head fixation, it should be placed in the "safe zone," away from articulation with the proximal ulna, between the radial styloid and Lister tubercle.
6. Comminuted fractures with more than three fragments benefit from radial head replacement using a metal, modular prosthesis.
7. Radial head excision alone is contraindicated in the presence of other destabilizing injuries.
8. Loose radial head prostheses with a rough surface can cause extensive proximal radial osteolysis.

Olecranon Fractures

1. The integrity of the extensor mechanism should be examined carefully.
2. The tension band technique is indicated for isolated, noncomminuted olecranon fractures proximal to the coronoid, without ligamentous instability. Failure to adhere to this principle may lead to failure of fixation.
3. Insertion of K-wires into the anterior cortex of the ulna distal to the fracture line enhances fixation strength and may help prevent backing out.
4. Plate fixation is preferred for comminuted fractures, fractures with coronoid extension, or fractures associated with elbow instability.
5. Nonsurgical treatment may be beneficial for elderly, low-demand patients, even in the presence of significant displacement.

Proximal Ulnar Fractures

1. Posterior fracture-dislocations of the proximal ulna are associated with a high incidence of radial head fractures and LCL injuries.
2. Type II (posterior radial head displacement) Monteggia fractures compose 70% to 80% of Monteggia fractures in adults.
3. Complex proximal ulnar fractures often contain a significant coronoid fragment, which is typically triangular and involves 50% to 100% of the coronoid process. This fragment is important for re-creating the anterior buttress of the greater sigmoid notch of the proximal ulna.
4. Coronoid reduction and fixation are critical components of elbow stability.
5. The proximal ulna has a natural dorsal angulation (PUDA), which should be taken into account when contouring plates for internal fixation.
6. The risk of proximal radioulnar synostosis is increased by multiple surgeries, extensive soft-tissue damage or dissection, and concomitant radial head injuries.
7. Ulnar fracture malreduction is the most common cause of residual radial head malalignment in a Monteggia fracture-dislocation.

Coronoid Fractures

1. The presence of a coronoid fracture is pathognomonic of an episode of elbow instability, and associated injuries are common.
2. A coronoid fracture is not typically an avulsion fracture but is caused by a shearing mechanism.
3. Anteromedial facet fractures occur from a primarily varus force, are often associated with an LCL injury, and represent a distinct subtype of injury.
4. Hinged external fixation may be used to help maintain stability in difficult or revision cases.
5. In the setting of a complex proximal ulnar fracture, the coronoid fragment is an important restraint against recurrent posterior subluxation. In these situations, the coronoid fragment should be repaired before the main ulnar fracture is reduced.

6. Larger coronoid fragments are important because they frequently include the insertion of the MCL.
7. Fixation of the coronoid fragment can be performed with cannulated screws from the posterior surface of the ulna or with suture fixation if the fragment is small.
8. Fractures involving the anteromedial facet can be repaired with a buttress plate for rigid fixation via a medial approach.

Bibliography

Bryan RS, Morrey BF: Extensive posterior exposure of the elbow: A triceps-sparing approach. *Clin Orthop Relat Res* 1982;166:188-192.

Doornberg JN, Ring DC: Fracture of the anteromedial facet of the coronoid process. *J Bone Joint Surg Am* 2006;88(10):2216-2224.

Duckworth AD, Clement ND, McEachan JE, White TO, Court-Brown CM, McQueen MM. Prospective randomised trial of non-operative versus operative management of olecranon fractures in the elderly. *Bone Joint J* 2017;99-B(7):964-972.

Duckworth AD, Clement ND, White TO, Court-Brown CM, McQueen MM. Plate versus tension-band wire fixation for olecranon fractures. *J Bone Joint Surg Am* 2017;99(15):1261-1273.

Flinkkilä T, Kaisto T, Sirniö K, Hyvönen P, Leppilahti J: Short- to mid-term results of metallic press-fit radial head arthroplasty in unstable injuries of the elbow. *J Bone Joint Surg Br* 2012;94(6):805-810.

Frankle MA, Koval KJ, Sanders RW, Zuckerman JD: Radial head fractures associated with elbow dislocations treated by immediate stabilization and early motion. *J Shoulder Elbow Surg* 1999;8(4):355-360.

Johnston GW: A follow-up of one hundred cases of fracture of the head of the radius with a review of the literature. *Ulster Med J* 1962;31:51-56.

Macko D, Szabo RM: Complications of tension-band wiring of olecranon fractures. *J Bone Joint Surg Am* 1985;67(9):1396-1401.

Marsh JP, Grewal R, Faber KJ, Drosdowech DS, Athwal GS, King GJ: Radial head fractures treated with modular metallic radial head replacement: Outcomes at a mean follow-up of eight years. *J Bone Joint Surg Am* 2016;98(7):527-535.

Mathew PK, Athwal GS, King GJ: Terrible triad injury of the elbow: Current concepts. *J Am Acad Orthop Surg* 2009;17(3):137-151.

McKee MD, Jupiter JB: Trauma to the adult elbow and fractures of the distal humerus, in Browner B, Jupiter J, Levine A, Trafton P: *Skeletal Trauma*, ed 3. Philadelphia, PA, WB Saunders, 2003, pp 1404-1480.

McKee MD, Pugh DM, Wild LM, Schemitsch EH, King GJ: Standard surgical protocol to treat elbow dislocations with radial head and coronoid fractures: Surgical technique. *J Bone Joint Surg Am* 2005;87(pt 1, suppl 1):22-32.

Moro JK, Werier J, MacDermid JC, Patterson SD, King GJ: Arthroplasty with a metal radial head for unreconstructible fractures of the radial head. *J Bone Joint Surg Am* 2001;83(8):1201-1211.

O'Driscoll SW, Jupiter JB, Cohen MS, Ring D, McKee MD: Difficult elbow fractures: Pearls and pitfalls. *Instr Course Lect* 2003;52:113-134.

Pollock JW, Brownhill J, Ferreira L, McDonald CP, Johnson J, King G: The effect of anteromedial facet fractures of the coronoid and lateral collateral ligament injury on elbow stability and kinematics. *J Bone Joint Surg Am* 2009;91(6):1448-1458.

Ring D: Fractures and dislocations of the elbow, in Bucholz RW, Heckman JD, Court-Brown CM, eds: *Rockwood and Green's Fractures in Adults*, ed 46. Philadelphia, PA, Lippincott Williams & Wilkins, 2001, pp 989-1049.

Ring D, Quintero J, Jupiter JB: Open reduction and internal fixation of fractures of the radial head. *J Bone Joint Surg Am* 2002;84(10):1811-1815.

Rouleau DM, Faber KJ, Athwal GS. The proximal ulna dorsal angulation: A radiographic study. *J Shoulder Elbow Surg* 2010 Jan;19(1):26-30.

Sanchez-Sotelo J, O'Driscoll SW, Morrey BF: Medial oblique compression fracture of the coronoid process of the ulna. *J Shoulder Elbow Surg* 2005;14(1):60-64.

Turner RG, King JWG: Proximal ulnar fractures and fracture-dislocations, in Galatz LM, ed: *Orthopaedic Knowledge Update: Shoulder and Elbow*, ed 3. Rosemont, IL, American Academy of Orthopaedic Surgeons, 2008, pp 517-529.

Chapter 93
TERRIBLE TRIAD INJURIES OF THE ELBOW

ROBERT Z. TASHJIAN, MD

I. OVERVIEW

A. Elbow dislocations are categorized as simple (no associated fracture) and complex (associated fracture).

B. Terrible triad injuries refer to complex elbow injuries that include posterolateral elbow dislocation, a radial head or neck fracture, and a coronoid process fracture. They are characterized by historically poor outcomes, secondary to persistent instability, stiffness, and arthrosis.

C. Generally, nonsurgical management has a limited role in the management of terrible triad injuries.

D. Surgical treatment using a standard protocol of coronoid fracture fixation, if possible, radial head fracture fixation or replacement, and lateral ligamentous repair can result in predictable results.

1. A standardized surgical protocol results in an average flexion arc of 112° and 77% good or excellent results.
2. Complications include stiffness, heterotopic bone formation, infection, ulnar neuropathy, persistent instability, nonunion, and malunion. Revision surgery is necessary in 20% to 25% of cases.

II. PATHOANATOMY AND BIOMECHANICS

A. The primary stabilizing components of the elbow involved with terrible triad injuries include the radial head, the coronoid, the ligamentous structures (the lateral and medial collateral ligaments), and the common extensor mechanism.

1. Coronoid process—An important anterior and varus stabilizer to the ulnohumeral joint
   a. Anatomic components of the coronoid process include the tip, body, anterolateral facet, and anteromedial facet. The O'Driscoll fracture classification is based on the fracture location of these subregions.
   b. Biomechanically, the coronoid process provides resistance to posterior subluxation beyond 30° of flexion. Small (<10% of height) fractures have been shown to have little effect on elbow stability.
   c. In radial head excision with intact ligaments, coronoid resection of 30% fully destabilizes the ulnohumeral joint, although stability is restored with radial head replacement. In larger coronoid defects (50% to 70% resection), stability cannot be restored by radial head replacement alone.
   d. The coronoid process fracture in this type of injury is typically simple, transverse, and small (O'Driscoll type 1; <30% of height); average height is 35% of total coronoid height. Based on biomechanical data on the restoration of joint stability, most should be repaired.
   e. The coronoid fragment always has some anterior capsule attached, which can be useful for soft-tissue repair of the fracture.
2. Radial head
   a. The radial head is an important secondary valgus stabilizer. It provides approximately 30% of valgus stability with intact medial ligaments.
   b. The radial head also is a primary restraint to posterolateral rotatory instability.

Dr. Tashjian or an immediate family member has received royalties from Shoulder Innovations, Wright Medical Technology, Inc., and Zimmer; serves as a paid consultant to or is an employee of Cayenne Medical and Mitek; and has stock or stock options held in Conextions, INTRAFUSE, and KATOR.

c. In biomechanical studies with intact ligaments, isolated radial head excision leads to increased rotatory laxity. Radial head excision and a fracture of 30% of the coronoid with intact ligaments results in subluxation even with intact ligaments. Clinically, it has been shown that radial head excision in terrible triad injuries without ligament repair results in 50% redislocation at 2 months.

d. Complete restoration of the radial head articular surface, with repair or replacement, is required to restore elbow stability in terrible triad injuries.

3. Lateral ligamentous complex (**Figure 1**)

a. The lateral collateral ligament (LCL) is always injured in a terrible triad injury and usually is avulsed off the lateral epicondyle with a portion of the extensor muscles.

b. The LCL complex is the primary restraint to posterolateral rotatory instability of the elbow; it prevents external rotation of the radius and ulna relative to the humerus.

c. The components of the LCL complex include the lateral ulnar collateral ligament (LUCL), the radial collateral ligament, and the annular ligament.

4. Medial collateral ligament (MCL, **Figure 1**)

a. The anterior bundle of the MCL is the most important stabilizer of valgus stress to the elbow.

b. In an incompetent MCL, the radial head becomes a very important secondary stabilizer to valgus instability.

c. In terrible triad injuries, excellent outcomes can be obtained without MCL repair if all articular fractures and the LCL are repaired or reconstructed. MCL repair may be performed in rare cases in which stability cannot be achieved.

B. Mechanism of injury

1. Typically, a fall on an outstretched arm with an axial force and valgus moment on a forearm in supination; the injury begins with disruption of the LCL, followed by anterior capsule disruption and possibly MCL disruption, with fractures of the radial head and coronoid.

2. Terrible triad injuries differ from anteromedial facet fractures of the coronoid, which also occur with a dislocation of the elbow. A varus deformity, posteromedially directed, creates LCL injury and fracture of the anteromedial facet of the coronoid. The radial head is preserved.

III. EVALUATION

A. History—Typically, the history reveals a fall on an outstretched arm; the dislocation can result from both high-energy and low-energy injuries.

B. Physical examination

1. Skin: Medial ecchymosis may suggest a medial-side injury.

2. Distal radioulnar joint: An Essex-Lopresti lesion must be ruled out.

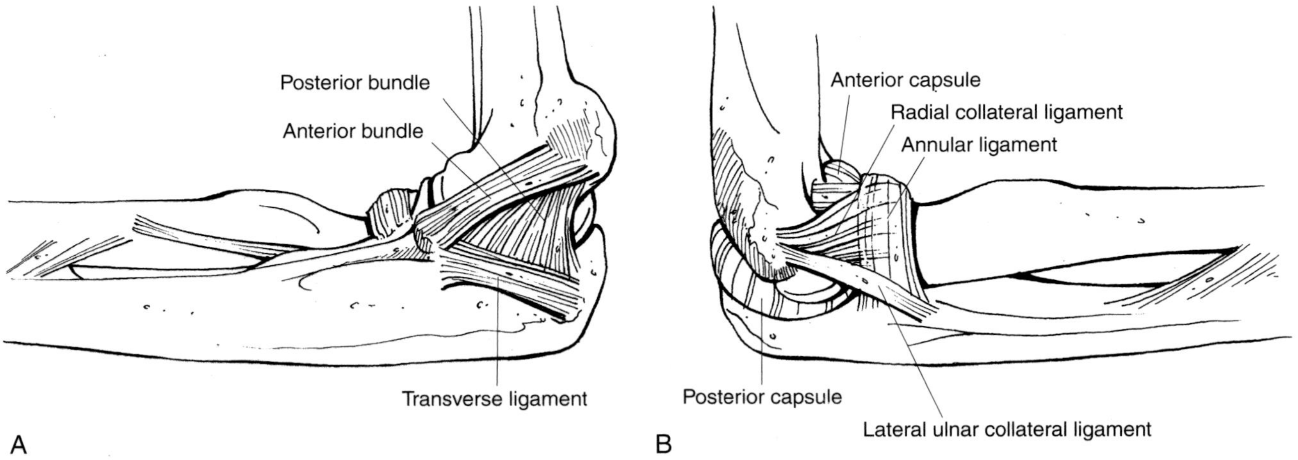

Figure 1 Illustration depicts the anatomy of the medial (**A**) and lateral (**B**) collateral ligaments of the elbow. (Reproduced from Tashjian RZ, Katarincic JA: Complex elbow instability. *J Am Acad Orthop Surg* 2006;14[5]:278-286.)

C. Imaging

1. AP and lateral radiographs of the elbow prereduction and postreduction; radiographs should be scrutinized for associated fractures of the capitellum and trochlea.
2. PA and lateral wrist and forearm radiographs when indicated.
3. Advanced imaging is obtained routinely, specifically CT with three-dimensional reconstruction to further classify the proximal radius and coronoid fractures.

IV. CLASSIFICATION

A. Classification systems have been developed for individual parts of the terrible triad, specifically the radial head and coronoid process fractures (**Figures 2** through **4**).

B. By definition, a terrible triad must include a posterolateral elbow dislocation, with fractures of the coronoid and the radial head.

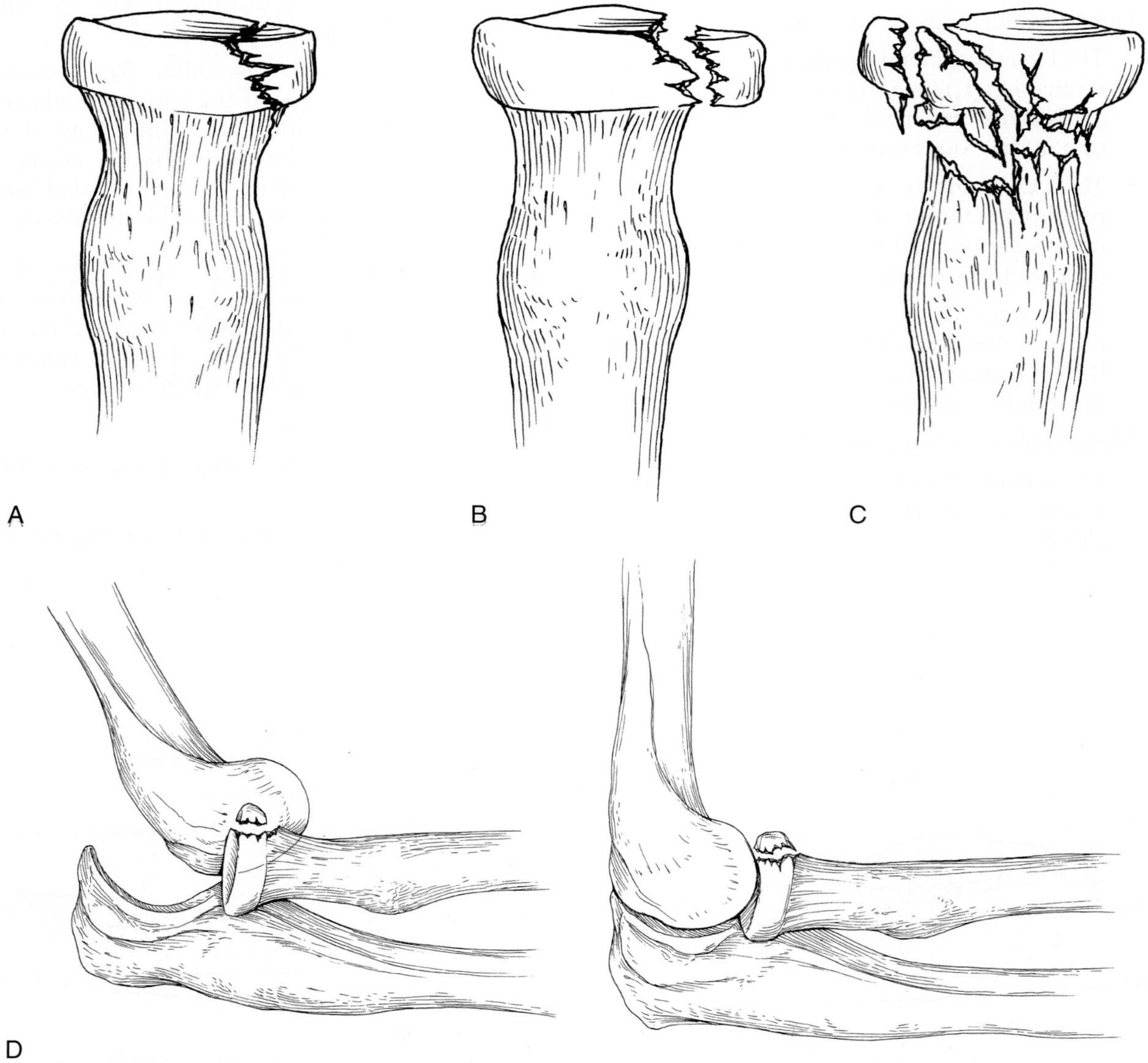

Figure 2 Illustrations demonstrate the Mason classification of radial head fractures. **A**, Type I, nondisplaced fracture. **B**, Type II, displaced partial articular fracture. **C**, Type III, comminuted fracture. **D**, A type IV injury indicating an associated ipsilateral ulnohumeral dislocation. (Reproduced from Mathew PK, Athwal GS, King GJW: Terrible triad injury of the elbow: Current concepts. *J Am Acad Orthop Surg* 2009;17[3]:137-151.)

TOP TESTING FACTS

1. Terrible triad injuries refer to complex elbow dislocations that include posterolateral elbow dislocation, a radial head or neck fracture, and a coronoid process fracture.
2. MCL repair is not required as part of a terrible triad injury repair unless persistent instability is present after coronoid fracture fixation, radial head repair or reconstruction, and LCL repair.
3. Anteromedial facet fractures of the coronoid typically are NOT associated with terrible triad injuries. The mechanism of elbow instability from an anteromedial facet injury results from a varus posteromedially directed force rather than the valgus posterolaterally directed force typically seen in a terrible triad injury.
4. Radial head fractures should be repaired or replaced unless they involve less than 25% of the articular surface and are not critical to elbow stability. The radial head should never be resected and left without replacement in a terrible triad repair.
5. Most coronoid process fractures should be repaired, with the possible exception of small tip fractures (<10% of height).
6. The LUCL ligament needs to be repaired to its isometric point, which is at the center of the capitellum, approximately 2 mm anterior to the lateral epicondyle.
7. Slight persistent ulnohumeral widening on the lateral radiograph can be monitored postoperatively.
8. Complications are very common, with over 25% of patients requiring revision surgery. The most common reasons are stiffness, heterotopic bone formation, and ulnar neuritis. Persistent instability, using contemporary fixation techniques and the surgical algorithm, is uncommon compared with that seen using historical procedures.
9. External fixation of the elbow can be used when repair of the bony injuries and the lateral and medial ligament complexes does not restore stability. This is usually an intraoperative decision based on stability during range of motion assessed fluoroscopically.
10. During rehabilitation with an intact MCL, many authors place the arm in pronation to protect the LCL repair. For a compromised MCL with a repaired LCL, the elbow should be placed in neutral rotation.

Bibliography

Chan K, MacDermid JC, Faber KJ, King GJ, Athwal GS: Can we treat select terrible triad injuries nonoperatively? *Clin Orthop Relat Res* 2014;472(7):2092-2099.

Cheung EV, Steinmann SP: Surgical approaches to the elbow. *J Am Acad Orthop Surg* 2009;17(5):325-333.

Cohen MS, Hastings H II: Rotatory instability of the elbow: The anatomy and role of the lateral stabilizers. *J Bone Joint Surg Am* 1997;79(2):225-233.

Doornberg JN, Linzel DS, Zurakowski D, Ring D: Reference points for radial head prosthesis size. *J Hand Surg Am* 2006;31(1):53-57.

Doornberg JN, Parisien R, van Duijn PJ, Ring D: Radial head arthroplasty with a modular metal spacer to treat acute traumatic elbow instability. *J Bone Joint Surg Am* 2007;89(5):1075-1080.

Doornberg JN, van Duijn J, Ring D: Coronoid fracture height in terrible-triad injuries. *J Hand Surg Am* 2006;31(5):794-797.

Egol KA, Immerman I, Paksima N, Tejwani N, Koval KJ: Fracture-dislocation of the elbow functional outcome following treatment with a standardized protocol. *Bull NYU Hosp Jt Dis* 2007;65(4):263-270.

Forthman C, Henket M, Ring DC: Elbow dislocation with intra-articular fracture: The results of operative treatment without repair of the medial collateral ligament. *J Hand Surg Am* 2007;32(8):1200-1209.

Garrigues GE, Wray WH III, Lindenhovius AL, Ring DC, Ruch DS: Fixation of the coronoid process in elbow fracture-dislocations. *J Bone Joint Surg Am* 2011;93(20):1873-1881.

Gupta A, Barei D, Khwaja A, Beingessner D: Single-staged treatment using a standardized protocol results in functional motion in the majority of patients with a terrible triad elbow injury. *Clin Orthop Relat Res* 2014;472(7):2075-2083.

Lindenhovius AL, Jupiter JB, Ring D: Comparison of acute versus subacute treatment of terrible triad injuries of the elbow. *J Hand Surg Am* 2008;33(6):920-926.

Mathew PK, Athwal GS, King GJ: Terrible triad injury of the elbow: Current concepts. *J Am Acad Orthop Surg* 2009;17(3):137-151.

McKee MD, Schemitsch EH, Sala MJ, O'driscoll SW: The pathoanatomy of lateral ligamentous disruption in complex elbow instability. *J Shoulder Elbow Surg* 2003;12(4):391-396.

Najd Mazhar F, Jafari D, Mirzaei A: Evaluation of functional outcome after nonsurgical management of terrible triad injuries of the elbow. *J Shoulder Elbow Surg* 2017;26(8):1342-1347.

Pugh DM, Wild LM, Schemitsch EH, King GJ, McKee MD: Standard surgical protocol to treat elbow dislocations with radial head and coronoid fractures. *J Bone Joint Surg Am* 2004;86-A(6):1122-1130.

Ring D, Jupiter JB, Zilberfarb J: Posterior dislocation of the elbow with fractures of the radial head and coronoid. *J Bone Joint Surg Am* 2002;84-A(4):547-551.

Schneeberger AG, Sadowski MM, Jacob HA: Coronoid process and radial head as posterolateral rotatory stabilizers of the elbow. *J Bone Joint Surg Am* 2004;86-A(5):975-982.

Shukla DR, Pillai G, McAnany S, Hausman M, Parsons BO: Heterotopic ossification formation after fracture-dislocations of the elbow. *J Shoulder Elbow Surg* 2015;24(3):333-338.

Tashjian RZ, Katarincic JA: Complex elbow instability. *J Am Acad Orthop Surg* 2006;14(5):278-286.

Zeiders GJ, Patel MK: Management of unstable elbows following complex fracture-dislocations—the "terrible triad" injury. *J Bone Joint Surg Am* 2008;90(suppl 4):75-84.

Zhang D, Tarabochia M, Janssen S, Ring D, Chen N: Risk of subluxation or dislocation after operative treatment of terrible triad injuries. *J Orthop Trauma* 2016;30(12):660-663.

Chapter 94
FOREARM TRAUMA AND DIAPHYSEAL FRACTURES

CHRISTOPHER M. McANDREW, MD, MSc

I. EPIDEMIOLOGY AND OVERVIEW

A. Of hand, wrist, and forearm fractures, 44% involve the radius and/or ulna.
   1. The most common age group affected is 5 to 14 years (34%).
   2. Fractures of the distal radius and/or ulna are more common than diaphyseal fractures.
   3. Common etiologies include falls at home (30%), highway accidents (14%), and sporting injuries (14%).

B. Nonsurgical care of the majority diaphyseal forearm fractures in adults produce poor results.
   1. The best report of closed treatment includes a loss of >50° of rotation for 30% of patients.
   2. Compression plating technique has resulted in reduced nonunion rates and better functional outcomes and is the standard of care.
   3. Treatment of adult diaphyseal fractures of the forearm with open reduction and plate fixation is considered the standard against which all other treatments are now compared.
   4. Imaging of forearm trauma and fractures generally consists of plain radiographs of the forearm, wrist, and elbow. MRI may be considered in some patterns with associated ligamentous injury, such as Essex-Lopresti and Galeazzi fractures.

II. ANATOMY AND BIOMECHANICS

A. Despite the diaphyseal nature of the central portions of the radius and ulna, the forearm is best considered a single articular unit composed of the proximal, middle, and distal radioulnar joints.

B. The axis of rotation for pronation/supination of the forearm extends from the center of the radial head through the ulnar styloid and is independent of elbow position.

C. The interosseous membrane (IOM) connects the ulna to the radius obliquely, 21° proximally to the transverse axis of the forearm (**Figure 1**).
   1. Axial load is transmitted from the distal radius to the proximal ulna via the IOM.
   2. The proportion of axial load is estimated to be 80% radius at the wrist, with an increasing amount of load borne proximally by the ulna, depending on elbow position.
   3. The central fibers are on maximal tension in neutral rotation.
   4. The distal fibers are on maximal tension in supination.

D. The radial bow accommodates pronation of the forearm.
   1. The bow is not purely in the sagittal or coronal plane.
   2. The mean maximal radial bow in the coronal plane is approximately 15 mm and is located 60% distally along the axis of the radius (**Figure 2**).
   3. Failure to restore this anatomic relationship results in loss of rotation and grip strength.
   4. Range of motion (ROM) of the forearm and wrist positively correlates with Disabilities of the Arm, Shoulder and Hand (DASH) scores following both-bone forearm fracture treatment.

III. SPECIFIC FOREARM FRACTURE TYPES

A. Isolated radial shaft fracture
   1. Defined as a radius shaft fracture with less than 5 mm of ulnar positive variance on injury radiographs.

Dr. McAndrew or an immediate family member serves as a paid consultant to or is an employee of Zimmer.

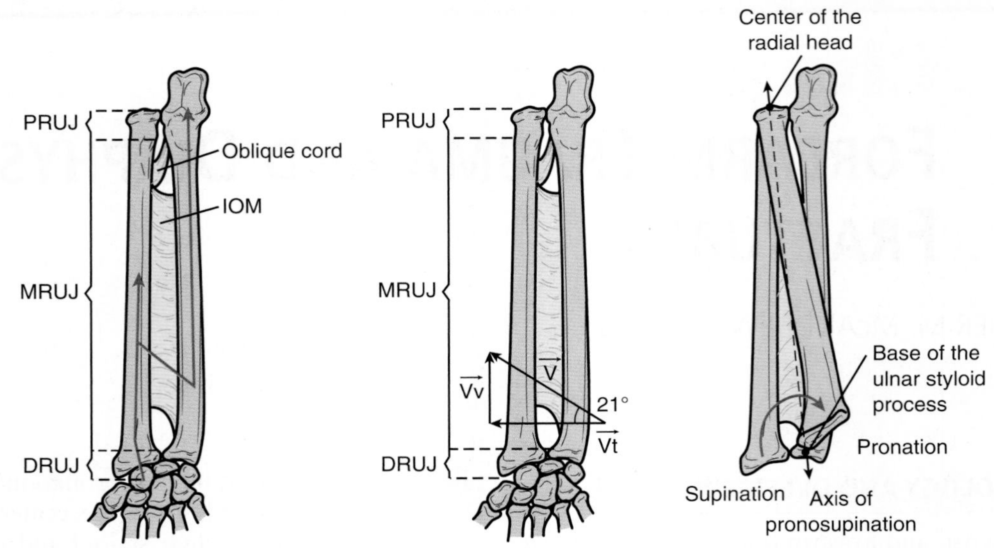
PRUJ
Oblique cord
IOM
MRUJ
DRUJ
Load transfer: radioulnar transfer through the IOM (MRUJ)
PRUJ
MRUJ
Vv
V
21°
Vt
DRUJ
The IOM stabilizes the MRUJ (V) in the vertical (Vv) and transverse (Vt) directions
Center of the radial head
Base of the ulnar styloid process
Pronation
Supination
Axis of pronosupination
The axis of rotation of the PRUJ, MRUJ and DRUJ corresponds to the axis of pronosupination: it joins the center of the radial head and the base of the ulnar styloid process

Figure 1 Illustrations show the relationship of the radius, ulna, and interosseous membrane (IOM). The orientation of the IOM transfers axial load from the distal radius to the proximal ulna. The axis of rotation of the forearm extends from the center of the radial head to the ulnar styloid. PRUJ = proximal radioulnar joint, MRUJ = middle radioulnar joint, DRUJ = distal radioulnar joint.

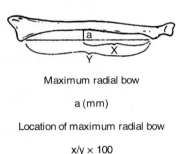

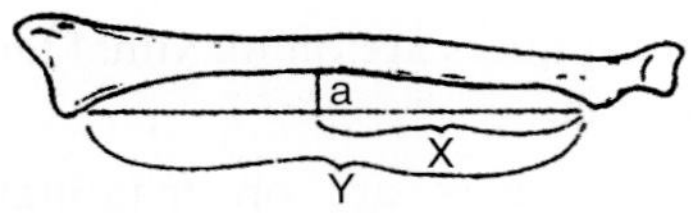
a
X
Y
Maximum radial bow
a (mm)
Location of maximum radial bow
x/y × 100

Figure 2 Illustration shows the measurement of the location and magnitude of the maximal radial bow in the coronal plane. The maximal bow measures a mean 15 mm (a) and 60% distal along the length of the radius (x/y × 100). (Reproduced with permission from Schemitsch EH, Richards RR: The effect of malunion on functional outcome after plate fixation of fractures of both bones of the forearm in adults. *J Bone Joint Surg Am* 1992;74:1068-1078.)

2. Epidemiology—Approximately three fourths of radial shaft fractures without associated ulnar shaft fracture have less than 5 mm of ulnar positive variance on injury radiographs.
3. Anatomy—Majority in the middle third of the radius.
4. Surgical approaches—The volar (Henry) or dorsal (Thompson) approach, as described in Section III.
5. Mechanism of injury—Likely, a direct blow to the radial side of the forearm without substantial rotational forces or axial load through the forearm.
6. Clinical evaluation—Includes examination of the distal neurovascular status and evaluation for compartment syndrome and associated joint injury of the elbow and wrist.
7. Radiographic evaluation—Includes orthogonal radiographs of the wrist, forearm, and elbow. If no subluxation of the elbow exists and the ulnar variance on premanipulation radiographs is less than 5 mm, the diagnosis is isolated radial shaft fracture.
8. Treatment and rehabilitation—Open reduction and internal fixation (ORIF), restoring the anatomic relationship of the radius and ulna, should be followed by early (less than 2 weeks) active ROM and no weight bearing until the fracture heals.
9. Complications—All reported complications relate to iatrogenic nerve palsy (of the PIN) and missed diagnoses of associated elbow pathology.

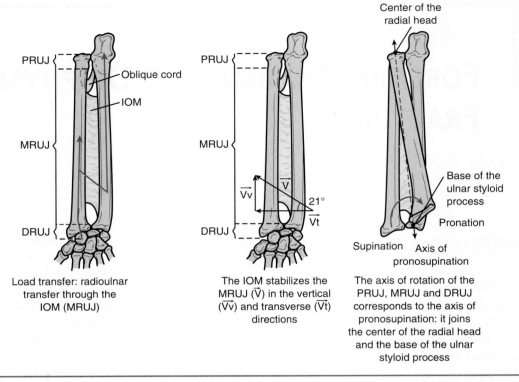

B. Galeazzi fracture

1. A radial shaft fracture associated with a distal radioulnar joint (DRUJ) injury, which may or may not include an ulnar styloid fracture.
2. Epidemiology—Approximately, one-fourth of radial shaft fractures, without ulnar shaft fracture, have an associated DRUJ injury.
3. Anatomy—More than one half of radial shaft fractures with associated DRUJ injury occur in the distal third and are associated with increased ulnar variance.
4. Surgical approaches
    a. Volar (Henry) or dorsal (Thompson) approach for internal fixation of the radius fracture, as described in Section III.
    b. Longitudinal approach over the extensor carpi ulnaris tendon sheath, with protection of the superficial transverse ulnar nerve branches, is used for reduction and fixation of displaced ulnar styloid fractures.
5. Mechanism of injury—Axial loading, usually through the outstretched hand.
6. Clinical evaluation—Includes examination of the distal neurovascular status and evaluation for compartment syndrome and associated joint injury of the elbow and wrist.
7. Radiographic evaluation—Includes evaluation of the wrist, forearm, and elbow.
8. Treatment
    a. ORIF of the radial shaft is the preferred method of treatment of this type of fracture. The DRUJ is stable in most cases after anatomic reconstruction of the radius.
    b. ORIF of the ulnar styloid through the extensor carpi ulnaris approach may be accomplished with fixation using headless screws or tension band wiring.
    c. If the DRUJ is not reduced after ORIF of the radius, the DRUJ should be explored to remove interposed soft tissues (most commonly the triangular fibrocartilage complex).
    d. Splinting of the unstable DRUJ in neutral or supinated rotation for 4 to 6 weeks is performed to treat DRUJ dislocation that is unstable in pronation after ORIF of the radius. If the DRUJ is still unstable, reduction and pinning with two Kirschner wires from the ulna to the radius in neutral is performed and maintained for 4 to 6 weeks.
9. Rehabilitation—After ORIF of the radius (and the ulnar styloid), early (less than 2 weeks) active ROM and no weight bearing is recommended until fracture healing occurs. Immobilization in a splint/cast or with pin fixation for 4 to 6 weeks is reserved only for an unstable DRUJ, with active ROM initiated immediately after splint or pin removal.
10. Complications—Usually are related to undiagnosed associated injuries to the elbow or a missed diagnosis of DRUJ instability. Long-term follow-up demonstrates equivalent subjective and objective outcomes in patients with and without DRUJ instability at the time of injury, when treated appropriately.

C. Ulnar shaft fracture

1. Historically, good results have been obtained with bracing treatment or compressive wraps and early ROM with proper patient selection (no associated injuries, "nightstick fractures").
2. Anatomy—Most are in the middle third of the ulna, but particular attention should be given to those fractures in the proximal third that have higher associations with elbow pathology (eg, Monteggia fracture-dislocations) and nonunion.
3. Surgical approach—Direct approach to the subcutaneous border between the flexor carpi ulnaris and extensor carpi ulnaris, described in Section III.C.
4. Mechanism of injury—Usually a direct blow to the ulnar forearm (defensive position); can occur with rotational stress, and these injuries (identified during the history) should alert the clinician to the possibility of associated elbow pathology.
5. Clinical evaluation—The distal neurovascular status, the soft-tissue envelope, and pain at the elbow and wrist should be evaluated. Exclusion of proximal radioulnar joint (PRUJ) injury is paramount.
6. Radiographic evaluation—Includes radiographs of the wrist, forearm, and elbow. Displacement of greater than 50% of the shaft width and angulation of greater than 10° have been associated with poor outcomes in function and nonunion and may warrant surgical treatment.
7. Treatment
    a. Nonsurgical treatment with short-term (2 weeks) immobilization followed by active ROM is recommended for minimally displaced fractures that have no evidence of wrist, elbow, or interosseous instability.

b. Surgical treatment has been advocated for fractures with more than 10° of angulation and/or greater than 50% shaft-width displacement to maximize forearm function and decrease nonunion. Special attention also should be given to proximal and extreme distal ulnar shaft fractures, which have a higher nonunion rate.

8. Rehabilitation—Early (2 weeks) active ROM should be encouraged for stable fractures with minimal displacement. Following surgical treatment, early active ROM also is encouraged (described in Section VI.)

9. Complications—When associated elbow injury is excluded, complication rates are low. Nonunion occurs in approximately 10% of cases treated nonsurgically, and appropriate patient/injury selection can reduce this rate.

D. Both-bone forearm fractures

1. The epidemiology has been described previously in Section I.A.

2. The anatomy has been described previously in Section II.

3. Surgical approaches have been described previously in Section III.

4. Mechanism of injury—High-energy transfer is required to fracture the diaphyseal section of both bones of the forearm. This commonly results from motor vehicle accidents and falls from heights onto the upper extremities, with bending moments and direct blows causing the fractures. Low-energy injuries with resulting fractures should alert the clinician to possible associated elbow and wrist pathology.

5. Clinical evaluation—Should include distal neurovascular examination, soft-tissue envelope evaluation, and exclusion of compartment syndrome. A thorough history includes handedness and employment/hobby expectations.

6. Radiographic evaluation—Includes orthogonal radiographs of the wrist, forearm, and elbow. Contralateral radiographs may assist the treating surgeon by providing a template for reconstruction.

7. Treatment is described in Section V. Surgical treatment is recommended for all both-bone forearm fractures in those older than 10 years, if the patient is able to tolerate surgery (**Figure 3**).

8. Rehabilitation is described in Section VI.

9. Outcomes

a. Mild losses in active ROM in pronation (7° less than normal), supination (9°), wrist flexion (11°), and wrist extension (5°) are expected after surgical fixation of both-bone forearm fractures with plate fixation with no complications.

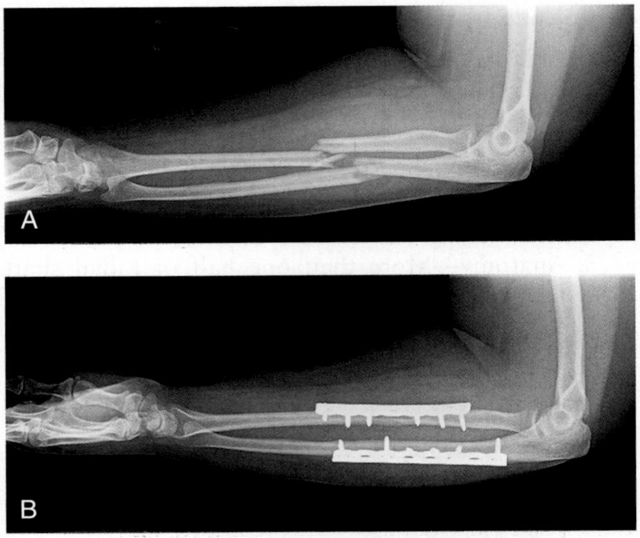

Figure 3 Preoperative (**A**) and postoperative (**B**) lateral forearm radiographs show a both-bone forearm fracture.

b. Reduced strength in pronation (70% of normal), supination (68%), wrist flexion (84%), wrist extension (63%), and grip (75%) are expected after uncomplicated surgical care of both-bone forearm fractures with plate fixation.

c. Good subjective results (average DASH scores of 12 to 18) can be achieved overall, but worse outcomes are associated with decreased ROM, strength, and pain.

d. Currently, nonunion is less than 3% overall but increases with open fracture and bone loss.

e. Malunion of the radius with failure to restore the magnitude and location of the bow to within 5% of the normal opposite side results in a 20% loss of forearm rotation and loss of grip strength.

f. Infection rates of less than 3% are reported following both-bone forearm fractures, including those open fractures treated with débridement and immediate ORIF.

g. Radioulnar synostosis was reported historically, occurring in 2% of adult forearm fractures. Risk factors include a single approach to both bones for surgical fixation, errant placement of bone graft, fractures closer to or involving the elbow, delay to surgical repair of fractures, associated head trauma, and high-energy mechanisms.

h. Rates of refracture after plate removal have ranged from 4% to 25%. An increased risk for refracture is reported with early (<1 year) removal of plates, use of large fragment (4.5-mm) screws, and delayed union.

E. Longitudinal radioulnar dissociation (Essex-Lopresti lesion)

1. Most commonly associated with radial head fracture, which allows proximal migration to occur if excision or inadequate reconstruction is performed.

2. Proximal migration of the radius results in dorsal displacement of the ulna distally, limiting forearm supination and wrist extension.

3. Recognition of the acute injury and treatment are paramount for optimal function because late reconstruction procedures result in limited success.

a. Restoration of radial length with anatomic reduction or reconstruction/arthroplasty is the first step to successful treatment.

b. Stabilization of the DRUJ in supination, possibly with pin fixation, is used if necessary.

IV. SURGICAL APPROACHES FOR FIXATION OF DIAPHYSEAL FRACTURES OF THE RADIUS AND ULNA

A. The volar approach to the radius (Henry approach) is most commonly used.

1. The skin incision is longitudinal from lateral to the biceps tendon to the radial styloid, with the length dictated by the necessary exposure of the radius.

2. The lateral antebrachial cutaneous nerve lies in the subcutaneous fat, paralleling the cephalic vein and running along the border of the brachioradialis.

3. The internervous plane between the brachioradialis (radial nerve) and pronator teres/flexor carpi radialis (median nerve) is used.

4. The radial artery is located deep to the brachioradialis proximally, and its radial branches are ligated to allow ulnar retraction.

5. The superficial radial nerve is located deep to the brachioradialis proximally and is gently retracted radially with the muscle.

6. Proximally, the radius is exposed lateral/radial to the biceps insertion (the radial artery is medial/ulnar to the tendon).

a. With the forearm in full supination, the insertion of the supinator muscle is identified and released.

b. Subperiosteal dissection from ulnar to radial protects the posterior interosseous nerve (PIN) within the supinator muscle.

7. In the middle third of the forearm, slight pronation exposes the insertion of the pronator teres muscle. Subperiosteal release of the pronator teres and flexor digitorum superficialis from radial to ulnar exposes the radius shaft.

8. Distally, the pronator quadratus and flexor pollicis longus are released from their radial origins ulnarly, exposing the distal radius. Distally, the superficial radial nerve lies between the brachioradialis and extensor carpi radialis longus tendons, becoming superficial 9 cm proximal to the radial styloid.

B. The dorsal approach to the radius (Thompson approach) also can be used.

1. The skin incision is longitudinal from the lateral epicondyle to the ulnar side of the Lister tubercle, with the length dictated by the necessary exposure of the radius.

2. The internervous plane between the extensor carpi radialis brevis (radial nerve location) and the extensor digitorum communis/extensor pollicis longus (PIN location) is used.

3. Proximally, the PIN must be identified and protected within the supinator.

a. The PIN can be found distal to the radiocapitellar joint after it pierces the supinator at a distance of 3.2 cm in supination, 4.2 cm in neutral, and 5.6 cm in pronation (**Figure 4**).

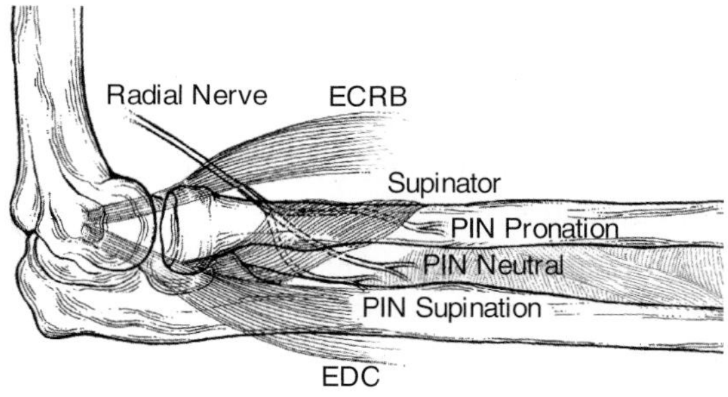

Figure 4 Illustration shows the relationship of the posterior interosseous nerve (PIN) to the radiocapitellar joint. With an intact radius, the distance from the radiocapitellar joint to the midaxial position of the PIN changes in supination (3.2 cm), neutral (4.2 cm), and pronation (5.6 cm). EDC = extensor digitorum communis tendon, ECRB = extensor carpi radialis brevis tendon. (Reproduced with permission from Calfee RP, Wilson JM, Wong AH: Variations in the anatomic relations of the posterior interosseous nerve associated with proximal forearm trauma. *J Bone Joint Surg Am* 2011;93[1]:81-90.)

7 | Trauma

b. Fracture or osteotomy reduces the effect of forearm pronation, and the PIN is found closer to the radiocapitellar joint in these situations.

4. The abductor pollicis longus and extensor pollicis brevis can be retracted distally (middle third) or proximally (distal third) to expose the radius.

C. Exposure of the ulna is performed along the subcutaneous border.

1. The interval between the extensor carpi ulnaris (PIN) and the flexor carpi ulnaris (ulnar nerve) is used.

2. The ulnar nerve and artery are volar to the flexor carpi ulnaris muscle and are placed at risk if this muscle is not carefully dissected directly off the ulna.

3. The dorsal cutaneous branch of the ulnar nerve extends from the ulnar nerve 6.4 cm from the distal end of the ulna and becomes subcutaneous 5.0 cm from the proximal edge of the pisiform.

V. SURGICAL PRINCIPLES OF DIAPHYSEAL FRACTURES OF THE RADIUS AND ULNA

A. ORIF with interfragmentary compression is the preferred method of treatment and the standard against which other approaches are compared.

1. Interfragmentary screw application with neutralization plating is appropriate for spiral and oblique fractures.

2. Compression plating with (oblique, **Figure 5**) or without (transverse) interfragmentary screw compression through the plate also can be used.

3. If the fracture is comminuted such that interfragmentary compression is not feasible, a bridge plating technique, with attention to reconstruction of the overall length, alignment, and rotation, is used (**Figure 6**). Contralateral radiographs of the uninjured elbow, forearm, and wrist are used as a template.

B. Intramedullary fixation has been studied in small case series and can produce comparable results in union rates and ROM.

1. The ulna is fixed antegrade, with an entry point in the olecranon process.

2. The radius is fixed retrograde, with an entry point just ulnar to the Lister tubercle.

C. External fixation may be used temporarily in emergent situations or if soft-tissue compromise prevents safe ORIF. Safe half-pin fixation can be applied through the subcutaneous border of the ulna and the dorsal/radial border of the radius, with blunt dissection and retraction to protect soft-tissue structures.

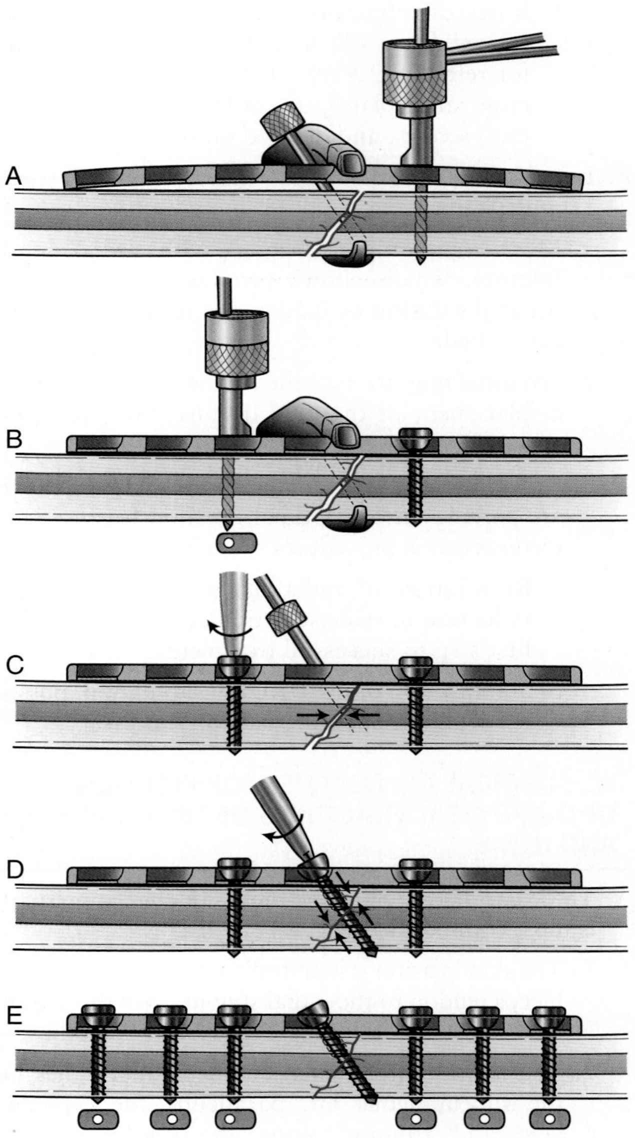

Figure 5 Illustrations demonstrate compression plate application using a dynamic compression plate. **A**, A plate with a slight concave bend is fixed to the fracture fragment to allow creation of an acute angle at the bone-plate interface (axilla). **B**, An eccentrically drilled (away from the fracture) hole is placed through the plate into the other fracture fragment, and compression at the fracture is achieved as the screw head articulates with the beveled surface of the plate hole. **C**, An overdrilled pilot hole is created perpendicular to the fracture, and the core diameter drill bit is placed through a drill sleeve inserted into the pilot hole to drill the far cortex in the same orientation. **D**, The interfragmentary screw is applied. **E**, Plate fixation is completed in both fracture fragments.

Nonsurgical care of adult both-bone forearm fractures is reserved only for patients whose comorbid conditions prevent safe surgical and anesthetic care.

3. Treatment
   a. Good joint alignment helps maintain mobility of the fourth and fifth CMC joints.
   b. Small marginal fractures (of the metacarpal or carpus) with no impaction are treated with closed reduction using longitudinal traction and K-wire fixation.
   c. More comminuted fractures may benefit from temporary external fixation or bridging plate fixation. Open reduction and internal fixation with disimpaction of articular surfaces and autogenous bone grafting can be considered.
   d. In patients with posttraumatic arthritis, arthrodesis is considered.

E. Fractures of the metacarpal head
   1. Evaluation—A Brewerton view (20° of MCP flexion) or CT scan may assist with visualization.
   2. Surgical treatment—A dorsal approach is preferred.

F. Fractures of the thumb metacarpal
   1. Extra-articular fractures
      a. Up to 30° of angulation is acceptable because of the mobility of the saddle joint.
      b. Fixation is usually accomplished with a percutaneous K-wire.
   2. Bennett fracture—Base of the first metacarpal fracture (**Figure 1**)
      a. Pathoanatomy—The volar oblique ligament is attached to the volar ulnar fragment of the base; the abductor pollicis longus displaces the distal metacarpal proximally, and the adductor pollicis displaces the metacarpal into adduction. The metacarpal base is displaced dorsally and rotated into supination.
      b. Evaluation—The fracture is best visualized on the true lateral and hyperpronated AP (Robert) views.
      c. Treatment
         - Closed reduction can be obtained with longitudinal traction and extension/abduction/pronation of the metacarpal, as well as ulnarward pressure on the base of the metacarpal. The reduction is stabilized with a percutaneous K-wire fixation from the thumb metacarpal into the trapezium and another wire joining the thumb and index metacarpals.
         - Open reduction is indicated if more than 2 to 3 mm of articular incongruity is present after closed reduction or notable central articular impaction.

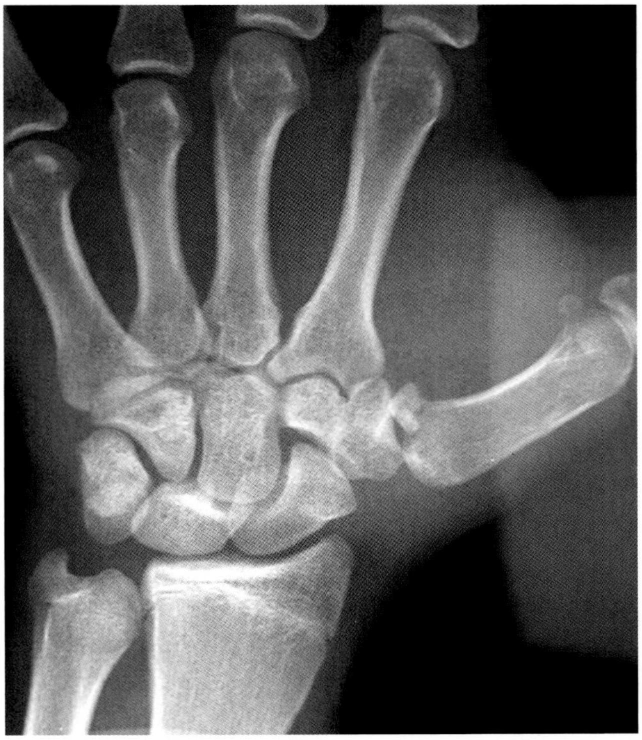

Figure 1 PA radiograph of the hand of an adolescent demonstrates a Bennett fracture.

   3. Rolando fracture
      a. Rolando fracture refers generally to more complex articular fractures of the base of the thumb metacarpal, although it is often described as specific to three-part Y or T intra-articular fractures (**Figure 2**).
      b. Treatment
         - ORIF with a plate and screws is possible for some simple fractures.
         - Alternative treatment includes external fixator and K-wires or an external traction device.
         - Bone graft may be helpful if realignment creates bone defects.

III. METACARPOPHALANGEAL DISLOCATIONS

A. Dorsal MCP dislocations—The most frequently involved digit is the index finger.

B. Simple dislocation (subluxation)
   1. Simple dislocations can be inadvertently converted to complex dislocation (interposed volar plate) during reduction.

7 | Trauma

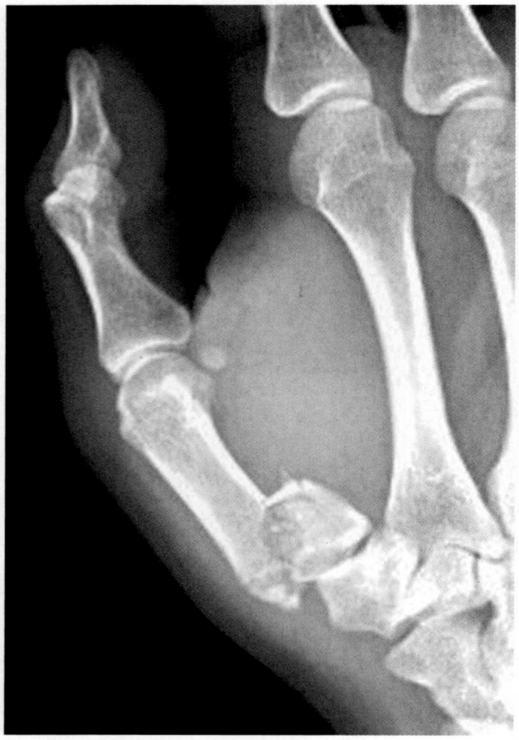

Figure 2 Oblique radiograph of a complete articular fracture of the base of the thumb metacarpal (eponym Rolando).

2. Traction and hyperextension *should not* be used to reduce MCP dislocations.
   a. Instead, the wrist and finger is flexed to take tension off the flexor tendons, and the base of the proximal phalanx is pushed volarly and distally to slide the displaced volar plate over the metacarpal head.
   b. To reduce thumb MCP dorsal dislocations, the interphalangeal joint of the thumb and the wrist are flexed while the proximal phalanx is pushed volarly.

C. Complex/irreducible dislocation
1. Evaluation—The patient presents with the digit held in slight extension and a prominence in the palm.
2. Pathoanatomy—The key aspect is the interposed volar plate. The flexor tendon, lumbrical, and A1 pulley also wrap around the metacarpal head, but this rarely prevents reduction.
3. Treatment
   a. A volar approach puts the digital nerves at risk of injury because they are displaced into a subcutaneous position by the metacarpal head.
   b. Dorsal approach—A longitudinal incision is made and the proximal part of the sagittal band is divided on the ulnar side. The joint capsule is divided if needed for better joint exposure. The volar plate is attached to the proximal phalanx and covers the metacarpal head, blocking closed reduction. To reduce the joint, the volar plate is split longitudinally. A Freer elevator is then used to push the volar plate palmarly.

IV. FRACTURES OF THE PROXIMAL AND MIDDLE PHALANX

A. Anatomy and biomechanics
1. Proximal phalanx
   a. Most transverse proximal phalanx fractures are apex palmar.
   b. The central extensor tendon pulls the distal fragment dorsal, and the interossei insertion flexes the proximal fragment.
   c. Proximal phalanx fractures have less stability than metacarpal fractures because they are not supported by adjacent bones as are the metacarpals. In addition, multiple tendon forces act on the fragments.
   d. Authors of cadaver studies estimate that shortening of the proximal phalanx produces an extensor lag at the proximal interphalangeal (PIP) joint, with each millimeter of bone loss equaling 12° of extensor lag, but the actual imbalance is more variable and multifactorial.
2. Fractures of the middle phalanx
   a. The angulation depends on the fracture position.
   b. Proximal middle phalanx fractures are apex dorsal because of the pull of the central slip.
   c. Distal middle phalanx fractures displace palmarly as a result of the pull of the superficialis insertion.
   d. Shortening of the middle phalanx following fracture may result in distal interphalangeal (DIP) joint extension lag.

B. Specific fractures
1. Fractures of the proximal phalanx base—Extra-articular base fracture
   a. Most proximal phalanx base fractures are unstable because of dorsal metaphyseal impaction.
   b. Closed reduction and cast immobilization can be attempted with stable fractures, and the MCP joint should be flexed >60°.

c. Nonsurgical treatment of unstable fractures is an option. It leads to residual deformity with good hand function.

d. Multiple options exist for better alignment with K-wire fixation; however, all risk tendon adhesions and stiffness.

e. With complex trauma, including flexor tendon laceration, internal fixation with a mini condylar plate may enable early mobilization.

2. Fractures of the diaphysis of the proximal and middle phalanges

a. The angulation is usually apex volar as a result of the pull of the central slip and lateral bands.

b. Treatment—The type of fracture determines the treatment.

3. Fractures of the neck of the proximal and middle phalanges

a. Epidemiology and pathoanatomy

- These fractures are uncommon in adults.
- In children, phalangeal neck fractures may displace and rotate 90° (apex dorsally).
- With complete displacement, the volar plate may become entrapped in the fracture.

b. Treatment—Closed reduction and a percutaneous K-wire

4. Condylar fractures of the proximal and middle phalanx

a. Angulation and malrotation are evaluated.

b. Treatment

- Displaced condylar fractures require reduction and fixation, which is sometimes possible to achieve percutaneously.
- If open reduction is necessary, screw fixation is attempted.
- The PIP joint can be exposed by incising between the lateral band and the central tendon or through a midaxial incision opening the capsule above the collateral ligament.

V. PROXIMAL INTERPHALANGEAL JOINT DISLOCATIONS AND FRACTURE-DISLOCATIONS

A. Epidemiology

1. Dorsal—These are the most common form of PIP joint dislocations. They are often associated with volar plate avulsion or fracture of the volar base of the middle phalanx.

2. Lateral—Sometimes associated with interposition of the collateral ligament.

3. Volar—Can be associated with injury to the central tendon.

B. Dorsal PIP joint dislocations and fracture-dislocations

1. Anatomy

a. The accessory collateral ligaments insert onto the volar plate.

b. The proper collateral ligaments insert onto the condyles.

c. Fracture-dislocations involving >40% of the volar base of the joint surface are unstable.

d. Boutonniere deformity involves compensatory hyperextension of the DIP joint (and an inability to flex the DIP joint actively) due to tightness in the lateral bands attempting to compensate for an inadequate central slip.

2. Treatment of PIP joint dislocations

a. Most dorsal PIP joint dislocations are stable after closed reduction under digital block, even if a small volar plate avulsion fracture exists.

b. The major risk is stiffness of the PIP joint. Treatment consists of immediate mobilization (with buddy straps for comfort as preferred) and stretching to maintain motion.

c. Swelling improves for 1 year and is partially permanent. Stiffness and soreness can last for months and are particularly noticeable first thing in the morning.

d. The unusual volar PIP dislocation should be evaluated for central slip injury and treated with extension splinting of the PIP joint for 4 to 6 weeks.

e. Incomplete reduction and collateral ligament instability can be a result of interposition of the collateral ligament or other soft-tissue structures and are treated with open reduction.

3. Treatment of dorsal fracture-dislocations

a. Stable—Dorsal extension block splint with the joint in 60° to 70° of flexion, decreasing flexion weekly over 2 to 3 weeks

b. Unstable—Treatment options include the following:

- Extension block pinning
- ORIF

- Volar plate arthroplasty (currently out of favor)
- Dynamic digital traction using force-couple splint fixation
- Hemihamate arthroplasty

VI. THUMB METACARPOPHALANGEAL LIGAMENT INJURIES AND DISLOCATIONS

A. Ulnar collateral ligament (UCL) disruption (gamekeeper's thumb or skier's thumb)

1. Pathoanatomy
   a. The UCL ruptures off the base of the proximal phalanx.
   b. The avulsed ligament, with or without a bony fragment, can become displaced above the adductor aponeurosis, preventing healing (the so-called Stener lesion).
2. Treatment
   a. Tears of the UCL of the thumb MCP joint without a Stener lesion are believed to heal with 4 to 6 weeks of immobilization.
   b. Injuries that are unstable (difficult to define, but usually 30° more opening with radial stress than the opposite uninjured side) are believed to have Stener lesions and are treated surgically.

B. Radial collateral ligament (RCL) disruption

1. Pathoanatomy
   a. The RCL ruptures from its origin, from its insertion, or at the midsubstance.
   b. RCL ruptures are frequently associated with dorsal or dorsoradial capsular tears and with extensor pollicis brevis avulsions or tears.
   c. No equivalent of the Stener lesion exists, but RCL ruptures seem susceptible to chronic instability.
2. Treatment—The optimal treatment is unclear; percutaneous K-wire immobilization with or without open repair are options.

C. MCP dislocation

1. Pathoanatomy—Both collateral ligaments and the volar plate are injured, but no Stener lesion is present, and healing of the ligaments is predictable.
2. Treatment—Reduction and 3 to 4 weeks of immobilization

7 | Trauma

VII. FRACTURES OF THE DISTAL PHALANX

A. Types of fractures

1. Tuft
2. Diaphyseal
3. Volar (profundus tendon avulsion)
4. Dorsal (mallet finger)
5. Epiphyseal injury (Seymour fracture)

B. Tuft fractures

1. Closed tuft fractures are treated symptomatically. The roles of decompression of a subungual hematoma and nail bed repair are debated.
2. Open tuft fractures are usually treated with simple irrigation, débridement, and suturing in the emergency department.

C. Displaced unstable transverse distal phalanx fractures and flexor profundus avulsion fractures may best be treated with reduction and K-wire fixation.

D. Epiphyseal fractures (Seymour fracture)

1. Open epiphyseal fractures occur in children (typical mechanism: finger caught in car door).
2. The fracture results in nail matrix disruption. The plate may be avulsed lying dorsal to the proximal nail fold. The nail bed also may become interposed in fracture, resulting in nonunion or osteomyelitis.

E. Mallet fracture—Indications for ORIF of mallet fractures

1. Subluxation of the distal phalanx (volar subluxation seen with dorsal articular fracture fragment)
2. Indications with some debate
   a. Articular fragment >40%
   b. Gap in articular surface >2 mm

F. Profondus tendon avulsions are treated with ORIF when the fracture is large, and tendon advancement and reattachment when the fragment is small.

TOP TESTING FACTS

1. Lag screws can be used without a plate when fracture length is at least twice the bone diameter.
2. Closed reduction and percutaneous pinning is favored for most closed, isolated fractures that can be adequately reduced. ORIF is generally reserved for fractures with associated soft-tissue injury or unstable articular fractures.
3. For metacarpal fractures, angular deformity is better tolerated at the neck than at the diaphyseal level and in the little and ring fingers compared with the index and long fingers.
4. The main deforming force for a little finger CMC fracture-dislocation is the extensor carpi ulnaris tendon.
5. Bennett fractures are best viewed on the Robert (hyperpronated) view.
6. The main deforming force in a thumb trapeziometacarpal fracture-dislocation (Bennett fracture) is provided by the abductor pollicis longus and the adductor pollicis longus.
7. In complex MCP dislocations, the volar plate remains attached to the proximal phalanx, becomes interposed between the metacarpal head and proximal phalanx, and prevents closed reduction.
8. The major risk of dorsal PIP joint dislocation is stiffness.
9. Dorsal PIP joint dislocations can usually be treated nonsurgically if the fracture of the volar base of the middle phalanx comprises less than 40% of the articular surface.

Bibliography

Caggiano NM, Harper CM, Rozental TD: Management of proximal interphalangeal joint fracture dislocations. *Hand Clin* 2018;34(2):149-165. doi:10.1016/j.hcl.2017.12.005. Review. PubMed PMID:29625635.

Lin JS, Samora JB: Surgical and nonsurgical management of mallet finger: A systematic review. *J Hand Surg Am* 2018;43(2):146-163.e2. doi:10.1016/j.jhsa.2017.10.004. Epub 2017 November 22. Review. PubMed PMID:29174096.

Liverneaux PA, Ichihara S, Hendriks S, Facca S, Bodin F: Fractures and dislocation of the base of the thumb metacarpal. *J Hand Surg Eur Vol* 2015;40(1):42-50. doi:10.1177/1753193414554357. Epub 2014 October 13. Review. PubMed PMID:25311936.

Salazar Botero S, Hidalgo Diaz JJ, Benaïda A, Collon S, Facca S, Liverneaux PA. Review of acute traumatic closed mallet finger injuries in adults. *Arch Plast Surg* 2016;43(2):134-144. doi:10.5999/aps.2016.43.2.134. Epub 2016 March 18. Review. PubMed PMID:27019806; PubMed Central PMCID:PMC4807168.

Wong VW, Higgins JP. Evidence-based medicine: Management of metacarpal fractures. *Plast Reconstr Surg* 2017;140(1):140e-151e. doi:10.1097/PRS.0000000000003470. Review. PubMed PMID:28654615.

Chapter 96
Wrist Fractures and Dislocations, Carpal Dissociation, and Distal Radius Fractures

DAVID C. RING, MD, PhD
STEVEN L. MORAN, MD
MARCO RIZZO, MD
ALEXANDER Y. SHIN, MD

7 | Trauma

I. CARPAL FRACTURES

A. Scaphoid fractures

1. Epidemiology—The scaphoid is the most frequently fractured carpal bone.
2. Anatomy
   a. More than one half of the bone is covered by articular cartilage.
   b. The blood supply to the scaphoid is limited. Proximal pole fracture fragments receive a limited blood supply from the scapholunate ligament and radioscapholunate ligament.
3. Evaluation
   a. Physical examination—The following findings are suggestive of a scaphoid fracture:
      - Tenderness of the scaphoid in the anatomic snuffbox
      - Pain with axial compression of the first metacarpal
      - Tenderness at the scaphoid tuberosity
   b. Imaging
      - Radiographs (PA in neutral and with the wrist in ulnar deviation [scaphoid view], lateral, and semisupinated and semipronated oblique) may initially appear normal.
      - Suspected scaphoid fracture. When there is tenderness of the scaphoid but the initial radiographs are normal (a suspected scaphoid fracture), the extremity can be splinted or casted, and one of the following options is then chosen. There is no consensus on the best management strategy for suspected scaphoid fractures.
        - MRI, CT, or bone scan either immediately or within a few days. Bone scans must be delayed a few days to allow for increased metabolic activity.
        - Repeat examination and radiographs 2 weeks later, with more sophisticated imaging used only for patients in whom scaphoid fracture is still suspected.
      - Diagnosis of displacement
        - On radiographs: More than 1 mm displacement or translation of the fracture;

Dr. Ring or an immediate family member has received royalties from Skeletal Dynamics and Wright Medical Technology, Inc. and serves as a board member, owner, officer, or committee member of the American Academy of Orthopaedic Surgeons and the Orthopaedic Trauma Association. Dr. Moran or an immediate family member has received royalties from Integra; serves as a paid consultant to or is an employee of Integra; and serves as a board member, owner, officer, or committee member of the American Board of Plastic Surgery. Dr. Rizzo or an immediate family member serves as a paid consultant to or is an employee of Zimmer; serves as an unpaid consultant to Synthes; and serves as a board member, owner, officer, or committee member of the American Association for Hand Surgery. Dr. Shin or an immediate family member has received royalties from Mayo Medical Ventures and Trimed.

more than 15° of dorsal angulation of the lunate

- On CT scans: Any gap, translation, or angulation

4. Treatment

   a. Nonsurgical

   - Nondisplaced scaphoid waist fractures—verification using CT should be considered; can be treated with cast immobilization.
   - Inclusion of the thumb and the elbow in the cast are debated.
   - The duration of cast immobilization is also debated—8 to 10 weeks is standard.
   - Distal scaphoid tubercle fractures can be treated symptomatically (ie, splint, ice, medication).

   b. Surgical

   - Displaced fractures merit surgery because the rate of nonunion is 50%. Scaphoid fractures associated with perilunate fracture-dislocations should also be repaired. Proximal pole fractures are increasingly considered for surgical treatment, even when they are nondisplaced.
   - The surgical exposure can be dorsal, volar, or arthroscopic assisted.
   - Internal fixation is usually performed with a single screw, typically one that has no head and generates compression via differential pitch in the screw threads.

B. Triquetral avulsion fractures

1. These injuries are considered wrist sprains and are treated symptomatically.
2. Stretching exercises help limit the potential for wrist stiffness.

C. Capitate fractures

1. Like the scaphoid bone, the capitate is covered mainly by cartilage. The blood supply is tenuous and can be compromised by transverse fractures.
2. Scaphocapitate syndrome refers to a greater arc injury pattern in which force passes from the scaphoid to the capitate neck, resulting in both scaphoid and capitate fractures. In this syndrome, the capitate head may be rotated 180°, requiring open reduction and internal fixation (ORIF) through a dorsal approach.

D. Hamate fractures

1. Fracture-dislocation of the ring and little metacarpal joints often result in fracture of the hamate.
   a. There is a shearing fracture of the dorsal part of the hamate with or without central articular impaction.
   b. Small fractures without articular impaction can be treated with closed reduction of the carpometacarpal joint and 4 weeks of Kirschner wire (K-wire) immobilization.
   c. Larger fractures and fractures with articular impaction are treated with open reduction and screw fixation.
2. Fracture of the hook of the hamate usually results from a direct blow from a golf club, baseball bat, or racket.
   a. Most hamate hook fractures are diagnosed months after injury as a nonunion causing tenderness with direct pressure.
   b. Acute fractures tend to heal, but often go undiagnosed.
   c. Surgery is elective and usually consists of excision of the hook of the hamate.

II. CARPAL LIGAMENT INJURY AND PERILUNATE DISLOCATION

A. Anatomy and biomechanics

1. The scapholunate interosseous ligament (SLIL) is the primary stabilizer of the scapholunate joint. It is composed of three distinct portions:
   a. The proximal or membranous portion, which has no significant strength
   b. The dorsal portion, which is the strongest portion and prevents translation
   c. The palmar portion, which acts as a rotational constraint
2. Distal scaphoid stabilizers include the scaphotrapezial interosseous ligaments (STIL).
3. The radioscapholunate ligament (ligament of Testut) is a volar intra-articular neurovascular structure and provides little mechanical stability.
4. The palmar stabilizers include the radioscaphocapitate ligament, long radiolunate ligament, and short radiolunate ligament. These ligaments are all thought to be secondary stabilizers of the scaphoid.

TABLE 1

Stages of Progressive Perilunate Instability and Reverse Perilunate Instability

Mayfield's Stages of Progressive Perilunate Instability	
Stage	**Characteristics**
I	Scapholunate dissociation or scaphoid fracture
II	Capitolunate dislocation
III	Lunotriquetral dissociation or triquetral fracture
IV	Lunate dislocation
Stages of Reverse perilunate instability	
Stage	**Characteristics**
I	Lunotriquetral dissociation
II	Capitolunate dislocation
III	Scapholunate dissociation

TABLE 2

Intercarpal Angles and Distances

Parameter	Mean Value	Abnormal Value/ Significance
Scapholunate angle	46°	<30° or >60°
Radiolunate angle	0°	>15° dorsal suggests DISI deformity. >15° palmar suggests VISI deformity.
Capitolunate angle	0° (range, 30° dorsal to 30° palmar)	>30° in either volar or dorsal direction
Intercarpal distance		>2 mm between the scaphoid and lunate Increased distance, or diastasis, between the scaphoid and lunate or lunate and triquetrum may indicate an SLIL or LTIL injury.

DISI = dorsal intercalated segmental instability, LTIL = lunotriquetral interosseous ligament, SLIL = scapholunate interosseous ligament, VISI = volar intercalated segmental instability

5. The dorsal stabilizers are the dorsal radiocarpal ligament and the dorsal intercarpal ligament.

B. Pathomechanics (**Table 1**)

1. Mayfield described the four classic stages of progressive perilunate instability of the wrist, starting with scapholunate ligament disruption.
2. Reverse perilunate instability is a spectrum that might include isolated lunotriquetral (LT) ligament injury.

C. Evaluation

1. Imaging

a. Radiographic abnormalities (**Table 2**)

- Dorsal tilt of the lunate greater than 15° on a true lateral radiograph.
- Volar tilt of the lunate on the lateral radiograph is highly variable and should be compared with the contralateral uninjured side.
- A gap of 4 mm or greater between the scaphoid and lunate on the PA view (sometimes with clenching of the hand or ulnar or radial deviation of the wrist) suggests scapholunate ligament injury.
- Ulnar translocation means the carpus is displaced ulnarward (>50% of the lunate lies ulnar to the lunate fossa).
- It can be very difficult to distinguish acute injuries from newly discovered old injuries. Radiographs with slight radioscaphoid arthritis (osteophyte or "beaking" of the radial styloid) represent old injuries. This is the earliest stage of the type of arthritis that occurs with the scapholunate ligament injury known as scapholunate advanced collapse (SLAC). Later stages of SLAC are scaphocapitate and capitolunate arthritis.
- Carpal arcs of Gilula—Gilula described three parallel arcs observed on PA radiographs. The first arc corresponds to the proximal articular surface of the proximal row, the second arc corresponds to the distal articular surface of the proximal row, and the third arc represents the proximal articular surface of the distal carpal row. Disruption of one of these arcs suggests a carpal fracture or ligamentous injury (**Figure 1**).
- Carpal height ratio—This ratio is calculated by dividing the carpal height by the length of the third metacarpal. The normal ratio is 0.54 ± 0.03. In disease processes such as scapholunate dissociation, SLAC, and Kienböck disease, collapse of the midcarpal joint produces a reduction in this ratio.

b. MRI and arthroscopy

- The roles of MRI and MRI with gadolinium arthrography are debated.
- Arthroscopy is considered the reference standard for the diagnosis of intercarpal ligament injuries.

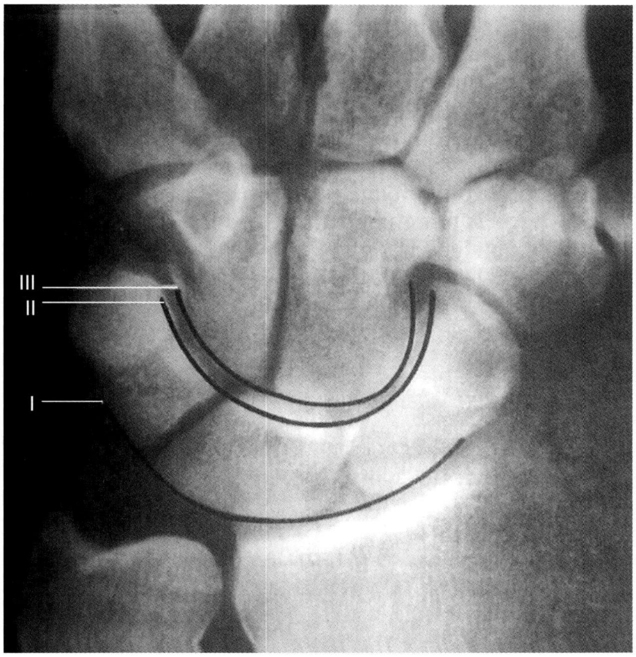

Figure 1 PA radiograph shows the carpal arcs of Gilula. I, smooth arc outlines the proximal surfaces of the scaphoid, lunate, and triquetrum. II, smooth arc outlines the distal surfaces of the scaphoid, lunate, and triquetrum. III, arc outlines the proximal surfaces of the capitate and hamate. (Reproduced from Blazar PE, Lawton JN: Diagnosis of acute carpal ligament injuries, in Trumble TE, ed: *Carpal Fracture-Dislocations*. Rosemont, IL, American Academy of Orthopaedic Surgeons, 2001, p 24.)

- The most common intercarpal ligament injury is disruption of the scapholunate interosseous ligament, which can be classified based on arthroscopic examination (**Table 3**).

D. Scapholunate (SL) ligament injuries

1. Epidemiology—SL ligament injuries are the most common form of interosseous carpal injury.
2. Pathomechanics
   a. Unopposed extension forces on the lunate imparted by the triquetrum, leading to dorsal intercalated segmental instability (DISI)
   b. Abnormal scaphoid motion and dorsal subluxation of the scaphoid from the radial fossa during wrist flexion, leading to SLAC wrist arthritis (**Figure 2**)
3. Evaluation
   a. Physical examination
      - Positive scaphoid shift test—The wrist is moved from ulnar to radial deviation. With the examiner's thumb pressing against the scaphoid tubercle, this maneuver will produce pain or a clunk, depending on the degree of instability.
      - This maneuver should be compared with the contralateral uninvolved wrist. Only

TABLE 3

Stages of Scapholunate Instability

Stage	Pathoanatomy	Findings
Predynamic instability	Partial tear or attenuation of SLIL	Radiographs normal
Dynamic instability	Partial or complete tear of SLIL	Stress radiographs abnormal Arthroscopy abnormal (Geissler type II or III)
Static instability	Early: Complete SLIL tear with attenuation or attrition of supporting wrist ligaments Late: Lunate extends as a result of its sagittal plane shape and the unopposed extension force of the intact LT interosseous ligament and becomes fixed in dorsiflexion	Early: Radiographs positive for scaphoid changes; scapholunate gap >3 mm, Scapholunate angle >60° Arthroscopy abnormal (Geissler type IV) Late: Lateral radiograph shows DISI deformity (radiolunate angle >15°)
SLAC wrist	With long-standing abnormal positioning of the carpal bones, arthritic changes occur. Arthritic changes are first seen at the styloscaphoid and radioscaphoid joints and move to the midcarpal joint in a standard progression	1. Stage 1: Arthritis noted at radial styloid 2. Stage 2: Arthritis noted at radiocarpal joint 3. Stage 3: Arthritis noted at capitolunate interface

DISI = dorsal intercalated segmental instability; LT = lunotriquetral; SLAC = scapholunate advanced collapse; SLIL = scapholunate interosseous ligament

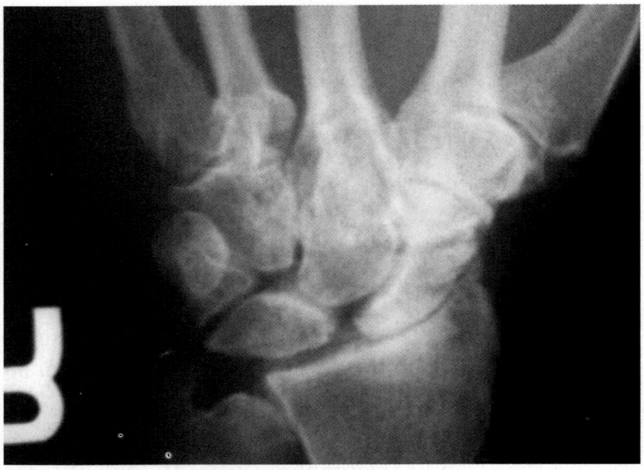

Figure 2 PA radiograph shows a patient with a scapholunate advanced collapse injury.

marked differences in laxity or clunk are reliable.

b. Radiographs—PA and lateral views should be obtained.
- Scapholunate angle—46° is the mean normal; greater than 60° is considered abnormal.
- Diastasis between the scaphoid and lunate—greater than 4 mm is abnormal.
- "Signet ring" sign—As the scaphoid flexes, the distal pole will appear as a ring on PA radiographs.
- Radiolunate angle—greater than 15° dorsal indicates a DISI deformity on a true lateral radiograph.
- Disruption of the Gilula lines suggests ligament injury.

4. Treatment

a. Acute injuries—Treatment options include open repair with suture anchors or drill holes through bone, temporary stabilization of the carpus using K-wires or screws, and cast immobilization.

b. Chronic injuries (dynamic or static)
- Indications for open repair—Satisfactory ligament remains for repair; the scaphoid and lunate remain easily reducible; no degenerative changes within the carpus
- Soft-tissue reconstruction (all with inconsistent and imperfect results)
  - Dorsal capsulodesis or tenodesis prevents dynamic or static scaphoid flexion.
  - Flexor carpi radialis tenodesis uses a strip of the muscle passed from volar to dorsal through a bone tunnel in the distal scaphoid and attached to the distal radius or lunate. Both link the scaphoid to the lunate and limit passive scaphoid flexion.
  - Ligament reconstruction—Attempts to reconstruct the SLIL with bone-ligament-bone constructs from the carpus, foot, and extensor retinaculum.
  - Arthrodesis—Scaphotrapezial or scaphocapitate arthrodesis can be used to stabilize the scaphoid.

c. Chronic injuries with arthritis (SLAC changes)—See **Table 4**.

E. LT ligament injuries

1. LT injuries are much less common and difficult to diagnose.

2. Anatomy of the LT ligament

a. Like the SL ligament, the LT interosseous ligaments are C-shaped ligaments, spanning the dorsal, proximal, and palmar edges of the joint surfaces.

b. The palmar region of the LT is the thickest and strongest region.

TABLE 4

Treatment of Scapholunate Advanced Collapse Changes

Stage	Characteristics	Treatment
I	Early arthritic changes, present only at radial styloid	STT fusion combined with radial styloidectomy for pain relief Scaphocapitate fusion with radial styloidectomy
II	Arthritis present at radioscaphoid joint	Four-corner fusion or proximal row carpectomy[a]
III	Arthritis present at the capitolunate joint	If the capitate is too arthritic to allow a proximal row carpectomy, options may be limited to the following: Four-corner fusion Total wrist fusion Total wrist arthroplasty

[a]Debate as to the benefits of four-corner fusion over proximal row carpectomy and vice versa is ongoing; however, no studies to date clearly show the superiority of one procedure over another.

STT = scaphotrapezial-trapezoid

c. The dorsal LT ligament region is most important in rotational constraint.

3. Most volar intercalated segmental instability on radiographs occurs in anatomically normal wrists. It is often associated with wrist laxity. It is important to compare radiographs of the symptomatic and asymptomatic sides.

4. Physical examination—The diagnostic performance characteristics of tests such as the LT ballottement, shear, and compression tests are uncertain. The low prevalence of LT pathology markedly decreases the accuracy and usefulness of all diagnostic tests, including imaging and arthroscopy.

5. Arthroscopy is the reference standard for LT injuries.

6. Treatment—Surgical treatment options include LT ligament repair, LT ligament reconstruction, and LT or capitate-hamate-lunate-triquetral arthrodesis.

F. Perilunate dislocations

1. Pathoanatomy

a. The lunate often remains bound to the carpus by stout radiolunate ligaments, and the carpus dislocates around it. The capitate may move dorsally to cause dorsal perilunate dislocation (common) or palmarly to cause palmar perilunate dislocation (rare).

b. Lunate dislocation occurs when the lunate dislocates from the radial fossa palmarly, resulting in palmar lunate dislocation (common), or dorsally, resulting in dorsal lunate dislocation (rare).

c. Fractures may pass through any bone found within the greater arc of the wrist, including the distal radius, scaphoid, trapezium, capitate, hamate, and triquetrum.

d. Lesser arc injuries pass only through ligamentous structures, with no corresponding fractures.

2. Evaluation

a. Diagnosis can be delayed because some radiographic findings may be subtle; 25% of these injuries are missed during the initial presentation.

b. The physical examination may reveal significant swelling, ecchymosis, and decreased range of motion.

c. The risk of acute carpal tunnel syndrome can be as high as 25% to 50%.

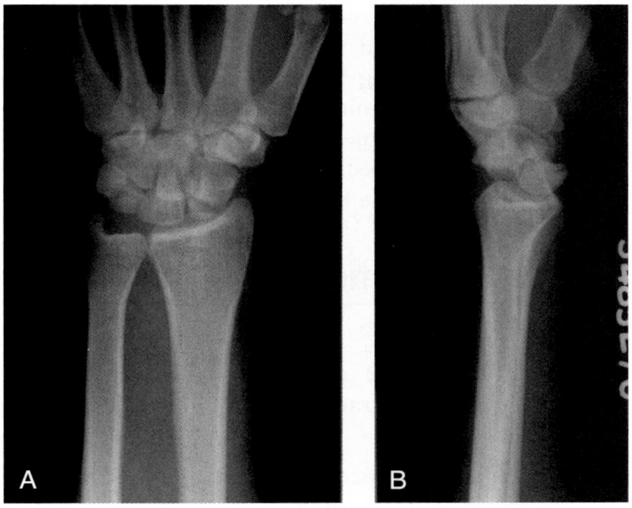

Figure 3 PA (**A**) and lateral (**B**) radiographs show a transscaphoid perilunate dislocation. Note the disruption of the carpal arcs of Gilula on the PA view.

d. Radiographs

- PA views may show a disruption of the carpal arcs of Gilula and overlapping of the carpal bones (**Figure 3**, A).
- Lateral views will show dislocation of the capitate or lunate bones (**Figure 3**, B).

e. CT and MRI are usually not necessary or helpful.

3. Treatment

a. Acute presentation

- Closed reduction may be performed initially for pain relief, but surgery is the definitive treatment.
- Lunate dislocations may require an extended carpal tunnel approach initially for lunate reduction if the lunate cannot be reduced by closed means.
- Beware of acute carpal tunnel syndrome and forearm compartment syndrome. Both can develop over hours to days.
- If the injury can be reduced closed and no acute carpal tunnel syndrome or ulnar translocation is present, a dorsal approach may be adequate, and it can be performed many days later.

b. Surgical treatment

- After the SL ligament is repaired, the repair can be protected with a temporary screw or K-wires across the SL interval.

- Most surgeons place wires across the LT interval and midcarpal joint as well, but results using SL and LT screws leaving the midcarpal joint free to move are comparable, and some surgeons do not treat the LT ligament specifically. More data are needed to determine the best treatment approach.

III. FRACTURES OF THE DISTAL RADIUS

A. Overview

1. Fractures of the distal radius are among the most common fractures seen in the emergency department.
2. Patients of advanced age with osteoporosis have an increased fracture risk during low-energy falls.
3. Fracture patterns vary depending on the mechanism of injury.
4. Principles of treatment—The goals of all treatment are to optimize comfort and function.

B. Management of distal radius fractures

1. Options include closed reduction and cast immobilization, closed reduction and percutaneous pinning with or without external fixation, and ORIF.
2. Most open fractures and volar shearing fractures are best treated operatively.
3. Surgical treatment indications relate to infirmity, functional demands, tolerance of deformity, and personal preferences. Injury and patient characteristics meriting a discussion of surgical treatment include the following:
   a. Loss of reduction, including ulnar variance 5 mm or more positive; dorsal articular tilt ≥15° (ie, volar apex angulation); and loss of radial inclination >10°
   b. Articular gap or step of 2 mm or more
   c. Unstable volar extra-articular fractures (Smith fracture)
   d. Fractures with associated neurovascular injuries
   e. Fractures with associated intercarpal ligament injuries
   f. Multiple trauma, such as bilateral distal radius fractures or the need to use crutches for a leg injury (relative indication)
4. Cast or splint immobilization
   a. The optimal reduction technique and immobilization are debated.
   b. Current best evidence suggests initial displacement determines the final alignment regardless of the time of immobilization, so wrist splints or short arm casts are usually used, and the elbow and forearm are usually left free unless there is severe radioulnar joint injury/disruption.
   c. Displaced fractures are immobilized for 4 to 6 weeks after acceptable closed reduction.
   d. It is important to encourage elevation, digital range of motion, and functional use of the limb to avoid stiffness of the fingers and forearm and to limit swelling.
   e. Nondisplaced distal radius fractures are associated with occasional extensor pollicis longus rupture, usually about 4 to 6 weeks after injury.
5. Surgical treatment
   a. Closed reduction and percutaneous pinning with or without external fixation—0.62-inch or 1.6-mm K-wires
   b. External fixator
      - Bridging external fixation can be used to protect pin fixation or to provide ligamentotaxis.
      - Full incisions over the radius and index metacarpal at the time of fixator pin placement minimize the risk of iatrogenic injury to the superficial branch of the radial nerve or tethering of the first dorsal interosseous muscle.
      - The fixator and pins typically remain in place for 6 to 8 weeks.
      - Bone graft or bone void fillers can be used to structurally support bone defects and perhaps allow earlier removal of the fixator.
   c. ORIF
      - Volar locking plates make it possible to stabilize dorsally displaced fractures from through the volar Henry approach (through the sheath of the flexor carpi radialis tendon).
      - Potential pitfalls include intra-articular screw placement, application to inappropriate fracture patterns with prominent implant placement which may lead to tendon rupture.
      - The most common tendon to rupture following application of a volar plate is the flexor pollicis longus, due to volar extension of the plate beyond the so-called watershed line, meaning the tendon may rub directly against the edge of the plate.

- Dorsal tendons such as the extensor pollicis longus and extensor digitorum communis can fray and rupture from prominent screw tips following volar insertion.
- Dorsal plates or constructs are now preferred for dorsal shearing fractures and complex articular fractures (in combination with volar plates).
- Distraction (or bridge) plate fixation is increasingly utilized for complex articular fracture, those with complex metaphyseal or diaphyseal fragmentation in particular. A distraction plate is applied between the index or long finger metacarpal and the shaft of the radius (as with external fixation), applied with distraction, and removed about 3 months after injury. Application of the bridge/distraction plate should not be a substitute for accurate ORIF.

C. Volarly displaced extra-articular fractures (Smith fractures) can be treated with reduction and casting if no comminution is present and a good reduction is obtained, but these relatively uncommon injuries are usually treated surgically with a volar plate and screws.

D. Fractures of the radial styloid (chauffeur fractures)

1. These fractures may be associated with SL ligament injuries because the intra-articular fracture line extends into the joint at that level. Therefore, in the setting of isolated radial styloid fractures, intercarpal ligament injuries must be suspected.
2. Treatment
   a. Nonsurgical—If the fracture is nondisplaced or minimally displaced, it may be treated nonsurgically.
   b. Surgical—Intra-articular displacement (or diastasis) greater than 2 mm is an indication for surgery. Compression screw fixation with partially threaded 3.5- or 4.0-mm cancellous screws can effectively compress the fragments and maintain the reduction. Alternative fixation options include K-wires and fragment-specific pin plate and screw fixation.

E. Distal radioulnar joint

1. The distal radioulnar joint is assessed following stabilization of the radius. Slightly greater laxity than the opposite uninjured wrist (based on preoperative examination) is to be expected.
2. Only frank dislocation with forearm rotation—very uncommon—merits surgery to stabilize the joint.
3. The presence of a displaced fracture at the base of the ulnar styloid is not in itself an indication for surgical fixation, and clinical stability of the DRUJ must be elucidated and compared with the normal contralateral side when possible.

TOP TESTING FACTS

1. Nondisplaced scaphoid waist fractures, as verified by CT, can be treated with cast immobilization or percutaneous (dorsal or volar) screw fixation.
2. A triquetral avulsion fracture is a simple wrist sprain and can be treated symptomatically.
3. Indications for surgical treatment of a scaphoid fracture include fracture displacement and perilunate ligamentous injuries.
4. The SLAC pattern of arthritis progresses from the radial styloid to the radioscaphoid joint, and to the capitolunate joint.
5. The potential for acute carpal tunnel syndrome with perilunate fracture-dislocations should always be considered.
6. Radiographic measures of alignment that prompt consideration of surgical treatment for distal radius fractures include shortening (≥5 mm), dorsal angulation (≥15°), loss of radial inclination (>10°), or articular displacement (≥2 mm).
7. Intra-articular volar shear fractures (Barton fractures) and unstable volar extra-articular fractures (Smith fractures) are treated with a volar plate and screws.
8. The tendon most at risk from a prominent volar plate is the flexor pollicis longus.
9. The tendon most at risk of rupture from a nondisplaced distal radius fracture is the extensor pollicus longus.
10. In the setting of isolated radial styloid fractures, scapholunate injury should be suspected.
11. The presence of a displaced fracture at the base of the ulnar styloid is not an indication for surgical fixation. Clinical examination of the DRUJ must be performed to rule out instability.

7 | Trauma

Bibliography

Costa ML, Achten J, Parsons NR, et al: Percutaneous fixation with Kirschner wires versus volar locking plate fixation in adults with dorsally displaced fracture of distal radius: Randomised controlled trial. *BMJ* 2014;349:g4807. doi:10.1136/bmj.g4807. PubMed PMID: 25096595; PubMed Central PMCID:PMC4122170.

Kalainov DM, Cohen MS: Treatment of traumatic scapholunate dissociation. *J Hand Surg Am* 2009;34(7):1317-1319.

Krief E, Appy-Fedida B, Rotari V, David E, Mertl P, Maes-Clavier C. Results of perilunate dislocations and perilunate fracture dislocations with a minimum 15-year follow-up. *J Hand Surg Am* 2015;40(11):2191-2197. doi:10.1016/j.jhsa.2015.07.016. Epub 2015 Aug 29. PubMed PMID:26328900.

Lang PO, Bickel KD: Distal radius fractures: Percutaneous treatment versus open reduction with internal fixation. *J Hand Surg Am* 2014;39(3):546-548.

Lee DJ, Elfar JC: Carpal ligament injuries, pathomechanics, and classification. *Hand Clin* 2015;31(3):389-398. doi:10.1016/j.hcl.2015.04.011. Review. PubMed PMID:26205700; PubMed Central PMCID:PMC4514919.

Ring D, Lozano-Calderón S: Imaging for suspected scaphoid fracture. *J Hand Surg Am* 2008;33(6):954-957.

Souer JS, Rutgers M, Andermahr J, Jupiter JB, Ring D: Perilunate fracture-dislocations of the wrist: Comparison of temporary screw versus K-wire fixation. *J Hand Surg Am* 2007;32(3):318-325.

Chapter 97
Pelvic, Acetabular, and Sacral Fractures

RAYMOND D. WRIGHT Jr, MD

I. PELVIC FRACTURES

A. Epidemiology

1. Most commonly occurs in men in their 40s
2. Considerable diversity in associated visceral and soft-tissue injuries
3. Morbidity and mortality rates range from 10% to 50%

B. Anatomy

1. Osseous
   a. The pelvic ring is formed by two innominate bones joined posteriorly through the sacrum and anteriorly by the symphysis pubis (**Figures 1** and **2**).
   b. Each innominate bone is formed by the confluence of the ilium, ischium, and pubis.
   c. The pelvic ring has no inherent bony stability.
      - Anterior stability comes from the symphysis pubis, a fibrocartilaginous disk between the anterior portion of the innominate bones and the surrounding ligamentous attachments.
      - Posterior stability comes from the anterior and posterior sacroiliac ligaments (posterior are stronger than anterior).
      - The sacrospinous and sacrotuberous ligaments provide stability to the pelvic floor. The iliolumbar ligaments form a broad connection between the transverse processes of L4, L5, and the posterior ilium.

2. Vascular
   a. The common iliac system begins near L4 at the bifurcation of the abdominal aorta.
      - The external iliac artery courses anteriorly along the pelvic brim to emerge as the common femoral artery distal to the inguinal ligament.
      - The internal iliac artery divides caudal and posterior near the sacroiliac joint. The posterior division gives rise to the superior gluteal artery and several other branches before exiting the posterior pelvis as the inferior gluteal and internal pudendal arteries. The anterior portion of the internal iliac artery becomes the obturator artery.
   b. The corona mortis is a connection between the obturator and iliac systems. One cadaver analysis demonstrated that the anastomosis is found a mean of 6.2 cm from the symphysis pubis in 84% of specimens and can be arterial, venous, or both. Traditionally, this structure is discussed in the context of retropubic dissection for acetabular fractures.
   c. A venous plexus in the posterior pelvis that results in the internal iliac system. Injury to this venous plexus and bony bleeding account for 90% of the hemorrhage associated with pelvic ring injuries.

3. Neurologic
   a. The lumbosacral plexus is created from nerve roots L1-S4 (**Figure 3**).
   b. The lateral femoral cutaneous nerve (L2-3) runs deep to the inguinal ligament near the anterior superior iliac spine.
   c. The obturator nerve (L2-4) runs along the quadrilateral surface and exits peripherally

Dr. Wright or an immediate family member serves as a paid consultant to or is an employee of Paid consultant and serves as a board member, owner, officer, or committee member of the Kentucky Orthopaedic Society.

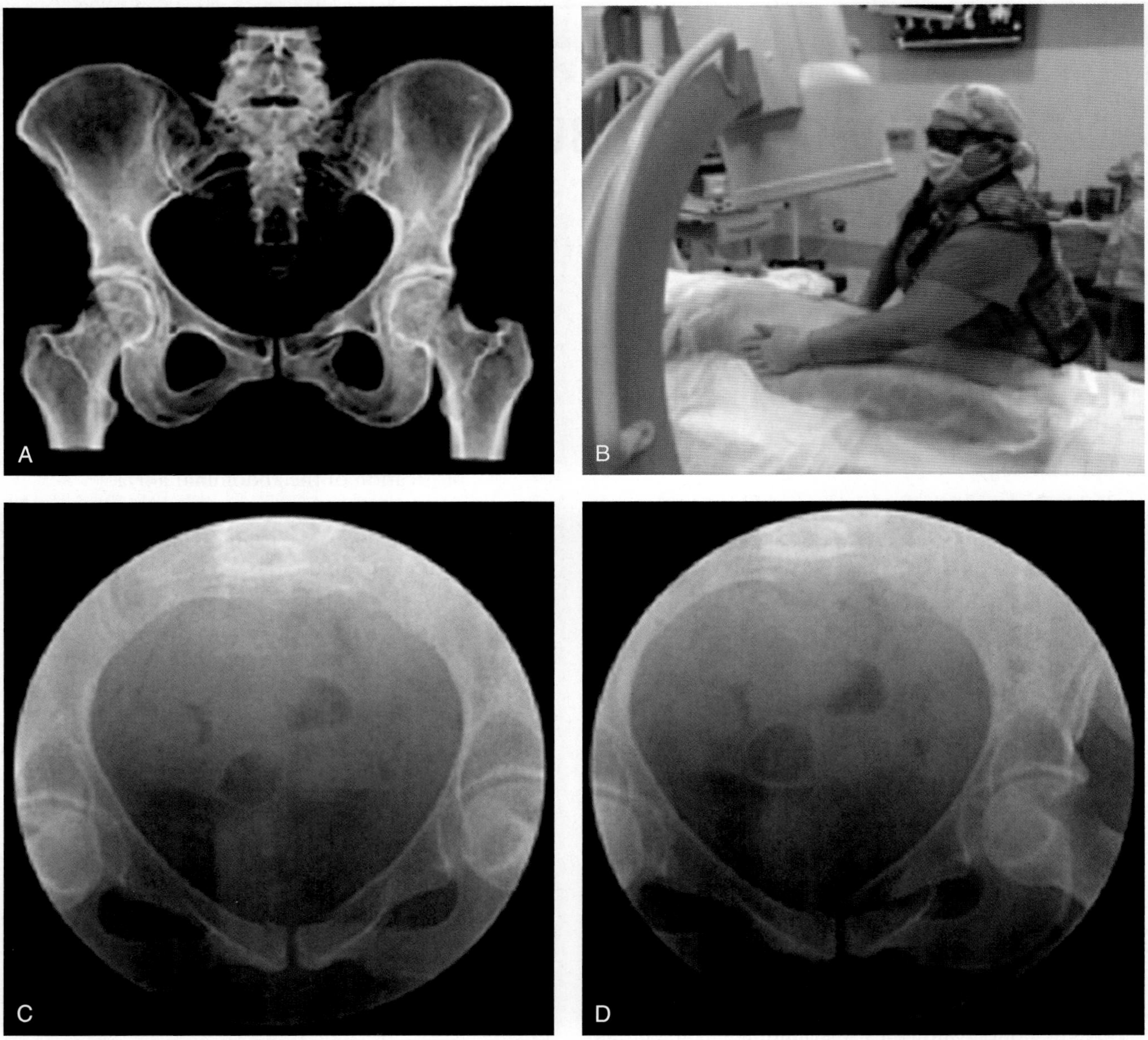

Figure 1 A 37-year-old female is involved in a T-bone motor vehicle crash. Pelvic radiograph demonstrates a left parasymphyseal fracture with a left sacral fracture (**A**). The patient was taken to the operating room for examination under anesthesia and fluoroscopy (EUAF) (**B**). The image at rest demonstrates very little displacement (**C**). However, with laterally directed manual force, gross instability of the pelvic ring is unmasked (**D**).

and cranially in the obturator canal at the obturator sulcus.

d. The femoral nerve (L2-4) travels with the iliopsoas tendon.

e. The sciatic nerve (L4-S3) exits the greater sciatic notch.

f. The L5 nerve root lies on the cranial anterior portion of the sacral ala 10 to 15 mm medial to the anterior portion of the sacroiliac joint.

C. Classification

1. AO Foundation/Orthopaedic Trauma Association (AO/OTA)

   a. Classification based on the Tile and Pennal classification system with an additional numeric modifier (**Figure 4**).

   b. The Tile classification system evaluated the potential instability of the pelvic ring injury.

   - Type A, stable

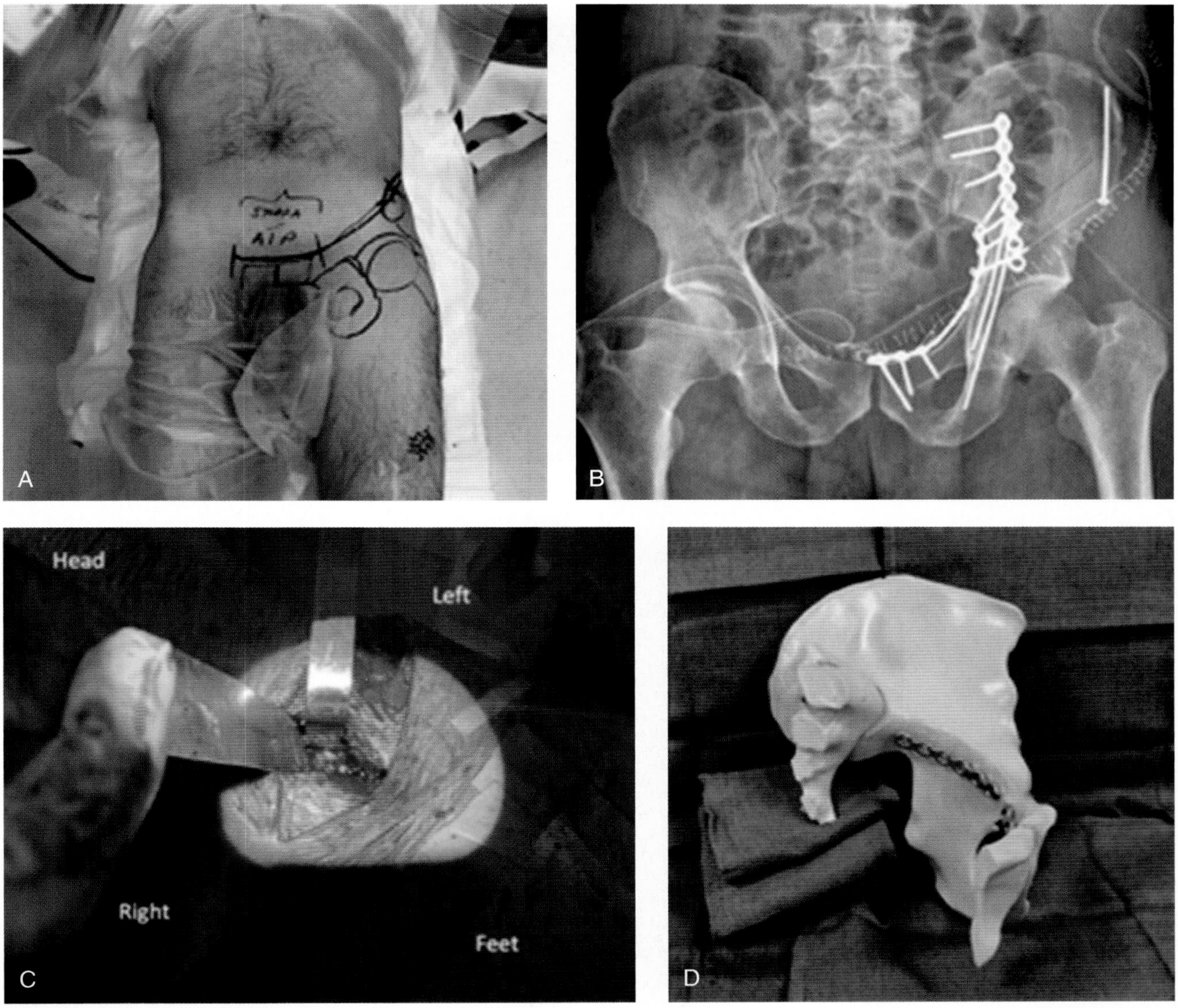

Figure 2 A 43-year-old male is treated operatively for an associated both-column (ABC) acetabulum fracture. (**A**) Clinical photograph showing that the patient is placed supine and an ilioinguinal exposure is employed. The Stoppa or AIP window may be used alone or as part of this ilioinguinal exposure. Radiograph showing implants inserted through ilioinguinal exposure including an infrapectineal plate (**B**). The infrapectineal view is best obtained with the surgeon standing on the opposite side of the injured hip (**C**). The position of the infrapectineal plate is demonstrated on the sawbones model (**D**).

- Type B, rotationally unstable, vertically stable
- Type C, rotationally and vertically unstable

2. Young-Burgess
   a. Classification based on mechanism of injury (**Figure 5**).
   b. Mechanisms divided into the following categories: lateral compression, anterior-posterior compression, vertical shear, and combined mechanical injury (**Table 1**).
3. Letournel
   a. This system is based on anatomic site of injury.
   b. The pelvis is divided into anterior and posterior portions.
   c. This classification system is purely descriptive and provides no estimation of injury severity or pelvic stability (**Figure 6**).

D. Mechanism of injury

1. Most frequently high-energy trauma

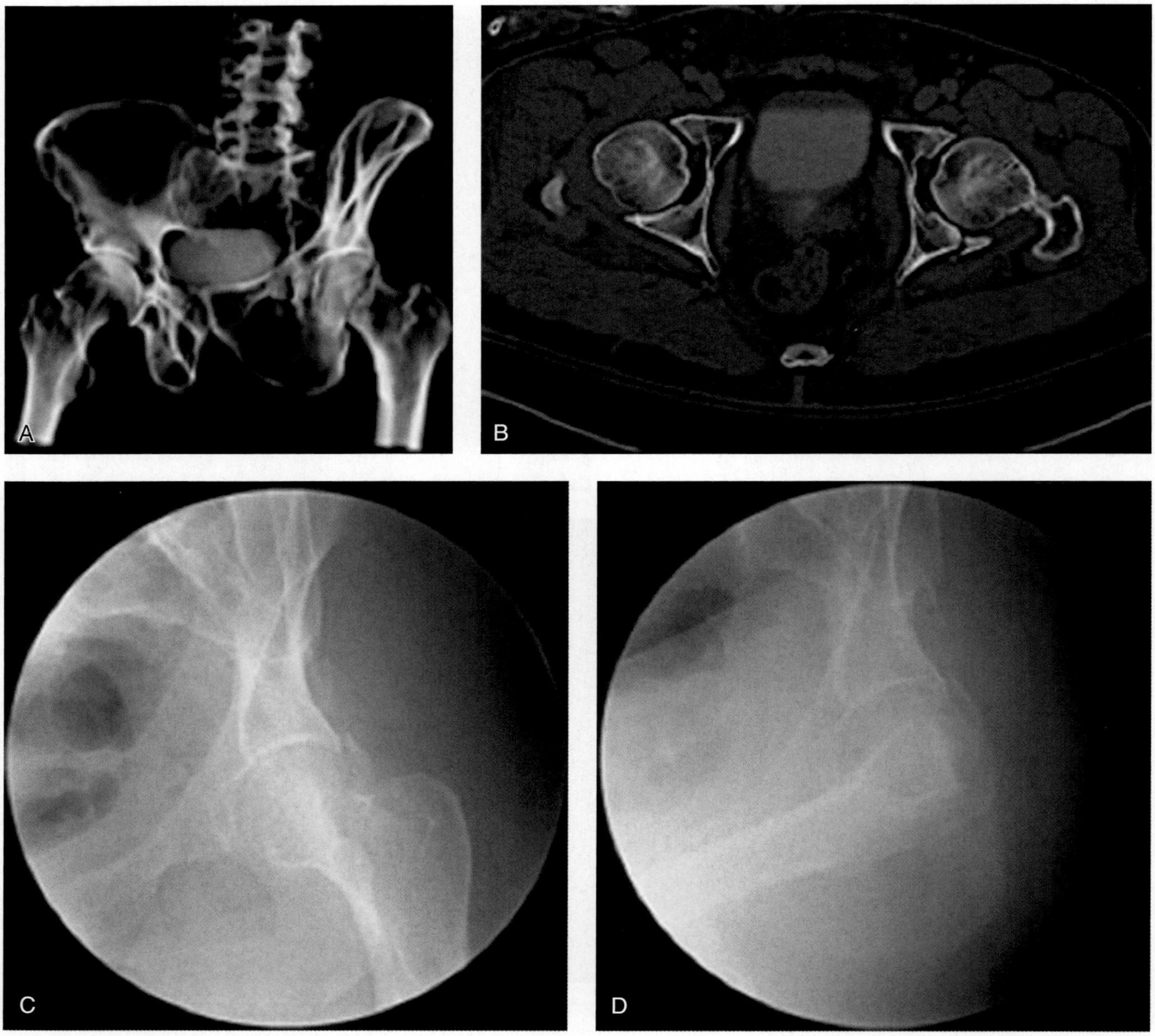

Figure 3 A 27-year-old male sustains a left posterior wall acetabulum fracture. The obturator oblique view (**A**) and CT scan slice (**B**) are shown. The patient underwent examination under anesthesia and fluoroscopy (EUAF). The surgeon stands on the side of the uninjured hip with the patient placed supine on a radiolucent table. The C-arm is placed on the side ipsilateral to the injured hip and rolled back to obtain an obturator oblique view (**C**). The hip is flexed, adducted, and internally rotated, and axial pressure is applied by the surgeon. In the obturator oblique view, the concentric femoro-acetabular articulation indicates stability (**D**).

2. Most common causes of injury (descending frequency):
   a. Motorcycle crashes
   b. Pedestrian-sustained automobile injuries
   c. Falls
   d. Motor vehicle crashes
   e. Crush injuries
3. Low-energy mechanisms may be possible in elderly patients with poor bone quality

E. Evaluation

1. Full advanced trauma life support (ATLS) workup because of high incidence of associated injuries.
2. The skin and soft tissues should be inspected for evidence of open injury including the perineum

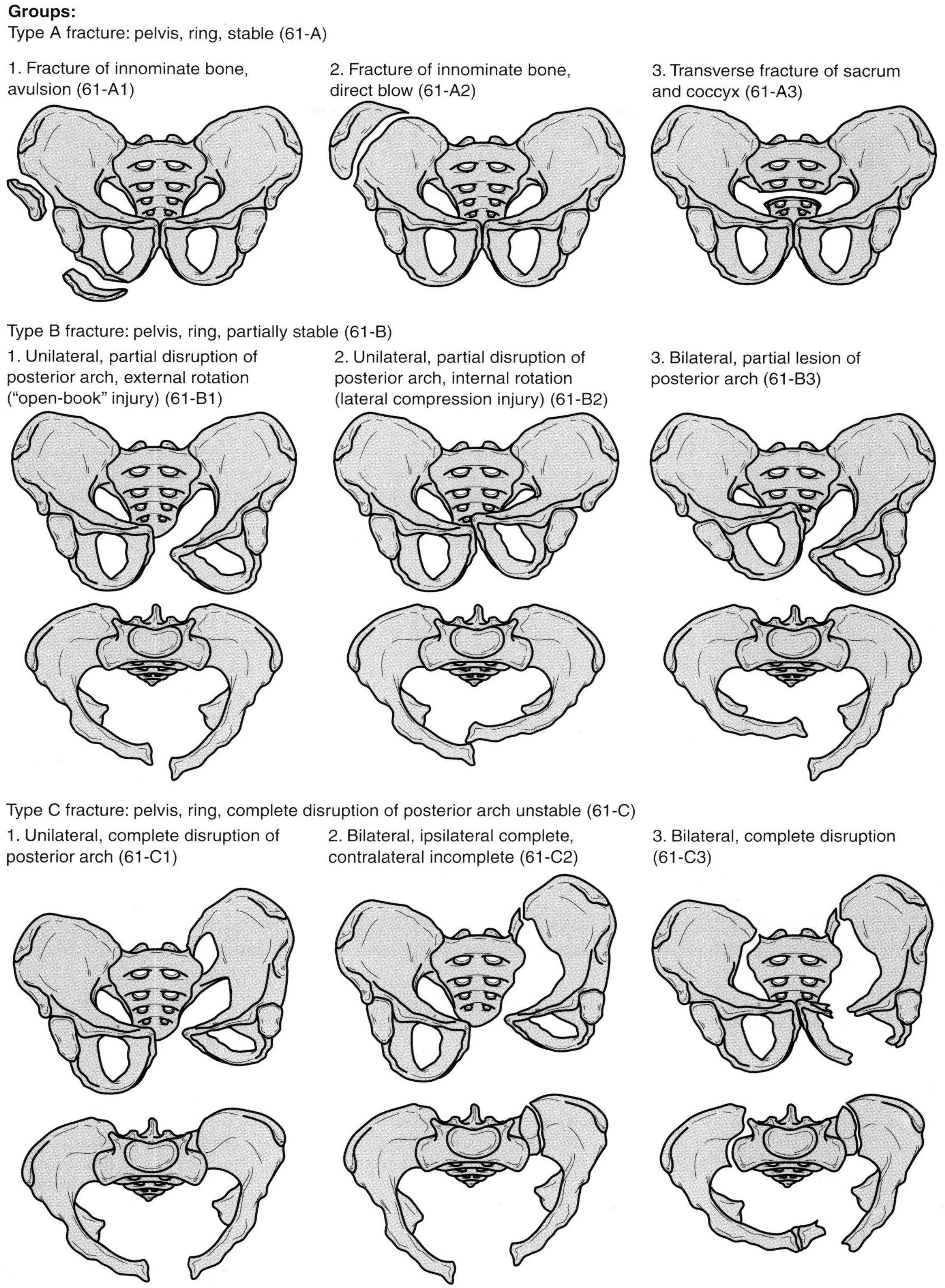

Figure 4 Illustrations demonstrating the AO/Orthopaedic Trauma Association fracture compendium for pelvic fractures. Type A fractures are considered stable. Type B fractures are rotationally unstable and vertically stable. Type C fractures are rotationally and vertically unstable.

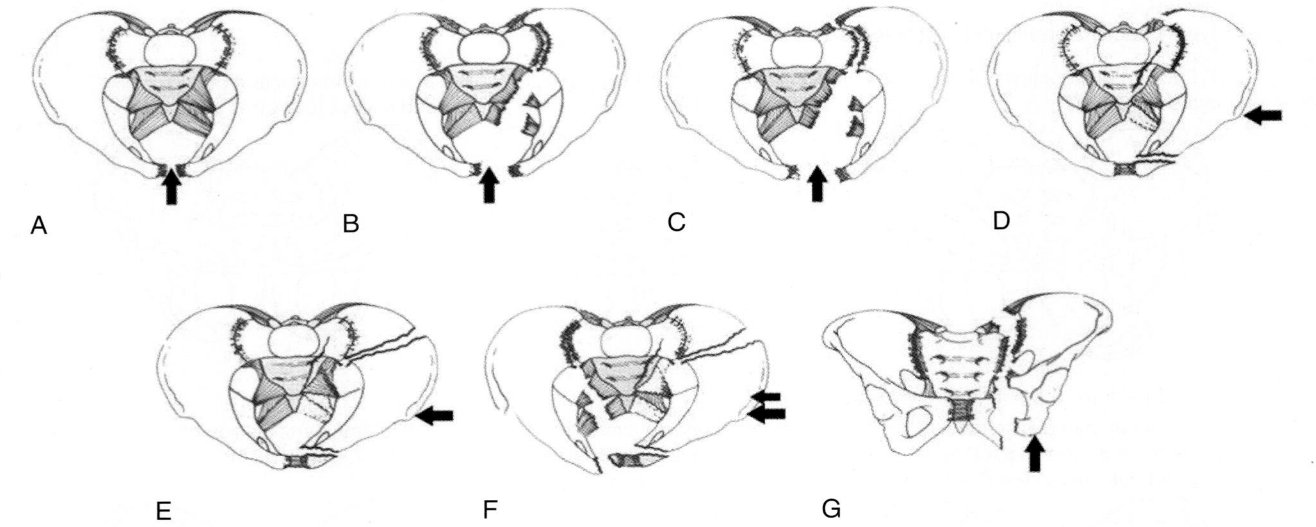

Figure 5 Diagrams show the Young-Burgess classification of pelvic fractures. **A**, Anterior-posterior compression type I. **B**, Anterior-posterior compression type II. **C**, Anterior-posterior compression type III. **D**, Lateral compression type I. **E**, Lateral compression type II. **F**, Lateral compression type III. **G**, Vertical shear. (Reproduced from Hak DJ, Smith WR, Suzuki T: Management of hemorrhage in life-threatening pelvic fracture. *J Am Acad Orthop Surg* 2009;17[7]:451.)

and gluteal folds; a rectal and vaginal examination should be performed.

3. The skin is inspected for closed internal degloving lesions (Morel-Lavallee). The resulting necrotic fat and hematoma can contaminate the surgical exposure and may require débridement.
4. Neurologic examination, including sacral nerve roots
5. Imaging
   a. AP pelvic radiograph as a screening study in patients suspected of having a pelvic ring injury (routine screening study for trauma patients) (**Figure** 7, A)
   b. Inlet pelvic view (**Figure** 7, B)
      - Variable amount of caudal tilt, which depends on individual patient anatomy; ideally, the beam is perpendicular to the S1 end plate

TABLE 1

Comparison of the Young-Burgess Classification Fracture Types

Mechanism	I	II	III	Comments
LC	Horizontal fractures in rami with sacral impaction	Posterior ligamentous disruption of SI joint or equivalent bony disruption of posterior ilium	LC pattern on side ipsilateral to injury with contralateral external rotation deformity	Deaths with increasing LC grades because of increasing incidence of brain injury with only modest increases in complications related to ARDS, sepsis, and shock
APC	Anterior symphyseal widening ≤ 25 mm, incomplete anterior SI injury	Anterior symphyseal widening ≥ 25 mm, disruption of anterior SI, sacrospinous, and sacrotuberous ligaments	Anterior symphyseal injury with complete dissociation of SI joint	Circulatory shock, sepsis, and ARDS are substantial causes of death in increasing APC grades. APC III injuries have the highest fluid requirements, hemorrhage, and mortality
VS	Total disruption of posterior ligamentous structures resulting in craniocaudal as well as rotational instability			Associated systemic injury pattern similar to LC group
CMI	Fracture pattern does not fit any single classification			Associated systemic injury pattern similar to APC group

APC = anteroposterior compression, ARDS = acute respiratory distress syndrome, CMI = combined mechanical injury, LC = lateral compression, SI = sacroiliac, VS = vertical shear

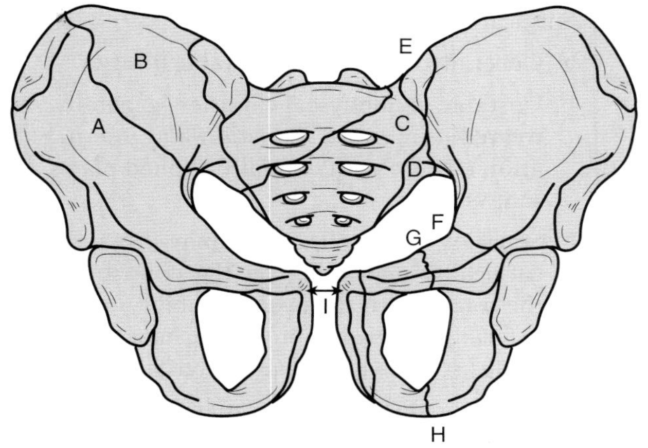

Figure 6 Illustration depicts the Letournel classification of pelvic fractures. This classification is descriptive and provides information about the location and types of injuries to the pelvic ring. A = iliac fracture, B = crescent fracture, C = sacral fracture, D = sacro-iliac joint disruption, E = crescent fracture/dislocation, F = pubic root fracture, G = mid-ramus fracture, H = inferior ramus fracture, I = symphysis disruption.

- Horizontal rotation as well as anterior or posterior translation of the injured hemipelvis can be visualized on this view

c. Outlet pelvic view (**Figure** 7, C)

- Variable amount of cranial tilt; ideally, the cranial portion of the symphysis pubis is centered at the level of the S2 body
- Demonstrates cranial-caudal displacement of the pelvic ring, sacral morphology

d. CT

- Improves detection and understanding of injury pattern; 30% of posterior injuries can be missed on plain radiographs.
- May evaluate sacral nerve root tunnels for presence of bony debris or stenosis from fracture.
- Soft tissue may be evaluated to detect hematoma formation, active arterial bleeding (in contrast-enhanced studies), and displacement of pelvic organs from hemorrhage.
- CT confirms diagnosis and provides fine detail of the pelvic ring injury and enables the clinician to detect occult injuries that may not be visible on plain radiographs.

e. Examination under anesthesia and fluoroscopy (EUAF)

- Patient is placed supine on a radiolucent table
- C-arm is set to give an inlet view of anterior pelvic ring
- Lateral compression stress is applied under live fluoroscopy to unmask occult instability (**Figure 1**, B).

F. Treatment

1. Initial management

a. Consideration of the patient's hemodynamic status and injury pattern determines initial management.

b. ATLS protocol is mandatory for all patients with osseous pelvic trauma.

c. Patients with unstable fracture patterns and hemodynamic instability may benefit from emergent skeletal stability to minimize intrapelvic hemorrhage.

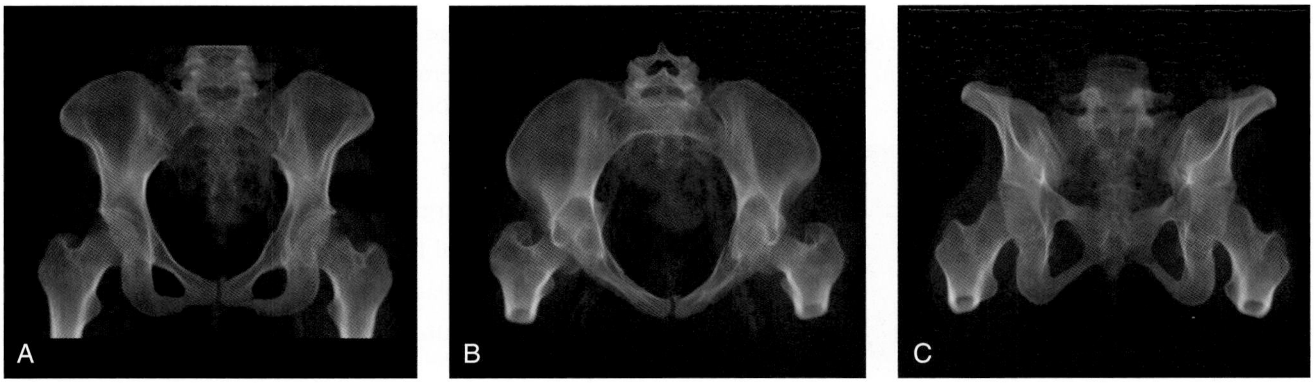

Figure 7 Images show the radiographic evaluation for pelvic fractures. **A**, The AP pelvic view is used to provisionally diagnose an injury and direct further workup. **B**, The inlet pelvic view is obtained so that the S1 and S2 bodies overlap and provides information regarding the anterior-posterior translation of one hemipelvis relative to the contralateral side. Additionally, horizontal plane rotation can be demonstrated with this view. **C**, The outlet pelvic view demonstrates the upper and second sacral segment morphology and can demonstrate craniocaudal translation of an injured pelvic segment.

d. Emergent osseous pelvic stability may be achieved by various means.
   - External fixation—Excellent anterior pelvic control; relatively little utility in pelvic fractures with complete posterior injury; may require fluoroscopy for safe placement; pins may contaminate definitive surgical incisions.
   - C-clamp—Excellent posterior ring control; requires fluoroscopy for safe placement; may contaminate posterior approaches or insertion of iliosacral screws
   - Pneumatic antishock garments—Application may diminish venous return, cause compartment syndrome, and cause injury to the skin and soft tissues.
   - Pelvic binders—Can provide stability to the entire pelvic ring; may be applied in the field.
   - Sheets—Readily available; strategic application requires Kocher clamps, towel clips, and so forth for application; portions of sheet may be cut out for vascular access, angiography, external fixator placement, and percutaneous fixation; skin needs to be monitored regularly (**Figures 8** and **9**).
   - Traction—May be used for fractures with potential cranial-caudal instability.

2. Nonsurgical treatment
   a. Indicated in patients with stable injuries or those in whom substantial medical comorbidities prohibit surgical intervention.
   b. Patients are usually mobilized with toe-touch or flatfoot weight bearing on the side of the posterior ring injury.
   c. Radiographs may be obtained after mobilization to determine if occult instability is unmasked with mobilization.

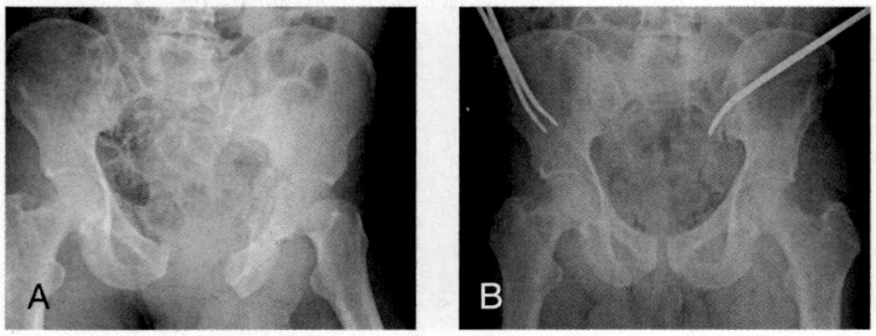

Figure 8 AP radiographs show an open pelvic fracture in a 52-year-old man. **A,** The symphysis pubis is widened with incomplete injury to the left anterior sacroiliac joint. **B,** The same pelvic ring injury after a sheet is applied to close the pelvic ring.

3. Surgical treatment
   a. Generally reserved for unstable injuries.
   b. Unstable symphyseal injuries generally are treated using open reduction and internal fixation (ORIF) with cranially applied plates and screws.
   c. Superior ramus fractures may be stabilized surgically, depending on the contribution of the fractures to the overall stability of the pelvic ring; surgical options include medullary ramus screws, plates, and external fixators.
   d. Posterior ilium fractures may be treated with ORIF or percutaneous fixation, depending on the displacement and location of the iliac injury.
   e. Sacroiliac disruptions may be treated percutaneously if incomplete or complete with displacement amenable to closed reduction; open reduction generally is required for complete injuries that do not reduce using closed or indirect means. Open reduction may be performed anteriorly through the lateral window of the ilioinguinal exposure or through posterior open exposure to the sacroiliac joint. Fixation methods include iliosacral screws, transsacral plates, transsacral bars, or a two-hole or three-hole plate applied across the anterior sacroiliac joint.
   f. Sacral fractures that are part of a pelvic ring injury may be treated using percutaneous fixation techniques if acceptable reduction is present; these techniques include iliosacral screws and posterior transiliac bars. ORIF may be performed through a direct posterior exposure. After open reduction is achieved, fixation may be achieved with iliosacral screws, transiliac, transsacral screws, transiliac bars, or a transiliac plate.
   g. Postoperative mobility is generally toe-touch or flatfoot weight bearing on the side of the posterior pelvic ring injury for approximately 6 weeks.

4. Specific surgical techniques
   a. External fixation
      - Pin placement options:
        - Gluteus medius pillar directed toward the pelvic brim
        - Anterior inferior iliac spine directed toward the sciatic buttress or posterior superior iliac spine
        - Fluoroscopy is required for safe, durable pin placement.

- Retroperitoneal packing also may be used to control hemorrhage as an adjunctive measure.

6. Rehabilitation
   a. Stable fractures treated nonsurgically
      - Patients may mobilize immediately with protected weight bearing after a stable fracture pattern is confirmed.
      - After radiographic healing occurs, patients may engage in quadriceps, hip, and core strengthening.

   b. Unstable fractures treated surgically
      - Patient mobility and weight bearing generally depend on the location of the posterior pelvic ring fracture.
      - Mobility includes weight-of-limb weight bearing ipsilateral to the posterior pelvic injury with full weight bearing on the contralateral side.
      - Patients with bilateral posterior injuries are mobilized with bed-to-chair transfers only, using the upper extremities to mobilize, if possible.
      - When radiographic healing has occurred, weight bearing may be advanced gradually, as well as lower extremity strengthening.

7. Complications
   a. Nonunion is rare in stable injuries but can occur in injuries that are treated closed with neglected instability.
   b. Malunion is more common than nonunion, especially in patients with craniocaudal instability.
   c. Sitting imbalance and limb-length discrepancy may result from cranial displacement of an unstable pelvic fracture.
   d. Thromboembolic phenomena
      - Incidence of deep vein thrombosis may be 35% to 50%
      - Incidence of pulmonary embolism in up to 10% of cases
      - Fatal pulmonary embolism in 2% of patients

   e. Chemical prophylaxis is recommended for patients with pelvic fracture; the duration and type are debatable.
   f. Patients with contraindications to deep vein thrombosis/pulmonary embolism prophylaxis may benefit from placement of an inferior vena cava filter.
   g. Iatrogenic neurovascular injury is possible while instrumenting the pelvis. A thorough understanding of the osseous fixation pathways and their respective radiographic correlates is mandatory before attempting surgical fixation of pelvic ring injuries.

II. ACETABULAR FRACTURES

A. Epidemiology

1. Acetabular fractures frequently occur with associated injuries.
2. One of the largest series of acetabular fractures demonstrated the following associated injuries:
   a. Extremity injury, 35%
   b. Head injury, 19%
   c. Chest injury, 18%
   d. Nerve palsy, 13%
   e. Abdominal injury, 8%
   f. Genitourinary injury, 6%
   g. Spine injury, 4%

B. Anatomy

1. Letournel described the acetabulum as being contained within an arch forming an inverted Y (**Figure 15**).
   a. Anterior column—Extends from the anterior portion of the iliac crest to the symphysis pubis; includes the iliac fossa, medius pillar, anterior superior iliac spine (ASIS), anterior inferior iliac spine, and superior ramus.

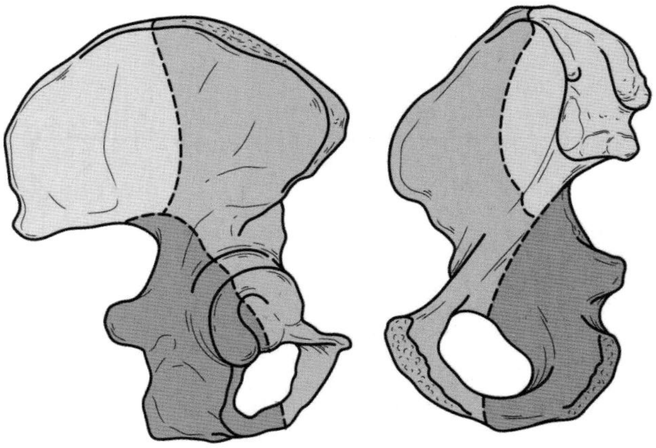

Figure 15 Illustrations show the columns of the acetabulum as described by Letournel. (Reproduced with permission from Letournel E: Acetabulum fractures: Classification and management. *Clin Orthop Relat Res* 1980;151:82.)

b. Posterior column—Cranial border is sciatic buttress; extends caudally to include ischial tuberosity, posterior wall, and quadrilateral surface

2. The column concept emphasizes the importance of osseous structures surrounding the articular surface for reduction, clamp application, and insertion of durable implants.

C. Classification

1. AO/OTA classification—Pelvis (bone 6); acetabular location (region 2) (**Figure 16**)

2. More commonly classified by Judet and Letournel as five elementary and five associated fracture patterns (**Figure 17**)

a. Elementary patterns—Anterior wall, anterior column, posterior wall, posterior column, and transverse (**Table 2**)

b. Associated patterns—Posterior column–posterior wall, transverse–posterior wall, T-shaped, anterior column–posterior hemitransverse, associated both-column (**Table 3; Figure 18**)

D. Surgical exposures

1. Kocher-Langenbeck (**Figure 19**)

a. Performed in the prone or lateral positions

b. Exposure hazards

- Sciatic nerve—Protected with visualization, knee flexion, and hip extension. Retractors should not be placed in the lesser sciatic notch.

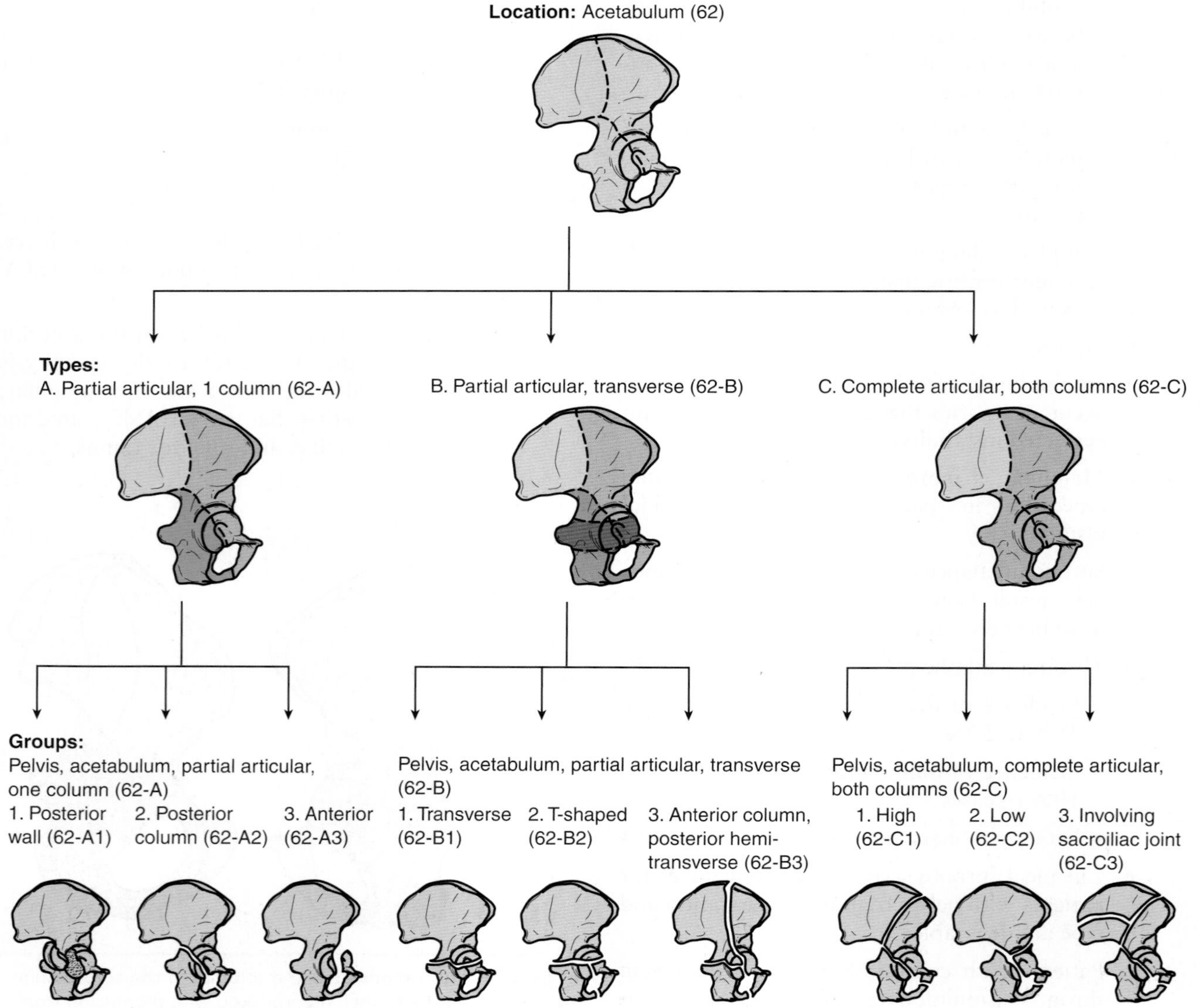

Figure 16 Diagram depicts the AO/Orthopaedic Trauma Association fracture compendium for the acetabulum.

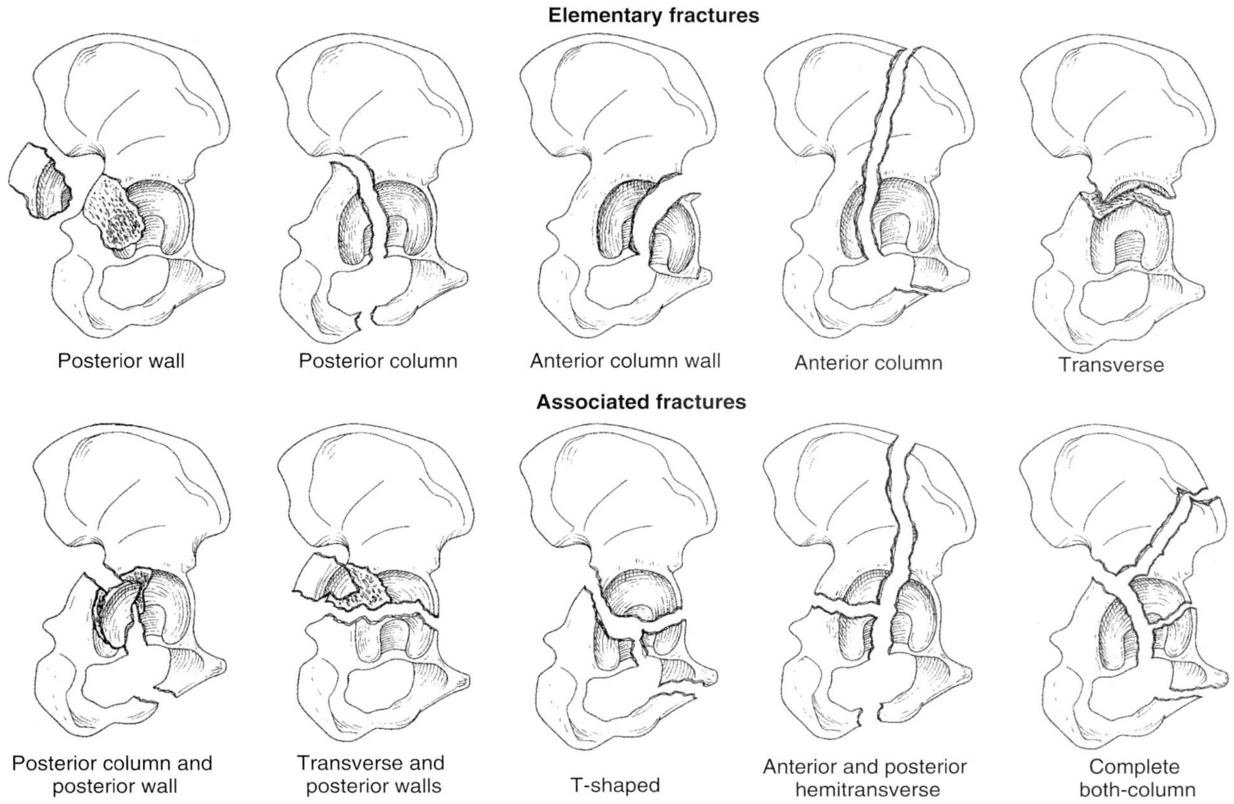

Figure 17 Diagram shows the acetabular subtypes as described by Letournel and Judet. (Reproduced from Webb LX: Open reduction and internal fixation of posterior wall acetabular fractures, in Flatow E, Colvin AC, eds: *Atlas of Essential Orthopaedic Procedures*. Rosemont, IL, American Academy of Orthopaedic Surgeons, 2013, p 385.)

- Ascending branch of medial femoral circumflex artery—Protected by performing tenotomy of the piriformis and the obturator internus 1 cm midline to their respective femoral insertions.
- Superior gluteal neurovascular branches—Between medius and minimus.

c. Useful for the following fractures
- Posterior wall
- Posterior column
- Posterior column–posterior wall
- Transverse
- Transverse–posterior wall
- Some T-shaped

2. Ilioinguinal (**Figure 20**)

a. Usually performed in the supine position; generally regarded as the most common exposure for associated both-column acetabulum fractures.

b. The skin incision classically is made along the iliac crest just posterior to the medius pillar and continued anterior to the ASIS. The incision is directed caudal and midline ending 2 cm cranial to the pubic symphysis in the midline. The lateral window is created by subperiosteal dissection of the iliacus muscle from the internal iliac fossa. The middle window is created by incising the external oblique aponeurosis and reflecting it distally, followed by splitting the inguinal ligament along its oblique course. The lateral femoral cutaneous nerve usually can be identified just deep to the inguinal ligament at the ASIS. The iliopectineal fascia divides the middle window into two portions: the lateral portion contains the iliopsoas tendon and the femoral nerve, and the medial portion contains the inguinal artery, vein, and lymphatics. The iliopectineal fascia is divided sharply and under direct visualization. The classic description of the medial window includes lateral mobilization of the spermatic cord or round

TABLE 2

The Elementary Acetabular Fracture Types

Elementary Fracture	Description	Comments
Posterior wall	Separation of posterior articular surface	Frequently associated with posterior hip dislocation High incidence of posttraumatic DJD despite simple pattern Marginal impaction may complicate reduction tactics
Posterior column	Cranial fracture is frequently near the apex of the greater sciatic notch; divides the articular and quadrilateral surfaces; and exits the inferior obturator ring	Superior gluteal neurovascular structures may be displaced or injured by fracture fragments
Anterior wall	Fracture line begins between the AIIS and iliopectineal eminence; involves varied amounts of anterior articular surface and the superior ramus	Fracture very infrequently encountered
Anterior column	Fracture through the innominate extends caudally to involve the articular surface and inferior obturator ring	Very low—cranial fracture limit at anterior horn articular surface Low—cranial fracture limit at psoas gutter Middle—cranial fracture limit at interspinous notch High—cranial fracture limit at iliac crest
Transverse	Divides the acetabulum into cranial and caudal segments	Only elementary fracture to include both columns Transtectal—traverses acetabular dome Juxtatectal—cranial portion of cotyloid fossa Infratectal—cotyloid fossa horizontally split

AIIS = Anterior inferior iliac spine, DJD = degenerative joint disease

ligament with transection of the rectus abdominus tendon.

c. Exposure hazards

- Iliac vessels—Protected with subperiosteal dissection in lateral window; keeping the patient's hip flexed while dissecting and working in the middle window removes tension from the vessels.
- Lateral femoral cutaneous nerve—This structure is identified deep to inguinal ligament, usually at the level of the ASIS, but its position may vary.

TABLE 3

The Associated Acetabular Fractures

Associated Fracture	Description	Comments
Posterior column–posterior wall	Association of posterior column and posterior wall fractures	Posterior column component is occasionally incomplete
Transverse–posterior wall	Extremely common fracture type	Often accompanied by a posterior hip dislocation
T-type	Transverse fracture associated with a vertical fracture that divides the ischiopubic segment	Also may be associated with a posterior wall fracture
Anterior-posterior hemitransverse	May be fracture of anterior wall or anterior column combined with the posterior portion of a transverse fracture	Common fracture pattern of the elderly after a fall onto the hip
Associated both column	Complete dissociation of acetabulum from axial skeleton	Radiographic "spur sign" (Figure 18) is diagnostic; represents the caudal portion of the intact ilium Secondary congruence results from medialization of anterior and posterior columns of acetabulum; may be indication for nonsurgical care in certain patients

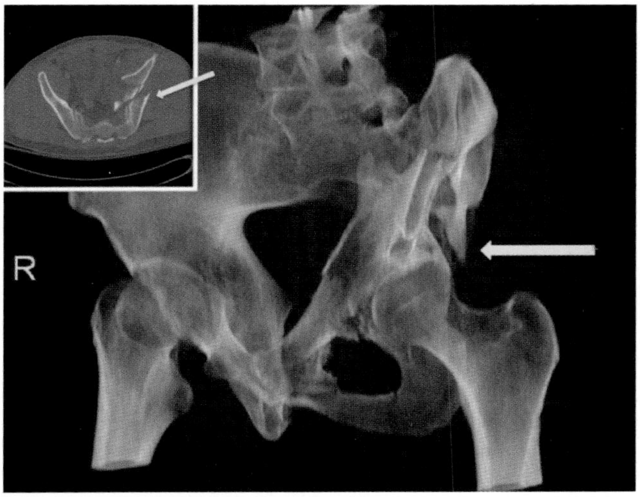

Figure 18 The obturator oblique view and corresponding axial CT scan cut (inset) of a left associated both-column acetabulum fracture. The spur sign (yellow arrows) is the radiographic representation of caudal portion of the intact ilium.

- Spermatic cord and ilioinguinal nerve—Careful dissection of external oblique aponeurosis.
- Corona mortis—Communication between the obturator and iliac systems; this may be arterial, venous, or both.

d. Useful for the following fractures:

- Anterior column
- Anterior column–posterior hemitransverse
- T-shaped
- Transverse
- Associated both-column

3. Extended iliofemoral
   a. Indicated by some authors for some complex acetabular fractures that contain a transtectal transverse component, comminution of the sciatic buttress, or associated both-column acetabulum fractures with comminution in the posterior column.
   b. This approach is classically indicated for surgical management of acetabular fractures that are at least 3 weeks old.
4. Stoppa/anterior intrapelvic (**Figure 2**, A)
   a. This approach may substitute for the medial window in the ilioinguinal exposure, or it can stand alone for certain acetabular fractures.
   b. Retropubic dissection is performed to expose the inner quadrilateral surface.
   c. This approach is useful for fracture visualization, reduction, clamp application, and intrapelvic plate placement.
   d. Used for associated both-column and anterior column fractures.
5. Smith-Petersen
   a. This exposure uses the internervous plane between the superior gluteal and femoral nerves.
   b. The interval may be useful for the surgical repair of select anterior wall fractures.

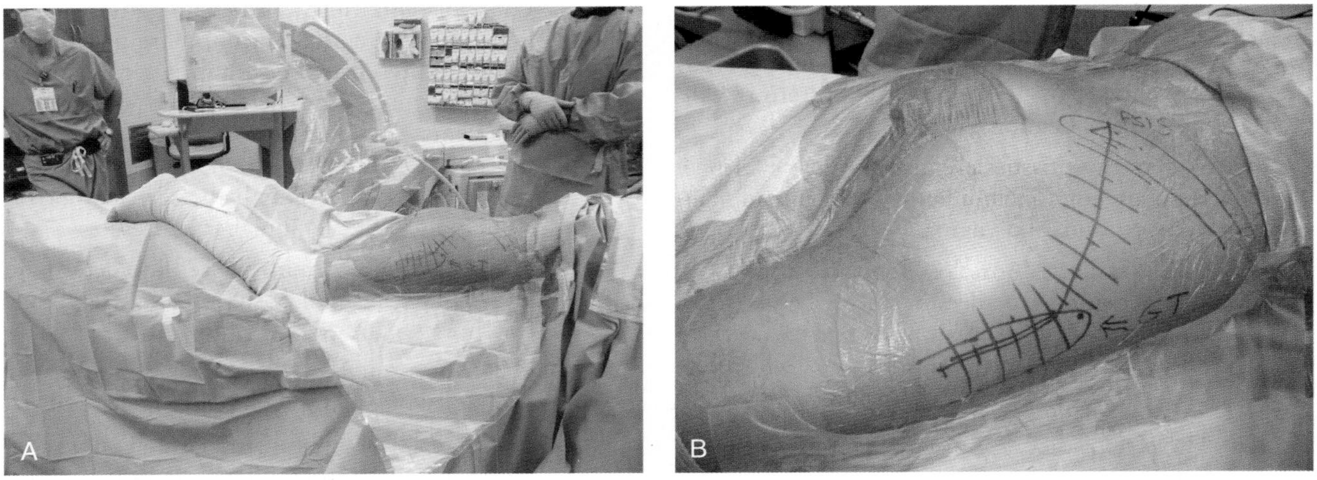

Figure 19 Photographs show the patient positioning and surgical marking of a patient undergoing open reduction and internal fixation for an acetabulum fracture via a prone Kocher-Langenbeck exposure. **A**, The patient is placed in the prone position with the ipsilateral limb prepared and draped circumferentially. **B**, The planned incision with pertinent landmarks.

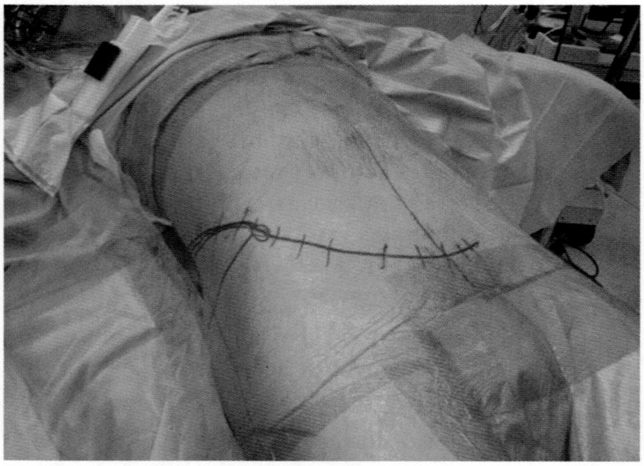

Figure 20 Photograph shows the surgical preparation and marking for open reduction and internal fixation of an acetabulum via an ilioinguinal exposure. The patient is in the supine position with the ipsilateral limb prepared and draped circumferentially.

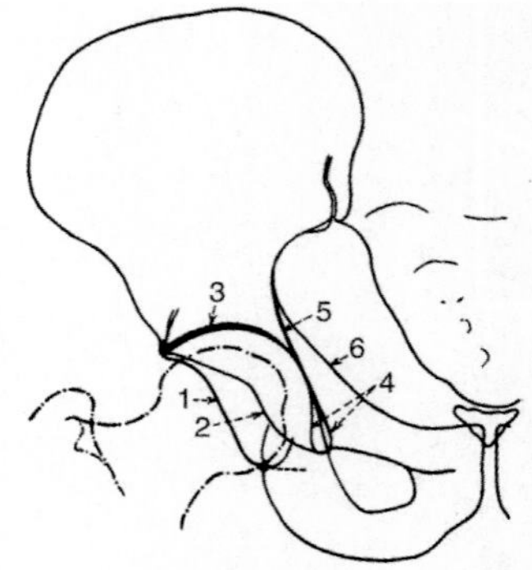

Figure 21 Illustration shows the radiographic lines described by Letournel to help evaluate acetabular fractures on plain pelvic radiographs. 1 = posterior border, 2 = anterior order, 3 = dome, 4 = teardrop, 5 = ilioischial line, 6 = iliopectineal line. (Reproduced from Bellino MJ: Acetabular fractures: Acute evaluation, in Baumgaertner MR, Tornetta P III, eds: *Orthopaedic Knowledge Update: Trauma*, ed 3. Rosemont, IL, American Academy of Orthopaedic Surgeons, 2005, p 264.)

E. Mechanism of injury
   1. Frequently high-energy injuries: motor vehicle collisions, falls from a height, motorcycle crashes
   2. Low-energy mechanism possible in patients with poor bone quality
   3. Fracture pattern determined by force vector and position of hip at time of impact
   4. Energy mechanism may be direct to pelvis or indirect, with axial force through the femoral head

F. Evaluation
   1. Physical examination
      a. Full ATLS evaluation warranted because of high incidence of associated injuries.
      b. Ipsilateral lower extremity is evaluated for fracture, ligamentous knee injury, sciatic nerve palsy (especially in posterior wall fracture-dislocation).
      c. Skin and soft tissues are inspected for evidence of open injury, including the perineum, gluteal folds, rectum, and vagina.
      d. Skin is inspected for closed internal degloving lesions (Morel-Lavallee); resulting necrotic fat and hematoma can contaminate surgical exposure and may require débridement.
   2. Imaging
      a. AP pelvic radiograph used as initial screening test
         - Six radiographic lines may be scrutinized to reach a provisional diagnosis of acetabular fracture as well as pattern (**Figure 21**; **Table 4**).
         - Lines are anatomy tangential to the radiographic beam and do not necessarily represent one particular anatomic structure.
      b. Judet views (45° oblique)—Iliac oblique and obturator oblique views (**Figure 22**)
         - Iliac oblique view allows visualization of posterior column, anterior wall, sciatic notch, and iliac fossa.
         - Obturator oblique view demonstrates the anterior column, posterior wall, and obturator sulcus.
         - When obtained properly, the iliac oblique view of one side has the obturator oblique view of the contralateral side on the same radiograph.
      c. CT scans confirm the articular pattern, highlight articular comminution, marginal impaction, and presence of occult ipsilateral femoral head fractures, and help detect loose bony fragments within the acetabulum. CT also can exclude the presence of associated pelvic ring injuries, which may be present in approximately 30% of acetabular fractures.
      d. Stress examination may be useful to determine hip stability in small posterior wall acetabular fractures
         - Patient is placed supine on a radiolucent table with C-arm on side ipsilateral to injured hip (**Figure 3**).
         - AP and obturator oblique views of the hip are obtained.
         - Surgeon stands on contralateral side while adducting, flexing, and internally rotating

TABLE 4

Description of the Radiographic Lines Used for Evaluating Acetabular Fractures

Radiographic Line	Anatomic Structure	Comment
Posterior border of acetabulum	Posterior wall	Usually peripheral to the anterior wall Inferiorly overlies the outline of the upper ischial tuberosity
Anterior border of acetabulum	Anterior wall	Peripherally more transverse than the posterior border Medially confluent with the lower border of the teardrop
Roof	Acetabular dome	Represents only 2-3 mm of the cranial dome Does not indicate overall dome integrity
Teardrop (radiographic U)	None	External limb—outer cotyloid fossa Internal limb—outer wall of the obturator canal merging to the quadrilateral surface Lower border—located in the ischiopubic notch; forms the superior border of the obturator foramen
Ilioischial line	Posterior column	Results from beam tangent to a segment of the ischial quadrilateral surface Cranially confluent with the iliopectineal line
Iliopectineal line (pelvic brim)	Anterior column	Between the symphysis and ilioischial line (anterior three-fourths of the pelvis), this line corresponds exactly with the anatomic brim Posterior one-fourth corresponds with a surface 1-2 cm caudal to the anatomic brim

the injured hip. Gentle axial force is applied while live fluoroscopy is used to assess for subluxation of the hip and/or joint incongruence.

G. Treatment

1. Surgical treatment

a. ORIF is indicated for fractures resulting in hip instability, at least 2 mm articular displacement, marginal impaction, or loose intra-articular fractures trapped within the joint.

b. Recent support for percutaneous management of minimally displaced acetabular fractures to facilitate mobility in multiply injured patients.

c. Total hip arthroplasty for select elderly patients.

2. Nonsurgical treatment

a. Indicated in minimally displaced (<2 mm) fractures.

b. Roof-arc angles—Fractures that do not involve the acetabular dome, defined as the

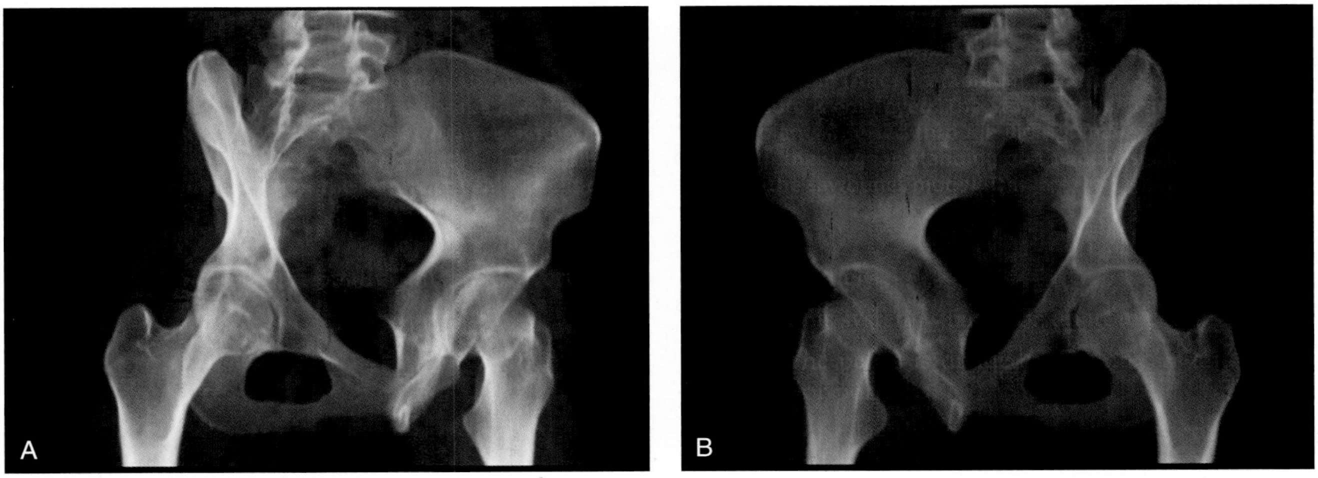

Figure 22 Judet views of the pelvis. **A**, Iliac oblique view demonstrates the anterior wall of the left acetabulum as well as the posterior column. **B**, Obturator oblique view demonstrates the anterior column of the left hip and a large displaced fracture of the left posterior wall. Notice that the iliac oblique of the injured hip also gives an obturator oblique of the contralateral hip, and vice versa.

area within a 45° roof arc or the cranial 10 mm of the acetabulum defined on CT.

c. Posterior wall acetabulum fractures may be treated nonsurgically in the absence of marginal impaction and with a negative stress examination performed under anesthesia with fluoroscopy.

d. Associated both-column acetabulum fractures may exhibit secondary congruence; anterior and posterior columns medialize and conform to the femoral head, resulting in acceptable alignment.

H. Rehabilitation

1. Weight-of-limb weight bearing is used on the side of the injured acetabulum.
2. Patients with bilateral acetabulum fractures practice bed-to-chair transfers only, using the upper extremities to mobilize.
3. Early postoperative continuous passive motion may be used to prevent joint stiffness.
4. Active knee and ankle motion may be initiated immediately.
5. Patients who undergo posterior exposure via a Kocher-Langenbeck procedure should be placed on posterior hip precautions for patient comfort, to protect the posterior repair, and to prevent redislocation.
6. After 6 to 10 weeks, or after radiographic healing has occurred, the patient may advance gradually from weight-of-limb weight bearing to full weight bearing.
7. Quadriceps, hip, and core strengthening should be introduced gradually as weight bearing is advanced.

I. Complications

1. Thromboembolic phenomena, same as seen in pelvic fractures
2. Heterotopic bone formation
   a. Most commonly occurs when patients undergo surgical fixation via a Kocher-Langenbeck procedure (**Figure 23**) or extended iliofemoral exposures; heterotopic bone formation after ilioinguinal exposure is rare.
   b. Patients who undergo more than one exposure to the acetabulum are also at increased risk for heterotopic bone formation.
   c. Prophylaxis options
      - Indomethacin 25 mg three times daily for 2 to 6 weeks
      - Radiation therapy (700 cGy); should be avoided in children or in women of childbearing age

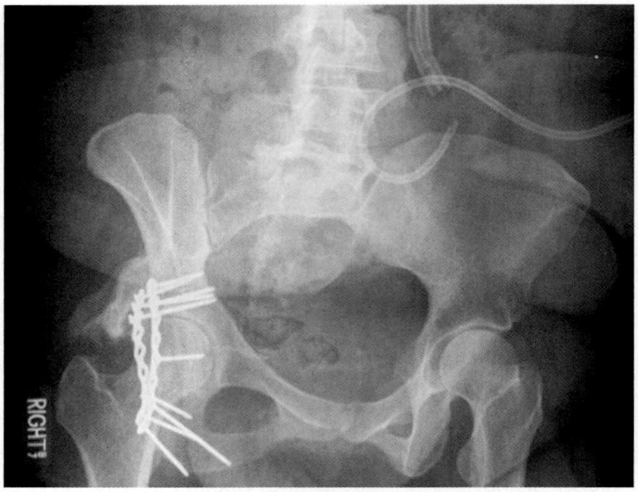

Figure 23 AP radiograph of a patient with heterotopic ossification following fixation for an acetabular fracture via a Kocher-Langenbeck exposure.

3. Femoral head aseptic necrosis
   a. Can occur most commonly when hip dislocation occurs in concert with acetabulum fracture.
   b. A dislocated femoral head should be reduced in an expedited fashion to minimize the thrombosis of vessels supplying the femoral head.
   c. Intraoperative dissection should avoid injury to the ascending branch of the medial femoral circumflex artery.
4. Nerve or vessel injury
   a. May be traumatic or iatrogenic.
   b. Careful handling of soft tissues is mandatory for preservation of nerve function (eg, keeping the hip extended and knee flexed during Kocher-Langenbeck exposure to protect the sciatic nerve).
   c. Retractors should be placed carefully. The use of self-retaining retractors should be sparse.

III. SACRAL FRACTURES

A. Epidemiology

1. Sacral fractures occur in 45% of injuries to the pelvic ring.
2. Some spare the pelvic ring and result from a direct blow (transverse sacral fracture, coccygeal fractures). These make up less than 5% of all sacral fractures.

B. Anatomy

1. The sacrum is roughly triangular in the coronal plane.

7 | Trauma

2. In the sagittal plane, the sacral anatomy varies but has some degree of lordosis, especially in the caudal segments.
3. Sacral nerve root tunnels arise from the sacral canal and proceed from midline, cranial, and posterior to lateral, caudal, and peripheral.

C. Fracture classification

1. Sacral fractures generally are organized into three categories.
    a. Fractures associated with pelvic ring injuries
    b. Fractures involving the lumbosacral junction
    c. Fractures intrinsic to the sacrum
2. Sacral fractures associated with pelvic fractures are frequently vertical in nature. They are described by the AO/OTA, Young-Burgess, or Letournel classification systems (see Section I.C).
3. Fractures involving the lumbosacral junction are best classified using the Isler system. This classification describes the fracture line in reference to the L5-S1 facet (**Figure 24**).
    a. Type I fractures are lateral to the facet.
        - These are unlikely to affect lumbosacral stability.
        - When combined with ramus fractures, they may affect pelvic ring stability.
    b. Type II fractures traverse the L5-S1 facet.
        - Extra-articular fractures of the lumbosacral junction
        - Articular dislocation with facet displacement
    c. Type III fractures are medial to the facet.
        - This fracture type has increased potential to result in substantial instability.
        - Bilateral fractures may result in lumbosacral dissociation.
4. Fractures intrinsic to the sacrum typically are classified according to the system of Denis. This system describes the fracture's relationship to the sacral nerve root tunnels (**Figure 25**).
    a. Zone I fractures are lateral to the sacral nerve roots.
        - This is the most common of the fracture locations (50% of the original series by Denis et al).
        - Nerve root deficits occurred in 6% of cases and involved the L5 root or sciatic nerve.
    b. Zone II fractures pass through the neural foramina.
        - Zone II fractures are the second most common fracture type (34% of fractures) in the series by Denis et al.

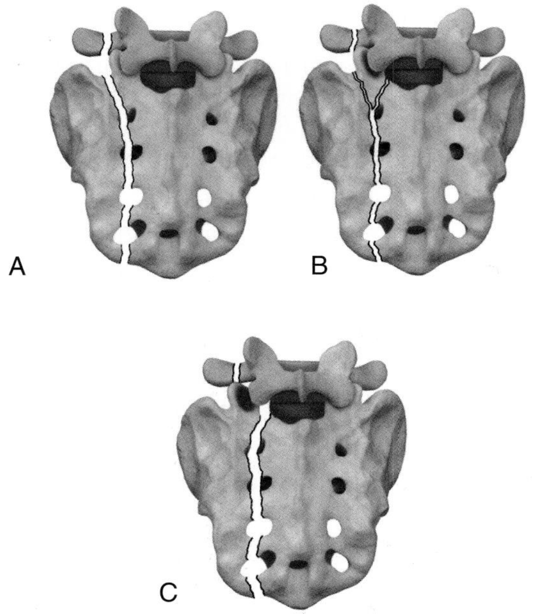

Figure 24 Illustrations depict the Isler classification system for sacral fractures. (**A**) Type I fracture, (**B**) Type II fracture, Type III fracture. (Reproduced with permission from Vaccaro AR, Kim DH, Brodke DS, et al: Diagnosis and management of sacral spine fractures: Instructional course lecture. *J Bone Joint Surg Am* 2004;86[1]:165-175.)

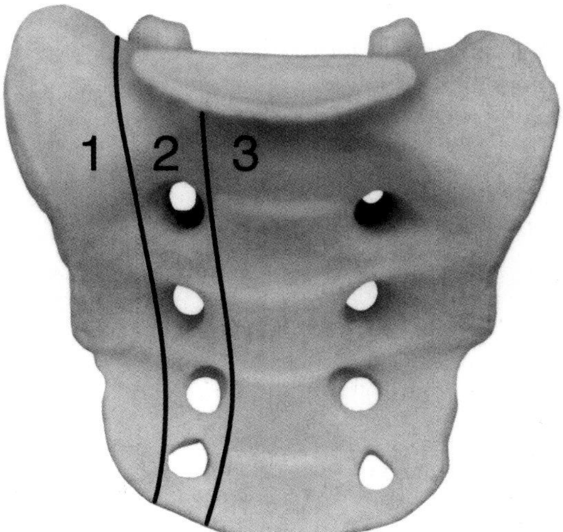

Figure 25 Illustration shows the sacral fracture classification system of Denis. 1= Zone I, 2 = Zone II, 3 = Zone III. (Reproduced with permission from Vaccaro AR, Kim DH, Brodke DS, et al: Diagnosis and management of sacral spine fractures: Instructional course lecture. *J Bone Joint Surg Am* 2004;86[1]:165-175.)

7 | Trauma

- Of these, 28% had unilateral L5, S1, or S2 injuries.
- Zone II fractures can be considerably unstable if a sheer component is present in the injury or if comminution is present in the fracture.

c. Zone III fractures are medial to the sacral nerve root tunnels.

- These fractures have the highest rate of neurologic deficits.
- Dysfunction of the bowel, bladder, and sexual organs occurs in 76% of patients with zone III fractures.
- A transverse component can exist within zone III fractures. These are often misdiagnosed as bilateral zone I or zone II fractures (which are actually quite rare). Strange-Vognsen and Lebach and Roy-Camille et al further classified the transverse portion of zone III injuries (**Figure 26**).

5. Fractures also can be classified by description of the letter they most closely resemble (**Figure 27**).

D. Mechanism of injury

1. Usually high energy: falls from a height, motor vehicle collisions, and motorcycle crashes. In patients with poor bone quality, sacral stress fractures may develop without supraphysiologic loading.
2. A direct blow or fall onto the sacrum may result in transverse fractures.
3. Insufficiency fractures may occur in patients with poor bone quality.

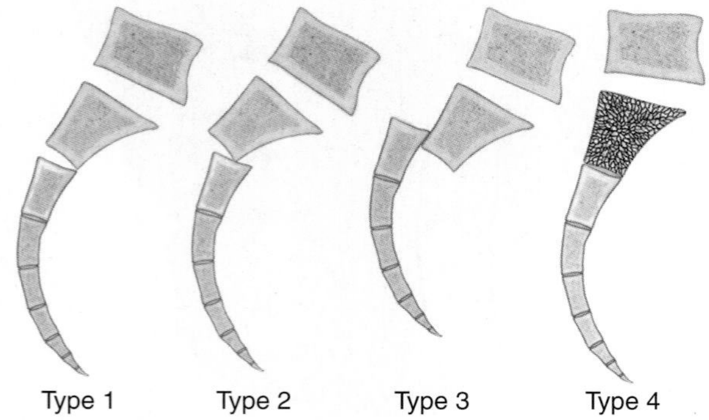

Figure 26 Illustrations show the subclassification of zone III injuries. (Reproduced with permission from Vaccaro AR, Kim DH, Brodke DS, et al: Diagnosis and management of sacral spine fractures: Instructional course lecture. *J Bone Joint Surg Am* 2004;86[1]:165-175.)

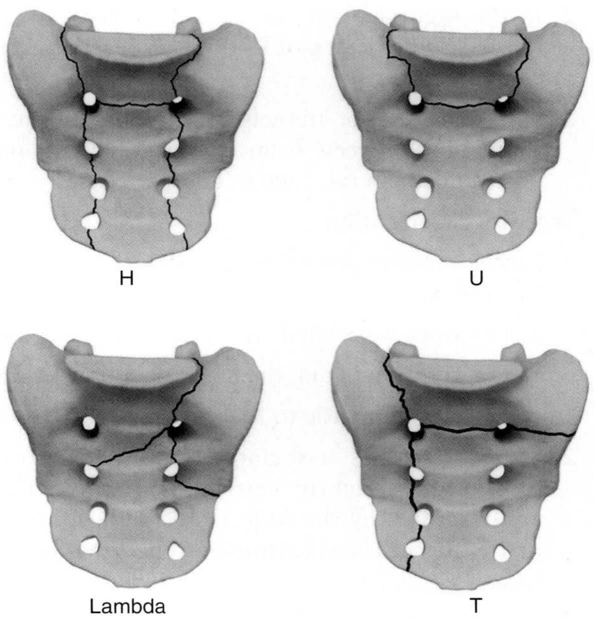

Figure 27 Illustrations show sacral fractures classified by the letter they most closely resemble. (Reproduced with permission from Vaccaro AR, Kim DH, Brodke DS, et al: Diagnosis and management of sacral spine fractures: Instructional course lecture. *J Bone Joint Surg Am* 2004;86[1]:165-175.)

E. Evaluation

1. Physical evaluation

a. Identical to that of pelvic ring injuries; pelvic stability should be assessed by manual stress examination; patient should undergo a full ATLS workup because of the high energy required to fracture the sacrum.

b. Sacral fractures can be missed at initial presentation, and up to 30% are diagnosed late.

c. Careful attention should be given to examination of the sacral nerve roots.

- A careful lower extremity examination, including motor function, sensory function, and reflexes, should be performed and documented.
- Neurologic examination includes a digital rectal examination.
  - This should document voluntary and spontaneous rectal sphincter contraction.
  - The presence of sensation to light touch and pinprick to concentric dermatomes of S2 to S5 should be documented.
- Reflexes including the bulbocavernosus and cremasteric should be examined.

d. Vascular examination of the bilateral lower extremities should be performed.

e. Soft tissues in the pelvic region and perineum should be thoroughly examined for occult open injuries. Closed internal degloving (Morel-Lavallee) lesions also may be present.

2. Imaging

a. AP, inlet, and outlet pelvic radiographs.

b. Sacral lateral view may be useful in transverse sacral body fractures or coccygeal fractures.

c. CT with coronal and sagittal reconstructions for evaluation of sacral nerve root tunnels and preoperative planning.

F. Treatment

1. When considering treatment options, sacral fractures may be categorized broadly into four subtypes.

a. Fractures associated with a pelvic ring injury

b. Fractures that also have a lumbosacral facet injury

c. Sacral fractures with an associated dislocation of the lumbosacral junction

d. Fractures with neurologic injury, persistent spinal cord injury, or cauda equina syndrome

2. For sacral fractures that are part of a pelvic ring injury, fracture treatment should coincide with treatment of the pelvic ring.

3. Fractures with lumbosacral facet injury

a. Stable injuries or those with minimal displacement may be treated nonsurgically.

b. Unstable injuries require surgical fixation to minimize the risk of residual facet incongruity.

4. Fractures with lumbosacral dislocation

a. Patients without debris in the nerve root tunnels or central canal may be treated with percutaneous fixation in situ.

b. Patients who have fractures with more displacement may require open treatment with decompression. Many techniques, including lumbopelvic fixation, have been described.

G. Rehabilitation

1. See Section I.F.6 on pelvic fractures for sacral injuries that are part of a pelvic fracture.

2. Additional spinal cord rehabilitation may be needed for patients with neurologic deficits.

H. Complications

1. Infection occurs in 5% to 50% of surgical cases.

2. The incidence of sacral fracture nonunion is 10% to 15%.

3. Of patients sustaining a sacral fracture, 30% will have chronic pain.

TOP TESTING FACTS

1. The radiographic workup of a patient with a pelvic fracture includes AP, inlet, and outlet pelvic views as well as CT, which should be a confirmatory study to evaluate the fine detail of the posterior ring and occult injuries.
2. The initial management of pelvic fractures includes measures to minimize hemorrhage, including pelvic binders, sheets, and skeletal traction.
3. Young-Burgess anterior-posterior compression type III injuries have the highest fluid requirements as well as risk of hemorrhage and mortality.
4. Identification of the dysmorphic upper sacral segment is important in planning for the surgical treatment of the posterior pelvic ring.
5. The sacral lateral view is mandatory for placement of iliosacral screws in the upper sacral segment to avoid injury to the L5 and S1 nerve roots.
6. Acetabular fractures are most often classified according to the system of Judet and Letournel. The fractures are divided into elementary and associated patterns.
7. Judet views of the pelvis allow detailed understanding of the acetabular injury pattern. The obturator oblique view demonstrates the anterior column and posterior wall, whereas the iliac oblique view demonstrates the posterior column and anterior wall.

8. CT should be obtained as part of the radiographic workup and will demonstrate marginal impaction, articular comminution, bony fragments contained within the joint, and impaction lesions of the femoral head.
9. Small or peripheral posterior wall acetabular fractures may be treated nonsurgically in the absence of marginal impaction and with a negative, fluoroscopically assisted stress examination performed under anesthesia.
10. Lumbopelvic fixation may be required in addition to decompression for sacral fractures with nerve root or central canal deficit and anatomic compromise.

Bibliography

Avilucea FR, Archdeacon MT, Collinge CA, Sciadini M, Sagi HC, Mir HR: Fixation strategy using sequential intraoperative examination under anesthesia for unstable lateral compression pelvic ring injuries reliably predicts union with minimal displacement. *J Bone Joint Surg Am* 2018;100(17):1503-1508.

Berger-Groch J, Thiesen DM, Grossterlinden LG, Schaewel J, Fensky F, Hartel MJ: The intra- and interobserver reliability of the Tile AO, the Young and Burgess, and FFP classifications in pelvic trauma. *Arch Orthop Trauma Surg* 2019;139(5):645-650.

Bruce B, Reilly M, Sims S: OTA highlight paper predicting future displacement of nonoperatively managed lateral compression sacral fractures: Can it be done? *J Orthop Trauma* 2011;25(9):523-527.

Burgess AR, Eastridge BJ, Young JW, et al: Pelvic ring disruptions: Effective classification system and treatment protocols. *J Trauma* 1990;30(7):848-856.

Butler BA, Lawton CD, Hashmi SZ, Stover MD: The relevance of the Judet and Letournel acetabular fracture classification system in the modern era: A review. *J Orthop Trauma* 2019;33(suppl 2):S3-S7.

Farrell ED, Gardner MJ, Krieg JC, Chip Routt ML Jr: The upper sacral nerve root tunnel: An anatomic and clinical study. *J Orthop Trauma* 2009;23(5):333-339.

Gardner MJ, Routt ML Jr: Transiliac-transsacral screws for posterior pelvic stabilization. *J Orthop Trauma* 2011;25(6):378-384.

Hermans E, Brouwers L, van Gent T, et al: Quality of life after pelvic ring fractures: Long-term outcomes. A multicentre study. *Injury* 2019. pii:S0020-1383(19)30174-3. doi:10.1016/j.injury.2019.04.002.

Koo H, Leveridge M, Thompson C, et al: Interobserver reliability of the Young-Burgess and tile classification systems for fractures of the pelvic ring. *J Orthop Trauma* 2008;22(6):379-384.

Letournel E: Acetabulum fractures: Classification and management. *Clin Orthop Relat Res* 1980;151:81-106.

Marsh JL, Slongo TF, Agel J, et al: Fracture and dislocation classification compendium – 2007: Orthopaedic Trauma Association classification, database and outcomes committee. *J Orthop Trauma* 2007;21(10, suppl):S1-S133.

Matta JM, Anderson LM, Epstein HC, Hendricks P: Fractures of the acetabulum: A retrospective analysis. *Clin Orthop Relat Res* 1986;205:230-240.

Mehta S, Auerbach JD, Born CT, Chin KR: Sacral fractures. *J Am Acad Orthop Surg* 2006;14(12):656-665.

Moed BR, Reilly MC: Acetabulum fractures, in Bucholz RW, Court-Brown CM, Heckman JD, Tornetta PT III, eds: *Rockwood and Green's Fractures in Adults*, ed 7. Philadelphia, PA: Lippincott, Williams, & Wilkins, 2010, pp 1463-1523.

Morellato J, Hogue M, O'Toole RV, Sciadini MF, Nascone J: Anterior intrapelvic approaches: Fracture patterns you may want to reconsider. *J Orthop Trauma* 2019;33(suppl 2):S21-S26.

Nork SE, Jones CB, Harding SP, Mirza SK, Routt ML Jr: Percutaneous stabilization of U-shaped sacral fractures using iliosacral screws: Technique and early results. *J Orthop Trauma* 2001;15(4):238-246.

Pastor T, Tiziani S, Kasper CD, Pape HC, Osterhoff G: Quality of reduction correlates with clinical outcome in pelvic ring fractures. *Injury* 2019. pii:S0020-1383(19)30246-3.

Pennal GF, Tile M, Waddell JP, Garside H: Pelvic disruption: Assessment and classification. *Clin Orthop Relat Res* 1980;151:12-21.

Routt ML Jr, Falicov A, Woodhouse E, Schildhauer TA: Circumferential pelvic antishock sheeting: A temporary resuscitation aid. *J Orthop Trauma* 2002;16(1):45-48.

Suzuki T, Smith WR, Hak DJ, et al: Combined injuries of the pelvis and acetabulum: Nature of a devastating dyad. *J Orthop Trauma* 2010;24(5):303-308.

Vaccaro AR, Kim DH, Brodke DS, et al: Diagnosis and management of sacral spine fractures. *Instr Course Lect* 2004;53:375-385.

Wendt H, Gottschling H, Schröder M, et al: Recommendations for iliosacral screw placement in dysmorphic sacrum based on modified in-out-in corridors. *J Orthop Res* 2019;37(3):689-696.

Chapter 98

Hip Dislocations and Femoral Head Fractures

JOHN A. SCOLARO, MD, MA

I. HIP DISLOCATIONS

A. Epidemiology

1. Posterior dislocations represent 90% of all hip dislocations.
2. Most dislocations are secondary to motor vehicle accidents (MVAs); falls from height and sporting injuries are other common mechanisms of injury.

B. Anatomy and surgical approaches

1. Anatomy
   a. Strong capsular ligaments—The anterior iliofemoral and posterior ischiofemoral ligaments run from the acetabulum to the femoral neck (**Figure 1**).
   b. The ligamentum teres runs from the acetabulum (cotyloid fossa) to the femoral head (fovea centralis).
   c. The main arterial blood supply comes from the superior and posterior cervical arteries, which are primarily derived from the medial circumflex artery (posterior); a lesser contribution (10% to 15%) is made via the artery of the ligamentum teres (**Figure 2**).
2. Surgical approaches—for dislocations and fracture-dislocations, approach is based on location of pathology.
   a. Anterior (Smith-Petersen, Hueter)—commonly used surgical approach for associated anterior acetabular lesions, femoral neck and head fractures, posterior fracture-dislocations, and irreducible fracture-dislocations. Anterior dislocation of the femoral head allows reduction and fixation of most lesions.
   b. Lateral (surgical dislocation)—allows visualization of the femoral head as well as the anterior and posterior acetabulum. Commonly used when there is an associated acetabular fracture that requires fixation.
   c. Posterior approach (Kocher-Langenbeck)—provides access to the posterior femoral neck, acetabulum, and soft tissues but limited access to the articular surface of the femoral head for fracture reduction and fixation.

C. Mechanism of injury

1. Anterior dislocations
   a. These dislocations result from an abduction and external rotation force.
   b. A flexed hip leads to an inferior (obturator) dislocation; an extended hip results in a superior (pubic) dislocation.
   c. Femoral head impaction or osteochondral fractures are commonly seen.
2. Posterior dislocations
   a. Posterior dislocations are most commonly seen after dashboard injuries, in which the knee strikes the dashboard, resulting in a posteriorly directed force through the femur.
   b. The presence of an associated fracture, as well as the location and extent of the fracture, is dictated by the flexion, abduction, and rotation of the hip joint at the time of the impact. Increased flexion and adduction favor a pure dislocation without fracture of the posterior wall.

Dr. Scolaro or an immediate family member has received royalties from Globus Medical and serves as a paid consultant to or is an employee of Globus Medical, Smith & Nephew, Stryker, and Zimmer.

This chapter is adapted from Ostrum RF: Hip dislocations and femoral head fractures, in Boyer MI, ed: *AAOS Comprehensive Orthopaedic Review*, ed 2. Rosemont, IL, American Academy of Orthopaedic Surgeons, 2014, pp 387-394.

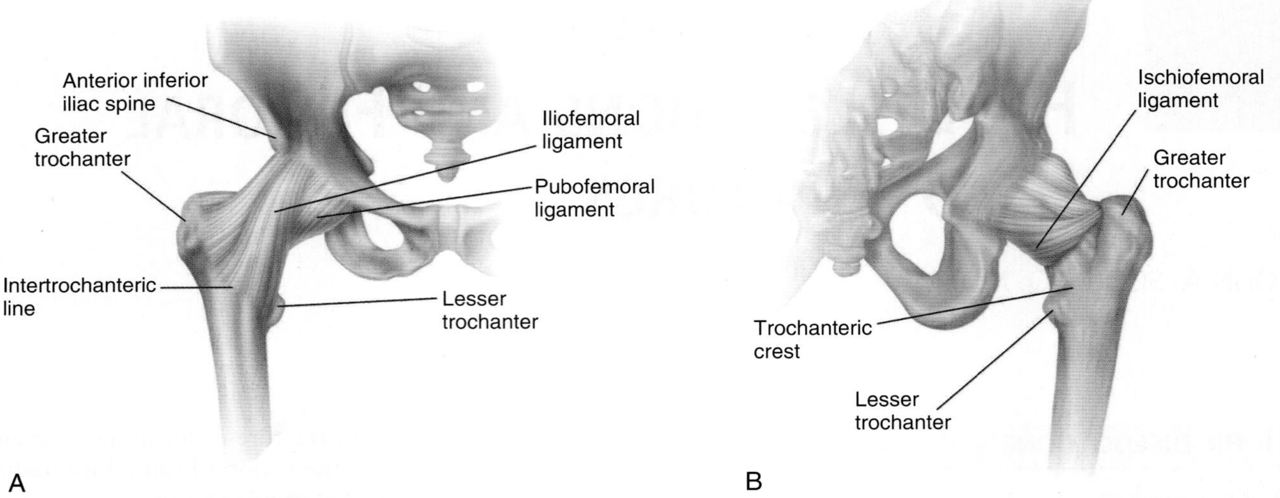

Figure 1 Illustrations show the hip capsule and its thickenings (ligaments) as visualized anteriorly (**A**) and posteriorly (**B**).

D. Clinical evaluation

1. Native hip dislocation is an orthopaedic surgical emergency and timely reduction is necessary.
2. Anterior hip dislocations present with the leg in a flexed (inferior) or extended (superior), abducted, and externally rotated attitude.
3. Posterior hip dislocations present with the limb in an adducted and internally rotated position.
4. In the setting of an irreducible fracture or fracture-dislocation, the hip and knee are commonly slightly flexed with the leg shortened and in neutral rotation.
5. Sciatic nerve injury may be seen in 8% to 20% of patients; prereduction and postreduction neurologic examinations should be documented.
6. A high percentage of patients sustain associated ipsilateral knee pathology.
   a. Examination of the knee should be performed following hip reduction.
   b. Advanced imaging should be performed, if necessary, for diagnosis. Knee effusion, osseous contusion, and meniscal pathology are most common.

E. Imaging evaluation

1. Standard AP radiographs show dislocation of the femoral head.
   a. The limb position and femoral head appearance can be used to distinguish an anterior from a posterior dislocation.
   b. In posterior dislocations, the femoral head appears smaller than the contralateral hip (if unaffected) on a standard AP radiograph and is located superiorly.
   c. In anterior dislocations, the femoral head appears larger and overlaps the medial acetabulum or the obturator foramen.
   d. Irreducible femoral head fracture-dislocations without an associated acetabular fracture are identified by close apposition of the proximal femoral head to the supra-acetabular lateral iliac cortical bone.
2. Judet views (iliac and obturator oblique)
   a. These views can provide additional information regarding the location of the dislocation and identify associated acetabular pathology.
   b. The obturator oblique provides information about posterior dislocations and the posterior wall, whereas the iliac oblique best shows an anterior dislocation and the anterior wall.
3. CT scans
   a. Should not delay hip reduction in simple dislocations and fracture-dislocations.
   b. Are performed following successful hip reduction and before surgical intervention for any irreducible dislocation.
   c. Provide important information about concentricity of reduction, bony or cartilaginous fragments within the joint, articular

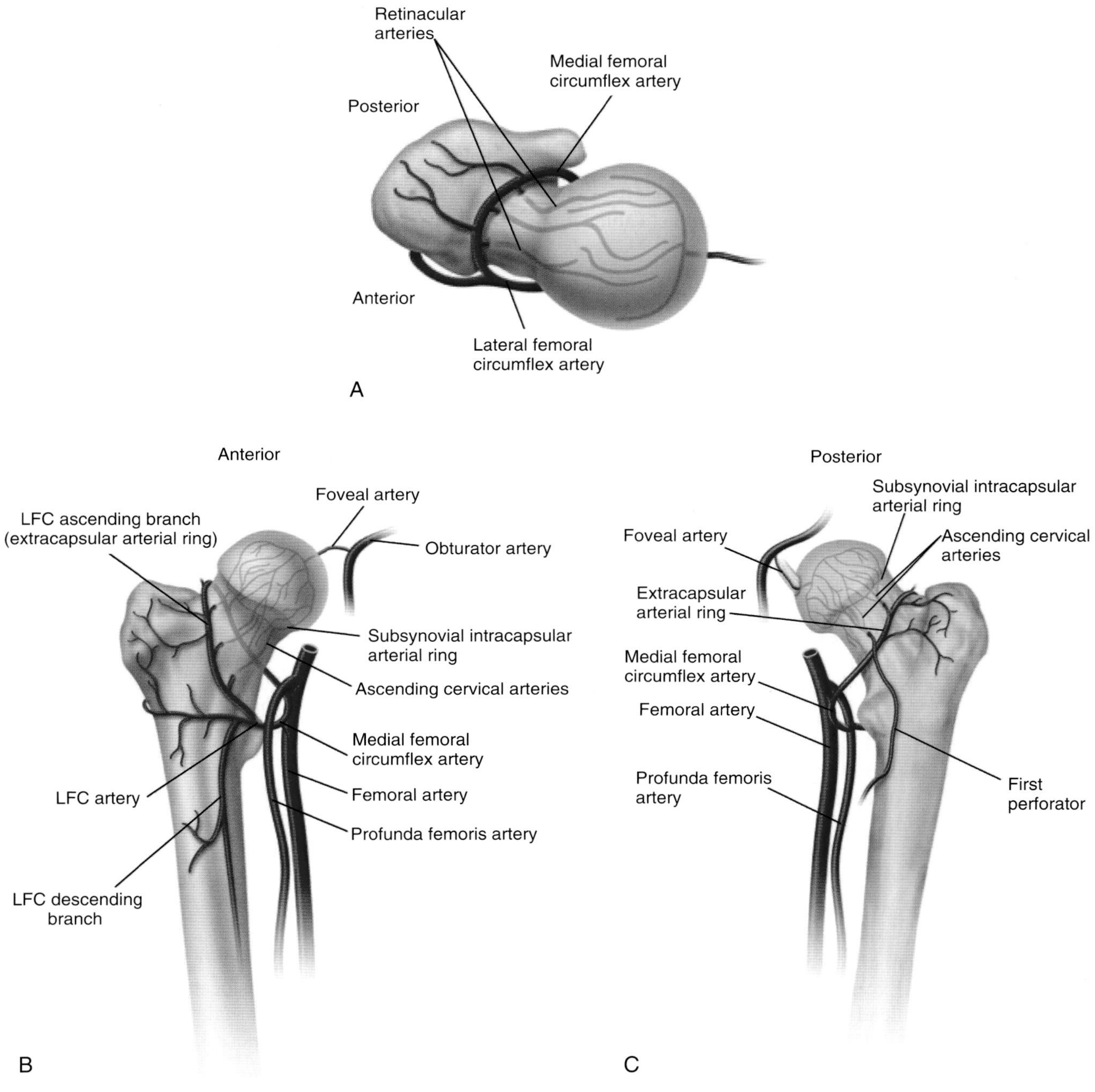

Figure 2 Axial (**A**), anterior (**B**), and posterior (**C**) illustrations depict the vascular supply to the femoral head, which arises from the medial and lateral circumflex vessels. These vessels create a ring, giving rise to the cervical vessels. A minor contribution comes from the obturator artery via the ligamentum teres. LFC = lateral femoral circumflex.

impaction of the femoral head or acetabulum, as well as acetabular, femoral head and/or neck fractures.

d. In the setting of an irreducible dislocation, valuable information can be obtained before surgery regarding a block to reduction or associated fracture of the femoral neck.

4. MRI

a. In the acute setting may have a role to identify damage to the hip labrum or the articular surface of the femoral head/acetabulum. In children and adolescents, MRI is effective in both identifying entrapped posterior soft tissues as well as unossified acetabular fragments following hip dislocation.

b. Commonly used in later follow-up to evaluate for osteonecrosis of the femoral head.

F. Classification

1. Hip dislocations are classified as anterior or posterior.
2. Thompson-Epstein classification is commonly used and also provides prognostic information (**Table 1**).

G. Treatment

1. Closed reduction

a. Prompt closed reduction is paramount and timing has been shown to affect the outcome.

b. Adequate sedation and pharmacologic muscle relaxation are necessary.

c. Reduction is performed by using inline traction on the lower extremity and re-creation of the position of the limb at the time of injury.

d. Several reduction maneuvers have been described for posterior dislocations. Commonly, with the patient in the supine position and pelvis stabilized, the hip is flexed, adducted, and internally rotated with constant inline traction. As the femoral reduces, the hip is externally rotated, extended, and abducted.

e. Following reduction of a posterior dislocation, the limb should be placed in extension, abduction, and external rotation. After reduction of an anterior dislocation, the limb is maintained in extension, abduction, and neutral or internal rotation. Traction is indicated for unstable injuries or for injuries with dome involvement.

f. If one or two closed reduction attempts with appropriate sedation/relaxation are unsuccessful, then an emergent open reduction is necessary. Excessive force, which can lead to femoral head or neck fractures, should be avoided.

TABLE 1

Thompson-Epstein Classification of Hip Dislocations

Type	Characteristics
I	Dislocation with or without minor fracture
II	Dislocation with single large fracture of the rim with or without a large major fragment
III	Dislocation with comminuted fracture of the rim with or without a large major fragment
IV	Dislocation with fracture of the acetabular floor
V	Dislocation with fracture of the femoral head

g. Irreducible dislocations are seen in up to 15% of patients. Irreducible anterior dislocations are due to interposed capsule or soft tissue. In posterior dislocations, reduction can be prevented by the capsule, labrum, adjacent short external rotators or, a bony fragment.

2. Surgical management

a. Indications include an irreducible dislocation, a nonconcentric hip joint due to entrapped soft tissue, cartilage or bone, hip instability, as well as otherwise operative femoral neck, head, or acetabular fractures.

b. Fluoroscopic examination under anesthesia can be used to determine hip stability following dislocation or to determine whether a dislocation with small associated femoral head or acetabular fracture requires surgical intervention.

c. Hip arthroscopy can be used to remove small entrapped osseous and cartilage fragments from within the hip joint, especially when surgical intervention is not otherwise indicated.

d. Open reduction and internal fixation of associated femoral or acetabular fractures should be performed through an approach from the direction of the dislocation.

- For posterior dislocations, the Kocher-Langenbeck approach is used.
- For anterior dislocations, an anterior (Smith-Petersen, Hueter), lateral, or anterolateral (Watson-Jones) approach is used.

H. Rehabilitation

1. Early mobilization and range of motion
2. Following posterior dislocations, hip hyperflexion, adduction and internal rotation is frequently avoided for 4 to 6 weeks.
3. Immediate or touchdown weight bearing is initiated for simple dislocations that do not require any surgical intervention.
4. Modified weight bearing is commonly implemented following operative or nonsurgical management of associated femoral or acetabular fractures.

I. Complications

1. Posttraumatic arthritis develops in 15% to 20% of patients because of cellular cartilage injury, nonconcentric hip reduction, or articular incongruity. Posttraumatic arthritis can develop years after the initial injury.

2. Osteonecrosis develops in approximately 2% to 10% of hips reduced within 6 hours.
   a. The rate of osteonecrosis increases with a delay in reduction.
   b. Osteonecrosis usually appears within 2 years after the injury but is commonly evident within a year.
3. Sciatic nerve injury
   a. More commonly affects the peroneal division.
   b. The injury is seen in 8% to 19% of posterior dislocations.
   c. It is more common with fracture-dislocations than with simple dislocations.
4. Recurrent instability is reported in 1% of patients.
5. Myositis and ectopic bone formation around the hip are uncommon unless other risk factors such as surgery, delayed reduction, or traumatic brain injury are present.

II. FEMORAL HEAD FRACTURES

A. Epidemiology
   1. Femoral head fractures occur in anywhere from 5% to 15% of patients with posterior hip dislocations.
   2. Commonly, femoral head fractures are produced by contact of the femoral head on the posterior rim of the acetabulum at the time of subluxation/dislocation.
   3. Anterior dislocations are more commonly associated with cranial and posterior impaction of the femoral head.
   4. Fractures can result from impaction, avulsions, or shear.
   5. Fracture size and location, as well as the degree of comminution, are determined by the force and direction of impact as well as the position of the femoral head at the time of dislocation.

B. Anatomy and surgical approaches—Similar to those for hip dislocations (Section I.B.3).

C. Mechanism of injury and clinical evaluation—Similar to those for hip dislocations.

D. Imaging evaluation—Similar to those for hip dislocations

E. Classification—The Pipkin classification system is used for femoral head fractures (**Figure 3**).

F. Treatment—Based on fragment location, size, displacement, and hip stability (**Table 2**).

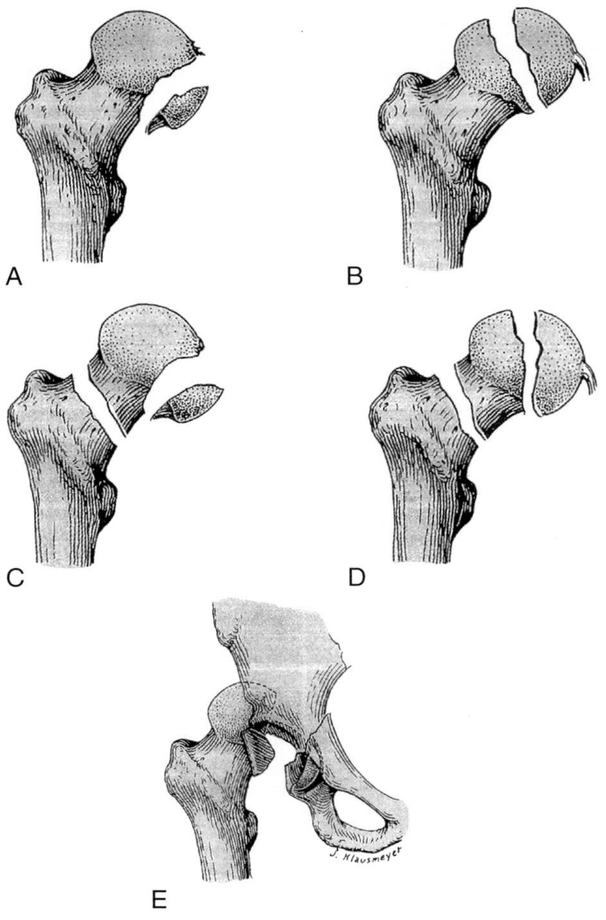

Figure 3 Illustration demonstrates the Pipkin classification of femoral head fractures. **A**, Intrafoveal fracture, Pipkin type I. **B**, Suprafoveal fracture, Pipkin type II. **C** and **D**, Intrafoveal fracture or suprafoveal fracture associated with femoral neck fracture, Pipkin type III. **E**, Any femoral head fracture configuration associated with an acetabular fracture, Pipkin type IV. (Reproduced with permission from Swionkowski MF: Intrascapular hip fractures, in Browner BD, Jupiter JB, Levine AM, Trafton PG, eds: *Skeletal Trauma: Basic Science, Management, and Reconstruction*, ed 2. Philadelphia, PA, WB Saunders, p 1756.)

1. Nonsurgical—reserved for small Pipkin I (infrafoveal) fractures where the hip joint is perfectly concentric and there is no concern that the fragment will block motion or become entrapped within the hip joint.
2. Fracture fragment excision—reserved for small Pipkin I (infrafoveal) fractures after closed reduction and for fragments unable to be fixed following open reduction and internal fixation of major femoral or acetabular fractures in Pipkin II–IV injuries.

TABLE 2

Treatment of Femoral Head Fractures Based on the Pipkin Classification

Type	Characteristics	Treatment
I	Infrafoveal, disruption of the ligamentum teres from the head fragment	Nonsurgical treatment is most common because this is not a weight-bearing fragment Non–weight bearing, hip precautions, progressive weight bearing May need excision of small fragments, fixation of large fragments because they can heal as a malunion and limit hip motion
II	Suprafoveal, ligamentum teres attached to head fragment	Countersunk screws for open reduction and internal fixation Usually Smith Petersen approach—optimizes fracture visualization and fixation, minimizes complication rate Periacetabular capsulotomy to preserve femoral head blood supply
III	Associated femoral neck fracture	Simultaneous open reduction and internal fixation of femoral head and neck through a Watson-Jones or Smith Petersen approach Consideration should be given to prosthetic replacement, especially in patients who are elderly, have osteoporosis, or have a comminuted fracture
IV	Associated acetabular fracture	Posterior Kocher-Langenbeck approach for acetabular fixation, excision of small infrafoveal fragments through this approach Small posterior wall fragments may be treated nonsurgically and suprafoveal fractures can then be treated through an anterior approach Use of anterior and posterior approaches together is controversial

3. Arthroscopic—can be used to excise small fragments; arthroscopically aided fixation of fracture fragments has also been described.
4. Internal fixation—commonly utilizes isolated small diameter headless compression screws or countersunk minifragment screws positioned below the articular surface.
5. Arthroplasty—should be considered for Pipkin III fractures as well as select patients with Pipkin IV fractures who may have severe preexisting arthritis, marginal impaction or who are elderly and would benefit from the ability to immediately bear full weight.

G. Rehabilitation

1. Immediate weight bearing may be allowed following nonsurgical management of small fracture fragments, isolated fragment excision, and arthroplasty.
2. Modified weight bearing for 6 to 8 weeks is usually recommended following femoral head fracture fixation or when fixation is performed of associated femoral or acetabular fracture.
3. Immediate early range of motion of the hip and strengthening of the abductors and quadriceps is important
4. Radiographs after 6 months to evaluate for osteonecrosis and arthritis

H. Complications

1. The anterior approach is associated with reduced surgical time, improved visualization, and fracture reduction, with decreased rates of osteonecrosis, but also with an increase in heterotopic ossification compared with the posterior approach. Heterotopic ossification is extra-articular, rarely bridges from pelvis to hip, and is rarely clinically significant.
2. Osteonecrosis
    a. Related to a delay in hip dislocation reduction.
    b. Occurs in up to 23% of patients, depending on the injury, dislocation, and time to relocation and definitive treatment.
    c. Patients should be counseled about this complication preoperatively.
    d. Most common following Pipkin III fractures.
3. Fixation failure is associated with osteonecrosis or nonunion.
4. Posttraumatic arthritis is a result of joint incongruity or initial cartilage damage.

Decreased range of motion—uncommonly clinically significant; decreased hip internal rotation most frequently identified.

TOP TESTING FACTS

Hip Dislocations and Femoral Head Fractures

1. Posterior hip dislocation is more common than anterior dislocation.
2. Delayed reduction of a hip dislocation, or fracture-dislocation, increases the risk of osteonecrosis and long-term sequelae.
3. The most common maneuver to reduce a posterior hip dislocation is flexion, adduction, and internal rotation.
4. Postreduction CT scan of the hip provides information about intra-articular fragments, reduction concentricity, and associated injuries.
5. Hip arthroscopy can be successfully performed to remove intra-articular osseous or free cartilage fragments within the hip, as well as infrafoveal femoral head fracture fragments.
6. Hip stability is best assessed in the operating room by performing a manipulation under anesthesia with fluoroscopic imaging.
7. In most patients, osteonecrosis is commonly seen by 1 year following injury; posttraumatic arthritis may develop at any point later.
8. The Smith Petersen approach and surgical dislocation are the most commonly used approaches to address femoral head fractures; approach is based on fracture location and whether an associated acetabulum fracture requires fixation.
9. Femoral head fixation is most commonly performed with headless compression or countersunk minifragment screws.
10. Pipkin III fractures have a high rate of osteonecrosis and fixation failure; arthroplasty should be considered for these injuries.
11. Non-bridging ectopic bone is commonly seen following fixation of femoral head fractures, especially following an anterior Smith-Petersen approach; it is rarely bridging or clinically significant.

Bibliography

Bastian JD, Turina M, Siebenrock KA, Keel MJ: Long-term outcome after traumatic anterior dislocation of the hip. *Arch Orthop Trauma Surg* 2011;131(9):1273-1278.

Khanna V, Harris A, Farrokhyar F, Choudur HN, Wong IH: Hip arthroscopy: Prevalence of intra-articular pathologic findings after traumatic injury of the hip. *Arthroscopy* 2014;30(3):299-304.

Mandell JC, Marshall RA, Banffy MB, Khurana B, Weaver MJ: Arthroscopy after traumatic hip dislocation: A systematic review of intra-articular findings, correlation with magnetic resonance imaging and computed tomography, treatments, and outcomes. *Arthroscopy* 2018;34(3):917-927.

Marecek GS, Scolaro JA, Routt ML Jr: Femoral head fractures. *JBJS Rev* 2015;3(11).

Scolaro JA, Marecek G, Firoozabadi R, Krieg JC, Routt MLC: Management and radiographic outcomes of femoral head fractures. *J Orthop Traumatol* 2017;18(3):235-241.

Tannast M, Pleus F, Bonel H, Galloway H, Siebenrock KA, Anderson SE: Magnetic resonance imaging in traumatic posterior hip dislocation. *J Orthop Trauma* 2010;24(12):723-731.

Thompson VP, Epstein HC: Traumatic dislocation of the hip; a survey of two hundred and four cases covering a period of twenty-one years. *J Bone Joint Surg Am* 1951;33(3):746-778.

Chapter 99
FRACTURES OF THE HIP

STEVEN J. MORGAN, MD

I. GENERAL CONSIDERATIONS

A. Epidemiology

1. Hip fractures occur most commonly in patients 70 years or older.
2. The risk of hip fracture increases with decreasing bone mass.
3. Hip fractures are more common in women.
4. Intertrochanteric femur fractures account for approximately 50% of all proximal femur fractures.
5. Femoral neck fractures are slightly less common and account for approximately 40% of proximal femur fractures.

B. Anatomy

1. Fractures of the proximal femur are distinguished by their anatomic location in relationship to the joint capsule.
   a. Femoral neck fractures are considered intracapsular fractures, which are at higher risk of nonunion. Because of the absence of a periosteal or extraosseous blood supply, no callus forms during healing. Fracture healing occurs by intraosseous bone healing.
   b. Intertrochanteric fractures are considered extracapsular fractures. Callus formation is common in these fracture patterns, and nonunion is rare because of the absence of synovial fluid and the presence of an abundant blood supply.
2. Vascular anatomy (**Figure 1**)
   a. The medial femoral circumflex artery is the main blood supply to the femoral head. This artery terminates in the posterior aspect of the extracapsular arterial ring.
   b. The lateral femoral circumflex artery gives rise to the anterior aspect of the arterial ring.
   c. The superior and inferior gluteal arteries also contribute branches to the ring.
   d. The ascending cervical arteries originate from the extracapsular arterial ring and are divided into four distinct groups based on their anatomic relationship to the femoral neck: lateral, medial, posterior, and anterior. The lateral group of ascending branches is the main blood supply to the femoral head.
   e. The ascending branches give off multiple perforator vessels to the femoral neck and terminate in the subsynovial arterial ring located at the margin of the articular surface of the femoral head. The lateral epiphyseal artery then penetrates the femoral head and is believed to be the dominant blood supply to the femoral head from this system. Fractures that disrupt the ascending blood flow to the lateral epiphyseal vessel have an increased risk of osteonecrosis.
   f. The artery of the ligamentum teres arises from either the obturator or medial femoral circumflex artery. It does not provide sufficient blood supply to maintain the viability of the femoral head.

C. Surgical approaches

1. The anterior lateral (Watson Jones) approach is used for the open reduction and internal fixation (ORIF) of femoral neck fractures or hemiarthroplasty.
   a. This approach is based on the interval between the gluteus medius and the tensor fascia lata. No internervous plane is present because both muscles are innervated by the superior gluteal nerve.
   b. The superior gluteal nerve can be damaged if the intermuscular plane is extended to the iliac crest.

Dr. Morgan or an immediate family member serves as a paid consultant to or is an employee of Acumed, LLC and has stock or stock options held in Johnson & Johnson.

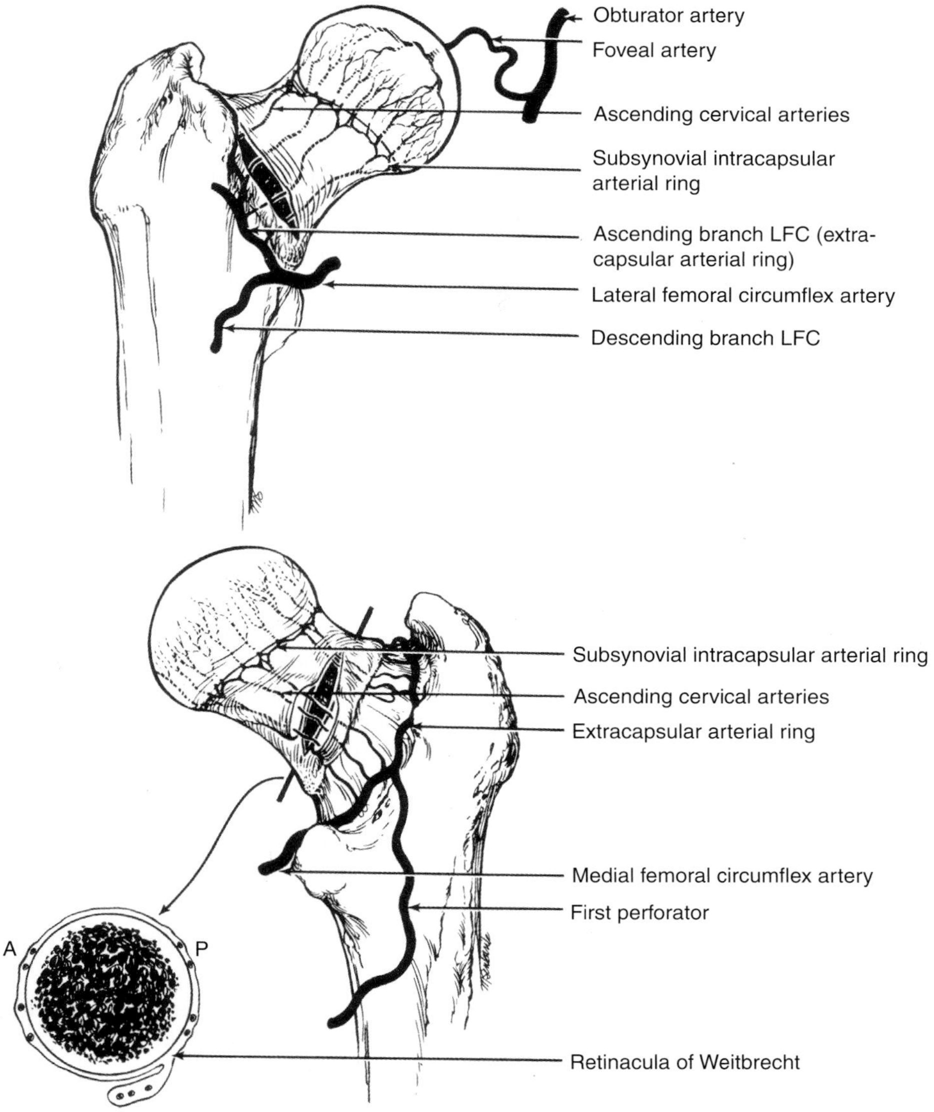

Figure 1 Illustrations depict the vascular anatomy of the femoral head and neck. LFC = lateral femoral circumflex artery. (Reproduced with permission from DeLee JC: Fractures and dislocations of the hip, in Rockwood CA Jr, Green DP, Bucholz RW, Heckman JD, eds: *Rockwood and Green's Fractures in Adults*, ed 4. Philadelphia, PA, Lippincott Williams & Wilkins, 2001, p 1662.)

2. The anterior (Smith-Petersen) approach can be used for ORIF of the femoral neck or hemiarthroplasty. If used for ORIF, a separate lateral approach to the proximal femur is required for fixation placement.
   a. The superficial dissection is between the tensor fascia lata (superior gluteal nerve) and the sartorius (femoral nerve).
   b. The deep dissection is between the gluteus medius (superior gluteal nerve) and the rectus femoris (femoral nerve).
   c. The lateral femoral cutaneous nerve is at risk with this approach.
   d. The ascending branch of the lateral femoral circumflex artery is encountered between the tensor and the sartorius and must be sacrificed.
3. The lateral (Hardinge) approach is used primarily for hemiarthroplasty. This approach splits both the gluteus medius and the vastus lateralis, reflecting the anterior third of these structures medially. The superior gluteal nerve and artery are at risk in this approach.
4. The posterior (Southern) approach is used primarily for partial or total hip arthroplasty (THA).
   a. The approach splits the gluteus maximus muscle (inferior gluteal nerve) and the fascia lata.

b. The tendons of the piriformis, obturator internus, and the superior and inferior gemelli are transected at their point of insertion and retracted posteriorly to protect the sciatic nerve.

c. The sciatic nerve is the main structure at risk with this exposure.

5. The lateral approach to the proximal femur is used for ORIF of intertrochanteric femur fractures.

a. This is a direct lateral approach that splits the fascia lata and either elevates the vastus lateralis from posterior to anterior or splits the muscle fibers.

b. No internervous plane is present; the vastus lateralis is innervated by the femoral nerve.

D. Hip biomechanics

1. The mean femoral neck-shaft angle in the adult is 130° ± 7°. The mean anteversion of the neck is 10° ± 7°.

2. Forces on the proximal aspect of the femur are complex. The osseous structure itself also is complex, consisting of both cortical and cancellous bone.

a. The two prime trabecular groups of the proximal femur are the principal tensile group and the principal compressive group. Secondary compressive and tensile trabecular groups (**Figure 2**) also exist. These trabecular bone patterns are the result of bone's response to stress, expressed as Wolff's law.

b. The weakest area in the femoral neck is located in the Ward triangle.

c. The calcar femorale is a medial area of dense trabecular bone that transfers stress from the femoral shaft to the inferior portion of the femoral neck.

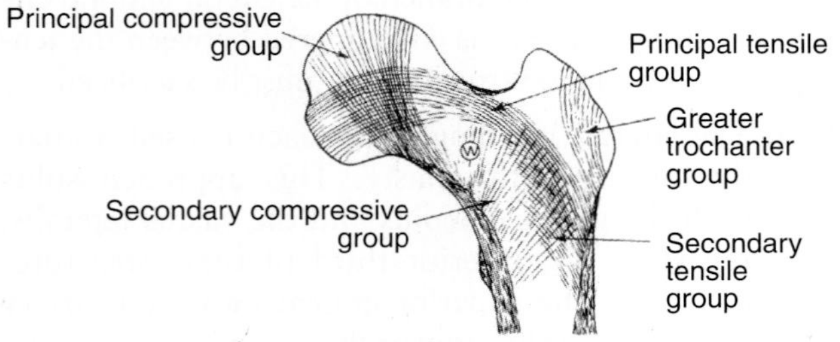

Figure 2 Illustration shows the trabecular groups of the proximal femur. W = the Ward triangle. (Adapted with permission from Singh M, Nagrath AR, Maini PS: Changes in trabecular pattern of the upper end of the femur as an index of osteoporosis. *J Bone Joint Surg Am* 1970;52:457-467.)

d. Fractures of the proximal femur follow the path of least resistance.

e. The amount of energy absorbed by the bone determines the degree of comminution.

3. Standing position

a. The center of gravity is located at the midpoint between the two hips.

b. The weight of the body is supported equally by both hips.

c. The force vector acting on the hip is vertical.

d. The Y ligament of Bigelow resists hyperextension. Minimal muscle forces are required for balance in a symmetric stance, and the joint reactive force or compressive force across the hip is approximately one-half the body weight.

4. Single-leg stance

a. The center of gravity moves away from the hip. To counter the eccentric lever arm created by the weight of the body, the hip abductors function as stabilizers of the contralateral hemipelvis, contracting to maintain the pelvis in a level position. Because the lever arm created by the lateral offset of the greater trochanter is shorter than the lever arm created by the entire body opposite the hip, the magnitude of the muscle contracture is greater than the weight of the body. This results in a compressive load across the hip of approximately four times the body weight.

b. The resulting force vector in the standing phase is oriented parallel to the compressive trabeculae of the femoral neck.

c. In repetitive load situations, the tensile forces can cause microfractures in the superior femoral neck.

- Failure of these microfractures to heal in conditions of repetitive loading results in stress fracture.
- The frequency and degree of load influence the fatigue process.

5. Trendelenburg gait

a. Trendelenburg gait is noted when the hip abductors are no longer sufficient to counter the forces in single-leg stance. Without compensation, the pelvis cannot be maintained in a level position. Weakness of the abductors can be caused by disuse, paralysis, or by a diminished lever arm resulting from decreased femoral offset.

Oakes DA, Jackson KR, Davies MR, et al: The impact of the garden classification on proposed operative treatment. *Clin Orthop Relat Res* 2003;409:232-240.

Ong BC, Maurer SG, Aharonoff GB, Zuckerman JD, Koval KJ: Unipolar versus bipolar hemiarthroplasty: Functional outcome after femoral neck fracture at a minimum of thirty-six months of follow-up. *J Orthop Trauma* 2002;16(5):317-322.

Parker MJ, Handoll HH: Gamma and other cephalocondylic intramedullary nails versus extramedullary implants for extracapsular hip fractures in adults. *Cochrane Database Syst Rev* 2010;9:CD000093.

Rizzo PF, Gould ES, Lyden JP, Asnis SE: Diagnosis of occult fractures about the hip: Magnetic resonance imaging compared with bone-scanning. *J Bone Joint Surg Am* 1993;75(3):395-401.

Szita J, Cserhati P, Bosch U, Manninger J, Bodzay T, Fekete K: Intracapsular femoral neck fractures: The importance of early reduction and stable osteosynthesis. *Injury* 2002;33(suppl 3):C41-C46.

Tanaka J, Seki N, Tokimura F, Hayashi Y: Conservative treatment of Garden stage I femoral neck fracture in elderly patients. *Arch Orthop Trauma Surg* 2002;122(1):24-28.

Taylor F, Wright M, Zhu M: Hemiarthroplasty of the hip with and without cement: A randomized clinical trial. *J Bone Joint Surg Am* 2012;94(7):577-583.

Trueta J, Harrison MH: The normal vascular anatomy of the femoral head in adult man. *J Bone Joint Surg Br* 1953;35-B(3):442-461.

Vaidya SV, Dholakia DB, Chatterjee A: The use of a dynamic condylar screw and biological reduction techniques for subtrochanteric femur fracture. *Injury* 2003;34(2):123-128.

Zuckerman JD, Skovron ML, Koval KJ, Aharonoff G, Frankel VH: Postoperative complications and mortality associated with operative delay in older patients who have a fracture of the hip. *J Bone Joint Surg Am* 1995;77(10):1551-1556.

Chapter 100
Fractures of the Femoral Shaft and Distal Femur

MARK J. GAGE, MD
RICHARD S. YOON, MD

I. Fractures of the Femoral Shaft

A. Anatomy (**Figure 1**)

1. The bony anatomy of the femoral shaft includes an anterior bow.
2. Compartments of the thigh
   a. Anterior compartment contains the quadriceps muscles
   b. Posterior compartment contains the hamstrings
   c. Adductor compartment
3. Deforming forces
   a. The abductors (gluteus medius and minimus) insert on the greater trochanter and abduct the proximal segment.
   b. The iliopsoas inserts on the lesser trochanter and flexes the proximal fragment.
   c. The adductor longus, adductor brevis, gracilis, and adductor magnus have a broad area of insertion on the distal femur and contribute to a varus force on the distal segment.

Dr. Gage or an immediate family member serves as a paid consultant to or is an employee of Arthrex, Inc. and has received research or institutional support from AO, Arthrex, Inc., and Foundation for Orthopaedic Trauma. Dr. Yoon or an immediate family member is a member of a speakers' bureau or has made paid presentations on behalf of Surgical Care Affiliates (SCA); serves as a paid consultant to or is an employee of Arthrex, Inc., DePuy, A Johnson & Johnson Company, LIfeNet Health, Orthobullets, ORTHOXEL, Synthes, and Use-Lab; serves as an unpaid consultant to BuiltLean; has stock or stock options held in Taithera Inc.; and has received research or institutional support from Biomet, Coventus, Synthes, and Wright Medical Technology, Inc.

B. Mechanisms of injury

1. Typical femoral shaft fractures often are high-energy injuries, such as from a motor vehicle or motorcycle accident. The most common mechanism in motor vehicle accidents is impact of the knee against the car's dashboard. Associated injuries include pelvis/acetabulum fractures, hip fractures and/or dislocations, and fractures of the femoral head, distal femur, patella, tibial plateau, and knee ligaments.
2. A small percentage of fractures occur as a result of repeated stress, such as that experienced by a young military recruit or runner following an increase in the intensity of physical training.
3. Pathologic fractures may be the first presentation of metastatic cancer. Radiographs should be used to evaluate for bony lesions, particularly when the injury is not consistent with the mechanism.
4. A fall from a standing height is a common mechanism in the elderly, underscoring the need for emphasis of osteoporotic fracture prevention.
5. Atypical femoral fractures may occur in the femur from the lesser trochanter to the supracondylar flare and are due to relatively low mechanisms of injury in patients who have a history of prolonged (>3-5 years) diphosphonate use (please refer to chapter 105 "Geriatric Fracture Care" for more information).
6. Bilateral femur fractures historically had a mortality rate of up to 25%. Recent studies demonstrate lower death rates, of less than 7%.

This chapter is adapted from Cannada LK: Fractures of the femoral shaft and distal femur, in Boyer MI, ed: *AAOS Comprehensive Orthopaedic Review*, ed 2. Rosemont, IL, American Academy of Orthopaedic Surgeons, 2014, pp 1159-1176.

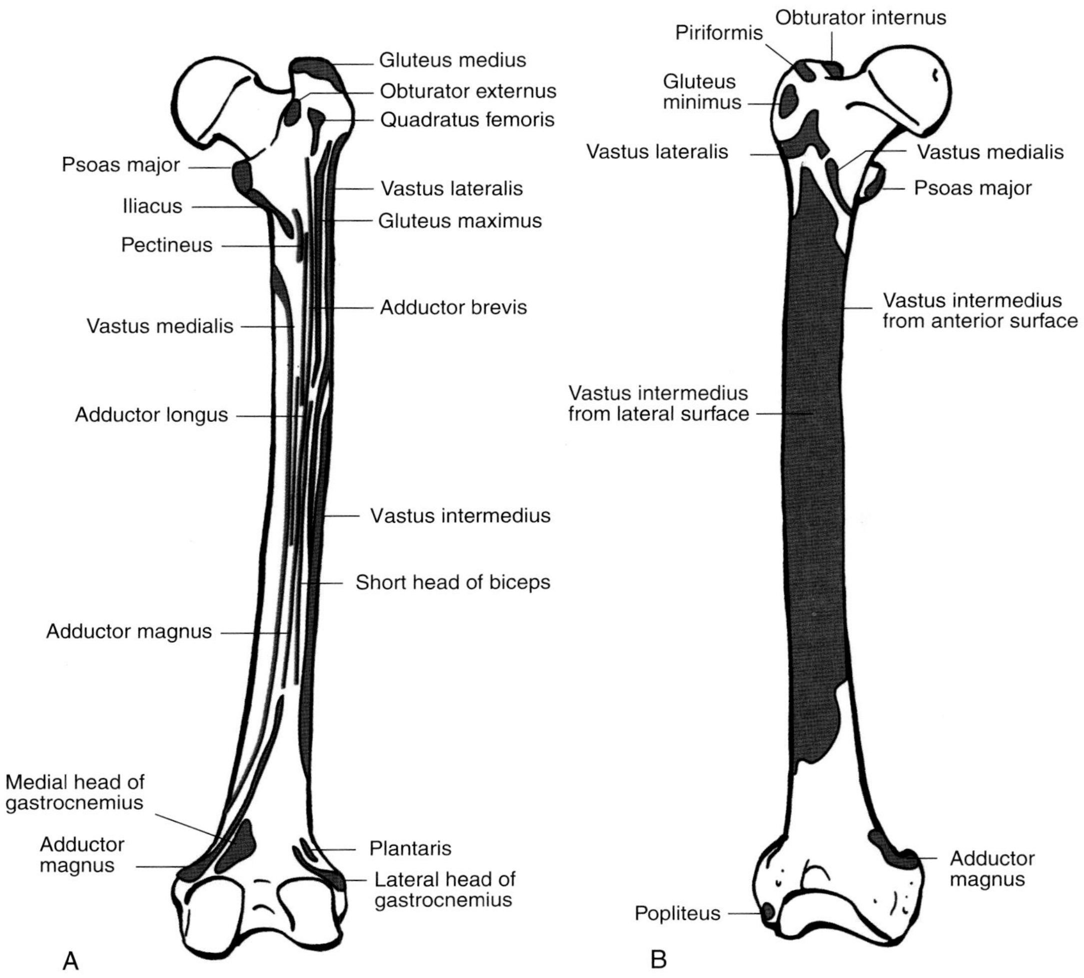

Figure 1 Illustrations depict the primary muscular attachments on the anterior (**A**) and posterior (**B**) aspects of the femur. (Adapted with permission from Nork SE: Fractures of the shaft of the femur, in Bucholz RW, Heckman JD, Court-Brown C, eds: *Rockwood and Green's Fractures in Adults*, ed 6. Philadelphia, PA, Lippincott Williams and Wilkins, 2001, p 1852.)

C. Clinical evaluation

1. Advanced Trauma Life Support principles should be initiated in patients with femoral shaft fractures.
2. Physical examination
   a. Obvious thigh deformity, with the limb shortened, rotated, and swollen compared with the contralateral extremity is a common presentation.
   b. The limb should be palpated for tenderness and deformity.
   c. The distal extremity should be evaluated for neurovascular integrity.
   d. The presence of pain to palpation, ecchymosis, crepitus, and deformity indicates that the patient should be examined for further injuries.
3. Additional injuries to the spine, pelvis, and ipsilateral lower extremity can occur, as can soft-tissue injuries, specifically ligamentous and/or meniscal injuries of the knee; therefore, patients with femur fractures always should be evaluated closely for associated injuries.
4. Ipsilateral femoral neck fracture occurs in about 5% of cases, but is still missed routinely (in up to 50% of patients).
   a. Initially, these fractures are nondisplaced or minimally displaced in up to 60% of patients.
   b. The femoral neck fracture often is vertically oriented.

D. Radiographic evaluation

1. An AP view of the pelvis and AP and lateral views of the femur, including the hip and knee joints, are indicated.

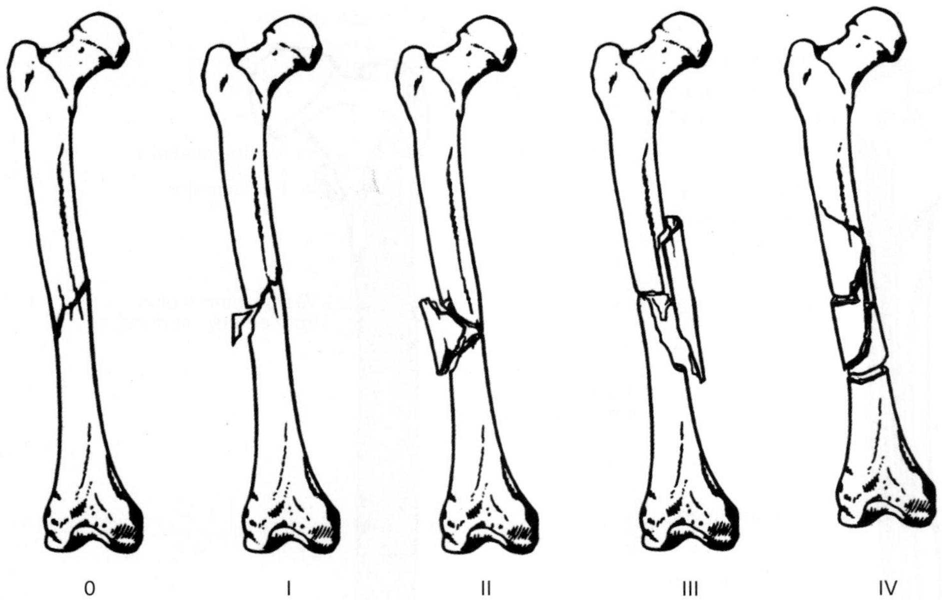

Figure 2 Illustrations show the Winquist and Hansen classification system of femoral shaft fractures. Type 0—no comminution; type I—minimal or no comminution; type II—at least 50% of the cortices intact; type III—comminution of at least 50% to 100% of the circumference of the bone; type IV—no cortical contact at the fracture site with circumferential comminution. (Reproduced from Poss R, ed: *Orthopaedic Knowledge Update*, ed 3. Park Ridge, IL, American Academy of Orthopaedic Surgeons, 1990, pp 513-527.)

2. The abdominal trauma CT may be used to evaluate the hip to detect associated nondisplaced femoral neck fracture following blunt trauma.

E. Fracture classification

1. The Winquist and Hansen classification system is based on the amount of comminution and has implications for weight-bearing status and the use of interlocking screws (**Figure 2**).
2. TheArbeitskinmeinshaftfurOsteosynthesisfragen/Orthopaedic Trauma Association (AO/OTA) Classification of Fractures and Dislocations is the internationally accepted system and useful in guiding treatment (**Figure 3**).

F. Nonsurgical treatment

1. Early stabilization (within the first 24 hours) of femur fractures minimizes the complication rates and can reduce the hospital length of stay.
2. Skeletal traction is a reasonable early treatment before skeletal stabilization.
3. A long period of bed rest may be detrimental, however, and patients should be monitored closely.
   a. Patients should be evaluated closely for pin tract infection and decubiti secondary to prolonged immobilization.
   b. Serial radiographs should be obtained to monitor for distraction at the fracture site during treatment.
   c. Mechanical and chemical deep vein thrombosis (DVT) prophylaxis should be instituted.

G. Surgical treatment

1. A statically locked, reamed intramedullary (IM) nail is the standard of care for femoral shaft fractures.
   a. Central placement of an IM nail within the femoral canal results in lower tensile and shear stresses on the implant.
   b. IM nailing has several benefits over plates and screws, including less extensive exposure and dissection, a lower infection rate, less quadriceps scarring, early functional use of the extremity, immediate full weight bearing, improved restoration of length and alignment with comminuted fractures, rapid fracture healing, and a low refracture rate.
   c. The starting point should be based on surgeon preference.
   d. At least two interlocking screws, one proximal and one distal, should be used for all fractures.
   e. For femur fractures with segmental comminution, multiple interlocking screws proximally and distally should be considered.
2. Retrograde approach
   a. Indications for this approach include multiple-system trauma; trauma to the ipsilateral extremity, pelvis/acetabulum, and/or spine; bilateral femur fractures; and morbid obesity.
   b. The overall union rate of retrograde nailing is comparable with that of antegrade nailing.

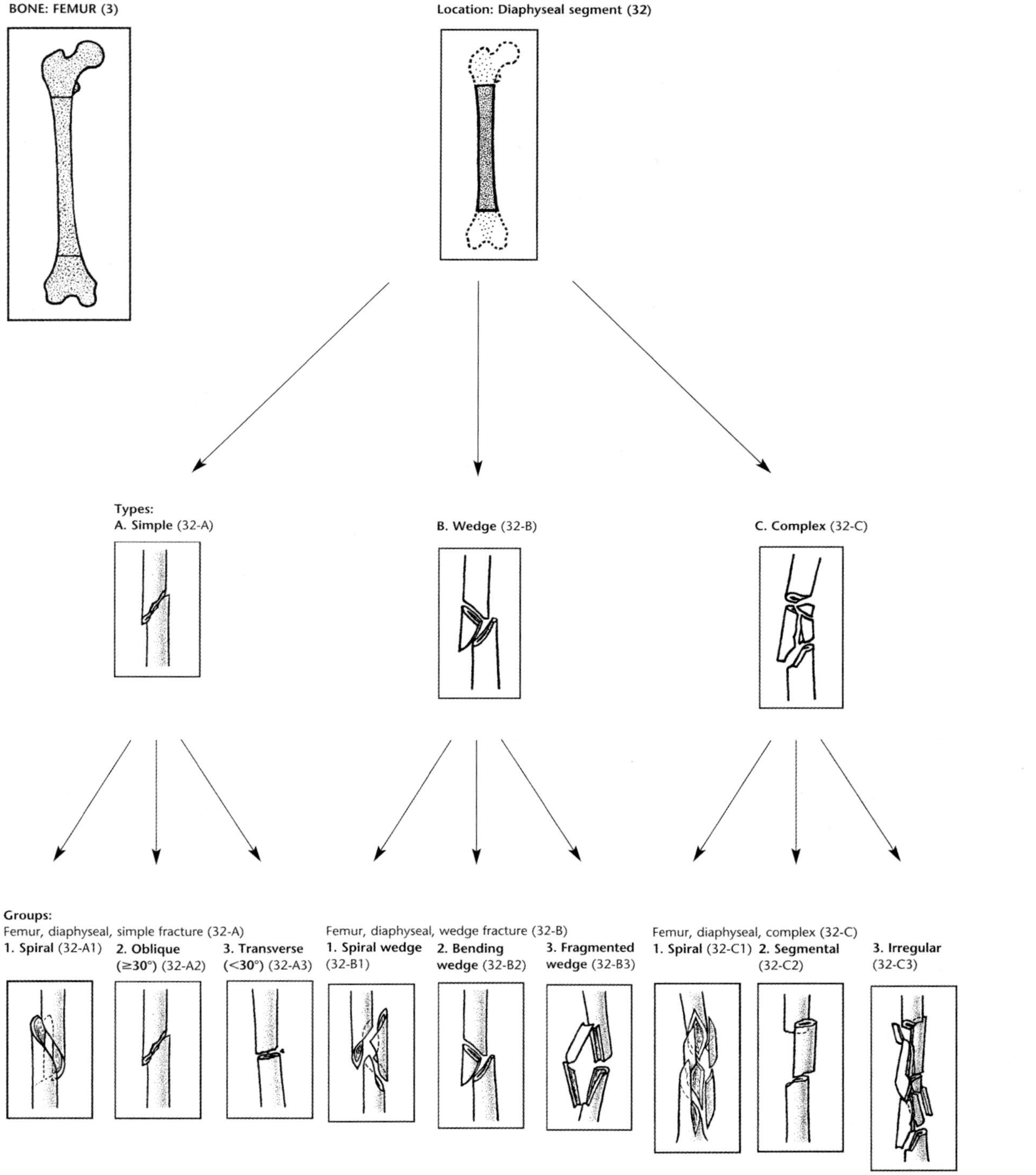

Figure 3 Diagram depicts the AO/OTA classification system of femoral shaft fractures.

c. The approach has several advantages, including ease of entry point, the potential for shorter surgical times, and the avoidance of using a fracture table.

d. The recommended starting point for retrograde nailing is 10 mm anterior to the posterior cruciate ligament in the intercondylar notch and in line with the femoral canal.

e. The optimum starting point in the lateral plane is just anterior to the Blumensaat line (**Figure 4**). The Blumensaat line can be visualized on the

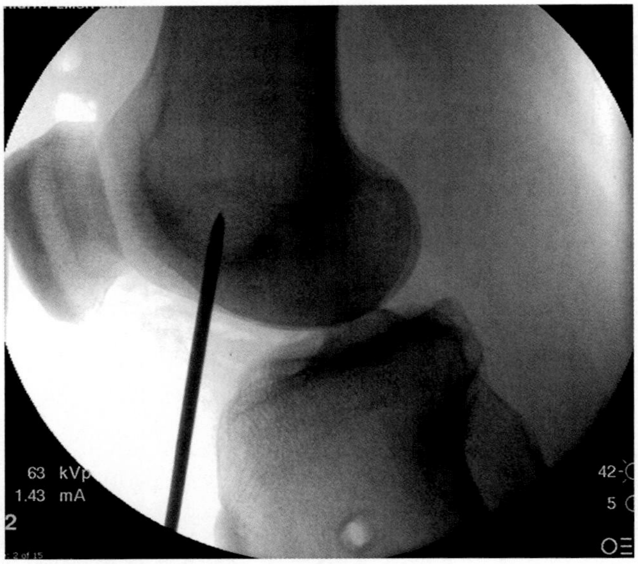

Figure 4 Fluoroscopic image demonstrates the lateral starting point for a retrograde intramedullary nail.

lateral view. The line represents the intercondylar notch roof.

f. A true lateral radiograph should be obtained preoperatively, with both femoral condyles overlapping and appearing as a single condyle. The radiograph should be reviewed preoperatively to assess for patella baja, which may interfere with a percutaneous incision and require an arthrotomy (rare).

g. Surgical pearls: A radiolucent triangle or bump should be strategically placed to assist with reduction; the prepatellar skin and patella should be protected during reaming by seating the reamer in bone before starting; before completion of surgery, in addition to fluoroscopic imaging of the femoral neck, an AP pelvis radiograph is recommended to rule out a femoral neck fracture. Limb rotation is best evaluated by comparing the lesser trochanter profile to the contralateral leg. In comminuted fractures, length should be evaluated and matched to the contralateral femur using a radio-opaque ruler. Finally, the knee should be checked for ligamentous injuries after skeletal stabilization of the femur.

h. Complications include malrotation and knee pain.

3. Antegrade—Piriformis entry point

a. This entry point is in line with the mechanical axis of the femur.

b. An excessively anterior entry point increases the risk for femoral neck fracture secondary to hoop stresses.

c. The piriformis entry point may result in more muscle and tendon damage and damage to the blood supply of the femoral head than the trochanteric entry point.

d. Using a piriformis entry point minimizes the risk of deformity, specifically varus, in proximal femoral fractures.

4. Antegrade—Trochanteric entry point

a. The main advantage over a piriformis entry point is that it is a more accessible starting point.

b. Potential complications include iatrogenic comminution with malreduction, anterior cortical penetration distally with nail curvature mismatch, and varus malreduction if the nail does not match the patient's anatomy. Modern implants with smaller radius of curvature are less likely to cause anterior cortical abutment.

H. Reamed versus nonreamed IM nailing

1. Reamed IM nailing is recommended over non-eamed nailing because it allows placement of a larger diameter nail with better cortical fit.

2. Reaming has been shown to improve rates of healing in femoral shaft fractures when compared with nonreamed nails.

3. Previous concerns with reaming included an increased incidence of acute respiratory distress syndrome (ARDS) and lung complications in patients who had associated pulmonary injury. A study comparing open reduction and internal fixation with reamed IM nailing in this patient population showed no increased incidence, however.

I. Flat table versus fracture table

1. Whether to use a fracture table or a fluoroscopic flat table is a decision to be made with all antegrade nailings. Studies support either choice.

2. Considerations include the fracture pattern, the patient's body habitus, the number of assistants available, associated injuries, and surgeon preference.

3. Multiple complications have been reported with the use of a fracture table, including pudendal nerve neurapraxia and compartment syndrome of the unaffected leg. Additionally, positioning a patient with multiple injuries on a fracture table can be difficult.

J. Plate and screw fixation
   1. Plate fixation of femur fractures is not used commonly and has few indications.
   2. Consider femoral plating for the following:
      a. Fracture involving the distal metaphyseal-diaphyseal junction of the femur
      b. Periprosthetic fracture
      c. Preexisting femoral deformity that would preclude passage of a nail
      d. Small or obliterated intramedullary canal
   3. Complications of compression plating
      a. Failure of fixation
      b. Infection
      c. Nonunion
      d. Devitalization of fracture fragments with excessive periosteal stripping
      e. Stress shielding with possible refracture

K. External fixation
   1. Most frequently used as temporizing skeletal stabilization as a form of orthopaedic damage control.
   2. Useful for the unstable trauma patient or in situations when the soft tissue envelope does not permit initial definitive fracture fixation.
   3. Facilitates greater mobilization and ease of care in the critically ill patient when compared with skeletal traction.
   4. Concerns regarding external fixation:
      a. Pin tract infection
      b. The timing of external fixation removal and conversion to IM nailing. The literature supports safe conversion to IM nailing within the first 2 weeks to minimize the risk for infection.

L. Ipsilateral femoral neck and shaft fractures
   1. Radiographic evaluation
      a. Most femoral neck fractures that are associated with an ipsilateral shaft fracture are vertically oriented and nondisplaced or minimally displaced, making radiographic detection difficult.
      b. Fine-cut CT may help detect femoral neck fractures before surgery.
   2. Treatment
      a. The timing of discovery of the femoral neck fracture has implications for its treatment.
      b. No matter when the fracture is discovered, it is essential to obtain an anatomic reduction and optimize femoral neck fracture stabilization.
      c. One device or two devices may be used. With one device, a cephalomedullary nail or a centromedullary nail with cannulated screws strategically placed around the nail may be used. With two devices, a retrograde nail with cannulated screws or a retrograde nail with a sliding hip screw construct is recommended.

M. Open femoral shaft fractures
   1. Open femoral shaft fractures should be treated with irrigation and débridement and primary IM nailing. This requires an incision that is adequate to allow visualization and débridement of the bone ends and the entire zone of injury.
   2. No increased rate of infection is seen with retrograde nailing of open femur fractures.
      a. Retrograde nailing does not increase risk of septic knee in the treatment of open femur fractures.
   3. The infection rate of open fractures of the femur is substantially lower than that of open tibia fractures.

N. Rehabilitation
   1. With stable fracture fixation, early mobilization and weight bearing are permitted. Most patients are allowed to bear weight to varying degrees, but associated injuries, the fracture pattern, implant selection, and surgeon preference dictate the exact postoperative rehabilitation orders.
   2. Early active motion of the hip and knee joint is encouraged.

O. Complications
   1. Fat embolism syndrome
      a. This usually occurs 24 to 72 hours after initial trauma in a small percentage of patients with long bone fractures.
      b. It can be fatal in up to 15% of patients.
      c. Diagnosis is based on the presence of at least one major and four minor criteria
      d. Major criteria: Hypoxemia, altered mental status, petechial rash, pulmonary edema
      e. Minor criteria: tachycardia, pyrexia, retinal emboli, fat in urine/sputum, thrombocytopenia, anemia

f. Treatment includes mechanical ventilation with high positive end-expiratory pressure levels.

g. Prevention involves early (within 24 hours) stabilization of long bone fractures.

2. Thromboembolism

a. DVT is a concern in trauma patients, especially those with long bone trauma, pelvic and acetabular fractures, and spine trauma. It may lead to a fatal pulmonary embolism (PE).

b. Duplex ultrasonography may be used to diagnose DVT.

c. In patients with suspected PE, a CT scan, ventilation-perfusion scan, or pulmonary angiogram (the benchmark) may be used for diagnosis.

d. The symptoms of a PE include acute-onset tachypnea, tachycardia, low-grade fevers, hypoxia, mental status changes, and chest pain.

e. Preventive measures include chemical prophylaxis (warfarin, subcutaneous heparin, low-molecular-weight heparin), sequential compression devices or foot pumps, and early surgical stabilization and subsequent mobilization, which are important, controllable measures.

3. Acute respiratory distress syndrome

a. ARDS is acute respiratory failure with pulmonary edema.

b. It can result from multiple etiologies and is known to occur after trauma and shock.

c. The patient may be difficult to ventilate secondary to decreased lung compliance.

d. Other signs and symptoms include tachypnea, tachycardia, and hypoxemia.

e. Treatment consists of high positive end-expiratory pressure.

f. The mortality rate can be as high as 50%.

g. Early stabilization of long bone fractures minimizes ongoing soft-tissue injury and helps reduce the incidence of ARDS.

4. Compartment syndrome

a. Compartment syndrome of the thigh is rare following femur fractures. It is important to rule out concomitant vascular injury and to consider the mechanism of injury; a crush injury or an injury involving a prolonged extrication, in which the dashboard console was crushing the leg compartments, should be followed up closely.

b. Compartment syndrome has been reported after IM nailing on the fracture table in the "well leg" holder.

5. Nerve palsy

a. In femur fractures stabilized on the fracture table, pudendal nerve palsy may occur as a result of excessive traction and/or improper positioning with the perineal post.

b. A peroneal nerve neurapraxia may occur secondary to excessive traction.

c. These injuries may be missed unless the clinician asks about them.

6. Nonunion, delayed union, malunion

a. The rate of nonunion after treatment of femoral shaft fractures with a locked IM nail is low.

b. Treatment often includes reamed exchange nailing with a larger IM nail.

c. For an infected nonunion (a rare complication), chronic suppressive antibiotic use until healing occurs is recommended, followed by implant removal.

d. Delayed unions may occur because of technical concerns. Removal of the interlocking screw may allow compression across the fracture and allow union to occur.

e. Up to 20% of patients may have limb rotational deformities.

f. Typically, rotational deformities of less than 20° are well tolerated.

7. Hardware failure and recurrent fracture

a. With reamed, statically locked IM nailing of femur fractures, the occurrence of hardware failure is low.

b. The closer a fracture is to the interlocking screw placement, the higher the stresses on the hardware.

8. Heterotopic ossification

a. The insertion site for an antegrade nail involves soft-tissue disruption of the abductors. Thus, heterotopic ossification about the hip may develop in some patients.

b. Heterotopic ossification of minimal clinical significance has been reported to occur in up to 26% of patients with fractures stabilized using a piriformis starting point. The occurrence rate associated with a trochanteric starting point has not yet been reported.

P. Others

1. Atypical femur fractures

a. With prolonged use of bisphosphonates, bone turnover rate decreases considerably. It has been hypothesized that these are insufficiency fractures that resulted from severely suppressed bone turnover and accumulation of skeletal microdamage.

b. Patients typically sustain these fractures from low-energy mechanisms (eg, giving way at standing height).

c. These fractures have a characteristic pattern.

- They tend to be simple transverse or oblique fractures.
- Cortical thickening occurs around the fracture site.
- Lateral or medial beaking occurs.
- The medial cortex of the distal segment tends to have a proximally oriented fracture line.

d. Treatment

- IM nailing (but watchfulness for compromised bone quality and healing capacity should be maintained).
- Delayed and nonunion may occur with any malreduction.
- Plate fixation with compression applied across the fracture.
- Discontinuation of bisphosphonates.
- Evaluation and monitoring of the contralateral femur for similar findings with radiographs and MRI

2. Interprosthetic/interimplant fractures of the femoral shaft

a. Interprosthetic fracture is a fracture between a hip prosthesis and a knee prosthesis.

b. Interimplant fractures can occur between a short hip nail and a knee prosthesis.

c. The incidence is increasing.

d. Most often, affected patients already have compromised bone quality, and this must be considered in formulating treatment plans.

e. Plate fixation is the treatment of choice. Intramedullary retrograde nailing with open-boxed knee replacements can supplement fixation in the patient with poor bone quality. Fixation should extend proximal to the distal extent of the hip implant and span the majority of the femur to avoid stress risers.

II. FRACTURES OF THE DISTAL FEMUR

A. Epidemiology

1. Distal femur fractures are bimodally distributed.
2. Incidence is higher in young, healthy males (often from high-energy trauma) and elderly females with osteopenia (from low-energy mechanisms).

B. Anatomy

1. The geometric cross-section of the femoral shaft transitions from cylindrical to trapezoidal.
2. The distal femur is trapezoidal and is composed of cancellous bone.
3. The distal femur is in physiologic valgus of approximately 9°.
4. The posterior half of both femoral condyles lies posterior to the femoral shaft.
5. Deforming forces of the distal femur after a fracture

a. The origin of the gastrocnemius characteristically pulls the distal fragment into extension, resulting in an apex posterior angulation.

b. The patient must be closely evaluated preoperatively for a coronal plane "Hoffa" fracture (**Figure 5**). Most often, they are unicondylar involving the lateral femoral condyle and are best detected using CT.

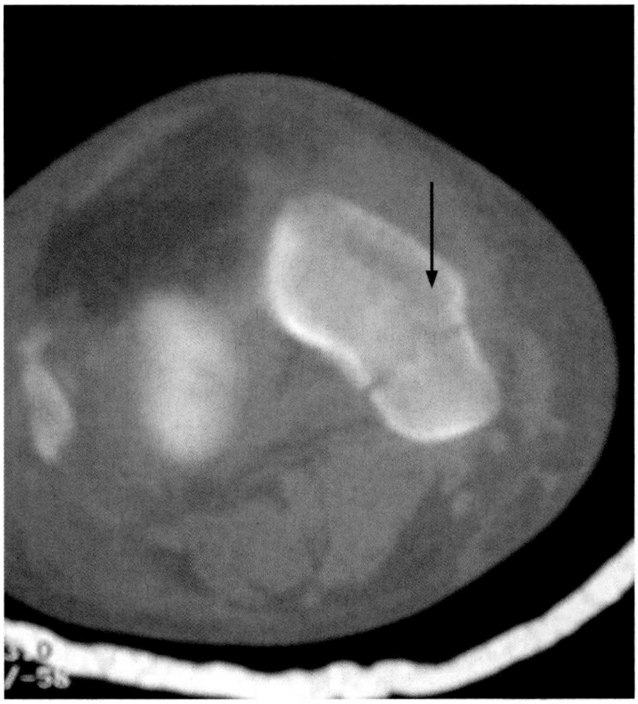

Figure 5 CT scan shows a Hoffa fracture (arrow).

C. Surgical approach

1. Depends on the choice of reduction type (indirect or direct) and plate
2. Minimally invasive surgical approaches include minimally invasive plate osteosynthesis.
   a. This approach is ideal for extra-articular fractures, which can be reduced indirectly.
   b. A lateral incision is made to facilitate plate placement, with small incisions proximally for diaphyseal screw placement.
3. Lateral parapatellar approach
   a. Affords excellent exposure of the femoral shaft and permits eversion of the patella.
   b. One disadvantage is that a different incision is needed for future total knee arthroplasties (TKAs).
   c. Allows for sufficient visualization of the joint surface.

D. Mechanism of injury

1. Fractures involving the supracondylar femur often result from the same high-energy mechanisms seen in fractures of the femoral shaft.
2. Low-energy mechanisms, such as minor falls, are common in the older population.

E. Clinical evaluation

1. Consider the mechanism of injury: in high-energy mechanisms, a full trauma evaluation should be completed.
2. The patient usually presents with pain, swelling, and deformity in the distal femur region.
3. Neurovascular structures lie close to these fractures, so the neurovascular status should be assessed thoroughly.
4. The skin should be examined closely for open wounds.
5. In the elderly patient, preexisting medical conditions and degenerative knee joint disease should be considered.

F. Imaging

1. AP and lateral radiographs of the distal femur are standard.
2. Radiographic evaluation of the ipsilateral lower extremity should be considered because of the risk of associated injuries.
3. Oblique views may help provide further details regarding the intercondylar anatomy; however, CT scanning often eliminates the need for these additional radiographs.
4. Traction radiographs are helpful but may be too uncomfortable for the patient.
5. CT provides details about intra-articular involvement and can identify coronal plane deformities with reconstruction views.

G. Classification—The AO/OTA classification is the universally accepted system for characterizing injuries of the distal femur (**Figure 6**).

1. Type A fractures are extra-articular injuries.
2. Type B fractures are partially articular and involve a single condyle.
3. Type C fractures are intercondylar or bicondylar intra-articular injuries with varying degrees of comminution.

H. Nonsurgical treatment—Nonsurgical treatment is indicated for nondisplaced distal femur fractures only. Nonsurgical treatment of displaced supracondylar and intercondylar femur fractures generally is associated with poor results and should be reserved for patients who represent an unacceptable surgical risk.

I. Surgical treatment

1. The goal of surgical treatment should be stable fixation to permit early mobilization and joint range of motion.
2. Successful surgical treatment is predicated on a biologically friendly surgical approach with preservation of periosteum and soft-tissue attachments.
3. Plate and screw constructs with precontoured plating has become a mainstay for these fractures.
   a. Modern plating systems allow for percutaneous placement, less periosteal disruption, and the application of locking screw fixation reducing the need for additional medial column plate stabilization.
   b. The locked nature of the screws in the femoral condyles allows the placement of multiple "internal external fixators" that have been shown to be axially superior to earlier fixation techniques.
   c. Another advantage of the newer design plates is the submuscular advancement of the plate to the bone, which minimizes periosteal stripping and preserves the blood supply. Unlike traditional plate and screw constructs with nonlocked screws, plates that use locking screws on either side of the fracture do not rely on direct contact of the plate to the bone for stability. This is particularly helpful in the distal

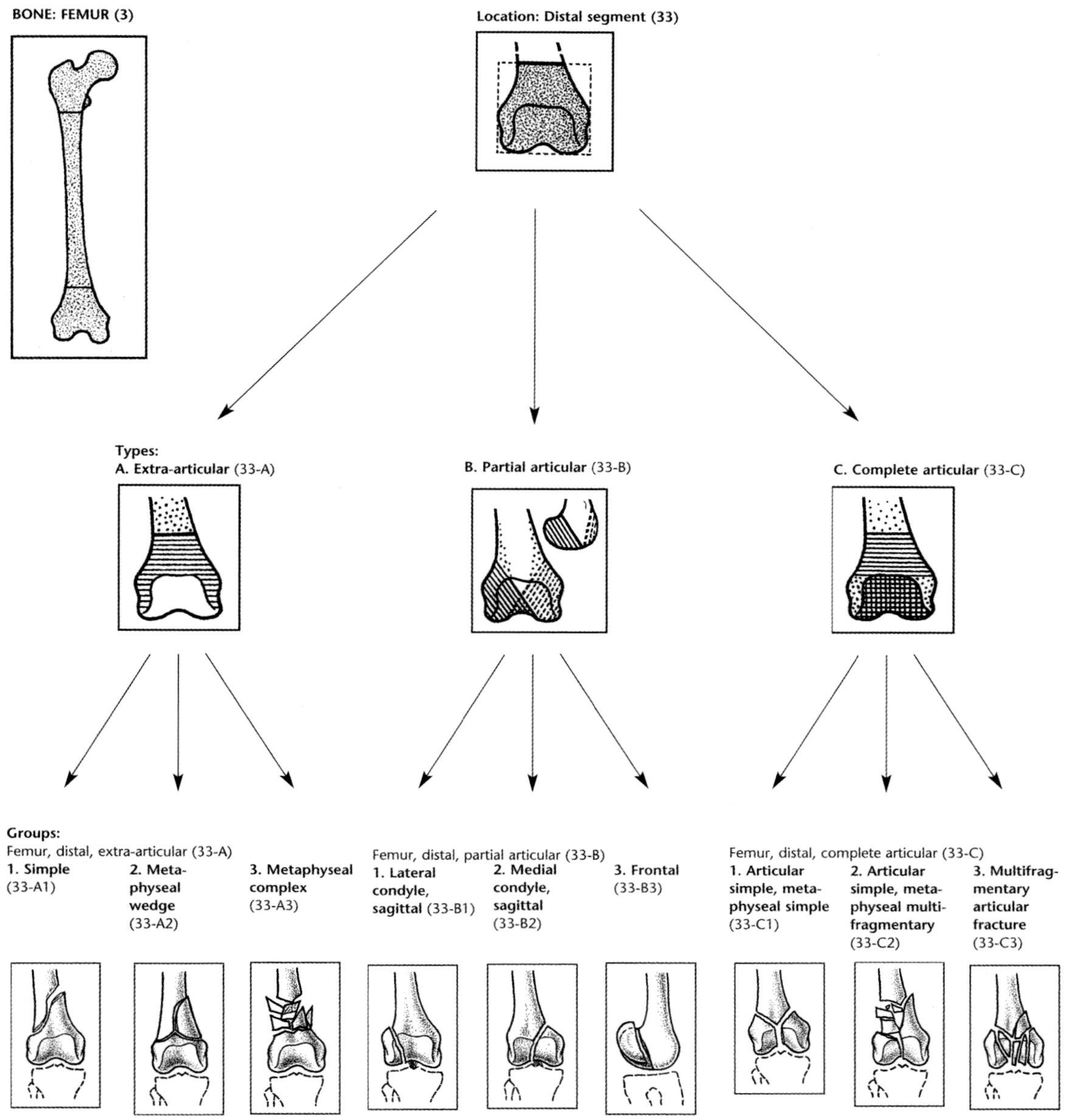

Figure 6 Diagram depicts the AO/OTA classification of distal femur fractures.

femur where bone morphology is variable and plate-bone mismatch can occur.

d. Constructs with too many stainless steel, bicortical locking screws on either side of the fracture can lead to an overly rigid construct and hinder bone healing. More recent studies discuss allowing for sufficient distance between the fracture and the first locked screw and different locking construct combinations that will decrease plate stiffness and facilitate healing.

J. Surgical technique

1. The patient should be positioned supine on a radiolucent table.
2. Open fractures should be treated in accordance with open fracture treatment principles. Temporizing knee-spanning external fixators should be used until the soft tissue permits the placement of internal fixation.
3. Once the soft tissues have been stabilized, the surgical approach and fixation tactic are dictated by the degree of articular involvement (**Table 1**).

TABLE 1

Possible Implants for Distal Femur Fractures as Determined by the AO/OTA Classification System

System
Type A or C1/C2 Fractures
Dynamic condylar screw
95° blade plate
Antegrade femoral nail
Retrograde femoral nail
Locked internal fixator (lateral plate with locked distal screws)
Type B Fractures
Screw and/or plate fixation
Type C3 Fractures
Standard condylar buttress plate
Locked internal fixator (lateral plate with locked distal screws)

Reproduced from Kregor PJ, Morgan SJ: Fractures of the distal femur, in Baumgaertner MR, Tornetta P III, eds: *Orthopaedic Knowledge Update: Trauma*, ed 3. Rosemont, IL, American Academy of Orthopaedic Surgeons, 2005, pp 397-408.

a. Type A fractures
- Plate fixation is a viable option and is associated with good results.
    - Traditional plating options include a dynamic condylar screw, a 95° blade plate, or most commonly, plate and screw construct with locking screw options. A dynamic condylar screw or blade plate requires surgical exposure the length of the plate to allow for application.
- Locked plating can be performed via a minimally invasive lateral approach to the distal femur, exposing only the portion of the distal lateral condyle necessary to facilitate placement of the implant.

b. Type B
- Partial articular fractures are often best treated with buttress plating.
- Articular surface should by anatomically reduced and compressed with lag screws.
- Coronal plane fractures may not be amenable to buttress plating and are best addressed with anterior-posterior lag screw fixation.

c. Type C fractures
- With significant articular surface involvement, open reduction is used to facilitate anatomic reduction.
- Lag screws at the articular surface allow absolute stability and primary bone healing. Modern implants allow for smaller caliber plates and screws to be used to increase density of fixation and stability for more complex articular injuries and reduce the risk of hardware failure and malunion.
- Length, alignment, and rotation should be restored at the metaphyseal component of the fracture. This may be achieved through a bridge plating construct across comminution or through lag screw and neutralization plating for more simple metaphyseal involvement.

K. IM nails
1. IM nailing is a viable option for distal femur fractures. Retrograde technique allows for easier manipulation of the distal segment to facilitate and maintain reduction.
2. When retrograde nailing of a distal femur fracture with articular involvement, the articular surface should be reduced and secured with Kirschner wires and/or lag screws before femoral canal preparation and nail placement.
3. Few indications exist for a short retrograde nail; any retrograde nails should be inserted proximally at least to the level of the lesser trochanter.

L. External fixation—Bridging external fixation may be advantageous as a temporizing measure in open fractures or in fractures with substantial comminution or soft-tissue compromise. When using bridging external fixation, the external fixator pins should be placed away from the footprint of the planned definitive fixation if possible.

M. Supracondylar fracture after TKA
1. It is important to evaluate the stability of the prosthesis. If it is stable, then fixation strategy can be planned.
2. Locking plate
    a. The locking plate is the fixation device of choice for distal fractures particularly in osteopenic bone.
    b. The literature supports good results for locking plate fixation of periprosthetic fractures proximal to a TKA.
3. Retrograde nailing represents an alternative treatment option. Before proceeding with this treatment, it is important to learn the details of

the TKA to assess if it will permit retrograde nail placement through the femoral prosthesis.

a. Start point through femoral implant may be too posterior and can lead to a recurvatum deformity of the fracture.

N. Rehabilitation

1. Postoperative treatment should include the administration of intravenous antibiotics for 24 hours following closure of all wounds and the routine use of mechanical and chemical prophylaxis for DVT.

2. Patients are mobilized as soon as possible after surgery. Weight-bearing restrictions are at the discretion of the surgeon and dependent on the fracture pattern and fixation construct.

3. Active-assisted range-of-motion exercises should be initiated in the early postoperative period to avoid knee stiffness.

O. Complications

1. Nonunion—rates improved with modern surgical soft tissue handling and percutaneous plate placement.

2. Symptomatic hardware—most commonly due to lateral plate irritation of the iliotibial band or medial screw irritation if length of screws are too long and not adequately assessed with view.

3. Malunion—most commonly valgus and recurvatum deformities. Distal articular block may be translated medially if plate does not match bone morphology or placement of plate is excessively posterior.

TOP TESTING FACTS—FEMORAL SHAFT AND DISTAL FEMUR FRACTURES

1. Bilateral femur fractures have a mortality rate of less than 7% with modern techniques.
2. Early stabilization (within the first 24 hours) of femur fractures reduces respiratory complications and can reduce the hospital length of stay.
3. A statically locked, reamed IM nail is the standard of care for femoral shaft fractures.
4. After surgical treatment of femoral shaft fractures, AP pelvic radiographic imaging should be performed to rule out a femoral neck fracture. Limb rotation and length should be evaluated, and the knee should be examined for ligamentous injuries.
5. No increased rate of knee infection is seen with retrograde nailing of open femur fractures.
6. The infection rate for open femur fractures is significantly lower than that of open tibia fractures.
7. Atypical femur fractures from diphosphonate use tend to be simple transverse or oblique fractures with cortical thickening around the fracture site and cortical beaking.
8. Imaging of distal femur fractures must be closely evaluated preoperatively for a coronal plane Hoffa fracture. These are most commonly found in the lateral femoral condyle.
9. High-energy distal femur fractures with significant displacement are associated with popliteal artery injuries
10. Articular fractures require anatomic reduction for good results frequently requiring open reduction through a parapatellar approach.
11. Poorly applied locking plates for the treatment of distal femur fractures can create an overly rigid construct. To avoid this problem, adequate spacing between fracture and locking screws is necessary to allow sufficient flexibility in the construct.
12. Recurvatum deformity is a concern during retrograde nailing of distal femur fracture around a total knee arthroplasty. This is due to the posterior start point allowed through the femoral implant of a knee replacement when addressing a periprosthetic fracture.

Bibliography

Bazylewicz DB, Egol KA, Koval KJ: Cortical encroachment after cephalomedullary nailing of the proximal femur: Evaluation of a more anatomic radius of curvature. *J Orthop Trauma* 2013;27(6):303-307.

Brumback RJ, Uwagie-Ero S, Lakatos RP, Poka A, Bathon GH, Burgess AR: Intramedullary nailing of femoral shaft fractures: Part II. Fracture-healing with static interlocking fixation. *J Bone Joint Surg Am* 1988;70(10):1453-1462.

Harvin WH, Oladeji LO, Della Rocca GJ, et al: Working length and proximal screw constructs in plate osteosynthesis of distal femur fractures. *Injury* 2017;48(11):2597-2601.

Kandemir U, Augat P, Konowalczyk S, Wipf F, von Oldenburg G, Schmidt U: Implant material, type of fixation at the shaft, and position of plate modify biomechanics of distal femur plate osteosynthesis. *J Orthop Trauma* 2017;31(8):e241-e246.

7 | Trauma

Koso RE, Terhoeve C, Steen RG, Zura R: Healing, nonunion, and re-operation after internal fixation of diaphyseal and distal femoral fractures: A systematic review and meta-analysis. *Int Orthop* 2018;42(11):2675-2683.

Marchand LS, Todd DC, Kellam P, Adeyemi TF, Rothberg DL, Maak TG: Is the lesser trochanter profile a reliable means of restoring anatomic rotation after femur fracture fixation? *Clin Orthop Relat Res* 2018;476(6):1253-1261.

Ostrum RF, Agarwal A, Lakatos R, Poka A: Prospective comparison of retrograde and antegrade femoral intramedullary nailing. *J Orthop Trauma* 2000;14(7):496-501.

Chapter 101

KNEE DISLOCATIONS AND PATELLAR FRACTURES

DAVID S. WELLMAN, MD
GREGORY S. DIFELICE, MD

I. KNEE DISLOCATIONS

A. Epidemiology

1. Knee dislocations represent less than 0.2% of all orthopaedic injuries.
2. The incidence reported in the literature is likely underrepresentative of the true incidence because 20% to 50% of knee dislocations spontaneously reduce in the field.

B. Anatomy

1. The stability of the knee joint is provided by bony articulations as well as dynamic and static soft-tissue stabilizers (**Table 1**).
2. The four major ligamentous stabilizers of the knee are the anterior cruciate ligament (ACL), the posterior cruciate ligament (PCL), the medial collateral ligament (MCL), and the fibular collateral ligament (FCL).
3. The posterolateral corner (PLC) and posteromedial corner (PMC) as well as the medial and lateral menisci confer additional stability to the knee.
4. The PLC is made up of the FCL, the iliotibial band, the popliteofibular ligament, the biceps femoris, and the popliteus tendon.
5. The relatively high incidence of neurovascular compromise in knee dislocation is explained by the anatomy of the knee (**Figure 1**).
   a. The popliteus artery travels through the adductor hiatus, where it is relatively immobile, and distally through the fibrous arch deep to the soleus muscle.
   b. The common peroneal nerve travels along the posterior edge of the biceps femoris and continues distally around the fibular neck. The tibial nerve, after branching from the sciatic nerve, courses distally through the center of the popliteus fossa.

TABLE 1

Soft-Tissue Stabilizers of the Knee

Structure	Function
ACL	Primary: Resists anterior translation of the tibia relative to the femur Secondary: Resists varus/valgus stresses in full extension
PCL	Primary: Resists posterior translation of the tibia relative to the femur Secondary: Resists tibial external rotation
MCL	Resists valgus stress
PMC	Resists valgus stress
FCL	Resists varus stress
PLC	Resists posterior translation, external rotation, and varus angulation of the tibia

ACL = anterior cruciate ligament, FCL = fibular collateral ligament, MCL = medial collateral ligament, PCL = posterior cruciate ligament, PLC = posterolateral corner, PMC = posteromedial corner

Dr. Wellman or an immediate family member is a member of a speakers' bureau or has made paid presentations on behalf of DePuy, A Johnson & Johnson Company; serves as a paid consultant to or is an employee of OrthoDevelopment; and has stock or stock options held in Imagen. Dr. DiFelice or an immediate family member has received royalties from Arthrex, Inc.; serves as a paid consultant to or is an employee of Arthrex, Inc.; and has received research or institutional support from Arthrex, Inc.

This chapter is adapted from Riehl JT, Langford J, Koval KJ: Knee dislocations and patellar fractures, in Boyer MI, ed: *AAOS Comprehensive Orthopaedic Review* 2. Rosemont, IL, American Academy of Orthopaedic Surgeons, 2014, pp 423-429.

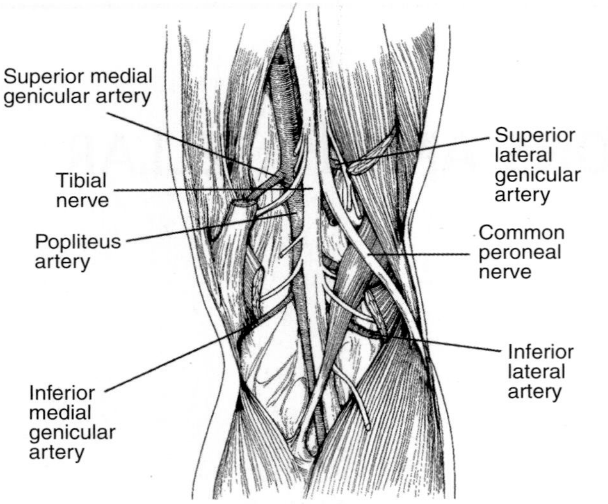

Figure 1 Illustration shows the posterior anatomy of the knee. Note the relationship between the popliteus artery and the tibial and common peroneal nerves. (Reproduced from Good L, Johnson RJ: The dislocated knee. *J Am Acad Orthop Surg* 1995;3:284-292.)

C. Mechanism of injury

1. High-energy injuries include those from motor vehicle collisions, falls from a height, and industrial accidents.
2. Low-energy injuries include sports-related injuries, often with a rotatory component.
3. Ultra-low–energy injuries include those occurring from seemingly trivial trauma in morbidly obese patients.

D. Clinical evaluation

1. In high-energy mechanisms, other life-threatening injuries can be present. Evaluation should follow Advanced Trauma Life Support (ATLS) protocols.
2. Knee dislocation should be suspected in patients with uncontained hemarthrosis about the knee, contusions, and gross laxity. Additionally, any patient with two or more ligamentous injuries or with certain fractures about the knee should be evaluated for a suspected knee dislocation.
3. A thorough neurovascular examination is of the utmost importance. Pulses are assessed for symmetry and, when symmetric, should be accompanied by the ankle-brachial index (ABI). If these tests are normal (ABI ≥ 0.9), serial and frequent neurovascular examinations should follow. Neurovascular examination should be performed both prereduction and postreduction. See Section F below for workup of an abnormal examination.
4. Ligamentous examination should proceed in a systematic fashion to identify disrupted and intact structures. **Table 2** lists the soft-tissue stabilizers of the knee, their function, and the corresponding tests. The soft-tissue stabilizers of the knee and the most sensitive clinical examination maneuvers that indicate disruption are listed below.
   a. ACL: Positive Lachman test
   b. PCL: Positive posterior drawer test
   c. MCL: Valgus laxity at 30° of knee flexion
   d. PMC: Positive posteromedial drawer test
   e. FCL: Varus laxity at 30° of knee flexion
   f. PLC: Positive posterolateral drawer test
   g. Differentiating PLC injuries from combined PLC/PCL injuries: Positive dial test (increased tibial external rotation at 30° of flexion indicates PLC injury; increased tibial external rotation at 30° and 90° of flexion indicates combined PLC/PCL injury)

TABLE 2

Soft-Tissue Stabilizers of the Knee and Clinical Tests for Stability

Structure	Test
ACL	Lachman: With the knee flexed 20°, the examiner translates the tibia anteriorly.
PCL	Posterior drawer test: With the knee flexed 90°, the examiner translates the tibia posteriorly.
MCL	Valgus stress test: With the knee flexed 30°, the examiner applies valgus stress.
PMC	Posteromedial drawer test: With the knee at 0° and 30° of flexion, the examiner applies valgus stress.
FCL	Varus stress test: With the knee flexed 30°, the examiner applies varus stress.
PLC	Posterolateral drawer test: With the knee flexed 90° and in 15° of external rotation and with the foot flat on table, the examiner applies posterior force to knee. Varus stress at 0° and 30°: With the knee at 0° and 30°, the examiner applies varus stress at respective positions. Dial test: With the knees flexed 30°, the tibias are bilaterally externally rotated; increased rotation of 10° to 15° from affected side indicates PLC injury. Increased tibial external rotation at both 30° and 90° of flexion indicates combined PLC/PCL injury.

ACL = anterior cruciate ligament, LCL = fibular collateral ligament, MCL = medial collateral ligament, PCL = posterior cruciate ligament, PLC = posterolateral corner, PMC = posteromedial corner

h. Collateral ligament, one or more cruciate ligaments, and capsular injury: Varus/valgus laxity at full knee extension

i. PCL, PMC, PLC, and posterior capsule: Positive supine heel-lift test

E. Associated injuries

1. Vascular injury
2. Neurologic injury
   a. Neurapraxia (stretch)
   b. Axonotmesis (axonal disruption, endoneurium intact)
   c. Neurotmesis (complete transection)
3. Chondral and meniscal injuries (incidence of 37% to 55% and 28% to 48%, respectively)
4. Capsular injury
   a. Prevents immediate arthroscopic reconstruction due to fluid extravasation concerns
   b. May result in severe swelling
5. Compartment syndrome
6. Fracture
7. Extensor mechanism disruption
   a. Reported in up to 8.6% of cases
   b. Associated patella dislocation in 5%

F. Vascular injury

1. Incidence in the literature ranges from 23 to 32%.
2. Signs of vascular injury (asymmetric pulses postreduction, active bleeding, expanding hematoma) warrant immediate vascular surgery consultation.
3. Injury range: transection, contusion, intimal tear, thrombus formation. Initial physical examination may be normal in the presence of an intimal flap tear, but such tears can propagate resulting in complete arterial occlusion.
4. Angiography is unnecessary when physical examination and ABIs are normal (≥ 0.9).
5. The main indication for angiography is clinical signs of vascular injury without limb-threatening ischemia. Ischemia should proceed directly to the operating room (OR) for evaluation with a vascular surgeon.
6. Warm limb ischemia durations longer than 6 hours warrant prophylactic fasciotomies.

G. Neurologic injury

1. Incidence ranges from 14% to 40%.
2. Common peroneal nerve injury occurs more often than tibial nerve injury, and it is most commonly associated with posterolateral dislocations.
3. If the peroneal nerve recovers, improvement usually begins by 3 months from injury and is accompanied by a positive Tinel sign.
4. Observation is the treatment of choice for incomplete peroneal nerve palsies.
5. If electromyographic (EMG) testing is performed, a baseline study can be obtained at approximately 4 to 6 weeks from injury; repeat EMG testing can be performed at 3 months.
6. Tibialis posterior transfer can be performed as a salvage procedure to restore active dorsiflexion.

H. Imaging

1. AP and lateral radiographs should be obtained in all cases of suspected knee dislocation. If this can be accomplished without significant delay, the radiographs should be obtained both before and after any reduction attempt.
2. Stress radiographs in the acute, chronic, and postoperative phases can provide useful information for treatment decisions.
3. MRI is used to evaluate ligamentous, capsular, meniscal, cartilaginous, and other soft-tissue lesions, helping to guide surgical treatment. It should be obtained as soon as logistically and safely possible.
4. Magnetic resonance angiography has been suggested by some authors as an alternative to traditional angiography in the acute setting. Likewise, CT angiography, because of its speed and accuracy, has been adopted by many centers for use in the acute evaluation of knee dislocations.

I. Classification—The most widely utilized classification scheme was developed by Schenck in 1994. The classification defines the extent of ligamentous injury while also taking into account associated fractures, arterial injuries, and nerve injuries (**Table 3**).

J. Closed reduction

1. Closed reduction is performed following neurovascular assessment and evaluation of plain radiographs.
2. The reduction maneuver is axial limb traction with translation of the tibia in the appropriate direction.
3. For posterolateral dislocations where the medial femoral condyle has "buttonholed" or perforated through the medial capsular structures (the dimple sign), it is recommended to avoid attempts at closed reduction but rather to proceed to the OR for emergent open reduction.

TABLE 3

Schenck Classification

Type	Description
KD I	Collateral ligament + single cruciate ligament
KD II	Bicruciate injury with both collateral ligaments intact
KD III	Bicruciate injury + single collateral Subtype M: MCL Subtype L: FCL
KD IV	Bicruciate injury + both collateral ligaments
KD V	MLI with associated periarticular fracture
+ N	Nerve injury
+ C	Arterial injury

FCL = fibular collateral ligament, KD = knee dislocation, MCL = medial collateral ligament, MLI = multi ligament instability

4. Following reduction, a knee immobilizer or splint is placed. If the reduction cannot be maintained in a splint, an external fixator is indicated along with inpatient admission for observation of limb neurovascular status.

K. Surgical treatment

1. Surgical treatment has been proven to lead to better patient reported outcomes.
2. Surgery is indicated in the acute setting in a physically active patient without medical comorbidities that prohibit surgery. In the chronic setting, surgical treatment is indicated for knee instability without significant arthrosis.
3. Treatment of associated PLC and PMC injuries is imperative to obtain good long-term results with ACL/PCL reconstructions.
4. Surgical options include repair verses reconstruction, with repairs reserved for acute avulsions of the collaterals. Some have begun to advocate for cruciate repairs in the proximal-type avulsion injuries in select patient populations.
5. Timing and materials for ligamentous reconstruction vary according to surgeon preference.
6. Several authors have reported good patient-reported outcome measures at follow-up durations greater than 2 years from surgery, but at the same duration of follow-up, the evidence of radiographic osteoarthritis has been reported to be as high as 42% to 87% in some series.

L. Nonsurgical treatment is indicated in patients unable to tolerate a surgical procedure and in less active patients.

M. Postoperative rehabilitation

1. Traditionally patients were kept non–weight bearing for 6 weeks, with the knee braced in full extension, but there has been a recent trend toward earlier motion and less weight-bearing restriction.
2. Progressive range of motion (ROM) and closed chain exercises are initiated around the 4 to 6 week mark.
3. Return to unrestricted activity (sports, heavy labor) can take up to 9 months or more.

N. Complications

1. Arthrofibrosis
   a. May be caused by heterotopic ossification (reported incidence of 26% to 43%) and scarring about the capsule.
   b. Terminal extension and 10° to 15° of terminal flexion are commonly lost.
   c. If the stiffness is severely limiting, manipulation under anesthesia or arthroscopic lysis of the adhesions may be indicated. If stiffness is caused by heterotopic bone, resection may be performed.
2. Residual instability (often related to failure to recognize and treat all components of the initial injury)
3. Medial femoral condyle osteonecrosis
4. Sensory and motor disturbances
5. Iatrogenic neurovascular injury or tibial plateau fracture due to tunnel convergence
6. Venous thromboembolic events (VTEs)

II. PATELLAR FRACTURES

A. Epidemiology

1. Fractures of the patella most commonly occur in people of age 20 to 50 years.
2. The male-to-female ratio is 2:1.
3. Patellar fractures make up 1% of all skeletal injuries.

B. Anatomy (**Figure 2**)

1. The patella is the largest sesamoid bone in the body.
2. The subcutaneous location of the patella and the large joint reactive forces it sustains make it prone to injury.
3. The patella has seven facets; the distal pole is termed the apex.

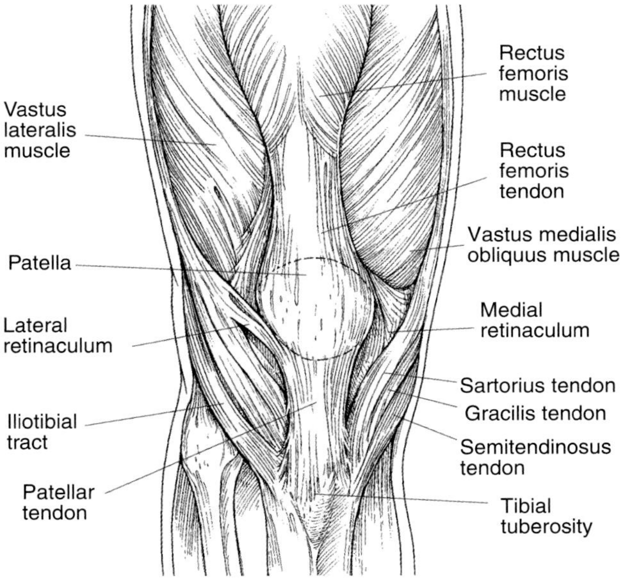

Figure 2 Illustration shows the anatomy of the extensor mechanism of the knee. (Reproduced from Matava MJ: Patellar tendon ruptures. *J Am Acad Orthop Surg* 1996;4:287-296.)

4. The proximal portion of the patella is covered with the thickest articular cartilage in the body. The distal pole is devoid of articular cartilage.
5. Bipartite patella most commonly involves the superolateral portion.
6. The patella increases the power of the extensor mechanism 30% by anteriorly displacing the extensor mechanism away from the knee center of rotation (increased moment arm).
7. The blood supply arises from the geniculate arteries which contribute to an arterial ring around the patella; the principle arterial supply enters the patella inferomedially.

C. Mechanism of injury
   1. Direct blow (eg, from a fall)—Results in a simple or comminuted fracture pattern.
   2. Indirect—Results from eccentric contraction; typically causes a transverse fracture pattern.

D. Clinical evaluation
   1. The soft tissues should be inspected carefully for lacerations, abrasions, and ecchymosis.
   2. Extensor lag and the ability to perform a straight leg raise should be evaluated.
   3. The examiner should palpate for an extensor mechanism defect.
   4. If pain limits the evaluation, intra-articular injection of local anesthetic can enable better assessment.

E. Radiographic evaluation
   1. AP and lateral radiographs should be obtained in each case. Oblique views also can be beneficial to evaluate the multiple facets. Additionally, an axial (sunrise) view can help evaluate longitudinal fracture lines.
   2. Bipartite patella can be differentiated from fracture by smooth, regular borders with sclerotic edges. Bipartite patella is often bilateral and involves the superolateral portion.

F. Fracture classification—Based on the fracture pattern, patellar fractures typically are classified as extra-articular, partial articular, or complete articular (**Figure 3**).

G. Treatment
   1. Anatomic reduction of the articular surface is paramount. Reduction may be assessed with palpation through retinacular defects, surgical arthrotomy, or fluoroscopy.
   2. Indications for surgical treatment include open fractures, extensor mechanism dysfunction, articular step-off of 2 mm, and articular gap of 3 mm.
   3. When nonsurgical treatment is chosen, the knee is kept in nearly full extension for 4 to 6 weeks. Isometric quadriceps exercises and straight leg raises are begun 1 week after injury.
   4. Fixation construct options
      a. Two longitudinal Kirschner wires (threaded or unthreaded) with 18-gauge stainless steel wires in a figure-of-8 fashion; a second wire may be placed around the patella in a cerclage configuration (**Figure 4**).
      b. Parallel cannulated screws with stainless steel wire in a figure-of-8 configuration. Screw tips must not extend beyond the edge of the patella. Best used in simple fracture patterns. Comminution, especially of the inferior pole, risks failure.
      c. Thin mesh plates with minifragment screws are beneficial for obtaining and maintaining reductions in highly comminuted patterns (**Figure 5**).
      d. Nonabsorbable suture placed into the patella tendon (similar to the technique for a patella tendon rupture) and then through drill holes in the proximal pole can be used in the setting of comminuted, extra-articular distal pole fractures.

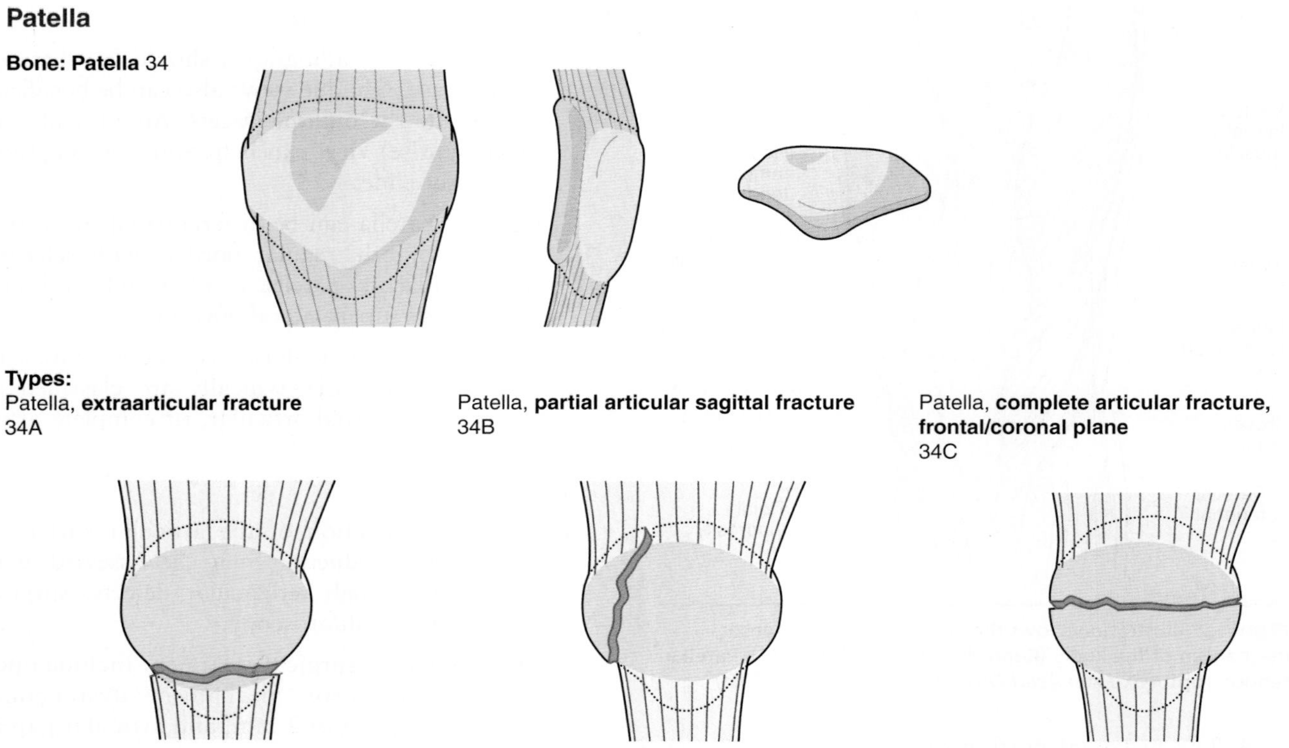

Figure 3 Illustrations demonstrate the classification of patellar fractures according to the AO/OTA system. (Reproduced from Kellam JF, Meinberg EG, Agel J, Karam MD, Roberts CS: Fracture and dislocation classification compendium-2018: International Comprehensive Classification of Fractures and Dislocations Committee. *J Orthop Trauma*. 2018.)

5. In cases of severe comminution, fixation may not be possible. It is important to save as much of the patella as is possible. Partial patellectomy is performed, with reattachment of the patellar or quadriceps tendon to the remaining fragment, along with retinacular repair (**Figure 6**).
   a. Indication for partial patellectomy: A large, salvageable fragment in the presence of smaller comminuted polar fragments that are unreconstructible.
   b. The tendon should be reattached close to the articular surface to prevent patellar tilt.
6. In some rare cases, total patellectomy is necessary. In one clinical series of total patellectomies, advancement of the vastus medialis obliquus was shown to improve outcomes.
7. Postoperative care includes splint immobilization in extension for 4 to 6 weeks followed by a ROM program with physical therapy. Weight bearing in full extension is allowed immediately.

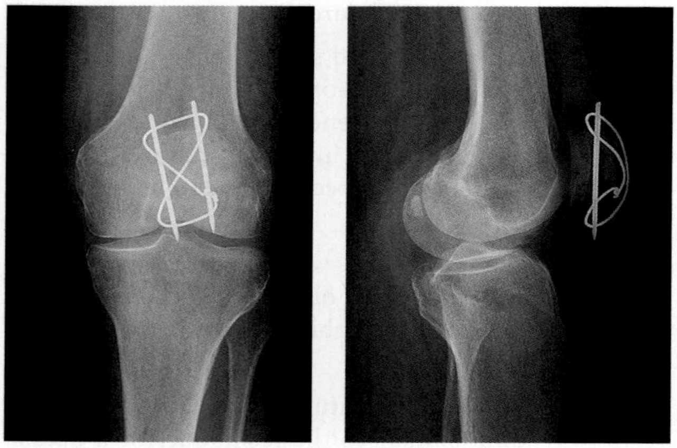

Figure 4 AP and Lateral radiographs demonstrating fully threaded Kirschner wires and a figure-of-8 18-gauge wire securing a simple transverse patella fracture.

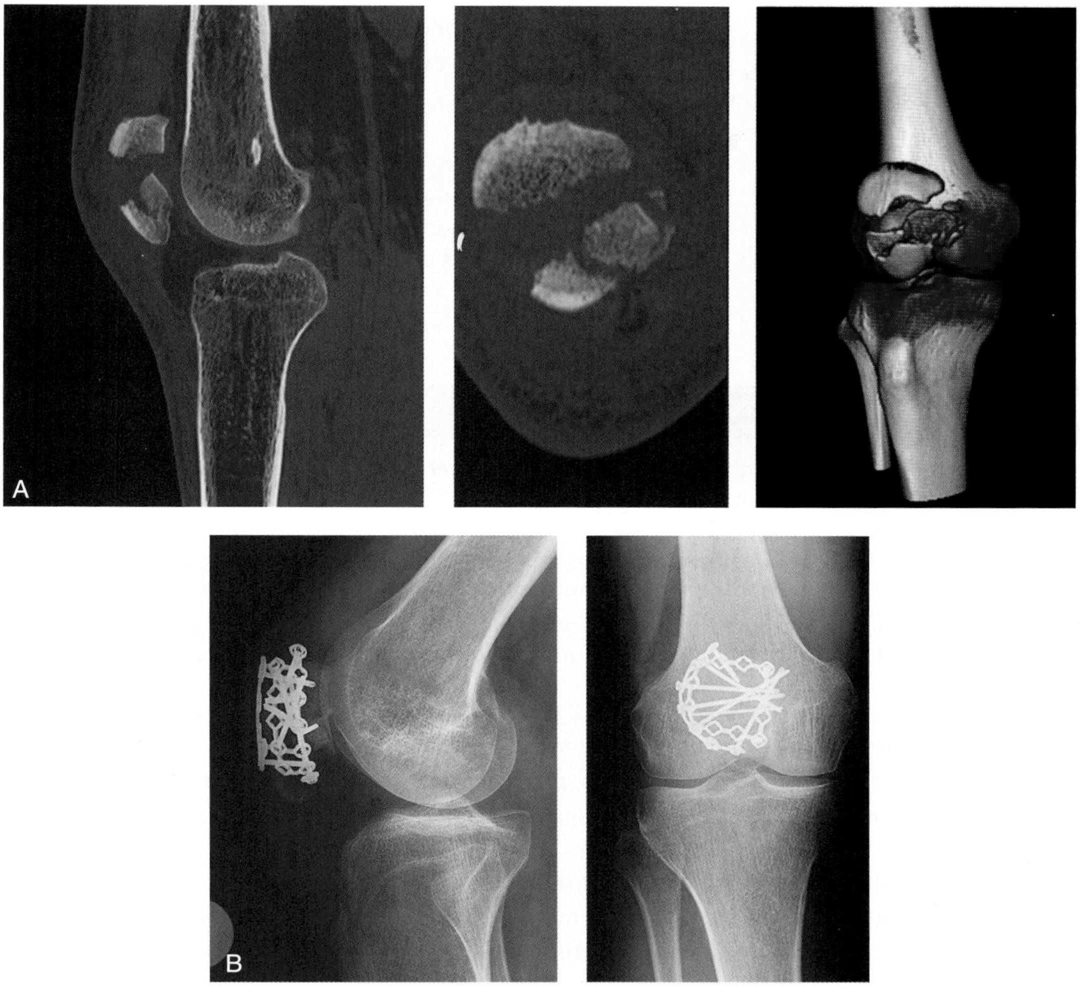

Figure 5 **A**, Sagittal, coronal, and 3-D reformatted CT images of a comminuted patella fracture in a 26 year old male. **B**, Postoperative AP and lateral knee radiograph demonstrating fracture healing. 2.4-mm minifragment plate provides multiplanar rigid fixation to a comminuted patella fracture. The fracture is approached with an anterior incision and a lateral parapatellar arthrotomy. The joint surface is visualized, and a mesh plate is cut and contoured to fit the lateral face of the patella. The arthrotomy is closed using the plate as an anchor to give soft tissue stability. Often, a Krakow stitch will be placed in the patella tendon and secured to the plate to give additional stability to the inferior pole in the setting of comminution.

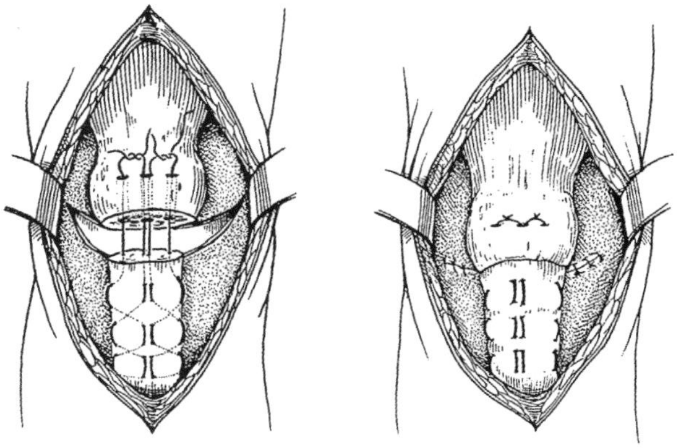

Figure 6 Illustrations demonstrate partial patellectomy. The ligament is sutured to the remaining patellar fragment. (Adapted from Cramer KE, Moed BR: Patellar fractures: Contemporary approach to treatment. *J Am Acad Orthop Surg* 1997;5:323-331.)

H. Complications

1. Painful implants (in some series, >50%) are the most likely reason for a return to the OR.
2. Decreased ROM (especially terminal knee flexion)
3. Infection (up to 11%)
4. Loss of reduction (around 10%); more common in osteoporotic bone
5. Posttraumatic osteoarthritis (50%)
6. Osteonecrosis
7. Nonunion (1% to 7%)

ACKNOWLEDGMENT

The authors would like to thank Dr. Joseph Ruzbarsky for his contributions to this chapter.

TOP TESTING FACTS

1. The popliteus artery travels through the adductor hiatus, where it is relatively immobile, and distally through the fibrous arch, deep to the soleus muscle.
2. The common peroneal nerve travels along the posterior edge of the biceps femoris and continues distally around the fibular neck. The tibial nerve branches at a variable level but courses down the middle of the popliteus fossa. This makes the peroneal nerve more immobile and therefore more susceptible to injury.
3. An ABI <0.9 warrants a vascular surgery consult and angiography (if no clinical ischemic signs are found). Ischemic findings on clinical examination should proceed to the OR with vascular surgery for emergent reperfusion.
4. The incidence of vascular injury may be as high as 32%; it can present in a delayed fashion as arterial injuries can propagate over time. Serial examinations are mandatory.
5. When warm ischemia time is longer than 6 hours, prophylactic fasciotomies should be performed.
6. Bipartite patella most commonly involves the superolateral portion and demonstrates smooth, regular borders on radiographs.
7. The patella increases the power of the extensor mechanism by 30%.
8. The dominant blood supply to the patella enters medially through the inferior pole.
9. Indications for surgical treatment of patellar fractures include open fractures, extensor mechanism dysfunction, articular step-off of 2 mm, and articular gap of 3 mm.
10. In cases of severe comminution, fixation may not be possible. It is important to save as much of the patella as is possible. Partial patellectomy is performed, with reattachment of the patellar or quadriceps tendon to the remaining fragment, along with retinacular repair.
11. Painful implants are the most likely reason for a return to the OR after surgical fixation of patellar fractures.

Bibliography

Bonnaig NS, Casstevens C, Archdeacon MT, et al: Fix it or discard it? A retrospective analysis of functional outcomes after surgically treated patella fractures comparing ORIF with partial patellectomy. *J Orthop Trauma* 2015;29(2):80-84.

Fanelli GC, Harris JD, Tomaszewski DJ, Riehl JT, Edson CJ, Reinheimer KN: Multiple ligament knee injuries, in DeLee JC, Drez D Jr, Miller MD, eds: *DeLee & Drez's Orthopaedic Sports Medicine: Principles and Practice*, ed 3. Philadelphia, PA, Saunders, 2009, pp 1747-1765.

Krych AJ, Sousa PL, King AH, Engasser WM, Stuart MJ, Levy BA: Meniscal tears and articular cartilage damage in the dislocated knee. *Knee Surg Sports Traumatol Arthrosc* 2015;23(10):3019-3025.

LaPrade RF, DePhillipo NN, Cram TR, et al: Partial controlled early postoperative weightbearing versus nonweightbearing after reconstruction of the Fibular (lateral) collateral ligament: A randomized controlled trial and equivalence analysis. *Am J Sports Med* 2018;46(10):2355-2365.

Lazaro LE, Wellman DS, Klinger CE, et al: Quantitative and qualitative assessment of bone perfusion and arterial contributions in a patellar fracture model using gadolinium-enhanced magnetic resonance imaging: A cadaveric study. *J Bone Joint Surg Am* 2013;95(19):e1401-e1407.

Lorich DG, Fabricant PD, Sauro G, et al: Superior outcomes after operative fixation of patella fractures using a novel plating technique: A prospective cohort study. *J Orthop Trauma* 2017;31(5):241-247.

Marom N, Ruzbarsky JJ, Roselaar N, Marx RG: Knee MLI injuries: Common problems and solutions. *Clin Sports Med* 2018;37(2):281-291.

Matthews B, Hazratwala K, Barroso-Rosa S: Comminuted patella Fracture in elderly patients: A systematic review and case report. *Geriatr Orthop Surg Rehabil* 2017;8(3):135-144.

Melvin JS, Mehta S: Patellar fractures in adults. *J Am Acad Orthop Surg* 2011;19(4):198-207.

Moatshe G, Chahla J, LaPrade RF, Engebretsen L: Diagnosis and treatment of multiligament knee injury: State of the art. *J ISAKOS* 2017;0:1-10.

Moatshe G, Dornan GJ, Løken S, Ludvigsen TC, Laprade RF, Engebretsen L: Demographics and injuries associated with knee dislocation: A prospective review of 303 patients. *Orthop J Sport Med* 2017;5(5):1-5.

Schenck R: Classification of knee dislocations. *Oper Tech Sport Med* 2003;11:193-198.

Werner BC, Gwathmey FW, Higgins ST, Hart JM, Miller MD: Ultra-low velocity knee dislocations: Patient characteristics, complications, and outcomes. *Am J Sports Med* 2014;42(2):358-363.

Chapter 102

TIBIAL PLATEAU AND TIBIAL-FIBULAR SHAFT FRACTURES

KENNETH A. EGOL, MD

I. TIBIAL PLATEAU FRACTURES

A. Epidemiology

1. Historically, tibial plateau fractures were more common in young patients after high-energy trauma; now, a larger percentage results from a low-energy fall in older patients with osteoporotic bone (as a result of an aging active population).

B. Anatomy

1. Tibial plateau

   a. The medial tibial plateau is larger than the lateral plateau and is concave in the sagittal and coronal planes. The lateral plateau is convex and extends higher than the medial plateau. Both articular surfaces are covered with hyaline cartilage.

   b. Both plateaus are covered by a fibrocartilaginous meniscus. The coronary ligaments attach the menisci to the plateaus, and the intermeniscal ligament connects the menisci anteriorly.

2. Tibial spines are attachment points for the anterior cruciate ligament (ACL), the posterior cruciate ligament (PCL), and the menisci.

3. Tibial shaft

   a. The tibial shaft is triangular in cross section.

   b. Proximally, the tibial tubercle is located anterolaterally about 3 cm distal to the articular surface; it is the point of attachment for the patellar tendon.

   c. Laterally on the proximal tibia is Gerdy's tubercle, which is the point of insertion for the iliotibial band. Medially is the pes anserinus, which is the point of insertion for the sartorius, gracilis, and semitendinosus muscles.

4. Soft-tissue structures

   a. The medial (tibial) collateral ligament inserts into the medial proximal tibia.

   b. The ACL and PCL provide anterior-posterior stability.

   c. The lateral (fibular) collateral ligament inserts into the fibular head.

5. Neurovascular structures

   a. The common peroneal nerve courses around the neck of the fibula distal to the proximal tibial-fibular joint before it divides into its superficial and deep branches.

   b. The trifurcation of the popliteal artery into the anterior tibial, posterior tibial, and peroneal arteries occurs posteromedially at the level of the proximal tibia.

   c. Vascular injuries to these structures are common following knee dislocation but also can occur in high-energy fractures of the proximal tibia.

6. Musculature

   a. The anterior compartment musculature attaches to the proximal lateral tibia.

Dr. Egol or an immediate family member has received royalties from Exactech, Inc.; is a member of a speakers' bureau or has made paid presentations on behalf of Smith & Nephew; serves as a paid consultant to or is an employee of Exactech, Inc.; serves as an unpaid consultant to Polypid; has received research or institutional support from Acumed, LLC and Synthes; and serves as a board member, owner, officer, or committee member of the Orthopaedic Trauma Association.

This chapter is adapted from Kubiak EN, Egol KA: Tibial plateau and tibial-fibular shaft fractures, in Boyer MI, ed: *AAOS Comprehensive Orthopaedic Review*, ed 2. Rosemont, IL, American Academy of Orthopaedic Surgeons, 2014, pp 431-441.

b. The proximal medial tibial surface is devoid of muscle coverage but serves as an attachment point for the pes tendons.

C. Mechanisms of injury

1. Tibial plateau fractures result from direct axial compression—usually with a valgus (more common) or varus (less common) moment—and indirect shear forces. Examples include the following:

a. High-speed motor vehicle accidents

b. Falls from a height

c. Collisions between the bumper of a car and a pedestrian ("bumper injury")

2. The direction, magnitude, and location of the force as well as the position of the knee at impact determine the fracture pattern, location, and degree of displacement.

3. Associated injuries

a. Meniscal tears are associated with up to 50% of tibial plateau fractures.

b. Associated injury to the cruciate or collateral ligaments occurs in up to 30% of patients.

c. Skin compromise is frequently present in high-energy fracture patterns.

D. Clinical evaluation

1. Physical examination

a. The examiner should palpate over the site of potential fracture or ligamentous disruption to elicit tenderness.

b. Hemarthrosis typically is present; however, capsular disruption may result in extravasation into the surrounding soft-tissue envelope.

c. Widening of the femoral-tibial articulation of more than 10° on varus or valgus stress examination, compared with the other leg, indicates instability.

2. Neurovascular examination

a. If pulses are not palpable, Doppler ultrasonographic studies should be performed. If the knee is subluxated, it should be reduced and the examination repeated.

b. The examiner should assess for signs and symptoms of an impending compartment syndrome (pain out of proportion to the injury, pain on passive stretch of the toes, pallor, pulselessness, or impaired neurologic status); out-of-proportion pain is the most sensitive predictor.

c. Compartment pressures should be measured directly if the patient is unconscious and has a tense, swollen leg.

d. Ankle-brachial index (ABI) less than 0.9 requires consultation with a vascular surgeon.

3. Radiographic evaluation

a. Plain radiographs—Should include a knee trauma series (AP, lateral, and oblique views) and a plateau view (10° caudal tilt).

b. CT—Provides improved assessment of fracture pattern, aids in surgical planning, and improves the ability to classify fractures; CT should be ordered when better visualization of the bone fragments is required or to confirm a suspected traumatic arthrotomy (air in the open joint) (**Figure 1**).

c. MRI—of limited use in the acute setting.

E. Fracture classification

1. The Schatzker classification is used most commonly (**Figure 2**).

2. The Moore classification accounts for patterns not described in the Schatzker classification (**Figure 3**) and represent a fracture-dislocation.

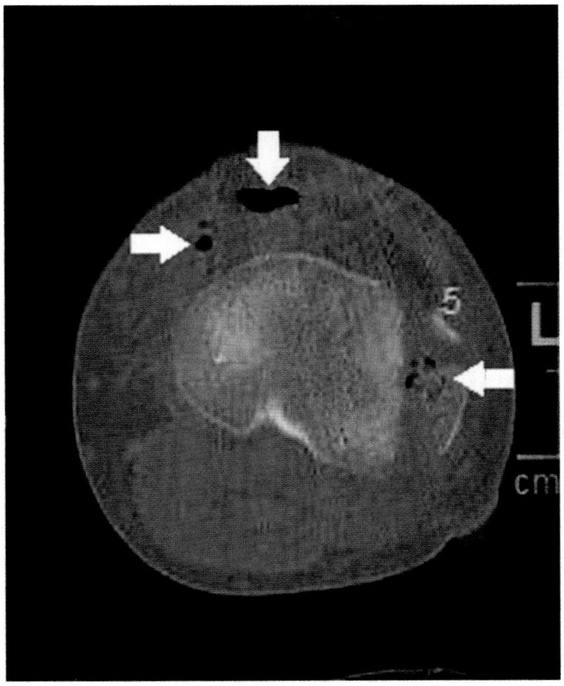

Figure 1 CT Scan demonstrating air in the joint (arrows) consistent with traumatic arthrotomy associated with a lateral tibial plateau fracture.

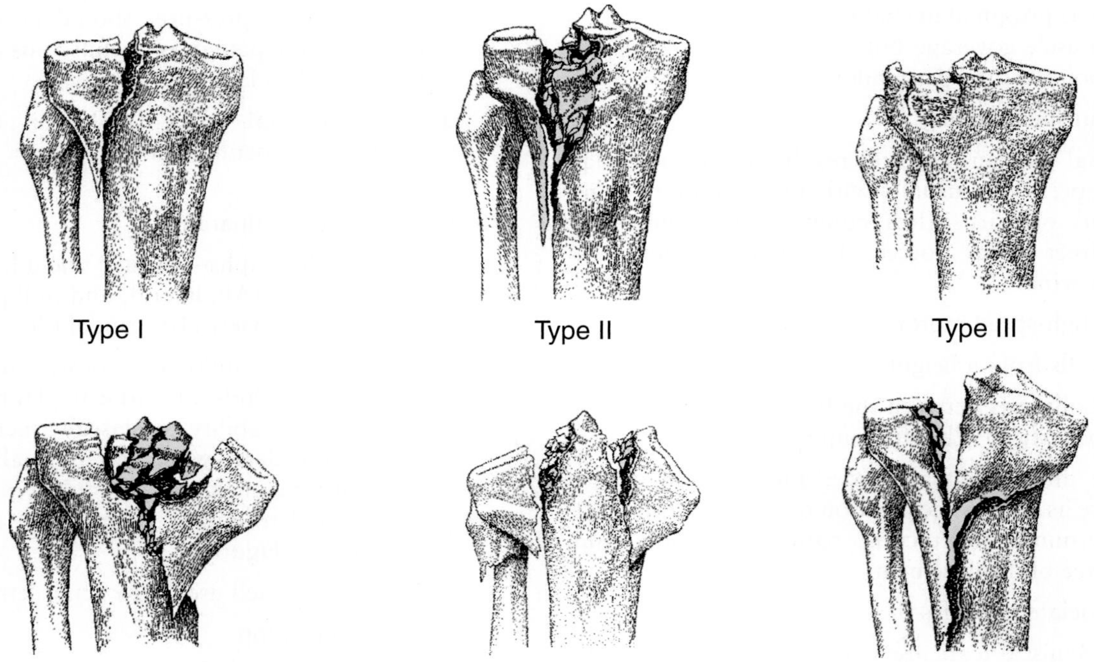

Figure 2 Illustrations depict the Schatzker classification of tibial plateau fractures. Type I: lateral plateau split; type II: lateral split-depression; type III: lateral depression; type IV: medial plateau fracture; type V: bicondylar injury; type VI: tibial plateau fracture with metaphyseal-diaphyseal dissociation. (Reproduced from Watson JT: Knee and leg: Bone trauma, in Beaty JH, ed: *Orthopaedic Knowledge Update*, ed 6. Rosemont, IL, American Academy of Orthopaedic Surgeons, 1999, p 523.)

3. The Orthopaedic Trauma Association (OTA) classification is the internationally accepted classification system (**Figure 4**).

F. Nonsurgical treatment

1. Nonsurgical treatment is indicated for:
   a. nondisplaced and stable fractures
   b. patient cannot undergo surgery for medical reasons
   c. knee with significant preexisting arthrosis.
2. Patients are placed in a hinged fracture brace, and early range-of-motion exercises are initiated.

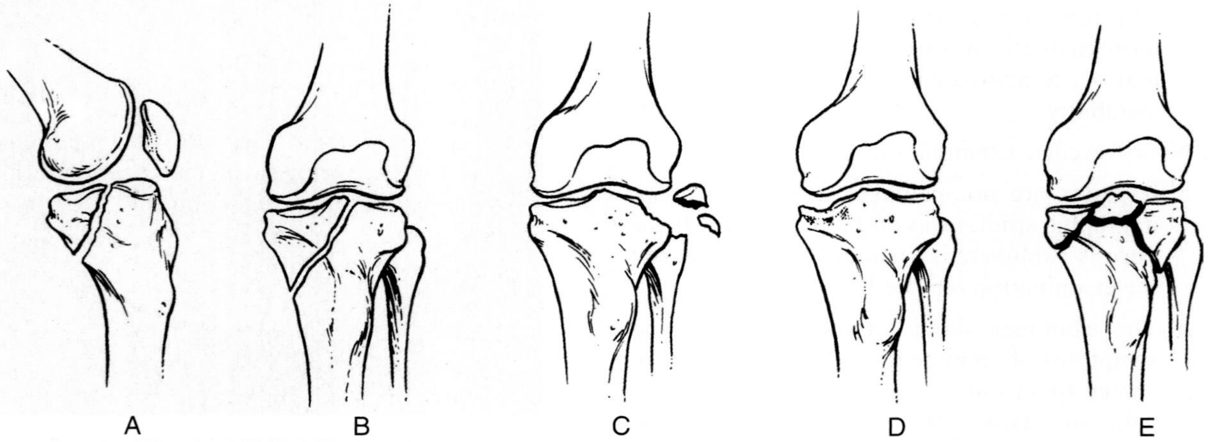

Figure 3 Illustrations show the Moore classification of tibial plateau fractures. **A**, Split fracture of the medial plateau in the coronal plane. **B**, Fracture of the entire condyle. **C**, Rim avulsion fracture. **D**, Pure compression fracture. **E**, Four-part fracture.

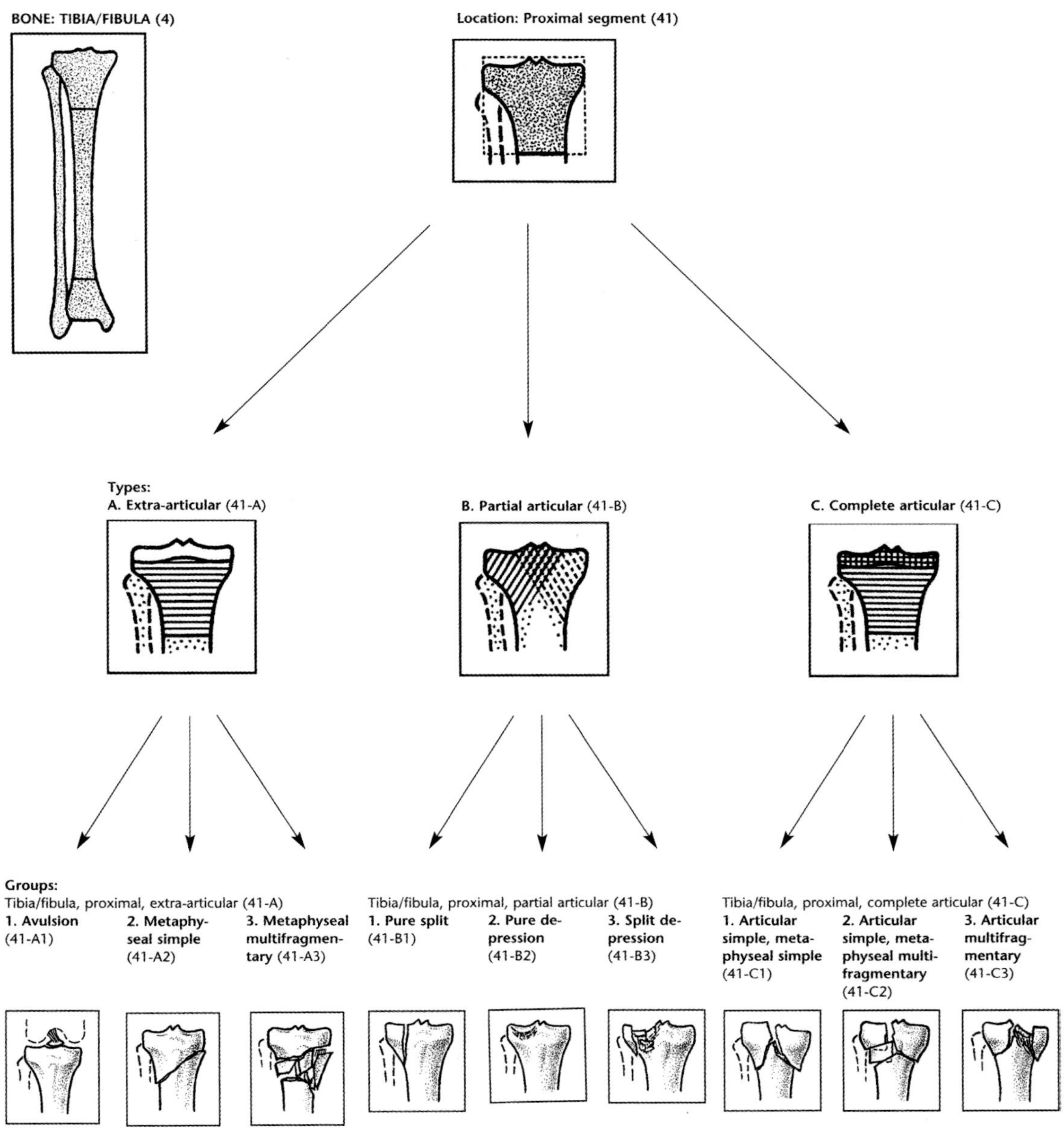

Figure 4 Illustration showing the OTA classification of proximal tibial/fibular fractures.

3. Partial weight bearing (30 to 50 lb) for 8 to 12 weeks is allowed, with progression to full weight bearing as tolerated thereafter.

G. Surgical treatment

1. Indications

a. For closed fractures: the range of articular depression considered to be acceptable varies from 2 mm or less to 1 cm. Instability greater than 10° of the nearly extended knee compared with the contralateral side is an accepted indication for surgical treatment of closed tibial plateau fractures.

b. For open fractures: irrigation and débridement is required, with either temporary fixation or immediate open reduction and internal fixation. Regardless of approach, the knee joint should not be left open.

c. For severe soft-tissue injury, temporary spanning external fixation should be considered if the limb is shortened or the joint is subluxated.

2. Reduction techniques

a. Indirect techniques have the advantage of minimal soft-tissue stripping and fragment devitalization. Centrally depressed articular fragments cannot be reduced indirectly by ligamentotaxis, however.

b. With direct techniques, depressed articular fragments may be elevated through, a split or a cortical window placed inferiorly through a metaphyseal osteotomy.

c. Arthroscopic-assisted reduction can be used in low-energy fractures; it also can be used as an adjunct to treatment by assessing the quality of fracture reduction.

3. Internal fixation techniques

a. Most low-energy fracture patterns are treated with a lateral approach and buttress plating.

b. A posteromedial approach is used to buttress posteromedial fragments.

c. Lag screws alone can be used for simple split fractures that are anatomically reduced in young patients with good quality bone, for depression fractures that are elevated percutaneously, or for securing simple avulsion fractures.

d. Plates may be applied submuscularly for fractures that extend to the metadiaphyseal region to secure the metaphysis to the diaphysis.

e. A submeniscal arthrotomy is performed to visualize the articular surface and repair as indicated. If torn, the meniscus should be repaired before closure.

f. Calcium phosphate cement is recommended to support metaphyseal defects due to a lower incidence of articular subsidence compared with autograft.

4. External fixation techniques

a. External fixation pins or wires should be placed 10 to 14 mm below the articular surface to avoid penetration of the synovial recess posteriorly.

b. A circular frame is an alternative to a long percutaneous plate.

5. Bicondylar tibial plateau fractures

a. Bicondylar fractures require dual-plate fixation or unilateral fixation with a locking plate. The use of a lateral locked plate is recommended only in the absence of medial comminution when the medial cortex is anatomically reduced.

b. An anterior midline incision should be avoided in bicondylar fractures because of the historically high rates of wound complications leading to the "dead bone sandwich" or high rates of wound complications.

H. Postoperative management

1. Early knee range of motion is encouraged.

2. Physical therapy should consist of active and active-assisted range-of-knee motion exercises, isometric quadriceps strengthening, and protected weight bearing.

3. Progressive weight bearing is generally initiated at 10 to 12 weeks postoperatively.

I. Complications

1. Early complications

a. Infection rates vary widely, from 1% to 38% of patients; superficial infections are more common (occurring in up to 38% of patients) than deep wound infections (occurring in up to 9.5%). Pin tract infections are common when external fixation is used.

b. Deep vein thrombosis develops in up to 10% of patients; pulmonary embolism may occur in 1% to 2%.

c. Knee stiffness may require secondary intervention. Associated with higher energy patterns and use of spanning external fixator.

2. Late complications

a. Painful hardware is a late complication.

b. Posttraumatic arthrosis may be related to chondral damage that occurs at the time of the injury. At follow-up, lateral articular incongruities appear to be well tolerated, whereas factors such as joint stability, coronal alignment, and retention of the meniscus may be more important in predicting arthrosis.

c. Nonunion is rare.

d. Loss of reduction, collapse, and/or malunion can occur if elevated fragments are not adequately buttressed.

II. TIBIAL-FIBULAR SHAFT FRACTURES

A. Epidemiology

1. These too have a bimodal incidence with most tibial shaft fractures resulting from low-energy mechanisms of injury. These fractures account for 4% of all fractures seen in the Medicare population. In younger patients, a high-energy injury such as a motor vehicle accident usually is the cause.

2. Isolated fibular shaft fractures are rare and usually are the result of a direct blow; they also can be associated with rotational ankle injuries (Maisonneuve fractures).

B. Anatomy
   1. Bony structures
      a. The anteromedial crest of the tibia is subcutaneous.
      b. The proximal medullary canal is centered laterally.
      c. The anterior tibial crest is composed of dense cortical bone.
      d. The fibular shaft is palpable proximally and distally. The fibula is the site of the muscular attachment for the peroneal musculature and the flexor hallucis longus. It contributes little to load bearing (15%).
   2. Musculature
      a. The anterior compartment contains the tibialis anterior, extensor digitorum longus, the extensor hallucis longus, the anterior tibial artery, and the deep peroneal nerve.
      b. The lateral compartment contains the peroneus longus and brevis and the superficial peroneal nerve.
      c. The superficial posterior compartment contains the gastrocnemius-soleus complex, the soleus, the popliteus, and the plantaris muscles.
      d. The deep posterior compartment contains the tibialis posterior, the flexor digitorum longus, the flexor hallucis longus, the posterior tibial artery, the peroneal artery, and the tibial nerve.

C. Mechanism of injury
   1. Most tibial-fibular shaft fractures result from a torsional (indirect) or bending (direct) mechanism.
      a. Indirect mechanisms result in spiral fractures.
      b. Direct mechanisms result in wedge or short oblique fractures (low energy) or increased comminution (higher energy).
      c. Stress fractures may occur in athletes and military recruits and are the result of fatigue failure (**Figure 5**).
   2. Associated injuries include open wounds, compartment syndrome, ipsilateral skeletal injury (ie, extension to the tibial plateau or plafond), and remote skeletal injury.

D. Clinical evaluation
   1. Physical examination
      a. The examiner should inspect the limb for gross deformity, angulation, and malrotation.

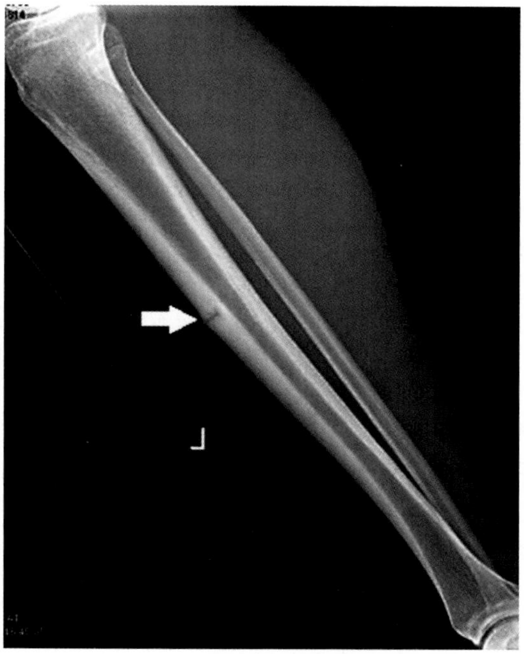

Figure 5 Lateral radiograph of a right tibia demonstrates a tibial stress fracture with the pathognomonic "dreaded black line" (arrow).

      b. Palpation for tenderness and swelling is important as well. The fact that the anterior tibial crest is subcutaneous makes identification of the fracture site easier.
   2. Neurovascular examination
      a. The examiner should assess for signs and symptoms of impending compartment syndrome (tense compartment, pain out of proportion to the injury, or pain on passive stretch of the toes).
      b. Compartment syndrome is more common following a pedestrian struck mechanism.
      c. Continuous intracompartmental monitoring is indicated in patients who are unable to communicate (eg, the intubated and sedated patient in the intensive care unit).
      d. Compartment release by fasciotomy is indicated if the patient has one or more of the signs and symptoms listed above and there is less than 30 mm Hg difference (ΔP) between the compartmental pressure and the diastolic pressure.
      e. After the diagnosis of compartment syndrome is made, all four compartments must be released.
      f. May be done through a single or double incision technique.

7 | Trauma

3. Radiographic evaluation
   a. Plain radiographs should include a tibia trauma series (AP, lateral, and oblique), with dedicated ankle or plateau views if the fracture extends to the surface of the joint. The entire tibia and fibula must be visualized, from knee to ankle.
   b. After any fracture manipulation, postreduction views must also be obtained.
   c. CT can be used to assess fracture healing or identify nonunion, but it plays no role in acute fracture management.

E. Fracture classification
1. Fractures are usually described based on the pattern, location, and amount of comminution.
2. The OTA classification includes types 42A (simple patterns—that is, spiral, transverse, or oblique), 42B (wedge), and 42C (complex, comminuted) (**Figure 6**).
3. Soft-tissue classification
   a. The Oestern and Tscherne classification is used for closed fractures (**Table 1**).
   b. The Gustilo-Anderson classification is used for open fractures (**Table 2**).
   c. The OTA Open Fracture Classification has recently been published.

F. Nonsurgical treatment
1. Indications—Nonsurgical treatment is indicated for low-energy stable tibial fractures (such as axially stable fracture patterns) and virtually all isolated fibular shaft fractures.
   a. Nonsurgical treatment is contraindicated for open fractures and fractures with an intact fibula.
2. Initial long leg casting is indicated, followed by functional bracing treatment in a patellar tendon–bearing brace or cast, with weight bearing as tolerated after 2 to 3 weeks. Cast-wedging may be used to correct deformity.
3. Following closed treatment, the mean shortening is 4 mm and mean angulation is less than 6°; nonunion occurs in 1.1% of patients.

G. Surgical treatment
1. Indications
   a. When acceptable reduction parameters cannot be maintained, including less than 50% displacement, less than 10° of angulation, less than 1 cm of shortening, and less than 10° of rotational malalignment
   b. In patients with open fractures, fractures with associated compartment syndrome, and inherently unstable patterns (segmental, comminuted, short, displaced), and in patients with multiple injuries (eg, floating knee)
   c. Stress fractures that have failed nonoperative treatment.
2. Intramedullary (IM) nailing
   a. Reamed IM nailing is the treatment of choice for unstable fracture patterns because it allows the use of a larger-diameter nail (with larger locking bolts) and paradoxically results in maintenance of periosteal perfusion. In addition, with tibial reaming, in contrast to femoral reaming, concern about embolization of the marrow contents is minimal.
      - Insertion of IM nails may be via a supra- or infrapatellar portal.
      - Recent studies suggest that suprapatellar nailing leads to reduced knee pain, visual analog score, sagittal angle, and fluoroscopy time. To date no differences have been reported in outcomes.
      - Suprapatellar nailing in the semi-extended position may allow for easier reduction of proximal and distal fractures.
   b. A nonreamed IM nail is looser fitting than a reamed nail and is associated with less cortical necrosis. It is also associated with a higher rate of locking screw breakage than is reamed IM nailing.
   c. Use of blocking screws, a unicortical plate, a lateral starting point, and IM nailing in a semi-extended position may help prevent displacement of proximal fractures into flexion and valgus.
   d. Use of blocking screws and/or fibular plating may help prevent displacement of distal fractures into valgus (if at the same level as a fibular fracture) or varus (if the fibula is intact).
   e. Contraindications to IM nailing include a preexisting tibial shaft deformity that may preclude IM nail passage and a history of previous IM infection.
3. Plates and screws
   a. Open plating techniques typically have been associated with wound problems and nonunion.
   b. Newer plate designs and minimally invasive techniques have allowed these implants to play

Chapter 103
FRACTURES OF THE ANKLE AND TIBIAL PLAFOND

CHRISTOPHER DEL BALSO, BSc, MSc, MBBS, FRCSC
DAVID W. SANDERS, MD, MSc, FRCSC
KENNETH A. EGOL, MD

I. ROTATIONAL FRACTURES OF THE ANKLE

A. Epidemiology

1. Rotational fractures of the ankle are among the most common injuries requiring orthopaedic care.
2. Ankle fractures vary from relatively simple injuries with minimal long-term effects to complex injuries with severe long-term sequelae.
3. Population-based studies have identified an increase in the incidence of ankle fractures. Data from Medicare enrollees suggest the rate of ankle fractures in the United States averages 4.2 fractures per 1,000 Medicare enrollees annually.
4. Rates of surgery vary depending on the type of fracture.
    a. For isolated lateral malleolar fractures, which account for two-thirds of rotational ankle fractures, the surgical intervention rate is approximately 11%.
    b. For trimalleolar fractures, the surgical intervention rate is 74%.
5. Risk factors for ankle fracture include age, increased body mass, and a history of ankle fracture.
6. The highest incidence of ankle fractures occurs in elderly women.

B. Anatomy of the lower leg

1. Osseous anatomy and ligaments of the ankle joint (**Figure 1**)
    a. The osseous anatomy of the ankle provides stability during weight bearing and mobility in plantar flexion.
    b. The ankle joint behaves like a true mortise in dorsiflexion.
    c. Stability is achieved by articular contact between the medial malleolus, the fibula, the tibial plafond, and the talus.
    d. The talar dome is wider anteriorly than posteriorly so that, as the ankle dorsiflexes, the fibula rotates externally through the tibiofibular syndesmosis to accommodate the talus.
    e. The lateral malleolus is surrounded by multiple strong ligaments.
        - These include the interosseous membrane and the tibiofibular ligamentous complex, consisting of the interosseous ligament and the syndesmotic ligaments (anterior inferior tibiofibular ligament [AITFL], posterior inferior tibiofibular ligament, inferior transverse tibiofibular ligament, inferior interosseous ligament).
        - These ligaments are responsible for the stability of the ankle in external rotation.
        - In addition, the lateral collateral ligaments of the ankle, including the anterior and

Dr. Sanders serves as a paid consultant to or is an employee of Stryker; has received research or institutional support from Arthrex, Inc. and Stryker; and serves as a board member, owner, officer, or committee member of the Orthopaedic Trauma Association. Dr. Egol or an immediate family member has received royalties from Exactech, Inc.; is a member of a speakers' bureau or has made paid presentations on behalf of Smith & Nephew; serves as a paid consultant to or is an employee of Exactech, Inc.; serves as an unpaid consultant to Polypid; has received research or institutional support from Acumed, LLC and Synthes; and serves as a board member, owner, officer, or committee member of the Orthopaedic Trauma Association. Neither Dr. Del Balso nor any immediate family member has received anything of value from or has stock or stock options held in a commercial company or institution related directly or indirectly to the subject of this chapter.

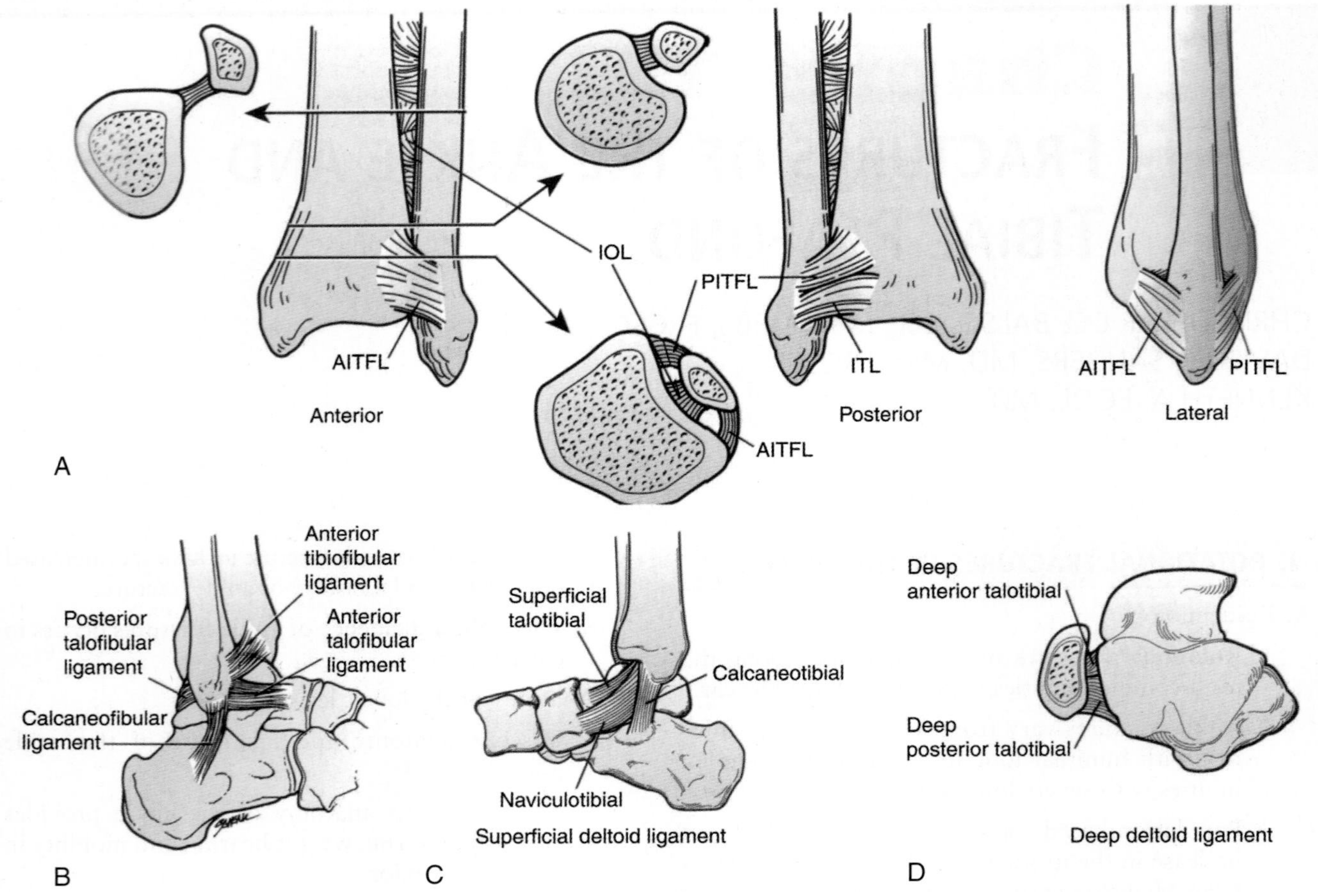

Figure 1 Illustrations show the osseous anatomy and ligaments of the ankle joint. **A**, Anterior, posterior, and lateral views of the tibiofibular syndesmotic ligaments. **B**, The lateral collateral ligaments of the ankle and the anterior syndesmotic ligament. Sagittal plane (**C**) and transverse plane (**D**) views of the medial collateral ligaments of the ankle. AITFL = anterior inferior tibiofibular ligament, IOL = interosseous ligament, ITL = inferior transverse ligament, PITFL = posterior inferior tibiofibular ligament. (Panels **A**, **C**, and **D** adapted with permission from Browner B, Jupiter J, Levine A, eds: *Skeletal Trauma: Fractures, Dislocations, and Ligamentous Injuries*, ed 2. Philadelphia, PA, WB Saunders, 1997. Panel **B** reproduced with permission from Marsh JL, Saltzman CL: Ankle fractures, in Bucholz RW, Heckman JD, Court-Brown CM, eds: *Rockwood and Green's Fractures in Adults*, ed 6. Philadelphia, PA, Lippincott Williams and Wilkins, 2006, pp 2147-2247.)

posterior talofibular ligaments and calcaneofibular ligaments, provide support and resistance to inversion and anterior translation of the talus relative to the fibula.

2. Medial malleolus
   a. The medial malleolar surface of the distal tibia has a larger surface anteriorly than posteriorly.
   b. The posterior border of the medial malleolus includes the groove for the posterior tibial tendon.
   c. The medial malleolus includes the anterior malleolus, which is larger than and extends approximately 0.5 cm distal to the posterior malleolus.
   d. The deltoid ligament provides medial ligamentous support of the ankle.
      - The important deep component of the deltoid ligament arises from the intercollicular groove and posterior malleolus.
      - The deep layer of the deltoid ligament is a short, thick ligament inserting on the medial surface of the talus.
      - The superficial deltoid ligament arises from the anterior malleolus of the medial malleolus.
3. Tendinous and neurovascular structures
   a. Posterior group
      - The posterior group includes the Achilles and plantaris tendons.

c. CT may assist in determining whether a fracture can be reduced percutaneously or an open approach is required.

d. If temporary external fixation is planned, CT done following application of the external fixator and realignment of the limb provides the best information. If definitive external fixation is selected, the CT should be obtained preoperatively.

H. Nonsurgical treatment

1. Nonsurgical care is less common for tibial plafond fractures than for ankle fractures.

2. Indications

a. Stable fracture patterns without displacement of the articular surface are treated nonsurgically; the nonsurgical treatment of fractures with articular displacement generally has yielded poor results.

b. Nonambulatory patients or patients with significant neuropathy may be treated nonsurgically as well.

3. Nonsurgical treatment consists of casting for 6 weeks followed by a fracture brace and range-of-motion exercises, versus early range-of-motion exercises.

a. Manipulation of displaced fractures is unlikely to result in the reduction of intra-articular fragments.

b. Loss of reduction is common.

c. The inability to monitor soft-tissue status and swelling is a major disadvantage.

I. Surgical treatment

1. Most treatment strategies for tibial plafond fractures currently are related to the safe management of the soft tissues.

2. External or internal fixation may be used.

3. External fixation

a. General issues

- As definitive treatment, external fixation uses limited approaches to reduce the articular surface with minimal internal fixation of the joint surface.
- It may bridge the ankle or may be localized to the distal tibia.
- External fixation that spans the ankle may involve less disruption of the zone of injury, but it has the disadvantage of rigidly immobilizing the ankle.
- Hybrid external fixation applied to a tibial side of the ankle joint allows greater motion at the ankle. The placement of pins and wires often disrupts the zone of injury.

b. Techniques for application of definitive external fixation

- In an ankle-bridging technique, pins are placed initially in the calcaneus and talar neck and proximal pins are placed in the medial subcutaneous border of the tibia.
- A fixator is then placed, and the articular surface is reduced provisionally with ligamentotaxis.
- Fracture reduction forceps or clamps can then be placed percutaneously directly over the fracture lines to reduce displaced fragments.
- Articular fragments are stabilized using lag screws.
- The external fixator is used to maintain length, alignment, and rotation of the extremity and to protect the joint as fracture healing occurs.
- This technique preserves soft tissues and can be staged if necessary when the zone of injury is not thought to be safe enough to tolerate the limited approaches required for reduction.

4. Internal fixation

a. General

- Internal fixation using definitive plate fixation of high-energy tibial plafond fractures continues to evolve.
- Initial successes using this technique, described by Rüedi and Allgöwer, were followed by many reports of failure, with the incidence of wound complications approaching 40% in a large series of patients with high-energy tibial plafond fractures.
- Staged treatment with early external fixation +/– fibular fixation followed by definitive reduction and fixation after soft-tissue healing has reduced the rate of wound complications to 0% to 6%,

b. Tips for minimizing complications

- Various techniques have been recommended for minimizing the complications of plating, including delaying definitive surgical treatment using spanning external fixation until the soft tissues have settled; using lower-profile implants; minimizing anteromedial incisions; indirect reduction techniques that minimize soft-tissue stripping; and patient selection based on the injury pattern as necessary.

- Previous guidelines suggested >7 cm distance between incisions about the ankle; it appears to be acceptable to place incisions closer to one another than previously believed. A prospective study found separation of as little as 5 cm was acceptable when good surgical technique was used.

c. Definitive internal fixation is performed in two stages.

- Stage 1—Fibular plating to regain lateral column length and application of a simple spanning external fixator.
  - Two proximal half-pins are placed on the anterior tibia.
  - Placing pins within or outside of the future zone of surgery is controversial and has not been definitively shown to affect complication rates.
  - A 5- or 6-mm centrally threaded pin can be placed across the calcaneus and attached to the proximal half-pins using a combination of struts. This technique is simple to perform and maintains stability and alignment. Extra care is necessary to avoid pressure from bony fragments on soft tissues, prevent shortening, and maintain forefoot positioning.
  - Typically, a delay of approximately 2 weeks is needed to allow the soft tissues to heal.
- Stage 2—Formal articular reduction and internal fixation
  - Once ORIF is performed, incisions are made only as large as required to anatomically reduce the articular surface. Periosteal stripping is performed only at the edges of the fracture to achieve visualization of the reduction while preserving the blood supply.
  - Precontoured plates may be useful; both anteromedial and anterolateral plates facilitate percutaneous placement.
  - Void filling with bone graft or substitutes to fill metaphyseal voids was once described as a standard step in fixation of a tibial plafond fracture; however, with less extensive dissection in the metaphyseal region, the indications for grafting have become less routine.

TABLE 3

Pearls for the Treatment of Tibial Plafond Fractures

Treatment Step	Pearls
Soft-tissue management	Avoid surgery when swollen Use spanning fixator to control alignment and soft tissues
Spanning fixator	Simple construct Tibial pins should avoid future surgical site Reestablish length and alignment
Definitive open reduction and internal fixation	Approach guided by CT Limited incisions, avoid periosteal stripping Restore alignment and anatomically reduce joint Use distractor intraoperatively to facilitate reduction. Low-profile implants

5. Pearls are described in **Table 3.**

J. Rehabilitation

1. Rehabilitation after tibial plafond fractures is prolonged. Patients should be counseled that weight bearing may be delayed for 3 months or more.
2. In patients treated by external fixation, the healing time is generally 12 to 16 weeks.
3. Tibial plafond fractures have a significant deleterious long-term effect on ankle function and quality of life. Worse outcomes are seen when complications occur.
4. When possible, motion of the ankle joint should be permitted and facilitated.
5. The use of a removable boot or brace may be of benefit as the patient transitions from immobilization and non–weight bearing to mobilization and protected weight-bearing status.

K. Complications

1. Malunion
   a. Malalignment of the tibia is relatively common.
   b. Articular malunion is probably even more common than recognized.
   c. Series using definitive external fixation have reported an increased incidence of fair or poor articular reduction compared with formal ORIF.
   d. Angular malalignment also may occur. Loss of alignment following treatment occurs in particular if union is delayed and implant failure occurs.

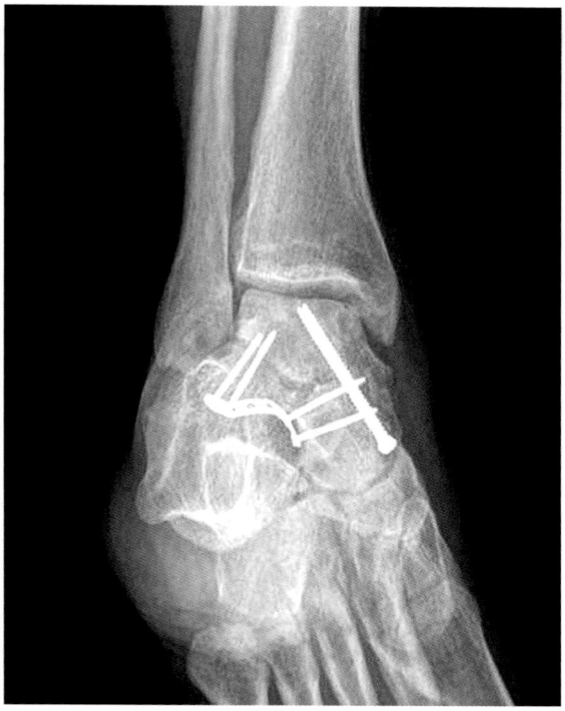

Figure 2 Postoperative radiograph of a fracture of the talus treated with medial screws and a lateral plate through two incisions.

6. Complications (**Table 1**)
   a. Posttraumatic arthritis is the most common complication of talar fractures and can affect the subtalar and/or tibiotalar joints.
   b. Osteonecrosis
      - The limited blood supply to the talus creates the risk of osteonecrosis with fractures of the talar neck.
      - The risk of osteonecrosis increases with each successive Hawkins type of fracture. Restricting weight bearing beyond that needed for the healing of a fracture does not decrease the risk of osteonecrosis.

TABLE 1

Complications of Talar Neck Fractures

Fracture Pattern	Osteonecrosis (%)	Posttraumatic Arthritis (%)	Malunion (%)
Type I	0-13	0-30	0-10
Type II	20-50	40-90	0-25
Type III/IV	80-100	70-100	18-27

Reproduced from Fortin PT, Balazsy JE: Talus fractures: Evaluation and treatment. *J Am Acad Orthop Surg* 2001;9:114-127.

      - The Hawkins sign, consisting of subchondral osteopenia seen at 6 to 8 weeks on plain radiographs, indicates revascularization of the talar body. It is 100% sensitive but only 58% specific for this and is therefore a reliable indicator of an intact blood supply when present, although its absence does not rule out an intact vascularity.
      - Osteonecrosis of the talus may be seen as early as 3 to 6 months postoperatively on plain radiographs, accompanied by sclerosis. MRI is sensitive for detecting osteonecrosis, with decreased signal intensity on T1-weighted MRI, but rarely guides treatment.
      - Osteonecrosis usually does not involve the entire talar body and often does not require further surgery. Tibiotalar fusion is an option for treating a talus damaged by osteonecrosis when nonsurgical treatment is unsuccessful.
      - Extensive osteonecrosis may require excision of the talar body with tibiotalocalcaneal fusion or Blair fusion, which involves resection of the talar body with fusion of the talar head to the tibia and bone grafting for repair of the osteonecrotic defect to maintain overall limb length.
   c. Varus malunion also can occur as a complication of untreated talar fractures and can limit eversion of the foot. It may be treated with a corrective osteotomy.

C. Fractures of the talar body
   1. Fractures involving large portions of the talar body are usually the result of high-energy injuries.
   2. CT provides the best visualization of fractures of the talar body and is used to identify fractures in the transverse, coronal, and sagittal planes.
   3. ORIF with a dual lateral and medial approach is required when the articular surfaces of the talus are displaced by more than 2 mm. Medial and/or lateral malleolar osteotomy may be required for ORIF.
   4. A posteromedial or posterolateral approach to fracture repair, with dorsiflexion and distraction, can expose most of the talar dome.
   5. Complications of fractures of the talar body include posttraumatic arthritis (occurring in as many as 88% of cases) and osteonecrosis. Posttraumatic osteoarthritis is the most common complication.

7 | Trauma

D. Fractures of the lateral process of the talus

1. These fractures occur with dorsiflexion–external rotation injuries. A common mechanism is a snowboarding injury.
2. AP radiographs may show the fracture, but a CT scan is needed to adequately visualize these injuries and for surgical planning.
3. Nondisplaced fractures of the lateral process of the talus can be treated with immobilization in a cast and non–weight bearing.
4. ORIF is indicated for fractures displaced by more than 2 mm. Comminuted fractures not amenable to ORIF can be treated with casting. Excision of the fracture fragment is an option if symptoms persist.
5. The most common complication of fractures of the lateral process is posttraumatic subtalar arthritis.

E. Fractures of the posterior process of the talus

1. The posterior process of the talus includes a posteromedial and a posterolateral tubercle. Plain radiographs may not clearly show the area of fracture, whereas CT is useful for identifying these fractures.
2. Fractures of the posteromedial tubercle result from avulsion of the posterior talotibial ligament or posterior deltoid ligament.
   a. Small fragments of fractures of the posteromedial tubercle are treated with immobilization followed by late excision if symptoms persist.
   b. Large, displaced fragments are treated with ORIF.
3. Fractures of the posterolateral tubercle result from avulsion of the posterior talofibular ligament. Pain is aggravated by flexion and extension of the flexor hallucis longus tendon.
   a. Initial nonsurgical management with late excision for symptomatic lesions is indicated for fractures with no subtalar involvement.
   b. ORIF is indicated for fractures with subtalar involvement.
4. Nonunion in fractures of the posterior process of the talus is difficult to distinguish from symptomatic os trigonum. Both conditions can be treated with excision.

IV. FRACTURES OF THE CALCANEUS

A. Intra-articular fractures

1. Mechanisms of injury
   a. The calcaneus is the most frequently fractured of the tarsal bones. Most (75%) of fractures of the calcaneus are intra-articular.
   b. Axial loading is the primary mechanism of fracture of the calcaneus, with falls from a height and motor vehicle accidents the most common causes of such loading.
   c. An oblique shear force causing fracture of the calcaneus results in a primary fracture line and two primary fragments:
      - The superomedial fragment includes the sustentaculum, which is stabilized by strong ligamentous and capsular attachments. This is called the constant fragment because it usually retains its anatomic position, making it a useful reference point for fracture reduction.
      - The superolateral fragment has an intra-articular component through the posterior facet and posterolateral tuberosity of the calcaneus.
   d. Secondary fracture lines signal whether there is joint depression or a tongue-type fracture. The two types of fracture are defined by whether or not the superolateral fragment and posterior facet of the calcaneus are separated from the posterolateral tuberosity. In tongue-type fractures, the superolateral fragment and posterior facet are attached posteriorly to the tuberosity.
2. Radiographic evaluation
   a. The lateral view of the foot and ankle can be used to determine the Böhler angle (normally 20° to 40°) and to assess loss of height. Double density of the posterior facet indicates subtalar incongruity.
   b. AP and oblique views can show the calcaneocuboid joint.
   c. The Broden view helps intraoperatively evaluate reduction of the posterior facet.
   d. The axial Harris view reveals widening, shortening, lateral translation, and varus positioning of the tuberosity fragment of a calcaneal fracture.
   e. An AP view of the ankle is useful for assessing extrusion of the lateral wall of the calcaneus with impingement against the fibula or peroneal tendons.

3. Sanders classification of calcaneal fractures (**Figure 3**)
   a. Used to guide treatment and to predict outcome of treatment of calcaneal fractures
   b. Based on CT visualization of the widest portion of the subtalar joint in the coronal oblique plane and the number of fracture fragments of the posterior facet of the calcaneus
      - Type I fractures: nondisplaced.
      - Type II fractures: the posterior facet is in two fragments.
      - Type III fractures: the posterior facet is in three fragments.
      - Type IV fractures: comminuted, with more than three articular fragments.
   c. Other important characteristics of calcaneal features according to the Sanders classification include the degrees of shortening, widening, and lateral wall impingement, which may result in pathology of the peroneal tendon.

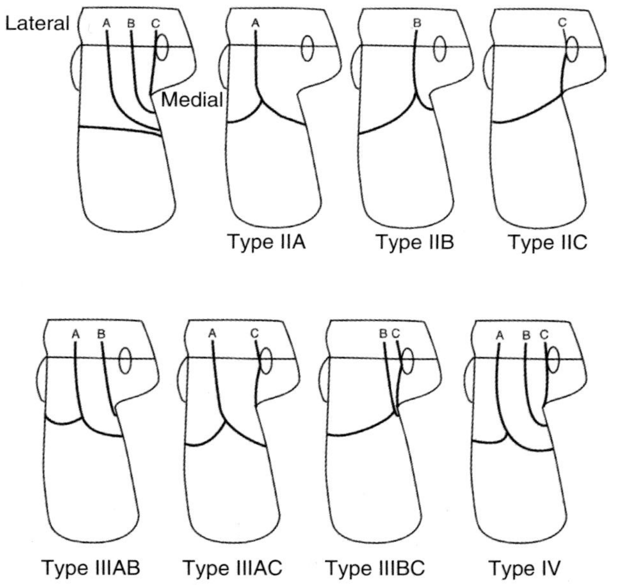

Figure 3 Illustrations showing CT-based classification of displaced intra-articular calcaneal fractures. The first drawing shows the lateral (**A**), central (**B**), and medial (**C**) fracture lines. Type I (not shown) = nondisplaced calcaneal fracture. Type II = displaced intra-articular calcaneus fractures (DIACF) with a single displaced primary fracture line in the posterior facet. Type III = DIACF with two displaced fracture lines into the posterior facet. Type IV = comminuted DIACF with three or more displaced fracture lines in the posterior facet. This classification is prognostic ($P = 0.06$). (Reproduced from Buckley RE, Tough S: Displaced intra-articular calcaneal fractures. *J Am Acad Orthop Surg* 2004;12[3]:172-178.)

4. Nonsurgical treatment
   a. Type I fractures are treated nonsurgically.
   b. Patients do not bear weight for 6 to 8 weeks.
   c. ROM exercises are initiated early, as soon as soft-tissue swelling allows.
5. Surgical treatment
   a. Treatment of type II and III fractures remains controversial. Both ORIF and nonsurgical management have been advocated; nonsurgical management is the same as that for type I fractures. Improved outcomes after surgery are associated with age younger than 40 years, female sex, and simple fracture patterns. Negative factors include smoking, diabetes, workers' compensation, carrying heavy physical workloads, and higher comminution of fracture.
   b. ORIF is generally delayed for 10 to 14 days until resolution of soft-tissue swelling (with the exception of fractures of the posterior tuberosity, which can cause skin necrosis and will benefit from early reduction and surgery) (**Figure 4**).
      - The sinus tarsi approach has increased in popularity and allows reduction and fixation early with lowered risk of wound complications. If chosen, this should be done early to allow ease of reduction.
      - An extensile lateral L-shaped incision is the most common approach in the ORIF of calcaneal fractures.
      - No-touch retraction techniques are used, a pin is placed in the tuberosity fragment to assist reduction, and a drain is inserted.
      - Bone grafting (autografting or allografting) has not been shown to be beneficial in treating calcaneal fractures. Injectable calcium phosphate cement has been shown to permit early weight bearing without loss of articular reduction.
   c. Type IV fractures can be treated with ORIF and primary fusion; ORIF alone (as well as nonsurgical treatment) is associated with poor results.
   d. Outcomes correlate with the accuracy of fracture reduction and the number of articular fragments. Type II fractures have better outcomes than type III fractures, whereas type IV fractures have the poorest outcomes.

7 | Trauma

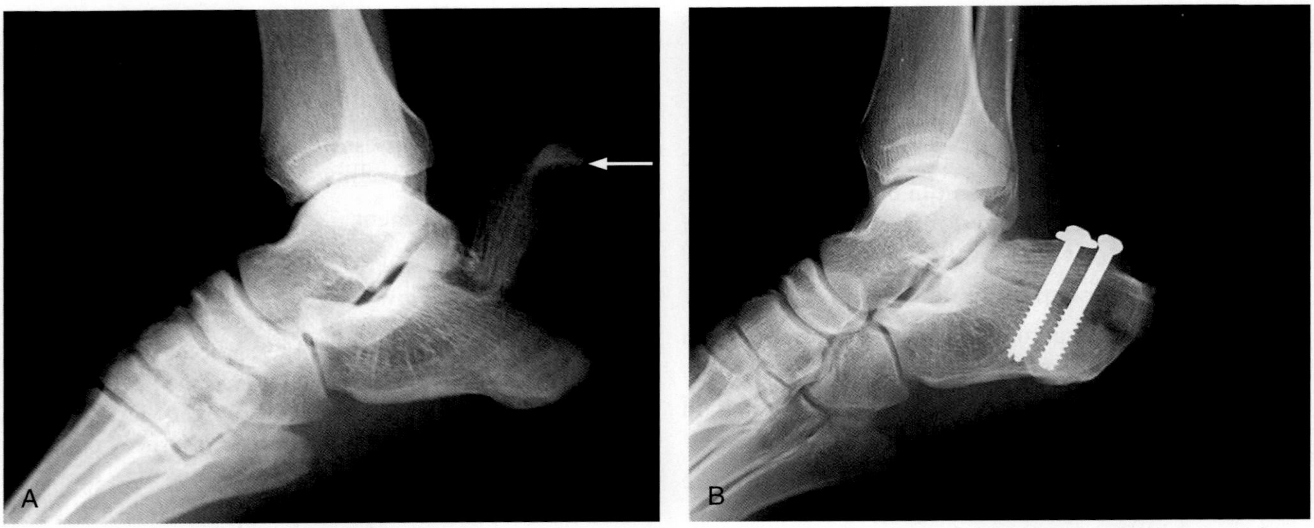

Figure 4 Lateral radiographs demonstrate avulsion of the calcaneal tuberosity requiring urgent reduction and fixation to prevent skin necrosis (arrow). Preoperative (**A**) and postoperative (**B**) views.

6. Complications
   a. A complication rate of up to 40% has been reported in fractures of the calcaneus. Factors that increase the risk of complications include falls from a height, early surgery, and smoking. Approximately 10% of patients have associated injuries of the lumbar spine.
   b. Wound-related complications are the most common complications of calcaneal fractures. Other potential complications include malunion, subtalar arthritis, and lateral impingement with pathology of the peroneal tendon.
   c. Compartment syndrome of the foot develops in up to 10% of patients and may lead to a claw toe deformity.
   d. Malunion can occur and result in loss of height and in widening of the heel and lateral impingement.
      - The talus may be dorsiflexed, with a decrease in the declination angle of the talus to less than 20°, which limits dorsiflexion of the ankle.
      - Impingement of the lateral wall associated with malunion may result in pathology of the peroneal tendon. Additionally, subtalar incongruity can result in subtalar arthritis. Difficulty with shoe wear also can occur, as a result of widening of the heel and loss of height. Malunions of the calcaneus are treated with lateral exostectomy. Fusion is also added to treat subtalar arthritis.

B. Extra-articular fractures (posterior tuberosity of the calcaneus)
   1. Mechanism of injury—Strong contraction of the gastrocnemius–soleus muscle complex and avulsion at its insertion on the posterior tuberosity of the calcaneus
   2. Treatment
      a. Early reduction is important because displaced fractures of the posterior tuberosity can cause pressure necrosis of the overlying skin.
      b. Full-thickness skin sloughing may require flap coverage.
      c. Small fracture fragments can be excised, but fractures with larger fragments require ORIF. Note, however, that screw fixation alone may fail in osteopenic bone but can be augmented with tension band fixation.

C. Fractures of the anterior process
   1. Mechanism of injury
      a. Inversion and plantar flexion.
      b. Fractures result from avulsion of the bifurcate ligament.
   2. Treatment
      a. Small extra-articular fragments are treated with immobilization.
      b. Larger fragments (>1 cm) can involve the calcaneocuboid joint and require ORIF if joint displacement is present.
      c. Late excision is used for chronically painful nonunion.

V. MIDFOOT FRACTURES

A. Fractures of the navicular bone

1. Anatomy
    a. The navicular bone articulates with the medial, intermediate, and lateral cuneiform bones, the cuboid bone, and the calcaneus and talus.
    b. The talonavicular articulation is critical to maintaining the ROM of inversion and eversion of the foot.
    c. The blood supply to the navicular bone is limited in its central watershed portion, making this area susceptible to fractures.
2. Radiographic evaluation
    a. Plain radiographs including AP, lateral, internal oblique, and external oblique images of the foot are used for the initial evaluation of navicular fractures.
    b. CT is useful for characterizing the fracture pattern. MRI can be used for the detection of stress fractures.
3. Avulsion fractures of the navicular bone
    a. Constitute one half of all navicular fractures; avulsion of the dorsal lip results from stress imposed by the deltoid ligament during eversion of the foot; medial avulsion results from stress imposed by the tibialis posterior muscle; plantar avulsion results from stress imposed by the spring ligament.
    b. Acute treatment consists of immobilization with delayed excision of painful fragments.
    c. ORIF is required for fractures with fragments involving more than 25% of the articular surface.
4. Fractures of the tuberosity of the navicular bone
    a. The principal mechanism of fracture is eversion and contraction of the posterior tibial tendon, which may result in the diastasis of a preexisting accessory navicular bone.
    b. Best visualized on an oblique radiograph and at 45° of internal rotation.
    c. Most avulsion fractures of the tuberosity can be managed with immobilization.
    d. Acute ORIF is indicated with more than 5 mm of diastasis or with large intra-articular fracture fragments.
    e. Symptomatic nonunion is treated with late excision and reattachment of the tibialis posterior tendon.
5. Fractures of the navicular body (**Figure 5**)
    a. Mechanism of injury is axial loading.
    b. The Sangeorzan classification of fractures of the body of the navicular bone is based on the plane of the fracture and the degree of comminution (**Table 2**).
    c. Minimally displaced type I and II fractures are treated nonsurgically.

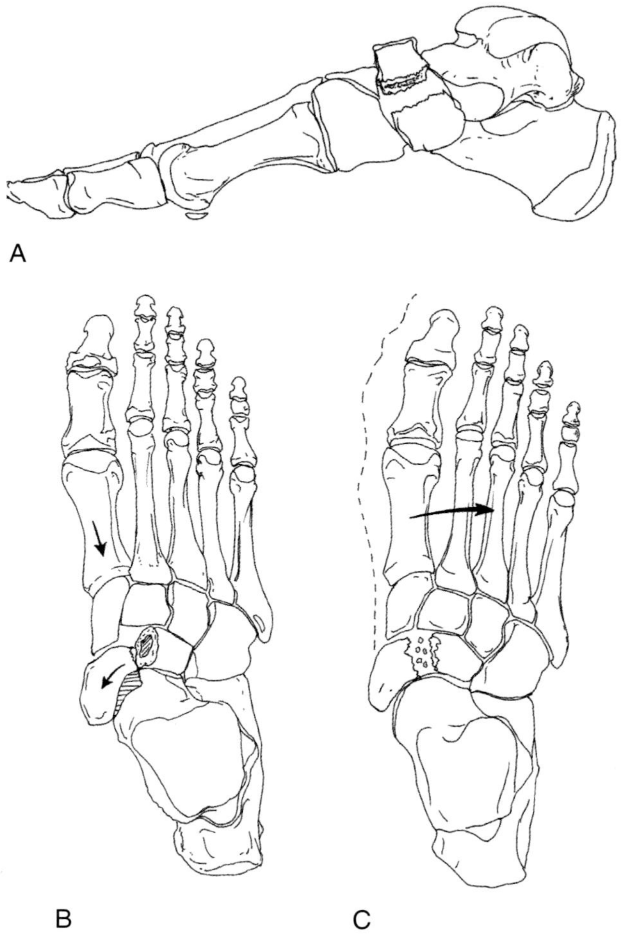

Figure 5 Illustrations showing navicular fractures. **A**, Lateral view of a type I navicular fracture (axial plane fracture line). **B**, AP view of a type II navicular fracture (sagittal plane fracture line). The arrows indicate the direction of applied force. Note the subluxation of the talonavicular joint and proximal migration of the first ray, a common component of type II fractures. **C**, AP view of a type III navicular fracture. Note the comminution, displacement, and incongruity of the talonavicular and naviculocuneiform joints. The arrow indicates the direction of applied force. (Reproduced from Stroud CC: Fractures of the midtarsals, metatarsals, and phalanges, in Richardson EG, ed: *Orthopaedic Knowledge Update: Foot and Ankle*, ed 3. Rosemont, IL, American Academy of Orthopaedic Surgeons, 2003, p 58.)

TABLE 2

Sangeorzan Classification of Navicular Fractures

Type	Features
I	Transverse Involves a dorsal fragment < 50% of the bone No associated deformity
II	Oblique Most commonly from dorsal-lateral to plantarmedial May be associated with forefoot adduction
III	Central or lateral comminution with abduction May be associated with cuboid or anterior process calcaneal fractures

d. ORIF through a medial incision is used for displaced type I and II fractures or with disruption of the talonavicular joint.

e. Type III fractures require ORIF. A spanning external fixator or plate may be used to maintain the length of the medial column of the foot after fixation of the primary fracture fragments.

6. Stress fractures of the navicular bone

a. Most common in runners and basketball players

b. When acute, these injuries can be treated either nonsurgically or surgically. Nonunion requires ORIF. Bone grafting may be used to encourage healing.

B. Tarsometatarsal (Lisfranc) fracture-dislocations

1. Anatomy

a. The bones of the midfoot include the navicular, cuboid, cuneiform bones, and bases of the metatarsal bones.

b. The midfoot has osseous stability through the recessed articulation of the base of the second metatarsal bone. The trapezoidal shape of the bases of the first three metatarsal bones contributes to stability of the foot, as do the plantar ligaments. The Lisfranc ligament runs from the base of the second metatarsal to the medial cuneiform bone.

c. The lateral tarsometatarsal joints (fourth and fifth metatarsal-cuboid joints) have 10° of motion in the sagittal plane. The medial three tarsometatarsal joints have limited motion.

d. Approximately 20% to 30% of tarsometatarsal fracture-dislocations may be missed in cases of multiple trauma.

2. Mechanisms of injury

a. Direct tarsometatarsal fracture-dislocations occur with dorsal force and may result in soft-tissue injuries and compartment syndromes. Involvement of both bony and soft-tissue components is common in direct injuries.

b. Indirect tarsometatarsal fracture-dislocations occur with axial loading and twisting on a loaded, plantarflexed foot. Patients commonly report a history of a fixed foot with rotation of the body around the midfoot.

3. Radiographic evaluation

a. Internal oblique, AP, and lateral views of the foot should be obtained.

b. Normal anatomic relationships should be maintained.

- The medial aspect of the second metatarsal should be aligned with the medial aspect of the middle cuneiform bone.
- The medial aspect of the fourth metatarsal should be aligned with the medial cuboid bone.
- Diastasis of greater than 2 mm between the base of the first and second metatarsal bones is pathologic.
- There should be no dorsal subluxation of the bases of the metatarsal bones on the lateral view.

c. The fleck sign is a small avulsed fragment of bone in the interval between the bases of the first and second metatarsal bones. This represents avulsion of the Lisfranc ligament from its insertion at the base of the second metatarsal.

d. Weight-bearing or stress radiographs can be obtained when the results of physical examination and plain radiography are equivocal.

4. Fracture classification—Tarsometatarsal injuries are divided into three categories (**Figure 6**).

a. Type A injuries: total incongruity of the midfoot joints. The most common direction of such incongruity is lateral, and homolateral injuries may be associated with compression fractures of the cuboid bone.

b. Type B injuries: partial incongruity of the midfoot joints. Common patterns include medial dislocation of the first metatarsal or lateral dislocation of some or all of the lateral rays.

B. Clinical evaluation
   1. The primary method of diagnosis of compartment syndromes of the foot is clinical.
   2. Loss of pulses and capillary refilling are unreliable signs of a compartment syndrome.
   3. Loss of two-point discrimination and light touch sensation are more reliable than loss of pinprick sensation as indicators of a compartment syndrome.
   4. Pain with passive dorsiflexion of the foot results from stretching of the intrinsic muscles of the foot. This decreases compartment volume and increases pressure.
   5. Pressure measurements can be helpful in clinically equivocal cases. Pressure thresholds exceeding 30 mm Hg or within 30 mm Hg of diastolic blood pressure have been advocated as indications for compartment release.

C. Treatment (**Figure 9**)
   1. Fasciotomy is indicated when clinical symptoms are consistent with a compartment syndrome.
   2. Medial and/or dorsal incisions can be used to release pressure in all nine compartments of the foot.
      a. Two dorsal incisions are commonly used.
   3. Closure should be delayed because primary skin closure can increase intracompartmental pressure. A split-thickness skin graft may be required for closure.
   4. Alternatively, "pie-crusting" dorsally may release hematoma and effectively decompress the dorsal compartments of the foot.

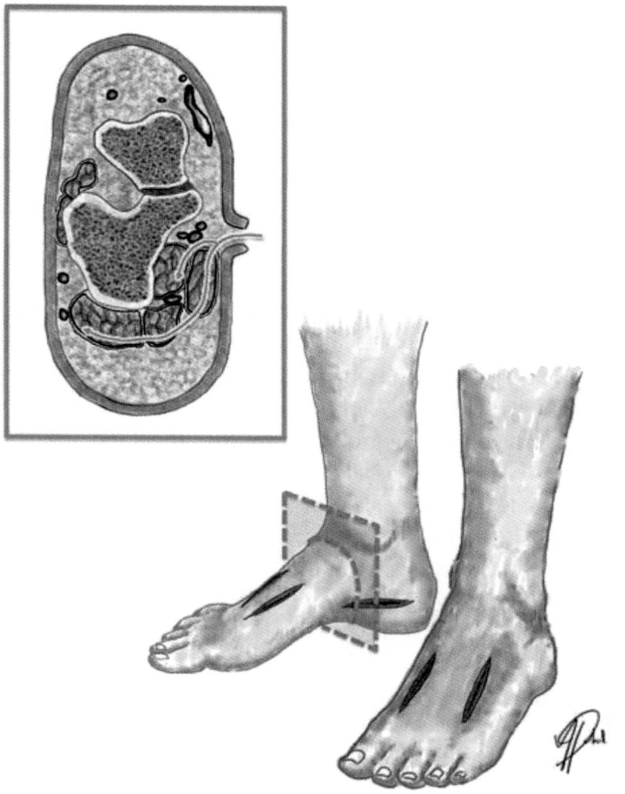

Figure 9 Illustration of the feet demonstrating incision sites for a three-incision fasciotomy. The blue panel indicates the level of the cross-section shown in the inset image. Inset, Cross-section of the medial, superficial central, deep central, and lateral compartments. The superior blue arrow indicates the entrance into the deep central compartment. The inferior blue arrow indicates the entrance into the medial, superficial, central, and lateral compartments (from medial to lateral). (Reproduced from Dodd A, Le I: Foot compartment syndrome: Diagnosis and management. *J Am Acad Orthop Surg* 2013;21[11]:657-664.)

TOP TESTING FACTS

Fractures of the Talus

1. The talus is 70% covered by cartilage, and the extensor digitorum brevis is the only muscle attaching to it.
2. The blood supply to the talar body is mostly from the artery of the tarsal canal, a branch of the posterior tibial artery.
3. The blood supply to the talar neck is mainly from the artery of the tarsal sinus, a branch formed from the anterior tibial and peroneal arteries.
4. The deltoid artery supplies the medial body of the talus.
5. ORIF is required for all displaced talar neck fractures. ORIF is usually performed through combined anterolateral and anteromedial approaches.
6. Osteonecrosis occurs with increasing frequency as the Hawkins classification for a talar neck fracture increases in severity.
7. The Hawkins sign consists of subchondral osteopenia seen on plain radiographs at 6 to 8 weeks after fixation of a talar neck fracture and indicates revascularization of the talar body.

8. Posttraumatic osteoarthritis is the most common complication of talar fractures.
9. Varus malunion can occur as a complication of a talar fracture.
10. CT provides the best visualization of fractures of the talar body and is used to identify fractures in the transverse, coronal, and sagittal planes.

Fractures of the Calcaneus

1. The calcaneus is the most frequently fractured of the tarsal bones.
2. An oblique shear force causing fracture of the calcaneus results in a primary fracture line and two primary fragments.
3. The axial Harris view reveals widening, shortening, lateral translation, and varus positioning of the tuberosity fragment of a calcaneal fracture.
4. Negative prognostic factors for the surgical treatment of Sanders type II and III fractures include severity, advanced age, male sex, obesity, bilateral fractures, multiple trauma, and workers' compensation.
5. Fixation can be done using the sinus tarsi approach (less invasive) or the extended lateral approach (higher soft-tissue complications).
6. Malunion of calcaneal fractures can result in shortening, widening, and lateral impingement. The symptoms include difficulty with shoe wear and peroneal tendon symptoms.
7. Malunions that result in talar dorsiflexion with loss of the talar declination angle to less than 20° can limit ankle dorsiflexion.
8. Malunions of the calcaneus are treated with lateral exostectomy. Fusion is also added to treat subtalar arthritis.
9. Tension band fixation can be used to avoid failure of screw fixation in avulsion fractures of the calcaneal tuberosity.
10. Fractures of the anterior process of the talus occur with inversion and avulsion of the bifurcate ligament.

Midfoot Fractures

1. The central navicular has a limited blood supply and is susceptible to stress fractures.
2. The tarsometatarsal joints are constrained by the recessed articulation of the second metatarsal bone.
3. The Lisfranc ligament runs from the base of the second metatarsal to the medial cuneiform bone.
4. Lisfranc fracture-dislocations can occur with direct application of force or indirectly through axial loading and twisting on a fixed, plantarflexed foot.
5. Plain radiographs may show a fleck of bone in the proximal first metatarsal interspace. This fleck sign represents the avulsed Lisfranc ligament and is associated with poorer prognosis.
6. Homolateral dislocation of the tarsometatarsal joints may be associated with a compression injury to the cuboid.
7. Up to 30% of Lisfranc injuries are missed acutely. Weight-bearing or stress radiographs can be used to rule out injury.
8. Fusion of the fourth and fifth tarsometatarsal joints is poorly tolerated, and resection arthroplasty is used in conjunction with fusion of the medial tarsometatarsal joints for missed or late reconstruction of Lisfranc injuries.

Metatarsal and Phalangeal Fractures

1. Fractures of the metatarsal neck in which there is severe angulation and plantar prominence may require reduction and fixation.
2. Fractures of the metatarsal head are rare and can generally be treated nonsurgically.
3. Stress fractures of the proximal metatarsals may be seen in dancers.
4. Avulsion of the long plantar ligament, the lateral band of the plantar fascia, or contraction of the peroneus brevis may result in type I fractures of the fifth metatarsal (pseudo-Jones fracture).
5. Jones fractures occur where the proximal fifth metatarsal has poor blood supply; at the metadiaphyseal junction 1.5 to 2.5 cm distal to the base.
6. Acute ORIF with screws, together with a prolonged restriction of activity, is often used in athletes to minimize the possibility of nonunion of a type II fracture.

7. Diaphyseal stress fractures of the fifth metatarsal can be caused by cavovarus foot deformities or peripheral neuropathies. Second metatarsal neck stress fractures are seen in athletes and military recruits.
8. Bone grafting and/or structural correction may be needed to achieve the healing of type III fractures and prevent their recurrence, particularly in cases of atrophic nonunion.
9. Medial sesamoidectomy for nonunion may result in hallux valgus deformity.
10. Lateral sesamoidectomy for nonunion may result in hallux varus deformity.

Dislocations of the Foot

1. Medial subtalar dislocations may be irreducible if the talar head buttonholes through the extensor digitorum brevis or with interposition of the peroneal tendons.
2. Lateral subtalar dislocations may be irreducible if buttonholed through the talonavicular capsule and the posterior tibial tendon is interposed.
3. Subtalar dislocations are reduced by flexing the knee to relax the gastrocnemius–soleus complex, re-creating the deformity, plantarflexing the foot, and pushing on the talar head.
4. Dislocations of the first MTP joint are usually dorsal and are uncommon because of the thick plantar ligamentous complex.
5. Midtarsal dislocation involving the talonavicular and calcaneocuboid articulations (Chopart joint) can occur through axial loading (longitudinal) or crush injury.
6. First MTP joint dislocations may be irreducible because of buttonholing through the sesamoid–short flexor complex. Irreducible first MTP joint dislocations are treated through a dorsal approach.
7. Lesser MTP joint dislocations may be irreducible because of buttonholing through the plantar plate.

Compartment Syndromes

1. The foot has a total of nine compartments divided into four main groups: the medial, lateral, four interosseous, and three central compartments.
2. Loss of pulses and capillary refilling are unreliable signs of a compartment syndrome.
3. Loss of two-point discrimination and light touch are more sensitive signs of compartment syndrome than loss of pinprick sensation.
4. Pain with passive dorsiflexion of the foot results from stretching of the intrinsic muscles of the foot. This decreases compartment volume and increases pressure.
5. Pressure measurements can be helpful in clinically equivocal cases. Pressure thresholds exceeding 30 mm Hg or within 30 mm Hg of diastolic blood pressure have been advocated as indications for compartment release.
6. Fasciotomy is indicated when clinical symptoms are consistent with a compartment syndrome.
7. Two dorsal incisions can be used to release pressure in all nine compartments of the foot.
8. Closure after incision to release pressure in the compartment of the foot should be delayed because primary skin closure can increase intracompartmental pressure. A split-thickness skin graft may be required for closure.
9. Dorsal pie-crusting may release hematoma and effectively decompress the dorsal compartments of the foot.

Bibliography

Buckley R, Tough S, McCormack R, et al: Operative compared with nonoperative treatment of displaced intra-articular calcaneal fractures: A prospective, randomized, controlled multicenter trial. *J Bone Joint Surg Am* 2002;84-A(10):1733-1744.

Canale ST, Kelly FB Jr: Fractures of the neck of the talus: Long-term evaluation of seventy-one cases. *J Bone Joint Surg Am* 1978;60(2):143-156.

Dubois-Ferrière V, Lübbeke A, Chowdhary A, et al: Clinical outcomes and development of symptomatic osteoarthritis 2 to 24 years after surgical treatment of tarsometatarsal joint complex injuries. *J Bone Joint Surg Am* 2016;98(9):713-720.

Kelly IP, Glisson RR, Fink C, Easley ME, Nunley JA: Intramedullary screw fixation of Jones fractures. *Foot Ankle Int* 2001;22(7):585-589.

Kuo RS, Tejwani NC, Digiovanni CW, et al: Outcome after open reduction and internal fixation of Lisfranc joint injuries. *J Bone Joint Surg Am* 2000;82-A(11):1609-1618.

Larson CM, Almekinders LC, Taft TN, Garrett WE: Intramedullary screw fixation of Jones fractures: Analysis of failure. *Am J Sports Med* 2002;30(1):55-60.

Ly TV, Coetzee JC: Treatment of primarily ligamentous Lisfranc joint injuries: Primary arthrodesis compared with open reduction and internal fixation. A prospective, randomized study. *J Bone Joint Surg Am* 2006;88(3):514-520.

Myerson MS: Experimental decompression of the fascial compartments of the foot—The basis for fasciotomy in acute compartment syndromes. *Foot Ankle* 1988;8(6):308-314.

Quill GE Jr: Fractures of the proximal fifth metatarsal. *Orthop Clin North Am* 1995;26(2):353-361.

Sanders R, Fortin P, DiPasquale T, Walling A: Operative treatment in 120 displaced intraarticular calcaneal fractures: Results using a prognostic computed tomography scan classification. *Clin Orthop Relat Res* 1993;290:87-95.

Schulze W, Richter J, Russe O, Ingelfinger P, Muhr G: Surgical treatment of talus fractures: A retrospective study of 80 cases followed for 1-15 years. *Acta Orthop Scand* 2002;73(3):344-351.

Shah SN, Knoblich GO, Lindsey DP, Kreshak J, Yerby SA, Chou LB: Intramedullary screw fixation of proximal fifth metatarsal fractures: A biomechanical study. *Foot Ankle Int* 2001;22(7):581-584.

Song JH, Kang C, Hwang DS, Kang DH, Park JW. Extended sinus tarsi approach for treatment of displaced intraarticular calcaneal fractures compared to extended lateral approach. *Foot Ankle Int*. 2019;40:167-177.

Teng AL, Pinzur MS, Lomasney L, Mahoney L, Havey R: Functional outcome following anatomic restoration of tarsal-metatarsal fracture dislocation. *Foot Ankle Int* 2002;23(10):922-926.

Thordarson DB, Triffon MJ, Terk MR: Magnetic resonance imaging to detect avascular necrosis after open reduction and internal fixation of talar neck fractures. *Foot Ankle Int* 1996;17(12):742-747.

Vallier HA, Nork SE, Barei DP, Benirschke SK, Sangeorzan BJ: Talar neck fractures: Results and outcomes. *J Bone Joint Surg Am* 2004;86-A(8):1616-1624.

Chapter 105

GERIATRIC TRAUMA

SANJIT R. KONDA, MD
PHILIPP LEUCHT, MD

I. EPIDEMIOLOGY

A. The growing middle-aged (55 to 64 years old) and geriatric (age > 65) population has led to a dramatic increase in the incidence of geriatric trauma.

B. The current geriatric population is approximately 43.1 million and is expected to double to 83.7 million by 2050.

C. It is estimated that the current burden of geriatric trauma in the overall trauma population is 12% and that number will continue to grow to an estimated 40% by 2040.

D. The expanding elderly trauma population will assuredly place a stress on hospital system resources and, as such, an understanding of the factors contributing to the care of elderly trauma is paramount to maintain quality care.

II. RISK PROFILING OF GERIATRIC TRAUMA PATIENTS

A. Mechanism of injury, comorbidities, injury profile, physiologic status

1. Geriatric trauma patients have a different physiologic profile compared with their younger counterparts. This profile is age dependent and continues to evolve along the age spectrum.
2. As patients get older they have increased number of comorbidities. These comorbidities affect all organ systems and, as a result, their ability to respond and compensate to traumatic injuries continues to decompensate with increasing age.
3. Additionally, mechanism of injury is an important factor is delineating the contribution of injuries, physiologic status, and comorbidities to mortality risk. Low-energy mechanism of injury is defined as a fall ≤ 2 steps, whereas high-energy mechanisms of injury are defined as falls >2 steps (fall from height), pedestrian struck, and motorcycle and motor vehicle accidents. See **Table 1** for factors that contribute to mortality risk in low- and high-energy mechanisms of injury in middle-aged and geriatric trauma patients.

B. Quantifying risk in geriatric trauma patients

1. Traditional risk assessment tools in trauma include the Injury Severity Score (ISS) and the Trauma Injury Severity Score.
2. The Injury Severity Score is a quantitative tool used to characterize the injury profile in a trauma patient. It comprises six subcomponents which are recorded as an Abbreviated Injury Scale (AIS) and are ordinal in value such that 0 denotes no injury and 6 denotes an injury that is not compatible with life. The subcomponents of the ISS include AIS-Head/Neck, AIS-Face, AIS-Chest, AIS Abdomen, AIS Extremity (including pelvis), and AIS-External (Skin). The ISS is calculated by taking the highest AIS value in the three most injured AIS subcomponents and squaring and then summing the values ($ISS = X^2 + Y^2 + Z^2$). Generally, ISS > 15 is considered at threshold for major trauma and has been shown to have an inpatient mortality rate of 10%. The ISS only takes into consideration a patient's injury profile and does not account for a patients age, physiologic status, or comorbidity status. Therefore, its ability to characterize mortality risk in the geriatric population is not as robust as in the younger adult population.

Dr. Konda or an immediate family member is a member of a speakers' bureau or has made paid presentations on behalf of Stryker and serves as a paid consultant to or is an employee of Stryker. Dr. Leucht or an immediate family member is a member of a speakers' bureau or has made paid presentations on behalf of Synthes; serves as a paid consultant to or is an employee of Ankasa Regenerative Therapeutics, Strykerm, and Synthes; has stock or stock options held in Ankasa Regenerative Therapeutics; and serves as a board member, owner, officer, or committee member of the American Academy of Orthopaedic Surgeons Biological Implants Committee and the Orthopaedic Trauma Association.

TABLE 1

Predictors of Inpatient Mortality for Low-Energy and High-Energy Geriatric Trauma Patients (Multivariate Logistic Regression)

	Low Energy (Falls)		High Energy (MVC, MCC, Pedestrians Struck, Falls Height)		All Patients	
	Odds Ratio	*P*	Odds Ratio	*P*	Odds Ratio	*P*
Age, years	1.06 (1.04-1.07)	<0.01	1.12 (1.08-1.15)	<0.01	1.07 (1.05-1.08)	<0.01
PECs						
Leukemia	3.83 (1.37-10.740)	0.01	—	—	2.87 (1.05-7.85)	0.04
Diabetes with end-organ damage	3.19 (1.08-9.41)	0.04	—	—	—	—
Moderate or severe renal disease	1.94 (1.18-3.18)	0.01	—	—	1.98 (1.26-3.12)	0.00
Dementia	0.39 (0.17-0.87)	0.02	—	—	—	—
Metastatic solid tumors	—	—	20.65 (1.60-267.12)	0.02	—	—
Vital Signs						
HR	1.01 (1.00-1.02)	0.05	—	—	1.01 (1.00-1.02)	0.03
BP	0.99 (0.99-1.00)	0.02	0.99 (0.98-1.00)	0.01	0.99 (0.99-1.00)	0.00
GCS	0.71 (0.68-0.74)	<0.01	0.73 (0.69-0.78)	<0.01	0.73 (0.70-0.75)	<0.01
Anatomic Injuries						
Injury blood vessel	7.99 (1.82-35.06)	0.01	3.93 (1.58-9.74)	<0.01	4.33 (1.93-9.71)	0.00
Injury to nerves and spinal cord	3.81 (1.25-11.58)	0.02	—	—	2.82 (1.09-7.29)	0.03
Intracranial injury	3.81 (2.56-5.67)	<0.01	3.07 (1.72-5.47)	<0.01	3.85 (2.80-5.28)	<0.01
Injury thorax	2.55 (1.08-6.03)	0.03	2.12 (1.18-3.83)	0.01	1.82 (1.13-2.93)	0.01
>2 fractures	—	—	3.34 (1.45-7.69)	<0.01	2.61 (1.31-5.22)	0.01

BP = blood pressure, GCS = Glasgow Coma Scale, HR = heart rate, MCC = motorcycle crash, MVC = motor vehicle crash, PECs = Preexisting conditions

This table demonstrates that if low- and high-energy patients are evaluated together (all patients) instead of separately, then some of risk factors for mortality change and/or the contribution of each risk factor to mortality changes (odds ratio).

Recreated with permission from Konda SR, Lack WD, Seymour RB, Karunakar MA: Mechanism of injury differentiates risk factors in geriatric trauma patients. *J Orthop Trauma* 2015;29(7):331-336.

3. The TRISS tool is a multivariate logistic regression algorithm that predicts a probability of inpatient survival that accounts for age as a dichotomous variable (<55 versus >55) as well as the injury profile via the ISS and a physiologic profile via the Glasgow Coma Scale (GCS), systolic blood pressure, and respiratory rate. This tool has been validated to assess survival and mortality risk in the postdischarge setting once a patient's ISS score has been calculated by trained trauma registrars. This tool does not account for a patient's comorbidity status or energy mechanism. Therefore, it also has been shown to have only moderate predictive utility in the low-energy geriatric trauma population.
4. To account for age, physiologic status, injury profile, and comorbidity status, a more robust tool for this population has been developed, the Score for Trauma Triage in the Geriatric and Middle-Aged (STTGMA), to predict inpatient mortality risk in patients ≥ 55 y/o. Similar to TRISS, the STTGMA tool is multivariate logistic regression algorithm. This score has been validated against the NTDB and have been used prospectively with great accuracy (**Table 2**).

TABLE 2

Comparison of Variables Found to Be Independent Predictors of Mortality in Middle-Aged and Geriatric Trauma Patients (Variables Compromising the STTGMA)

	$STTGMA_{LE}$ OR (95% CI)	*P*	$STTGMA_{HE}$ OR (95% CI)	*P*
Age	1.05 (1.03-1.07)	<0.01	1.08 (1.03-1.17)	<0.01
CCI	1.28 (1.14-1.44)	<0.01	—	—
GCS	0.72 (0.69-0.76)	<0.01	0.69 (0.64-0.75)	<0.01
AIS-HN	1.67 (1.49-1.87)	<0.01	1.77 (1.44-2.21)	<0.01
AIS-CHS	1.52 (1.19-1.92)	<0.01	1.51 (1.20-1.90)	<0.01
AIS-EXT	—	—	1.59 (1.14-2.21)	<0.01

AIS = Abbreviated Injury Score, CCI = Charlson Comorbidity Index, CHS = Chest, EXT = Extremity, GCS = Glasgow Coma Scale, HE-GMTP = high-energy geriatric and middle-aged trauma patient, HN = Head and neck, LE-GMTP = low-energy geriatric and middle-aged trauma patient, STTGMA = Score for Trauma Triage in the Geriatric and Middle-Aged

Recreated with permission from Lott A, Haglin J, Saleh H, Hall J, Egol KA, Konda SR: Using a validated middle-age and geriatric risk tool to identify (<48 hours) hospital mortality and associated cost of care. *J Orthop Trauma* 2018;32(7):349-353.

III. PREOPERATIVE CONSIDERATIONS IN THE EVALUATION OF THE GERIATRIC TRAUMA PATIENT

A. Acute versus chronic comorbidities

1. Evaluation of a geriatric trauma patient's comorbidities is essential to determining a patient's risk profile.
2. Comorbidities can be classified as chronic-stable, chronic-unstable, and newly diagnosed (**Table 3**).
3. Chronic-stable conditions are unrelated to the trauma but need to be evaluated before surgery to maintain the comorbidity in a stable condition.
4. A chronic-unstable condition can be directly related to the geriatric trauma and needs to be evaluated before surgery to optimize the patient's medical condition before surgery can be safely performed.

B. Comorbidity classification

1. To account for the major medical comorbidities that affect a patient's perioperative morbidity and mortality, the Charlson Comorbidity Index (CCI) is a validated and widely used tool that can be used. It is simple to calculate (many online calculators exist) and has been shown to predict 1, 5, and 10-year mortality risk. It comprises 19 comorbid conditions that are assigned a value of 1 through 6 based on the mortality risk of each illness (**Table 4**).

TABLE 3

Classification of Comorbidities Based on Chronicity and Disease Stability

Comorbidity Classification	Relationship to Orthopaedic Injury	Intervention Required for Medical Optimization Before Surgery
Chronic-stable	Unrelated	Obtain medical records from primary care physician. Obtain routine preoperative medical evaluation.
Chronic-unstable (acute exacerbation of known preexisting comorbidity)	May have led to injury	Obtain medical records from primary care physician. Obtain medical evaluation to stabilize acute exacerbation of disease. Consider admission to medical service.
Newly diagnosed	May have led to injury	Obtain medical evaluation to determine extent of newly diagnosed comorbidity. Patient may benefit from extensive medical workup before surgery. Consider admission to medical service.

From Konda SR: *Perioperative and postoperative considerations in the geriatric patient*, in: *AAOS Orthopaedic Knowledge Update: Trauma*, ed 5. Chapel Hill, NC, American Academy of Orthopaedic Surgeons, 2016, p 599.

TABLE 4

Charlson Comorbidity Index

Comorbidity	Point Value
AIDS	6
Metastatic solid tumor	6
Moderate or severe liver disease	3
Any nonmetastatic solid tumor	2
Malignant lymphoma	2
Leukemia	2
Diabetes with end-organ damage	2
Moderate or severe renal disease	2
Hemiplegia	2
Diabetes without end-organ damage	1
Mild liver disease	1
Ulcer disease	1
Connective tissue disease	1
Chronic pulmonary disease	1
Dementia	1
Cerebrovascular disease	1
Peripheral vascular disease	1
Congestive heart failure	1
Myocardial infarction	1

Online calculator available for 1-yr mortality after admission available at Charlson ME, Pompei P, Ales KL, Mackenzie CR. A new method of classifying prognostic comorbidity in longitudinal studies: Development and validation. *J Chronic Dis* 1987;40(5):373-383. PMID: 3558716. http://www.pmidcalc.org/?sid=3558716&newtest=Y. Accessed January 19, 2019.

2. It is essential to capture a patient's comorbidity profile on admission to develop a risk profile for the patient that can be used to guide care.
3. Comorbidities in this index can be either chronic-stable, chronic-unstable, or newly diagnosed.

C. Preoperative physical and functional status assessment

1. Preoperative physical status assessment is another key component to the preoperative risk assessment of the geriatric trauma patient. Physical status refers to the systemic nature of the comorbidity.
2. A widely used and accepted physical status classification system is the American Society of Anesthesiology (ASA) Physical Status Classification System. ASA status is classified from 1 to 6 with 1 denoting a normal healthy patient, 2 denoting a patient with mild systemic disease, 3 denoting a patient with severe systemic disease, 4 denoting a patient with a severe systemic disease that is a constant threat to life, 5 denoting a moribund patient who is not suspected to survive without the operation, and 6 denoting a brain-dead person. See **Table 5** for specific examples of comorbidities that would qualify for each ASA class. Note that ASA class alone has been shown to correlate with risk of complications, readmission, and inpatient mortality.
3. Preoperative functional status assessment is key to determining a patient's perioperative cardiac risk. Functional status is a measure of a patient's ability to perform routine physical activity without decompensating.
4. A tool used to stratify functional status is the Metabolic Equivalent (MET). A MET is the resting metabolic rate (amount of oxygen consumed at rest), when sitting quietly in a chair is approximately 3.5 mL O_2/kg/min (1.2 kcal/min for 70 kg person). This means that work at 2 METs requires twice the metabolism and so forth. 1 MET is the ability to do basic tasks to take care of oneself such as eating, dressing, or toileting; 4 METs equates to walking up a flight of stairs; and 10 METs is the ability to perform strenuous activity like football or swimming. See **Table 6** for a description of different gradations of METs from 1 to 10.

D. Preoperative cardiac risk assessment

1. Preoperative cardiac risk assessment can be performed following guidelines set forth by the American College of Cardiology/American Heart Association. These guidelines, if followed can minimize the use of unnecessary and resource intensive cardiac testing.
2. A baseline resting 12-lead electrocardiogram (ECG) is routinely obtained on all geriatric trauma patients.
3. Additional cardiac testing is warranted only if a patient has cardiac risk factors, poor functional capacity (METs $\leq$ 4), or abnormalities on the baseline ECG.
4. Advanced cardiac testing (echocardiogram, stress testing, 24-hour ambulatory monitoring) is only indicated if it would have been performed in the absence of the proposed surgery.
5. In the event that preoperative stress testing is positive, studies have shown no improvement in outcome if prophylactic revascularization is performed before proposed surgery.

TABLE 5

American Society of Anesthesiologists Physical Status Classification

Classification	Definition	Examples
ASA I	A normal healthy patient	Healthy, nonsmoking, no or minimal alcohol use
ASA II	A patient with mild systemic disease	Mild disease only, with no substantive functional limitations; examples include (but are not limited to) current smoker, social alcohol drinker, pregnancy, obesity (30 < BMI <40) well-controlled DM/HTN, mild lung disease
ASA III	A patient with severe systemic disease	Substantive functional limitations; one or more moderate to severe diseases, examples include but are not limited to poorly controlled DM or HTN, COPD, morbid obesity (BMI ≤40), active hepatitis, alcohol dependence or abuse, implanted pacemaker, moderate reduction of ejection fraction, ESRD undergoing regularly scheduled dialysis, history (>3 mo) of MI, CVA, TIA, or CAD/stents.
ASA IV	A patient with severe systemic disease that is a constant threat to life	Examples include but are not limited to recent (<3 mo) MI, CVA, TIA, or CAD/stents, ongoing cardiac ischemia or severe valve dysfunction, severe reduction of ejection fraction, sepsis, DIC, ARD, or ESRD not undergoing regularly scheduled dialysis
ASA V	A moribund patient who is not expected to survive without the operation	Examples include but are not limited to ruptured abdominal/thoracic aneurysm, massive trauma, intracranial bleed with mass effect, ischemic bowel in the face of substantial cardiac pathology, or multiple organ/system dysfunction
ASA VI	A declared brain-dead patient whose organs are being removed for donor purposes	

ARD = acute respiratory distress, ASA = American Society of Anesthesiologists, BMI = basal metabolic index, CAD = coronary artery disease, COPD = chronic obstructive pulmonary disease, CVA = cerebrovascular accident, DIC = diffuse intravascular coagulopathy, DM = diabetes mellitus, ESRD = end-stage renal disease, HTN = hypertension, MI = myocardial infarction, TIA = transient ischemic attack

Reproduced with permission from American Society of Anesthesiologists. Available at: http://www.asahq.org/resources/clinical-information/asa-physical-status-classification-system. Accessed January 19, 2019.

TABLE 6

Estimated Energy Requirements for Various Activities

1 MET	Can you ... Take care of yourself?	4 METs	Can you ... Climb a flight of stairs or walk up a hill?
↓	Eat, dress, or use the toilet?	↓	Walk on level ground at 4 mph (6.4 kph)?
	Walk indoors around the house?		Run a short distance?
	Walk a block or 2 on level ground at 2 to 3 mph (3.2-4.8 kph)?		Do heavy work around the house such as scrubbing floors or lifting or moving heavy furniture?
4 METs	Do light work around the house like dusting or washing dishes?		Participate in moderate recreational activities such as golf, bowling, dancing, doubles tennis, or throwing a baseball or football?
		Greater than 10 METs	Participate in strenuous sports such as swimming, singles tennis, football, basketball, or skiing?

kph = kilometers per hour, MET = metabolic equivalent, mph = miles per hour

Recreated with permission from: Fleisher LA, Fleischmann KE, Auerbach AD, Barnason SA, Beckman JA, Bozkurt B, et al. ACC/AHA 20014 guidelines on perioperative cardiovascular evaluation and care for noncardiac surgery: A report of the American College of Cardiology/American Heart Association Task Force on Practice Guidelines. *J Am Coll Cardiol*. 2014;64(22):e77-e137.

E. Preoperative pulmonary risk assessment

1. Preoperative pulmonary risk assessment is routinely performed on all geriatric trauma patients as age is an independent predictor of postoperative pulmonary complications. Minimum workup involves obtaining a plain XR of the chest for all trauma patients >50 years old.
2. The American College of Physicians only recommends preoperative pulmonary function testing (PFT) such as spirometry in patients with COPD or asthma whose baseline airflow cannot be established or optimized. A forced vial capacity (FVC) <70% of the predictive value and an FEV1/FVC ratio <65% are predictive of postoperative pulmonary complications.
3. There is no role for routine preoperative arterial blood gas (ABG) analysis to risk stratify postoperative pulmonary complications. ABGs should be obtained only if clinically indicated.

F. Interdisciplinary patient care in perioperative setting

1. The role of interdisciplinary care for geriatric trauma patients has been adopted by the American College of Surgeons.
2. Preoperative optimization of the geriatric trauma patient with significant medical comorbidities is recommended to be performed in conjunction with a medical specialist or a geriatrician (ACS TQIP Best Practice Guidelines).
3. Co-management of orthopaedic geriatric trauma patients is becoming more common. This concept refers to the practice of admitting patients to the orthopaedic service but having the consulting medical specialist takes "ownership" of the patient. This implies the medical consultant will continue to manage ongoing medical issues and continue to the follow the patient postoperatively as an inpatient and outpatient.
4. Co-management of the geriatric trauma patient by an orthopaedic surgeon and geriatrician has been shown to lower length of stay, decrease readmission rates, decrease time to surgery, lower complication rates, and lower inpatient mortality rates.

IV. POSTOPERATIVE CONSIDERATIONS IN THE MANAGEMENT OF THE GERIATRIC TRAUMA PATIENT

A. Altered postoperative mental status

1. Altered postoperative mental status is associated with an increased risk of postoperative mortality.
2. It can be classified as either postoperative delirium (POD) or postoperative cognitive dysfunction (POCD).
3. POD is defined as an acute change in mental status characterized by waxing and waning status of mental alertness. It can be caused by a host of factors including but not limited to: infection, dehydration, hypoperfusion, medications, hypoxia, and hypoglycemia, baseline dementia, vision impairment, and use of physical restraints.
4. Treatment for POD includes treatment the underlying etiology and medical treatment can include haloperidol and/or low-dose lorazepam.
5. POCD on the other hand is not treatable. It presents as an impairment of memory and concentration anywhere from a few days to weeks after index surgery and has been loosely associated with general anesthesia. Patients with POCD may require long-term care for their impaired mental status.

B. Postoperative pulmonary complications

1. Postoperative pulmonary complications are common in patients with shoulder girdle and/or rib fracture as well as lower extremity injuries that leave them immobile and recumbent.
2. The common complications are atelectasis and pneumonia.
3. Atelectasis usually manifests between postoperative day 2 and 5. Clinically patients have increased work of breathing and hypoxemia. Treatment consists of continuous positive airway pressure, suctioning, and chest physiotherapy.
4. Pneumonia can present from postoperative day 0 to 5 and is associated with fever and new infiltrates on chest radiography. Treatment consists of sputum and blood cultures and initiation of broad-spectrum antibiotics with tailoring of organism-specific antibiotics when culture results finalized.

C. Postoperative cardiac complications

1. Postoperative cardiac complications can be risk stratified via the Revised Cardiac Risk Index (RCRI) (**Table 7**).
2. The RCRI predicts risk of a major cardiac event in the setting of a major noncardiac surgery.
3. Major cardiac events include myocardial infarctions, arrhythmias (eg, atrial fibrillation), and heart failure.
4. RCRI 0 correlates with a 0.4% chance of a major cardiac event and RCRI > 3 correlates with an 11% chance of a major cardiac event.

TABLE 7

Revised Cardiac Risk Index

1. History of ischemic heart disease
2. History of congestive heart failure
3. History of cerebrovascular disease (stroke or transient ischemic attack)
4. History of diabetes requiring preoperative insulin use
5. Chronic kidney disease (creatinine >2 mg/dL)
6. Undergoing suprainguinal vascular, intraperitoneal, or intrathoracic surgery
Risk for cardiac death, nonfatal myocardial infarction, and nonfatal cardiac arrest
0 predictors = 0.4%
1 predictor = 0.9%
2 predictors = 6.6%
≥ 3 predictors = >11%

From Konda SR: *Perioperative and postoperative considerations in the geriatric patient*, in: *AAOS Orthopaedic Knowledge Update: Trauma*, ed 5. Chapel Hill, NC, American Academy of Orthopaedic Surgeons, 2016, p 605.

5. Patients with preexisting cardiac disease or intraoperative lability of vital signs may benefit from a postoperative ECG to evaluate for a major cardiac event especially if they have an elevated RCRI.
6. Postoperative myocardial infarction may present as a "silent MI" in elderly patients with cardiac risk factors as only one-third of these patients present with classic chest pain. Workup should include serial troponins every 8 hours for up to 24 hours. An elevated and/or continuously rising troponin should prompt an urgent medical evaluation to determine if a myocardial infarction is occurring.
7. Postoperative atrial fibrillation, the most common arrhythmia, is problematic because it can cause mental status changes and syncope. Patients can be symptomatic with heart palpitations or asymptomatic. Diagnosis is performed via ECG and treatment focuses on a rate-control strategy, which has shown a trend toward reduction in all-cause mortality.
8. Acute postoperative heart failure should warrant suspicion for myocardial ischemia or infarction as the root cause in the geriatric trauma patients. Signs of heart failure include pulmonary edema with hypoxia, and treatment includes diuretics and vasodilators in patients without hypotension.

D. Postoperative gastrointestinal complications

1. Common postoperative gastrointestinal complications include GI bleeds, postoperative ileus, and clostridium difficile colitis.
2. GI prophylaxis to minimize the risk of stress ulcers/bleeds should be limited to specific high-risk populations in the ICU setting. First-line treatment includes H2 receptor antagonists and proton pump inhibitors.
3. The presence of GI bleed in the elderly requires urgent workup as mortality rates range from 10 to 25%.
4. Evaluation and treatment involves upper or lower GI endoscopy and patients should be aggressively resuscitated.
5. Postoperative ileus is the stagnation of the bowel causing the inability to tolerate oral feeds. Risk factors include obesity, pelvic surgery, acute blood loss anemia, and opioid use. Evaluation is either an abdominal radiography or CT abdomen/pelvis, which will show dilated bowel loops.
6. Medical or surgical evaluation is warranted to evaluate for any mechanical causes of bowel obstruction that would require surgical intervention.
7. *Clostridium difficile* colitis occurs when the use of perioperative antibiotics alters normal gut flora and replaced it with *C. difficile* resulting in a pseudomembranous colitis. Empiric therapy with oral metronidazole (nonsevere) or IV vancomycin (severe) should be started pending final culture results of the stool. Criteria for surgical consultation for possible colectomy include white blood cell count >20,000 cells/μL and/or plasma lactate between 2.2 and 4.0.

V. CONCLUSION

A. The incidence of geriatric trauma is increasing and surgeons need to be aware of the perioperative factors that will improve these patient's outcomes.

B. Risk profiling of this elderly population requires accounting for energy mechanism, age, physiologic status, injury profile, and comorbidity status.

C. Preoperative optimization of comorbidities should be managed in an interdisciplinary fashion following best-practice guidelines to optimize efficiency and value-based care.

D. Postoperative complications in the geriatric trauma patient will adversely affect outcomes of surgery. Therefore, it is imperative to continue the interdisciplinary management of these injured elderly patients until safe hospital discharge.

TOP 10 TESTING FACTS

1. Of all trauma in the United Status, the burden of geriatric trauma is expected to grow to 40% by 2040.
2. The Injury Severity Score (ISS) is calculated by taking the highest Abbreviated Injury Scale (AIS) value in the three most injured AIS subcomponents and squaring and then summing the values ($ISS = X^2 + Y^2 + Z^2$). Generally, ISS > 15 is considered at threshold for major trauma and has been shown to have an inpatient mortality rate of 10%.
3. ASA status is classified from 1 to 6 with 1 denoting a normal healthy patient, 2 denoting a patient with mild systemic disease, 3 denoting a patient with severe systemic disease, 4 denoting a patient with a severe systemic disease that is a constant threat to life, 5 denoting a moribund patient who is not suspected to survive without the operation, and 6 denoting a brain-dead person.
4. A MET is the resting metabolic rate (amount of oxygen consumed at rest), when sitting quietly in a chair is approximately 3.5 mL O_2/kg/min (1.2 kcal/min for 70 kg person). This means that work at 2 METs requires twice the metabolism and so forth. 1 MET is the ability to do basic tasks to take of self such as eating, dressing, or toileting; 4 METs equates to walking up a flight of stairs; and 10 METs is the ability to perform strenuous activity such as football or swimming.
5. Additional cardiac testing is warranted only if a patient has cardiac risk factors, poor functional capacity (METs ≤ 4), or abnormalities on the baseline ECG. Advanced cardiac testing (echocardiogram, stress testing, 24-hour ambulatory monitoring) is only indicated if it would have been performed in the absence of the proposed surgery
6. Co-management of the geriatric trauma patient by an orthopaedic surgeon and geriatrician has been shown to lower length of stay, decrease readmission rates, decrease time to surgery, lower complication rates, and lower inpatient mortality rates
7. Altered postoperative mental status is associated with an increased risk of postoperative mortality.
8. Atelectasis usually manifests between postoperative day 2 to 5. Clinically patients have increased work of breathing and hypoxemia. Treatment consists of continuous positive airway pressure, suctioning, and chest physiotherapy.
9. The Revised Cardiac Risk Index (RCRI) predicts risk of a major cardiac event in the setting of a major noncardiac surgery. Major cardiac events include myocardial infarctions, arrhythmias (eg,, atrial fibrillation), and heart failure. RCRI 0 correlates with a 0.4% chance of a major cardiac event and RCRI >3 correlates with an 11% chance of a major cardiac even.
10. The presence of GI bleed in the elderly requires urgent workup as mortality rates range from 10% to 25%.

Bibliography

American Society of Anesthesiologists. Available at: http://www.asahq.org/resources/clinical-information/asa-physical-status-classification-system. Accessed January 19, 2019.

Auerbach A, Goldman L: Assessing and reducing the cardiac risk of noncardiac surgery. *Circulation* 2006;113(10):1361-1376.

Campbell JW, Degolia PA, Fallon WF, et al: In harm's way: Moving the older trauma patient toward a better outcome. *Geriatrics* 2009;64:8-13.

Charlson Morbidity Index Calculator. Available at: https://www.mdcalc.com/charlson-comorbidity-index-cci. Accessed January 19, 2019.

Fleisher LA, Fleischmann KE, Auerbach AD, et al: ACC/AHA 2014 guidelines on perioperative cardiovascular evaluation and care for noncardiac surgery: A report of the American College of Cardiology/American Heart Association Task Force on practice guidelines. *J Am Coll Cardiol* 2014;64(22):e77-e137.

Konda SR, Lack WD, Seymour RB, Karunakar MA: Mechanism of injury differentiates risk factors in geriatric trauma patients. *J Orthop Trauma* 2015;29(7):331-336.

Konda SR, Seymour R, Manoli A, Gales J, Karunakar MA: Carolinas Trauma Network Research Group. Development of a middle-age and geriatric trauma mortality risk score: A tool to guide palliative care consultations. *Bull Hosp Joint Dis (2013)* 2016;74(4):298305.

Konda SR, Lott A, Saleh H, Gales J, Egol KA: Use of the STTGMA tool to risk stratify 1-year functional outcomes and mortality in geriatric trauma patients. *J Orthop Trauma* 2018;32(9):461-466.

Lott A, Haglin J, Saleh H, Hall J, Egol KA, Konda SR: Using a validated middle-age and geriatric risk tool to identify (<48 hours) hospital mortality and associated cost of care. *J Orthop Trauma* 2018;32(7):349-353.

McMahon DJ, Schwab CW, Kauder D: Comorbidity and the elderly trauma patient. *World J Surg* 1996;20:1113-1119; discussion 9-20.

Orthopaedic Trauma. Available at: https://www.facs.org/. Accessed December 1, 2018.

Ortman J, Velkoff V, Hogan H: An aging nation: The older population in the United States. Population estimates and projections. *Curr Popul Rep* 2014:P25-P1140.

Chapter 106
ACUTE COMPARTMENT SYNDROME

ADAM K. LEE, MD

I. EPIDEMIOLOGY

A. 200,000 cases per year, usually traumatic
B. Most common cause of malpractice suits
C. 75% with associated fractures
   1. 36% of these are tibia shaft fractures
   2. Overall incidence in tibial shaft fractures 2% to 24%
D. Risk factors
   1. Young, male, prolonged decreased BP
   2. Complex/butterfly/segmental tibia shaft fractures
   3. Bicondylar tibial plateau fractures
   4. Crush injuries
   5. Prolonged ischemia

II. ANATOMY/PATHOPHYSIOLOGY

A. Fascial compartment volume fixed (low compliance)
B. Vicious cycle
   1. Injury → inflammation → increased compartment pressure → decreased circulation (inflow, outflow, lymphatics) → ischemia/tissue damage → increased edema/vascular permeability → further increase in pressure
C. Time from injury important
   1. 4 hours—reversible ischemia
   2. 6 hours—permanent damage (muscle fibrosis, dysesthesias, foot drop)
      a. Volkmann contracture in forearm (decreased motion/strength, clawing)
   3. Prolonged—extensive muscle death → rhabdomyolysis → renal failure → amputation/death (rare)

Neither Dr. Lee nor any immediate family member has received anything of value from or has stock or stock options held in a commercial company or institution related directly or indirectly to the subject of this chapter.

III. EVALUATION

A. General
   1. High index of suspicion necessary
   2. Clinical diagnosis
   3. Six P's generally low sensitivity, so repeat exams are key
      a. Pain out of proportion/with passive stretch
         - Most reliable
         - Generally, if findings other than pain are present, the diagnosis has been delayed
      b. Paresthesias (late finding)
      c. Pallor
      d. Poikilothermia
      e. Pulselessness (more relevant for vascular injuries)
      f. Paralysis (late finding)
B. History
   1. Mechanism, time of injury, relevant medical history
   2. Increasing pain or analgesia requirements
C. Physical Examination—most important diagnostic tool
   1. Compressibility
      a. Unreliable at detecting increased compartment pressure in examiners of all experience levels
   2. Pain with passive stretch (may be affected by adjacent fractures)
D. Special tests (for equivocal examination findings, obtunded patients)
   1. Compartment pressure measurements
      a. Varies within compartment
      b. Should be evaluated within 5 cm of fracture

c. Absolute, one-time pressures >30 to 40 mm Hg overestimate diagnosis

d. Pressure difference (ΔP) more reliable

- ΔP = diastolic blood pressure − compartment pressure
- Consistent values <30 mm Hg raise concern for compartment syndrome
  - For an anesthetized patient, presedation diastolic blood pressure should be used
  - Continuous monitoring with indwelling catheter may further improve accuracy

IV. TREATMENT

A. Acute compartment syndrome

1. Emergent fasciotomies—goal is to alleviate pressure before irreversible damage occurs. Skin left open with sterile dressing

2. Return to OR 48 to 72 hours to débride nonviable tissue

3. Primary closure (1 to 5 days), split thickness skin graft (STSG) (>7 days)

   a. Prioritize closure of incisions to cover exposed bone (eg, medial leg wound)

4. Leg (**Figure 1**)

   a. Four compartments (anterior, lateral, superficial posterior, deep posterior)

   b. Anterior compartment almost always involved, lateral compartment second most common

   c. Single and dual-incision equivalent outcomes

   - Dual-incision fasciotomy (**Figure 2, A**)
     - Medial incision (superficial and deep posterior)
     - Lateral incision (anterior and lateral)
   - Single-incision fasciotomy (**Figure 2, B**)
     - Lateral incision, access all compartments laterally by raising a flap, release deep posterior compartment from fibular attachment

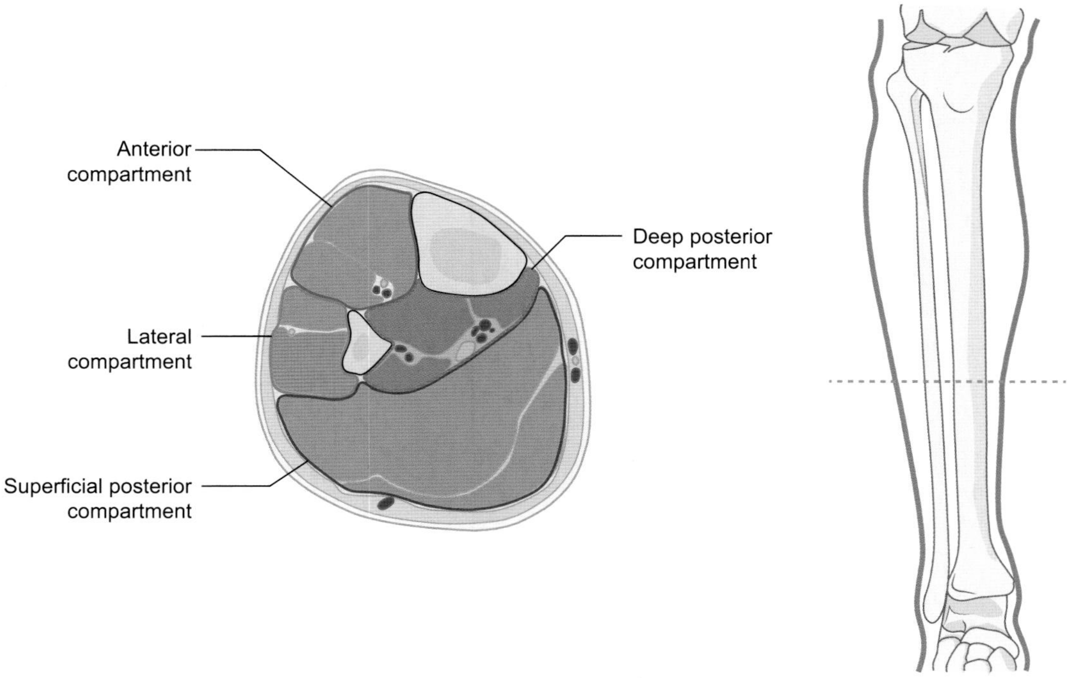

Figure 1 Cross-section of leg compartments. (AO Surgery Reference, www.aosurgery.org. Copyright by AO Foundation, Switzerland.)

5. Forearm (**Figure 3**)
   a. Three compartments (volar, dorsal, lateral/mobile wad)
   b. Volar most commonly involved
   c. Fractures (distal radius, both-bone forearm), narcotic overdose, IV infiltration
   d. Volar incision (volar compartment and carpal tunnel) and dorsal incision (dorsal compartment and mobile wad)
6. Thigh
   a. Three compartments (anterior, medial, posterior)
   b. High-energy femur fractures
   c. Single lateral incision (anterior and posterior compartments), additional medial Incision (may be required for the medial compartment)
7. Foot (**Figure 4**)
   a. Nine compartments (controversial)
   b. Surgical release controversial due to morbidity of release
      - Release changes foot morphology, infection risk, wound healing issues
      - Nonsurgical may result in paresthesias and toe clawing

B. Missed/late compartment syndrome (>48 hours with no function)
   1. Generally nonsurgical—goal is to decrease morbidity (increased rate of infection, wound healing problems) associated with surgery
   2. Surgical débridement of necrotic muscle if systemic issues

V. OUTCOMES AND COMPLICATIONS

A. Overall worse health outcomes

B. Patients with fasciotomy
   1. Increased length of stay, infection rate, time to healing (skin and bone), cost of care

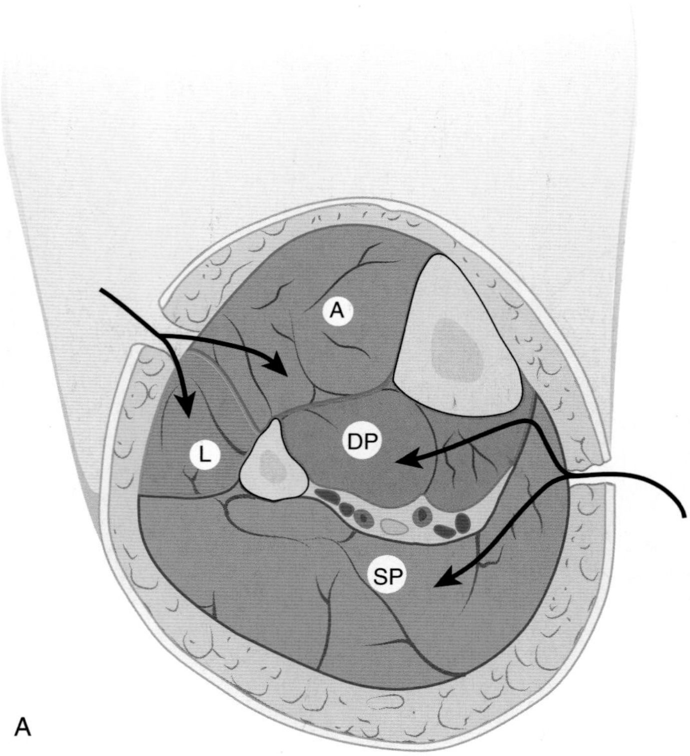

A

Figure 2 Leg fasciotomies. **A**, Dual-incision. **B**, Single-incision.

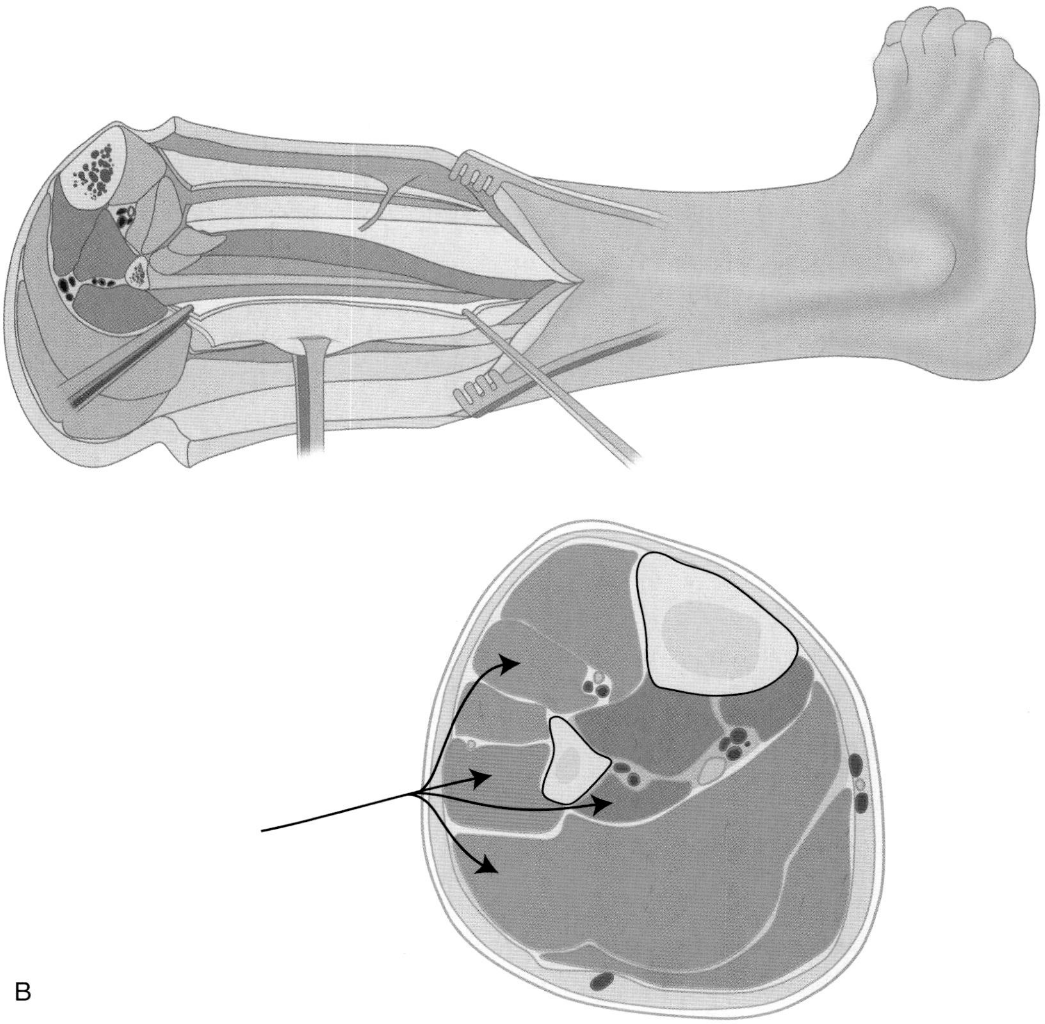

Figure 2 Cont'd

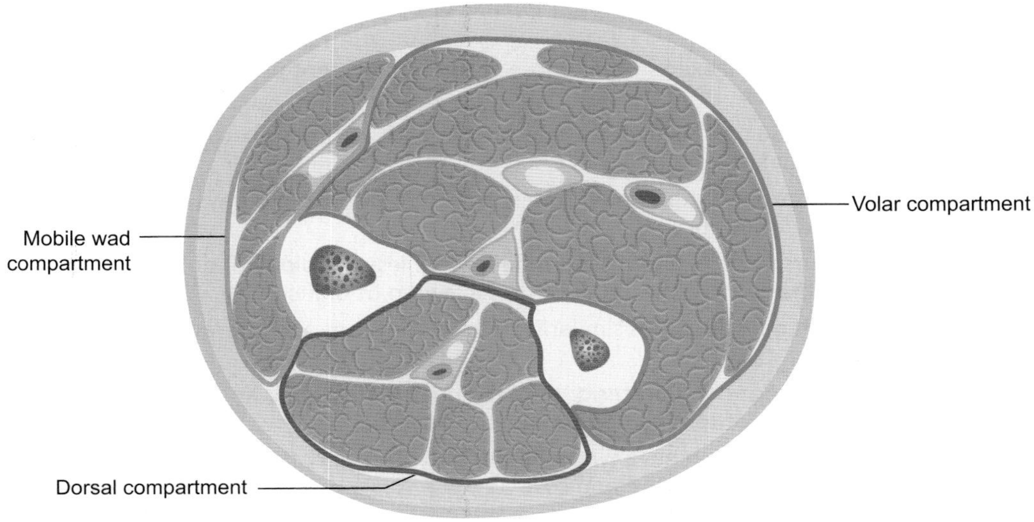

Figure 3 Cross-section of forearm compartments.

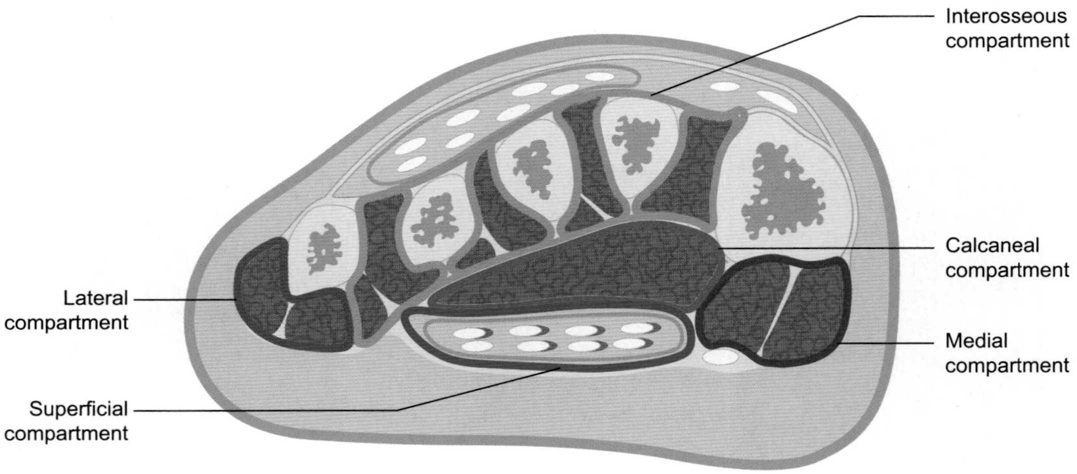

Figure 4 Cross-section of foot compartments.

C. Complications
 1. Rhabdomyolysis, renal failure, infection, amputation, death

VI. AAOS CLINICAL PRACTICE GUIDELINES

A. www.orthoguidelines.org/

B. No strong recommendations

C. Moderate recommendations
 1. Pressure monitoring assists in diagnosis
 2. Serial/continuous pressure monitoring and ΔP >30 mm Hg assist in ruling out acute compartment syndrome

D. All other recommendations limited or consensus

TOP TESTING FACTS

1. Common problem with high morbidity if missed; most associated with trauma/fracture
2. Risk factors: complex tibia shaft fractures, bicondylar tibial plateau fractures, young males, prolonged hypotension
3. Vicious cycle leading to progressively increasing compartment pressures in fixed volume compartments leading to tissue ischemia and necrosis
4. High index of suspicion with serial exams to diagnose with compartment pressure monitor to supplement (especially in obtunded patients)
5. ΔP (DPB – compartment P) <30 mm Hg over time consistent with acute compartment syndrome, continuous monitoring may be more reliable
6. Treatment is emergent fasciotomy with skin left open; return to OR in 2 to 3 days to débride unviable tissue; primary closure early versus STSG late
7. Late presentation (>48 hours) compartment syndrome may be less morbid with nonsurgical management; sequelae include muscle fibrosis, dysesthesias, foot drop/clawing of digits
8. Single versus dual-incision leg fasciotomies similarly effective, anterior and lateral compartments most often involved
9. Lateral incision to release anterior and posterior thigh compartments; volar and dorsal incisions to release forearm compartments; release of foot compartments controversial
10. Patients with compartment syndrome have worse health outcomes and after fasciotomy an increased length of stay, infection rate, risk of wound issues, and cost

Bibliography

Auld TS, Hwang JS, Stekas N, et al: The correlation between the OTA/AO classification system and compartment syndrome in both bone forearm fractures. *J Orthop Trauma* 2017;31(11):606-609. doi:10.1097/BOT.0000000000001020. PubMed PMID: 29053544.

Beebe MJ, Auston DA, Quade JH, et al: OTA/AO classification is highly predictive of acute compartment syndrome after tibia fracture: A cohort of 2885 fractures. *J Orthop Trauma* 2017;31(11):600-605. doi:10.1097/BOT.0000000000000918. PubMed PMID:28614149.

Bible JE, McClure DJ, Mir HR: Analysis of single-incision versus dual-incision fasciotomy for tibial fractures with acute compartment syndrome. *J Orthop Trauma* 2013;27(11):607-611. doi:10.1097/BOT.0b013e318291f284. PubMed PMID:23515126.

Blair JA, Stoops TK, Doarn MC, et al: Infection and nonunion after fasciotomy for compartment syndrome associated with tibia fractures: A matched cohort comparison. *J Orthop Trauma* 2016;30(7):392-396. doi:10.1097/BOT.0000000000000570. PubMed PMID:26978131.

Challa ST, Hargens AR, Uzosike A, Macias BR: Muscle microvascular blood flow, oxygenation, pH, and perfusion pressure decrease in simulated acute compartment syndrome. *J Bone Joint Surg Am* 2017;99(17):1453-1459. doi:10.2106/JBJS.16.01191. PubMed PMID:28872527; PubMed Central PMCID:PMC5685422.

Collinge CA, Attum B, Lebus GF, et al: Acute compartment syndrome: An expert survey of orthopaedic trauma association members. *J Orthop Trauma* 2018;32(5):e181-e184. doi:10.1097/BOT.0000000000001128. PubMed PMID:29432322.

Crespo AM, Manoli A III, Konda SR, Egol KA: Development of compartment syndrome negatively impacts length of stay and cost after tibia fracture. *J Orthop Trauma* 2015;29(7):312-315. doi:10.1097/BOT.0000000000000253. PubMed PMID:25463427.

Dodd A, Le I: Foot compartment syndrome: Diagnosis and management. *J Am Acad Orthop Surg* 2013;21(11):657-664. doi:10.5435/JAAOS-21-11-657. Review. PubMed PMID:24187035.

Kakar S, Firoozabadi R, McKean J, Tornetta P III: Diastolic blood pressure in patients with tibia fractures under anaesthesia: Implications for the diagnosis of compartment syndrome. *J Orthop Trauma* 2007;21(2):99-103. PubMed PMID:17304064.

Maheshwari R, Taitsman LA, Barei DP: Single-incision fasciotomy for compartmental syndrome of the leg in patients with diaphyseal tibial fractures. *J Orthop Trauma* 2008;22(10):723-730. doi:10.1097/BOT.0b013e31818e43f9. PubMed PMID:18978549.

McQueen MM, Duckworth AD, Aitken SA, Court-Brown CM: The estimated sensitivity and specificity of compartment pressure monitoring for acute compartment syndrome. *J Bone Joint Surg Am* 2013;95(8):673-677. doi:10.2106/JBJS.K.01731. PubMed PMID:23595064.

McQueen MM, Court-Brown CM: Compartment monitoring in tibial fractures. The pressure threshold for decompression. *J Bone Joint Surg Br* 1996;78(1):99-104. PubMed PMID:8898137.

Ojike NI, Roberts CS, Giannoudis PV: Compartment syndrome of the thigh: Asystematic review. *Injury* 2010;41(2):133-136. doi:10.1016/j.injury.2009.03.016. Epub 2009 Jun 24. Review. PubMed PMID:19555950.

von Keudell AG, Weaver MJ, Appleton PT, et al: Diagnosis and treatment of acute extremity compartment syndrome. *Lancet* 2015;386(10000):1299-1310. doi:10.1016/S0140-6736(15)00277-9. Review. Erratum in: *Lancet*. 2015;386(10006):1824. Appelton, Paul T [corrected to Appleton, Paul T]. *Lancet*. 2015;386(10006):1824. PubMed PMID:26460664.

Chapter 107
Rib Cage Fractures and Flail Chest

PAUL M. LAFFERTY, MD

I. EPIDEMIOLOGY

A. Most fractures are relatively benign and heal without significant morbidity.

1. Rib fractures can be a marker of severe injury, and an increased number of fractured ribs correlates with increased morbidity and mortality.
2. As many as 300,000 people are evaluated annually for rib fracture, and 7% of these will require hospitalizations for medical and/or surgical management.
3. Rib fractures occur in up to 10% of hospitalized trauma patients and may be associated with a mortality of 3% to 13%.
4. Flail chest, typically defined as three or more consecutive ribs fractured and/or dislocated in two or more locations, causes paradoxical movement of the affected flail chest wall segment.
   a. Flail chest carries a mortality rate of up to 15%. Rib fractures and flail chest can cause severe pain and are frequently associated with concomitant injuries such as pneumothorax, hemopneumothorax, and/or pulmonary contusions.
   b. The seventh through tenth ribs are the most common ribs fractured. Patients with advanced age, osteoporosis, or osteopenia are at increased risk and typically have higher numbers and increased severity of fractures.

II. ANATOMY

A. The thoracic cage consists of 12 pairs of ribs. The ribs are numbered 1 to 12 based on the corresponding thoracic vertebrae to which they connect posteriorly (**Figure 1**)

1. The posterior end is called the head. The articulations of the heads of the ribs (costocentral articulations) constitute a series of gliding or arthrodial joints and are formed by the articulation of the heads of the typical ribs with the facets on the contiguous margins of the bodies of the thoracic vertebrae and with the intervertebral fibrocartilages between them.
2. The first, eleventh, and twelfth ribs each articulate with a single vertebra.

B. Lateral to the head is the narrowed neck.

1. A small eminence located on the posterior rib surface is the tubercle, which articulates with the facet located on the transverse process of the same numbered vertebra.

C. The remainder of the rib is the body or shaft. Just lateral to the tubercle is the angle, the point at which the rib has its greatest degree of curvature.

D. The osseous components of ribs do not extend anteriorly to the sternum. Rather, the anterior end of each rib ends with costal cartilage. These are made of hyaline cartilage and can extend for several centimeters. Most ribs are attached, directly or indirectly, to the sternum via their costal cartilage.

III. EVALUATION

A. History

1. Most patients with rib fractures present with an obvious high-energy mechanism of injury, such as a motor vehicle collision.
2. Patients with rib fractures who have not sustained high-energy trauma typically describe a history of minor or moderate blunt trauma to the chest wall or a specific repetitive activity that resulted in insidious onset of pain.

Neither Dr. Lafferty nor any immediate family member has received anything of value from or has stock or stock options held in a commercial company or institution related directly or indirectly to the subject of this chapter.

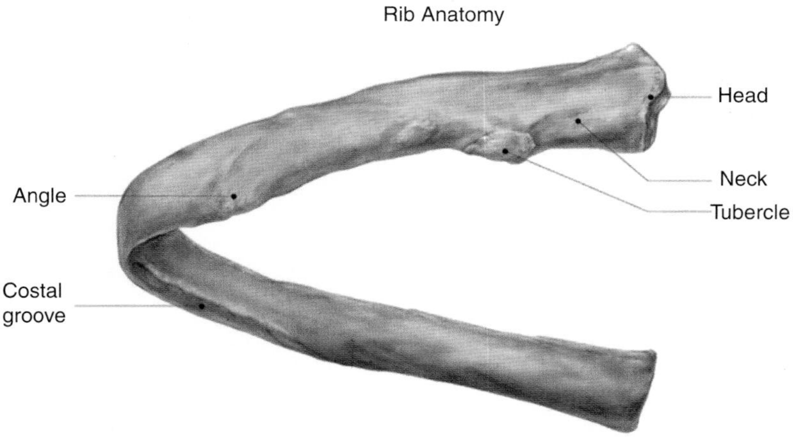

Figure 1 Illustration showing rib anatomy. (Studyblue.com)

3. The most common symptom of rib fractures is pain. In the case of stress fractures, it can also be elicited with reproduction of the inciting activity. bearing down, sneezing, or laughing.

B. Physical examination
  1. Visible bruising around the fractured rib may be present but is not common.
  2. Examination findings strongly suggestive of rib fracture include point tenderness on a specific rib or focal tenderness caused by compression of the rib cage distant from the site of pain. Bony crepitus and ecchymosis may be present.
  3. Pneumothorax may present as diminished breath sounds and possibly subcutaneous crepitus resulting from subcutaneous emphysema.

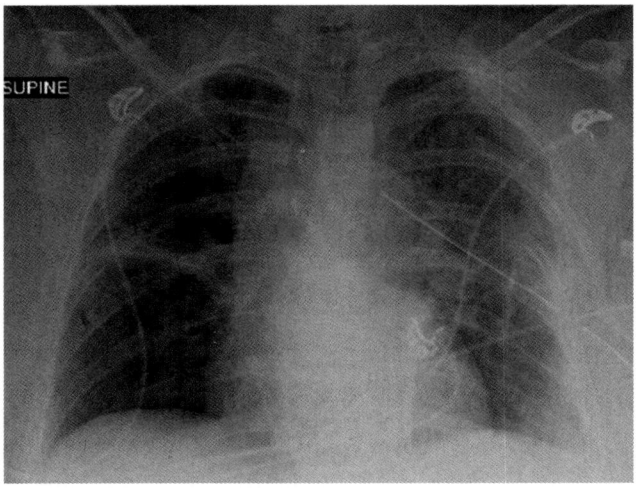

Figure 2 PA chest radiograph of a 58-year-old female who presented following a high-speed motorcycle crash with segmental fractures of ribs 3 through 11 resulting in a flail chest.

4. Flail chest occurs when three or more adjacent ribs are each fractured in at least two places, creating one floating segment comprised of several ribs and the soft tissues between them; this unstable section of chest wall exhibits paradoxical motion, moving in the opposite direction of uninjured, normal-functioning chest wall with breathing.
5. Rib stress fractures present with a gradual onset of activity-related chest wall pain, similar to stress fractures of other bones. Often the pain first occurs only with the inciting activity, then progresses to pain with deep breathing or simple movements, such as rolling over in bed or reaching overhead.

C. Imaging:
  1. Standard PA and lateral chest radiographs are adequate to identify some rib fractures, but overall sensitivity is poor (**Figure 2**)
  2. The sensitivity of dedicated rib films for rib fracture is higher, as these radiographs use a bone exposure (entailing higher levels of radiation) than standard chest radiographs. These include oblique views of the chest wall not included with a standard chest series (**Figure 3, A** and **B**).
  3. Rib fractures are commonly identified on CT studies obtained to assess trauma patients for internal injuries. Patients suspected of having sustained intrathoracic and/or intra-abdominal injury are usually evaluated with a CT scan of the chest/abdomen/pelvis.
  4. Both two-dimensional (2D) and three-dimensional (3D) (**Figure 4**) reconstructions are also valuable in assessing the amount of fracture displacement and chest wall deformity and are therefore helpful in making decisions regarding treatment. Caution should be exercised when assessing the coronal, sagittal, and 3D

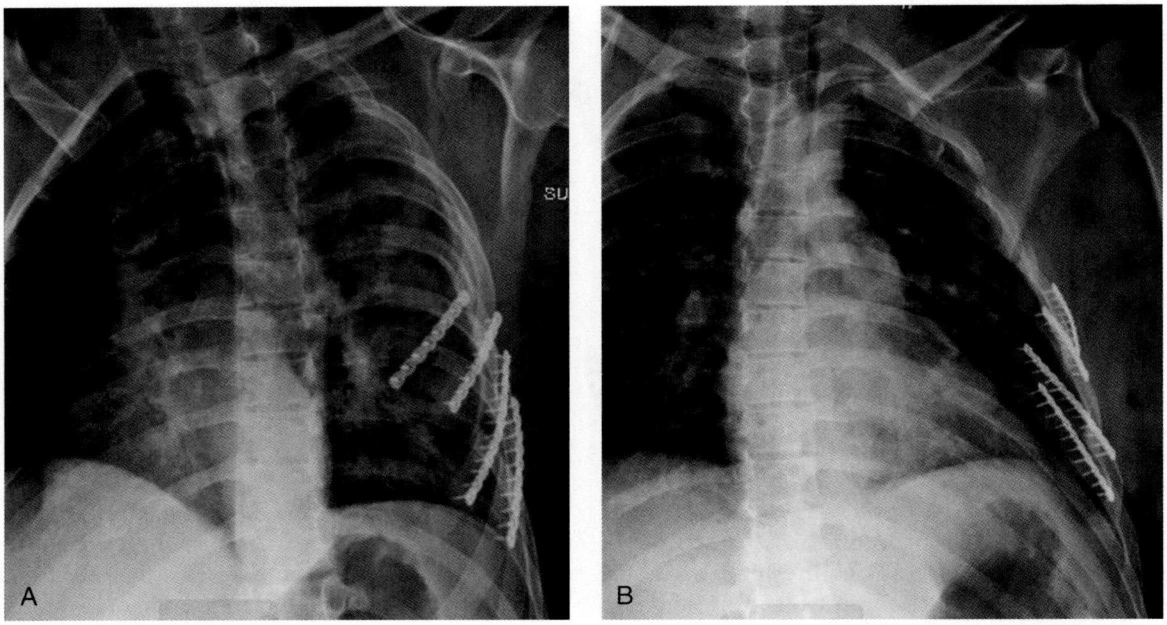

Figure 3 **A** and **B**, Rib series status-post surgical fixation in a 32-year-old male who was pedestrian struck by a motor vehicle. Patient sustained displaced left first through twelfth rib fractures with flail segments involving first through seventh ribs. Fixation of ribs 4 through 7 was performed to restore chest wall anatomy.

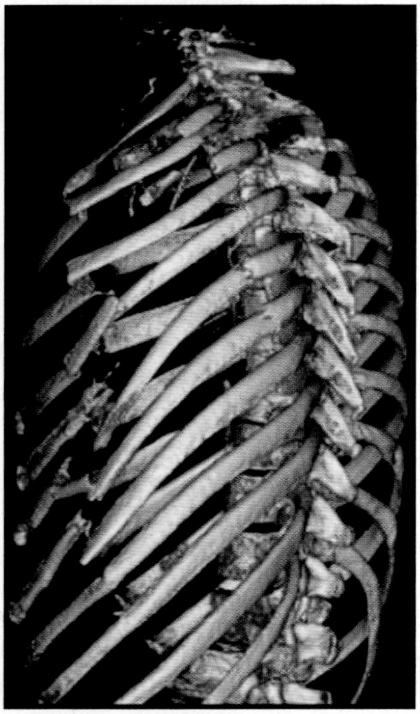

Figure 4 Three-dimensional CT reconstruction of the 58-year-old female shown in **Figure 2**. Again noted are segmental fractures of ribs 3 through 11.

reconstructions, as volume averaging can lead to smoothening out of fracture lines, with the ultimate risk of missing certain fractures. Therefore, conventional axial slices of the CT scan should always be scrutinized.

D. Associated injuries

1. Rib fractures and flail chest injuries sustained by patients as a result of more high-energy trauma often have associated injuries.
2. Fractures of ribs 1, 2, or 3 may be associated with mediastinal injury, particularly to the aorta, as well as injury to the brachial plexus and subclavian vessels, and they are associated with increased mortality in some observational studies.
3. First rib fractures are associated with greater overall injury severity (Injury Severity Score >15) and life-threatening internal injury (including injuries to the brain, spine, lungs, and pelvis), independent of mechanism, age, or gender.
4. Intra-abdominal organ injuries are more common in patients with fractures of the ninth through twelfth ribs, with hepatic and splenic injuries being most common.

Section 8

Foot and Ankle

Section Editors TAN
MC CORMICK

Chapter 108

Anatomy and Biomechanics of the Foot and Ankle

VINCENT JAMES SAMMARCO, MD
ROSS TAYLOR, MD

I. ANATOMY

A. Bones and ligaments

1. The ankle joint (**Figure 1**)

   a. The ankle joint includes the tibia, talus, and fibula.

   b. It is a ginglymus (hinge) joint.

   c. The talar dome is biconcave with a central talar sulcus.

   d. The radius of curvature is greater laterally.

   e. Viewed axially, the joint is trapezoidal and wider anteriorly than posteriorly.

   f. The talus is the only tarsal bone without muscular or ligamentous insertions.

   g. The medial malleolus and lateral malleolus have osseous grooves for the posterior tibial tendon (PTT) and peroneal tendons, respectively.

   h. Lateral ankle ligaments—The lateral ankle ligamentous complex is composed of three ligaments.

   - Anterior talofibular ligament (ATFL)—The ATFL extends from the anterior aspect of the distal fibula to the body of the talus. Strain in the ATFL increases with plantar flexion, inversion, and internal rotation.
   - Calcaneofibular ligament (CFL)—The CFL extends from the tip of the fibula posterior to its insertion on the lateral wall of the calcaneus. It runs deep to the peroneal tendons and crosses the subtalar joint. The CFL is under increased strain with dorsiflexion and inversion.
   - Posterior talofibular ligament (PTFL)—The PTFL originates broadly at the posterior fibula and inserts mainly at the posterolateral tubercle of the talus. It is a broad, strong ligament that is congruous with the posterior capsule of the ankle and subtalar joint.

   i. Deltoid ligament

   - The deltoid ligament is a triangle-shaped ligament with the apex at the medial malleolus and with fibers extending to the calcaneus, talus, and navicular.
   - The ligament is divided into superficial and deep components. The superficial component has three parts, extending anteriorly to the navicular, inferiorly to the sustentaculum, and posteriorly on the talar body. The deep deltoid ligament extends in two bands from the medial malleolus to the talar body just inferior to the medial facet.
   - Syndesmosis—The tibiofibular articulation is composed of the tibial incisura fibularis and its corresponding fibular facet. It has three ligamentous structures that are variably responsible for its support: the anterior inferior tibiofibular ligament (35%), the interosseous ligament (22%), and the PTFL (43%).

Dr. Sammarco or an immediate family member has received royalties from Extremity Medical; is a member of a speakers' bureau or has made paid presentations on behalf of Extremity Medical; serves as a paid consultant to or is an employee of Extremity Medical, Integra, and Synthes; and serves as a board member, owner, officer, or committee member of the American Academy of Orthopaedic Surgeons. Neither Dr. Taylor nor any immediate family member has received anything of value from or has stock or stock options held in a commercial company or institution related directly or indirectly to the subject of this chapter.

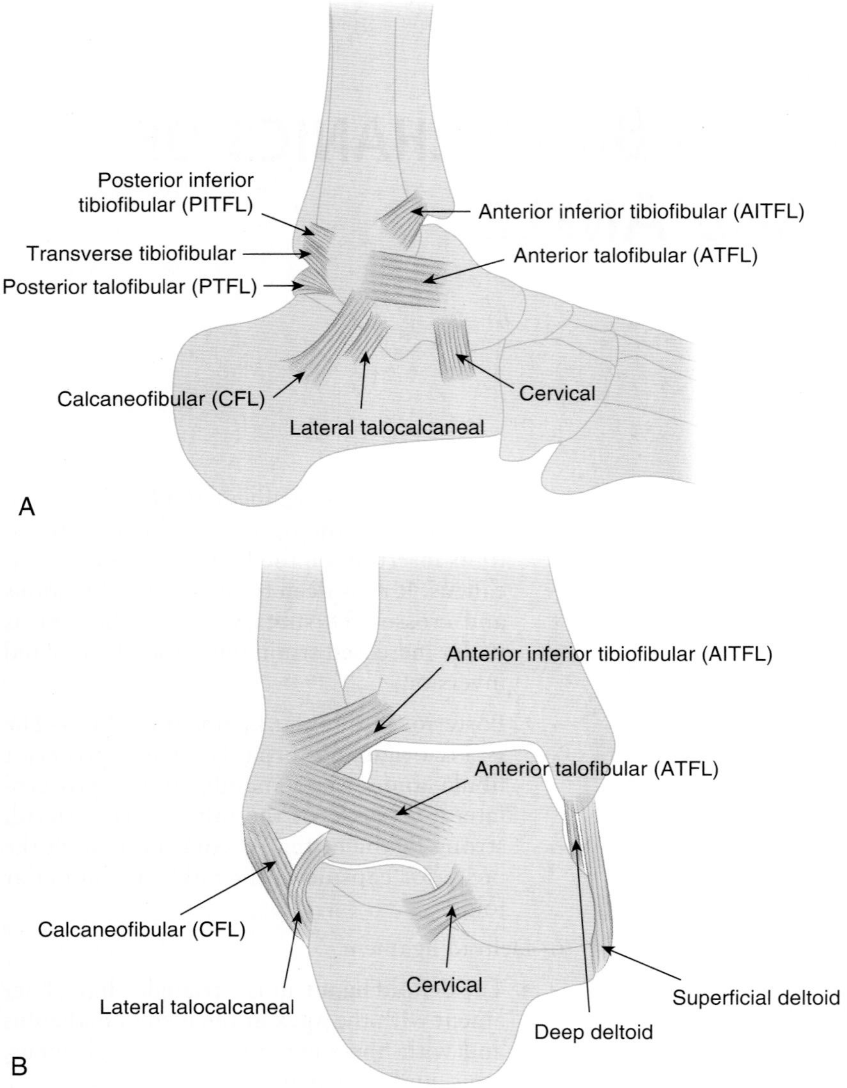

Figure 1 Illustrations show the lateral ankle and subtalar ligaments viewed laterally (**A**) and anteriorly (**B**). (Reproduced from Katcherian D: Soft-tissue injuries of the ankle, in Lutter LD, Mizel MS, Pfeffer GB, eds: *Orthopaedic Knowledge Update: Foot and Ankle*. Rosemont, IL, American Academy of Orthopaedic Surgeons, 1994, pp 241-253.)

2. Hindfoot and midfoot
   a. The subtalar joint has three facets: one posterior, one in the middle, and one anterior.
      - The posterior facet is the largest.
      - The middle facet rests on the sustentaculum of the calcaneus and is located medially.
      - The anterior facet is often continuous with the talonavicular joint.
   b. The transverse tarsal joint (Chopart joint) is composed of the talonavicular and calcaneocuboid joints and acts in concert with the subtalar joint to control foot flexibility during gait.
      - The talonavicular joint is supported by the spring ligament complex, which has two separate components: the superior medial calcaneonavicular ligament and the inferior calcaneonavicular ligament.
      - The calcaneocuboid joint is saddle shaped. It is supported plantarly by the inferior calcaneocuboid ligaments (superficial and deep) and superiorly by the lateral limb of the bifurcate ligament.
   c. The naviculocuneiform and intercuneiform joints are connected by dense ligamentous structures that allow little motion between the joints.
   d. The tarsometatarsal (TMT) joint is made up of the first, second, and third metatarsocuneiform joints and the fourth and fifth metatarsocuboid joints.

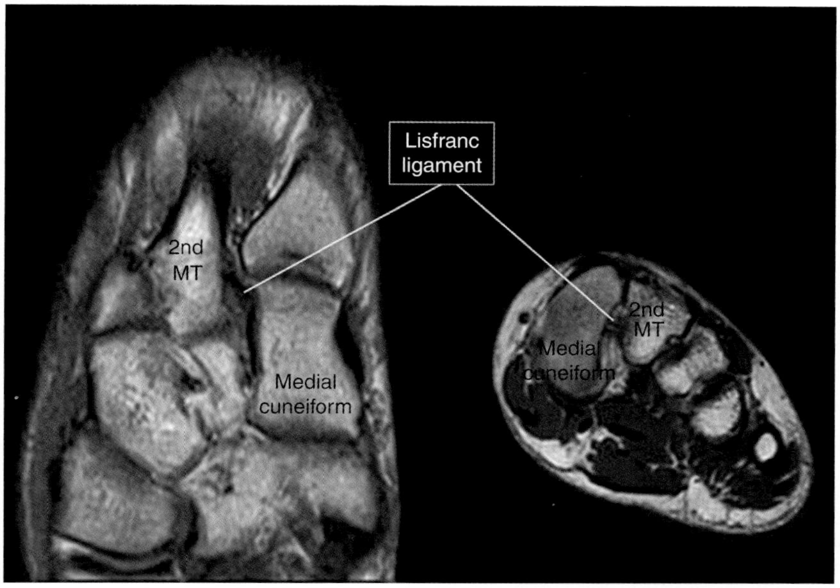

Figure 2 Lisfranc ligament as seen in coronal and axial MRI images coursing between the medal cuneiform and the base of the second metatarsal.

- The osseous anatomy functions as a transverse Roman arch in the axial plane with the dorsal surface wider than the plantar surface.
- The second metatarsal base functions as the keystone.
- The ligamentous support of the TMT joint has three layers. The strongest layer is the interosseous layer, which includes the Lisfranc ligament (**Figure 2**). This ligament originates from the plantar aspect of the medial cuneiform and extends to the base of the second metatarsal. The plantar layer is the next strongest, and the dorsal layer is the weakest.

3. Forefoot
   a. The plantar aspect of the first metatarsophalangeal (MTP) joint is made up of the dense phalangeosesamoidal complex, or plantar plate (**Figure 3**).
   b. The conjoined tendon of the adductor hallucis muscles has a broad insertion over the lateral aspect of the lateral sesamoid and at the lateral aspect of the base of the proximal phalanx.
   c. The plantar fascia originates from the medial calcaneal tuberosity and inserts distally on the base of the fifth metatarsal (lateral band), as well as the plantar plate and the bases of the five proximal phalanges.

B. Muscles and tendons (**Figure 4**)

1. Compartments of the leg (**Table 1**)
   a. The anterior compartment contains the tibialis anterior, extensor hallucis longus (EHL), extensor digitorum longus (EDL), and peroneus tertius muscles, as well as the anterior tibial artery and deep peroneal nerve (DPN). Deep to the extensor retinaculum of the ankle, the anterior tibial artery and DPN lie between the tibialis anterior and EHL tendons.
   b. The superficial posterior compartment contains the gastrocnemius-soleus complex and the plantaris muscle.
      - Two heads of the gastrocnemius muscle originate from the medial and lateral femoral condyles and act as knee flexors as well as ankle plantar flexors.
      - The soleus originates on the tibia and fibula. It runs deep to the gastrocnemius and joins it distally to form the Achilles tendon.
      - The Achilles tendon fibers twist medially 90° so that the superficial fibers at the myotendinous junction insert laterally on the calcaneus.
      - The plantaris is absent in 7% of individuals.
   c. The deep posterior compartment contains the PTT, flexor digitorum longus (FDL), and flexor hallucis longus (FHL), which become entirely tendinous as they enter the ankle.
      - Posterior to the medial malleolus, the posterior compartment structures enter the fibro-osseous tarsal tunnel.
      - Oriented from anteromedial to posterolateral in the tarsal tunnel are the PTT, FDL tendon, posterior tibial artery, tibial nerve, and FHL tendon.

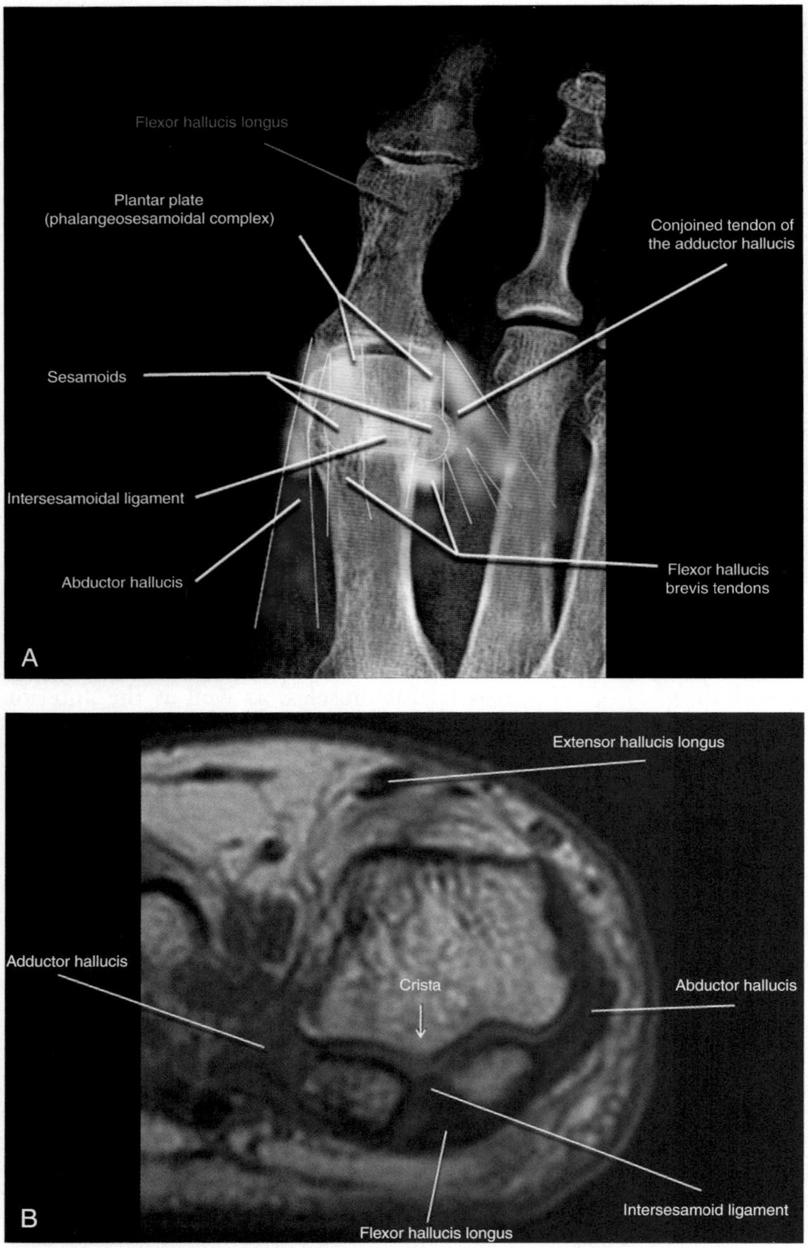

Figure 3 **A**, AP radiograph with soft-tissue structures drawn for illustration. **B**, Cross-section MRI of the hallux metatarsophalangeal joint. (Reproduced with permission from Mann RA, Coughlin MJ: Adult hallux valgus, in Mann RA, Coughlin MJ, eds: *Surgery of the Foot and Ankle*, ed 6. St. Louis, MO, Mosby, 1993, vol. 1, pp 167-296.)

- The FHL and FDL have interconnections at the knot of Henry in the plantar midfoot.

d. The lateral compartment contains the peroneus longus and peroneus brevis muscles, the superficial peroneal nerve (SPN), and the peroneal artery.

- The tendons enter a system of fibro-osseous tunnels posterior to the fibula to the level of their insertion.
- The superior peroneal retinaculum is located at the distal 3 cm of the fibula; the inferior peroneal retinaculum is contiguous with the inferior extensor retinaculum dorsally and inserts on the peroneal tubercle of the calcaneus, which divides the peroneal tendon sheath into separate compartments for the peroneus brevis (dorsal) and peroneus longus (plantar).

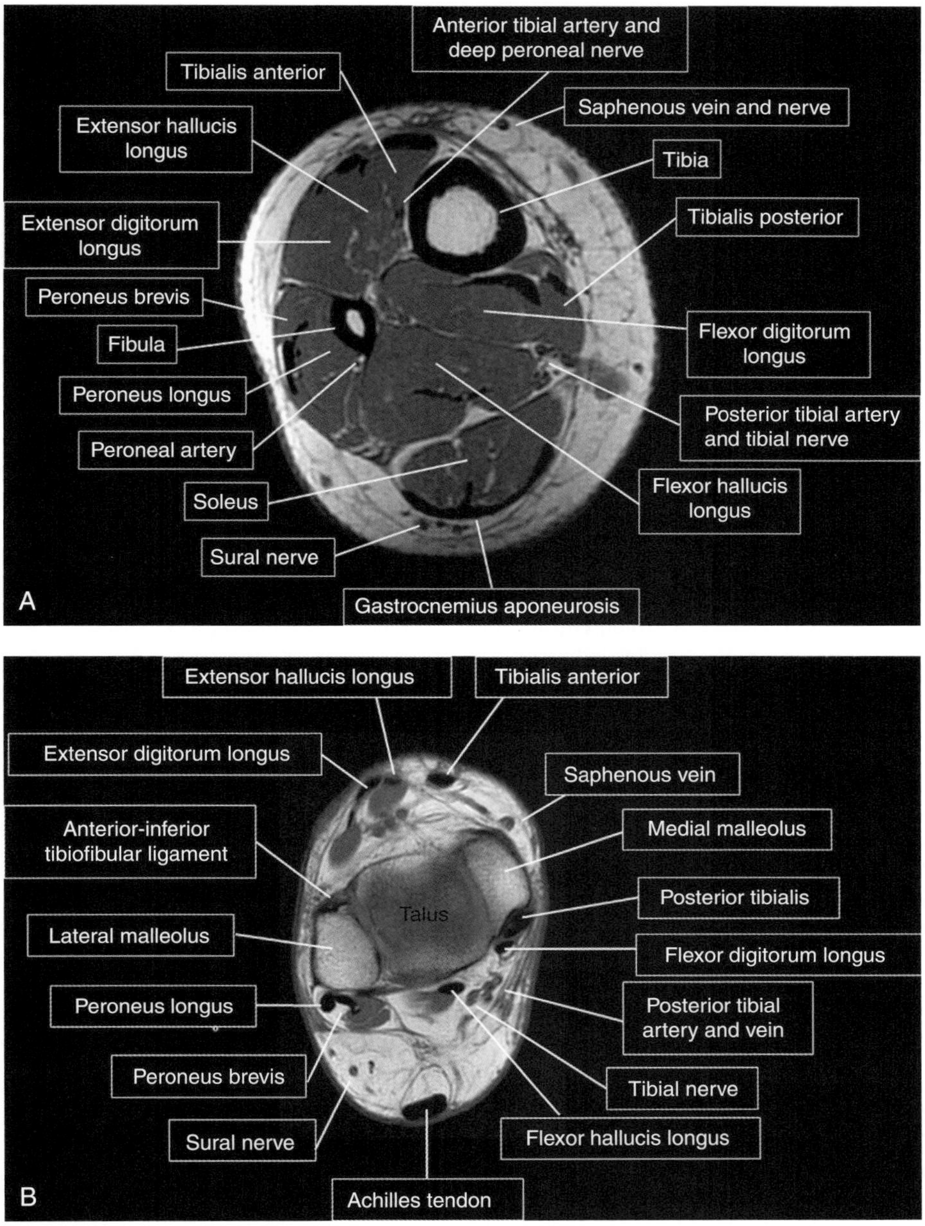

Figure 4 Axial MRI images of the leg at the level of **A**, the distal third of the leg and **B**, the level of the ankle joint.

- The peroneus brevis inserts at the base of the fifth metatarsal.
- The peroneus longus curves sharply beneath the cuboid, where it crosses plantarly to insert medially at the base of the first TMT joint. An osseous groove is present at the plantar cuboid, and an os peroneum is present in 5% to 26% of individuals.
- Accessory peroneals (including the peroneus quartus) are present in 12% of individuals and can contribute to pathology (**Figure 5**).

2. Muscles of the plantar foot
   a. First layer—The first layer is the most superficial of the plantar layers. It contains the flexor digitorum brevis (FDB), abductor hallucis, and abductor digiti minimi (ADM) muscles.
   b. Second layer—This layer contains the quadratus plantae (QP) and lumbrical muscles as well as the FDL and FHL tendons. On the plantar surface of the layer lie the medial and lateral plantar arteries and nerves.

TABLE 1

The Compartments and Muscles of the Leg

Compartment	Muscle	Origin	Insertion	Innervation	Action
Anterior	Tibialis anterior	Tibia, IOM	Medial cuneiform and first metatarsal	DPN	DF, INV
Anterior	Extensor hallucis longus	Fibula, IOM	Distal phalanx hallux	DPN	DF hallux
Anterior	Extensor digitorum longus	Tibia and fibula, IOM	Middle and distal phalanx lesser toes	DPN	DF toes
Anterior	Peroneus tertius	Fibula	Base of fifth metatarsal	DPN	DF, EV
Superficial posterior	Gastrocnemius	Medial and lateral femoral condyles	Calcaneus through Achilles	Tibial	Ankle PF, knee flexor
Superficial posterior	Soleus	Tibia and fibula	Calcaneus through Achilles	Tibial	PF
Superficial posterior	Plantaris	Lateral femur	Calcaneus	Tibial	PF
Deep posterior	Posterior tibialis	Tibia, IOM	Navicular and plantar surface of second, third, and fourth metatarsals, cuboid, sustentaculum talus	Tibial	PF, INV
Deep posterior	Flexor hallucis longus	Fibula, IOM	Distal phalanx hallux	Tibial	PF hallux
Deep posterior	Flexor digitorum longus	Tibia	Distal lesser phalanges	Tibial	PF lesser toes
Lateral	Peroneus longus	Tibia and fibula	Medial cuneiform, base of first metatarsal	SPN	EV, PF
Lateral	Peroneus brevis	Fibula	Base of fifth metatarsal	SPN	EV, PF

DF = dorsiflexion, DPN = deep peroneal nerve, EV = eversion, INV = inversion, IOM = interosseous membrane, PF = plantar flexion, SPN = superficial peroneal nerve

c. Third layer—The third layer contains the oblique and transverse heads of the adductor hallucis, flexor hallucis brevis, and flexor digiti minimi brevis muscles.

d. Fourth layer—This layer is the deepest. It contains the fibro-osseous tunnels along which the posterior tibial and peroneus longus tendons travel to their final insertions. It contains the four dorsal interossei, three plantar interossei, and four lumbrical muscles.

3. Muscles of the dorsal foot

a. Laterally, the extensor digitorum brevis (EDB) arises from the anterior process of the calcaneus.

b. Medially, the extensor hallucis brevis (EHB) is variably present.

c. Each of these muscles contributes tendinous slips to the long extensor tendons or directly to the base of each proximal phalanx.

d. Deep to these muscles course the dorsalis pedis artery and DPN.

C. Arteries

1. Three major arteries typically supply the ankle and foot.

a. Posterior tibial artery—This artery bifurcates into the medial and lateral plantar arteries beneath the sustentaculum.

b. Peroneal artery—The peroneal artery arises from the tibioperoneal trunk and forms a perforating artery that pierces the interosseous membrane at the distal third of the leg.

c. Anterior tibial artery—This artery arises from the popliteal artery below the knee and descends through the anterior compartment of the leg. It combines variably with the perforating branch of the peroneal artery to form the dorsalis pedis artery.

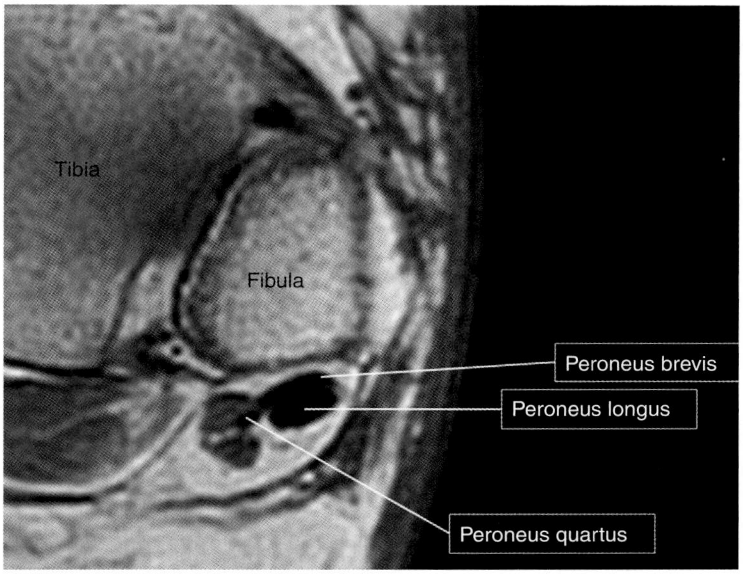

Figure 5 Magnetic resonance image showing the relationship of peroneus longus, peroneus brevis, and an accessory peroneal muscle (peroneus quartus) at the level of the distal fibula.

2. Plantar arcades—The medial plantar artery and lateral plantar artery typically branch to give superficial and deep branches, which undergo anastomosis distally in the midfoot to give the superficial plantar arcade and deep plantar arch.

3. Osseous vascular supply of interest
   a. Talus (**Figure 6**)
      - Of the talar surface, 60% is covered with articular cartilage, limiting the potential sites for arterial supply to five bony regions: the tarsal canal, the sinus tarsi, the superior neck, the medial body, and the posterior tubercle.

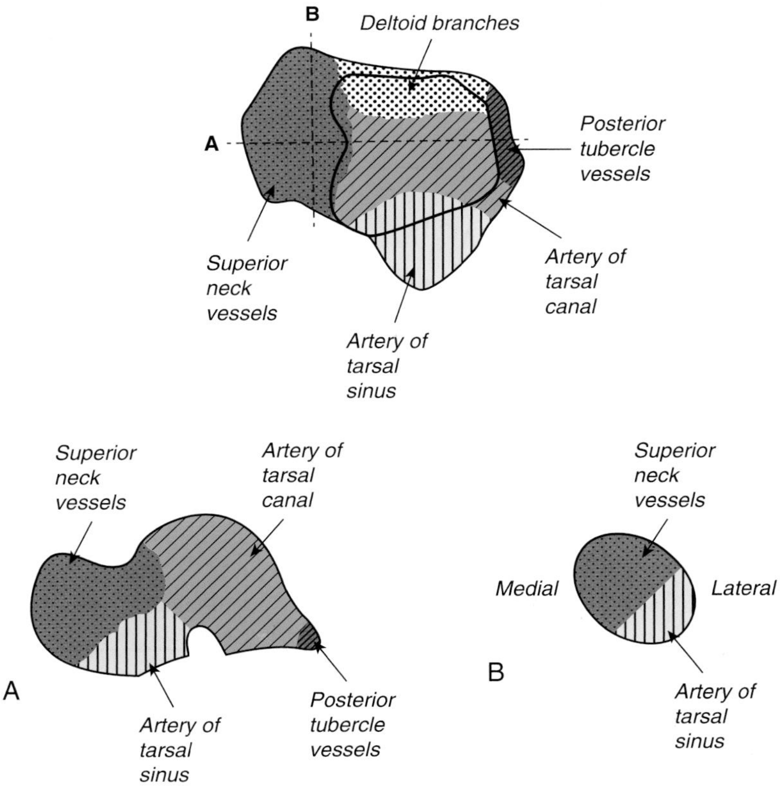

Figure 6 Drawing of the vascular supply and watershed areas of the talus. Axial and (**A**) sagital views are represented. **B** shows a coronal cross section of the talar neck. (Reproduced with permission from Gillerman RN, Mortensen WW: The arterial supply of the talus. *Foot Ankle* 1983;4:64-72.)

- Injection studies have demonstrated that the talar neck is well vascularized by an anastomotic ring of vessels that receives blood dorsally from the dorsalis pedis artery, laterally from the perforating peroneal artery through the lateral tarsal artery, and inferiorly through the artery of the tarsal canal.
- The talar body receives most of its blood supply retrograde through the artery of the tarsal canal, which predisposes it to osteonecrosis and nonunion following talar neck fractures and talar dislocations.
- Recent studies using gadolinium-enhanced MRI have demonstrated that the posterior tibial artery is the dominant arterial supply to the talus, providing antegrade flow through the posterior tubercle and potentially accounting for lower rates (30% to 50%) of traumatic osteonecrosis observed in contemporary studies.

b. Navicular

- The periphery is well vascularized, but the central third is less vascular.
- The navicular is prone to stress fracture in the dorsal third, where the compression forces are concentrated.

c. Fifth metatarsal

- Penetrating the fifth metatarsal medially at the junction of its proximal and middle thirds, the main nutrient vessel to the fifth metatarsal then divides into proximal and distal vessels.
- The proximal blood supply to the fifth metatarsal is through the tuberosity, creating a watershed area at the proximal metaphyseal/diaphyseal junction, which is prone to stress fractures and nonunion.

D. Nerves of the foot (**Figure 7** and **Table 2**)

1. Tibial nerve—The tibial nerve travels in the deep posterior compartment of the leg and has three major branches.

   a. Medial calcaneal nerve—This nerve innervates the plantarmedial heel.

   b. Medial plantar nerve—This nerve supplies sensory innervation to the plantarmedial foot, the plantar aspect of the first, second, and third toes and the medial half of the fourth toe. It

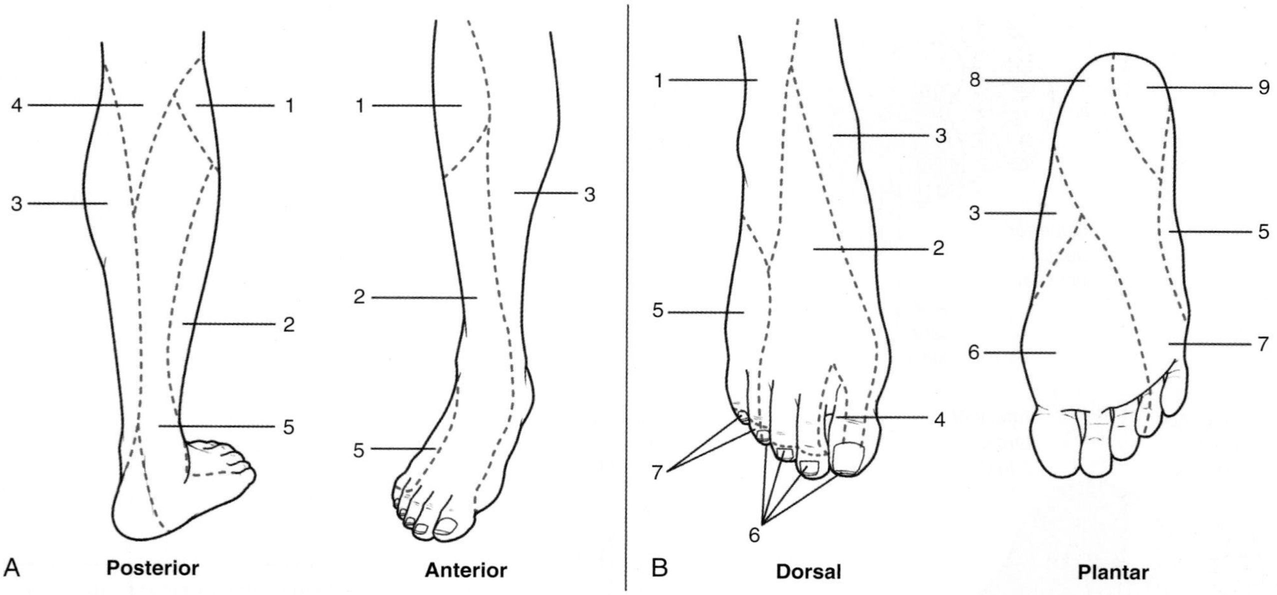

Figure 7 Illustrations show the nerves of the leg and foot. **A**, Posterior and anterior views show the cutaneous innervation of the leg and ankle. 1 = lateral sural cutaneous nerve, 2 = superficial peroneal nerve, 3 = saphenous nerve, 4 = posterior femoral cutaneous nerve, 5 = sural nerve. **B**, Dorsal and plantar views depict the cutaneous innervation of the dorsal and plantar foot. 1 = peroneal cutaneous nerve, 2 = saphenous nerve, 3 = superficial peroneal nerve, 4 = deep peroneal nerve, 5 = sural nerve, 6 = medial plantar nerve, 7 = lateral plantar nerve, 8 = medial calcaneal nerve, 9 = first calcaneal nerve.

TABLE 2

Nerves at Risk During Surgery of the Foot

Procedure	Nerve at Risk	Anatomic Location
ORIF of the fibula	SPN	Crosses fibula 7-11 cm proximal to tip
Anterolateral arthroscopy portal	SPN	Plantar flexion of fourth toe will allow visualization below skin
Anteromedial arthroscopy portal, ORIF of the medial malleolus	Saphenous	Medial to tibialis anterior
Anterior approach to ankle, anterior central arthroscopy portal	DPN	Deep to and between tibialis anterior and EHL
ORIF of the medial malleolus, posteromedial arthroscopy portal	Tibial	Deep to tibialis posterior and FDL, superficial to FHL
Peroneal reconstruction, ORIF of the calcaneus, lateral ligament reconstruction, posterolateral arthroscopy portal	Sural	Anterolateral to Achilles, often crosses field distal to fibula
ORIF of the fifth metatarsal	Sural	Dorsal, medial to base of fifth metatarsal
ORIF of the Lisfranc sprain	DPN	Runs deep to EHB over dorsum of 1-2 metatarsal bases with DPA
Bunion—medial approach	Medial dorsal cutaneous nerve of the hallux	Subcutaneous tissue dorsal medial first metatarsal and first metatarsal head
Sesamoids	Digital nerve of the hallux	Immediately plantar to sesamoids
Plantar fascia release	Medial calcaneal	May exit through abductor hallucis fascia or plantar fascia at level of release

DPA = dorsalis pedis artery, DPN = deep peroneal nerve, EHB = extensor hallucis brevis, EHL = extensor hallucis longus, FDL = flexor digitorum longus, FHL = flexor hallucis longus, ORIF = open reduction and internal fixation, SPN = superficial peroneal nerve

provides motor innervation to the FHB, AbH, FDB, and the first lumbrical.

c. Lateral plantar nerve—This nerve provides sensation to the plantarlateral foot, the lateral fourth toe, and the fifth toe. Motor innervation is provided to the remaining plantar muscles not innervated by the medial plantar nerve.
   - The first branch of the lateral plantar nerve (Baxter nerve) courses anterior to the medial calcaneal tuberosity between the QP and the FDB, terminally innervating the ADM.
   - The Baxter nerve is implicated in heel pain but provides no cutaneous innervation.

2. SPN—The SPN divides into medial and intermediate dorsal cutaneous nerves of the foot proximal to the ankle.
3. DPN—The DPN travels in the anterior compartment, where it innervates the tibialis anterior, EDL, EHL, and courses between the tibialis anterior and EHL tendons. It innervates the EDB and EHB muscles in the foot and provides sensation to the first dorsal web space.
4. Sural nerve—The sural nerve has a variable origin from confluent branches of the tibial and common peroneal nerves. It provides sensation to the dorsolateral foot and dorsal fourth and fifth toes.
5. Saphenous nerve—The saphenous nerve is the terminal branch of the femoral nerve and supplies sensation to the medial side of the foot.

II. BIOMECHANICS

A. Ankle and syndesmosis
1. The ankle joint is composed of the tibia, fibula, and talus.
   a. Its primary motion is dorsiflexion and plantar flexion.
   b. With the foot fixed, dorsiflexion is accompanied by internal tibial rotation, and plantar flexion is accompanied by external tibial rotation.
2. The bimalleolar axis runs obliquely at 82° (±4°) in the coronal plane and defines the main motion of the ankle.

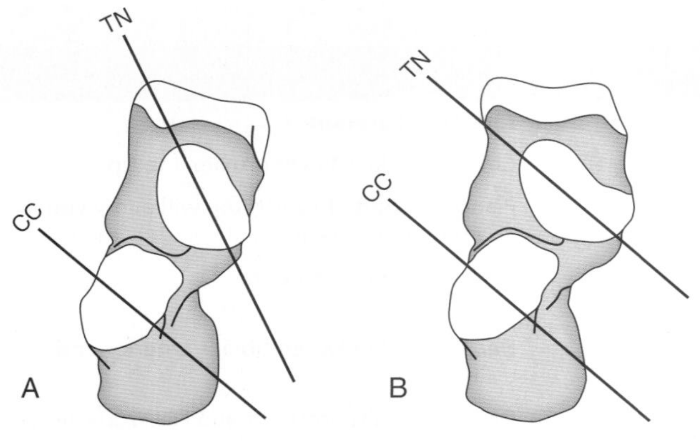

Figure 8 Illustrations show the inversion (**A**) and eversion (**B**) of the subtalar joint, which locks and unlocks the transverse tarsal joint by aligning or deviating the major joint axes of the talonavicular (TN) and calcaneocuboid (CC) joints. (Adapted with permission from Mann RA, Haskell A: Biomechanics of the foot and ankle, in Coughlin MJ, Mann RA, Saltzman CL, eds: *Surgery of the Foot and Ankle*, ed 8. Philadelphia, PA, Mosby, 2007, p 21.)

a. The talus is wider anteriorly than posteriorly, and the contact area of the dome of the talus increases and moves anteriorly with dorsiflexion.

b. Increased load transmission in the malleoli also occurs with dorsiflexion.

c. The fibula transmits approximately 10% to 15% of the axial load.

3. The tibiofibular syndesmosis allows rotation and proximal and distal migration of the fibula with the tibia but little motion in the sagittal or coronal planes.

B. Hindfoot—Subtalar joint and transverse tarsal (Chopart) joint

1. These joints act through a series of coupled motions to create inversion and eversion of the hindfoot and to lock and unlock the midfoot.
2. The transverse tarsal joint is made up of the talonavicular and calcaneocuboid articulations.
3. Inversion of the subtalar joint locks the transverse tarsal joint; eversion unlocks the joint (**Figure 8**).
4. The joints are parallel during heel strike, when the calcaneus is in eversion, allowing the midfoot to be flexible for shock absorption as the foot accepts the body's weight.
5. The joint axes are deviated as the subtalar joint moves to inversion (eg, during push-off), making the foot inflexible so that it provides a rigid lever arm for push-off.
6. The relationships of the tendons as they cross the ankle and subtalar joints are shown in **Figure 9**.

C. TMT and midfoot joints

1. Little motion occurs through the intercuneiform and naviculocuneiform joints.

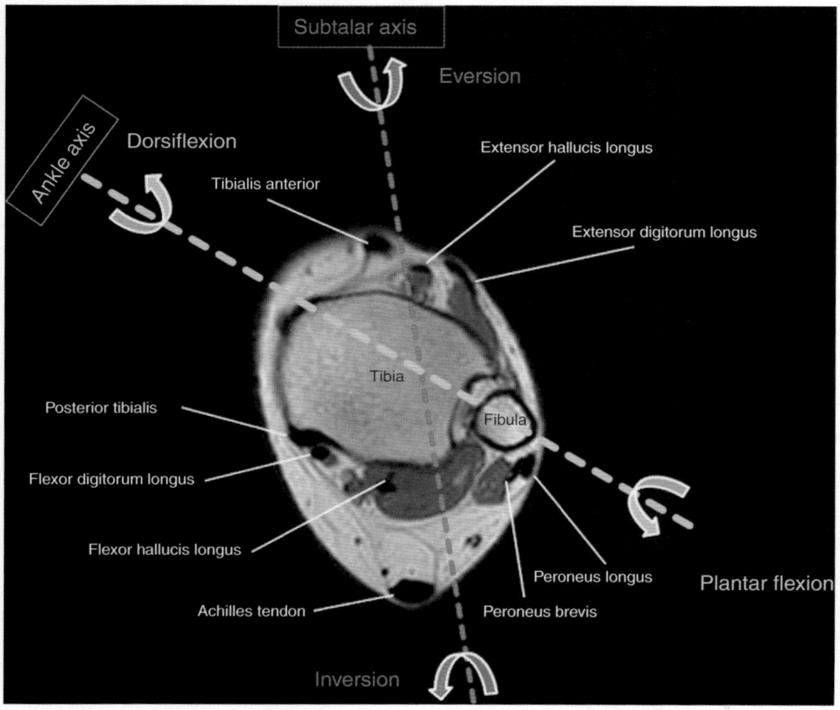

Figure 9 Illustration shows the relationships of the tendons that cross the ankle joint to the axes of the subtalar and tibiotalar articulations. Tendons anterior to the ankle axis create a dorsiflexion moment, whereas tendons posterior to the ankle axis create a plantar flexion moment. Tendons medial to the subtalar axis cause inversion; tendons lateral to the subtalar axis cause eversion.

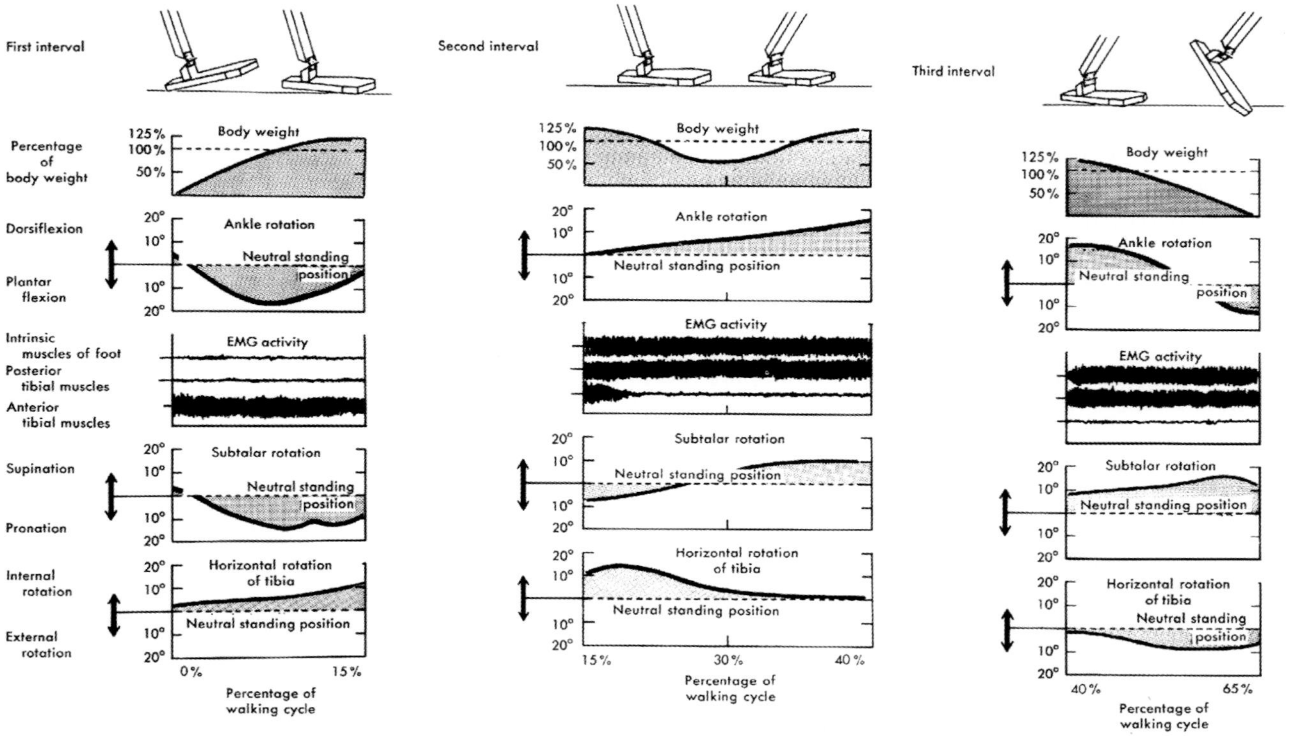

Figure 10 Illustrations summarize the kinematics and electromyographic (EMG) activity during the three intervals of the stance phase. (Reproduced with permission from Mann RA: Biomechanics of the foot and ankle, in Mann RA, Coughlin MJ, eds: *Surgery of the Foot and Ankle*, ed 6. St Louis, MO, Mosby, 1993, pp 29-31.)

2. The fourth and fifth TMT joints are the most mobile, with a range of motion of 5° to 17°. The second TMT is the least mobile, with 1° of motion.

D. MTP joints

1. The hallux MTP joint has a normal range of motion of 30° to 90°.
2. Dorsiflexion of the MTP joints during push-off tightens the plantar fascia through a windlass effect, raising the longitudinal arch and inverting the heel.

III. GAIT

A. The phases of the gait cycle are described in Chapter 17.

B. Motions and muscle activity at the ankle during the three intervals of stance phase are shown in **Figure 10**.

TOP TESTING FACTS

1. The ATFL is under increased strain in plantar flexion, inversion, and internal rotation; the CFL is under increased strain in dorsiflexion and inversion.
2. The spring ligament complex, which supports the talonavicular joint, comprises the superomedial calcaneonavicular ligament and the inferior calcaneonavicular ligaments.
3. The Lisfranc ligament originates at the plantar aspect of the medial cuneiform and continues to the central portion of the lateral base of the second metatarsal metaphysis.
4. The conjoined tendon of the adductor hallucis muscle inserts at the lateral proximal phalanx and lateral sesamoid.

5. The Achilles tendon fibers rotate 90° toward their insertion. The superficial fibers of the Achilles tendon at the myotendinous junction insert laterally on the calcaneus.
6. The peroneus brevis tendon lies dorsal and the peroneus longus tendon lies plantar to the peroneal tubercle of the calcaneus at the inferior peroneal retinaculum.
7. The talar body receives most of its blood supply retrograde from the talar neck, making it susceptible to nonunion and osteonecrosis when the talar neck is fractured.
8. The nerves at risk during placement of portals for ankle arthroscopy are anterolateral–superficial peroneal nerve, anteromedial–saphenous nerve, anterior central–deep peroneal nerve, posterolateral–sural nerve, posteromedial–tibial nerve.
9. Inversion of the subtalar joint causes the talonavicular and calcaneocuboid joint axes of the transverse tarsal (Chopart) joint to deviate, decreasing motion and locking the midfoot.
10. The second TMT joint has the least motion; the fourth and fifth have the most.

Bibliography

Esquenazi A: Biomechanics of gait, in Vaccaro AR, ed: *Orthopaedic Knowledge Update*, ed 8. Rosemont, IL, American Academy of Orthopaedic Surgeons, 2005, pp 377-386.

Mann RA: Biomechanics of the foot and ankle, in Mann RA, ed: *Surgery of the Foot*, ed 7. St Louis, MO, Mosby, 1999, pp 2-35.

Miller AN, Prasarn ML, Dyke JP, Helfet DL, Lorich DG: Quantitative assessment of the vascularity of the talus with gadolinium-enhanced magnetic resonance imaging. *J Bone Joint Surg Am* 2011;93(12):1116-1121.

Resch S: Functional anatomy and topography of the foot and ankle, in Myerson MS, ed: *Foot and Ankle Disorders*. Philadelphia, PA, WB Saunders, 2000, pp 25-49.

Sammarco VJ, Acevedo JI: Clinical biomechanics of the foot and ankle, in Richardson EG, ed: *Orthopaedic Knowledge Update: Foot and Ankle*, ed 3. Rosemont, IL, American Academy of Orthopaedic Surgeons, 2004, pp 207-218.

Sarrafian SK: *Anatomy of the Foot and Ankle*. Philadelphia, PA, JB Lippincott, 1983.

Warfel JH: *The Extremities: Muscles and Motor Points*, ed 6. Philadelphia, PA, Lea & Febiger, 1993.

Chapter 109
Regional Anesthesia for Foot and Ankle Surgery

RANDALL J. MALCHOW, MD
RAJNISH K. GUPTA, MD

I. REGIONAL ANESTHESIA TECHNIQUES

A. Innervation to the foot and the ankle is provided by the sciatic nerve (branching into the superficial peroneal, deep peroneal, tibial, and sural nerves) and the saphenous nerve (originating from the femoral nerve; **Figure 1**).

B. Sciatic block (classic or infragluteal)

1. Usually performed in the lateral "Sims" position (lateral recumbent position with dependent leg straight, and nondependent hip and knee flexed).
2. Typically performed using a nerve stimulator and/or ultrasonography.
3. Although more technically challenging, continuous catheters can be placed.

C. Popliteal sciatic nerve block (**Figure 2**)

1. Can be performed with the patient positioned prone, lateral, or supine, with the leg propped up in a leg holder (**Figure 3**).
2. Nerve localization can be performed using nerve stimulation and/or ultrasonography.
3. Continuous catheters can be placed at this location to allow prolonged analgesia for up to 5 days.

D. Saphenous nerve block

1. The saphenous nerve provides cutaneous innervation to the anteromedial leg and ankle, as well as periosteal branches to the medial malleolus and joint capsule.
2. Because the saphenous nerve is a branch of the femoral nerve, the block can be performed by blocking the femoral nerve at the groin or the saphenous nerve independently, either in the adductor canal along the midthigh, or as part of the ankle block, described in Section I.E.
3. The femoral block is performed with either nerve stimulation and/or ultrasonography, whereas the adductor canal block is typically performed using ultrasonography alone because nerve stimulation of the sensory saphenous nerve is unreliable.
4. A continuous nerve catheter can be placed at either location.

E. Ankle block

1. Complete blockade of the five distal peripheral nerves of the foot and the ankle.
2. Continuous nerve catheters cannot be placed for an ankle block.
3. Paresthesias are common and may help identify nerve location but also may indicate that the needle is too close to the nerve.
4. Two deep nerves
   a. Posterior tibial nerve—injection midway between the Achilles tendon and the medial malleolus through the flexor retinaculum just posterior to the posterior tibial artery (**Figure 4**).
   b. Deep peroneal nerve—injection between the anterior tibial artery and the extensor hallucis longus tendon just deep to the extensor retinaculum (**Figure 5**).
   c. Ultrasonography is very useful in identifying anatomy, visualizing spread, and improving success for these two deep nerve blocks of the ankle.

Neither of the following authors nor any immediate family member has received anything of value from or has stock or stock options held in a commercial company or institution related directly or indirectly to the subject of this chapter: Dr. Malchow and Dr. Gupta.

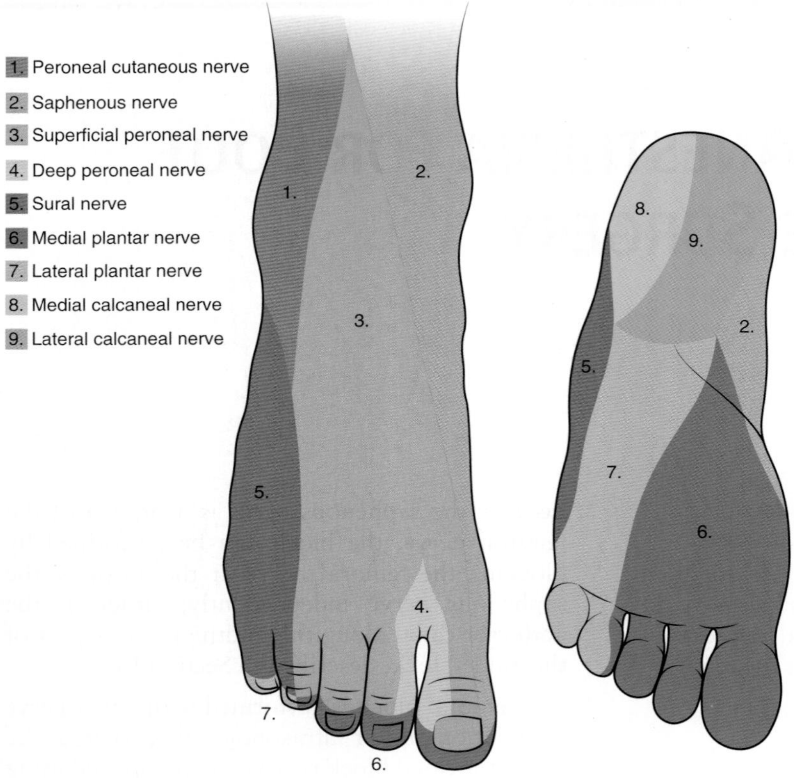

Figure 1 Drawings show the cutaneous sensory distribution of the foot and the ankle.

5. Three superficial nerves require subcutaneous infiltration above or below the intermalleolar line.
   a. Saphenous nerve—injection from the tibialis anterior tendon to the medial malleolus.
   b. Superficial peroneal nerve—injection from the tibialis anterior tendon laterally across the dorsum of the foot.
   c. Sural nerve—injection from the lateral malleolus to the Achilles tendon.

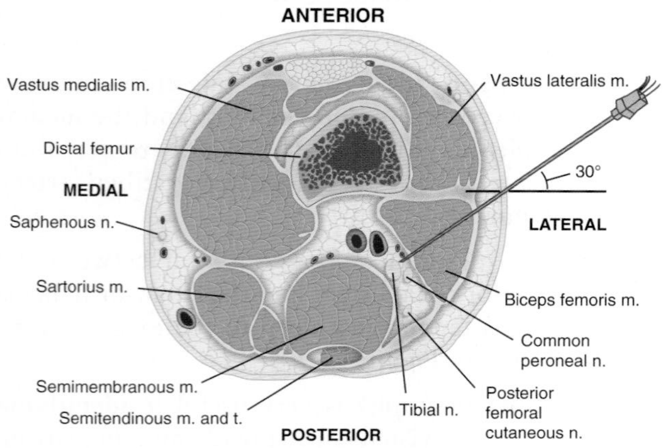

Figure 2 Cross-sectional diagram of the distal thigh shows the needle approach for a lateral popliteal nerve block.

F. General nerve block considerations
   1. A time-out procedure should be performed before all nerve blocks to ensure verification of patient identification, correct laterality and surgical site, and any relevant allergies.
   2. Preoperative blocks allow a significant decrease or avoidance of general anesthesia and opioids; however, blocks may be performed postoperatively to allow nerve examination, when necessary.
   3. No weight bearing is allowed if a popliteal block and/or a femoral nerve block is present.
   4. A postoperative knee immobilizer should be provided to help prevent falls after a femoral nerve block due to quadriceps weakness.

II. CONTINUOUS PERINEURAL CATHETERS

A. Typically involve a lower concentration local anesthetic—ie, more sensory block, less motor block.

B. Continuous peripheral nerve catheters are used following inpatient surgery or at home following ambulatory surgery (managed by the patient or a home health worker).

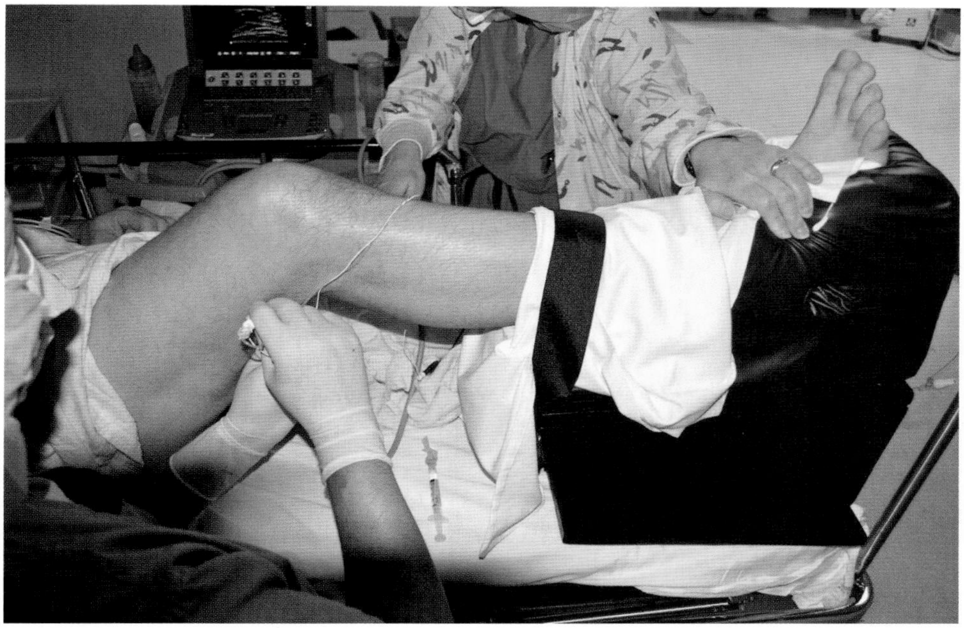

Figure 3 Photograph demonstrates the leg position for an ultrasound-guided lateral popliteal nerve block using a leg holder.

C. Appropriate analgesia may require using two simultaneous catheters if substantial sciatic and saphenous distributions are involved at the surgical site. Local anesthetic toxicity can be avoided by limiting total volume and concentration.

D. Infusion pumps

1. Electronic pumps are reprogrammable, refillable, and reusable; however, they can be expensive and bulky.

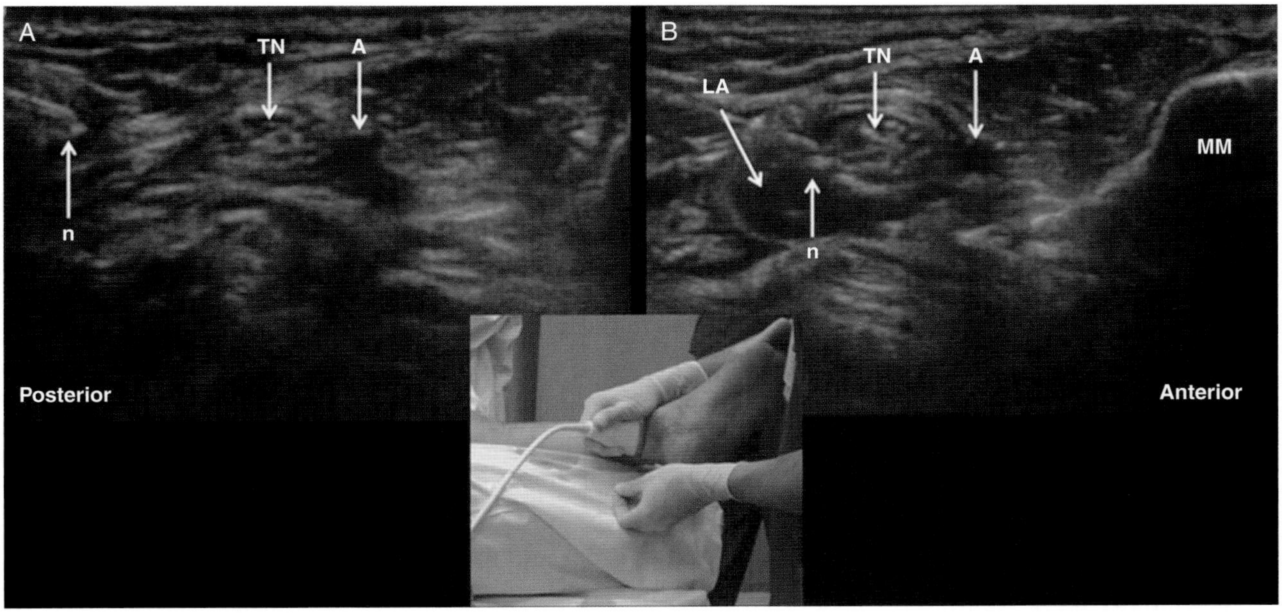

Figure 4 Tibial nerve block at the ankle. Transverse preinjection view (**A**) and postinjection view (**B**) of the tibial nerve (TN) lying posterior to the posterior tibial artery (A) and the medial malleolus (MM). The foot is elevated on a bolster, and the block needle (n) is inserted in-plane in a posterior-to-anterior direction to inject local anesthetic (LA) around the nerve. (From Chin KJ, Wong NWY, Macfarlane AJR, Chan VWS: Ultrasound-guided versus anatomic landmark-guided ankle blocks. *Reg Anesth Pain Med* 2011;36:611-618.)

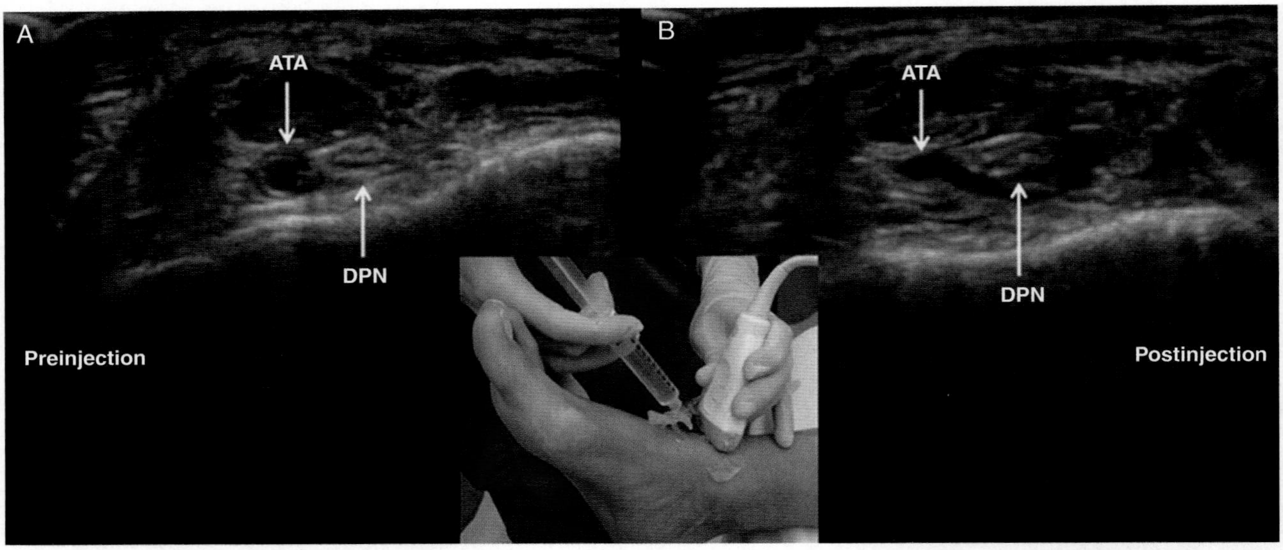

Figure 5 Deep peroneal nerve block at the ankle. Transverse preinjection view (**A**) and postinjection view (**B**) of the anterior tibial artery (ATA) and the adjacent deep peroneal nerve (DPN), lying superficial to bone (hyperechoic line). The needle has been inserted out-of-plane in this case. (From Chin KJ, Wong NWY, Macfarlane AJR, Chan VWS: Ultrasound-guided versus anatomic landmark-guided ankle blocks. *Reg Anesth Pain Med* 2011;36:611-618.)

2. Elastomeric/disposable pumps are cheaper, lighter, and easier to use for the patient but can have somewhat inconsistent flow rates.

III. PROCEDURE-SPECIFIC REGIONAL ANESTHESIA OPTIONS AND CONSIDERATIONS

A. Blocks for minimal to moderate invasiveness (**Table 1**)—Require anesthesia and analgesia for the distal sciatic nerve branches but usually do not require long-acting analgesia in the saphenous nerve distribution.

1. Popliteal sciatic nerve block at the knee
   a. Pros—Blocks movement of the foot for surgical akinesis
   b. Cons—Causes postoperative motor block
   c. If a catheter is present, it may end up in the surgical field if the patient's lower extremity is prepared above the knee or the tourniquet is placed on the thigh.
   d. Alternatives—Proximal sciatic nerve block or ankle block
2. Saphenous nerve block
   a. Options for a saphenous block from proximal to distal include a femoral nerve block, an adductor canal block, or a saphenous nerve block at the ankle. Subcutaneous saphenous blocks immediately above or below the knee generally are unreliable.
   b. Considerations—Adductor canal and saphenous blocks at the ankle do not provide analgesia for thigh pain from the tourniquet, whereas a femoral nerve block does.
   c. Saphenous blocks at the ankle are easier and quicker to perform than adductor canal blocks but are appropriate only for procedures of the midfoot or forefoot.
3. Ankle block
   a. Indicated for relatively minor surgery involving the forefoot only.
   b. Patient retains movement of the foot and ankle and limited weight bearing is possible.

B. Blocks for high invasiveness (**Table 1**)—Require potent anesthesia and long-acting analgesia in both the sciatic and saphenous nerve distributions.

1. Popliteal or proximal sciatic nerve block and/or catheter
   a. This is the primary block for the painful stimulus.
   b. A proximal sciatic block should be considered if a preoperative popliteal catheter will be in the surgical prep field or could interfere with the thigh tourniquet.
   c. Proximal sciatic blocks reduce knee flexion strength, which complicates ambulation with crutches.

TABLE 1

Regional Anesthesia Options for Specific Procedures

Surgical Procedure	Ankle	Popliteal	Saphenous	Femoral	Popliteal Catheter	General Anesthesia
Minimal to Moderate Invasiveness[a]						
Plantar fascia endoscopy/ESWT						X
Hammer toe	X	X				
Toenail	X					
Hallux rigidus	X	X	X			
Morton neuroma	X					
Toe amputation	X					
Phalangeal/metatarsal ORIF	X	X	X			
Ankle arthroscopy		X		X		
Achilles tendon repair		X		X		
High Invasiveness[b]						
Malleolar ORIF		X	X		X	
Hallux valgus	X	X	X		X	
Ankle reconstruction			X	X	X	
Ankle arthrodesis			X	X	X	
Transmetatarsal amputation			X	X	X	
Tarsal/calcaneal ORIF			X		X	

ESWT = extracorporeal shockwave therapy, ORIF = open reduction and internal fixation
[a]Minimal to moderate postoperative pain.
[b]Severe postoperative pain possible.

2. A femoral block or adductor canal block with or without a catheter will be necessary for complete regional anesthesia of the foot and ankle, as described previously.

IV. PHARMACOLOGY

A. Mild to moderate sedation—While judicious sedation is useful for anxiolysis, the patient is kept responsive enough to report paresthesias.
   1. Benzodiazepines (such as midazolam), opioids (such as fentanyl), and/or ketamine.
   2. Propofol can be used in extreme situations; general anesthesia is currently only used in pediatrics for akinesis during the block.

B. Local anesthetics
   1. Short-acting
      a. Examples (lidocaine, mepivacaine)
      b. Rapid onset in 10 to 15 minutes
      c. Duration of 3 to 6 hours
   2. Long-acting
      a. Examples (bupivacaine, ropivacaine, levobupivacaine)
      b. Slower onset in 15 to 45 minutes
      c. Duration of 10 to 16 hours
      d. All long-acting local anesthetics have greater systemic toxicity than short-acting local anesthetics.
      e. Catheter infusions—typically use low concentration long-acting local anesthetics (sensory greater than motor effect).
   3. Combinations of short-acting and long-acting local anesthetics have intermediate durations (8 to 12 hours).

C. Additives are considered in single-shot blocks but not usually in catheter infusions. (Additives in nerve blocks are generally considered an off-label use.)
   1. Epinephrine
      a. Serves as a marker for intravascular injection during bolus, but also can prolong the block.

b. A potential concern exists about vasoconstriction causing nerve ischemia, especially in high-risk patients.

2. Clonidine—can extend a block 2 to 3 hours and may be neuroprotective.
3. Dexmedetomidine—can extend a block 2 to 3 hours and may be neuroprotective.
4. Dexamethasone—can extend a block 4 to 6 hours with some blocks lasting up to 30 hours. Recommend using preservative-free version.
5. Buprenorphine—may extend block 2 to 4 hours and enhance quality of analgesia.
6. Bicarbonate—Can reduce pain on injection and quicken onset; should be avoided with bupivacaine or ropivacaine as it can cause precipitation.
7. Combination of clonidine and dexamethasone is not advised as this combination has been associated with neurapraxia.

V. INTRAOPERATIVE MANAGEMENT

A. Choices include general anesthesia or conscious sedation.

B. Management depends on the completeness of the block for the surgical site, the block coverage for the tourniquet site, patient position on the OR table, and patient comfort or anxiety.

VI. COMPLICATIONS

A. Failed block—Requires alternative anesthesia or analgesia plan

B. Wrong-side block—Prevented with appropriate time-out procedures and site marking

C. Bleeding/hematoma—Is rare and typically resolves with compression unless the patient has a severe bleeding diathesis (medical or pharmacologic)

D. Postoperative neurologic symptoms (PONS)

1. Time course
   a. In the initial 2 weeks, 7% to 10% of patients experience residual PONS from a variety of causes.
   b. The incidence of PONS is less than 0.2% at 9 months.
   c. Permanent injury is rare.
2. Substantial dysesthesia or neurapraxia with motor block should be urgently referred to a neurologist and/or a chronic pain specialist; early imaging studies should be considered, as well as early and late electromyographic/nerve conduction velocity studies if motor involvement is present.
3. Oral medications may be used for symptom control.
   a. NSAIDs and acetaminophen
   b. Anticonvulsants (eg, gabapentin or pregabalin)
   c. Tricyclic antidepressants (eg, amitriptyline or duloxetine), muscle relaxants
   d. Opioids should be the last option. Nerve pain is not well managed with opioids.

E. Local anesthetic systemic toxicity (LAST)

1. Prevention is key. Appropriate regional technique and drug dosing should be used.
2. Risk is traditionally 1:1,500; incidence decreases significantly with ultrasound use.
3. Usually presents as seizure but rarely can cause life-threatening cardiac arrhythmias.
4. Treatment
   a. Airway control and advanced cardiac life support
   b. Intravenous administration of 20% lipid emulsion therapy as antidote
   c. Stop seizure with benzodiazepines or propofol
   d. Arrhythmia management with amiodarone and/or pacing

F. Catheter-related complications

1. Inadequate analgesia—requires a supplemental analgesia plan
2. Catheter problems—leaking, dislodgement, and kinking
3. Pain/paresthesias on removal—patient should get assistance from an anesthesiologist; rarely, may require surgical removal.
4. Infusion pump failures
5. Inadequate patient education—follow-up may be by phone contact
6. Infection—rare; depends on catheter duration (increased risk >5 days)
   a. Higher risk of infection in patients who are immunocompromised.
   b. Superficial infection—can be treated with oral antibiotics; monitor after the catheter is removed.
   c. Deep infections—consider advanced imaging (such as MRI), antibiotics, and possible surgical drainage.

VII. MEDICATION MANAGEMENT

A. Medication management for postoperative pain can be used in place of or along with regional anesthesia.

B. Minimizing opioid use by using nonopioid medications, reducing opioid dose, and reducing opioid duration is advisable.

C. Acetaminophen

1. Useful, primarily as a scheduled analgesic, to accentuate other analgesics.
2. Be mindful that manufacturers of acetaminophen are now recommending a maximum daily dose of 3,000 mg (including combination medications).
3. Decrease dosing in patients with hepatic or renal impairment, malnutrition, starvation, and hypovolemia.

D. Nonsteroidal anti-inflammatory drugs (NSAIDs)

1. Very useful as an analgesic and anti-inflammatory medication.
2. Examples—ibuprofen, naprosyn, diclofenac, meloxicam, celecoxib
3. Be mindful of patients with renal dysfunction or peptic ulcer disease.
4. Although controversial, concerns about NSAID-induced nonunion have generally been refuted. Most studies that showed elevated nonunion rates with NSAIDs were in small, poorly performed studies. Subsequent, higher quality studies have shown no significant difference in nonunion rates with short courses of NSAIDs.

E. Anticonvulsants

1. Examples—gabapentin, pregabalin
2. Useful for neuropathic pain, patients with chronic pain or opioid tolerance, and as an opioid-reduction strategy.
3. Can cause delirium, especially in elderly. Can cause withdrawal when stopping suddenly if the patient is on high dose. Consider tapering.

TOP TESTING FACTS

1. The deep peroneal nerve provides sensation to the deep medial foot and web space of the first and second interspace; the tibial nerve provides sensation to the deep structures of the foot and ankle and the plantar aspect of the foot.
2. The saphenous nerve is the sensory extension of the femoral nerve below the knee, innervating the deep and superficial structures of the anteromedial foot and ankle.
3. The advantages of the popliteal block compared with the ankle block include motor block for surgical akinesis, single injection for sciatic blockade, calf tourniquet analgesia, and possible catheter placement.
4. The saphenous nerve can be blocked successfully as part of a femoral nerve block (with resultant quadriceps weakness), or as a sensory-only adductor canal block or subcutaneously at the anteromedial ankle.
5. Popliteal sciatic catheters can extend analgesia for up to 5 days, are used successfully in inpatients and outpatients, and allow more invasive procedures to be performed in the ambulatory setting.
6. Short-acting local anesthetics (eg, lidocaine, mepivacaine) provide 3 to 6 hours of analgesia, whereas long-acting agents (eg, bupivacaine, ropivacaine) provide 10 to 16 hours of analgesia.
7. Although PONS can occur following surgery and anesthesia, permanent nerve injury is rare.
8. Local anesthetic systemic toxicity (LAST) involving seizures and/or cardiac complications usually can be prevented; however, 20% lipid emulsions have provided a silver bullet for the treatment of cardiac arrest resulting from LAST and should be available immediately.
9. Popliteal catheter complications include failure, leaking, dislodgment, infection, kinking, and neurapraxia.
10. Judicious use of NSAIDs, especially with short courses, has recently been shown to have no significant impact on postoperative bone healing, as previously thought.

Bibliography

Boezaart AP: *Atlas of Peripheral Nerve Blocks and Anatomy for Orthopaedic Anesthesia*. Philadelphia, PA, Saunders Elsevier, 2008.

Borgeat A, Blumenthal S: Nerve injury and regional anaesthesia. *Curr Opin Anaesthesiol* 2004;17(5):417-421.

Buckenmaier CC III, Bleckner LL: Anaesthetic agents for advanced regional anaesthesia: A North American perspective. *Drugs* 2005;65(6):745-759.

Capdevila X, Choquet O: Regional anesthesia and patient outcomes. *Tech Reg Anesth Pain Manag* 2008;12(4):161-210.

Casalia AG, Carradori G, Moreno M: Blockade of the sciatic nerve in the popliteal fossa. *Tech Reg Anesth Pain Manag* 2006;10(4):173-177.

Chin KJ, Wong NWY, Macfarlane AJR, Chan VWS. Ultrasound-guided versus anatomic landmark-guided ankle blocks. *Reg Anesth Pain Med* 2011;36:611-618.

Clendenen SR, Whalen JL. Saphenous nerve innervation of the medial ankle. *Local Reg Anesth* 2013;6:13-16.

Concepcion M: Ankle block. *Tech Reg Anesth Pain Manag* 1999;3:241-246.

Dodwell ER, Latorre JG, Parisini E, et al. NSAID exposure and risk of nonunion: A meta-analysis of case-control and cohort studies. *Calcified Tissue Int* 2010;87(3):193-202.

Enneking FK, Chan V, Greger J, Hadzić A, Lang SA, Horlocker TT: Lower-extremity peripheral nerve blockade: Essentials of our current understanding. *Reg Anesth Pain Med* 2005;30(1):4-35.

Monkowski DP, Egidi HR: Ankle block. *Tech Reg Anesth Pain Manag* 2006;10(4):183-188.

Malchow RJ, Gupta RK, Shi Y, Shotwell MS, Jaeger LM, Bowens C: Comprehensive analysis of 13,897 consecutive regional anesthetics at an ambulatory surgery center. *Pain Med* 2018;19(2):368-384.

Neal JM, Bernards CM, Hadzic A, et al: ASRA practice advisory on neurologic complications in regional anesthesia and pain medicine. *Reg Anesth Pain Med* 2008;33(5): 404-415.

Redborg KE, Antonakakis JG, Beach ML, Chinn CD, Sites BD: Ultrasound improves the success rate of a tibial nerve block at the ankle. *Reg Anesth Pain Med* 2009;34(3):256-260.

Williams BA, Matusic B, Kentor ML: Regional anesthesia procedures for ambulatory knee surgery: Effects on in-hospital outcomes. *Int Anesthesiol Clin* 2005;43(3):153-160.

Vieira PA, Pulai I, Tsao GC, Manikantan P, Keller B, Connelly NR: Dexamethasone with bupivacaine increases duration of analgesia in ultrasound-guided interscalene brachial plexus blockade. *Eur J Anaesthesiol* 2010;27(3):285-288.

Chapter 110

Disorders of the First Ray

THOMAS PADANILAM, MD

I. HALLUX VALGUS

A. Epidemiology and overview

1. Hallux valgus is defined as lateral deviation of the proximal phalanx on the first metatarsal head.
2. It is frequently associated with medial deviation of the first metatarsal.
3. Hallux valgus is more common in women than in men.

B. Etiology

1. Hallux valgus is commonly related to wearing shoes that have a narrow toe box.
2. Metatarsus primus varus and pes planus have been implicated.
3. Of patients with hallux valgus, 70% have a family history of the condition, which suggests a hereditary component.
4. Other causes include rheumatoid arthritis, connective tissue disorders, and cerebral palsy.
5. The metatarsal articular surface may have a valgus (lateral) orientation, as measured by the distal metatarsal articular angle (DMAA), which can contribute to development of a hallux valgus deformity.

C. Pathoanatomy

1. With valgus deviation of the great toe, the metatarsal assumes a varus position.
2. The sesamoid complex assumes a lateral position relative to the first metatarsal head, which is moved medially.
3. The medial capsule of the hallux metatarsophalangeal (MTP) joint becomes attenuated, and the lateral capsule contracts.
4. The adductor tendon, through its insertion on the proximal phalanx and the fibular sesamoid, becomes a deforming force.
5. With progression, the windlass mechanism is lost, resulting in a loss of weight bearing under the first metatarsal and transfer to the lesser metatarsals (transfer metatarsalgia).

D. Evaluation

1. History and physical examination
   a. A bony prominence may be noted along the medial aspect of the first MTP joint.
   b. The patient may report pain along the prominence with shoe wear.
   c. Swelling and redness can occur as a result of bursal inflammation.
   d. Nerve symptoms may be present with compression of the digital nerve.
   e. The patient's activity level and expectations should be considered.
   f. Because of the stress transfer laterally, hallux valgus is frequently associated with other deformities, such as hammer toe and calluses.
2. Imaging
   a. Plain radiographs are used to assess hallux valgus.
   b. Weight-bearing AP and lateral views are the most commonly obtained radiographs. A sesamoid view also may be helpful.
   c. The angular measurements that are used in the evaluation of hallux valgus are shown in **Table 1** and **Figure 1**. These measurements are made on the AP radiographic view.
   d. A congruent joint has no lateral subluxation of the proximal phalanx on the metatarsal head. An incongruent joint shows lateral subluxation of the proximal phalanx on the metatarsal head (**Figure 2**).

Neither Dr. Padanilam nor any immediate family member has received anything of value from or has stock or stock options held in a commercial company or institution related directly or indirectly to the subject of this chapter.

TABLE 1

Important Radiographic Angles in the Evaluation of Hallux Valgus

Angle	Location	Importance	Normal
HVA	Between long axes of first proximal phalanx and first metatarsal, bisecting their diaphysis	Identifies the degree of deformity at the MTP joint	≤15°
IMA	Between long axes of first and second metatarsals, bisecting shafts of first and second metatarsals	Not influenced by overresection of medial eminence; not accurate for postoperative evaluation of distal osteotomies	≤9°
DMAA	Angle of line bisecting metatarsal shaft with line through base of distal articular cartilage cap	Offset of angle is predisposing factor in development of hallux valgus	≤15°
PPAA	Articular angle of base of proximal phalanx in relation to longitudinal axis	Offset of angle is predisposing factor in development of hallux valgus	≤10°

DMAA = distal metatarsal articular angle, HVA = hallux valgus angle, IMA = intermetatarsal angle, MTP = metatarsophalangeal, PPAA = proximal phalangeal articular angle

Adapted from Campbell JT: Hallux valgus: Adult and juvenile, in Richardson EG, ed: *Orthopaedic Knowledge Update: Foot and Ankle*, ed 3. Rosemont, IL, American Academy of Orthopaedic Surgeons, 2004, pp 3-15.

e. The degree of arthritic changes in the MTP joint should be considered.

f. These radiologic parameters guide surgical treatment decisions.

E. Treatment

1. Nonsurgical

a. Nonsurgical treatment includes shoe-wear modifications, including changing to shoes with a wide toe box and soft uppers.

b. Occasionally, pads or cushions over the prominence can relieve hallux valgus–related pain.

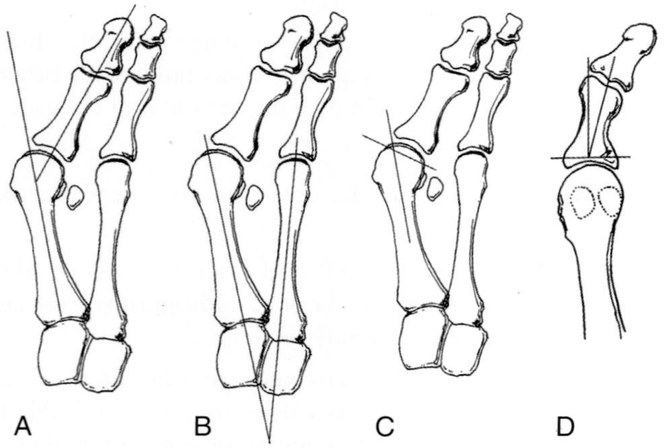

Figure 1 Illustrations show the angular measurements of hallux valgus deformity. **A**, Hallux valgus angle. **B**, First-second intermetatarsal angle. **C**, Distal metatarsal articular angle. **D**, Proximal phalangeal articular angle. (Reproduced from Campbell JT: Hallux valgus: Adult and juvenile, in Richardson EG, ed: *Orthopaedic Knowledge Update: Foot and Ankle*, ed 3. Rosemont, IL, American Academy of Orthopaedic Surgeons, 2004, pp 3-15.)

c. Orthoses may be helpful in patients with pes planus or symptoms of metatarsalgia.

2. Surgical

a. Surgical procedures, indications, and pearls/pitfalls are shown in **Table 2**.

b. All components of the deformity must be addressed when choosing a procedure.

c. A procedure to correct a congruent joint should be an distal osteotomy to correct the deformity and to maintain joint congruency.

d. In the presence of arthritis in the MTP joint fusion should be considered.

e. With increased intermetatarsal angle a proximal osteotomy is required.

f. Sesamoid reduction is correlated with maintenance of correction (**Figure 3**).

II. JUVENILE HALLUX VALGUS

A. Epidemiology

1. Juvenile hallux valgus occurs more commonly in girls than in boys.

B. Pathoanatomy

1. Typically, the angular deformity associated with hallux valgus is less severe in children than it is in adults.

2. Large medial prominences are rare.

3. A congruent joint with an increased DMAA is more common in juvenile hallux valgus than in the adult condition.

4. Juvenile hallux valgus is sometimes associated with other deformities, such as metatarsus adductus.

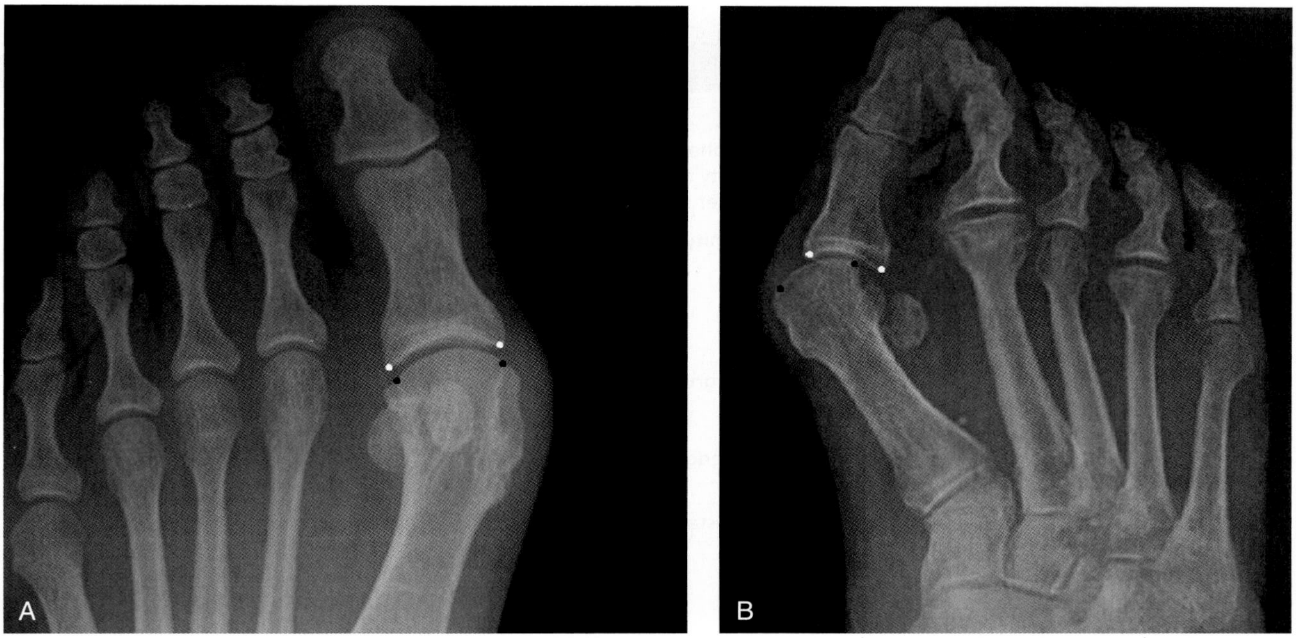

Figure 2 AP radiographs. The black dots represent the borders of the articular surface of the metatarsal head and the white dots the articular surface of the proximal phalanx. **A,** A congruent joint where there is no subluxation of the joint. **B,** An incongruent joint with lateral subluxation of the proximal phalanx on the metatarsal head.

5. Generalized ligamentous laxity may be more common in children with hallux valgus than in the general population.

C. Treatment

1. Nonsurgical treatment includes shoe-wear modification and education.
2. Surgical
   a. Indications for surgery are shown in **Table 2.**
   b. Open physes at the base of the proximal phalanx or first metatarsal may preclude the use of osteotomies or fusion in those areas to avoid growth arrest.
   c. Surgical options are similar to those for adults except that, in the presence of open physes, an increased intermetatarsal angle (IMA) is corrected with a medial opening wedge cuneiform osteotomy rather than a proximal metatarsal osteotomy or fusion.
   d. Increased DMAA can be addressed with a distal biplanar chevron first metatarsal osteotomy.
3. Recurrence rates of up to 50% have been noted with surgical treatment.

III. HALLUX VARUS

A. Epidemiology and overview

1. Hallux varus is defined as a hallux valgus angle (HVA) measuring 0° or less.
2. The condition can be associated with an extension deformity of the MTP joint and flexion of the interphalangeal (IP) joint. Supination of the hallux may be seen as well.

B. Etiology

1. The most common cause of hallux varus is iatrogenic deformity resulting from hallux valgus repair (2% to 10% incidence), which can result from excessive tightening of the medial joint capsule, excessive resection of the medial eminence, overcorrection of the IMA, excision of the fibular sesamoid, or excessive lateral capsular release.
2. Hallux varus may be associated with inflammatory conditions, such as rheumatoid arthritis, or neurologic conditions, such as Charcot-Marie-Tooth disease.

C. Evaluation

1. History and physical examination
   a. Hallux varus is principally asymptomatic.

TABLE 2

Surgical Treatment of Hallux Valgus

Procedure	Indications	Pearls/Pitfalls
Akin Closing wedge osteotomy of the proximal phalanx	Hallux valgus interphalangeus Congruent deformity Combined with other surgical procedures	Performed when the proximal phalangeal articular angle is >10° Minimal ability to correct hallux valgus
Distal soft-tissue release Combines a release of the lateral structures with medial eminence resection and exostectomy	Incongruent deformity IMA < 11° HVA < 35°	Avoid fibular sesamoid excision to decrease the risk of hallux varus Combined with proximal procedures for larger deformities. Rarely done as isolated procedure
Distal metatarsal osteotomy (chevron) A lateral translation of the metatarsal head after osteotomy	Congruent or incongruent deformity IMA < 13° HVA < 30° Biplanar (closing wedge) used for DMAA > 15°	Avoid an extensive lateral capsular release to minimize the risk of osteonecrosis
Proximal metatarsal osteotomy The metatarsal shaft is brought laterally to reduce the IMA	Combined with a distal soft-tissue release HVA > 25° IMA > 13°	Multiple methods such as crescentic, proximal chevron, and oblique osteotomies can be used Overcorrection of IMA can lead to hallux varus Dorsiflexion at osteotomy can result in transfer metatarsalgia
Metatarsal cuneiform fusion (Lapidus procedure)	Combined with a distal soft-tissue release Hypermobility of the first ray	10%-15% nonunion rate noted; however, many are asymptomatic Must avoid shortening and dorsiflexion at fusion, which can result in metatarsalgia
Keller arthroplasty Resection of the base of the proximal phalanx	Elderly, low-demand patients with mild deformity and/or arthritic changes in the joint	Can lead to a cock-up toe deformity Transfer metatarsalgia can also be seen
Metatarsophalangeal fusion	Severe deformities (HVA > 40°) Arthritic changes in the joint Inflammatory conditions such as rheumatoid arthritis Neurologic conditions such as cerebral palsy	Should attempt to fuse in 10°-15° of valgus and 10°-15° of dorsiflexion relative to the first metatarsal
Medial eminence resection (Silver procedure)	Rarely indicated Reserved for elderly patients with minimal functional demands	Medial eminence incision places the dorsomedial cutaneous nerve, a branch of the superficial peroneal nerve, at risk

DMAA = distal metatarsal articular angle, HVA = hallux valgus angle, IMA = intermetatarsal angle

b. The most commonly reported symptom is difficulty with shoe wear because of a prominent IP joint.

c. Transfer lesions may develop along the lesser metatarsals.

d. It must be determined whether the MTP and IP joint deformities are fixed or passively correctable.

2. Imaging—Weight-bearing radiographs can help determine the degree of arthrosis.

D. Treatment

1. Nonsurgical—Most cases of hallux varus can be managed nonsurgically.

a. Taping the toe

b. Placing pads over prominent areas

c. Wearing shoes that have extra depth and a wide, flexible toe box

2. Surgical procedures

a. Passively correctable deformities can be treated with medial capsular release/lengthening and a tendon transfer.

b. Historically, the entire extensor hallucis longus tendon was rerouted under the intermetatarsal ligament to the base of the proximal phalanx; this required fusion of the IP joint.

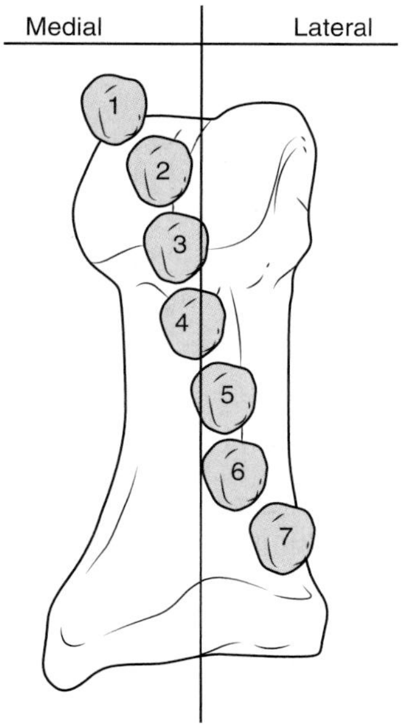

Figure 3 Position of the medial sesamoid is noted in relation to a line drawn down the midaxis of the first metatarsal. Those whose postoperative sesamoid is in position 5 to 7 have a much higher recurrence of deformity compared with those with a more medial position for the sesamoid. (Used from Smith J, Bluman E: Hallux valgus and hallux varus, in Chou L, ed: *Orthopaedic Knowledge Update: Foot and Ankle*, ed 5. Rosemont, IL, American Academy of Orthopaedic Surgeons, 2014, pp 186, Figure 3.)

c. Methods for maintaining IP joint motion include a split transfer of the extensor hallucis longus tendon and rerouting of the extensor hallucis brevis tendon.

d. Fixed deformities or those with substantial arthrosis require fusion of the MTP joint for correction.

IV. HALLUX RIGIDUS

A. Refer to Arthritides of the Foot and Ankle Chapter

V. TURF TOE INJURIES

A. Epidemiology and overview

1. Turf toe injury is defined as an injury of varied severity to the periarticular structures surrounding the hallux MTP joint.

2. The flexibility of shoes used on artificial turf and the shoe-surface interface have been suggested as causative factors.

3. The most common mechanism of turf toe injury is hyperextension of the MTP joint from an axial load applied to a plantarflexed foot.

4. "Sand toe" injuries are hyperflexion injuries frequently seen in beach volleyball players.

B. Evaluation

1. History and physical examination

a. Determining the location of the tenderness can help identify injured structures. Tenderness proximal to the sesamoids suggest a low-grade injury and distal to sesamoids suggest a more serious injury.

b. The capability and comfort associated with weight bearing can indicate the severity of injury.

c. An intrinsic minus position of the hallux with the MTP joint extended and the IP joint flexed indicates a severe injury.

2. Imaging

a. Radiographic evaluation with weight-bearing AP, lateral, oblique, and sesamoid views is indicated.

b. Proximal migration of the sesamoids on an AP radiograph indicates a complete rupture of the plantar plate. The distal sesamoid-to-joint distance should be no greater than 3 mm compared with those on the contralateral side.

c. Dorsiflexion stress lateral view: If the distance between the proximal phalanx and sesamoid increase by 3 mm on a lateral view with dorsiflexion of the hallux a significant injury to the plantar plate has occurred.

d. Dorsal MTP dislocations are classified based on the status of the sesamoids.

- I: dorsal dislocation of proximal phalanx and sesamoids with intact intersesamoid ligament
- IIa: Dislocation with rupture of the intersesamoid ligament (widening of space between sessamoids)
- IIb: Dislocation with transverse fracture through the sesamoids

C. Treatment

1. Nonsurgical

a. Most injuries can be treated with rest and analgesics.

b. More severe injuries may require a walker boot or short leg cast until the joint is stable.

c. Joint mobilization is begun once the injury is stable.

d. The severity of the injury varies substantially and determines the time needed for recovery. Severe injuries may require up to 12 weeks to heal before the patient can return to activity.

2. Surgical

a. Surgical treatment is rarely needed.

b. Surgery is indicated when retraction of the sesamoids, sesamoid fracture with diastasis, traumatic bunions, or loose fragments in the joint are present.

c. If plantar plate or flexor tendons cannot be restored, an abductor hallucis tendon transfer may be needed.

d. Type I dorsal dislocations are often irreducible closed due interposition of volar plate and may require open treatment.

VI. SESAMOID DISORDERS

A. Epidemiology and overview

1. The sesamoids, which sit within the flexor hallucis brevis tendon, absorb and transmit weight-bearing pressure, reduce friction, protect the flexor hallucis longus tendon, and help increase the mechanical force of the flexor hallucis brevis tendon. The flexor hallucis longus tendon glides between the two sesamoids.

2. The tibial sesamoid is bipartite in approximately 10% of the population; in 25% of persons with bipartite sesamoid, the condition is bilateral. The medial (tibial) sesamoid is larger and more affected by weight bearing; thus, it is more commonly injured.

B. Evaluation

1. History—Patients present with pain along the plantar aspect of the metatarsal head.

2. Physical examination—A plantarflexed first ray with a cavus deformity may be noted on examination.

3. Imaging

a. AP and lateral radiographs may reveal the presence of fractures or degenerative changes.

b. Individual oblique views can help isolate the sesamoids, and an axial view can help evaluate the articulation with the metatarsal head.

c. A bone scan may be helpful but should be interpreted with caution because 25% to 30% of asymptomatic patients may show increased uptake. A substantial difference in uptake between the injured and uninjured sides is helpful in confirming injury.

d. MRI can be helpful in evaluating sesamoids for variety of pathologic changes such as fractures, osteonecrosis, and arthritic changes.

C. Treatment

1. Nonsurgical

a. Reduced weight bearing under the first metatarsal and limitation of activities are the mainstays of nonsurgical treatment.

b. Pads, rocker soles, and metatarsal bars also may be effective.

c. Shaving of keratotic lesions can reduce symptoms.

d. Controversy exists in the treatment of acute fractures. Some authors recommend using a short leg cast with a toe extension; others use a stiff-soled shoe or boot with a pad around the sesamoid.

2. Surgical

a. Indications—Surgery is indicated after failed nonsurgical treatment.

b. Procedures

- Bone grafting of sesamoid nonunions has been reported to have good results in a small study.
- Dorsiflexion osteotomy should be considered for the patient with a cavus foot deformity with a plantarflexed first ray.
- Excision of the sesamoid may be required when nonsurgical treatment fails.

c. Complications

- Tibial sesamoid excision may result in hallux valgus.
- Fibular sesamoid excision may result in hallux varus.
- Excision of both sesamoids should be avoided because a cock-up deformity of the toe may result.

TOP TESTING FACTS

Hallux Valgus

1. To reduce the risk of hallux varus, fibular sesamoid excision should be avoided during distal soft-tissue release.
2. To minimize the risk of osteonecrosis, an extensive lateral capsular release should be avoided during (chevron) distal metatarsal osteotomy.
3. Patients with an IMA greater than 13° require proximal metatarsal osteotomy combined with distal soft-tissue release to correct the deformity.
4. A DMAA greater than 15° can be corrected with biplanar (closing wedge) distal metatarsal osteotomy (chevron).
5. An increased DMAA angle is more frequent in juveniles and males with hallux valgus.
6. MTP fusion is recommended for patients with inflammatory conditions, such as rheumatoid arthritis, or neurologic disorders, such as cerebral palsy.
7. Medial eminence incision places the dorsomedial cutaneous nerve, a branch of the superficial peroneal nerve, at risk.
8. Shortening or dorsiflexion of the first metatarsal postoperatively can lead to transfer metatarsalgia.
9. Failure to reduce the sesamoid position with surgical correction increases the risk of recurrence of hallux valgus.

Juvenile Hallux Valgus

1. A congruent joint with an increased DMAA is more common in juvenile hallux valgus than in the adult condition.
2. Recurrence rates of up to 50% have been reported after the surgical treatment of hallux valgus in juveniles.

Hallux Varus

1. The most common cause of hallux varus is iatrogenic deformity resulting from hallux valgus repair (2% to 10% incidence), which can be due to excessive tightening of the medial joint capsule, excessive resection of the medial eminence, overcorrection of the IMA, excision of the fibular sesamoid, or excessive lateral capsular release.
2. Hallux varus is principally asymptomatic, and most patients can be treated nonsurgically.
3. If the painful deformity is passively correctable, a soft-tissue procedure with tendon transfer can be performed.
4. If the painful deformity is fixed or significant arthrosis is present, then fusion of the MTP joint is recommended.

TOP TESTING FACTS

Turf Toe Injuries

1. Turf toe is a common term used to lump together a variety of injuries to the first MTP joint.
2. The most common mechanism of turf toe injury is hyperextension of the MTP joint with an axial load applied to a plantarflexed foot.
3. Determining the location of tenderness can help identify injured structures. The capability and comfort associated with weight bearing can indicate the severity of injury.
4. An intrinsic minus position of the hallux, with the MTP joint extended and the IP joint flexed, indicates a severe injury.
5. An AP radiograph of the foot showing proximal migration of the sesamoids indicates a complete rupture of the plantar plate.
6. The severity of the injury varies substantially and determines the time needed for recovery. Severe injuries may require a walker boot or short leg cast until the joint is stable.
7. Surgery is indicated when retraction of the sesamoids, sesamoid fracture with diastasis, traumatic bunions, or loose fragments in the joint are present.
8. Hallux dorsal MTP dislocation with intact intersesamoid ligament and sesamoids often require open reduction.

Sesamoid Disorders

1. The sesamoids sit within the flexor hallucis brevis tendon and help increase its mechanical force.
2. The flexor hallucis longus tendon glides between the two sesamoids.
3. The tibial sesamoid is bipartite in approximately 10% of the population. In 25% of persons with bipartite sesamoid, the condition is bilateral.
4. The medial (tibial) sesamoid is larger and more affected by weight bearing; thus, it is more commonly injured.
5. A plantarflexed first ray with a cavus deformity may be noted on examination and may need correction with a dorsiflexion osteotomy of the metatarsal.
6. Radiographs may reveal the presence of fracture or degenerative changes of the sesamoids.
7. A bone scan may be helpful but should be interpreted with caution because increased uptake may be seen in 25% to 30% of asymptomatic patients.
8. Tibial sesamoid excision may lead to hallux valgus and fibular sesamoid excision may lead to hallux varus. Excision of both sesamoids should be avoided, because a cock-up deformity of the toe may result.

Bibliography

Barg A, Harmer J, Presson A, Zhang C, Lackey M, Saltzman C: Unfavorable outcomes following surgical treatment of hallux valgus deformity. A systematic literature review. *J Bone Joint Surg Am* 2018;100:1563-1573.

Campbell JT: Hallux valgus: Adult and juvenile, in Richardson EG, ed: *Orthopaedic Knowledge Update: Foot and Ankle*, ed 3. Rosemont, IL, American Academy of Orthopaedic Surgeons, 2004, pp 3-15.

Harb Z, Kokkinakis M, Ismail H, Spence G: Adolescent hallux valgus: A systemic review of outcomes following surgery. *J Child Orthop* 2015; 9:105-112.

Juliano PJ, Campbell MA: Tendon transfers about the hallux. *Foot Ankle Clin* 2011;16(3):451-469.

Kadakia AR, Molloy A: Current concepts review: Traumatic disorders of the first metatarsophalangeal joint and sesamoid complex. *Foot Ankle Int* 2011;32(8):834-839.

Mason L, Molly A: Turf Toe and disorders of the sesamoid complex. *Clin Sport Med* 2015;34:725-739.

Padanilam TG: Disorders of the first ray, in Richardson EG, ed: *Orthopaedic Knowledge Update: Foot and Ankle*, ed 3. Rosemont, IL, American Academy of Orthopaedic Surgeons, 2004, pp 17-25.

Park C, Lee W: Recurrence of hallux valgus can be predicted from immediate postoperative non-weight-bearing radiographs. *J Bone Joint Surg Am* 2017;99:1190-1197.

Smith J, Bluman E: Hallux valgus and hallux varus, in Chou L, ed: *Orthopaedic Knowledge Update: Foot and Ankle*, ed 5. Rosemont, IL, American Academy of Orthopaedic Surgeons, 2014, pp 183-191.

Smyth N, Aiyer A: Introduction: Why are there so many different surgeries for hallux valgus? *Foot Ankle Clin* 2018;23:171-182.

Waldrop N, Zirker C, Wijdicks C, LaPrade R, O'Clanton T: Radiographic evaluation of plantar plate injury: An in vitro biomechanical study. *Foot Ankle Int* 2013;34(3): 430-408.

Chapter 111
FOREFOOT DISORDERS

STEVEN M. RAIKIN, MD

I. INTRODUCTION

A. Epidemiology

1. Deformities of the lesser (second through fifth) toes can present in isolation or in association with hallux deformities.
2. The metatarsophalangeal (MTP) joint region is the most frequently affected, followed by the proximal interphalangeal (PIP) and distal interphalangeal (DIP) joints.

B. Contributing factors

1. Fashion in women's footwear
    a. High heels and narrow, pointed toe boxes
    b. Inappropriately small shoe size
2. Cortisone injections
3. Advancing age
4. Neuromuscular disorders
5. Congenital deformities
6. Inflammatory arthropathies
7. Repetitive trauma to the forefoot region
8. Variations in bony anatomy of the forefoot
    a. Associated valgus alignment of the hallux
    b. Relatively long lesser metatarsal
    c. Irregularly shaped bony phalanx

II. SECOND MTP JOINT SYNOVITIS

A. Overview and epidemiology

1. Second MTP joint synovitis is a monoarticular synovitis.
2. The second MTP joint is the joint most frequently affected in MTP synovitis.
3. Predisposing factors are an elongated second metatarsal relative to the first metatarsal (Morton foot) or an associated hallux valgus deformity.

B. Pathoanatomy

1. The synovitis stretches the capsuloligamentous apparatus of the MTP joint, resulting in frontal and axial plane instability and deformity.
2. Subsequent attenuation of the plantar plate results in extension at the MTP joint and sagittal plane deformity.
3. The resulting conditions include MTP instability and potential subsequent dorsal dislocation as well as a predisposition to developing hammer toe deformities.

C. Evaluation

1. History and physical examination
    a. Patients present with pain, warmth, palpable fullness, and tenderness to palpation in the second MTP joint region in the absence of trauma or systemic inflammatory conditions.
    b. Clinical examination reveals a swollen, warm, and tender second toe at the level of the MTP joint.
    c. Tenderness may be greater plantarly (over the plantar plate), dorsally (over the dorsal capsule), or globally around the MTP joint.
    d. In the predislocation stages, the deformity is frequently passively correctable, but range of motion, particularly plantar flexion, is usually reduced.
    e. Instability of the second MTP joint may be present.
        - The instability is clinically reproducible via the dorsal drawer test. In this test, the metatarsal head and phalanx are individually stabilized and a dorsal translation stress is applied.

Dr. Raikin or an immediate family member has received research or institutional support from Zimmer.

- Attenuation of the plantar plate results in abnormal dorsal subluxation of the joint.

f. Progressive deformity may result in the toe crossing over one of the adjacent toes in either varus or valgus if one of the collateral ligaments is disrupted in addition to the plantar plate. This condition is known as crossover toe deformity.

g. Many patients have tenderness within the second web space that is secondary to inflammation or extrinsic pressure on the interdigital nerve from the MTP synovitis. This can result in neuritic symptoms that mimic a Morton neuroma. Care must be taken to differentiate second MTP joint synovitis from an interdigital neuroma because corticosteroid injections to treat an interdigital neuroma may further weaken the capsuloligamentous structures at the MTP joint, resulting in progressive deformities.

2. Imaging

a. Radiographs

- Weight-bearing AP radiographs should be obtained and assessed for widening or medial-lateral joint space imbalance of the MTP joint, which is consistent with synovitis, and dorsal subluxation of the MTP joint, which may result in the joint space appearing narrowed or the base of the proximal phalanx overlapping the metatarsal head. The toe may be seen deviating into varus or valgus if a crossover toe has developed.
- Lateral radiographs may demonstrate hyperextension of the MTP joint or dorsal subluxation of the proximal phalanx.

b. MRI or ultrasonography may be performed when the diagnosis is unclear or to quantify the extent of the ligamentous or plantar plate disruption.

D. Treatment

1. Nonsurgical

a. Initial treatment includes activity and footwear modifications, NSAIDs, and external support of the MTP joint.

b. External support is achieved with a crossover taping of the MTP joint or with the application of a commercially available Budin-type toe splint.

c. Nonsurgical treatment should be continued for 10 to 12 weeks, followed by the avoidance of shoe wear that can predispose to the condition.

2. Surgical

a. Indications—If nonsurgical treatment is unsuccessful or a fixed deformity cannot be accommodated with modifications in shoe wear, surgery may be indicated.

b. Surgical procedures

- If no deformity is present, a synovectomy of the joint is indicated.
- In the presence of a long second metatarsal, a joint-preserving shortening osteotomy should be performed. This is a short oblique osteotomy at the junction of the metatarsal head and neck that allows the metatarsal head to be slid proximally, rebalancing the metatarsal cascade. This also allows the capsuloligamentous structures and plantar plate to be relaxed and rebalanced in appropriate alignment (**Figure 1**).
- In the absence of a long second metatarsal, sagittal plane deformities are corrected with a soft-tissue reconstruction such as a flexor digitorum longus (FDL)–to–extensor digitorum longus (EDL) tendon transfer (Girdlestone-Taylor procedure) or an MTP capsular release and extensor tendon lengthening. Crossover toe deformities are corrected with an extensor digitorum brevis transfer.

c. Complications—During surgical correction of a chronically dislocated MTP joint, vascular compromise of the toe may occur as a result of vascular stretching during reduction of the joint. In this situation, the procedure may need to be reversed to save the digit.

III. FREIBERG INFRACTION

A. Overview

1. Infraction of the metatarsal head was first described by Freiberg in 1914.
2. The term infraction is a combination of the terms "infarction" and "fracture."
3. The second metatarsal head is most commonly involved, predominantly in the dorsal aspect. As the condition progresses, the metatarsal head undergoes collapse.
4. The condition may result from recurrent microtrauma or osteonecrosis of the metatarsal head, leading to subchondral collapse.

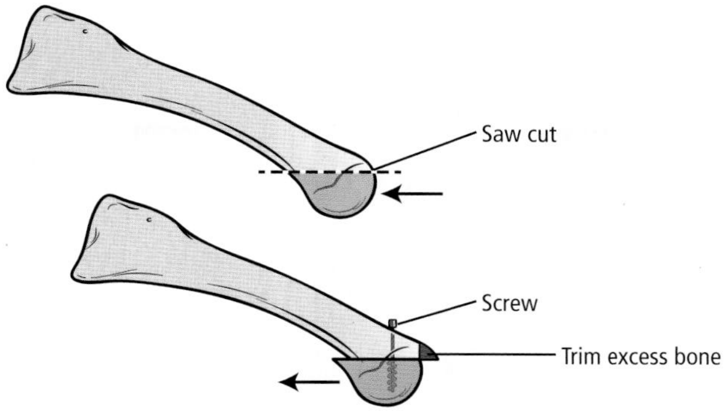

Figure 1 Schematic lateral view of the distal oblique shortening osteotomy of the lesser metatarsal stabilized with screw fixation. (Reproduced with permission from Deland JT: Angular deformities of the second toe, in Nunley JA, Pferrer GB, Sanders RW, Trepman E, eds: *Advanced Reconstruction of the foot and ankle*. Rosemont, IL, AAOS, 2004, pp 77-84.)

B. Evaluation

1. History and physical examination—Patients present with localized pain, swelling, and stiffness of the MTP joint that is exacerbated by weight-bearing activities.
2. Imaging
    a. Radiographs
        - In the precollapse stage, initial radiographs may be normal.
        - Collapse is initially seen radiographically as flattening of the metatarsal head and subchondral sclerosis. Progression of the condition results in the development of arthritic changes on both sides of the MTP joint.

    b. MRI—Before radiographic changes are noted, the diagnosis can be made using MRI, which reveals patchy edema in the metatarsal head and precollapse changes that are consistent with osteonecrosis.
3. Classification—The Smillie classification of Freiberg infraction is shown in **Table 1**.

C. Treatment

1. Nonsurgical
    a. Initial treatment includes unloading and protecting the second metatarsal head.
    b. A short leg cast extended to the toes or a fracture boot, worn for a 4- to 6-week period and followed by several months in a stiff-soled shoe with a metatarsal bar, may reverse early stage 1 involvement or quell the inflammatory process that causes early-phase symptoms.
2. Surgical
    a. Surgery is indicated for recalcitrant cases.
    b. A dorsal closing-wedge osteotomy of the metatarsal head is commonly used. The procedure resects the collapsed dorsal diseased bone and cartilage and brings the less affected plantar cartilage into contact with the articular cartilage of the proximal phalanx. At the same time, the metatarsal is shortened (via the closing wedge), unloading the predisposing stress on the metatarsal head (**Figure 2**).
    c. An isolated débridement of the joint may be performed in mild and moderate symptomatic cases.
    d. A partial head resection (DuVries arthroplasty) may be required when stage 4 and 5 involvement is present or when the plantar cartilage is not adequate to reconstruct the metatarsal head. Consideration may be given to adding a capsular interposition after joint débridement.

TABLE 1

Smillie Classification of Freiberg Infraction

Stage	Characteristics
1	Subchondral fracture, visible only on MRI or bone scan
2	Dorsal collapse of the articular surface, visible on plain radiographs
3	Progressive collapse of the metatarsal head, with the plantar articular portion remaining intact
4	Collapse of the entire metatarsal head, with early arthritic changes and joint space narrowing
5	Severe arthritic changes with joint space obliteration

Data from Smillie IS: Freiberg's infraction (Kohler's second disease). *J Bone Joint Surg Br* 1957;39(3):580.

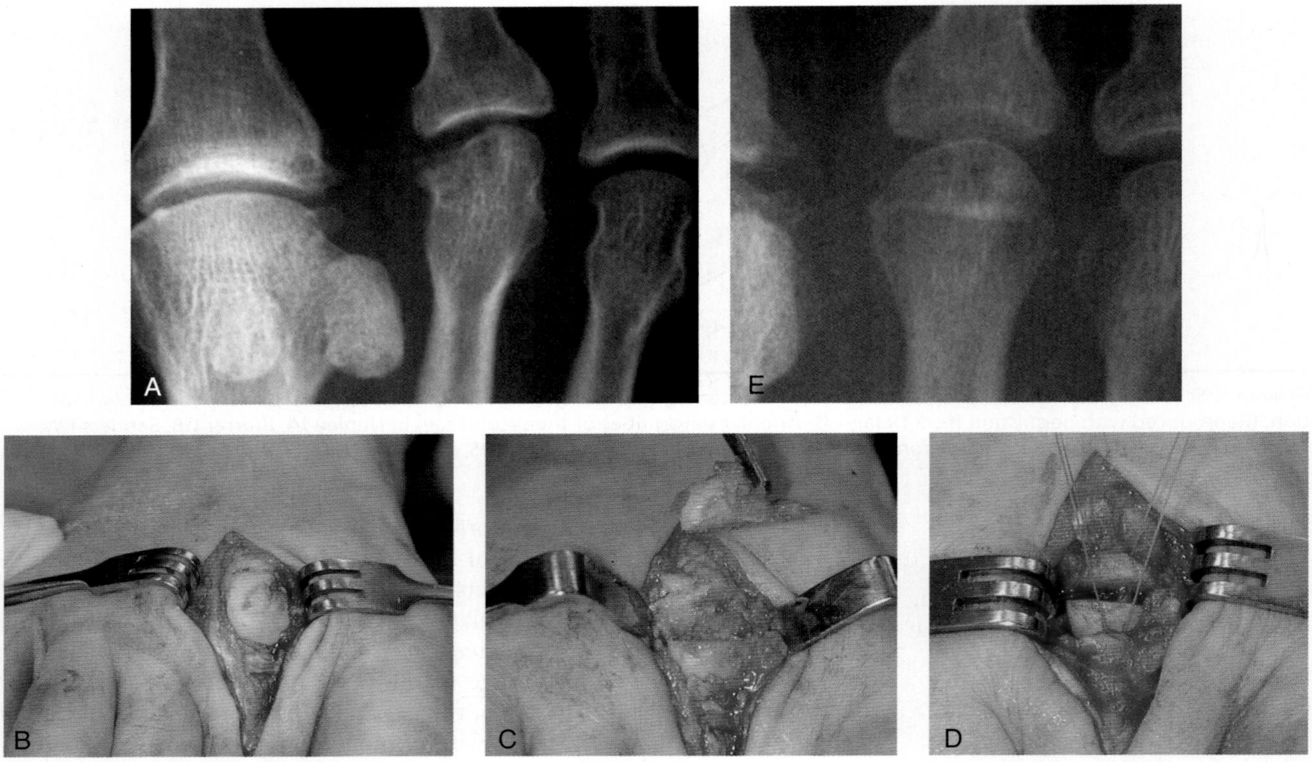

Figure 2 Sequence of correction of Freibergs Infraction. **A**, Preoperative radiograph demonstrating collapse of the metatarsal head; **B**, intraoperative view of collapsed MT head; **C**, intraoperative removal of dorsal wedge of collapsed bone and cartilage from MT head; **D**, intraoperative suture used to close the osteotomy and reconstruct the MT head; **E**, postoperative radiograph demonstrating the repaired rounded MT head.

e. In advanced cases, an osteochondral autograft from the ipsilateral knee, or an osteochondral metatarsal head allograft can be considered.

IV. DEFORMITIES OF THE LESSER TOES

A. Overview

1. Deformities of the lesser toes result from an imbalance between the intrinsic and extrinsic musculotendinous units of the toes.
2. With hyperextension at the MTP joint, the strong flexors overpower the intrinsic extensors of the interphalangeal (IP) joints. This results in flexion deformities at the IP joints and extension deformities at the MTP joints.
3. Lesser MTP deformity starts with dysfunction of the plantar plate.
4. **Table 2** summarizes the deformities of the lesser toes and the involvement of the MTP, PIP, and DIP joints.

B. Mallet toe deformity

1. Definition—Mallet toe is a hyperflexion deformity at the DIP joint (**Figure 3**). The deformity may be flexible or fixed.
2. Evaluation and clinical presentation
   a. Pain and callosities at the dorsum of the DIP joint will be present.
   b. Frequently, "tip calluses" (painful calluses that form at the distal tip of the toe as it impacts the ground) also will be present.
3. Treatment
   a. Nonsurgical—Treatment includes wearing shoes with high toe boxes and using foam or silicone gel toe sleeves or crest pads.
   b. Surgical
      - Surgical correction depends on the flexibility of the deformity.
      - A flexible deformity can be corrected with a percutaneous release of the FDL tendon at its insertion into the base of the distal phalanx.

- The Coleman block test distinguishes between fixed and flexible hindfoot varus.
  - If the hindfoot varus deformity is flexible, a first metatarsal dorsiflexion osteotomy may be used in isolation.
  - If the hindfoot is fixed, a Dwyer or lateralizing calcaneal osteotomy should be considered in addition to a dorsiflexion first metatarsal osteotomy.
- Treatment—nonsurgical treatment consists of physical therapy focusing on isometric and resistance exercises, peroneal strengthening, proprioception, and range of motion. Bracing treatment or taping can help prevent further inversion injuries. Surgical treatment requires demonstrable mechanical instability in the presence of functional instability as well as failure of nonsurgical treatment.
  - Anatomic repair (preferred)
    - Broström—direct repair of attenuated ligaments
    - Karlsson—direct repair of attenuated ligaments with reattachment to fibula
    - Modified Broström—direct ligament repair with augmentation using the inferior extensor retinaculum (**Figure 1**)
  - Nonanatomic repair techniques—most restrict subtalar mobility (**Figure 2**)
    - Nilsonne (popularized by Evans)—simple tenodesis of the peroneal brevis to the fibula; limits inversion, but does not restrict anterior translation; therefore, is seldom used
    - Elmslie—fascia lata graft to reconstruct the anterior talofibular ligament and CFL
    - Watson-Jones
      - Peroneus brevis is routed through the fibula from posterior to anterior, then into talus.
      - Limits anterior translation and inversion.
      - Keeps same angle to fibula as Evans; thus severely limits inversion
    - Chrisman-Snook–modified Elmslie technique using split peroneus brevis tendon routed through talus, through fibula from anterior to posterior, then to calcaneus
  - Anatomic reconstruction with graft
    - Reserved for conditions of generalized ligamentous laxity or failed Broström procedure, obesity, or patients with high functional demands
    - Can be used to augment the modified Broström technique
  - Additional pathology should be treated concomitantly (**Table 3**).

8 | Foot and Ankle

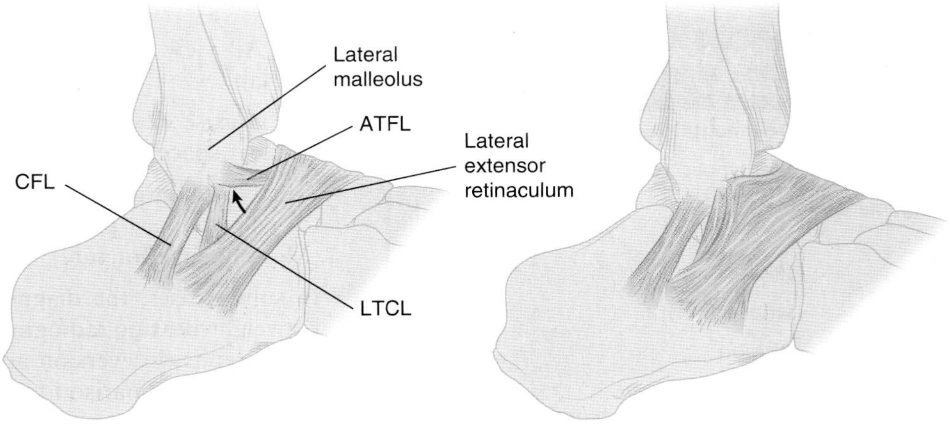

Figure 1 Illustrations show the Gould modification of the Broström technique to repair chronic lateral ankle instability. The ligament repair is reinforced by suturing the lateral extensor retinaculum and lateral talocalcaneal ligament to the distal fibula. The lateral talocalcaneal ligament is variable and may not be repairable. ATFL = anterior talofibular ligament, CFL = calcaneofibular ligament, LTCL = lateral talocalcaneal ligament. (Reproduced from Colville MR: Surgical treatment of the unstable ankle. *J Am Acad Orthop Surg* 1998;6:368-377.)

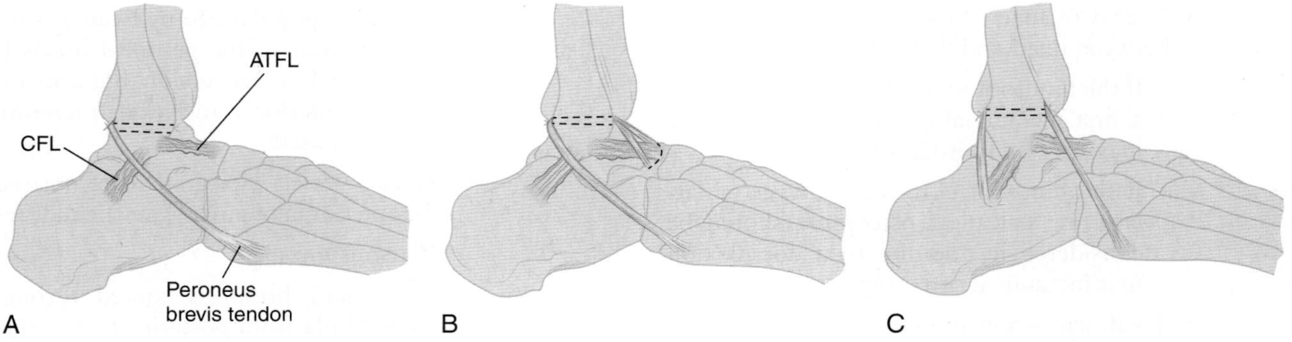

Figure 2 Illustrations depict types of augmented reconstruction to repair chronic lateral ankle instability. **A**, The Evans reconstruction technique uses a tenodesis of the peroneus brevis tendon to the fibula. **B**, The Watson-Jones procedure reconstructs the anterior talofibular ligament and addition to a tenodesis of the peroneus brevis tendon. **C**, The Chrisman-Snook procedure uses a split peroneus brevis tendon to reconstruct the anterior talofibular ligament and the calcaneofibular ligament. ATFL = anterior talofibular ligament, CFL = calcaneofibular ligament. (Reproduced from Colville MR: Surgical treatment of the unstable ankle. *J Am Acad Orthop Surg* 1998;6:368-377.)

IV. SYNDESMOTIC INSTABILITY

A. Pathomechanics

1. A combination of dorsiflexion and external rotation forces result in syndesmotic injuries.
2. Severe injuries are associated with deltoid ligament disruption and fibula fracture.
3. Instability results in lateral and rotatory displacement of the talus.
4. Expect longer recuperation with these high ankle sprains.

TABLE 3

Chronic Lateral Ankle Instability: Associated Pathology and Treatment Options

Associated Pathology	Treatment Options
Peroneal tenosynovitis	Tenosynovectomy
Anterolateral impingement lesion	Excision
Attenuated SPR	SPR reefing
Synovitis	Synovectomy
Loose bodies	Excision
Peroneal tears	Repair Débridement with tendon transfer
Osteochondral lesions of the talus	Curettage and drilling Osteoarticular transfer

SPR = superior peroneal retinaculum

B. Evaluation

1. History and physical
   a. Acute injury with twisting mechanism
   b. If instability is present, patient usually cannot bear weight
   c. Tenderness near the syndesmosis and deltoid ligament
   d. Pain with external rotation
   e. Positive squeeze test (pain at syndesmosis when compressing the tibia and fibula at midcalf)
   f. Swelling and ecchymosis
2. Imaging
   a. Plain radiography
      - The AP view shows decreased tibiofibular overlap.
      - The mortise view shows increased tibiofibular clear space.
      - Tibial radiographs should be obtained to rule out a proximal fibula fracture (Maisonneuve fracture).
      - In subtle cases, the diagnosis is confirmed by weight-bearing radiographs and by stress radiographs (in eversion and external rotation), with comparison to the opposite side (**Figure 3**).
   b. CT may help evaluate the syndesmotic space, especially in chronic cases.
   c. MRI may show subtle syndesmotic ligament injury.

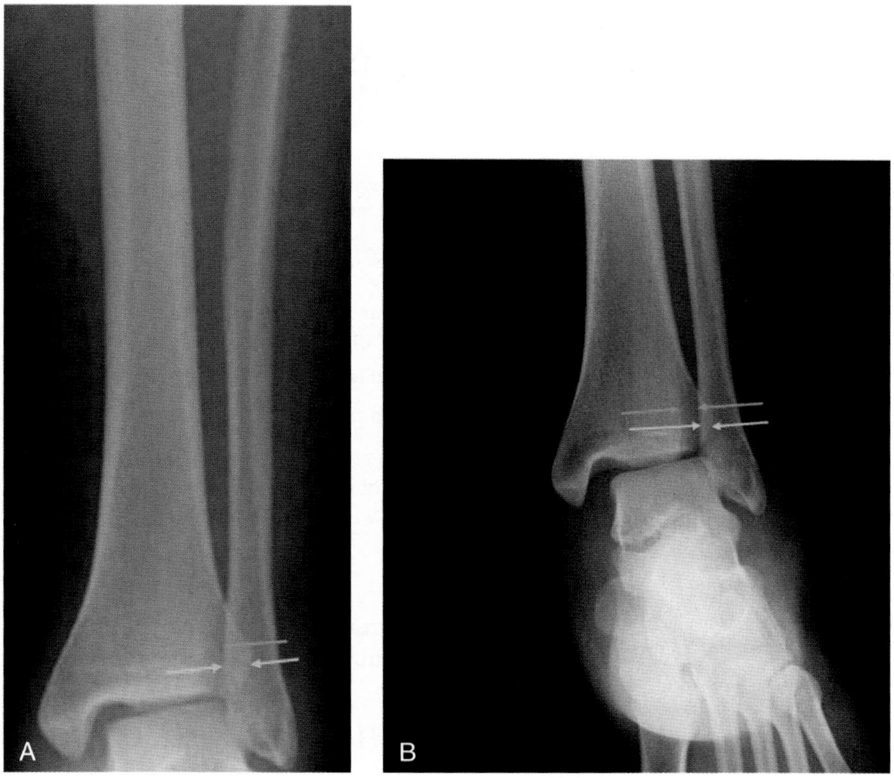

Figure 3 **A** and **B**, Blue arrows demonstrate the normal and abnormal tibiofibular clear space. Normal is less than 6 mm on either the AP or mortise ankle. Yellow arrows demonstrate normal and abnormal tibiofibular overlap. Normal is greater than 6 mm on AP and greater than 1 mm on mortise.

C. Treatment

1. Stable injuries
   a. Initial treatment is a period of RICE.
   b. A brief period of immobilization, until pain and swelling are controlled, is followed by immobilization in a functional brace.
   c. Weight bearing is delayed until the patient is pain-free.
   d. Recovery tends to be prolonged—at least twice that of a standard ankle sprain.
2. Unstable injuries
   a. Open reduction and internal fixation with the syndesmotic screws is required.
   b. If the fibula is fractured, open reduction and internal fixation of the fibula restores length and rotation and facilitates syndesmotic reduction.
   c. The size of the screw, the number of cortices engaged, using suture button fixation, weight-bearing restrictions, and the need for screw removal remain controversial.
   d. Late presentations or chronic injuries can be managed with ligament reconstruction and syndesmotic fixation.

V. DELTOID LIGAMENT INSTABILITY

A. Pathomechanics

1. Deltoid ligament injury occurs with the pronation mechanism.
2. Rupture of the deep deltoid ligament renders the medial aspect of the ankle unstable; this rarely occurs without a lateral injury.
3. When associated with Maisonneuve injuries or fibula fractures, anatomic reduction and internal fixation of the bony and syndesmotic components ensures the proper restoration of alignment, and the deltoid injury can be expected to heal itself.
4. In patients with chronic deltoid insufficiency, malalignment must be ruled out. The most common malalignment deformity is pes valgus (flatfoot).

B. Evaluation

1. History and physical examination
   a. Pronation injury
   b. Instability
   c. Progressive deformity
   d. Medial tenderness
   e. Valgus instability
   f. Valgus ankle deformity

2. Imaging
   a. Weight-bearing mortise and lateral radiographs reveal a valgus ankle deformity.
   b. Varus and valgus stress ankle radiographs confirm the diagnosis and determine whether deformity is fixed or dynamic.

C. Treatment
1. In the presence of genu valgum and pes planus, corrective surgery should include the restoration of proper limb alignment to remove the stress from the deltoid ligament.
2. Direct ligament repair and ligament augmentation procedures have been described.
3. The efficacy of one technique over another has not been scientifically evaluated.
4. Ankle fusion is a salvage procedure.

VI. OSTEOCHONDRAL LESIONS OF THE TALUS

A. Pathophysiology
1. Osteochondral lesions of the talus may result from acute trauma or repetitive microtrauma.
2. These lesions are bilateral in 10% of patients with no history of trauma.
3. Medial lesions are most commonly nontraumatic and tend to be larger and deeper than lateral lesions.
4. Medial lesions are more common than lateral lesions.
5. Lateral lesions more often have a traumatic etiology and tend to be smaller and shallower than medial lesions.

B. Evaluation
1. History—symptoms include swelling, pain, catching, or locking
2. Imaging—radiographs may be normal or show subtle radiolucency or bone fragmentation

C. Classification
1. The Berndt and Harty radiographic classification is shown in **Table 4.**
2. The Ferkel and Sgaglione CT classification is shown in **Table 5.**
3. The Hepple and associates MRI classification is shown in **Table 6.**

D. Treatment
1. Recommend surgical treatment based on lesion size
   a. Less than 1 cm—excision and curettage or drilling

TABLE 4

Berndt and Harty Radiographic Staging System for Osteochondritis Dissecans of the Talus

Stage	Radiographic Finding
1	Small area of subchondral compression
2	Partial fragment detachment
3	Complete fragment detachment without displacement
4	Plate fragment detachment with displacement

Reproduced with permission from Berndt AL, Harty M: Transchondral fracture (osteochondritis dissecans) of the talus. *J Bone Joint Surg Am* 1959;41:988-1020.

TABLE 5

Ferkel and Sgaglione CT Staging System for Osteochondritis Dissecans of the Talus

Stage	CT Finding
1	Cystic lesion within dome of talus with an intact roof on all views
2a	Cystic lesion with communication to talar dome surface
2b	Open articular surface lesion with overlying nondisplaced fragment
3	Nondisplaced lesion with lucency
4	Nondisplaced fragment

Reproduced with permission from Ferkel RD, Sgaglione NA: Arthroscopic treatment of osteochondral lesions of the talus: Long-term results. *Orthop Trans* 1993;17:1011.

TABLE 6

Hepple and Associates MRI Staging System for Osteochondritis Dissecans of the Talus

Stage	MRI Finding
1	Articular cartilage edema
2a	Cartilage injury with underlying fracture and surrounding bony edema
2b	Stage 2a without surrounding bony edema
3	Detached but nondisplaced fragment
4	Detached and displaced fragment
5	Subchondral cyst formation

Reproduced with permission from Hepple S, Winson IG, Glew D: Osteochondral lesions of the talus: Revise classification. *Foot ankle Int* 1999;20:789-793.

b. Greater than 1 cm and cartilage cap intact—retrograde drilling and/or bone grafting

c. Greater than 1 cm and displaced—open reduction and internal fixation versus osteochondral grafting

- Osteochondral grafting
  - Autologous chondrocyte implantation—autograft harvested, grown in a laboratory over the course of several weeks, and replanted
  - Autologous chondrocyte transplantation—harvested and replanted during the same procedure
  - Osteochondral allograft—fresh or fresh frozen
  - Cartilage allograft—juvenile chondrocyte allograft or extracellular matrix cartilage allograft
  - The results of arthroscopic versus open techniques are comparable

VII. SUBTALAR INSTABILITY

A. Pathophysiology

1. Subtalar instability is difficult to directly differentiate from ankle instability because the CFL contributes to both ankle and subtalar stability.
2. Subtalar instability may coexist with ankle instability.

B. Evaluation—the diagnosis is made clinically and using stress Broden inversion radiographs compared with the contralateral limb.

C. Treatment—surgical treatment with the Chrisman-Snook or modified Broström procedure is used because these repairs cross the subtalar joint.

TOP TESTING FACTS

1. MRI should be considered if pain persists 8 weeks after an acute ankle sprain. It is important to rule out osteochondral lesions, peroneal pathology, occult fractures of the talus or anterior calcaneus, tarsal coalition, bone bruise, and impingement lesions.
2. 90% of acute ankle sprains resolve with RICE and early functional rehabilitation.
3. Malalignment associated with chronic lateral ankle instability must be corrected when considering a lateral ligament stabilization. Coleman block testing helps to distinguish between fixed and flexible hindfoot varus.
4. Chronic lateral ankle instability is best treated with physical therapy and bracing treatment, followed by direct anatomic repair if nonsurgical treatment fails.
5. In chronic lateral ankle instability, a tendon graft should be considered to supplement repair in patients whose prior surgery failed, and those with generalized ligamentous laxity and high functional demands.
6. Subtalar stiffness is a common complication after tendon rerouting reconstruction for chronic ankle instability.
7. Syndesmotic injury requires surgical stabilization when the medial ankle has been disrupted (eg, deltoid rupture or medial malleolar fracture).
8. Chronic deltoid insufficiency usually is associated with planovalgus foot deformity.
9. Subtalar instability is difficult to distinguish from ankle instability because the calcaneofibular ligament contributes to the stability of both joints.

Bibliography

Andersen MR, Diep LM, Frihagen F, Hellund JC, Madsen JE, Figved W: The importance of syndesmotic reduction on clinical outcome after syndesmosis injuries. *J Orthop Trauma* 2019;33(8):397-403. doi:10.1097/BOT.0000000000001485.

Brodell JD Jr, MacDonald A, Perkins JA, Deland JT, Oh I: Deltoid-spring ligament reconstruction in adult acquired flatfoot deformity with medial peritalar instability. *Foot Ankle Int* 2019;40(7):753-761. doi:10.1177/1071100719839176.

DiGiovanni BF, Fraga CJ, Cohen BE, Shereff MJ: Associated injuries found in chronic lateral ankle instability. *Foot Ankle Int* 2000:21(10):809-815.

Fortin PT, Guettler J, Manoli A II: Idiopathic cavovarus and lateral ankle instability: Recognition and treatment implications relating to ankle arthritis. *Foot Ankle Int* 2003;23(11):1031-1037.

Grass R, Rammelt S, Biewener A, Zwipp H: Proteus longus ligamental plasty for chronic instability of the distal tibiofibular syndesmosis. *Foot Ankle Int* 2003;24(5):392-397.

Honeycutt MW, Riehl JT: The effect of a dynamic fixation construct on syndesmosis reduction: A cadaveric study. *J Orthop Trauma* 2019;33(9):460-464. doi:10.1097/BOT.0000000000001506.

Karlsson J, Bergsten T, Lansinger O, Peterson L: Reconstruction of the lateral ligaments of the ankle for chronic lateral instability. *J Bone Joint Surg Am* 1988;70(4):581-588.

Keffe DT, Haddad SL: Subtalar instability: Etiology, diagnosis and management. *Foot Ankle Clin* 2002;7(3):577-609.

Krips R, van Dijk CN, Halasi PT, et al: Long-term outcome of anatomical reconstruction versus tenodesis for the treatment of chronic anterolateral instability of the ankle joint: A multicenter study. *Foot Ankle Int* 2001;22(5): 415-421.

Krips R, Brandsson S, Swenson C, van Dijk CN, Karlsson J: Anatomical reconstruction and Evans tenodesis of the lateral ligaments of the ankle: Clinical and radiological findings after follow-up for 15-30 years. *J Bone Joint Surg Br* 2002;84(2):232-236.

Leardini A, O'Conner J, Catani F, Giannini S: The roll of passive structures in the mobility and stability of the human ankle joint: A literature review. *Foot Ankle Int* 2000;21(7):602-615.

Lynch SA, Renstrom PA: Treatment of acute lateral ankle ligament rupture in the athlete: Conservative versus surgical treatment. *Sports Med* 1999;27(1):61-71.

Messer TM, Cummins CA, Ahn J, Kelikian AS: Outcome of the modified Broström procedure for chronic lateral ankle instability using suture anchors. *Foot Ankle Int* 2000;21(12):996-1003.

Nihal A, Rose DJ, Trepman E: Arthroscopic treatment of anterior ankle impingement syndrome in dancers. *Foot Ankle Int* 2005;26(11):908-912.

Nikolopoulos CE, Tsirikos AI, Sourmelis S, Papachristou G: The accessory anteroinferior tibiofibular ligament as a cause of talar impingement: A cadaveric study. *Am J Sports Med* 2004;32(2):389-395.

Shimozono Y, Yasui Y, Ross AW, Kennedy JG: Osteochondral lesions of the talus and the athlete: Up to date review. *Curr Rev Musculoskelet Med* 2017;10(1):131-140.

Thornes B, Shannon F, Guiney AM, Hession P, Masterson E: Suture-button syndesmosis fixation: Accelerated rehabilitation and improved outcomes. *Clin Orthop Relat Res* 2005;431:207-212.

Tol JL, van Dijk CN: Etiology of the anterior ankle impingement syndrome: A descriptive anatomical study. *Foot Ankle Int* 2004;25(6):382-386.

Yamamoto H, Yagishita K, Ogiuchi T, Sakai H, Shinomiya K, Muneta T: Subtalar instability following lateral ligament injuries of the ankle. *Injury* 1998;29(4):265-268.

Chapter 113

ARTHROSCOPY OF THE ANKLE

BENEDICT F. DIGIOVANNI, MD, FAOA
JESSICA M. KOHRING, MD

I. ANKLE ARTHROSCOPY

A. Anterior ankle arthroscopy

1. Setup/patient positioning

a. Appropriate patient positioning, the use of small joint arthroscope, small joint arthroscopic instruments, and noninvasive distraction are keys to efficient and successful ankle arthroscopic procedures

b. Positioning

- The patient is placed supine on a flat-top OR table. If the patient is taller than 6 feet, a table extension may be added to foot of table to allow noninvasive distraction to be applied to table.
- The thigh leg support is used, with care taken to keep the popliteal fossa free of pressure, and attached to the table at the level of midthigh. A thigh tourniquet is typically used, but a sterile pneumatic calf tourniquet may be used for large legs. The heel should rest just off of the bed (**Figure 1, A**).

c. Small joint arthroscope and instruments (**Figure 1, B**)

- 2.5/2.7 mm, 30° arthroscope
- 2.9 mm shaver blades (full radius, teeth, toothless), and baskets
- Ring curettes, angled chondral picks, micro vector drill guide

d. Noninvasive ankle distraction system

- Different systems are available. The authors prefer a noninvasive ankle strap and distractor (**Figure 1, C**).
- The aim is to place the ankle in distraction and in a plantarflexed position to allow improved access to the mid and posterior talar dome lesions as needed, and attempt to avoid malleolar osteotomies whenever possible. Gross and then fine distraction is applied to a point where slack is eliminated in the system while still being able to easily dorsiflex/plantarflex the ankle during the procedure.

2. Overview

a. Thorough knowledge of the surface anatomy of the foot and ankle is required to perform safe, successful ankle arthroscopy.

b. It is necessary to have good working knowledge of the interrelationships between the bony landmarks and the tendons, arteries, veins, and superficial and deep nerves of the ankle.

c. Many potential complications are possible with ankle arthroscopy. Most complications can be avoided if the surgeon becomes familiar with the surface anatomy of the region, uses small joint instruments, and incorporates contemporary noninvasive distraction techniques.

- Complications occur in about 5% to 7% of patients.
- The most common complication is neurologic injury (approximately 80%), with approximately half of those involving the superficial peroneal nerve, and the others possibly related to the distraction.
  - Limit the amount of time the ankle is distracted to help decrease the risk of nerve irritation.
- A synovial cutaneous fistula is more common with ankle arthroscopy than with

Dr. DiGiovanni or an immediate family member serves as a board member, owner, officer, or committee member of the American Board of Orthopaedic Surgery, Inc. and the American Orthopaedic Foot and Ankle Society. Neither Dr. Kohring nor any immediate family member has received anything of value from or has stock or stock options held in a commercial company or institution related directly or indirectly to the subject of this chapter.

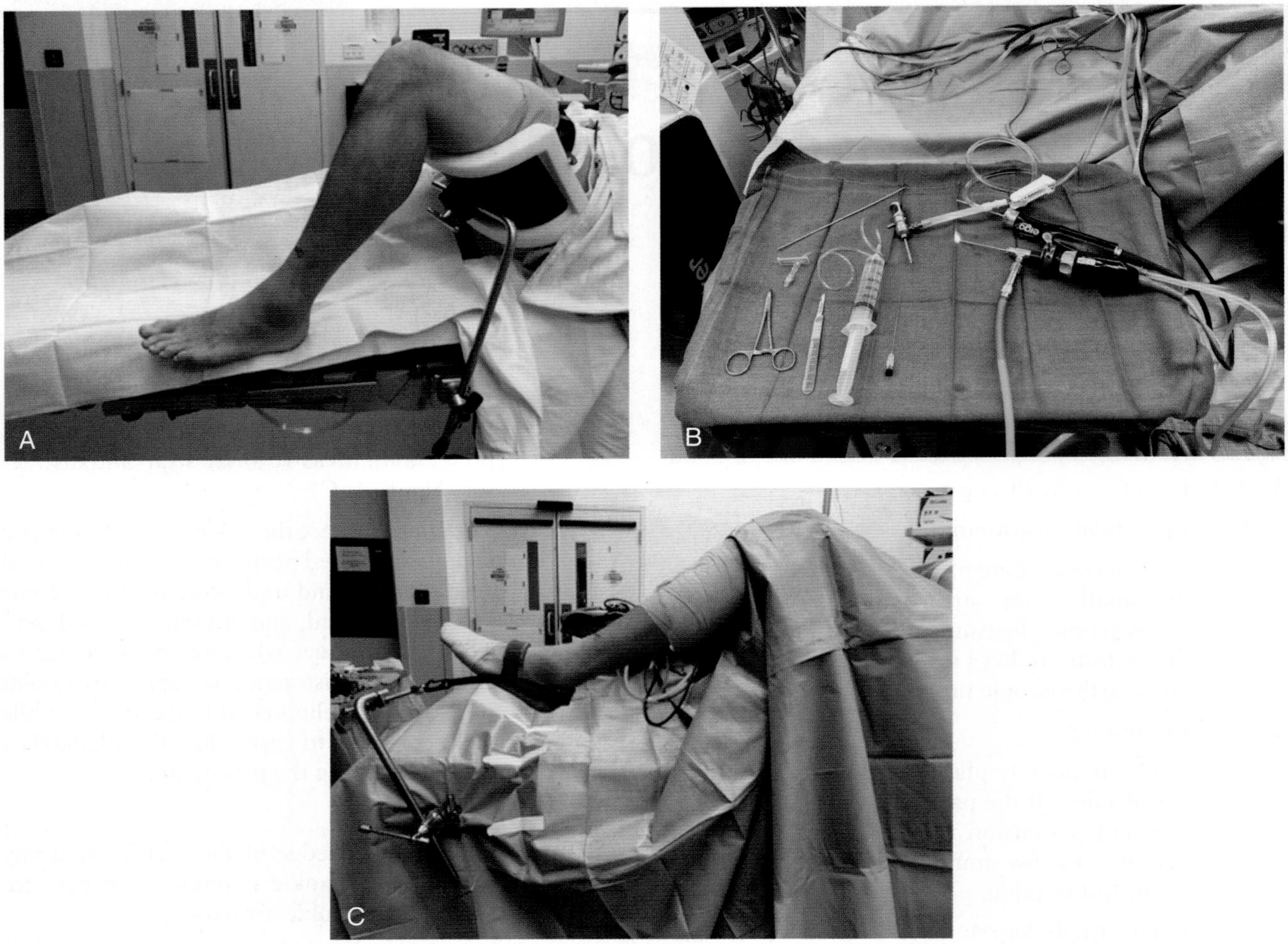

Figure 1 **A**, The patient is positioned supine on a flat-top table and a thigh tourniquet is placed. The surgical leg is placed in a thigh support leg holder with padding underneath the posterior thigh. The foot should barely touch the table with the knee resting in a flexed position. **B**, Example of the setup for a small joint arthroscope and instruments including arthroscope, cannula, 22-gauge spinal needle, and probe. **C**, Once the patient is prepped a sterile, noninvasive distractor is then placed over the dorsal midfoot and around the posterior heel and tensioned to bring the ankle into a plantarflexed position.

arthroscopy of other joints. A short period of immobilization is recommended (5 to 7 days) to decrease the incidence of draining fistula formation.

   d. The workhorse portals for anterior ankle arthroscopy are the anteromedial, anterolateral, and the optional posterolateral portals.

3. Portal placement

   a. Anteromedial portal

      - The anteromedial portal is placed just medial to the tibialis anterior tendon, at the lateral tip of the medial malleolus (**Figure 2**).
      - Injection of the ankle joint with saline, using a 22-gauge spinal needle, helps identify the correct portal location and distends the joint to facilitate placement of the arthroscope.
      - The most common error with anteromedial portal location is placement too far medially. If this occurs, the medial malleolus blocks full manipulation of the arthroscope and compromises joint visualization.
      - The structures that are most at risk during anteromedial portal placement are the greater saphenous nerve and the saphenous vein. Use a small hemostat to bluntly dissect soft tissue at the portal site in a transverse and longitudinal direction to mobilize the structures and to allow free passage of instruments without entrapping neurovascular structures.

   b. Anterolateral portal

      - The anterolateral portal is placed at the level of the ankle joint, medial to the lateral

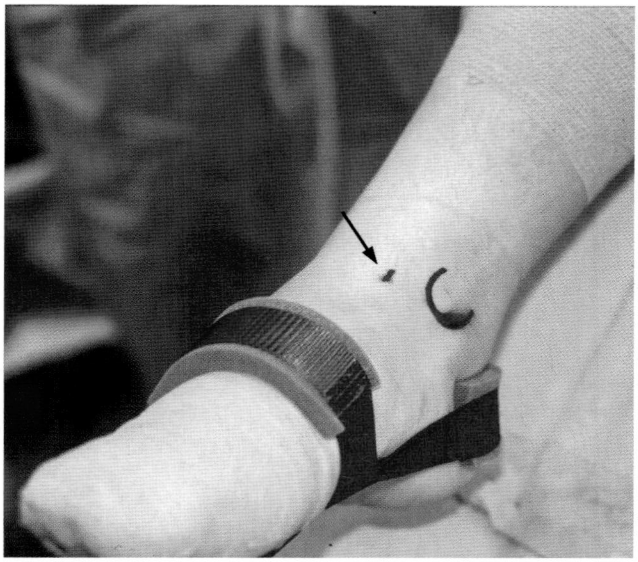

Figure 2 Intraoperative photograph shows the location of the anteromedial ankle portal (arrow). Note that portal placement is a fair distance away from the medial malleolus and close to the medial course of the tibialis anterior tendon. This position ensures that visualization is not obscured by the medial malleolus.

malleolus and in the soft spot just lateral to the peroneus tertius tendon (**Figure 3**).

- The anterolateral portal is made under direct visualization with the arthroscope in the anteromedial portal. A 22-gauge needle aids in atraumatic identification of an appropriate position parallel to the tibiotalar joint surface and is used as a temporary outflow.
- The most common error with anterolateral portal location is placement too far distally. The portal should be located approximately 5 to 10 mm proximal to the anteromedial portal site.
- The structure that is at greatest risk during placement of the anterolateral portal is the intermediate dorsal cutaneous branch of the superficial peroneal nerve (**Figure 4**).
  - Transillumination of the anterolateral skin using the arthroscope can help to identify the crossing nerve branches.
  - Use blunt dissection with a hemostat in the portal incision to keep the nerve branch from being injured during portal placement and avoid being entrapped during instrument passage (**Figure 5**).

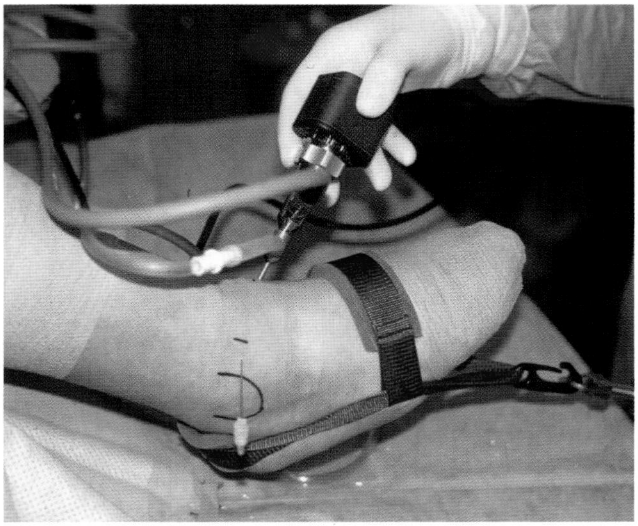

Figure 3 Intraoperative photograph depicts the position of the anterolateral ankle portal. This portal is located proximal to the tip of the fibula and approximately 5 to 10 mm proximal to the anteromedial portal.

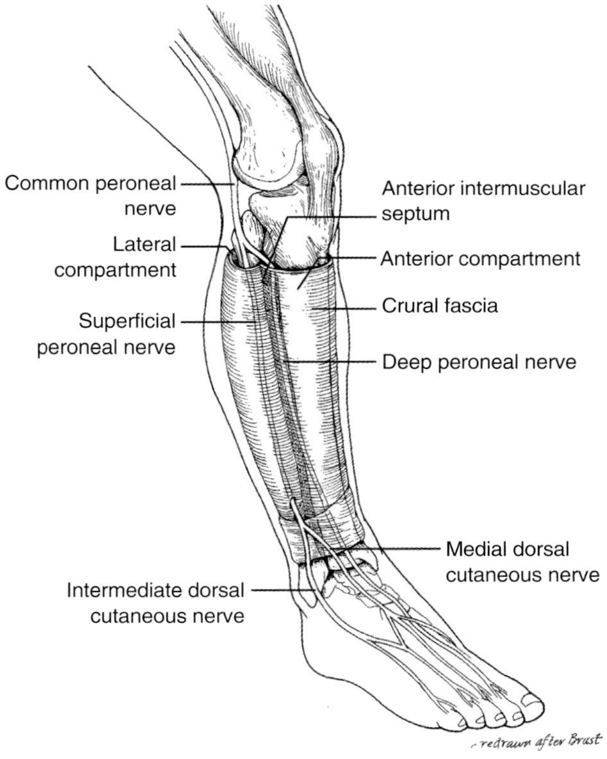

Figure 4 Illustration shows the surface anatomy of the lower leg. Note the course of the superficial peroneal nerve and its distal branches. Because of the branching pattern, the intermediate dorsal cutaneous branch of the superficial peroneal nerve is at risk of injury during anterolateral portal placement. (Reproduced from Stetson WB, Ferkel RD: Ankle arthroscopy: I. Technique and complications. *J Am Acad Orthop Surg* 1996;4[1]:17-23.)

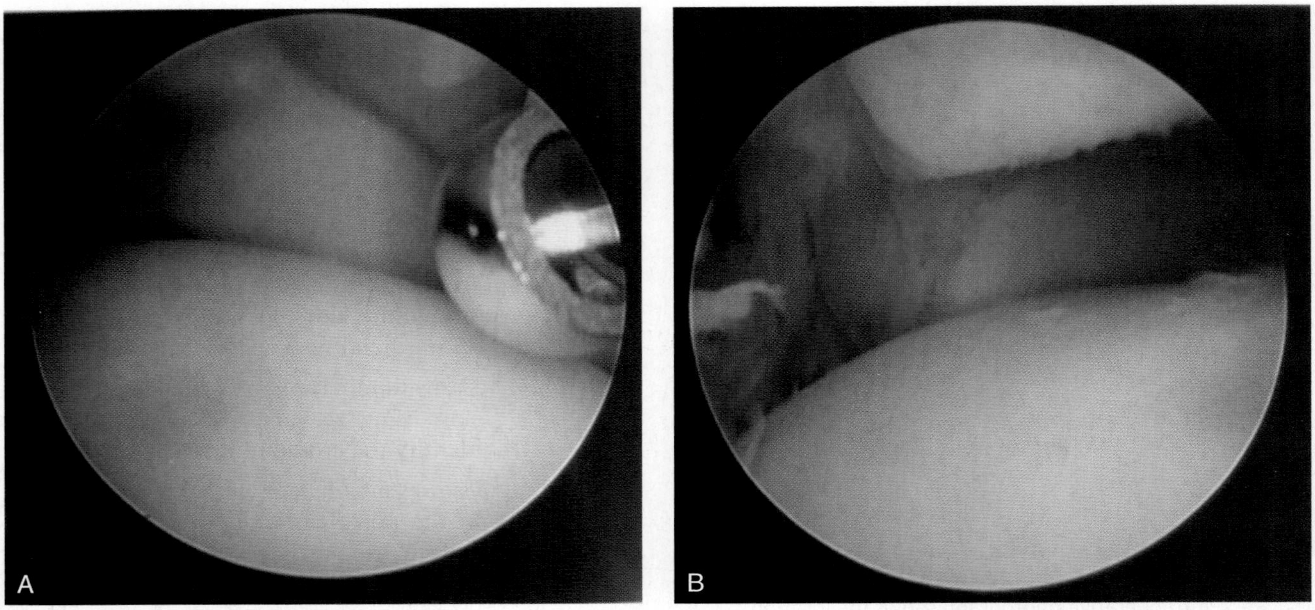

Figure 5 The intraoperative photograph on the left (**A**) shows the normal anatomy of the medial aspect of the tibiotalar joint viewed from the anterolateral portal. The lateral aspect of the tibiotalar joint is depicted in the picture on the right (**B**) where the fibula and syndesmotic ligaments can be seen.

c. Posterolateral portal

- The posterolateral portal is optional and is used for improved visualization of the posterior third of the tibiotalar joint not fully seen from the anterior portals.
- The posterolateral portal is placed 2 cm proximal to the tip of the lateral malleolus, medial to the peroneal tendons, and lateral to the Achilles tendon.
- A 22-gauge needle can be used to identify the correct location while using the arthroscope in the anteromedial portal for visualization. Another option is to place a switching stick (a smooth metal rod) from the anteromedial portal. The switching stick is inserted through the capsule, and the cannula is placed over the rod through the posterolateral portal.
- The most common error with the posterolateral portal location is placement too far distally, which obscures visualization.
- The structures that are at greatest risk during placement of the posterolateral portal are the sural nerve and the lesser saphenous vein.

B. Posterior ankle arthroscopy

1. Overview

a. Posterior ankle arthroscopy provides access to at least 50% of the posterior talar dome and allows for treatment of a variety of posterior ankle and hindfoot disorders both intra- and extra-articular in nature. These conditions include a symptomatic os trigonum, a prominent posterior talar process, or posterior process fracture.

b. The patient is placed in a prone position. The use of a soft-tissue distraction device or tensioned wire placed through the calcaneus can aid in joint visualization (**Figure 9**).

c. It can be helpful to use fluoroscopy when making the portals to visualize the direction of instrumentation.

2. Complications

a. Nerve injuries are the most common complications and occur in about 4% of patients. They include plantar numbness, tibial nerve injury, and sural neuritis.

3. Portal placement

a. Posterolateral

- The posterolateral portal is made adjacent to the Achilles tendon just above the level of the lateral malleolus. Direct a clamp anteriorly in the direction of the first webspace until it hits the tibia. Use this same path when inserting the arthroscope.
- The incision should only be made through the skin, then use blunt dissection to avoid injuring the sural nerve.

b. Posteromedial

- The posteromedial portal is made at the same level as the posterolateral portal just above the tip of the medial malleolus. An incision is made on the medial aspect of the Achilles tendon. It can be helpful to use a clamp to make this portal before inserting instruments.
- Orient the clamp toward the arthroscope at a 90° angle, aiming in the direction of the third webspace. Once the clamp touches the arthroscope, redirect it anteriorly toward the ankle joint until it reaches bone.
- The flexor hallucis longus is the key landmark in posterior ankle arthroscopy (**Figure 10**). Instruments should always be lateral to this structure to avoid the neurovascular bundle including the tibial nerve and posterior tibial artery and veins.

II. SYNOVITIS

A. Pathophysiology

1. The ankle joint synovial lining can become inflamed, resulting in generalized hypertrophic synovitis.
2. Diffuse ankle swelling and pain can result from several different processes.
   a. Inflammatory arthropathies include rheumatoid arthritis, psoriatic arthritis, infection, and gout.
   b. Other processes that result in complex diffuse synovitis include pigmented villonodular synovitis and synovial chondromatosis.
   c. Overuse and trauma also can cause generalized inflammation of the ankle joint synovium.

B. Evaluation

1. If concern for possible septic arthritis exists, joint aspiration with fluid analysis should be performed. Open débridement is an option, but arthroscopic irrigation, synovectomy, and débridement are useful, less invasive procedures.
2. The diagnostic workup is typically negative. MRI may show synovial signal changes, especially with pigmented villonodular synovitis.

C. Arthroscopic treatment

1. Partial synovectomy with lysis of adhesions often provides substantial pain relief for patients with inflammatory arthropathy and in cases of overuse or trauma.
2. For patients with pigmented villonodular synovitis or synovial chondromatosis, synovectomy with the removal of loose bodies can provide marked improvement.

III. ANTEROLATERAL SOFT-TISSUE IMPINGEMENT

A. Pathophysiology

1. Anterolateral soft-tissue impingement is a common cause of chronic pain after one or more lateral ankle sprains (**Figure 6**).
   a. It is characterized by a hypertrophic synovium, inflamed/enlarged capsular tissues, and scarring.
   b. It has been noted to occur with or without associated lateral ankle instability.
2. Anterolateral soft-tissue impingement occurs primarily at two sites.
   a. The most common site of impingement is at the superior portion of the anterior talofibular ligament.
   b. Impingement also occurs along the distal portion of the anterior-inferior tibiofibular ligament.

B. Evaluation

1. Patients with anterolateral soft-tissue impingement typically report a history of persistent anterolateral ankle pain with activity.
2. Physical examination notes well-localized tenderness at the anterolateral ankle joint.

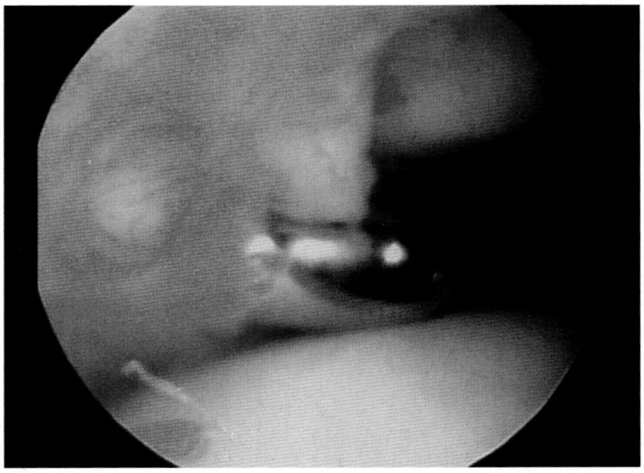

Figure 6 Arthroscopic view shows the typical appearance of an anterolateral soft-tissue impingement lesion. Note the hypertrophic synovium and scarring at the anterolateral corner of the ankle.

8 | Foot and Ankle

3. A physical examination test specific for anterolateral soft-tissue impingement involves reproduction of the pain with plantar flexion of the ankle, followed by thumb pressure at the anterolateral ankle joint, and dorsiflexion of the ankle. This test has been reported to be reproducible and accurate.
4. Diagnosis is based primarily on the history and physical examination. Conventional MRI has a reported sensitivity and specificity of less than 50% for anterolateral soft-tissue impingement of the ankle, whereas higher sensitivity (94%) and specificity (75%) have been noted with clinical examination.
5. A tibiotalar joint injection with anesthetic and/or steroid can aid in diagnosis of differentiating between intra- and extra-articular pathology that may be contributing to impingement symptoms.

C. Arthroscopic treatment

1. Small-joint power shavers or basket forceps are used to débride hypertrophic synovitis and scar tissue.
2. Chondromalacia of the talus is sometimes noted, especially in long-standing lesions.
3. Postoperative treatment typically involves a brief period of immobilization followed by nonimpact exercises at 2 weeks and impact exercises at 4 weeks.
4. Good to excellent results have been reported in 80% to 95% of patients.

IV. SYNDESMOTIC IMPINGEMENT

A. Pathophysiology

1. The ankle syndesmosis is composed of three main structures: the anterior-inferior tibiofibular ligament, the posteroinferior tibiofibular ligament, and the interosseous membrane.
2. Injury to the ankle syndesmosis can result in persistent pain and dysfunction secondary to syndesmotic impingement.
   a. This injury and associated syndesmotic impingement most often involves the anterior tibiofibular ligament, with resulting synovitis and scarring along this ligament.
   b. At times, the presence of a separate anterior-inferior tibiofibular ligament fascicle (the Bassett ligament) is noted and may contribute to impingement.

B. Evaluation

1. Patients with syndesmotic impingement have localized tenderness along the anterior syndesmosis.
2. Dorsiflexion and external rotation of the ankle increase the symptoms.
3. Patients may have tenderness during the squeeze test.

C. Arthroscopic treatment

1. Arthroscopic treatment of syndesmotic impingement involves débridement of the synovitis and scarring at the anterior-inferior tibiofibular ligament, with removal of the Bassett ligament, if present.
2. Only approximately 20% of the syndesmotic ligament is intra-articular. If the syndesmosis complex is competent, excision of this portion, if needed, will not cause mechanical problems.
3. Postoperative treatment typically involves a brief period of immobilization followed by nonimpact exercises at 2 weeks and impact exercises at 4 weeks.

V. ANTERIOR BONY IMPINGEMENT

A. Pathophysiology—Degenerative changes, repetitive overuse injuries (eg, in dancers and football players), and trauma all can result in anterior ankle bone spurs, resulting in bony impingement.

B. Evaluation

1. The typical clinical presentation of anterior bony impingement is localized anterior ankle tenderness with swelling, limited ankle dorsiflexion, and persistent symptoms.
2. A lateral radiograph of the ankle will show osteophytes on the distal tibia, with or without dorsal talus spurring.
3. Improved detail of anteromedial bone spurs can be obtained with oblique radiographs.
4. A weight-bearing lateral radiograph may show the area of bony impingement.
5. CT can be used to show more bony detail, if needed.

C. Classification—A classification system for anterior ankle osteophytes based on the size of the spur and the presence of associated arthritis has been developed (**Figure 7**). Treatment and recovery were found to correlate with the grade of impingement.

D. Arthroscopic treatment

1. Arthroscopic treatment of anterior bony impingement is a valuable tool, but caution must be exercised to avoid iatrogenic injury.
2. Adequate visualization is necessary before using a burr or shaver along the anterior distal tibia, to avoid injury to dorsal neurovascular tissues.

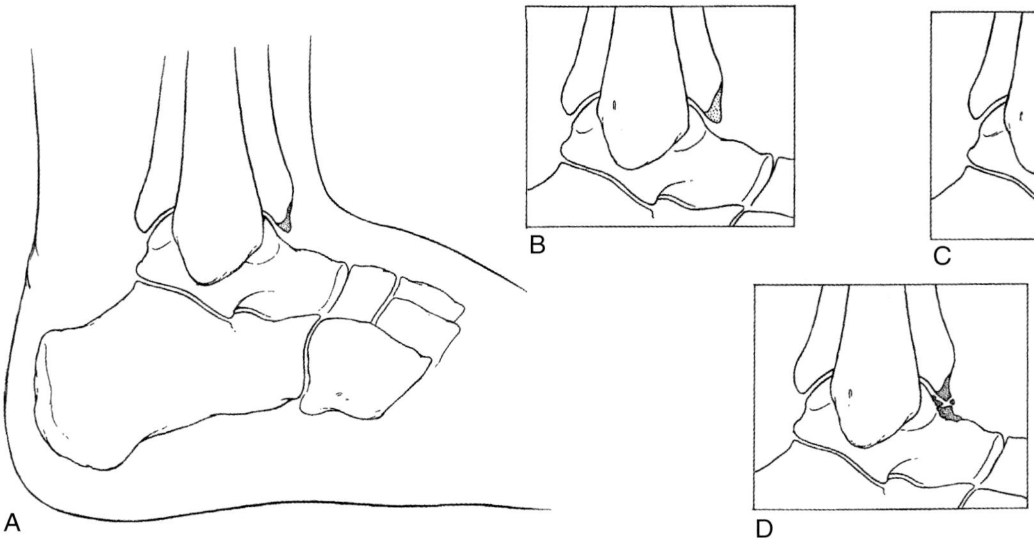

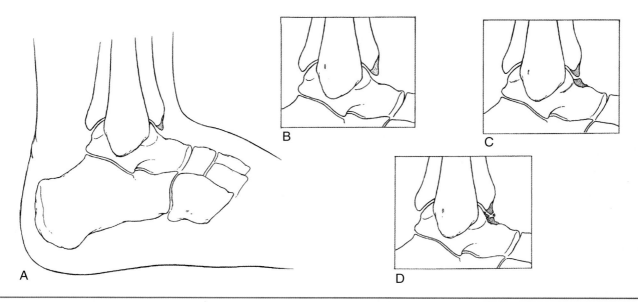

Figure 7 Illustration shows the classification system for anterior ankle osteophytes based on the size of the spur and the presence of associated arthritis. **A**, Grade I, synovial impingement, a tibial spur of up to 3-mm. **B**, Grade II, tibial spur greater than 3 mm. **C**, Grade III, substantial tibial exostosis with or without fragmentation; secondary spur formation on the dorsum of the talus. **D**, Grade IV, pantalocrural arthritic destruction (not a suitable candidate for arthroscopic débridement). (Reproduced with permission from Scranton PE, McDermott JE: Anterior tibiotalar spurs: A comparison of open versus arthroscopic débridement. *Foot Ankle* 1992;13[3]:125-129.)

3. A curved osteotome can be used through the anteromedial or anterolateral portal to detach bone spurs followed by removal via the portals.
4. Electrothermal probes can be used to simultaneously cut and coagulate soft-tissue scar/synovitis and bone spurs.
5. Excellent or good results can be expected approximately 75% of the time with the arthroscopic removal of anterior ankle bone spurs and scar/synovitis when joint-space narrowing is not present.
6. Postoperative treatment typically involves a brief period of immobilization followed by nonimpact exercises at 2 weeks and impact exercises at 4 weeks.

VI. POSTERIOR ANKLE IMPINGEMENT SYNDROME

A. Pathophysiology

1. Like anterior bony impingement, posterior ankle impingement syndrome is due to chronic overuse or acute trauma when the ankle is forced into a plantarflexed position.
2. It presents most often in ballet dancers, soccer and football players, and downhill runners.

B. Evaluation

1. The typical clinical presentation of posterior ankle impingement is when the patient experiences pain in the hindfoot with the ankle forced into a plantarflexed position.
2. The forced hyperplantar flexion test is used in diagnosis. The ankle is passively hyperflexed using quick repetitive movements in slight external and internal rotation. The examiner grinds the posterior talar process or os trigonum between the tibia and calcaneus. Patient pain or discomfort and reproduction of symptoms are positive findings.
3. The lateral radiograph and CT scan will show an os trigonum, hypertrophic posterior talar process, or a posterior talar process fracture.

C. Arthroscopic treatment

1. Arthroscopic treatment of posterior bony impingement involves resection of a symptomatic os trigonum or removal of a prominent posterior talar process. Additionally, there may be a soft-tissue component in addition to bone impingement that can be removed arthroscopically.

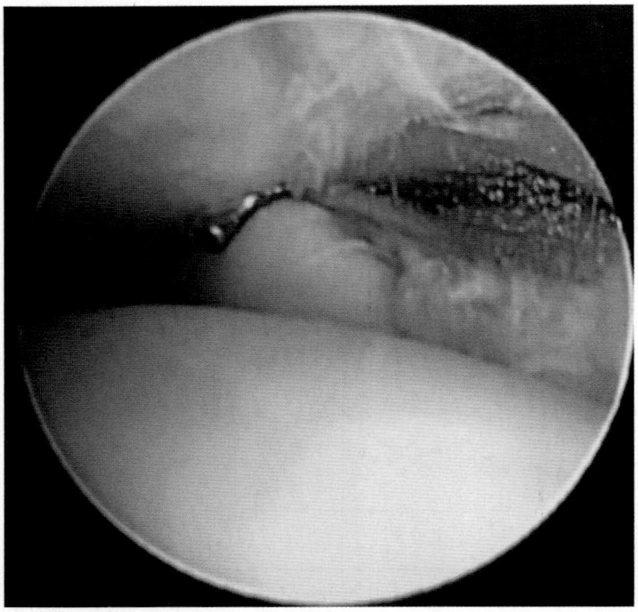

Figure 8 Arthroscopic view of the lateral ankle joint shows a probe in the syndesmosis to assess for instability.

2. The posterior talar process or os trigonum is often entrapped in scar tissue and must be freed before removal.
   a. Identification of the flexor hallucis longus tendon medially is an important landmark to prevent injury to the medial neurovascular bundle. It is important to remain lateral to this structure to prevent iatrogenic injury.
   b. Partial detachment of the posterior talofibular ligament, flexor retinaculum, and posterior talocalcaneal ligament may be required for adequate resection of bony impingement.
3. If a large os trigonum is present and unable to be removed arthroscopically, enlargement of the posterolateral portal may be required to fully resect the bone fragment via direct visualization and open removal.
4. Postoperative treatment includes weight bearing as tolerated after surgery and early range of motion exercises as soon as possible to limit scar formation.

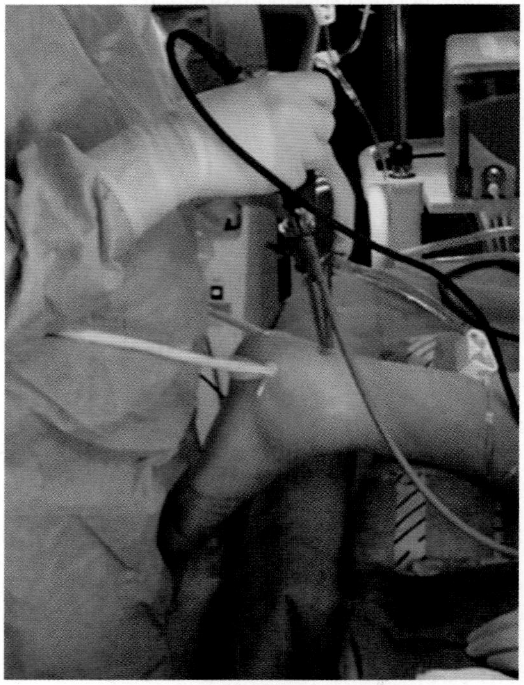

Figure 9 Posterior arthroscopy on a right ankle. A smooth Steinmann pin is passed from medial to lateral across the calcaneal tuberosity. A single sterile roll of kerlix is wrapped around the medial and lateral sides of the pin at the midportion of the kerlix roll. The slack from the medial and lateral sides is then passed behind the surgeon to a nonsterile surgical assistant. The nonsterile surgical assistant then ties the kerlix snuggly behind the surgeon (behind the surgeon is no longer sterile). The surgeon can lean back on the kerlix "belt" to create traction at the ankle. When the arthroscopy is complete, a sterile scissors cuts the sterile end of the kerlix from the medial and lateral sides of the calcaneus. The Steinmann pin is removed.

VII. ACUTE TRAUMATIC ANKLE INJURIES

Surgical treatment of rotational ankle fractures and their associated injuries can be aided by the use of ankle arthroscopy.

A. Pathophysiology

1. Syndesmosis disruption is common and occurs in up to 11% of all ankle injuries.
2. In rotational ankle fractures, 30% to 39% have a concomitant syndesmotic injury.

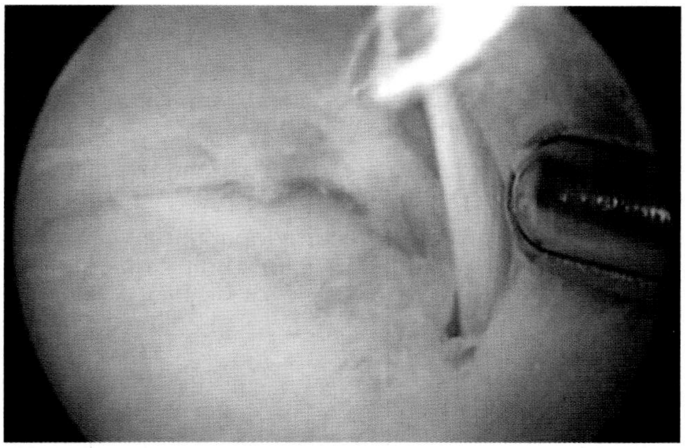

Figure 10 Posterior arthroscopy of a left ankle. An arthroscopic shaver has exposed the FHL (flexor hallucis longus muscle) at the posteromedial aspect of the ankle. The FHL should be the medial most extent of the posterior ankle débridement. Any débridement further medial than the FHL should be performed judiciously with concern for injury to the neurovascular bundle.

3. Osteochondral defects (OCDs) and other chondral injuries may be present in 57 to 90% of patients with ankle fractures.

B. Evaluation

1. The benchmark for assessment of syndesmotic instability is an intraoperative stress test including the Cotton test or external rotation stress test.
2. Osteochondral defects can oftentimes be identified on plain radiographs. MRI is the best imaging study to evaluate the size, location, and presence of instability of OCDs.

C. Arthroscopic evaluation

1. In recent years, ankle arthroscopy has been increasingly used to assess for syndesmotic instability and osteochondral defects at the time of ankle fracture fixation.
   a. It has the highest sensitivity and specificity for diagnosing syndesmotic injuries missed on plain and stress view radiographs.
2. Arthroscopic diagnosis of syndesmotic instability includes disruption of the deep portion of the posterior tibiofibular ligament, rupture of the interosseous ligament with a syndesmotic gap > 2 mm, or a fracture of the posterolateral portion of the tibial plafond (**Figure 8**).
3. Concurrent ankle arthroscopy at the time of open reduction and internal fixation of ankle fractures provides both better visualization and less disruption to the surrounding soft tissues to view fracture reduction as well as intra-articular pathology including OCDs and loose bodies.

TOP TESTING FACTS

1. The workhorse portals for ankle arthroscopy are the anteromedial, anterolateral, and the optional posterolateral portals.
2. Complications of arthroscopic ankle surgery using small joint instruments and contemporary noninvasive distraction techniques occur in about 5% to 7% of patients. The most common complication is neurologic injury (approximately 80%), with approximately half involving the intermediate dorsal cutaneous branch of the superficial peroneal nerve.
3. A synovial cutaneous fistula is a more common complication with ankle arthroscopy than with arthroscopy of other joints.
4. The structure that is at greatest risk of injury during placement of the anterolateral portal is the intermediate dorsal cutaneous branch of the superficial peroneal nerve.
5. The structures that are at greatest risk of injury during placement of the posterolateral portal are the sural nerve and the lesser saphenous vein.
6. The structures that are at greatest risk of injury during placement of the posteromedial portal during posterior ankle arthroscopy are the tibial nerve and posterior tibial artery and veins.
7. Anterolateral soft-tissue impingement is a common cause of chronic ankle pain after one or more lateral ankle sprains. It has been noted to occur with or without associated lateral ankle instability.
8. A physical examination test specific for anterolateral soft-tissue impingement involves reproduction of the pain with plantar flexion of the ankle, followed by thumb pressure at the anterolateral ankle joint, and dorsiflexion of the ankle. This test has been reported to be reproducible and accurate.

9. Injury to the ankle syndesmosis can result in persistent pain and dysfunction secondary to syndesmotic impingement.
10. Excellent or good results can be expected approximately 75% of the time with arthroscopic removal of anterior ankle bone spurs and scar/synovitis when joint-space narrowing is not present.
11. Treatment for posterior ankle impingement including os trigonum syndrome, a prominent posterior talar process, or posterior process fracture can be effectively treated via posterior ankle arthroscopy.
12. Ankle arthroscopy at the time of open reduction and internal fixation for ankle fractures and injuries can aid in fracture reduction, and diagnosis of syndesmotic instability and allows for identification and treatment of chondral injuries, OCDs, and loose bodies without significant soft-tissue dissection.

Bibliography

Branca A, Di Palma L, Bucca C, Visconti CS, Di Mille M: Arthroscopic treatment of anterior ankle impingement. *Foot Ankle Int* 1997;18(7):418-423.

Carreira DS, Vora AM, Hearne KL, Kozy J: Outcome of arthroscopic treatment of posterior impingement of the ankle. *Foot Ankle Int* 2016;37(4):394-400.

Da Cunha RJ, Karnovsky SC, Schairer W, Drakos MC: Ankle arthroscopy for diagnosis of full-thickness talar cartilage lesions in the setting of acute ankle fractures. *Arthroscopy* 2018;34(6):1950-1957.

Feller R, Borenstein T, Fantry AJ, Kellum RB: Arthroscopic quantification of syndesmotic instability in a cadaveric model. *Arthroscopy* 2017;33(2):436-444.

Ferkel RD, Small HN, Gittins JE: Complications in foot and ankle arthroscopy. *Clin Orthop Relat Res* 2001;391:89-104.

Hsu AR, Gross CE, Lee S: Extended indications for foot and ankle arthroscopy. *J Am Acad Orthop Surg* 2014;22(1):10-19.

Kim SH, Ha KI: Arthroscopic treatment for impingement of the anterolateral soft tissues of the ankle. *J Bone Joint Surg Br* 2000;82(7):1019-1021.

Liu SH, Nuccion SL, Finerman G: Diagnosis of anterolateral ankle impingement: Comparison between magnetic resonance imaging and clinical examination. *Am J Sports Med* 1997;25(3):389-393.

Lui TH, Ip K, Chow HT: Comparison of radiologic and arthroscopic diagnoses of distal tibiofibular syndesmosis disruption in acute ankle fracture. *Arthroscopy* 2005;21:1370.

Maquirriain J: Posterior ankle impingement syndrome. *J Am Acad Orthop Surg* 2005;13(6):365-371.

Massri-Pugin J, Lubberts B, Vopat BG, Guss D, Hosseini A, DiGiovanni CW: Effect of sequential sectioning of ligaments on syndesmotic instability in the coronal plane evaluated arthroscopically. *Foot Ankle Int* 2017;38(12):1387-1393.

Molloy S, Solan MC, Bendall SP: Synovial impingement in the ankle: A new physical sign. *J Bone Joint Surg Br* 2003;85(3):330-333.

Nickisch F, Barg A, Saltzman CL, Beals TC: Postoperative complications of posterior ankle and hindfoot arthroscopy. *J Bone Joint Surg Am* 2012;94(5):439-446.

Stetson WB, Ferkel RD: Ankle arthroscopy: I. Technique and complications. *J Am Acad Orthop Surg* 1996;4(1):17-23.

Tol JL, Verheyen CP, van Dijk CN: Arthroscopic treatment of anterior impingement in the ankle. *J Bone Joint Surg Br* 2001;83(1):9-13.

Tol JL, Verhagen RA, Krips R, et al: The anterior ankle impingement syndrome: Diagnostic value of oblique radiographs. *Foot Ankle Int* 2004:25(2):63-68.

Young BH, Flanigan RM, DiGiovanni BF: Complications of ankle arthroscopy utilizing a contemporary noninvasive distraction technique. *J Bone Joint Surg Am* 2011;93(10):963-968.

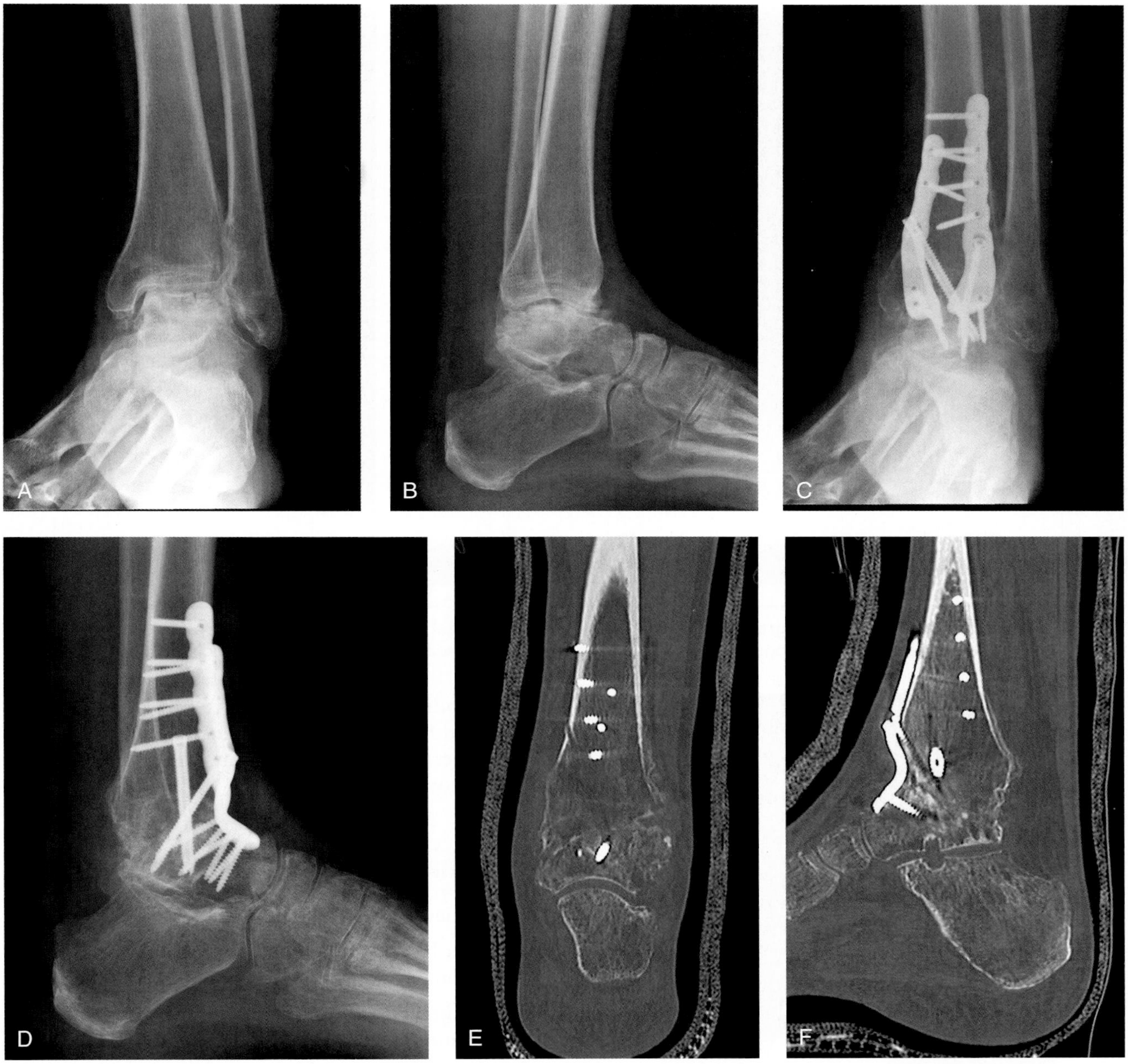

Figure 6 Imaging studies of a 42-year-old man with left ankle arthritis and osteonecrosis limited to the talar dome. Preoperative oblique (**A**) and lateral (**B**) weight-bearing ankle radiographs. Postoperative oblique (**C**) and lateral (**D**) weight-bearing radiographs obtained at 4-month follow-up. Progression to fusion confirmed with coronal (**E**) and sagittal (**F**) metal-suppression CT scans obtained at 4-month follow-up.

- Absolute contraindications for TAA include active infection and inadequate bone stock. Inadequate bone stock is defined as bone unable to support the TAA components. This can include osteonecrosis of the talus or distal tibia from prior fracture or systemic reasons or large cystic areas.
- Both mobile-bearing and fixed-bearing implants exist. There is no known difference in outcomes. However, a mobile-bearing implant should not be used if there is anterior talar translation or coronal plane deformity.
- Long-term follow-up of modern implants (particularly complication rates) is warranted to determine advantages over ankle arthrodesis (**Figure 8**).

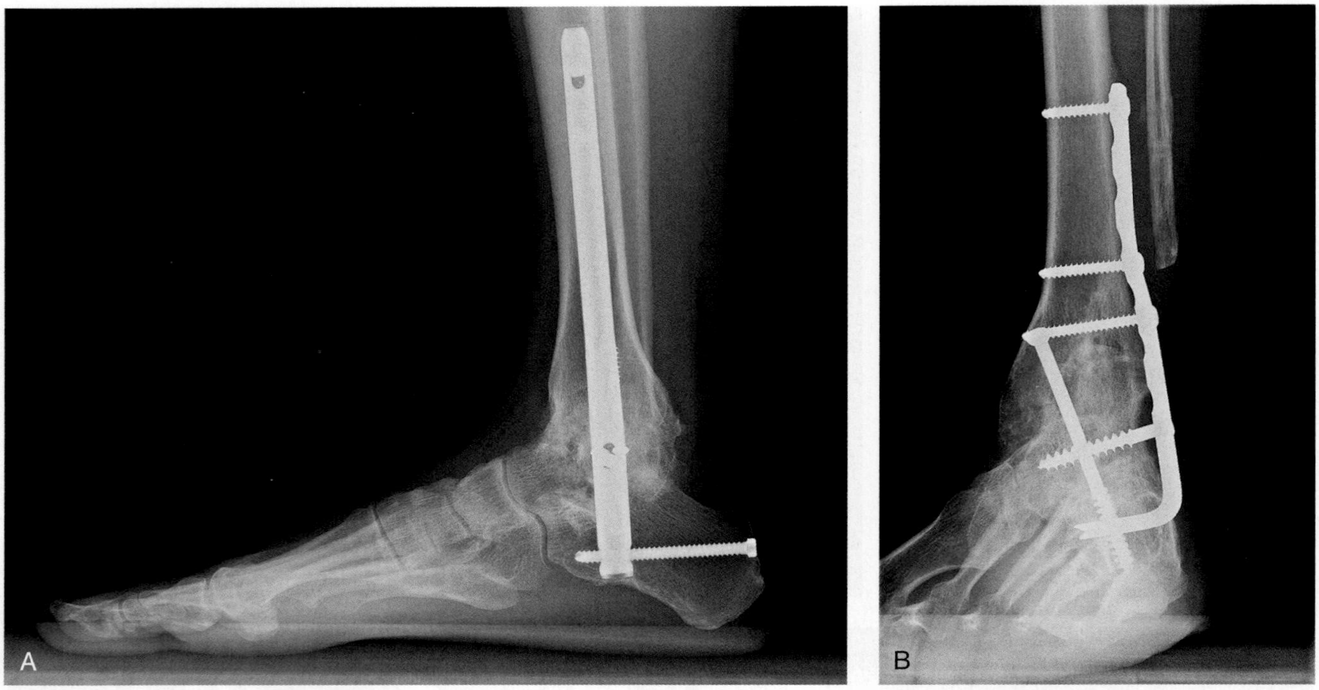

Figure 7 **A**, Postoperative lateral radiograph demonstrating a tibiotalocalcaneal arthrodesis utilizing a retrograde intramedullary nail. **B**, Postoperative oblique ankle radiograph demonstrating a tibiotalocalcaneal arthrodesis accomplished with a 90° blade plate.

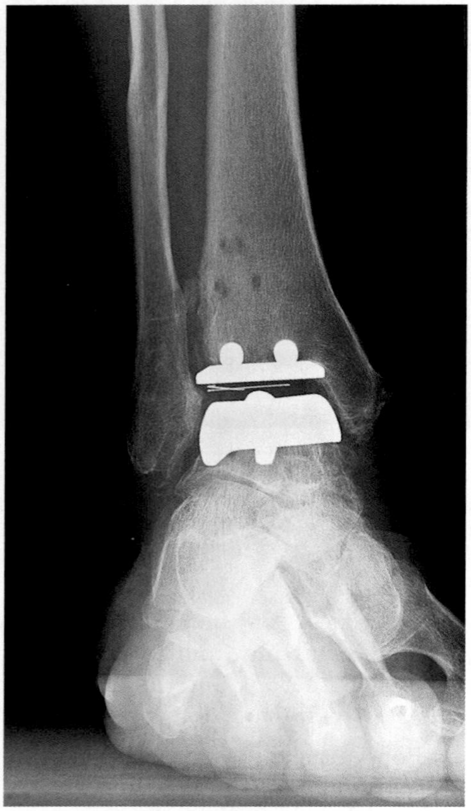

Figure 8 Postoperative oblique radiograph obtained after total ankle arthroplasty with a mobile-bearing implant.

D. Rehabilitation—Postoperative physical therapy is procedure-dependent. In general, ankle arthrodesis necessitates a minimum of 8 weeks of protected weight bearing.

II. ARTHRITIDES OF THE HINDFOOT

A. Overview

1. The hindfoot articulations include the subtalar, talonavicular, and calcaneocuboid joints.
2. Arthritides of the hindfoot may develop from trauma (calcaneus or talus fractures), inflammatory arthritides, primary arthritis (OA), end-stage tibialis posterior tendon disorders, tarsal coalitions, or neurologic disorders that are associated with long-standing cavovarus foot posture.
3. Arthritides of the hindfoot are most often posttraumatic in origin.
4. Hindfoot arthritis secondary to posterior tibial tendon dysfunction is often associated with Achilles tendon contracture.
5. Isolated talonavicular joint arthritis is associated with inflammatory arthropathy (rheumatoid arthritis [RA]).

B. Evaluation

1. History and physical examination

a. Patients with hindfoot arthritis generally report pain and/or swelling at the sinus tarsi, particularly when walking on uneven surfaces.

b. Inversion and eversion of the hindfoot reproduce pain.

c. Motion is typically limited when compared with the uninvolved side.

d. The patient should be examined while bearing weight to identify potential malalignment.

2. Imaging

a. Weight-bearing radiographs demonstrate loss of joint space and malalignment of the bones in the hindfoot (**Figure 9, A**).

b. Although Broden and Harris radiographic views may better define the extent of subtalar arthritis than standard radiographic views, CT may be warranted to provide greater detail of hindfoot arthritides.

C. Treatment

1. Nonsurgical

a. NSAIDs

b. Activity modification

c. Shoe modifications (stiff, rocker soles)

d. Bracing treatment that protects the hindfoot

- University of California Biomechanics Laboratory (UCBL) orthosis
- Rigid or hinged AFOs

e. Corticosteroid injections

f. Selective (fluoroscopically guided) anesthetic/corticosteroid injections are sometimes therapeutic, but they typically serve to identify the symptomatic hindfoot articulations.

2. Surgical

a. Arthrotomy (or, in select cases, arthroscopy) may prove successful to débride hindfoot articulations and remove symptomatic exostoses or loose bodies.

b. Lateral calcaneus exostectomy after calcaneal fracture is often effective in relieving subfibular impingement.

c. Arthrodesis

- Arthrodesis is typically recommended for hindfoot arthritis (**Figure 9, B**).
- Selective arthrodesis of a hindfoot articulation is indicated for isolated arthritis.
- Isolated calcaneocuboid, subtalar, and talonavicular joint arthrodeses limit hindfoot motion by approximately 25%, 40%, and 90%, respectively, prompting many surgeons to recommend triple arthrodesis when talonavicular joint arthrodesis is warranted.
- Triple arthrodesis is the recommended treatment of stage III tibialis posterior tendon dysfunction that is unresponsive to nonsurgical treatment.
- Some authors recommend subtalar bone block distraction arthrodesis to reestablish physiologic hindfoot alignment when associated loss of heel height and anterior ankle impingement are present.

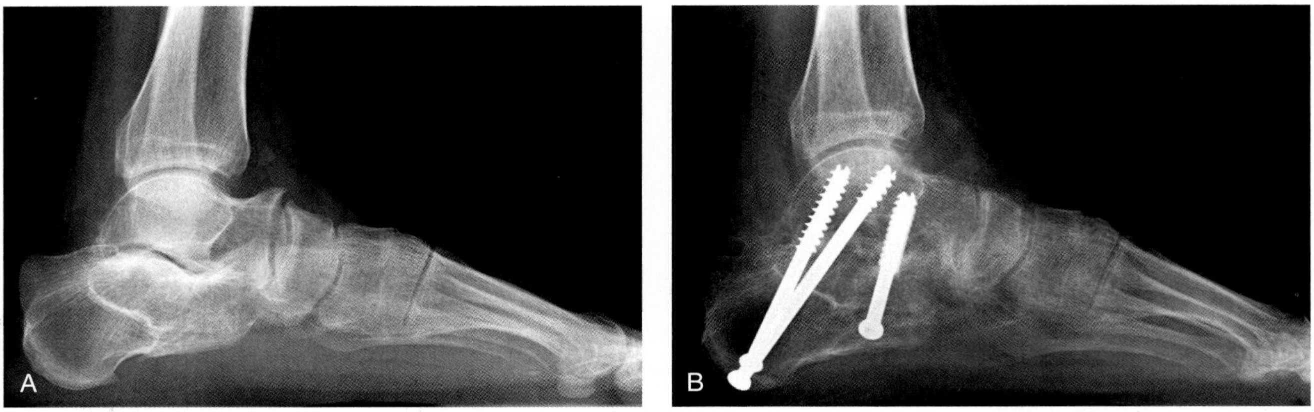

Figure 9 Lateral radiographs of the foot in a patient with posttraumatic subtalar arthritis, subtalar coalition, and calcaneal malunion. **A**, Preoperative view. **B**, Radiograph obtained after subtalar arthrodesis and calcaneal osteotomy to realign the hindfoot and restore hindfoot height.

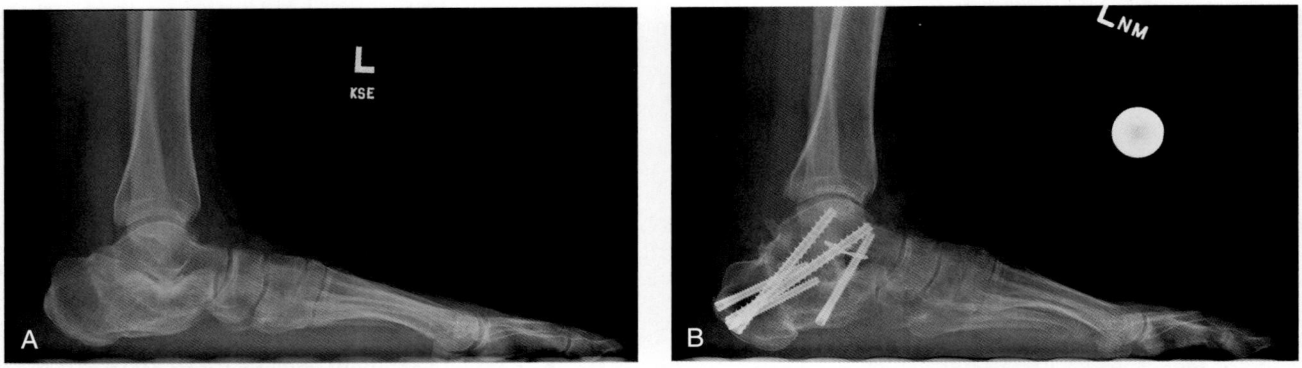

Figure 10 **A**, Lateral radiograph of a patient with prior calcaneus fracture with loss of heel height and subtalar arthritis. The inclination of the talus is decreased to a more horizontal position. **B**, A bone block distraction subtalar arthrodesis was performed, restoring the position of the talus.

- Loss of heel height typically occurs after a tuberosity fracture of the calcaneus.
- The resultant deformity is a relatively horizontal talus, thereby limiting ankle dorsiflexion.
- Despite the history of calcaneus fracture, patients typically complain of anterior ankle pain and limited ankle motion.
- A distraction subtalar bone block arthrodesis can restore the inclination of the talus, decrease anterior ankle pain, and increase ankle motion (**Figure 10**).

- Techniques for hindfoot arthrodesis include internal fixation with screws and/or staples.
- The recommended position for hindfoot arthrodesis maintains or reestablishes a plantigrade foot, with approximately 5° of hindfoot valgus and a radiographically congruent talus–first metatarsal axis (Meary line) on both AP and lateral weight-bearing radiographs.
- The desired position for triple arthrodesis is 5° to 7° of hindfoot valgus and a congruent talus–first metatarsal angle on the AP and lateral radiographs (0°).
- The union rate for isolated subtalar arthrodesis is 88% to 96%. In a triple arthrodesis, the most common joint not fused is the talonavicular joint.
- There is a 40% nonunion rate for subtalar arthrodesis in the setting of a previous ankle arthrodesis.

III. ARTHRITIDES OF THE MIDFOOT

A. Overview

1. The midfoot articulations include the naviculocuneiform and metatarsocuneiform/cuboid joints.
2. Midfoot joints may be viewed as nonessential joints, and if fused in anatomic alignment, physiologic foot function is generally anticipated.
3. The etiology of midfoot arthritis can be primary, inflammatory, or posttraumatic.
4. Primary OA of the midfoot is the most common type of midfoot arthritis.
5. Untreated tarsometatarsal (TMT) joint (Lisfranc) fracture-dislocation typically leads to loss of the longitudinal arch and forefoot abduction.

B. Evaluation

1. History and physical examination
   a. Patients report midfoot/arch pain with weight bearing, particularly with push-off during gait.
   b. Pain is elicited with palpation or stress.
   c. Bony prominences of the midfoot may be present.
   d. Loss of the longitudinal arch (sometimes associated with forefoot abduction) is frequently seen with weight bearing and with radiographic alignment. Midfoot arthritis is the second most common cause of longitudinal arch loss behind posterior tibial tendon dysfunction.
   e. Secondary hindfoot valgus, Achilles tendon contracture, and hallux valgus may also be present.

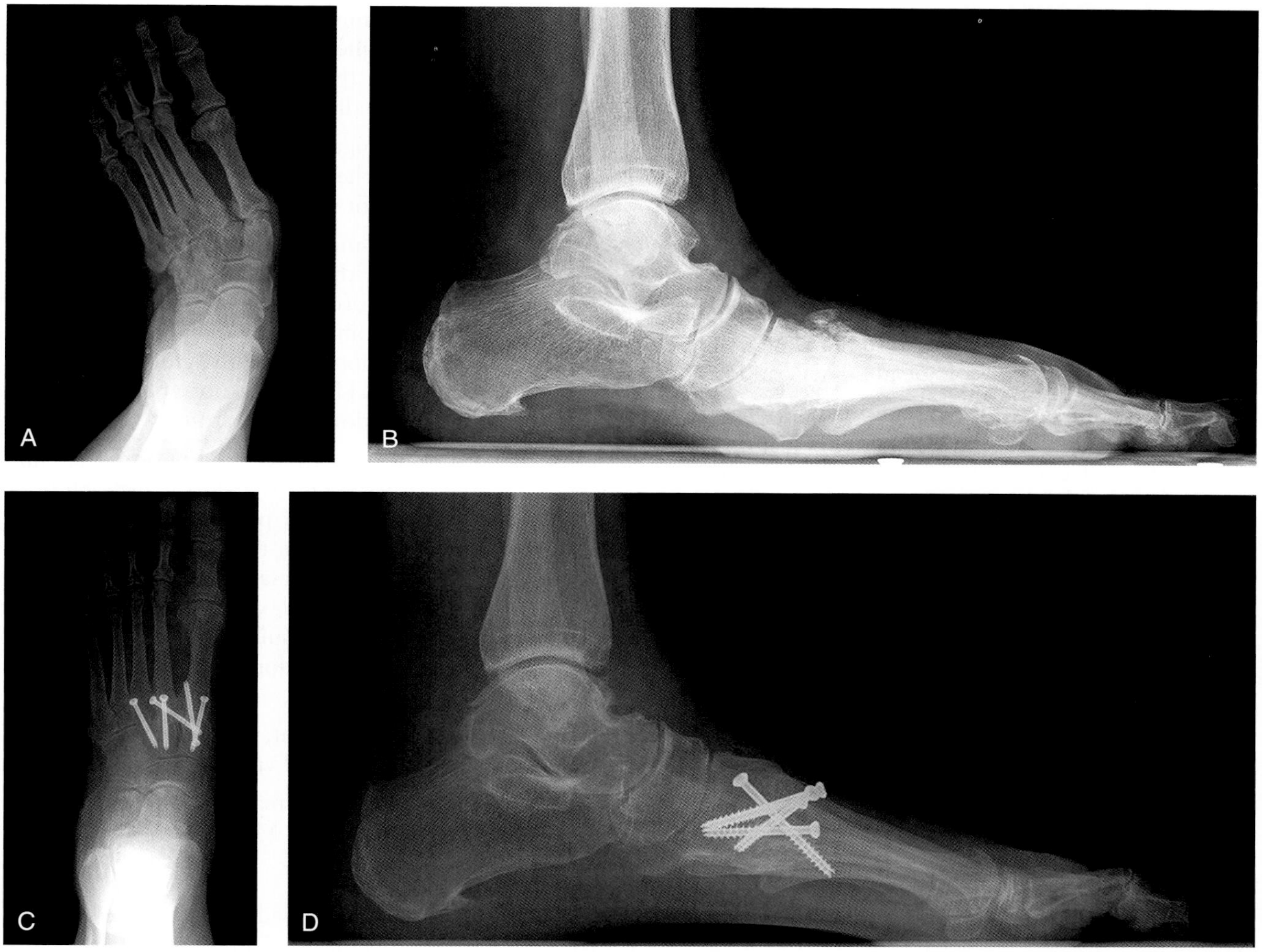

Figure 11 Preoperative AP (**A**) and lateral (**B**) radiographs demonstrating midfoot arthritis with deformity. AP (**C**) and lateral (**D**) radiographs obtained following midfoot fusion with realignment.

2. Imaging—AP, oblique, and lateral radiographs are needed.
    a. As with other arthritis, joint space narrowing, subchondral sclerosis, and dorsal foot osteophytes are seen in affected joints.
    b. Weight-bearing radiographs of the foot demonstrate a nonlinear talus–first metatarsal relationship with the apex of the deformity at the midfoot. This deformity produces a loss of the longitudinal arch and forefoot abduction (**Figure 11, A** through **D**).

C. Treatment

1. Nonsurgical
    a. NSAIDs
    b. Activity modification
    c. Longitudinal arch supports with rigid inserts
    d. Shoe modifications (rocker soles)
    e. Fixed-ankle bracing treatment in combination with shoe modifications (rocker soles) may further unload the midfoot during gait.
    f. Fluoroscopically guided corticosteroid injections are diagnostic and potentially therapeutic.
2. Surgical
    a. Near-full physiologic foot function, in particular during push-off, can be reestablished with successful realignment and arthrodesis of the first through third TMT and/or naviculocuneiform joints. The fourth and fifth TMT joints are not fused, to preserve the accommodation function of the foot.

b. Internal fixation of the midfoot articulations has evolved to include screws, staples, and plates specifically indicated for midfoot arthrodesis.

3. Pearls and pitfalls

a. Select cases of symptomatic fourth and fifth TMT joint arthritis diagnosed using selective corticosteroid joint injections may be treated with interposition arthroplasty, which maintains the lateral column and accommodates gait.

b. TMT joints are 2 to 3 cm deep; full joint preparation must extend to the plantar surface to optimize physiologic alignment and fusion.

c. Care must be taken to not malposition the second and third TMT joints during arthrodesis. Excessive plantar flexion will cause metatarsalgia of the involved ray, and excessive dorsiflexion will cause transfer metatarsalgia of the adjacent rays.

d. Severe deformity may warrant a biplanar midfoot osteotomy in conjunction with arthrodesis, particularly in nonbraceable Charcot midfoot deformity.

e. Given the high prevalence of midfoot arthritis following Lisfranc injury, primary arthrodesis may be considered especially in the setting of associated metatarsal base fractures.

f. Surgical management of arthritides of the midfoot may warrant simultaneous Achilles tendon lengthening and hindfoot realignment.

IV. ARTHRITIDES OF THE FOREFOOT

A. Overview

1. Arthritides of the forefoot most commonly affect the first metatarsophalangeal (MTP) joint (hallux rigidus). The most likely etiology is repetitive trauma, but metabolic (gout) or inflammatory conditions (eg, RA) also may be contributing factors.

2. Arthritis of the forefoot involving the lesser MTP joints is typically inflammatory (eg, RA) and rarely occurs secondary to osteonecrosis of the lesser metatarsal head (Freiberg infraction).

3. Hallux rigidus refers to degenerative joint disease of the first MTP joint.

B. Evaluation

1. History and physical examination

a. Patients with hallux rigidus typically report pain along a dorsal prominence over the MTP joint of the great toe, swelling of the great toe, and pain during push-off.

b. Physical examination demonstrates a tender dorsal prominence, dorsal erythema, dorsal impingement (pain with forced dorsiflexion), and limited hallux range of motion.

c. First MTP range of motion is the most important part of the physical examination and is very important for surgical decision making.

- Pain at the midrange of the motion arc, particularly with severe limitation of motion, suggests more advanced arthritis of the hallux MTP joint. This finding influences treatment decisions. Typically, global arthritis of the first MTP joint is not effectively managed with dorsal cheilectomy.
- Pain only at extreme motion indicates limited arthritis and the dorsal osteophyte is the main cause of pain. Pain with extreme dorsiflexion is due to the phalanx abutting the dorsal metatarsal osteophyte. Pain with extreme plantar flexion is likely secondary to the dorsal capsule and extensor hallucis longus (EHL) tendon being draped over the dorsal osteophyte.

d. When RA is present, the lesser MTP joints develop clawing and valgus deviation.

e. Freiberg infraction creates an isolated stiffness in the affected lesser MTP joint.

2. Imaging

a. Radiographs are used to stage the arthritis (**Figure 12, A** and **B**; **Table 1**).

- The AP and oblique films can be used to judge joint space narrowing.
- The lateral view demonstrates the dorsal metatarsal osteophyte and can reveal a dorsal proximal osteophyte of the proximal phalanx.

b. Lesser MTP joints may demonstrate periarticular erosions, dorsal and lateral deviation, and, frequently, dislocation.

c. Freiberg infraction manifests as a destructive single metatarsal head deformity, with characteristics similar to femoral head osteonecrosis (**Figure 13**).

C. Treatment

1. Nonsurgical

a. NSAIDs

b. Corticosteroid injections

c. Activity modification

d. Orthotic shoe inserts

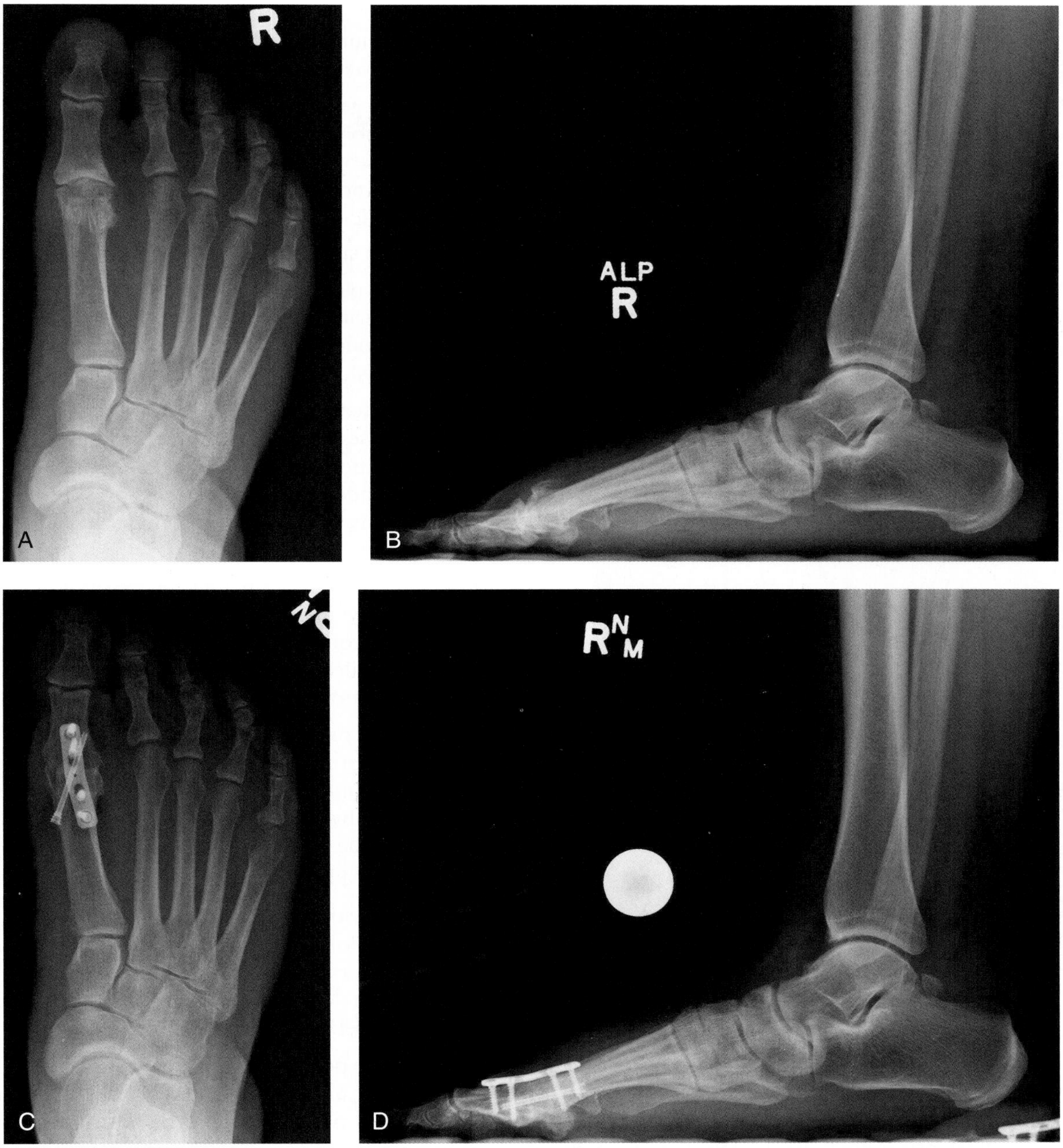

Figure 12 Preoperative AP (**A**) and lateral (**B**) radiographs demonstrating severe first metatarsophalangeal (MTP) joint arthritis. AP (**C**) and lateral (**D**) radiographs obtained following first MTP joint arthrodesis.

- Morton extension (stiff insert limiting hallux dorsiflexion)
- Stiffer insert that supports the entire forefoot
- These inserts must be used for the correct symptomatology. If the patient has minimal pain with range of motion but reports of dorsal joint pain with shoe wear, inserts in the plantar aspect of the foot will only increase the patient's symptoms as the foot will be elevated up against the dorsum of the shoe.

e. Shoe modifications include
   - Deeper toe box
   - Softer leather
   - Leather stretching
   - Stiffer sole
   - Rocker soles

TABLE 1

Classification of Arthritis of the Forefoot

Stage	Severity	Characteristics
I	Mild	MTP joint space maintained; dorsal osteophyte
II	Moderate	MTP joint space narrowing; large dorsal, medial, and lateral osteophytes
III	Severe	Complete loss of MTP joint space

MTP = metatarsophalangeal

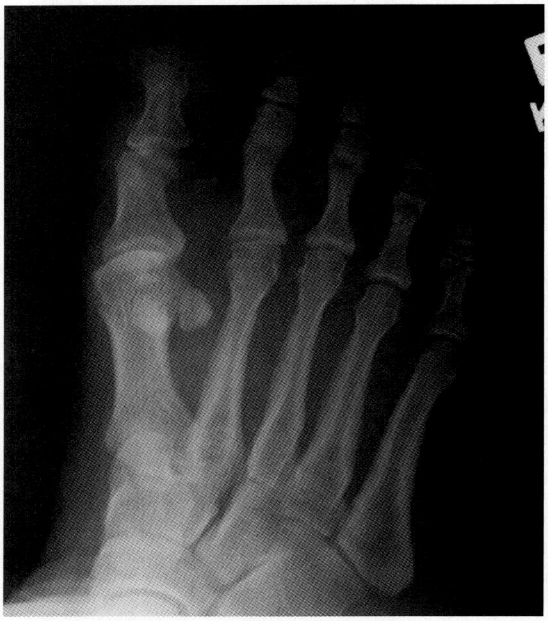

Figure 13 AP radiograph demonstrating flattening of the second metatarsal head, consistent with Freiberg infraction.

2. Surgical
   a. Surgical procedures are largely based on the location of pain in the motion arc and the amount of arthritis seen on radiographs.
   b. Joint débridement with a dorsal cheilectomy
      - Mild to moderate hallux rigidus typically responds to joint débridement with a dorsal cheilectomy.
         - Typically chosen for patients that do not have midrange motion pain and mild to moderate radiographic joint space narrowing.
      - Results may be enhanced with simultaneous microfracture of the first metatarsal head cartilage, plantar capsular release, or, most commonly, a dorsiflexion osteotomy of the proximal phalanx (Moberg osteotomy).
      - In general, dorsal cheilectomy will result in poor outcome, with pain at the midrange of the motion arc and complete loss of MTP joint space on radiographs (both characteristic of advanced arthritis).
   c. Joint sparing options
      - Typically chosen for patients with pain during the entire motion arc with mild to moderate joint space narrowing who do not wish to have an arthrodesis.
      - Interposition arthroplasty—In select cases, interposition arthroplasty using the patient's native extensor hallucis brevis tendon, dorsal capsule, or skin substitute may relieve symptoms while preserving hallux motion.
      - Synthetic implants. A recently developed polyvinyl alcohol implant has been used in conjunction with joint débridement and cheilectomy to treat symptoms and preserve motion.
         - Comparison of this implant to MTP arthrodesis demonstrated pain relief and functional outcomes were equivalent with obviously greater preserved motion with the use of the implant.
   d. First MTP joint arthrodesis
      - Advanced arthritis (pain during the entire arc of motion and severe joint space loss on radiographs) is best managed with first MTP joint arthrodesis (**Figure 12, C** and **D**).
      - The position of the great toe is important for gait and proper shoe wear. The first proximal phalanx should be positioned in about 25° of dorsiflexion and 15° of valgus relative to the first metatarsal (**Figure 12, C** and **D**). Alternatively, when referencing the position of the great toe, it should not be too far into valgus to crowd the second toe. Also, it should be dorsiflexed about 15° from the plantar border of the foot. Although this will change based on the anatomy of the arch (flatfoot versus cavus).
      - Biomechanical testing suggests that the combination of a compression screw and dorsal plate is the most stable construct for first MTP joint arthrodesis, albeit with a loss in push-off power during gait.

C. Acute paratenonitis/tendinitis

1. Pathoanatomy

a. Overuse can cause inflammation within the paratenon.

b. Inflammation also may occur within the retrocalcaneal bursa.

c. Less commonly, inflammatory arthropathy (eg, ankylosing spondylitis) and the use of fluoroquinolones have been linked to acute tendinitis.

2. Evaluation

a. Patients frequently report a recent change in their activity, such as increased intensity or type of activity, terrain, or a change of shoe wear.

b. Symptoms include pain, swelling, and warmth.

c. Physical examination reveals mild fusiform swelling, warmth, crepitus, and pain with palpation throughout the entire range of motion.

3. Treatment

a. Nonsurgical treatment is 65% to 90% successful and consists of diminished intensity of activities, physical therapy with eccentric strengthening and modalities (eg, iontophoresis, phonophoresis, ultrasonography), NSAIDs, ice, heel lifts, night splints, and, at times, immobilization (cast or removable boot) in severe cases.

b. Surgical débridement of a scarred or inflamed paratenon is 70% to 100% successful and is indicated only when nonsurgical treatment has failed. The most common complication of surgery is problems with wound healing.

D. Chronic tendinitis/tendinosis

1. Pathoanatomy

a. Chronic tendinitis and tendinosis are characterized by chronic degenerative changes within the tendon.

b. The exact pathway resulting in tendon degeneration is unknown, but the degeneration is believed to develop after prolonged acute tendinitis.

c. The Achilles tendon can be affected at its insertion as well as within the midsubstance, typically 2 to 6 cm from its insertion.

d. Patients with chronic tendinitis or tendinosis are typically older than those with acute paratenonitis or tendinitis.

e. Risk factors include hypertension, obesity, steroid use (oral or local injection), and estrogen use.

2. Evaluation

a. Patients have longer history of symptoms of pain with increased use.

b. Typical physical examination findings

- Nodular thickening in the tendon that moves with range of motion of the ankle, indicating pathology within the Achilles tendon
- Pain that is usually localized only over the swollen site if no acute paratenonitis is present

c. The diagnosis is clinical, but radiographs can reveal calcifications within the tendon with long-standing disease. MRI (**Figure 1**) and ultrasonography may delineate the exact location and the percentage of degeneration within the tendon.

3. Treatment

a. The initial treatment is the same as for acute tendinitis, consisting of diminished intensity of activities, physical therapy with eccentric strengthening and modalities (eg, iontophoresis, phonophoresis, and ultrasonography), NSAIDs, ice, heel lift, night splint, and, at times, immobilization (cast or removable boot) in severe cases.

b. Surgical treatment

- Chronic insertional tendinosis—The diseased portion of the tendon and retrocalcaneal bursa is excised. Often, a bony decompression of a prominent portion of the posterior calcaneus is performed. The

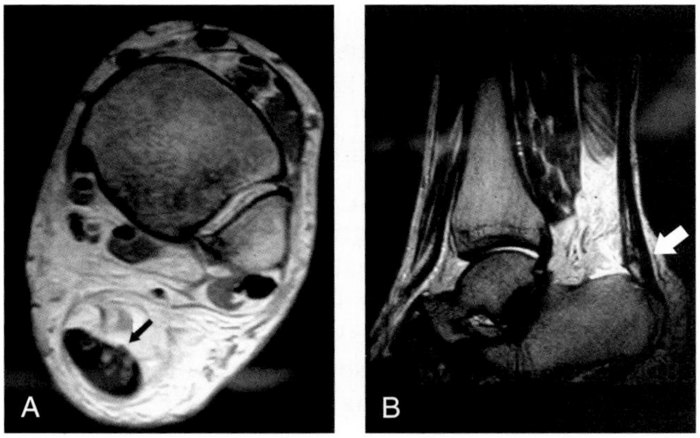

Figure 1 Chronic tendinosis of the Achilles tendon. **A**, Axial T1-weighted MRI shows substantial degenerative changes in the anterior aspect of the Achilles tendon (arrow). **B**, Sagittal T1-weighted MRI of the same ankle demonstrates greater than 50% involvement of the tendon (arrow).

8 | Foot and Ankle

calcific spurring at the insertion of the tendon is removed, and the tendon is reattached to the calcaneus.

- Midsubstance chronic tendinopathy—The diseased portion of the tendon is excised, and the tendon is primarily repaired, if possible.
- In both insertional tendinosis and midsubstance tendinopathy, a tendon transfer should be considered when more than 50% of the tendon is involved and in older patients (>55 years) with poor tissue quality. The most direct route of transfer and the most common tendon used is the flexor hallucis longus (FHL), but use of the flexor digitorum longus (FDL) or peroneus brevis (PB) tendon also has been described. The tendon can be woven through the defect or directly inserted into the calcaneus to reinforce the repair. Additionally, the use of an allograft to reinforce the repair has been described.

E. Noninsertional acute ruptures

1. Pathoanatomy

a. Acute ruptures most commonly occur between the ages of 30 and 40 years.

b. They are most common in men and in poorly conditioned and episodic athletes, up to 15% of whom may have prodromal symptoms.

c. Most ruptures occur 4 to 6 cm from the Achilles tendon insertion in the calcaneus, in the anatomically hypovascular region. Degenerative changes have been found at the tendon ends in patients with acute ruptures.

2. Evaluation

a. Most ruptures (75%) occur during sporting activities. The patient reports a "pop" or the sensation of being kicked in the heel during the injury. Afterward, the patient has weakness, ecchymosis, and difficulty walking.

b. Examination with the patient in the prone position is more accurate and reliable. Physical examination reveals increased resting dorsiflexion with the knees flexed (**Figure 2**), a palpable gap, weak plantar flexion, and an abnormal Thompson test (lack of plantar flexion when squeezing the calf).

c. The diagnosis is clinical, but MRI or ultrasonography can verify the presence and location of the rupture in cases of delayed presentation or can verify tendon apposition for nonsurgical treatment.

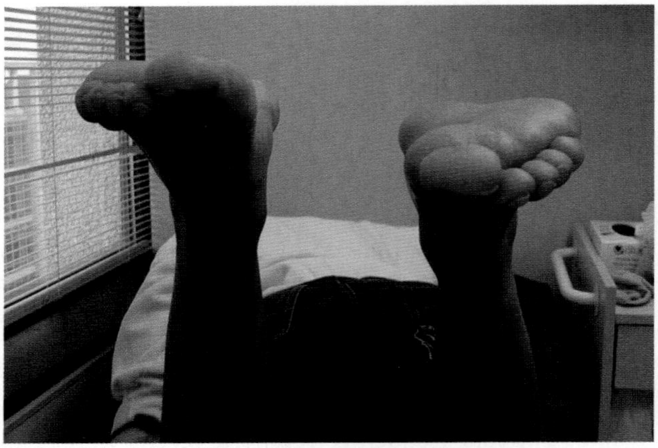

Figure 2 Clinical photograph shows decreased resting tension in the patient's right ankle, indicating an acute or even a chronic Achilles tendon rupture.

3. Treatment

a. Nonsurgical treatment

- Nonsurgical treatment should consist of functional rehabilitation, which includes immobilization initially in resting gravity equinus or a 20° plantarflexed position followed by early physical therapy with appropriate protection and gradual dorsiflexion to a neutral position (sample functional rehabilitation protocol provided in **Table 2**).
- Functional rehabilitation with early motion and use of a removable boot walker results in faster return to mobility and return to work compared with casting for 8 weeks. Similarly, functional rehabilitation results in lower rates of rerupture compared with traditional immobilization.

b. Surgical treatment

- Surgical treatment goals are to restore appropriate tension and repair the musculotendinous unit.
- Traditionally performed through a posterior midline approach with the patient in a prone position. Alternatively, it can be performed through a posteromedial approach which has the advantage of being through an area of higher vascularity and enabling the supine position. There is no evidence of a difference in wound complications between these two approaches. Overall rate of wound complications for open procedures is estimated at 7% to 8%.

TABLE 2

Sample Functional Rehabilitation Protocol for Use After Surgical or Nonsurgical Management of Acute Achilles Tendon Ruptures

Postoperative Week	Protocol
0-2	Posterior slab/splint Non–weight bearing with crutches immediately postoperatively in patients who undergo surgical treatment or immediately after injury in nonsurgically treated patients
2-4	Controlled ankle motion walking boot with 2-cm heel lift[a,b] Protected weight bearing with crutches Active plantar flexion and dorsiflexion to neutral, inversion/eversion below neutral Modalities to control swelling Incision mobilization if indicated[c] Knee/hip exercises with no ankle involvement (eg, leg lifts from sitting, prone, or side-lying position) Non–weight-bearing fitness/cardiovascular exercises (eg, bicycling with one leg) Hydrotherapy (within motion and weight-bearing limitations)
4-6	Weight bearing as tolerated[a,b] Continue protocol of week 2-4
6-8	Remove heel lift Weight bearing as tolerated[a,b] Slow dorsiflexion stretching Graduated resistance exercises (open and closed kinetic chain exercises and functional activities) Proprioceptive and gait training Ice, heat, and ultrasonography therapy, as indicated Incision mobilization if indicated[c] Fitness/cardiovascular exercises (eg, bicycling, elliptical machine, walking and/or running on treadmill) with weight bearing as tolerated Hydrotherapy
8-12	Wean out of boot Return to crutches and/or cane as necessary; gradually wean off the use of crutches and/or cane Continue to progress range of motion, strength, and proprioception
>12	Continue to progress range of motion, strength, and proprioception Retrain strength, power, and endurance Increase dynamic weight-bearing exercises, including plyometric training Sport-specific retraining

[a]Patients are required to wear the boot while sleeping.
[b]Patients are allowed to remove the boot for bathing and dressing but should adhere to the weight-bearing restrictions.
[c]If, in the opinion of the physical therapist, scar mobilization is indicated (ie, the scar is tight), the physical therapist can attempt to mobilize the scar with the use of friction or ultrasonography therapy instead of stretching.
Adapted from Willits K, Amendola A, Bryant D, et al. Operative versus nonsurgical treatment of acute Achilles tendon ruptures: A multicenter randomized trial using accelerated functional rehabilitation. *J Bone Joint Surg Am* 2010;92(17):2767-2775.

- A desire to decrease wound complications has also led to the development of new repair techniques with smaller incision size and decreased soft-tissue damage.
  - Percutaneous procedures may have lower rates of wound complications
  - Percutaneous procedures appear to have higher rates of sural nerve injury
  - Percutaneous and open procedures have similar return to work/activity rates, patient-reported outcome scores, rerupture rates, calf/ankle diameter, and plantar flexion strength
  - Limited open repair is a technique bridging the gap between open and percutaneous techniques wherein a limited open incision is made to visualize tendon apposition, but the suture repair is performed through percutaneous stab wounds. This technique is increasing in popularity.

c. Comparisons between surgical and nonsurgical management
  - Historically, rerupture was thought to be higher among nonsurgically managed patients compared with surgically managed patients. However, when accelerated

functional rehabilitation is used as the comparison to surgical intervention, rerupture rates appear to be similar.

- The most recent randomized trials, which have fully embraced functional rehabilitation as the nonsurgical method of choice, suggest few clinically significant differences between surgical and nonsurgical intervention.
  - The only consistently noted difference is an increased rate of complications in the surgical group—primarily soft-tissue complications related to the surgical approach.
  - At least one study suggests earlier strength recovery in the surgical group, the advantage of which diminishes by one year and is likely clinically insignificant in the long term.
- Overall, functional rehabilitation is a reasonable choice for the management of acute noninsertional Achilles ruptures, not just among the sedentary or elderly, but even among young, healthy, active individuals. Appropriate functional rehabilitation is key.

F. Insertional acute ruptures

1. Pathoanatomy—An avulsion of the Achilles sleeve from the calcaneus, sometimes with a small bony fragment from calcific tendinosis. An overuse injury that tends to occur in patients with retrocalcaneal bursitis, calcaneal edema, and/or chronic calcific insertional tendinosis. A Haglund deformity is often present, which exacerbates the condition through mechanical impingement.
2. Treatment
   a. In contrast to midsubstance tears, surgical repair is recommended in virtually all cases to restore function. These injuries require repair of the gastrocnemius soleus complex to bone.
   - One described technique includes the prone position and a 4 to 5 cm longitudinal posteromedial incision over the distal Achilles and calcaneal tuberosity. These authors excised any prominent posterosuperior calcaneal tuberosity, excised diseased tendon and any avulsed bone, and used either transosseous bone tunnels or suture anchors for repair.
   - FHL transfer is recommended when more than 50% of the width of the Achilles tendon insertion is débrided intraoperatively.

   b. Results of repair have been favorable with high patient satisfaction and good clinical outcomes in both high-level athletes and the general population.

G. Chronic (>3 months) midsubstance Achilles ruptures

1. Pathoanatomy—Missed or neglected ruptures are diagnosed the same way as an acute tear.
2. Evaluation
   a. Physical examination findings are more subtle in the chronic setting.
   - Less swelling is evident, the palpable gap is less apparent, and the Thompson test may be more equivocal.
   - Resting equinus in the prone position will often be asymmetric.
   - Calf atrophy with weakness is more likely in the chronic setting than in the acute setting.
   - Patients will exhibit increased ankle dorsiflexion on the affected side due to overlengthening of the Achilles complex.

   b. The diagnosis is clinical, but MRI or ultrasonography aids in verification and localization of the tendon ends.
3. Treatment
   a. Nonsurgical treatment consists of physical therapy and an ankle-foot orthosis (AFO), which may be articulated but should include a dorsiflexion stop.
   b. A primary repair can be attempted up to 3 months from the original injury.
   - Surgical repair after 3 months consists of a reconstruction, including a turndown procedure or V-Y advancement (**Figure 3**) for defects less than 4 cm, versus augmentation for defects greater than 5 cm of the existing tendon, and/or tendon transfers (FHL/FDL/PB) after excision of the degenerative tendon ends.
   - Wound healing issues remains the most common complication of any of the surgical procedures because of the extensive surgical incision.

II. TIBIALIS POSTERIOR TENDON DISORDERS

A. Anatomy

1. The tibialis posterior muscle is innervated by the posterior tibial nerve (L4-L5) and originates from the posterior fibula, tibia, and interosseous membrane.

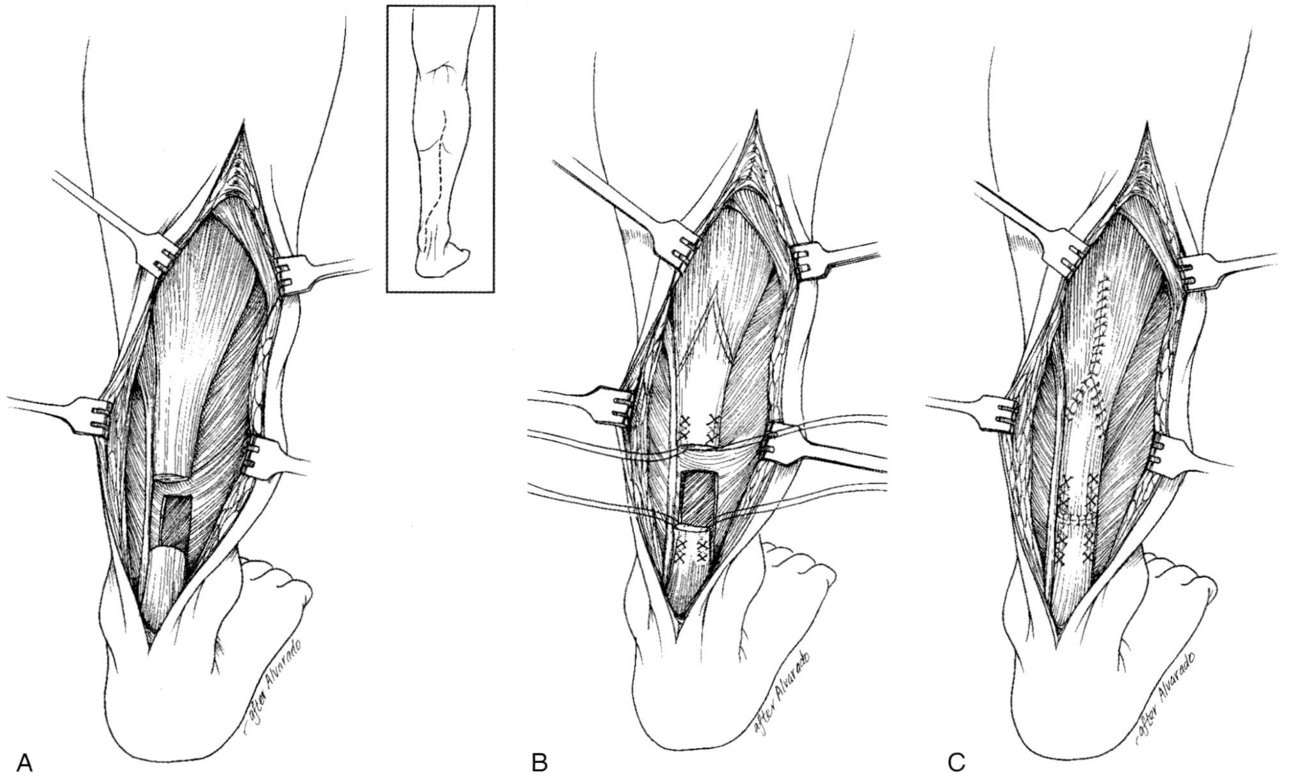

Figure 3 Illustrations demonstrate technique for V-Y lengthening of the triceps surae. **A**, A medial incision is extended proximally in a gently curving S (inset). The tendon ends are débrided, and the repair site is prepared by windowing the deep posterior fascia. **B**, A V cut is made in the triceps surae aponeurosis. **C**, After approximation of the tendon ends, the aponeurosis is closed. (Reproduced from Saltzman CL, Tearse DS: Achilles tendon injuries. *J Am Acad Orthop Surg* 1998;6[5]:316-325.)

2. The tendon travels distally, running posterior to the medial malleolus before dividing into three limbs.
    a. The anterior limb inserts into the tuberosity of the navicular and the first cuneiform.
    b. The middle limb inserts into the second and third cuneiforms, the cuboid, and second through fifth metatarsals.
    c. The posterior limb inserts on the sustentaculum tali anteriorly.
3. The tibialis posterior tendon lies in an axis posterior to the ankle joint and medial to the axis of the subtalar joint. It acts as an invertor of the hindfoot and adducts and supinates the forefoot during the stance phase of gait. It also acts as a secondary plantar flexor of the ankle.
4. Activation of the tibialis posterior tendon allows locking of the transverse tarsal joints, creating a rigid lever arm for the toe-off phase of gait. It also contracts eccentrically during the stance phase to diminish forces on the supporting ligaments of the medial arch (spring ligament).
5. The major antagonist to the tibialis posterior tendon is the PB.
6. The normal excursion of the tendon is relatively small (2 cm).

B. Classification—The stage (from I to IV) of tibialis posterior tendon dysfunction is assigned by assessing pain, deformity, flexibility, the ability to perform a single-limb heel rise, subtalar arthritis, and ankle valgus (**Table 3**).

C. Pathoanatomy
1. Tibialis posterior tendon dysfunction is the most common cause of an adult acquired flatfoot deformity.
2. The exact etiology is unknown, but the disease is found more commonly in obese women in the sixth decade of life and those with inflammatory arthropathy.
3. Degeneration of the tendon occurs in the watershed region, distal to the medial malleolus.

TABLE 3

Staging of Posterior Tibial Tendon Dysfunction

Stage	Pain	Deformity	Flexibility	Ability to Perform Single-Limb Heel Rise	Subtalar Arthritis	Ankle Valgus
I	Medial	Absent	Normal	Yes	No	No
II[a]	Medial and/or lateral	Pes planovalgus	Normal	Difficult or unable	No	No
III	Medial and/or lateral	Pes planovalgus	Decreased or fixed	Unable	Possible	No
IV	Medial and/or lateral	Pes planovalgus	Decreased or fixed	Unable	Possible	Yes

[a]In stage IIa, there is a lack of significant forefoot abduction (defined as talar head uncoverage<40%); in stage IIb, there is significant forefoot abduction (defined as talar head uncoverage≥40%).

4. The presence of an accessory navicular has a high correlation with developing posterior tibial tendon dysfunction.
   a. Type 1: Sesamoid bone in substance of tendon
   b. Type 2: Separate accessory bone attached to native navicular through a synchondrosis
   c. Type 3: Bony enlargement of the native navicular

D. Evaluation

1. Classic findings of prolonged involvement (**Figure 4**)
   a. Collapse of the medial longitudinal arch
   b. Hindfoot valgus
   c. Forefoot abduction and varus (the "too many toes" sign)
   d. Achilles/gastrocnemius contracture
      - Differentiate Achilles and gastrocnemius soleus contracture using the Silfverskiold test, which is based on the fact that the gastrocnemius crosses the knee and ankle, but the soleus does not.
        - If contracture is similar with knee extended and flexed (<10° difference), Silfverskiold test is negative and Achilles lengthening is appropriate
        - If contracture is worse with knee extended than flexed (≥10° difference), Silfverskiold test is positive and isolated gastrocnemius recession is preferred over an Achilles lengthening
2. Earlier stages are associated with varied degrees of physical findings.

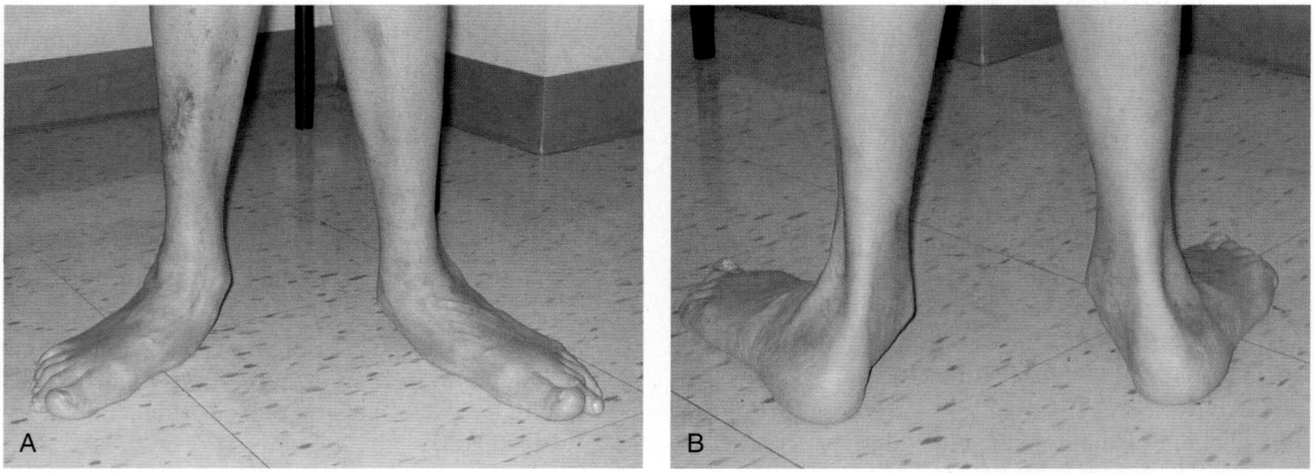

Figure 4 Anterior (**A**) and posterior (**B**) photographs show a patient with long-standing tibialis posterior tendon insufficiency. Note the classic physical findings: a collapsed medial longitudinal arch, hindfoot valgus, forefoot abduction, and varus (the "too many toes" sign).

3. In the later stages, the hindfoot and/or forefoot deformity may become fixed.
4. The patient also loses the ability to perform a single-limb heel rise for two reasons:
   a. Inability to lock the transverse tarsal joints to create a rigid lever arm
   b. Valgus displacement of the calcaneus that results in a weakened Achilles tendon moment arm
5. Plain radiographs reveal
   a. Loss of the Meary (talar–first metatarsal) angle
   b. Loss of calcaneal pitch
   c. Variable degrees of peritalar subluxation
   d. Talonavicular under coverage angle (**Figure 5**)
6. MRI demonstrates varied degrees of degenerative changes in the tendon and in the talonavicular, subtalar, and tibiotalar joints.
7. Ultrasonographic evaluation has gained an increasing role in evaluating pathology within the tibialis posterior tendon.

E. Treatment

1. Nonsurgical treatment is possible at any stage.
   a. After an initial period of immobilization, a custom-molded in-shoe orthosis or hindfoot stabilizing orthosis UCBL (University of California Biomechanics Laboratory–type with medial posting), a double upright AFO, and physical therapy have been shown to be effective in treating stage I and II disease.
   b. Stage III and IV disease requires bracing treatment that crosses the ankle (AFO, Marzano or Arizona brace). Nonsurgical treatment of stage III and IV disease is reserved for patients who cannot tolerate surgical intervention and those who are sedentary or low demand.
2. Surgical—If nonsurgical treatment fails, surgery is indicated. Surgical options depend on the stage of the disease. An Achilles tendon or gastrocnemius lengthening may be performed concomitantly in any stage when a contracture is present.
   a. A symptomatic accessory navicular without development of a flatfoot deformity can be treated with isolated excision of the accessory navicular and advancement of the posterior tibial tendon.
   b. Stage I disease should be treated with a tenosynovectomy.

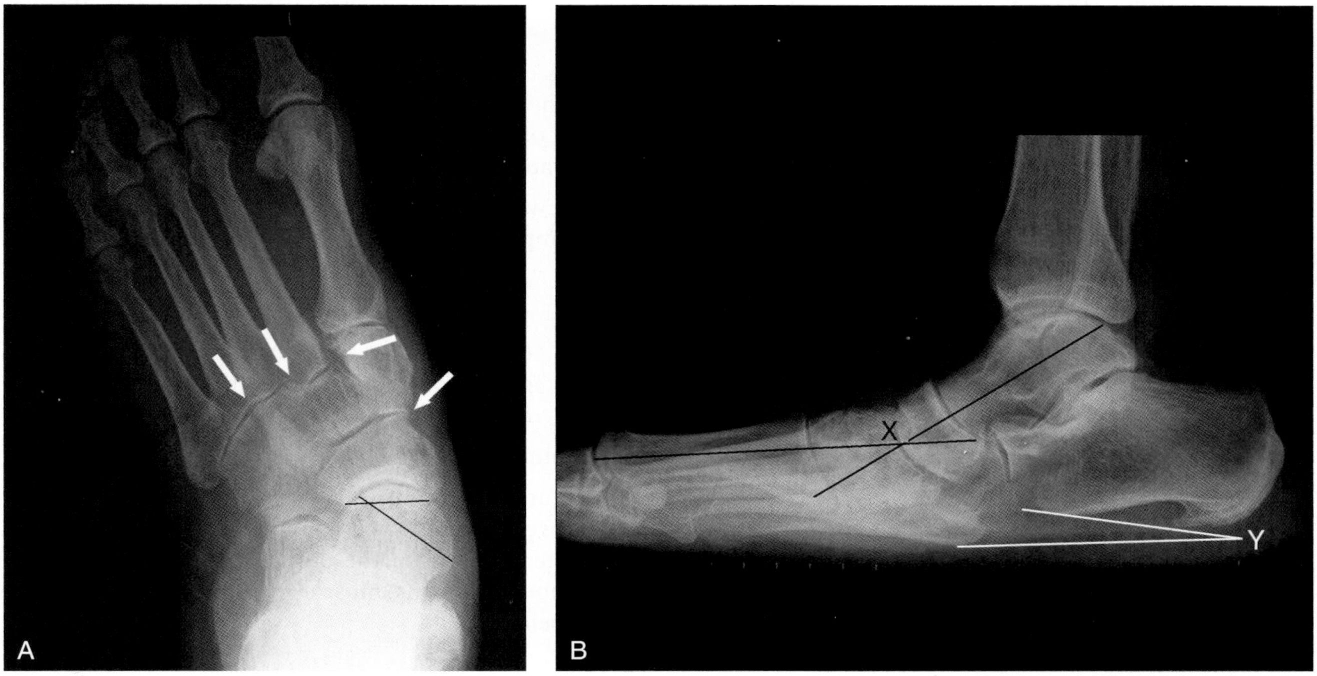

Figure 5 Tibialis posterior tendon dysfunction. **A,** Weight-bearing AP radiograph of the foot shows peritalar subluxation. Note the loss of the expected parallel lines of the talonavicular coverage angle. Also note the forefoot abduction and the associated degenerative changes of the adjacent metatarsal-cuneiform and cuneiform-navicular joints (arrows). **B,** Weight-bearing lateral radiograph of the foot shows loss of parallelism between the talus and first metatarsal (X), as well as almost completely absent calcaneal pitch (Y).

c. Stage II
   - Stage IIa: Typically a combination of a tendon transfer and a bony realignment procedure
     - The posterior tibial tendon is débrided and, if viable (excursion), may be utilized to supplement the tendon transfer
     - Most commonly an FDL tendon transfer, but FHL has also been used.
     - Medial displacement calcaneal osteotomy.
   - Stage IIb: To correct the forefoot abduction, typically a lateral column lengthening is added to the treatments for stage IIa, most commonly in the form of an Evans opening wedge osteotomy of the anterior process of the calcaneus
   - Finally, using a flat plate to simulate weight bearing intraoperatively after hindfoot corrections evaluate for forefoot varus/supination. If present, addition of plantar flexion into first ray is required:
     - If medial column is stable (metatarsal and navicular are colinear on lateral radiograph), then add Cotton osteotomy (opening wedge dorsal osteotomy of the first cuneiform).
     - If medial column is unstable (plantar sag at naviculocuneiform or first tarsometatarsal joint), then perform medial column fusion (tarsometatarsal and/or naviculocuneiform fusion depending on the apex of deformity).
   - Consideration for a spring ligament reconstruction to be used as a supplement.

d. Stage III disease is treated with a hindfoot arthrodesis, most commonly a triple arthrodesis. Recent literature supports limited arthrodesis of the talonavicular and subtalar joints in patients with deformity but an uninvolved calcaneocuboid joint.

e. Limited scientific data are available to guide treatment of stage IV disease. When the tibiotalar joint is preserved, hindfoot arthrodesis with a deltoid reconstruction has been reported as a treatment option. Alternatively, with tibiotalar arthritis in stage IV disease, reported options include a pantalar arthrodesis versus a hindfoot arthrodesis/reconstruction followed by a total ankle arthroplasty.

III. DISORDERS OF THE PERONEAL TENDONS

A. Anatomy

1. The peroneus longus (PL) and PB tendons are innervated by the superficial peroneal nerve (S1) and originate from the fibula and interosseous membrane.
2. The tendons run in a sulcus called the peroneal groove formed posteriorly in the fibula, and are further stabilized by a fibrocartilaginous rim and the superior peroneal retinaculum (SPR).
   a. Within the groove, the PB tendon is anterior and medial to the PL tendon.
   b. Both tendons curve anteriorly around the tip of the fibula, with the peroneal tubercle separating the two tendons at the level of the calcaneus.
   c. The PB tendon then runs distally to insert onto the tuberosity of the fifth metatarsal.
   d. The PL tendon makes a 90° turn medially at the cuboid groove before inserting into the base of the first metatarsal and medial cuneiform.
3. The primary function of the peroneal tendons, particularly the PB is to evert the hindfoot. In addition, they both secondarily plantarflex the ankle and the PL plantarflexes (pronates) the first ray.
4. A vascular watershed region just posterior to the fibula is the most common area of injury. Compression from the PL on the PB is also implicated in this region.
5. Two important anatomic variations have been implicated in tendon tears and instability:
   a. A low-lying PB muscle belly
   b. The presence of a peroneus quartus muscle (13% to 22%), which also may be seen in the groove and contributes to crowding of the fibro-osseous tunnel

B. Acute tendinitis

1. Pathoanatomy—Acute tendinitis may result from overuse, predisposition from a varus hindfoot, or stenosis within the peroneal tunnel from a peroneus quartus muscle or low-lying PB muscle belly.
2. Evaluation
   a. Patients report swelling and pain in the lateral hindfoot/ankle.

b. Physical examination reveals swelling and pain with palpation and may reveal reduced strength.

c. MRI reveals fluid within the peroneal tendon sheath.

3. Treatment

a. Initial treatment

- A short period of immobilization (cast or boot)
- NSAIDs
- Ice
- A lateral heel wedge for mild heel varus
- Physical therapy

b. Conditions that do not respond to nonsurgical measures are treated with tenosynovectomy.

C. Tendon tears or ruptures

1. Pathoanatomy

a. Tears may be the result of inversion injuries or injury causing tendon subluxation or dislocation.

- Most tendon tears occur in the PB tendon, at the level of the fibular groove.
- Less common are tears of the PL tendon, which usually occur at the peroneal tubercle.
- The PB and PL tendon tears are often longitudinal in the tendon and typically are seen in chronic situations.

b. Etiologic factors

- Compression of the PB between the PL tendon and the posterior fibula
- Subluxation/dislocation of the tendons
- Diminished blood supply (watershed region)
- Acute change in direction around the fibula
- Ankle instability/varus heel

2. Evaluation

a. Symptoms are similar to those of tendinitis.

b. Physical examination results are also similar, but subluxation or dislocation also may be provoked during examination with eversion against resistance.

c. MRI reveals longitudinal tears in the tendon, but these can be confused with a peroneus quartus muscle.

3. Treatment

a. Nonsurgical—Initial nonsurgical treatment is the same as for acute tendinitis. The success rate is poor.

b. Surgical—Patients in whom nonsurgical treatment fails are candidates for surgery.

- Acute partial rupture
  - Débridement and repair of the tear.
  - Tenodesis to the healthy tendon if ruptured or if more than 50% of the affected tendon is abnormal.
  - If heel varus is present, a lateral slide calcaneal osteotomy can be added to the procedure.
- Complete rupture
  - Complete rupture is rare.
  - The patient presents with severe limitation of eversion strength.
  - Treatment in the acute setting is an end-to-end repair.
- Chronic disease
  - One healthy and one unhealthy tendon: Tenodesis unhealthy tendon to healthy tendon.
  - Both tendons unhealthy:
    - Peroneal excursion present: Allograft tendon interposition
    - Peroneal excursion absent: Single stage flexor tendon transfer (FHL and FDL are both options but FHL may be superior donor given greater relative work capacity and closer proximity)

D. Dislocation/subluxation of the tendons

1. Pathoanatomy

a. A shallow peroneal groove and overcrowding of the fibular groove are predisposing factors.

b. Dislocation or subluxation occurs during an inversion injury to a dorsiflexed ankle with rapid reflexive contraction of the PL and PB tendons. A disruption of the SPR or fibrocartilage ridge results.

c. Acute longitudinal tendon tears also may occur in this setting.

d. Patients describe a "pop" or snapping sensation, followed by pain and swelling.

2. Evaluation

a. Physical examination reveals variable pain and swelling depending on the acuteness of the injury. Dislocation or subluxation may be elicited with ankle rotation or with forcing the foot from a position of inversion and plantar flexion to a position of eversion and dorsiflexion.

b. Radiographs may reveal an avulsion fracture of the distal fibula (rim fracture) at the insertion of the SPR. The diagnosis is clinical; additional studies are often not needed.

3. Treatment

a. Consideration of treatment of acute injuries with cast immobilization to allow the SPR to heal; however, results typically have been poor. In high-level athletes or active individuals, acute SPR repair, with or without a groove-deepening procedure, is a reasonable option.

b. Chronic injuries require a tendon débridement/repair/reconstruction and SPR repair with or without a groove-deepening procedure (**Figure 6**).

IV. TIBIALIS ANTERIOR TENDON DISORDERS

A. Overview

1. The tibialis anterior muscle is innervated by the deep peroneal nerve (L4) and originates primarily from the anterolateral tibia.

2. The tibialis anterior tendon passes underneath the superior and inferior extensor retinaculum and inserts on the medial aspect of the base of the first metatarsal and medial cuneiform.

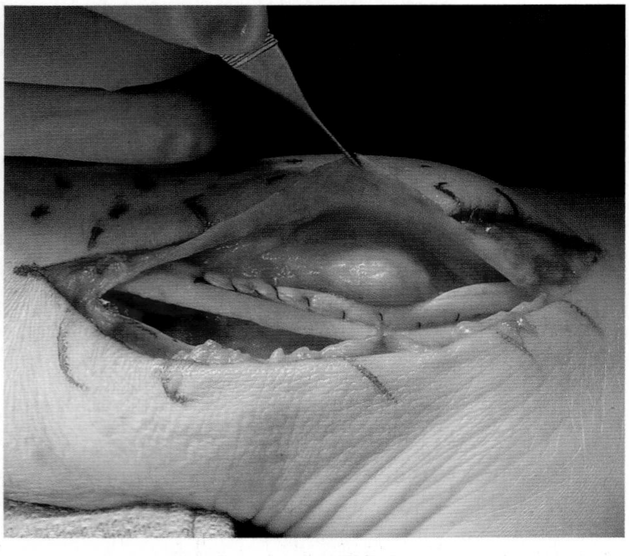

Figure 6 Intraoperative photograph shows a chronic peroneal tendon dislocation. Note the fibrotic and thickened paratenon and superior peroneal retinaculum (held by the Adson forceps) that is not adherent to the fibula at this level. Also note the repair of the peroneus brevis tendon with a running suture tubularizing the remaining tendon.

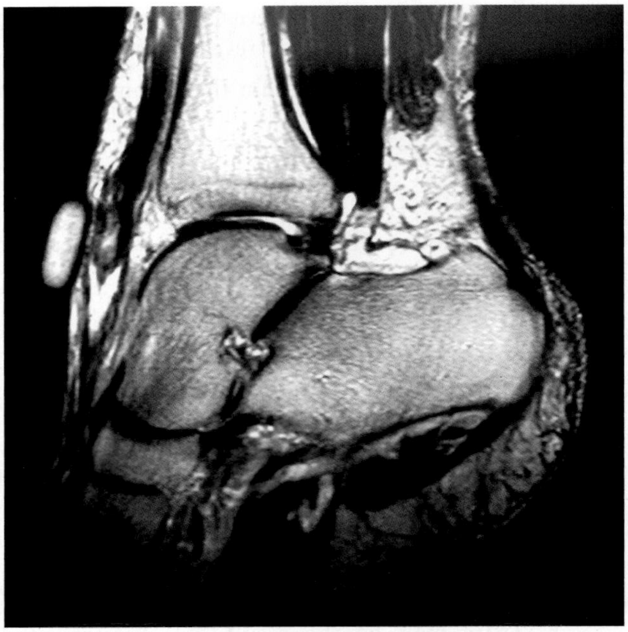

Figure 7 Sagittal T1-weighted MRI shows the "empty sheath" of a retracted ruptured tibialis anterior tendon (marked by a gel tablet).

3. It acts as the primary dorsiflexor of the ankle and also inverts the hindfoot.

4. The muscle dorsiflexes the foot in preparation for heel strike during the late swing phase of gait and eccentrically contracts after heel strike to slow progression to foot flat.

B. Laceration or rupture

1. Pathoanatomy

a. The most common types of tendon pathology include lacerations and closed ruptures (**Figure 7**).

b. Closed ruptures are the result of either strong eccentric contraction in younger individuals or attritional ruptures in older patients with diabetes, inflammatory arthritis, or previous local steroid injection.

2. Evaluation

a. Patients with chronic tibialis anterior tendon injuries report difficulty in clearing the foot during gait.

b. In the acute setting, the patient reports a "pop" followed by swelling in the anterior ankle.

c. Physical examination reveals swelling anteriorly in the acute setting, but this may be minimal in the chronic setting.

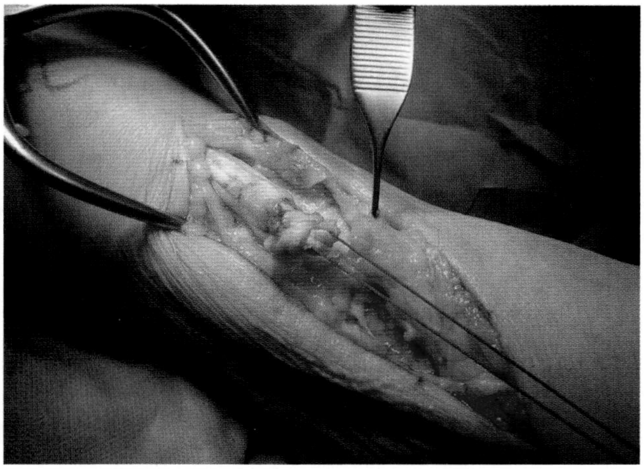

Figure 8 Intraoperative photograph shows a ruptured tibialis anterior tendon secured with a grasping stitch before repair.

d. A steppage pattern gait similar to footdrop is observed.

e. Weakness in dorsiflexion and the lack of a palpable tendon during resisted dorsiflexion are also seen on physical examination.

3. Treatment

a. Complete ruptures

- In the acute setting, an end-to-end repair is performed if the tendon is normal.
- The injury is typically an avulsion from the tendon insertion and may require suture anchors or bone tunnels for appropriate fixation (**Figure 8**).
- In the low-demand patient, benign neglect or bracing treatment with an AFO is acceptable.
- Débridement, V-Y lengthening, and repair are best if a healthy tendon is available to repair.
- To restore active dorsiflexion to the ankle in the setting of an insufficient tibialis anterior tendon in chronic rupture or attritional disease, free allograft interposition if good muscle excursion remains or extensor hallucis longus (EHL) tenodesis if muscle excursion is limited.

b. Partial ruptures or lacerations can be treated with casting alone.

V. FLEXOR HALLUCIS LONGUS TENDON DISORDERS

A. Anatomy

1. The FHL muscle is innervated by the posterior tibial nerve (S1) and originates from the posterior fibula.

2. The FHL tendon runs through a fibro-osseous tunnel posterior to the hindfoot formed by the posterolateral and posteromedial tubercles of the talus. The FHL tendon then travels underneath the sustentaculum tali and within the foot and crosses dorsal to the FDL at the knot of Henry. Multiple interconnections exist between the FHL and FDL tendons. Distally, the FHL tendon remains dorsal to the FDL tendon and neurovascular bundle and inserts onto the distal phalanx of the great toe.

3. The function of the muscle is primarily to plantarflex the interphalangeal (IP) and metatarsophalangeal joints of the great toe and secondarily to plantarflex the ankle.

B. Acute laceration

1. Pathoanatomy—Acute laceration is the most common form of FHL tendon injury.

2. Evaluation

a. Physical examination reveals a loss of active IP joint flexion.

b. MRI can confirm retracted ends of the tendon in equivocal cases.

3. The treatment

a. The treatment of isolated lacerations is controversial.

b. Repair is indicated in combined laceration of the FHL and flexor hallucis brevis.

C. Tenosynovitis

1. Pathoanatomy

a. Stenosing tenosynovitis commonly occurs in the fibro-osseous tunnel posterior to the talus.

- In patients with chronic tenosynovitis, a nodule may form, which causes triggering.
- Stenosing tenosynovitis is most common in dancers and gymnasts (activities involving maximal plantar flexion).

b. Tenosynovitis may coexist with posterior ankle impingement and the finding of an os trigonum.

2. Evaluation

a. Symptoms include posteromedial ankle pain and triggering or crepitus.

b. Physical examination reveals pain with resisted IP joint flexion and triggering with active or passive range of motion. Forceful plantar flexion also may elicit pain by recreating posterior ankle impingement.

c. MRI may demonstrate fluid around the tendon and/or signal change within the tendon.

3. Treatment
   a. Nonsurgical
      - Initial treatment is nonsurgical.
      - It includes relative rest, ice, NSAIDs, and physical therapy.
   b. Surgical
      - If symptoms persist, surgery may be performed.
      - Surgical procedures include surgical release, tenosynovectomy and/or débridement, and tendon repair.

VI. EXTENSOR DIGITORUM LONGUS AND EXTENSOR HALLUCIS LONGUS TENDON DISORDERS

A. Anatomy
1. The extensor digitorum longus (EDL) and EHL tendons are both innervated by the deep peroneal nerve (L5).
2. The tendons travel underneath the superior and inferior extensor retinaculum before inserting onto the base of the distal phalanx of the respective toes.

B. Pathoanatomy
1. The superficial location of the EDL and EHL tendons predisposes them to lacerations and closed rupture, although the latter is extremely rare. Rupture is either attritional or a result of high-energy eccentric contraction.
2. Attritional ruptures have been reported in
   a. Middle-aged patients
   b. Patients with repetitive microtrauma
   c. Patients who have received previous steroid injections

C. Evaluation—Physical examination reveals an inability to extend the IP joints of the toes actively.

D. Treatment
1. Acute EHL lacerations that are proximal to the extensor hood should undergo an end-to-end repair.
2. Partial lacerations or lacerations at or distal to the extensor hood may be treated closed, with immobilization of the hallux in extension.
3. Chronic EHL injuries or acute attritional ruptures can be treated with the following:
   a. Débridement and repair
   b. Free tendon grafting
   c. Tenodesis to a healthy extensor tendon
4. Treatment of EDL injuries is controversial.
   a. Repair is more commonly done in younger, active individuals.
   b. Authors who favor repair cite preventing future formation of a claw toe deformity as the rationale for surgery.

TOP TESTING FACTS

1. A vascular watershed region in the Achilles tendon is found 2 to 6 cm above the calcaneal insertion. This is the typical location of a majority of Achilles tendon pathology, particularly acute ruptures.
2. Acute Achilles tendinitis is typically associated with younger, more active patients, whereas patients with chronic Achilles tendinosis are typically older and more sedentary.
3. Skin problems (eg, infection, necrosis, and adhesions) are the most common complications associated with the surgical treatment of Achilles tendon disorders.
4. Functional rehabilitation is a reasonable choice for the management of acute noninsertional Achilles ruptures, not just among the sedentary or elderly, but even among young, healthy, active individuals.
5. The tibialis posterior tendon acts primarily as an invertor of the hindfoot and supinator of the forefoot during the stance phase of gait. Activation of the tibialis posterior tendon during the toe-off phase of gait locks the transverse tarsal joints, thus creating a rigid lever arm for push off.
6. Tibialis posterior tendon dysfunction is the most common cause of an adult acquired flatfoot deformity. Collapse of the medial longitudinal arch, hindfoot valgus, and forefoot abduction is the classic triad of foot deformity associated with tibialis posterior tendon insufficiency. The "too many toes" sign and the inability to perform a single-limb heel rise are additional classic findings of tibialis posterior tendon insufficiency.
7. Nonsurgical treatment for tibialis posterior tendon dysfunction consists of a UCBL-type orthosis for stage II disease and an AFO or Marzano or Arizona brace for stage III or IV disease.

8. Surgical treatment of stage II disease consists most commonly of FDL transfer in conjunction with a bony procedure, most commonly a medial calcaneal displacement osteotomy or a lateral column lengthening, while surgical treatment of stage III disease is a hindfoot arthrodesis, most commonly a triple arthrodesis.
9. Complete ruptures of the peroneal tendons are rare; tears are often longitudinal in the tendon and typically seen in chronic situations. Most peroneal tendon tears are in the PB tendon at the level of the fibular groove. They often are caused by inversion injuries and chronic compression from the PL.
10. Patients with chronic peroneal tendon injuries are treated with tenodesis to the healthy tendon or transfer of the FHL when both tendons are involved.
11. Dislocation or subluxation occurs during an inversion injury to a dorsiflexed ankle with rapid reflexive contraction of the PL and PB tendons. A disruption of the SPR or fibrocartilage ridge results.
12. Closed tibialis anterior tendon ruptures are either the result of strong eccentric contraction in younger individuals or attritional ruptures in older patients with musculoskeletal compromise.
13. The FHL runs through its fibro-osseous tunnel, lateral to the posteromedial tubercle of the talus, under the sustentaculum tali and through the knot of Henry, before inserting onto the base of the proximal phalanx of the great toe. Stenosing tenosynovitis of the FHL commonly occurs in the fibro-osseous tunnel posterior to the talus. It is most common in dancers and gymnasts and may coexist with posterior ankle impingement and the presence of an os trigonum.

Bibliography

Carr AJ, Norris SH: The blood supply of the calcaneal tendon. *J Bone Joint Surg Br* 1989;71(1):100-101.

Chadwick C, Whitehouse SL, Saxby TS: Long-term follow-up of flexor digitorum longus transfer and calcaneal osteotomy for stage II posterior tibial tendon dysfunction. *Bone Joint J* 2015;97-B(3):346-352.

Cho J, Kim JY, Song DG, Lee WC: Comparison of outcome after retinaculum repair with and without fibular groove deepening for recurrent dislocation of the peroneal tendons. *Foot Ankle Int* 2014;35(7):683-689.

Frey C, Shereff M, Greenidge N: Vascularity of the posterior tibial tendon. *J Bone Joint Surg Am* 1990;72(6):884-888.

Harkin E, Pinzur M, Schiff A: Treatment of acute and chronic tibialis anterior tendon rupture and tendinopathy. *Foot Ankle Clin* 2017;22(4):819-831.

Jockel JR, Brodsky JW: Single-stage flexor tendon transfer for the treatment of severe concomitant peroneus longus and brevis tendon tears. *Foot Ankle Int* 2013;34(5):666-672.

Khan RJ, Fick D, Keogh A, Crawford J, Brammar T, Parker M: Treatment of acute achilles tendon ruptures: A meta-analysis of randomized, controlled trials. *J Bone Joint Surg Am* 2005;87(10):2202-2210.

Lever CJ, Bosman HA, Robinson AH: The functional and dynamometer-tested results of transtendinous flexor hallucis longus transfer for neglected ruptures of the Achilles tendon at six years' follow-up. *Bone Joint J* 2018;100-B(5):584-589.

Lim CS, Lees D, Gwynne-Jones DP: Functional outcome of acute achilles tendon rupture with and without operative treatment using identical functional bracing protocol. *Foot Ankle Int* 2017;38(12):1331-1336.

Myerson MS: Achilles tendon ruptures. *Instr Course Lect* 1999;48:219-230.

Pellegrini MJ, Glisson RR, Matsumoto T, et al: Effectiveness of allograft reconstruction vs tenodesis for irreparable peroneus brevis tears: A cadaveric model. *Foot Ankle Int* 2016;37(8):803-808.

Petersen W, Bobka T, Stein V, Tillmann B: Blood supply of the peroneal tendons: Injection and immunohistochemical studies of cadaver tendons. *Acta Orthop Scand* 2000;71(2):168-174.

Puddu G, Ippolito E, Postacchini F: A classification of Achilles tendon disease. *Am J Sports Med* 1976;4(4):145-150.

Röhm J, Zwicky L, Horn Lang T, Salentiny Y, Hintermann B, Knupp M: Mid- to long-term outcome of 96 corrective hindfoot fusions in 84 patients with rigid flatfoot deformity. *Bone Joint J* 2015;97-B(5):668-674.

Romanelli DA, Almekinders LC, Mandelbaum BR: Achilles ruptures in the athlete: Current science and treatment. *Sports Med Arthrosc* 2000;8:377-386.

Sammarco GJ, Cooper PS: Flexor hallucis longus tendon injury in dancers and nondancers. *Foot Ankle Int* 1998;19(6):356-362.

Sammarco VJ, Magur EG, Sammarco GJ, Bagwe MR: Arthrodesis of the subtalar and talonavicular joints for correction of symptomatic hindfoot malalignment. *Foot Ankle Int* 2006;27(9):661-666.

Schipper ON, Anderson RB, Cohen BE: Outcomes after primary repair of insertional ruptures of the achilles tendon. *Foot Ankle Int* 2018;39(6):664-668.

Sobel M, Geppert MJ, Olson EJ, Bohne WH, Arnoczky SP: The dynamics of peroneus brevis tendon splits: A proposed mechanism, technique of diagnosis, and classification of injury. *Foot Ankle* 1992;13(7):413-422.

Steginsky B, Riley A, Lucas DE, Philbin TM, Berlet GC: Patient-reported outcomes and return to activity after peroneus brevis repair. *Foot Ankle Int* 2016;37(2):178-185.

Wilcox DK, Bohay DR, Anderson JG: Treatment of chronic achilles tendon disorders with flexor hallucis longus tendon transfer/augmentation. *Foot Ankle Int* 2000;21(12):1004-1010.

Willits K, Amendola A, Bryant D, et al: Operative versus nonoperative treatment of acute achilles tendon ruptures: A multicenter randomized trial using accelerated functional rehabilitation. *J Bone Joint Surg Am* 2010;92(17):2767-2775.

Wong JC, Daniel JN, Raikin SM: Repair of acute extensor hallucis longus tendon injuries: A retrospective review. *Foot Ankle Spec* 2014;7(1):45-51.

Chapter 116
HEEL PAIN

DAVID R. RICHARDSON, MD
E. GREER RICHARDSON, MD

I. OVERVIEW AND EPIDEMIOLOGY

A. General characteristics—Heel pain (subcalcaneal pain syndrome) is the most common foot-related symptom leading patients to seek medical care for the feet.

B. Epidemiology
   1. Heel pain may occur at any age. The peak incidence occurs between ages 40 and 60 years.
   2. Middle-aged women appear to have the highest incidence of heel pain.
   3. Race and ethnicity play no role in this entity.
   4. Stress fractures are more common in women than in men; they are also more common in military recruits than in the general population.

C. Etiology—Heel pain has various etiologies, including trauma, disease, and the degenerative processes of aging.

D. Evaluation
   1. History and physical examination
      a. The history and physical examination are extremely important when evaluating heel pain because imaging and laboratory studies may be of limited value.
      b. The foot should be examined for the point of maximal tenderness (**Figure 1**).
   2. Differential diagnosis (**Table 1**)
      a. Plantar fasciitis is the most common cause of heel pain.
      b. Calcaneal stress fracture, entrapment of the first branch of the lateral plantar nerve and fat pad atrophy, also should be high in the differential. Tarsal tunnel syndrome may also cause heel pain. This will be discussed in a subsequent chapter.
      c. A high index of suspicion is needed to diagnose the less common causes of heel pain syndrome, such as tumor or infection.
      d. Heel pain in the elderly and patients with atypical presentations should be investigated to rule out insufficiency fractures and tumors.

Dr. Richardson or an immediate family member serves as a board member, owner, officer, or committee member of the American Academy of Orthopaedic Surgeons. Neither Dr. E. Greer Richardson nor any immediate family member has received anything of value from or has stock or stock options held in a commercial company or institution related directly or indirectly to the subject of this chapter.

II. PLANTAR FASCIITIS

A. Overview and epidemiology
   1. Females 45 to 64 years old have the highest incidence of plantar fasciitis.
   2. Risk factors include limited ankle dorsiflexion due to tightness of the Achilles tendon, obesity (body mass index >30), and prolonged weight bearing.

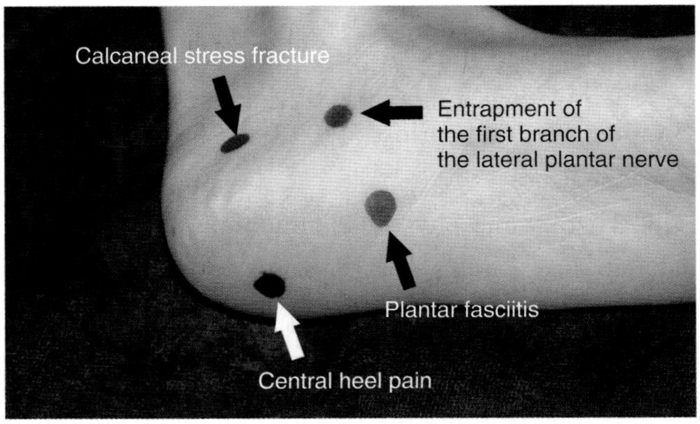

Figure 1 Clinical photograph shows the points of maximal tenderness in relation to the most common causes of heel pain. The foot is shown with the toes to the right and the medial aspect of the foot and ankle at the top.

8 | Foot and Ankle

TABLE 1

Differential Diagnosis of Heel Pain

Plantar fasciitis
Plantar fascia rupture
Fat pad atrophy
Fat pad contusion
Calcaneal stress fracture
Entrapment of the first branch of the lateral plantar nerve
Calcaneal apophysitis (Sever disease)
Tumor (eg, osteoid osteoma)
Tarsal tunnel syndrome
Gout
Inflammatory arthropathies (eg, psoriatic arthritis)
Spondyloarthropathies (eg, Reiter syndrome)
Infection
Radiculopathy
Paget disease
Neuropathy
Foreign body reaction

3. Plantar fasciitis also may be associated with anatomic variations (eg, pes planus, pes cavus, or excessive femoral anteversion).
4. A heel pain triad of tibialis posterior tendon dysfunction, plantar fasciitis, and tarsal tunnel syndrome has been described.
5. Although 50% of patients with plantar fasciitis have a plantar heel spur, typically located in the origin of the flexor hallucis brevis, heel spurs are not considered the cause of heel pain in such patients.

B. Pathogenesis—The etiology of plantar fasciitis is repetitive microtrauma to the plantar fascia causing microtears and periostitis.

C. Evaluation

1. History and physical examination
   a. The patient with plantar fasciitis will most often report "start-up" inferior heel pain and may prefer to walk on the toes for the first few steps.
   b. The pain usually lessens with ambulation and then increases with activity, especially on hard surfaces.
   c. A traumatic tear of the plantar fascia may occur in the midfoot region.
   d. The point of maximal tenderness is located at the proximal medial origin of the plantar fascia (**Figure 1**).
   e. Palpation of the plantar fascia with the toes and ankle in dorsiflexion increases the sensitivity of the examination.
   f. The ankle should be examined for tightness of the Achilles tendon.
2. Imaging and other studies
   a. Radiographs—Weight-bearing lateral and axial views of the hindfoot may be used to assess for arthritic changes, structural abnormalities, or bony pathology. They are not necessary on the initial visit.
   b. A bone scan may help quantitate inflammation and guide treatment.
   c. CT is not necessary.
   d. MRI may be beneficial before surgical release.
   e. Laboratory studies are not necessary unless other etiologies are suspected (eg, inflammatory arthritis, infection).

D. Treatment

1. Nonsurgical
   a. NSAIDs, stretching exercises (weight bearing and non–weight bearing), night splints, over-the-counter heel cups, and reduced activity all may be used initially.
   b. A non–weight-bearing, plantar fascia–specific stretching exercise program (**Figure 2**) and Achilles tendon stretching appear to be more effective than the traditional program of weight-bearing Achilles tendon stretching exercises.
   c. A short leg cast worn for 8 to 10 weeks may be necessary.
   d. Corticosteroid injections should be used sparingly because they may increase the risk for plantar fascia rupture or fat pad atrophy.
   e. The FDA has approved the use of electrohydraulic and electromagnetic extracorporeal shock wave therapy for chronic plantar heel pain that lasts longer than 6 months and when other treatment options have failed; however, the efficacy of such therapy remains controversial. It is a safe treatment option, with several studies supporting its use and showing improvement in patients' pain scales.

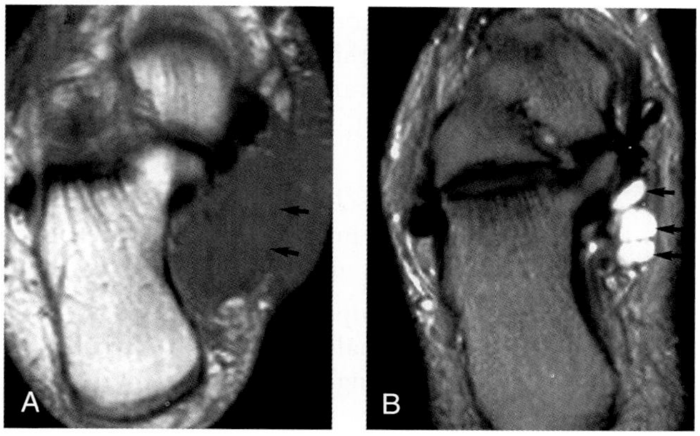

Figure 4 Space-occupying lesions of the tarsal tunnel. **A**, T1-weighted axial magnetic resonance image demonstrates an area of intermediate signal intensity (arrows) within the tarsal tunnel, representing a lymphoma. **B**, T2-weighted axial magnetic resonance image demonstrates a multiseptate area of high signal intensity (arrows) within the tarsal tunnel, representing a ganglion. (Reproduced from Recht MP, Donley BG: Magnetic resonance imaging of the foot and ankle. *J Am Acad Orthop Surg* 2001; 9[3]:187-199.)

b. Immobilization in a removable boot or cast is recommended after steroid injections to prevent iatrogenic rupture of the tibialis posterior tendon.

c. Off-the-shelf or custom orthoses may be beneficial if mechanical malalignment is present.

2. Surgical—Patients in whom nonsurgical treatment has failed are candidates for surgical decompression.

a. Procedure

- The tibial nerve should be identified proximal to the tarsal tunnel and decompressed, including releasing the flexor retinaculum.
- The medial plantar, lateral plantar, and medial calcaneal nerves should be identified and decompressed.
- Distal tarsal tunnel release is indicated when patients have associated chronic plantarmedial heel pain.
- The first branch of the lateral plantar nerve (Baxter nerve, or nerve to the abductor digiti minimi quinti) should be decompressed by releasing the deep fascia of the abductor hallucis.

b. Results

- The best results after tarsal tunnel release occur in patients with symptoms in the distribution of the tibial nerve, a positive nerve compression sign, positive electrodiagnostic studies, and space-occupying masses.
- The overall results after tarsal tunnel surgery vary greatly as measured in various studies, with successful outcomes in 50% to 90% of patients. The causes of suboptimal results include the presence of double crush syndrome, inadequate release, postoperative hematoma formation, scarring around the nerve, and improper diagnosis.
- Revision tarsal tunnel release is associated with less successful outcomes than primary release. The best results are seen in patients in whom previous decompression of the nerve was inadequate.
- Wrapping the nerve with autologous veins or commercially available nerve wraps may help prevent scar formation in revision cases.

IV. CHARCOT-MARIE-TOOTH DISEASE

A. Epidemiology and overview

1. Charcot-Marie-Tooth disease (cavovarus foot) is the most common inherited neuropathy, affecting approximately 1 in 2,500 persons.
2. Life expectancy is normal.
3. Males are affected more frequently, but females are affected more severely.
4. Pathologic evaluation demonstrates degenerative changes in the motor nerve roots. The primary abnormality in hereditary motor sensory neuropathy is in the peripheral nervous system.
5. The most common form of inheritance is autosomal dominant with a duplication of the peripheral myelin protein (PMP) gene on chromosome 17.

B. Etiology and pathoanatomy

1. Initially, intrinsic muscle weakness and contracture results in a high arch and clawing of the toes. The weak intrinsic muscles are overpowered by the intact extrinsic toe flexors and extensors.

a. The tibialis anterior is affected next, and its antagonist, the peroneus longus causes plantar flexion of the first ray. Initially, the hindfoot assumes a compensatory varus posture to balance the forefoot valgus (**Figure 5**).

2. Subsequently, the peroneus brevis weakens and hindfoot varus develops because the weakened peroneus brevis cannot oppose the intact tibialis posterior. Hindfoot varus is no longer compensatory at this stage.

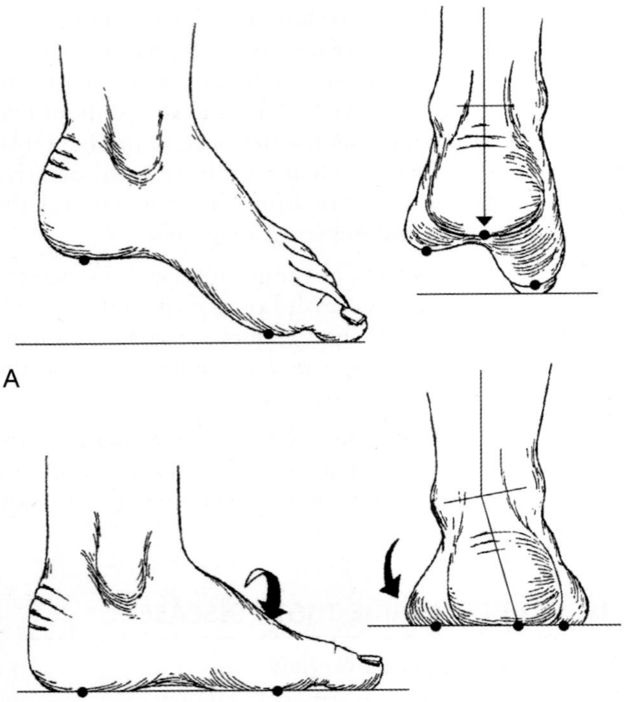

Figure 5 Illustrations demonstrate hindfoot varus deformity, when the plantarflexed first ray strikes the ground (**A**), the heel is forced into varus (**B**). (Reproduced with permission from Richardson EG: The foot and ankle: Neurogenic disorders, in Canale ST, ed: *Campbell's Operative Orthopaedics*, ed 10. St. Louis, MO, Mosby, 2003.)

3. Elevation of the arch (pes cavus) occurs because of tightening of the windlass mechanism, resulting from an imbalance between the weakened intrinsic muscle and the extrinsic muscles.
4. Claw toes develop as a result of loss of intrinsic function, resulting in hyperextension at the MTP joint and plantar flexion at the interphalangeal joints. Long toe extensors are recruited for ankle dorsiflexion and contribute to the hyperextension deformity of the MTP joint, whereas the long toe flexors are relatively spared and contribute to flexion deformities of the interphalangeal joints.
5. Ankle equinus is a result of the unopposed pull of the gastrocnemius-soleus complex against the weakened tibialis anterior.

C. Evaluation

1. History and physical examination
    a. Approximately 94% of patients with Charcot-Marie-Tooth disease have a foot deformity; a high arch and claw toes are common findings.
    b. Symptom onset commonly occurs during the first, second, or third decade of life and can include muscle cramps, shoe-wear problems, difficulty running, metatarsalgia, and ankle instability.
    c. The intrinsic muscles of the feet are affected first, followed by involvement of the peroneus brevis and tibialis anterior.
    d. The posterior compartment of the leg and peroneus longus usually are spared (tibial nerve innervation) during the developmental stages; however, atrophy of the entire calf usually occurs, resulting in "stork legs."
    e. Sensory changes can occur; these include dysesthesias, decreased vibration sense, and decreased proprioception.
    f. Inspection of the foot and ankle demonstrates callus formation under the metatarsal heads and lateral border of the foot with a cavovarus foot deformity.
    g. The initial finding usually is a plantarflexed first ray (forefoot valgus) as a result of overpull of the intact peroneus longus, which is not neutralized by the weakened tibialis anterior.
    h. Hindfoot varus deformity initially is flexible, but with time, it becomes fixed.
        - The Coleman block test is used to determine whether the hindfoot is flexible and whether the deformity is solely a result of the plantarflexed first ray (**Figure 6**).
        - In this test, the hindfoot and lateral forefoot are placed on a block and the patient is asked to stand. If the hindfoot corrects to neutral or everts, the cavovarus deformity is a result of the plantarflexed ray. If it does not correct, both the forefoot and hindfoot are involved and need to be addressed.
2. Imaging
    a. Radiographs of the foot and ankle demonstrate forefoot adduction, a plantarflexed first ray, and increased calcaneal inclination. The fibula will appear posterior to the tibia because of external rotation of the tibia. A double density of the talar dome often is a subtle sign of hindfoot varus.
    b. Axial views (Harris, Saltzman, and hindfoot alignment) will demonstrate hindfoot varus.

D. Treatment—The goals of any treatment, surgical or nonsurgical, are to preserve function, reduce pain, and protect the foot and ankle from further injury.

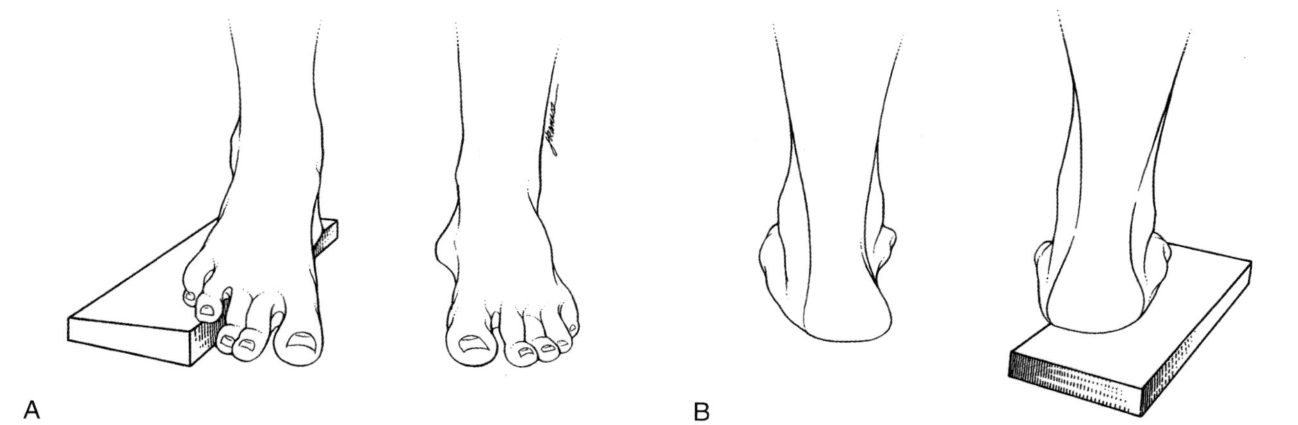

Figure 6 Illustrations show the Coleman lateral block test as viewed from the front (**A**) and the back (**B**). Note that the hindfoot varus corrects to neutral, indicating that the cavovarus deformity is the result of a plantarflexed first ray. (Reproduced from Alexander IJ: Pes cavus, in Nunley JA, Pfeffer GB, Sanders RW, Trepman E, eds: *Advanced Reconstruction: Foot and Ankle*. Rosemont, IL, American Academy of Orthopaedic Surgeons, 2004, pp 495-502.)

1. Nonsurgical
   a. The treatment should focus on mobilization and strengthening of the weakened muscles and using an accommodative insert. Patients are often deconditioned, and an exercise program geared to improving their function is important.
   b. Nonimpact conditioning with a stationary bike and swimming are preferred to prolonged walking and running. Progressive resistance exercises have to be performed prudently to avoid injury to the weakened muscles. Stretching exercises can help to minimize the development of fixed deformities.
   c. The most commonly used orthotic device is the molded ankle-foot orthosis.
      - The advantages of plastic braces over double-upright metal braces are lighter weight and better cosmetic appearance.
      - The plantarflexed first ray can be accommodated by elevating the heel and lateral forefoot.
2. Surgical
   a. Surgery should be delayed until progression of the deformity begins to cause symptoms or weakness of the muscle units results in contractures of the antagonistic muscle units. Patients who remain symptomatic despite nonsurgical treatment are candidates for surgery.
   b. Soft-tissue procedures are indicated if the deformity is flexible.
      - Transferring the peroneus longus to the peroneus brevis eliminates strong plantar flexion of the first ray and restores some eversion power to the foot and ankle.
      - Capsulotomies of the talonavicular joint and medial subtalar joint, in addition to posterior tibial tendon lengthening, may assist in correcting hindfoot varus.
      - Transfer of the tibialis posterior tendon to the dorsum of the foot through the interosseous membrane decreases the varus moment and may assist in ankle dorsiflexion.
      - Transfer of the tibialis posterior tendon around the ankle to the cuboid also has been described.
      - Release of the plantar fascia is necessary to help treat the cavus deformity.
      - Clinically, the Achilles tendon appears tight; however, close inspection reveals that the hindfoot is in calcaneus. Lengthening of the Achilles tendon can result in an increase in calcaneus and should be avoided until other procedures are done.
      - Flexor-to-extensor transfer (Girdlestone-Taylor procedure) of the lesser toes is useful for flexible claw toes.
      - The clawed great toe is treated with the Jones procedure, which includes interphalangeal joint fusion and transfer of the extensor hallucis longus (EHL) tendon to the metatarsal neck.

- In skeletally immature patients with a flexible forefoot and hindfoot, plantar fascia lengthening and tibialis posterior tendon transfer often are sufficient.

c. Most adult patients need some form of osseous surgery in addition to soft-tissue procedures.
   - For patients in whom Coleman block testing reveals overcorrection into slight valgus, dorsiflexion osteotomy of the first metatarsal, plantar fascial release, and peroneus longus to brevis transfer is appropriate (**Figure 7**).
   - Hindfoot varus is addressed with a lateral displacement osteotomy of the calcaneus or lateral closing wedge osteotomy of the calcaneus. This osteotomy is also useful because it corrects the foot during heel strike and lateralizes the force of the Achilles vector during toe-off (**Figure 8**).
   - Lateral ankle ligament reconstruction is useful in patients with ankle instability
   - For patients with severe rigid deformities, triple arthrodesis is the salvage procedure of choice. Correction of the deformity occurs through the bone resections.

d. After a stable plantigrade foot is achieved, most patients will require some type of orthotic device to correct the weakness of the tibialis anterior muscle. Although tibialis posterior tendon transfer through the interosseous membrane may restore some degree of active dorsiflexion, it typically is not enough to correct the footdrop.

e. Although some patients may have true equinus due to imbalance between the intact gastrocnemius-soleus complex and weakened tibialis anterior, caution should be exercised in performing an Achilles tendon lengthening. In many patients, the calcaneal inclination angle is abnormally steep, and Achilles lengthening can result in a calcaneus gait.

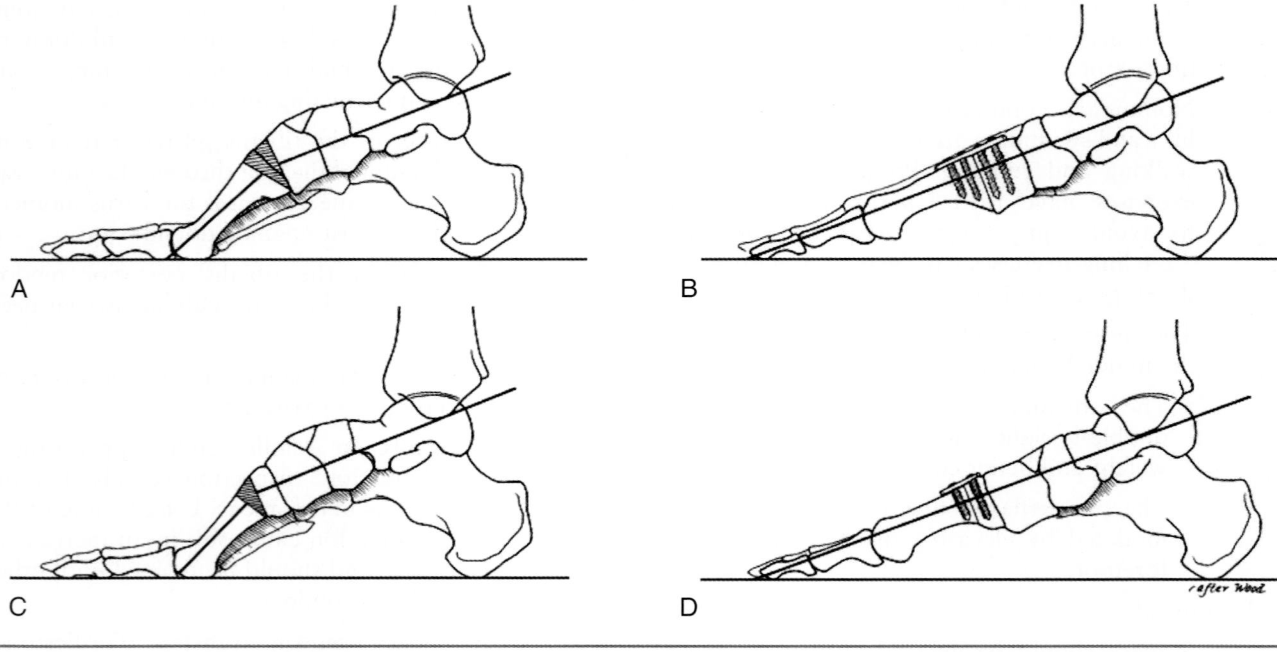

Figure 7 Illustrations demonstrate first metatarsal osteotomy for correction of a fixed first metatarsal cavus deformity. **A**, Medial view shows a plantarflexed first ray with the deformity in the first metatarsal. The shaded area depicts the wedge to be removed from the first tarsometatarsal joint. **B**, The wedge is closed and fixed with a four-hole one-quarter tubular plate and 2.7-mm or 3.5-mm cortical screws. **C**, In an alternative technique, bone from the proximal metatarsal metaphysis (shaded area) is removed. Alignment of the foot is corrected in a manner similar to that shown in panel B. **D**, Fixation is performed with a two- or three-hole one-third tubular plate and 3.5-mm cortical screws. (Adapted with permission from Hansen ST Jr, ed: *Functional Reconstruction of the Foot and Ankle*. Philadelphia, PA, Lippincott Williams and Wilkins, 2000, p 369.)

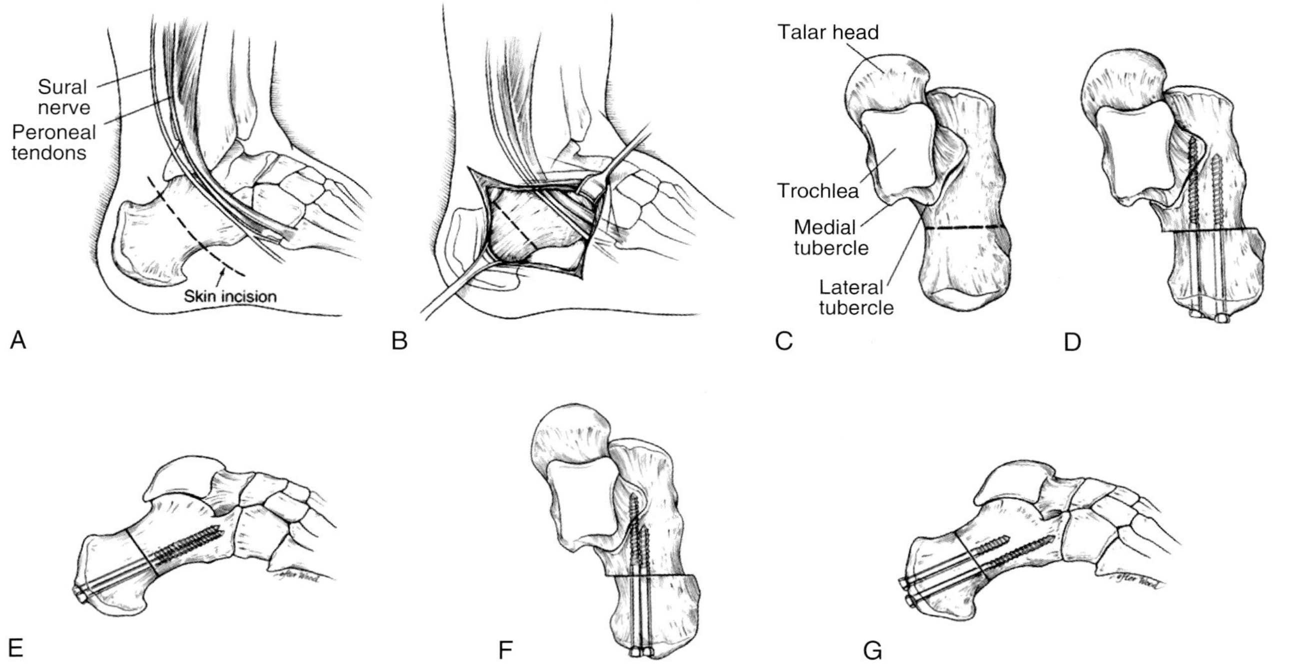

Figure 8 Illustrations demonstrate a lateralizing sliding calcaneal osteotomy. **A**, A posterior lateral incision is made. **B**, After the soft tissues have been retracted, the calcaneus is cut using a saw. **C**, The medial cut should not penetrate close to the sustentaculum tali. **D and E**, The osteotomy is held with two proximal-distal transcalcaneal screws. **F and G**, Alternative screw positions are shown. (Adapted with permission from Hansen ST Jr, ed: *Functional Reconstruction of the Foot and Ankle*. Philadelphia, PA, Lippincott Williams and Wilkins, 2000, p 369.)

V. NERVE ENTRAPMENT

A. Deep peroneal nerve

1. Pathoanatomy

a. Compression of the deep peroneal nerve in the region of the anterior ankle and dorsal foot results from entrapment under the superior and inferior extensor retinacula.

b. Compression under the inferior extensor retinaculum has been referred to as "anterior tarsal tunnel syndrome."

c. The deep peroneal nerve travels with the anterior tibial artery in the interval between the extensor digitorum longus and the EHL. Just proximal to the ankle, the nerve bifurcates into a lateral branch, which innervates the EDB, and a medial branch, which supplies sensation to the first dorsal web space.

d. Compression of the nerve can occur as a result of osteophytes (on the tibia and/or talus), avulsion fractures, an enlarged muscle belly of the EDB, ganglion cysts, synovitis, and tumors. Traction injuries can occur from ankle sprains (**Figure 9**).

2. Evaluation

a. History and physical examination

- Patients report a burning pain on the dorsum of the foot with paresthesias in the first dorsal web space. This pain usually is exacerbated by activities and relieved by rest.
- Nocturnal pain is common because the plantarflexed foot places the nerve on stretch. Shoes with a high heel can induce this plantarflexed posture, reproducing symptoms. Tight-fitting shoes or boots can cause external compression.
- Positive findings include weakness and/or atrophy of the EDB, reduced sensation in the first dorsal web space, and a positive Tinel sign over the area of compression.

b. Imaging

- Radiographs of the ankle and foot should be obtained to assess for osteophytes of the distal tibia, dorsal talus, or dorsal talonavicular joint.
- Electrodiagnostic studies may show a delay in latency and denervation of the EDB; however, normal results are common.

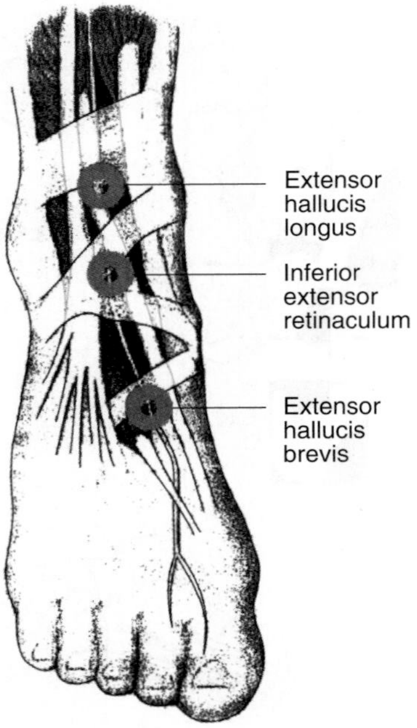

Figure 9 Illustration shows the points of compression of the deep peroneal nerve: under the hypertrophied extensor hallucis brevis (proximal circle); at the inferior edge of the inferomedial extensor retinaculum—the classic anterior tarsal tunnel syndrome (middle circle); and under the tendon of the extensor hallucis longus at the superior edge of the inferior extensor retinaculum (distal circle). (Reproduced with permission from Hirose CB, McGarvey WC: Peripheral nerve entrapments. *Foot Ankle Clin* 2004;9[2]:255-269.)

3. Treatment
   a. Nonsurgical
      - Reducing pressure over the nerve by avoiding tight-fitting shoes and high heels is recommended.
      - If patients have chronic edema, a diuretic is useful.
      - Corticosteroid and local anesthetic injection helps confirm the diagnosis and direct treatment. If the patient does not experience relief during the initial effect of the local anesthesia, the diagnosis should be reassessed.
   b. Surgical
      - When nonsurgical treatment fails, neurolysis is indicated.
      - Decompression of the nerve is begun just proximal to the superior extensor retinaculum and extends to the base of the first and second tarsometatarsal joint.
      - Osteophytes should be resected, and hypertrophied muscles can be debulked.
      - Approximately 80% of patients have a satisfactory result.

B. Superficial peroneal nerve
   1. Pathoanatomy
      a. The superficial peroneal nerve (SPN) branches from the common peroneal nerve at the level of the fibular neck and proceeds distally in the lateral compartment between the peroneus brevis and peroneus longus muscles.
      b. This purely sensory nerve becomes superficial in the distal third of the leg and, approximately 10 cm above the tip of the distal fibula, branches into the medial dorsal cutaneous nerve and intermediate dorsal cutaneous nerve (**Figure 10**).
         - The intermediate dorsal cutaneous nerve provides dorsal sensation to the third, fourth, and fifth toes.
         - The medial dorsal cutaneous nerve passes lateral to the EHL and provides sensation to the medial aspect of the dorsal foot.

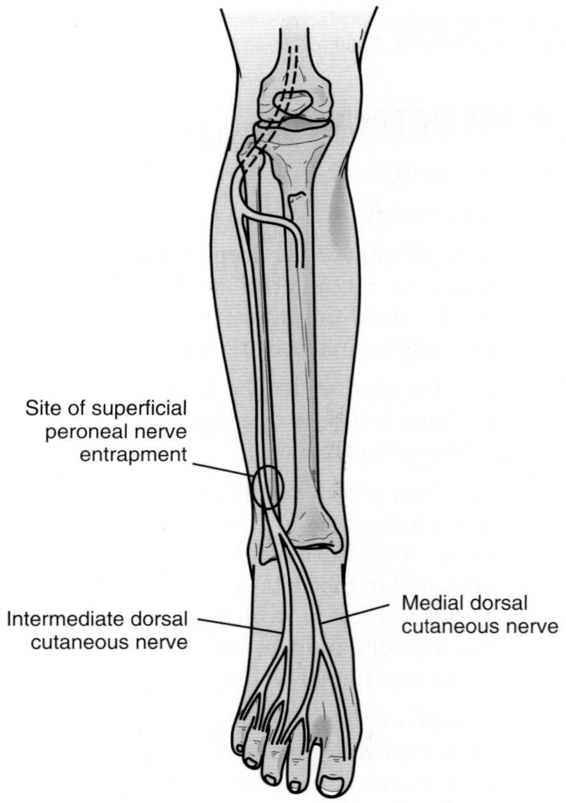

Figure 10 Illustration depicts superficial peroneal nerve entrapment.

c. Compression of the SPN can be seen anywhere along its course and usually is posttraumatic in nature. Iatrogenic injury can occur during open treatment of distal fibula fractures and placement of the anterolateral ankle portal for arthroscopy.

2. Evaluation

a. History and physical examination

- Compression of the SPN typically causes anterolateral distal leg and ankle pain as well as dorsal foot pain.
- The pain occurs in a distribution similar to the L5 distribution and may be associated with sensory dysfunction in this distribution. The most common site of compression is where the nerve pierces the leg fascia and becomes superficial.
- Motor findings are normal unless compression occurs proximally.
- Pain can be reproduced by plantar flexion and inversion and with direct compression of the nerve. The Tinel sign is useful for determining the site of compression.
- The differential diagnosis includes lateral ankle sprains that do not heal, chronic compartment syndrome, fascial defects, muscle herniations, and proximal nerve entrapment.
- Sensory nerve conduction velocities may be prolonged, although electrodiagnostic testing is most useful for excluding a more proximal cause of nerve compression.

b. Imaging

- Radiographs help evaluate for osseous impingement (exostosis or spurs); however, the diagnosis usually is made based on clinical examination.
- MRI may be useful for evaluating soft-tissue masses, which may cause compression.

3. Treatment

a. Nonsurgical

- Nonsurgical measures include injections of local anesthetic and steroids, as well as orthoses to prevent inversion of the ankle and foot.
- Physical therapy can be used to strengthen the muscles about the foot and ankle, as well as to desensitize the nerve.

b. Surgical

- If nerve entrapment does not respond to nonsurgical measures, neurolysis is indicated.
- Surgical decompression should begin at the level at which the nerve exits the fascia.
- The area of compression usually can be isolated preoperatively by using the Tinel sign; neurolysis must proceed distal to the site of compression.
- If associated muscle herniation or chronic compartment syndrome is present, concurrent fasciotomy is recommended.
- Approximately 80% of patients experience clinical improvement, although patient satisfaction is not universal.

C. Sural nerve

1. Pathoanatomy

a. The sural nerve is a purely sensory nerve that is formed by branches of the peroneal and tibial nerves.

b. At the musculotendinous junction of the gastrocnemius muscle, the sural nerve lies at the midline and then descends distally lateral to the Achilles tendon.

c. As the nerve progresses distally, it lies posterior to the peroneal tendons and then supplies branches to the lateral hindfoot. It then proceeds distally and crosses the base of the fifth metatarsal.

d. Sural nerve entrapment can result from fractures of the calcaneus, talus, or fifth metatarsal. Iatrogenic injury may occur during gastrocnemius recession or open reduction and internal fixation of fractures involving the calcaneus or base of the fifth metatarsal.

2. Evaluation

a. History and physical examination

- Patients typically report lateral foot and ankle pain that radiates proximally, as well as associated numbness in that distribution.
- A positive percussion test typically reproduces paresthesias in the lateral foot.
- The differential diagnosis includes lumbosacral radiculopathy, popliteal artery entrapment, disorders of the Achilles tendon, and chronic pain from lateral ankle sprains.
- NCV studies may demonstrate an increase in distal latency or a decrease in the nerve action potential, but they rarely are helpful.

b. Imaging
- Radiographs are useful for excluding fractures and exostosis.
- MRI is beneficial for diagnosing soft-tissue lesions such as ganglion cysts, which may cause compression.

3. Treatment

a. Nonsurgical
- Accommodative shoe wear may relieve pressure on the sural nerve.
- Injections of local anesthetic and corticosteroids can be diagnostic and therapeutic.

b. Surgical
- If nonsurgical treatment fails, neurolysis may be beneficial, especially if ganglions or malreduced fractures are present.
- If a true posttraumatic neuroma is present, resection and burying of the proximal stump is recommended.

D. Saphenous nerve

1. The saphenous nerve provides sensation to the medial ankle and a portion of the dorsomedial foot.
2. The nerve follows the greater saphenous vein and can be injured during anteromedial arthroscopic portal placement.
3. Saphenous nerve entrapment is rare in the foot and ankle and usually occurs proximally, at the medial aspect of the knee.
4. If a true neuroma is present, resection and burying of the proximal stump is recommended because of its subcutaneous location.

VI. CEREBROVASCULAR ACCIDENT AND TRAUMATIC BRAIN INJURY

A. Epidemiology and overview

1. Approximately 750,000 Americans experience cerebrovascular accidents (CVAs, or strokes) each year, and approximately 33% of these patients die. Most CVAs result from thrombosis, but hemorrhage and emboli are also causative.
2. Ten percent of patients who survive a CVA achieve a full recovery, 80% experience varied degrees of recovery, and 10% do not improve.
3. Two million traumatic brain injuries (TBIs) occur in the United States each year, resulting in nearly 50,000 deaths.
4. Neurologic deficits from CVAs and TBIs cause impairment of locomotion and difficulties with personal hygiene, behavior, emotion, and cognition.
5. CVA is the leading cause of hemiplegia in older adults; TBI is the most common cause in young adults. Intracranial disease is the most proximal cause of neuromuscular disease, resulting in foot and ankle pathology.

B. Pathoanatomy

1. Deformities of the foot and ankle caused by CVA or TBI result from upper motor neuron involvement.
2. Patients who have sustained a CVA have hyperreflexia, spasticity, increased tone, and minimal atrophy.
3. Neurologic recovery can take 6 to 18 months in CVA patients; in TBI patients, recovery can take several years.
4. After a CVA, 25% of patients regain normal ambulation, and 75% regain some level of ambulation.
5. Even in patients who cannot ambulate, the ability to stand is important for wheelchair transfers, dressing, and personal hygiene. Upright posture requires that a plantigrade foot be achieved.

C. Evaluation

1. History and physical examination

a. The typical physical finding in patients who have had a CVA is spastic equinovarus deformity of the foot and ankle (**Figure 11**).

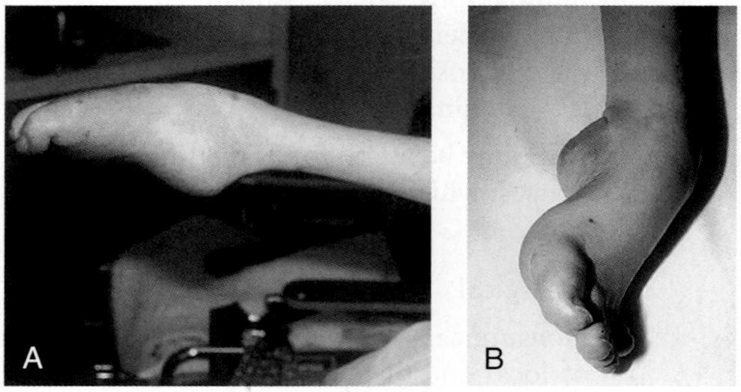

Figure 11 Photographs of equinovarus deformities in patients with acquired spasticity. **A**, Fixed equinus deformity and toe flexion. **B**, Substantial toe flexion and associated varus foot deformity. (Reproduced from Botte MJ: Equinovarus deformity, in Nunley JA, Pfeffer GB, Sanders RW, Trepman E, eds: *Advanced Reconstruction: Foot and Ankle*. Rosemont, IL, American Academy of Orthopaedic Surgeons, 2004, p 487.)

Coughlin MJ, Pinsonneault T: Operative treatment of interdigital neuroma: A long-term follow-up study. *J Bone Joint Surg Am* 2001;83(9):1321-1328.

Hirose CB, McGarvey WC: Peripheral nerve entrapments. *Foot Ankle Clin* 2004;9(2):255-269.

McCrory P, Bell S, Bradshaw C: Nerve entrapments of the lower leg, ankle and foot in sport. *Sports Med* 2002;32(6):371-391.

Patel AT, Gaines K, Malamut R, et al: Usefulness of electrodiagnostic techniques in the evaluation of suspected tarsal tunnel syndrome: An evidence-based review. *Muscle Nerve* 2005;32(2):236-240.

Sammarco GJ, Chang L: Outcome of surgical treatment of tarsal tunnel syndrome. *Foot Ankle Int* 2003;24(2):125-131.

Stamatis ED, Myerson MS: Treatment of recurrence of symptoms after excision of an interdigital neuroma: A retrospective review. *J Bone Joint Surg Br* 2004;86(1):48-53.

Younger AS, Hansen ST Jr: Adult cavovarus foot. *J Am Acad Orthop Surg* 2005;13(5):302-315.

Chapter 118
The Diabetic Foot and Ankle

TERRENCE PHILBIN, DO
GREGORY C. BERLET, MD
DAVID GOSS JR, DO
ADAM HALVERSON, DO

I. DIABETIC PERIPHERAL NEUROPATHY

A. Overview and epidemiology

1. Diabetic neuropathy manifests in the somatic and/or autonomic parts of the peripheral nervous system.
2. Of all patients with diabetes mellitus, 10% have some form of sensory, motor, or autonomic dysfunction at the time of diagnosis; neuropathy develops in 50% of these patients within 25 years of diagnosis.
3. No single etiologic pathway has been confirmed as responsible for all diabetic neuropathy. Metabolic factors (glycosylation of proteins, reduced availability of nerve growth factors, and immunologic factors) combined with a microvascular insufficiency likely result in the final common pathway of neuropathic changes.

B. Sensory neuropathy

1. Sensory neuropathy is the most prevalent and obvious nerve dysfunction seen in patients with diabetes, affecting as many as 70%.
2. In one study, the critical triad of sensory neuropathy, trauma, and foot deformity was present in 63% of patients with lower extremity ulcers.
3. Pain is associated with 25% to 33% of neuropathies. The pain can be superficial (burning, tingling, or allodynia), shooting or electric-like, or cramping and aching.
4. Sensory disturbances show a length-related pattern, with stocking and glove distribution due to a "dying-back" distal axonopathy.
5. Sensory neuropathy can be assessed using the Semmes-Weinstein monofilament test. Protective sensation is indicated by the ability to perceive a 5.07 (10 g) monofilament applied perpendicular to the skin.

C. Motor neuropathy

1. Motor neuropathy is most clinically apparent in the foot, as evidenced by the development of claw toes from intrinsic muscle weakness and equinus contracture of the Achilles tendon. These factors transfer stress to the forefoot, resulting in focal high pressures and resultant skin breakdown.
2. Claw toes occur because of the dysfunction of intrinsic muscles that cause hyperextension of the metatarsophalangeal joints and flexion of the proximal and distal interphalangeal joints.

Dr. Philbin or an immediate family member has received royalties from Arthrex, Inc., Biomet, Crossroads, Paragon 28, and Wright Medical Technology, Inc.; is a member of a speakers' bureau or has made paid presentations on behalf of Arthrex, Inc., Crossroads, DJ Orthopaedics, Medline, Tissue Tech, and Zimmer Biomet; serves as a paid consultant to or is an employee of Artelon, Arthrex, Inc., Crossroads, DJ Orthopaedics, Medline, Tissue Tech, and Zimmer Biomet; has stock or stock options held in Tissue Tech; has received research or institutional support from Biomimetic, DJ Orthopaedics; has received nonincome support (such as equipment or services), commercially derived honoraria, or other non–research-related funding (such as paid travel) from Springer; and serves as a board member, owner, officer, or committee member of the American Osteopathic Academy of Orthopedics board of directors. Dr. Berlet or an immediate family member has received royalties from Bledsoe Brace, Stryker, Wright Medical Technology, Inc., and ZimmerBiomet; is a member of a speakers' bureau or has made paid presentations on behalf of Wright Medical Technology, Inc.; serves as a paid consultant to or is an employee of Artelon, DJ Orthopaedics, Stryker, Wright Medical Technology, Inc., and ZimmerBiomet; has stock or stock options held in Bledsoe technologies, Ossio, Tissue Tech, and Wright Medical Technology, Inc.; and has received research or institutional support from DJ Orthopaedics, Tissue Tech, Zimmer. Neither of the following authors nor any immediate family member has received anything of value from or has stock or stock options held in a commercial company or institution related directly or indirectly to the subject of this chapter: Dr. Goss and Dr. Halverson.

TABLE 1

Recommendations for the Diabetic Foot at Risk

Risk Category	Description of Foot	Neuropathy	Deformity	Recommendations
1	Normal	Present	None	• Over-the-counter pressure-dissipating insoles • Accommodative laced shoes • Follow-up every 6 mo
2	Deformity without presence or history of ulcer	Present	Present	• Custom pressure-dissipating insoles • Extra-depth laced shoes • Follow-up every 4 mo
3	Deformity and history of ulcer	Present	Present	• Custom pressure-dissipating insoles • Extra-depth laced shoes • Follow-up every 2 mo • Evaluation of new onset skin/nail problems • Orthopaedic evaluation

3. Skin compromise occurs secondary to pressure placed on the dorsal surface as the toes contact the toe box of the shoe and increased pressure occurs beneath the metatarsal heads. Achilles tendon contracture displaces excessive pressure to the front of the foot, resulting in increased risk of ulceration.

D. Autonomic neuropathy

1. Autonomic neuropathy is the most overlooked manifestation of peripheral neuropathy. It occurs when the autonomic system cannot control the blood vessel tone and the sweat (eccrine and apocrine) glands in the foot.
2. Sweat gland dysfunction allows the skin to dry out and crack, thus allowing the ingress of microbes.
3. Standing foot pressure can be as high as 400 kPa, which necessitates fine regulation of the blood vessels to ensure adequate oxygenation of tissues and avoid local anoxia.

E. Treatment options—No proven method exists to reverse peripheral neuropathy associated with diabetes.

1. Decompression—When compression neuropathy is superimposed on peripheral neuropathy, decompression at the anatomic sites of pressure may be indicated.
2. Medical treatment
   a. Focuses on the symptoms of neuropathy (pain and burning)
   b. Medications from the gabapentin lineage, antidepressant medications, and topical anesthetics have been shown to relieve pain to varied degrees.
3. Protection from mechanical trauma—The key is to accommodate and protect the foot at risk secondary to neuropathy and associated deformities (**Table 1**).

II. FOOT ULCERATION

A. Overview and epidemiology

1. Affects approximately 12% of patients with diabetes
2. Responsible for approximately 85% of lower extremity amputations in patients with diabetes mellitus; most common medical complication for which patients with diabetes seek treatment
3. Factors associated with the inability of a diabetic foot ulcer to heal
   a. Persistently uncontrolled hyperglycemia
   b. Inability to unload the affected area effectively
   c. Diminished circulation
   d. Infection
   e. Poor nutrition
4. The accepted wound-healing levels are a serum albumin level of 3.0 g/dL and a total lymphocyte count greater than 1,500/mm^3.

B. Microbiology

1. Diabetic infections are usually polymicrobial.
2. The most common pathogens are aerobic gram-positive cocci (especially *Staphylococcus aureus*); gram-negative rods may be present in patients with chronic wounds or those recently treated with antibiotics.

3. Obligate anaerobic pathogens may cause infection in patients with foot ischemia or gangrene.
4. Deep cultures and bacterial biopsy are sometimes necessary to make a diagnosis.

C. Evaluation

1. History and physical examination—A comprehensive evaluation should include the foot and ankle and pay special attention to
   a. Tobacco use
   b. Prior treatments
   c. Medical comorbidities
   d. Assessment of Achilles tendon tightness
2. Vascular evaluation
   a. More than 60% of diabetic ulcers have diminished blood flow secondary to peripheral vascular disease.
   b. Physical examination of the lower extremity vascular system includes
      - Assessment of the dorsalis pedis and tibialis pulses
      - Examination of the condition of the skin, noting the absence of hair on the feet and toes
   c. When the physical examination indicates further evaluation, the ankle-brachial index (ABI), Doppler ultrasonography with digital arterial pressures, transcutaneous toe oxygen measurement, and arteriography can be used.
      - An ABI of at least 0.45 and toe pressures greater than 40 mm Hg are necessary to heal an ulcer in the diabetic foot.
      - Transcutaneous oxygen measurement greater than 30 mm Hg indicates that blood flow is adequate for healing.
3. Ulcer classification—The Wagner ulcer classification system (**Table 2**) and the Brodsky depth-ischemia classification (**Table 3**) are commonly used.
4. Physical examination—Key features of the ulcer evaluation include
   a. Depth of ulcer
   b. Presence of infection
   c. Nonviable tissue (gangrene)
   d. Pressure at location of ulcer
5. Imaging
   a. Weight-bearing AP, lateral, and oblique radiographs of the foot and ankle are obtained.

TABLE 2

Wagner Ulcer Classification System

Grade	Description
0	Skin intact
1	Superficial
2	Deeper, full-thickness extension
3	Deep abscess formation or osteomyelitis
4	Partial gangrene of the forefoot
5	Extensive gangrene

Adapted with permission from Wagner FW: A classification and treatment program for diabetic neuropathic and dysvascular foot problems. *Instr Course Lect* 1979;28:143-165.

   b. Nuclear studies using technetium Tc-99m, gallium Ga-67, or indium In-111 may help differentiate between soft-tissue infection and osteomyelitis, Charcot arthropathy, or a combination of infection and Charcot arthropathy.
   c. MRI also can help but may not distinguish between Charcot arthropathy and infection with high specificity.

D. Ulcer treatment

1. Nonsurgical
   a. Débridement—Sharp débridement of necrotic tissue down to a clean tissue base often results in healing.
   b. Wound care—The dressing should accomplish the following goals.
      - Provide a moist environment
      - Absorb exudates
      - Act as a barrier
      - Off-load pressure
      - Provide antibiosis (occasionally required)
   c. Total contact casting (TCC) and mechanical relief.
      - TCC is the benchmark for off-loading plantar ulcerations.
      - Patients with grade 3 or higher ulcers should undergo incision and drainage and antibiotic therapy, with wound improvement before TCC application.
      - Casts should be changed every 2 to 4 weeks until erythema and edema have resolved and the temperature of the affected limb has decreased and becomes similar to that of the contralateral limb. Ulcers should be

TABLE 3

The Brodsky Depth/Ischemia Classification of Diabetic Foot Lesions

Grade	Definition	Treatment
Depth Classification		
0	The at-risk foot. Previous ulcer or neuropathy with deformity that may cause new ulceration	Patient education, regular examination, appropriate footwear and insoles
1	Superficial ulceration, not infected	External pressure relief using total contact cast, walking brace, or special footwear
2	Deep ulceration exposing tendon or joint (with or without superficial infection)	Surgical débridement, wound care, pressure relief if closed and converts to grade 1; antibiotics as needed
3	Extensive ulceration with exposed bone and/or deep infection (osteomyelitis or abscess)	Surgical débridement, ray or partial foot amputation, intravenous antibiotics, pressure relief if wound converts to grade 1
Ischemic Classification		
A	Not ischemic	Adequate vascularity for healing
B	Ischemia without gangrene	Vascular evaluation (Doppler ultrasonography with assessment of digital arterial pressures, transcutaneous toe oxygen measurement, and arteriography), vascular reconstruction as needed
C	Partial (forefoot) gangrene of foot	Vascular evaluation, vascular reconstruction (proximal and/or distal bypass or angioplasty), partial foot amputation
D	Complete foot gangrene	Vascular valuation, major extremity amputation (transtibial or transfemoral) with possible proximal vascular reconstruction

Adapted from Brodsky JW: The diabetic foot, in Mann RA, Coughlin MJ, eds: *Surgery of the Foot and Ankle*, ed 7. St Louis, MO, Mosby-Year Book, 1999.

evaluated, and débridement should be performed at the time of cast changes.

- Radiographs should be repeated every 4 to 6 weeks—more often if an acute change occurs.

d. Pneumatic walking brace—As an alternative to TCC, a prefabricated pneumatic walking brace can be used to reduce forefoot and midfoot plantar pressure.

- Advantages—Permits more frequent wound surveillance; allows several types of dressings; easy to apply
- Disadvantages—Severe foot deformity makes using a pneumatic walking brace difficult, and patient compliance may be suboptimal.

e. Therapeutic Shoe Bill

- Congress signed into law in 1998 after studies showed potential net Medicare savings by preventing diabetic foot complications.
- Qualified patients include those being medically treated for diabetes with history of neuropathy with callous, past ulcerations, foot deformity, past amputation, or poor circulation.
- Bill annually covers one pair of "custom-molded shoes" with a total of three inserts or one pair of qualifying "depth shoes" with three inserts.
- Participants require certifying statement signed by the physician medically treating their diabetes and a prescription from a physician knowledgeable in shoe fitting.
- Shoes must be furnished by a Medicare registered provider or supplier of prescription footwear.
- Medicare pays 80% with 20% charged to the approved patient or their supplemental insurance.

2. Surgical
   a. Soft-tissue management—Drainage of deep infections often is necessary to prevent tissue necrosis, rid the area of infection, and achieve wound healing without tension.
   b. Management of deformity
      - Ostectomy or realignment arthrodesis may be needed to remove the internal pressure caused by bony prominences.
      - Achilles tendon lengthening can help reduce plantar forefoot pressure.
   c. Osteomyelitis
      - Before antibiotic treatment is begun, specimens for culture should be obtained by biopsy, ulcer curettage, or aspiration, rather than by wound swab.
      - Osteomyelitis is present in 67% of ulcers that can be probed to bone.

III. AMPUTATION

A. Overview and epidemiology
1. More than 80,000 diabetes-related amputations of the lower extremity are performed in the United States each year.
2. Medical and surgical advances, as well as improvements in orthotic and prosthetic devices, help many of these patients achieve functional and ambulatory levels similar to preoperative levels. Approximately 30% of amputees undergo amputation of the contralateral limb within 3 years; however, after amputation of a leg, the 5-year mortality rate is approximately 66%.
3. Multidisciplinary care
   a. A multidisciplinary diabetic foot care team should be involved to help minimize the likelihood of major amputations and improve the patient's quality of life.
   b. Multidisciplinary care must include proper patient education to help patients avoid complications by controlling their blood glucose, blood pressure, and serum lipid levels.
   c. The American Diabetes Association (ADA) reports that multidisciplinary foot care programs, along with comprehensive patient education, can reduce lower extremity amputation rates as much as 45% to 60%.

B. General amputation considerations (**Figure 1**)
1. Great toe (hallux) amputation—Results in increased pressures under the first metatarsal, lesser metatarsal heads, and remaining toes, increasing the risk of reulceration and further amputation.
2. Lesser toe amputation—Amputation of the second toe may result in hallux valgus deformity.
3. Ray amputation
   a. In general, forefoot stability is preserved if no more than two rays are resected.
   b. Preserving the bases of the metatarsals allows the Lisfranc joint to remain stable. Typically, patients tolerate partial lateral foot amputations better than partial medial amputations.
   c. First ray amputations can increase load to the adjacent rays. In addition, losing the anterior tibialis insertion can weaken ankle dorsiflexion, resulting in pronation of the foot.
   d. Fifth ray amputations are the most common.
   e. Ray amputations are generally more durable and functional than transmetatarsal amputations (TMAs).
4. TMA
   a. The patient requires less energy for ambulation after a TMA than after a transtibial amputation, and a TMA leaves a patient with a distal weight-bearing residual limb.

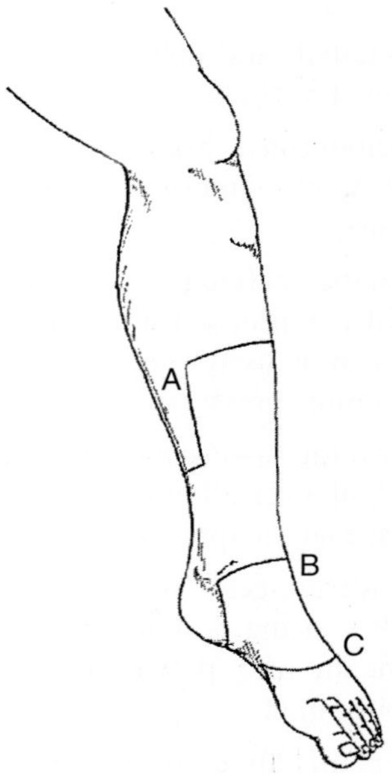

Figure 1 Illustration shows the surgical levels for transtibial (**A**), Syme (**B**), and transmetatarsal (**C**) amputations. (Courtesy of Peter Maurus, MD, Columbus, OH.)

b. Careful patient selection is required, including an assessment of muscle balance to determine the need for Achilles tendon lengthening and/or tendon transfer.

5. Lisfranc amputation—Preferred over TMA when substantial soft-tissue loss of the forefoot is present.

6. Chopart amputation

a. Disadvantages—Chopart amputation at the level of the transverse tarsal joints results in a shortened anatomic lever arm, reduced push-off, difficulty with stability, and possible equinovarus deformity.

b. Advantages—Retains the tibiotalar joint and a functional residual limb, in contrast to a more proximal amputation; Achilles tendon lengthening is usually necessary as well as transfer of the extensors to the dorsal talus to prevent equinovarus deformity.

7. Syme amputation

a. The primary advantage of a Syme amputation over more proximal amputations is its potential for achieving a full-load–bearing residual limb that is nearly normal in length and requires less energy expenditure during walking.

b. Candidates for a Syme amputation are patients with good potential for ambulation with a prosthesis following surgery, a viable heel pad, no infection at the heel pad level, and adequate vascularity.

c. The Syme amputation can be performed in two stages approximately 6 weeks apart; however, most surgeons use the single-stage technique because the results are essentially the same, but the cost and the risk of perioperative complications are lower with only one procedure. Successful healing was reported in 84.5% of patients treated with single-stage amputation.

d. Heel pad migration after a Syme amputation can be avoided by anchoring the heel pad to the distal tibia.

IV. CHARCOT ARTHROPATHY OF THE FOOT AND ANKLE

A. Overview and epidemiology

1. Up to 7.5% of patients with diabetes and neuropathy have Charcot arthropathy of the foot and ankle (also called Charcot foot); of those, 9% to 35% have bilateral involvement.

2. The pathogenesis of Charcot foot has been explained using two major theories.

a. The neurotraumatic theory attributes bony destruction to the loss of pain sensation and proprioception, combined with repetitive and mechanical trauma to the foot.

b. The neurovascular theory suggests that joint destruction is secondary to an autonomic stimulated vascular reflex causing hyperemia and periarticular osteopenia with contributory trauma.

B. Classification

1. The classic classification system for Charcot arthropathy is that of Eichenholtz (**Table 4**).

2. Brodsky created an anatomic-based classification system for the Charcot foot (**Figure 2**).

a. Type 1 involves the midfoot and accounts for approximately 60% of Charcot arthropathy.

b. Type 2 involves the hindfoot and accounts for 30% to 35% of Charcot arthropathy.

c. Type 3 involves the ankle or calcaneal tuberosity and accounts for the remaining 5% to 10% of Charcot arthropathy.

C. Evaluation

1. Early Charcot arthropathy often is confused with infection, despite the lack of a substantially elevated white blood cell count or fever.

2. In patients with diabetes, blood glucose levels usually fluctuate during a substantial infection; therefore, normal blood glucose levels should discount infection in the differential diagnosis.

TABLE 4

The Eichenholtz Classification of Charcot Arthropathy

Stage	Characteristics
0: Acute inflammatory phase	Foot is swollen, erythematous, warm, hyperemic; radiographs reveal periarticular soft-tissue swelling and varying degrees of osteopenia
I: Developmental or fragmentation stage	Periarticular fracture and joint subluxation with risk of instability and deformity
II: Coalescence stage; subacute Charcot	Resorption of bone debris and soft-tissue homeostasis
III: Consolidation or reparative stage; chronic Charcot	Restabilization of the foot with fibrous or bony arthrodesis of the involved joints

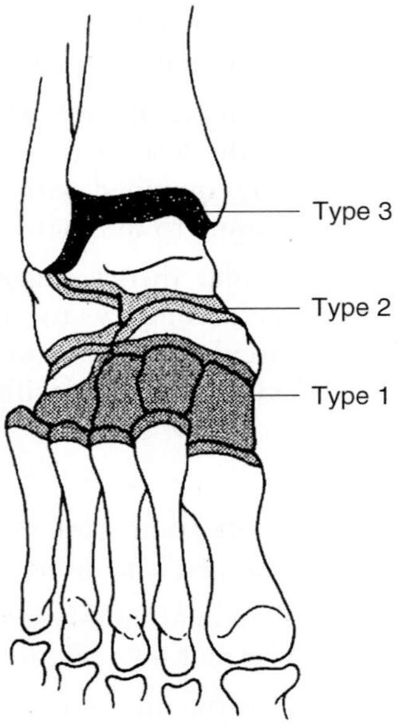

Figure 2 Illustration shows the Brodsky anatomic classification system for Charcot arthropathy of the foot. Type 1 involves the tarsometatarsal and naviculocuneiform joints. Type 2 involves the subtalar, talonavicular, or calcaneocuboid joint. Type 3 involves the tibiotalar joint. (Reproduced with permission from Brodsky JW: The diabetic foot, in Mann RA, Coughlin MJ, eds: *Surgery of the Foot and Ankle*, ed 7. St Louis, MO, Mosby-Year Book, 1999, p 949.)

3. Physical examination—The examiner should look for signs that indicate the stages of the Eichenholtz classification system.
   a. Stage 0 (acute): hyperemia of the foot with increased warmth and swelling. Radiographs can show fracture or joint subluxation (**Figure 3**, A).
   b. Stages 1 to 4: soft tissues stabilize and swelling subsides; skin color improves. The foot may develop deformity and instability (**Figure 3**, B). Serial radiographs can monitor disease progression.
   c. Stage 4 (consolidation): foot stability may increase via arthrodesis or fibrous union.
4. Imaging
   a. Radiographs will show obvious bone dissolution, joint dislocations, and deformity progression.
   b. Bone scanning can be misleading.
   c. MRI is the best modality for differentiating abscess from soft-tissue swelling, but it can be difficult to differentiate infection from Charcot arthropathy on MRI.

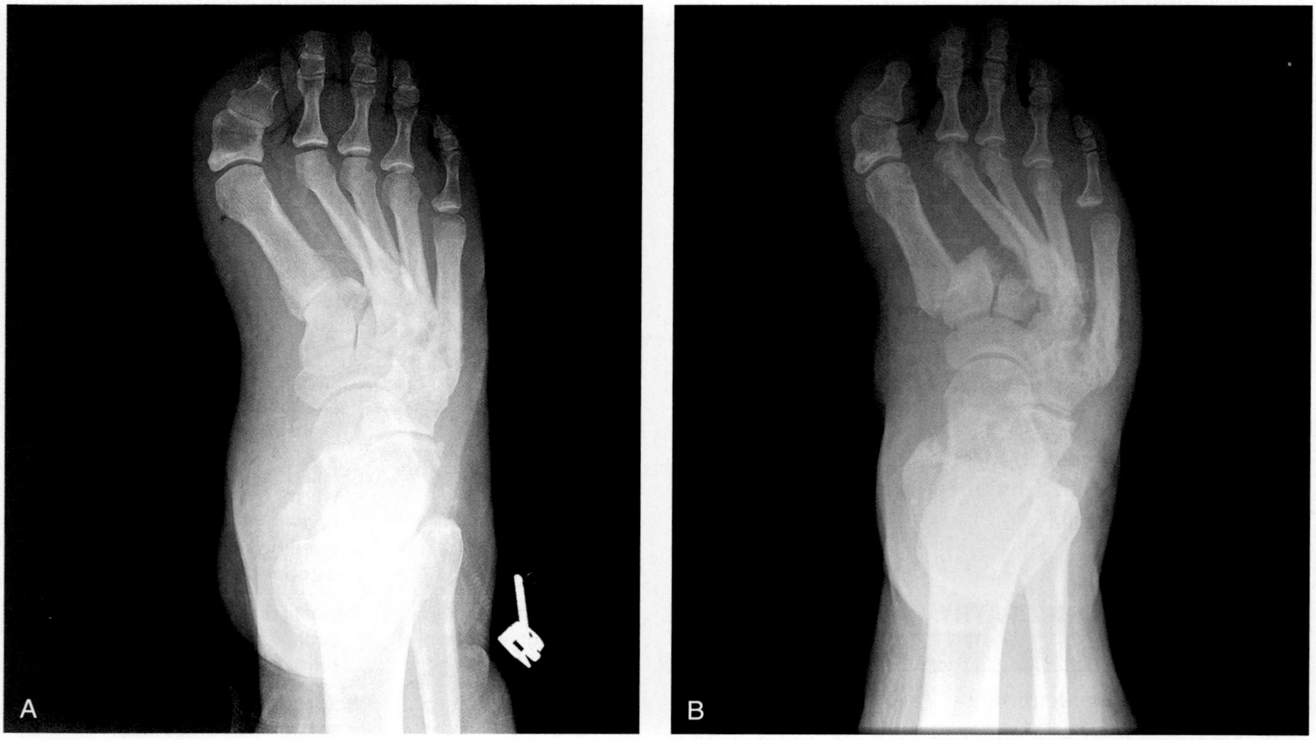

Figure 3 **A**, AP radiograph shows patient with Stage 0 Charcot arthropathy. No substantial joint or bone changes can be seen. **B**, AP radiograph shows Charcot arthropathy followed over time through the stages shows the progressive bone and joint changes that result in substantial deformity.

D. Treatment

1. The goals of treatment for Charcot arthropathy are a plantigrade, stable foot that can fit into a shoe, and the absence of recurrent ulceration.
2. Total contact casting and Charcot restraint orthotic walker (CROW)
   a. Most cases of acute Charcot arthropathy can be treated effectively with pressure-relieving methods such as TCC, the benchmark of treatment.
   b. TCC permits an even distribution of foot pressures across the plantar surface of the foot.
   c. TCC with guarded ambulation has yielded a mean healing rate of 75%.
   d. Casts are changed every 2 to 4 weeks until erythema and edema resolve, the temperature of the affected limb diminishes and is similar to that of the contralateral limb, and radiographs show stabilization, representing progress from Eichenholtz stage 0 to stage 2 (**Table 4**).
   e. TCC is commonly continued for up to 4 months.
   f. When the active disease phase has ended, the patient is fitted with a CROW and, later, with a custom shoe with orthoses.
      - CROW is a boot comprised of a two-piece rigid clamshell with rocker bottom and custom-molded removable insole.
      - Goal of insole is to evenly distribute weight and to support the ankle joint. Custom molding allows even pressure on an abnormally shaped collapsed foot.
      - Patients recovered from Charcot arthropathy subsequently qualify for shoe and insert provisions of the Therapeutic Shoe Bill to prevent recurrence and ulceration.
3. Acute surgical correction
   a. Limited indications exist for early stabilization of a Charcot joint.
   b. Surgery performed in the inflammatory phase of Charcot results in a high rate of nonunion, infection, wound complications, late deformity, and eventual amputation.
   c. Limited studies reveal that early surgical stabilization or intervention may successfully stabilize the foot deformity and prevent the complications associated with the residual Charcot deformity, such as foot instability and ulceration.
   d. The more proximal the deformity, the more difficult is stabilization with casting or bracing treatment. Such Charcot joints may benefit from early reconstruction.
4. Late surgical correction
   a. When deformity develops, the surgeon must decide whether accommodative, nonsurgical care with a combination of inlay depth shoes, foot orthoses, and ankle-foot orthoses is adequate.
   b. If a plantigrade weight-bearing surface cannot be achieved, surgical reconstruction is best performed in Eichenholtz stage 3, when the inflammatory process has resolved.
   c. Surgical indications for Charcot arthropathy of the foot include recurrent ulcers and instability not controlled by a brace. Surgical options are exostectomy or reconstruction with osteotomy and fusion.
   d. Surgical treatment may be indicated in up to 50% of patients.
   e. Exostectomy may be performed to excise bony prominences that cause ulcers.
   f. Reconstruction with osteotomy and fusion may be considered for correction of fixed deformity and severe instability that precludes successful bracing treatment.
      - Patients with complicated diabetes with associated neuropathy or peripheral artery disease have a 10-fold increase in postoperative infection complications.
      - Complicated diabetes yields union rates as low as 50%.

V. DIABETIC ANKLE FRACTURES

A. Overview and epidemiology

1. Intentional and deliberate evaluation and treatment of diabetic ankle fractures is paramount.
2. Owing to the increasing prevalence of diabetes, surgeons are treating more diabetic ankle fractures each year.
3. These patients present a unique clinical challenge due to increased risk of complications, regardless of surgical or nonsurgical treatment.
4. Delayed fracture and wound healing, soft-tissue compromise, vasculopathy, and neuropathy all need to be considered when formulating a treatment plan.

5. Diabetic patients with comorbidities (vasculopathy, neuropathy, Charcot arthropathy) have a higher risk of complications compared with diabetics without comorbidities.

B. Evaluation

1. A thorough neurologic and vascular history and examination is required when evaluating diabetic patients with ankle fractures.
2. Monofilament examination should be performed on diabetic patients to assess for presence of sensory neuropathy.
3. Patients with diminished or absent pulses warrant additional workup and potential intervention with a vascular consultation to optimize outcomes.

C. Treatment

1. Treatment is dictated by fracture pattern, stability, and patient comorbidities.
2. Isolated, stable, nondisplaced fractures can be treated by closed means. However, close follow-up with radiographic and clinical evaluation is essential for successful treatment. Any displacement or loss of reduction should be treated with surgical stabilization.
3. Higher complication rates are seen in unstable ankle fractures regardless of surgical or nonsurgical treatment; however, surgical treatment is more likely to result in a stable, functional ankle.
4. Nonoperative treatment of displaced ankle fractures is associated with up to 21-fold increased odds of complications compared with operative intervention.
5. In patients without associated diabetic comorbidities, standard ankle fracture fixation principles can be used.
6. When comorbidities are present, additional supplemental fixation (ie, multiple syndesmotic screws, bicortical medial malleolar screws, transarticular fixation, or supplemental external fixation devices) can be added to surgical constructs with the goal of enhanced stability. However, the current literature is inconclusive regarding the best way to achieve enhanced stability in these patients.
7. Prolonged non–weight bearing is recommended regardless of surgical or nonsurgical treatment of diabetic ankle fractures.

TOP TESTING FACTS

Diabetic Peripheral Neuropathy

1. Of all patients with diabetes, 10% have some form of sensory, motor, or autonomic dysfunction at the time of diagnosis; neuropathy develops in 50% of these patients within 25 years of diagnosis.
2. Sensory neuropathy is the most obvious and prevalent nerve dysfunction seen in patients with diabetes, affecting as many as 70%.
3. Motor neuropathy is clinically evident in the foot by the development of claw toes, which result from intrinsic muscle weakness and equinus contracture of the Achilles tendon.
4. Treatment of peripheral neuropathy usually focuses on the symptoms (pain and burning). Gabapentin, antidepressants, and topical anesthetic medications have been shown to relieve pain to varied degrees.

Ulcerations

1. An estimated 12% of patients with diabetes have foot ulcers.
2. Foot ulcers are responsible for approximately 85% of lower extremity amputations in patients with diabetes.
3. The accepted wound-healing levels for diabetes-related ulcerations of the foot and ankle are a serum albumin level of 3.0 g/dL and a total lymphocyte count greater than 1,500/mm^3.
4. An ABI of at least 0.45 and toe pressures greater than 40 mm Hg are necessary to heal a diabetes-related foot ulcer.
5. TCC is the benchmark nonsurgical treatment for the off-loading of plantar ulcerations. It permits an even distribution of pressure across the plantar surface of the foot.
6. Before antibiotic treatment of diabetes-related ulcerations is initiated, wound culture specimens should be obtained by biopsy, ulcer curettage, or aspiration (rather than by wound swab) to confirm or rule out the presence of osteomyelitis.

Amputation

1. More than 80,000 diabetes-related amputations are performed in the United States each year.
2. Approximately 30% of patients who have undergone diabetes-related amputation of a lower extremity undergo amputation of the contralateral limb within 3 years of the first amputation.
3. The ADA reports that multidisciplinary foot care programs, along with comprehensive patient education, can reduce diabetes-related lower extremity amputation rates as much as 45% to 60%.
4. In general, forefoot stability is preserved if no more than two rays are resected.
5. Achilles tendon lengthening is likely to be necessary for patients undergoing transmetatarsal amputations.
6. Syme amputation is advantageous because the potential exists for achieving a full-load–bearing residual limb that is nearly normal in length.

Charcot Arthropathy

1. Up to 7.5% of patients with diabetes and neuropathy have Charcot arthropathy of the foot and ankle, and 9% to 35% of those have bilateral involvement.
2. Early Charcot arthropathy often is confused with infection despite the lack of a substantially elevated white blood cell count or fever.
3. Surgical indications for Charcot arthropathy of the foot include recurrent ulcers and instability not controlled by a brace. Surgical options are exostectomy or reconstruction with osteotomy and fusion.
4. The anatomic location of the Charcot arthropathy affects its frequency, prognosis, and treatment.
5. The goal of treatment of Charcot arthropathy is a plantigrade foot without recurrent ulceration.

Diabetic Ankle Fractures

1. Diabetic ankle fractures need to be recognized, evaluated, and uniquely treated based on patient comorbidities.
2. Unstable diabetic ankle fractures require additional supplemental rigid fixation to enhance stability.
3. Diabetic ankle fractures should have prolonged non–weight bearing regardless of treatment modality.

Bibliography

Aksoy DY, Gürlek A, Cetinkaya Y, et al: Change in the amputation profile in diabetic foot in a tertiary reference center: Efficacy of team working. *Exp Clin Endocrinol Diabetes* 2004;112(9):526-530.

American Diabetes Association: *Statistics about diabetes: Data from the 2011 National Diabetes Fact Sheet (released January 26, 2011)*. February 12, 2014. www.diabetes.org/diabetes-basics/statistics. Accessed March 28, 2014.

Brodsky JW: The diabetic foot, in Mann RA, Coughlin MJ, eds: *The Diabetic Foot*, ed 6. St. Louis, MO, Mosby-Year Book, 1992, pp 1361-1467.

Early JS: Transmetatarsal and midfoot amputations. *Clin Orthop Relat Res* 1999;361:85-90.

Eichenholtz SN: *Charcot Joints*. Springfield, IL, CC Thomas, 1966.

Janisse DJ: The therapeutic shoe bill: Medicare coverage for prescription footwear for diabetic patients. *Foot Ankle Int.* 2005; 26(1):42-45.

Keeling JJ, Shawen SB, Andersen RC: *Transtibial amputation: Traumatic and dysvascular*, in *Orthopaedic Knowledge Update: Foot and Ankle*, ed 4. Rosemont, IL, American Academy of Orthopaedic Surgeons, 2008, pp 373-385.

Johnson JE: Operative treatment of neuropathic arthropathy of the foot and ankle. *J Bone Joint Surg Am* 1998;80:1700-1709.

Lavery LA, Lavery DC, Quebedeax-Farnham TL: Increased foot pressures after great toe amputation in diabetes. *Diabetes Care* 1995;18(11):1460-1462.

Lipsky BA, Berendt AR, Deery HG, et al: Diagnosis and treatment of diabetic foot infections. *Plast Reconstr Surg* 2006;117(7, Suppl)2125-2385.

Lovy AJ, Dowdell J, Keswani A, et al: Nonoperative versus operative treatment of displaced ankle fractures in diabetics. *Foot Ankle Int* 2017;38(3):255-260.

Myers TG, Lowery NJ, Frykberg RG, Wukich DK: Ankle and hindfoot fusions: Comparison of outcomes in patients with and without diabetes. *Foot Ankle Int* 2012;33(1):20-28.

Myerson M, Papa J, Eaton K, Wilson K: The total-contact cast for management of neuropathic plantar ulceration of the foot. *J Bone Joint Surg Am* 1992;74(2):261-269.

Pecoraro RE, Reiber GE, Burgess EM: Pathways to diabetic limb amputation: Basis for prevention. *Diabetes Care* 1990;13(5):513-521.

Philbin TM, Leyes M, Sferra JJ, Donley BG: Orthotic and prosthetic devices in partial foot amputations. *Foot Ankle Clin* 2001;6(2):215-228, v.

Pinzur MS, Slovenkai MP, Trepman E; The diabetes committee of the American orthopaedic foot and ankle society: Guidelines for diabetic foot care. *Foot Ankle Int* 1999;20(11):695-702.

Pinzur MS, Smith D, Osterman H: Syme ankle disarticulation in peripheral vascular disease and diabetic foot infection: The one-stage versus two-stage procedure. *Foot Ankle Int* 1995;16(3):124-127.

Pinzur MS, Stuck RM, Sage R, Hunt N, Rabinovich Z: Syme ankle disarticulation in patients with diabetes. *J Bone Joint Surg Am* 2003;85-A(9):1667-1672.

Quill G, Myerson M: *Clinical, Radiographic, and Pedobarographic Analysis of the Foot After Hallux Amputation. Paper Presented at the 58th Annual Meeting of the American Association of Orthopedic Surgeons.* Anaheim, CA, 1991.

Sanders LJ, Dunlap G: Transmetatarsal amputation: A successful approach to limb salvage. *J Am Podiatr Med Assoc* 1992;82(3):129-135.

Schon LC, Easley ME, Weinfeld SB: Charcot neuroarthropathy of the foot and ankle. *Clin Orthop Relat Res* 1998;349:116-131.

Simon SR, Tejwani SG, Wilson DL, Santner TJ, Denniston NL: Arthrodesis as an early alternative to nonoperative management of charcot arthropathy of the diabetic foot. *J Bone Joint Surg Am* 2000;82-A(7):939-950.

Smith DG: Amputation: Preoperative assessment and lower extremity surgical techniques. *Foot Ankle Clin* 2001;6(2):271-296.

Wagner FW Jr: Management of the diabetic neurotrophic foot: Part II. A classification and treatment program for diabetic, neuropathic, and dysvascular foot problems. *Instr Course Lect* 1979;28:143-165.

Wukich DK, Kline AJ: The management of ankle fractures in patients with diabetes. *J Bone Joint Surg Am* 2008;90(7):1570-1578.

Wukich DK, Lowery NJ, McMillen RL, Frykberg RG: Postoperative infection rates in foot and ankle surgery: A comparison of patients with and without diabetes mellitus. *J Bone Joint Surg Am* 2010;92(2):287-295.

Chapter 119

Tumors and Infections of the Foot and Ankle

KATHLEEN S. BEEBE, MD
VALERIE A. FITZHUGH, MD

I. Plantar Fibromatosis (Ledderhose Disease)

A. Overview and epidemiology

1. Plantar fibromatosis (Ledderhose disease) is a nodular fibrous proliferation associated with the plantar aponeurosis.
2. The incidence of plantar fibromatosis increases with advancing age, but it can be found in children and young adults.
3. Plantar fibromatosis is bilateral in up to 50% of patients who have the condition.

B. Evaluation

1. History and physical examination
   a. Plantar fibromatosis presents as a subcutaneous thickening or mass that is adherent to the underlying skin.
   b. It is usually asymptomatic or causes limited pain with activities.
   c. Patients with plantar fibromatosis may present with other forms of superficial fibromatosis such as palmar fibromatosis (Dupuytren disease) and penile fibromatosis (Peyronie disease). Unlike palmar fibromatosis, plantar fibromatosis rarely causes contracture of the digits.
2. Pathologic evaluation—Plantar fibromatosis must be histologically differentiated from fibrosarcoma, which is highly cellular and has more mitotic figures.
3. Imaging—MRI will reveal a mass associated with the plantar aponeurosis, most commonly on the medial portion.

C. Treatment

1. Nonsurgical—In most cases, simple observation is sufficient.
2. Surgical—Excision is associated with a high local recurrence rate and is rarely indicated or performed.

II. Subungual Exostosis

A. Overview and epidemiology—A subungual exostosis is a benign bony outgrowth that can occur in a subungual location.

B. Evaluation

1. History and physical examination—Subungual exostoses are generally found on the dorsal or medial aspect of the great toe and occasionally on the lesser toes, often after trauma or infection (**Figure 1**).
2. Imaging
   a. Radiographs—Plain radiographs reveal an exostotic tumor that arises from the tip of the dorsal aspect of the distal phalanx (**Figure 2**).
   b. The lesion may or may not be attached to the underlying bone.

Neither of the following authors nor any immediate family member has received anything of value from or has stock or stock options held in a commercial company or institution related directly or indirectly to the subject of this chapter: Dr. Beebe and Dr. Fitzhugh.

This chapter is adapted from Beebe K, MD, Lin SS, MD: Tumors and infections of the foot and ankle, in Boyer MI, ed: *AAOS Comprehensive Orthopaedic Review*, ed 2. Rosemont, IL, American Academy of Orthopaedic Surgeons, 2014, pp 1555-1560.

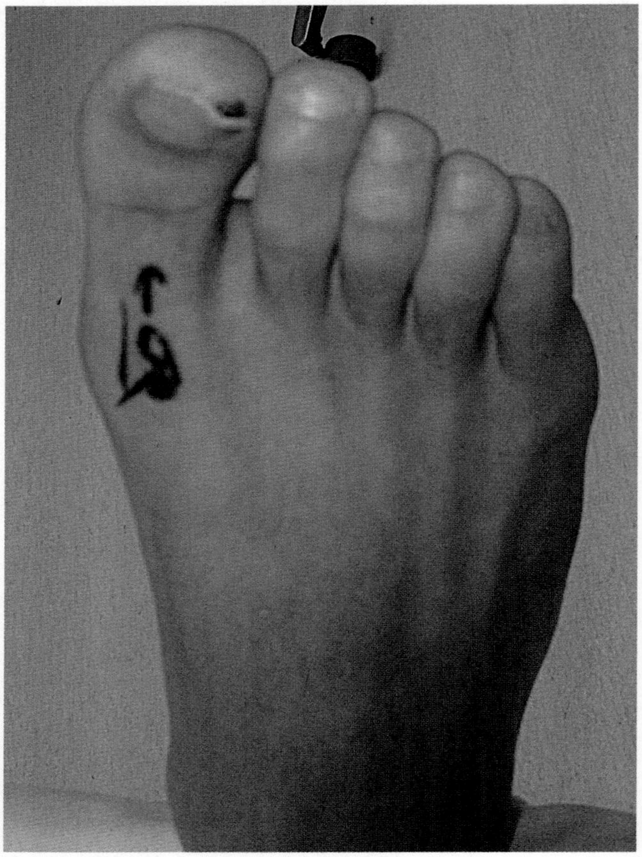

Figure 1 Clinical photograph shows a subungual exostosis on the great toe.

c. Radiographs can help differentiate a subungual exostosis from an osteochondroma, which grows away from the epiphysis.

C. Treatment is primarily surgical. It involves excision of the exostosis, often with complete excision of the nail.

III. GANGLION

A. Overview and epidemiology—A ganglion is a cystic mass that is often associated with a tendon, bursa, or joint.

B. Evaluation

1. History and physical examination

a. Patients typically present with a superficially located mass. Although ganglia are most commonly found on the dorsal surface of the wrist, they may be located on the dorsum of the foot and toes or on the ankle (**Figure 3**).

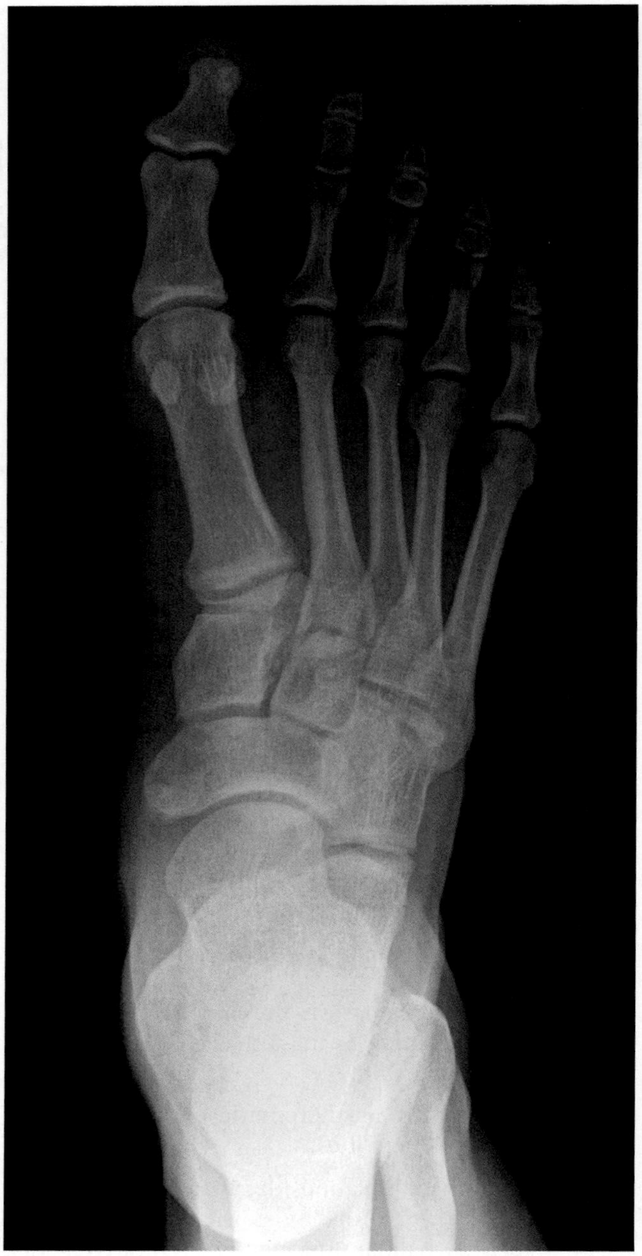

Figure 2 AP radiograph of the foot demonstrates an exostotic tumor arising from the tip of the dorsal aspect of the distal phalanx of the great toe.

b. Ganglia may or may not be associated with pain. They often increase and decrease in size, depending on activity.

2. Pathologic evaluation—Ganglia are composed of a viscous paucicellular material with a myxoid stroma, which may be diagnosed by aspiration or tissue culture.

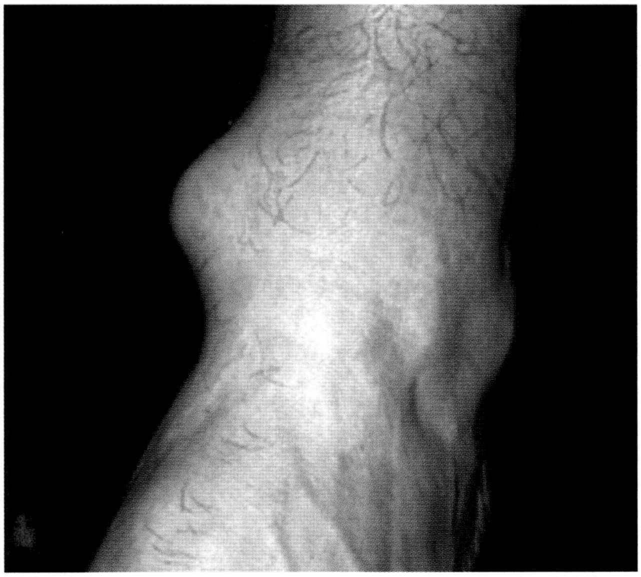

Figure 3 Photograph shows a ganglion cyst of the medial ankle. (Reproduced from Sarwark JF, ed: *Essentials of Musculoskeletal Care*, ed 4. Rosemont, IL, American Academy of Orthopaedic Surgeons, 2010, p 868.)

C. Treatment

1. Nonsurgical—If a ganglion causes mechanical pain or nerve compression, aspiration can be attempted.
2. Surgical
   a. If symptoms persist, surgical excision is performed.
   b. Excision must include the stalk of the ganglion to keep recurrence to a minimum.

IV. MELANOMA

A. Overview and epidemiology

1. Melanoma is a cutaneous malignancy that is characterized by an uncontrolled proliferation of melanocytes.
2. It is the most common malignant tumor of the foot.
3. Melanoma is not common among people with darker skin, but they are susceptible to disease in areas not in direct exposure to the sun, such as nail beds and soles of the feet.

B. Evaluation

1. History and physical examination—Melanoma usually presents as a macular lesion with an irregular border and color variegation. In general, lesions that are asymmetric and have irregular borders and color variegation, as well as lesions that have a diameter greater than 5 mm or that demonstrate an increase in size, should raise suspicion.
2. Pathologic evaluation—All subungual lesions that are growing or have not resolved after 4 to 6 weeks should undergo biopsy along with removal of the nail. The risk of death increases with each millimeter of increasing depth and with ulceration of the lesion.
3. Imaging—Radiographic evaluation of the primary lesion in melanoma is generally not indicated.
4. Histology—Malignant melanocytes with large nuclei containing prominent nucleoli within eosinophilic cytoplasm. Cytoplasm may contain pigment. Mutations in BRAF (V600E), NRAS, and C-KIT have been described (**Figure 4**).

C. Treatment

1. The standard treatment of melanoma is surgical excision.
2. The presence of ulceration and the depth of the lesion clearly affect the prognosis. Metastasis, which is most often noted in the lymph nodes and the lungs, also affects the prognosis.

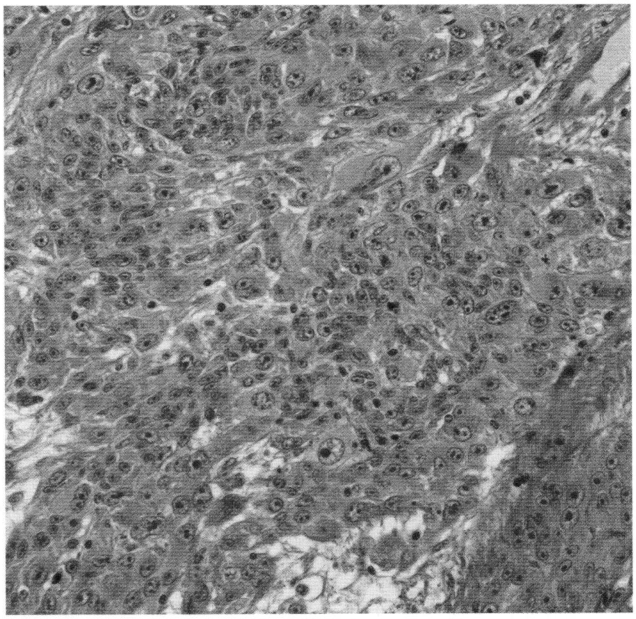

Figure 4 Photomicrograph of melanoma demonstrating sheets of large cells containing prominent cherry red nucleoli. The cells are invested within eosinophilic cytoplasm. Foci of melanin pigment deposition are also seen (Hematoxylin and eosin, 40×).

V. SYNOVIAL SARCOMA

A. Overview and epidemiology

1. Synovial sarcoma is a malignant soft-tissue tumor that often affects the lower extremities.
2. Most commonly, it affects the thigh and knee regions, followed by the foot and lower leg/ankle regions.

B. Evaluation

1. History and physical examination—The patient presents with a soft-tissue mass that may be painful. Regional lymph nodes may be enlarged.
2. Imaging—Plain radiographs are useful in the evaluation of synovial sarcoma because calcifications are noted within the mass approximately 15% to 20% of the time. Although synovial sarcomas may be in close proximity to a joint, they are rarely intra-articular.
3. Advanced imaging studies—MRI will reveal a heterogeneous mass that may or may not involve the underlying bone. MRI is most useful for defining the anatomic location and extent of the tumor. Because of the propensity of synovial sarcoma to metastasize to the lungs, evaluation of the lungs is recommended and can be performed using plain radiography or, more commonly, CT scanning. In addition, lymph node metastasis is noted in 10% of patients with metastatic disease, and evaluation should be performed to assess the regional and systemic lymph nodes.
4. Histology—monophasic and biphasic subtypes. Pathognomonic translocation for X:18 (SS-18 translocated to SSX-1, SSX-2, or SSX-4) (**Figure 5, A** and **B**).

C. Treatment

1. Surgical excision with a wide margin is the mainstay of treatment.
2. Radiation therapy is often used to improve local control.

VI. FOOT INFECTIONS IN THE NONDIABETIC PATIENT

A. Cellulitis

1. Overview and epidemiology—Cellulitis is an infection of the skin and subcutaneous tissue that is characterized by pain, erythema, swelling, and tenderness.
2. Pathoanatomy—*Staphylococcus aureus* and β-hemolytic streptococci are the most common causes of cellulitis in the nonimmunocompromised host.

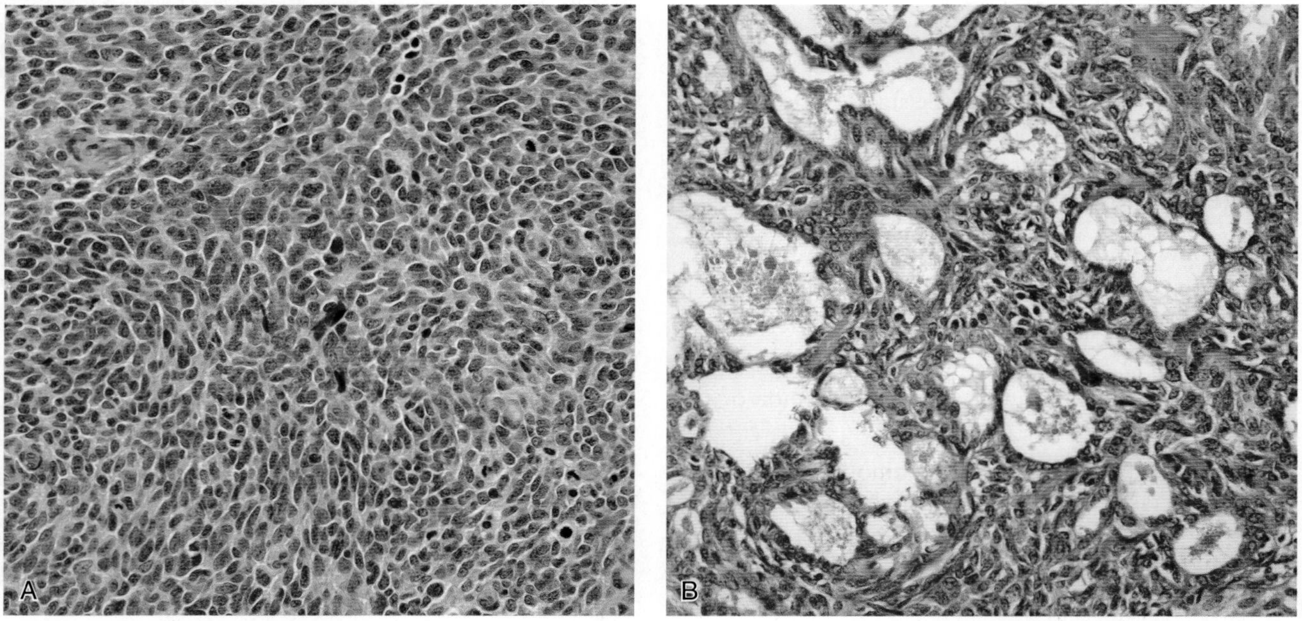

Figure 5 **A**, Photomicrograph of monophasic synovial sarcoma demonstrating well-oriented, plump spindled cells. The nuclei are ovoid and darkly staining. Mitotic figures are present (Hematoxylin and eosin, 40×). **B**, Photomicrograph of biphasic synovial sarcoma demonstrating glandular elements within a well-oriented, plump spindle cell stroma (Hematoxylin and eosin, 40×).

Section 9

Sports Medicine

Section Editors | KURT SPINDLER, MD
SETH GAMRADT, MD

Chapter 120

Anatomy and Biomechanics of the Knee

ERIC C. McCARTY, MD
DAVID R. McALLISTER, MD
JAMES P. LEONARD, MD

I. Anatomy

A. Bone anatomy

1. Distal femur

   a. The medial femoral condyle is larger and projects farther posteriorly and distally than the lateral condyle.

      - The medial epicondyle is the most anterior and distal osseous prominence.
      - The adductor tubercle is proximal and posterior to the medial epicondyle.
      - The gastrocnemius tubercle is slightly distal and posterior to the adductor tubercle.

   b. The lateral femoral condyle projects farther anteriorly and is wider in the medial-lateral direction than is the medial femoral condyle.

   c. The sulcus terminalis is a small ridge on the lateral femoral condyle just distal to the intercondylar notch; it separates the patellofemoral and tibiofemoral articular surfaces.

   d. The trochlear groove separates the two condyles anteriorly and constitutes the patellofemoral articulation.

   e. The intercondylar notch is of variable width and is the site of attachment of the cruciate ligaments.

2. Proximal tibia

   a. The tibial articular surface slopes 7° to 10° in the sagittal plane.

   b. The medial tibial plateau is larger than the lateral plateau and is concave in its frontal and sagittal planes.

   c. The lateral tibial plateau is smaller and more circular than the medial plateau. It is concave in the frontal plane and convex in the sagittal plane.

   d. The medial and lateral tibial plateaus are separated by the intercondylar eminence and its medial and lateral spinous processes.

   e. The tibial tuberosity is the site of attachment of the patellar tendon. It is typically located in the midline anteriorly but may be slightly lateral.

   f. Gerdy's tubercle is the insertion site of the iliotibial band and is located 2 to 3 cm lateral to the tibial tubercle on the proximal tibia.

   g. The proximal fibula articulates with a facet of the lateral cortex of the tibia and is not part of the knee articulation.

3. Patella

   a. The patella is the largest sesamoid bone in the body.

   b. It averages 2.5 cm in thickness.

   c. It has the thickest articular surface in the body, approximately 5 mm in the midportion and 2 mm on the sides.

Dr. McCarty or an immediate family member has received royalties from Biomet and Zimmer; serves as a paid consultant to or is an employee of Biomet; has received research or institutional support from Arthrex, Inc., Biomet, Breg, Mitek, Ossur, Smith & Nephew, and Stryker Smith & Nephew; and serves as a board member, owner, officer, or committee member of the American Orthopaedic Society for Sports Medicine and the International Society of Arthroscopy, Knee Surgery, and Orthopaedic Sports Medicine. Dr. McAllister or an immediate family member has received royalties from Biomet; serves as a paid consultant to or is an employee of Biomet and Musculoskeletal Transplant Foundation, Conmed and serves as a board member, owner, officer, or committee member of the American Orthopaedic Society for Sports Medicine and the International Society of Arthroscopy, Knee Surgery, and Orthopaedic Sports Medicine. Dr. Leonard or an immediate family member serves as a board member, owner, officer, or committee member of the American Orthopaedic Society for Sports Medicine.

d. The articular surface contains a vertical, central ridge that separates the broader lateral facet from the medial facet, and a smaller, more medial facet called the odd facet.

B. Vascular anatomy

1. The blood supply to the knee is formed from an anastomosis around the knee derived from the following arterial branches:

   a. Descending geniculate artery (branch of femoral artery)

   b. Medial and lateral superior geniculate arteries (branches of popliteal artery)

   c. Medial and lateral inferior geniculate arteries (branches of popliteal artery)

   d. Middle geniculate artery (branch of popliteal artery)

   e. Anterior tibial recurrent arteries

2. The middle geniculate artery supplies both the anterior and posterior cruciate ligaments.

3. The inferior geniculate arteries pass deep to their respective collateral ligaments.

4. The blood supply of the patella is derived from the geniculate artery complex with some contribution from the anterior tibial recurrent artery and primarily exists in the middle to inferior portions of the patella.

C. Nerve anatomy

1. The knee is innervated by branches of the femoral nerve (L2, L3, L4), obturator nerve (L2, L3, L4), and sciatic nerve (L4, L5, S1, S2).

2. The largest nerve providing innervation of the intra-articular knee is the posterior articular branch of the tibial nerve. This nerve supplies the infrapatellar fat pad, the synovial covering over the cruciate ligaments, and the periphery of the meniscus.

3. Nerves to the cruciate ligaments contain vasomotor and pain fibers as well as mechanoreceptors that may be involved in proprioception.

4. The infrapatellar branch of the saphenous nerve arises proximal to the knee joint medially and crosses distal to the patella to innervate the skin over the region of the anterior knee and proximal tibia.

D. Ligament anatomy

1. Anterior cruciate ligament (ACL) (**Figure 1**)

   a. The ACL is composed of 90% type I collagen and 10% type III collagen.

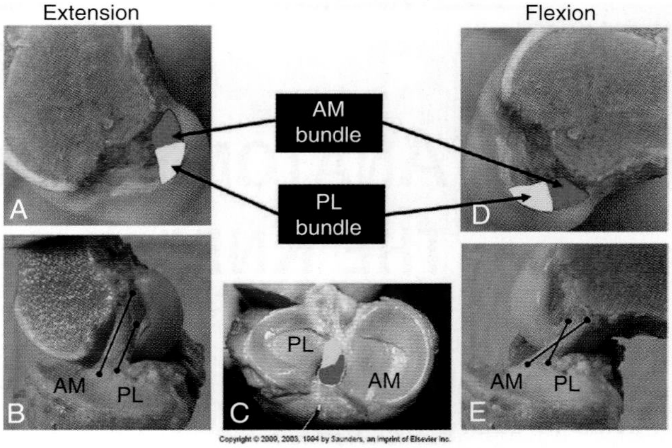

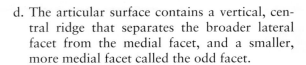

Figure 1 Photographs show the anterior cruciate ligament (ACL) anatomy. **A**, With the knee in extension, the anteromedial (AM) and posterolateral (PL) femoral insertions of the ACL are oriented vertically about the posterior aspect of the medial femoral condyle. **B**, The AM and PL bundles are parallel to each other, with the PL bundle taut. **C**, The AM and PL bundles are named according to their tibial sites of insertion. Note the close approximation to the anterior and posterior horns of the lateral meniscus. **D**, With the knee flexed, the insertions of the AM and PL bundles are oriented horizontally. **E**, The bundles cross each other, with the AM bundle taut. (Reproduced with permission from Honkamp NJ, Shen W, Okeke N, Ferretti M, Fu FH: Anterior cruciate ligament injuries, in DeLee JC, Drez D Jr, Miller MD, eds: *Orthopaedic Sports Medicine*. Philadelphia, PA, WB Saunders, 2010, vol 2, p 1646.)

   b. The mean length of the ACL is 33 mm; the mean midsubstance width is 11 mm.

   c. The femoral attachment is a semicircular area (20 mm long and 10 mm wide) on the posteromedial aspect of the lateral femoral condyle.

   d. The tibial attachment is a broad, irregular, oval-shaped area (30 mm long and 10 mm wide) slightly medial and anterior to the midline and between the medial and lateral tibial spinous processes.

2. Posterior cruciate ligament (PCL) (**Figure 2**)

   a. The mean length of the PCL is 38 mm; the mean midsubstance width is 13 mm.

   b. The femoral attachment is a broad, crescent-shaped area anterolateral on the medial femoral condyle (30 mm long and 5 mm wide).

   c. The tibial attachment is in a central sulcus on the posterior aspect of the tibia, 10 to 15 mm below the articular surface.

   d. The meniscofemoral ligaments are present 70% of the time; they originate from the posterior horn of the lateral meniscus and insert

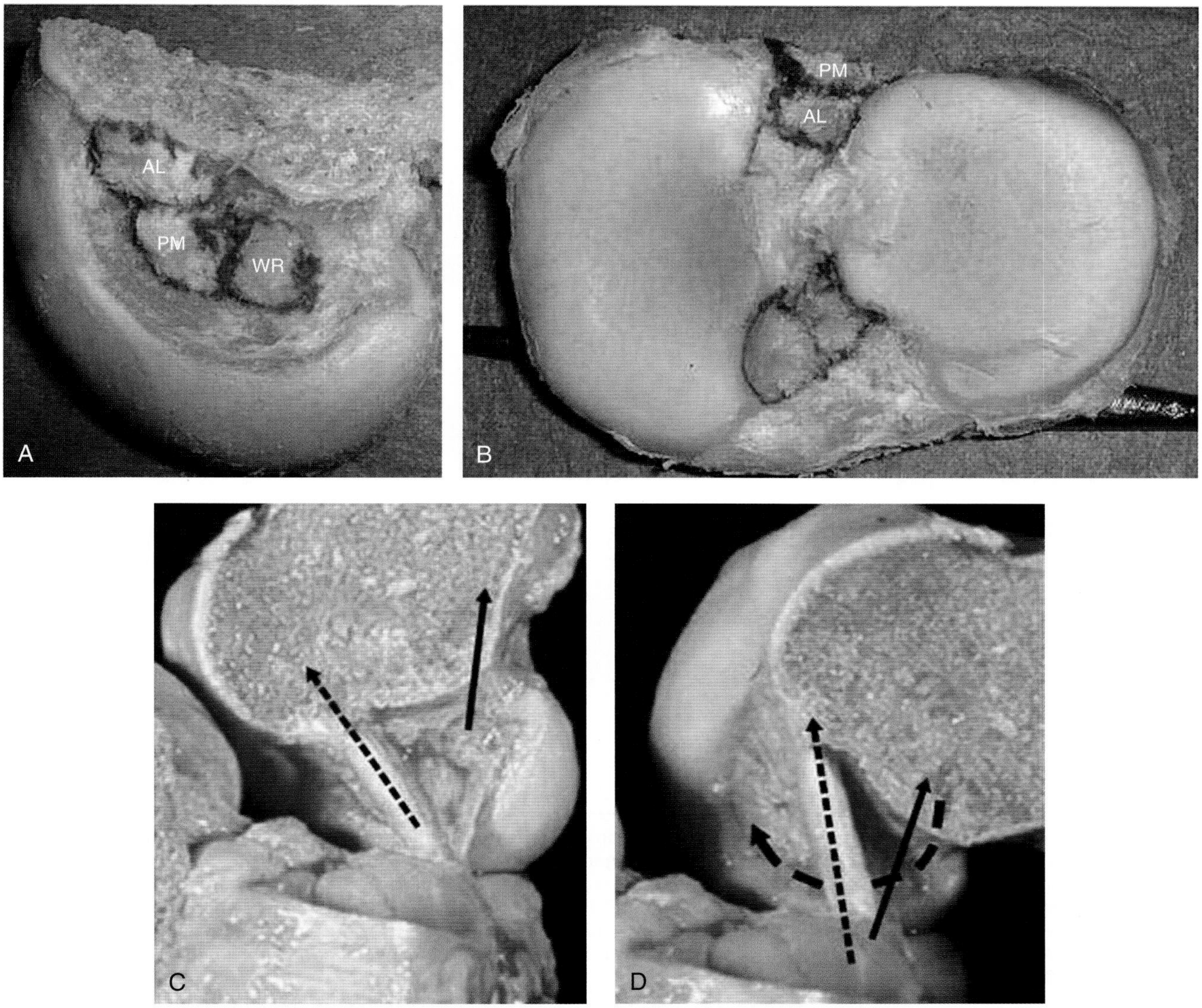

Figure 2 Photographs show posterior cruciate ligament (PCL) anatomy. **A**, Sagittal cross-section of the lateral femoral condyle showing the origins of the anterolateral (AL) and posteromedial (PM) bundles of the PCL and the ligament of Wrisberg (WR). **B**, Axial view of the tibial plateau showing the insertion sites of the AL and PM bundles of the PCL. As with the anterior cruciate ligament, the bundles of the PCL are named according to their tibial insertions. **C**, With the knee in extension, the AL bundle is loose (dashed arrow), whereas the PM bundle is taut (solid arrow). **D**, Flexion of the knee increases the tightness of the AL bundle (dashed arrow), also loosening of the PM bundle (solid arrow) as it passes between the AL bundle and the medial femoral condyle (curved dashed arrow). (Panels **A** and **B** reproduced with permission from Takahashi M, Matsubara T, Doi M, Suzuki D, Nagano A: Anatomic study of the femoral and tibial insertions of the anterolateral and posteromedial bundles of the human posterior cruciate ligament. *Knee Surg Sports Traumatol Arthrosc* 2006;14[11]:1055-1059. Panels **C** and **D** reproduced with permission from Amis AA, Gupte CM, Bull AMJ, Edwards A: Anatomy of the posterior cruciate ligament and the meniscofemoral ligaments. *Knee Surg Sports Traumatol Arthrosc* 2006;14:257-263.)

into the substance of the PCL and the medial femoral condyle.

- The ligament of Humphrey is anterior to the PCL.
- The ligament of Wrisberg is posterior to the PCL.

3. Medial structures of the knee (**Figure 3**)
   a. Organization (**Table 1**)
      - The medial side of the knee can be divided into three anatomic layers, from superficial to deep.

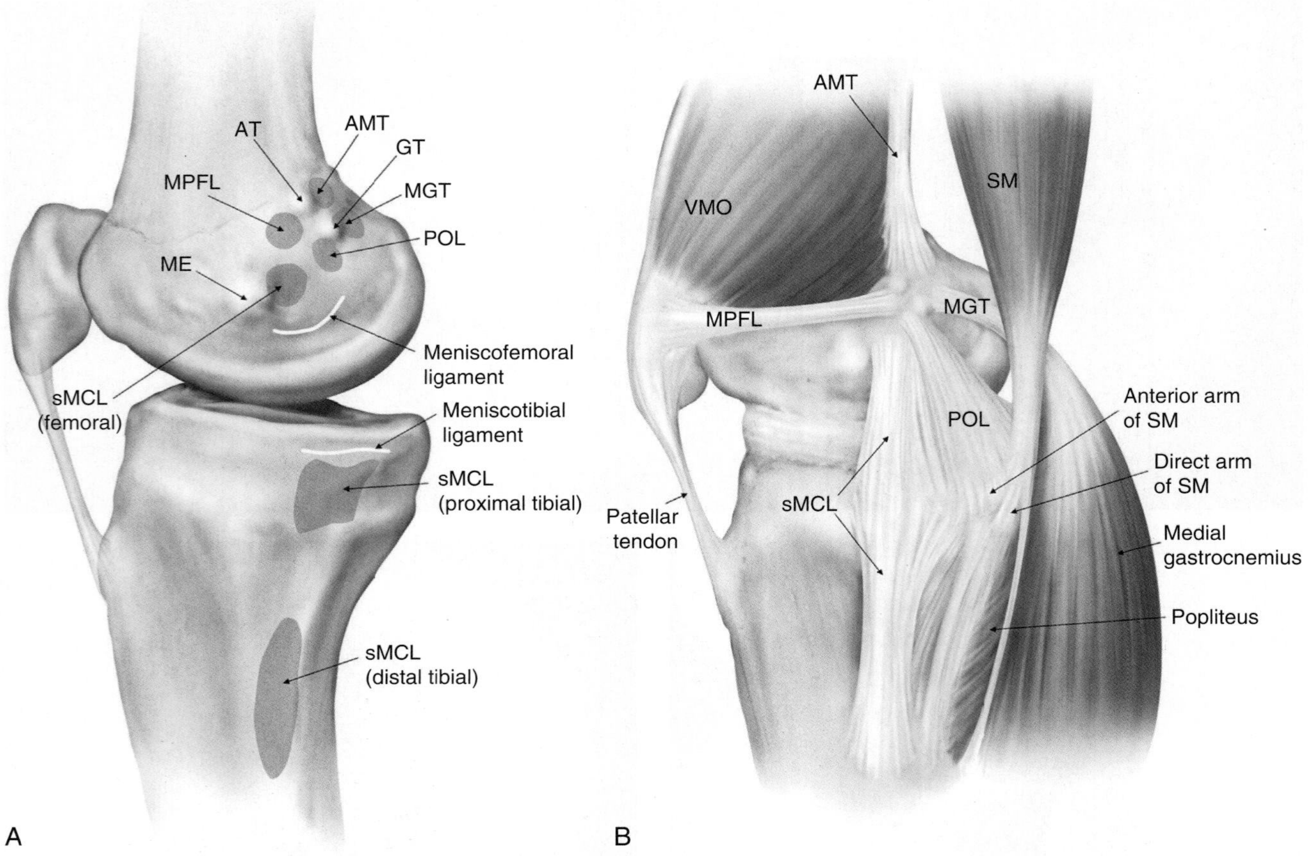

Figure 3 Illustrations of the medial structures of the knee demonstrate the bony origins and insertions of medial ligamentous and tendinous structures on the femur and tibia (**A**) and important ligamentous, tendinous, and muscular structures of the medial knee (**B**). AT = adductor tubercle, AMT = adductor magnus tendon, GT = gastrocnemius tubercle, ME = medial epicondyle, MGT = medial gastrocnemius tendon, MPFL = medial patellofemoral ligament, POL = posterior oblique ligament, SM = semimembranosus muscle, sMCL = superficial medial collateral ligament, VMO = vastus medialis obliquus muscle. (Reproduced with permission from LaPrade RF, Engebretsen AH, Ly TV, Johansen S, Wentorf FA, Engebretsen L: The anatomy of the medial part of the knee. *J Bone Joint Surg Am* 2007;89[9]:2000-2010.)

- The medial side of the knee can be classified into three functional groups. These groups are described from anterior to posterior.

b. Medial collateral ligament (MCL)

- The superficial MCL, also known as the tibial collateral ligament, lies deep to the gracilis and semitendinosus tendons. It originates from the medial femoral epicondyle and inserts onto the periosteum of the proximal tibia, deep to the pes anserinus and approximately 4.6 cm distal to the joint line.
- The deep MCL, also referred to as the medial capsular ligament, is a capsular thickening that originates from the femur and blends with the fibers of the superficial MCL distally. It is intimately associated with the

TABLE 1

Organization of the Medial Structures of the Knee

Layer	Anterior	Middle	Posterior
I (superficial)	Medial retinaculum	Sartorial fascia	Sartorial fascia
II (middle)	Medial patellofemoral ligament	Superficial medial collateral ligament	Posteromedial corner
III (deep)	No significant ligamentous structure	Deep medial collateral ligament	Posteromedial corner

medial meniscus through attachments to the coronary ligaments.

c. Medial patellofemoral ligament (MPFL)
   - The MPFL is a thickening of the medial retinaculum.
   - It originates from the adductor tubercle and inserts onto the superomedial border of the patella.

d. Posteromedial corner
   - The posteromedial corner of the knee consists of the posterior oblique ligament, the various insertions of the semimembranosus tendon, the oblique popliteal ligament, and the posterior horn of the medial meniscus.
   - The posterior oblique ligament originates from the medial surface of the femur distal to the adductor tubercle and posterior to the origin of the superficial MCL, inserting at the posteromedial corner of the tibia.
   - The oblique popliteal ligament is a thickening of the most posterior aspect of the capsule of the knee joint. It extends from the inferomedial aspect of the posterior knee at the site of insertion of the semimembranosus muscle on the tibia and travels superolaterally, inserting into the capsule behind the lateral femoral condyle.

4. Lateral structures of the knee (**Figure 4**)
   a. The lateral side of the knee comprises three layers:
      - Layer I consists of the iliotibial band and biceps femoris.

9 | Sports Medicine

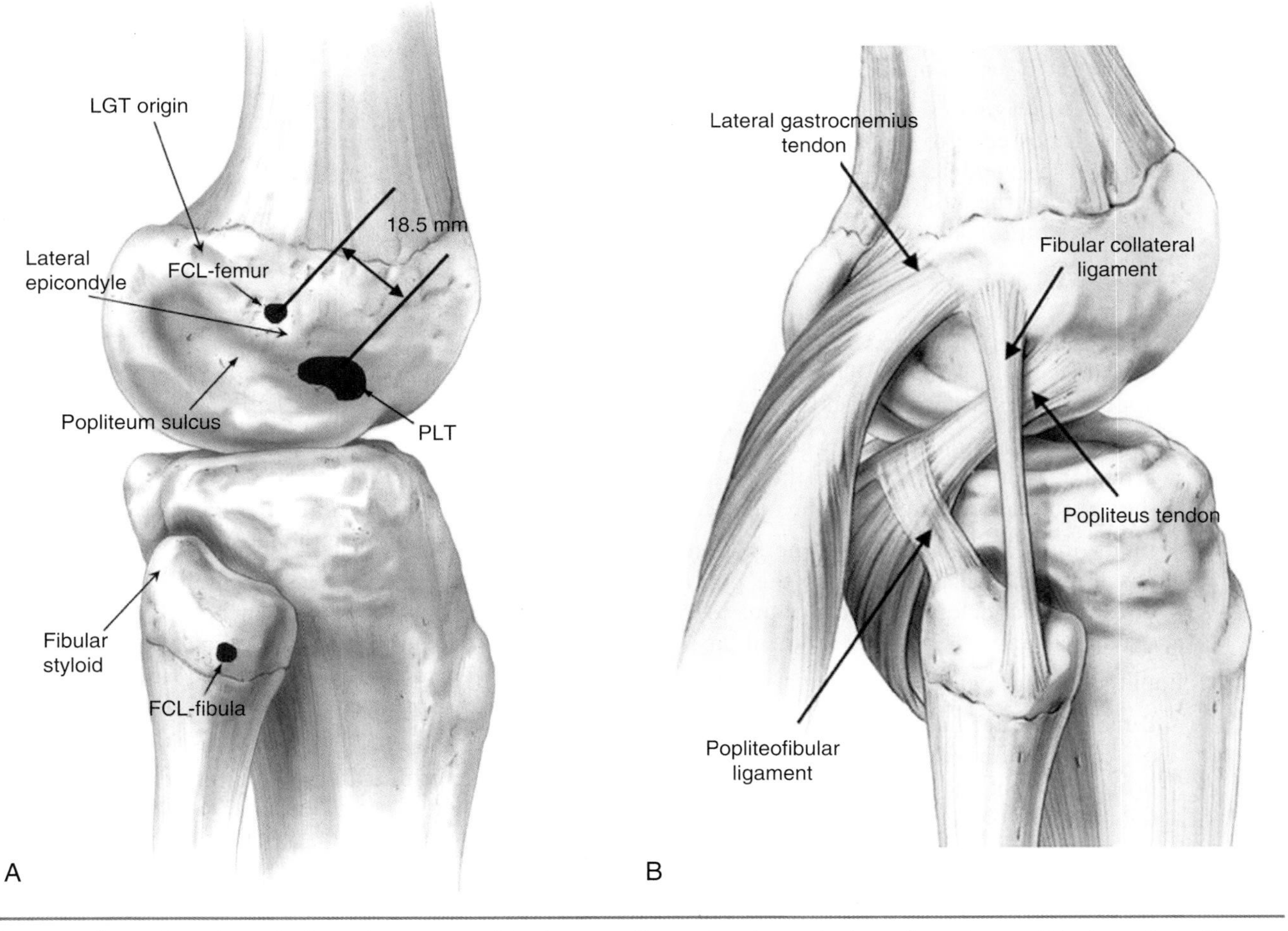

Figure 4 Illustrations show the lateral structures of the knee. **A**, Illustration shows the lateral structures of the knee, including bony attachments of key structures of the posterolateral corner: the lateral collateral ligament (fibular collateral ligament, FCL), popliteus tendon (PLT), and lateral gastrocnemius tendon (LGT). The mean distance between the origins of the FCL and PLT is 18.5 mm. **B**, Illustration shows the FCL, PLT, and popliteofibular ligament, the main structures of the posterolateral corner. (Reproduced with permission from LaPrade RF, Ly TV, Wentorf FA, Engebretsen L: The posterolateral attachments of the knee. *Am J Sports Med* 2003;31[6]:854-860.)

- Layer II consists of the quadriceps retinaculum and lateral patellofemoral ligaments.
- Layer III consists of the posterolateral corner and lateral side of the knee capsule.

b. The peroneal nerve runs between layers I and II.

c. The anatomy of the posterolateral corner is complex and highly variable.

- The lateral collateral ligament (LCL), popliteus tendon, and popliteofibular ligament are the main contributors to static stabilization.

d. Lateral collateral ligament

- The LCL is also known as the fibular collateral ligament.
- It lies between the second and third of the three layers of lateral structures of the knee.
- Its shape is tubular, with a diameter of 3 to 4 mm and a length of 66 mm.
- The LCL originates 1.4 mm proximal and 3.4 mm posterior to the ridge of the lateral femoral epicondyle and is posterior and superior to the insertion of the popliteus. It inserts on the lateral aspect of the fibular head.

e. Popliteus

- The popliteus originates on the back of the tibia and inserts medial, anterior, and approximately 18.5 mm distal to the LCL.
- It is intracapsular and becomes intra-articular as it passes through the hiatus in the peripheral attachment of the meniscus.
- In its intra-articular course, the popliteus has three branches, known as the popliteomeniscal fascicles, that contribute to the dynamic stability of the lateral meniscus.

f. Popliteofibular ligament

- Runs from the musculotendinous junction of the popliteus to the posterosuperior prominence of the fibula head adjacent to the insertion of the LCL.

g. The anterolateral complex of the knee consists of the layers of the iliotibial band and the anterolateral joint capsule.

- The middle third of the lateral capsular ligament is a thickening of the lateral capsule of the knee and is divided into meniscofemoral and meniscotibial components.
- A Segond fracture, which is pathognomonic of an injury to the ACL, results from an avulsion injury of the meniscotibial component.

h. The anterolateral ligament (ALL) refers to either the midthird capsular ligament, the deep, capsule-osseous layer of the iliotibial band, or a combination of both

- Originates in the lateral femoral epicondylar region and courses anterodistally to the anterolateral tibia, halfway between Gerdy's tubercle and the anterior margin of the fibula head approximately 5 to 10 mm distal to joint line.

E. Menisci (**Figure 5**)

1. The medial and lateral menisci of the knee are crescent-shaped fibrocartilaginous structures that each have a triangular cross section (**Table 2**).
2. Microstructure
   a. The menisci are composed mostly of type I collagen.
   b. The superficial layer contains a mesh network of fibers.
   c. Most collagen fibers of the menisci are oriented circumferentially along the length of the meniscus.
   d. Radial fibers act to tie the circumferential fibers together.
3. The transverse intermeniscal ligament connects the anterior horns of the medial and lateral menisci.
4. Vascular supply
   a. The superior and inferior geniculate arteries supply blood to the menisci.
   b. These vessels form a premeniscal capillary plexus with radial branches to peripheral portions of the menisci. Vascular penetration of the medial meniscus is 10% to 30%; of the lateral meniscus, 10% to 25%.
   c. Most of the adult meniscus is avascular and receives nutrition through diffusion.
5. Nerve supply
   a. The nerve supply is similar to the vascular supply (ie, concentrated in the periphery of the meniscus).
   b. Sensory fibers play a role in pain production.
   c. Mechanoreceptors supply proprioceptive feedback during joint motion.

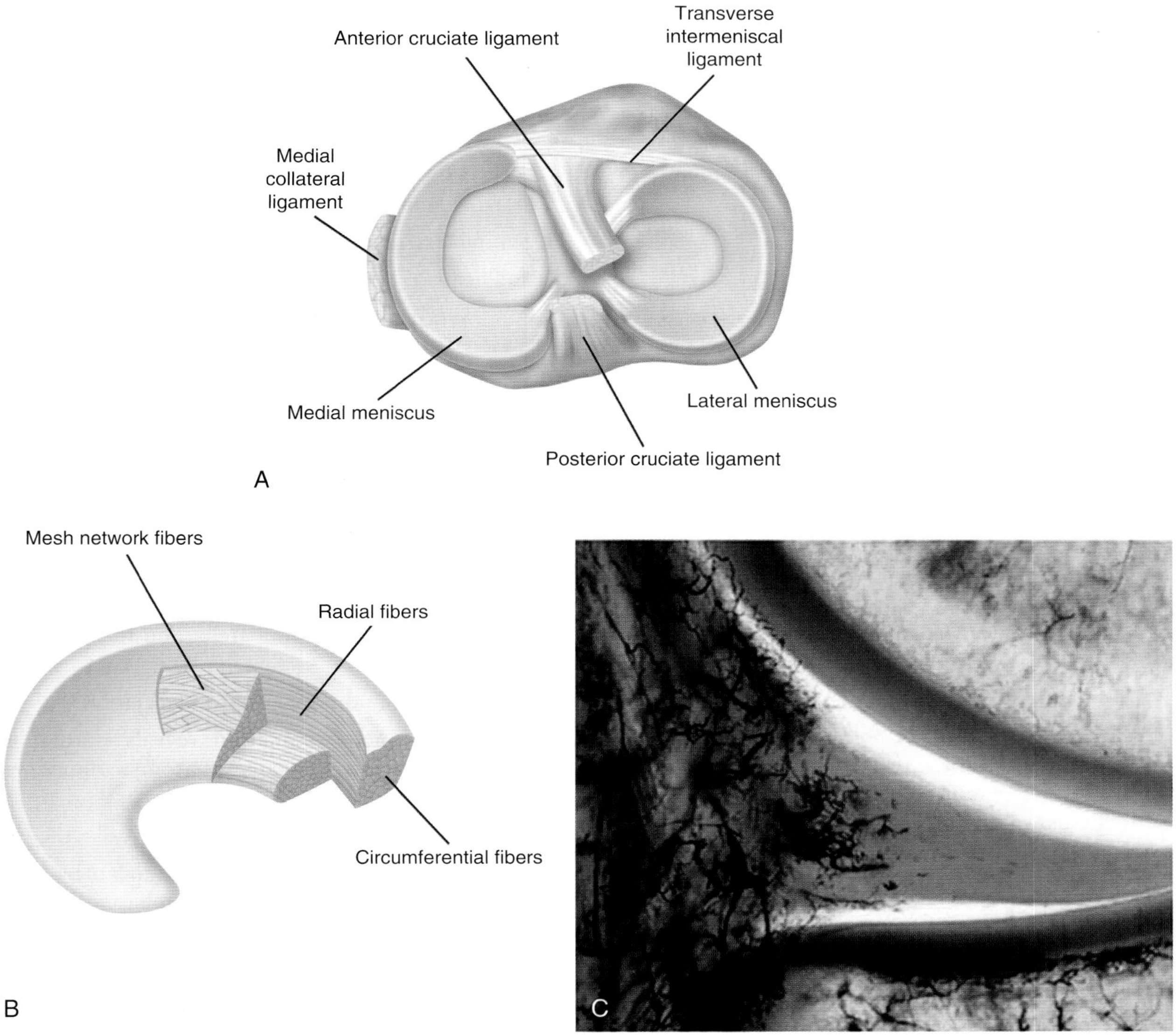

Figure 5 Meniscal anatomy. **A**, Illustration shows the axial anatomy of the menisci. The lateral meniscus is more circular in shape than the medial meniscus and has a close approximation to the insertion of the ACL on the tibia. **B**, Microstructure of a meniscus. The meniscus consists of circumferential, radial, and oblique fibers. **C**, Micrograph demonstrating the vascularity of the periphery of the meniscus. Only the peripheral one-fourth to one-third of the meniscus is vascularized. (Adapted with permission from Arnoczky SP, Warren RF: Microvasculature of the human meniscus. *Am J Sports Med* 1982;10:90-95.)

TABLE 2

Comparison of the Medial and Lateral Menisci

Medial Meniscus	Lateral Meniscus
C-shaped	Circular shaped
Mean width, 9-10 mm; mean thickness, 3-5 mm	Mean width, 10-12 mm; mean thickness, 4-5 mm
Covers 50% of the medial tibial plateau	Covers 70% of the lateral tibial plateau
Anterior and posterior horns are separated from each other and far from the anterior cruciate ligament	Anterior and posterior horns are close to each other and near the insertion of the anterior cruciate ligament
Solidly attached to the medial joint capsule through the coronary and meniscotibial ligaments	Loosely attached to the lateral joint capsule through the popliteomensical fascicle and coronary and meniscotibial ligaments

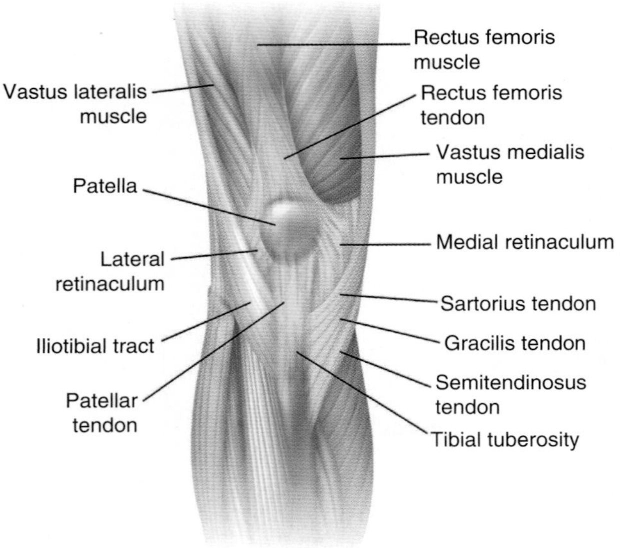

Figure 6 Illustration shows the anatomy of the extensor mechanism. The quadriceps mechanism includes the rectus femoris, vastus medialis, vastus intermedius, and vastus lateralis muscles and is continuous with the quadriceps tendon and medial and lateral retinaculum.

F. Extensor mechanism (**Figure 6**)

1. The quadriceps or extensor mechanism of the leg involves four muscles: the rectus femoris, vastus medialis, vastus lateralis, and vastus intermedius.
2. The medial and lateral retinacula are extensions of the quadriceps tendon.
3. The patellofemoral ligaments are discrete thickenings in the retinaculum.
4. The patella is invested in this retinacular layer of the extensor mechanism, which continues distally, investing and comprising the superficial portion of the patellar tendon before ultimately becoming continuous with the tibial periosteum.
5. The patellar tendon extends from the distal pole of the patella and inserts onto the tibial tuberosity. The patellar tendon ranges from 3.0 to 3.5 cm in width.

G. Popliteal fossa

1. The popliteal fossa contains the popliteal neurovascular structures.
   a. The popliteal artery and vein are separated from the underlying posterior joint capsule by a thin layer of fat.
   b. The tibial nerve is the most superficial of popliteal neurovascular structures. Next most superficial is the popliteal vein. The popliteal artery is the deepest structure, closest to the posterior joint capsule.
2. The popliteal fossa is formed proximally by the biceps femoris laterally and the semimembranosus and pes anserinus muscles medially.
3. It is formed distally by the two heads of the gastrocnemius muscle.

H. Synovial structures

1. Plicae
   a. Synovial plicae are variable-appearing folds of synovial tissue in the knee, thought to represent embryologic remnants.
   b. A plica may be medial (most common), lateral, suprapatellar, and/or infrapatellar, and plicae may occur in more than one of these locations.
   c. The medial plica originates in the synovium superiorly and laterally to the patella and inserts into the anterior fat pad.
2. Fat pads—Three extrasynovial structures located above and below the patella and in front of the distal femur.

I. Arthroscopic and portal anatomy (**Figure 7**)

1. Arthroscopic examination reveals normal and pathologic intra-articular anatomy of knee, with most structures evident.
2. Standard arthroscopic portals
   a. An anterolateral portal and an anteromedial portal just inferior to the patella
   b. A superomedial and a superolateral portal; often used for irrigation inflow
   c. A midpatellar tendon portal and a posteromedial and posterolateral portal; used less often
3. Structures potentially at risk of injury
   a. Infrapatellar branch of the saphenous nerve, with any anterior subpatellar portal
   b. Saphenous nerve, with posteromedial portal
   c. Peroneal nerve, with superolateral portal

II. BIOMECHANICS

A. Knee alignment (**Figure 8**)

1. Anatomic axis
   a. The anatomic axis of the knee is the angle formed by the intersection of lines drawn down the center of the tibia and femur on radiographs.
   b. The mean anatomic axis is 6° of valgus angulation.

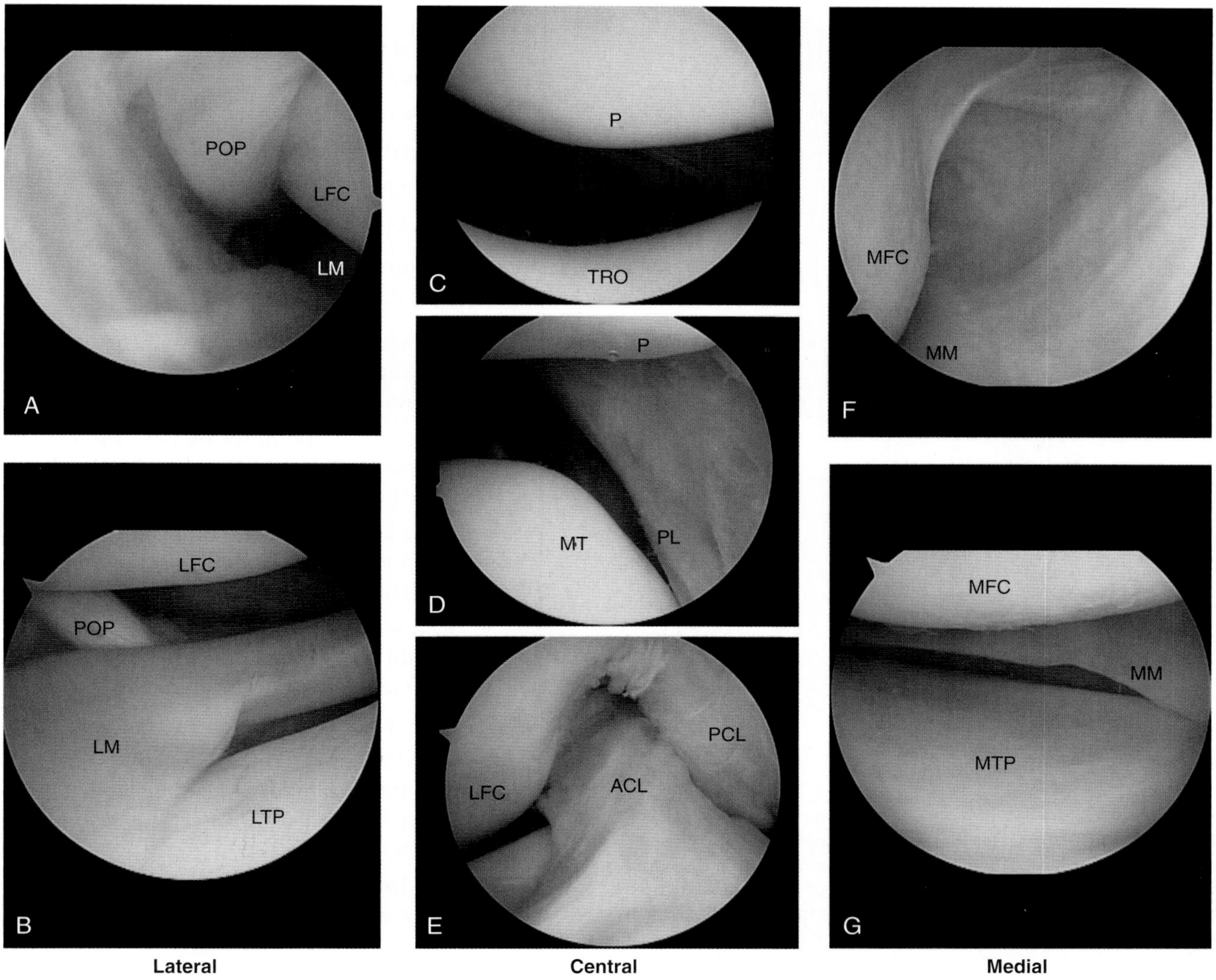

Figure 7 Arthroscopic views of the knee. **A**, The lateral gutter. **B**, The lateral compartment. **C**, The patellofemoral compartment. **D**, The medial plica. **E**, The notch. **F**, The medial compartment. **G**, The medial compartment. ACL = anterior cruciate ligament, LFC = lateral femoral condyle, LM = lateral meniscus, LTP = lateral tibial plateau, MFC = medial femoral compartment, MM = medial meniscus, MT = medial trochlea, MTP = medial tibial plateau, P = patella, PCL = posterior cruciate ligament, PL = plica, POP = popliteus tendon, TRO = trochlea

2. Mechanical axis
    a. The mechanical axis of the leg is determined by drawing a line from the center of the femoral head to the center of the ankle on a radiograph.
    b. Normally, this axis should pass through the medial part of the femoral notch or the lateral part of the medial compartment.
3. Q angle
    a. The Q angle is the angle formed by a line drawn from the anterior superior iliac spine to the midpatella and a line drawn from the midpatella to the tibial tuberosity.
    b. Normal Q angle in males is 14° ± 3°; normal Q angle in females is 17° ± 3°.
    c. Considerable disagreement exists about the reliability and validity of clinical Q angle measurement because of the lack of a standard measurement procedure.

B. Knee articulations
1. Tibiofemoral articulation
    a. Motion
        - The knee is more than a simple, pinned hinge (ginglymus) joint.

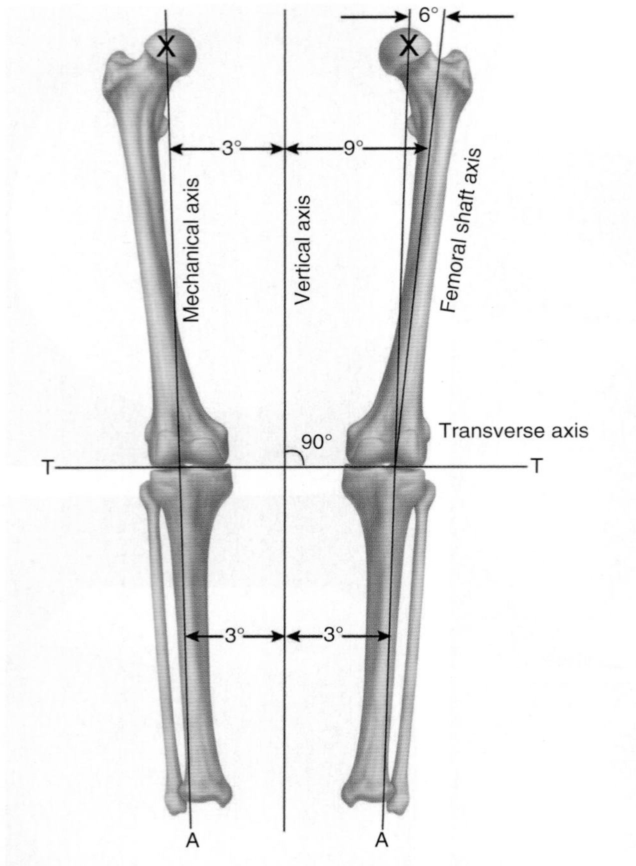

Figure 8 Illustrations demonstrate the measurement of lower extremity alignment. The mechanical axis of the left extremity is defined as a line drawn from the center of the femoral head to the center of the ankle. On average, the mechanical axis makes a 3° angle with a vertical line. The anatomic axis of the right extremity has a 6° average valgus angulation between the anatomic axis of the femur and the anatomic axis of the tibia. The anatomic axis of the femur makes a 9° angle with a vertical line and a 6° angle with the mechanical axis of each lower extremity. The anatomic axis of the tibia makes a 3° angle with a vertical line. A = anatomic, T = transverse

- The knee allows motion with six degrees of freedom (three translational and three rotational).
- The contact point of the femur with the tibia moves posteriorly as the knee flexes and anteriorly as the knee extends (posterior femoral roll back).
- The tibia rotates externally by approximately 10° during the last 20° of knee extension because of different sizes and curvatures of the femoral condyles. This rotation "locks" the knee in extension by tensioning the collateral and cruciate ligaments (screw-home mechanism).
- The popliteus "unlocks" the knee by rotating the knee internally during the initiation of knee flexion.

b. Reactive forces of knee joint

- Normal walking = 3× body weight
- Stair climbing = 4× body weight
- Deep knee bends = 7× body weight

2. Patellofemoral articulation

a. Patellar tracking

- The distal portion of the patella first engages the femoral trochlea at a knee flexion angle of almost 20°.
- As the knee continues to flex, the contact area moves from the distal to proximal pole of the patella.
- As the knee flexes, the patella also translates laterally and tilts medially within the trochlear groove.
- Deep in flexion, the quadriceps tendon and the odd facet and lateral facet of the patella all articulate with the trochlea.

b. Patellar stability

- The MPFL is the primary passive soft-tissue restraint to lateral patellar instability, providing 50% to 60% of lateral restraint at flexion of 0° to 30°.
- The lowest force required to laterally displace the patella occurs at 30° of flexion. At this position, the vastus medialis obliquus muscle is the most effective constraint.
- With further flexion, the bony constraint of the trochlear groove on the patella provides the primary constraint to lateral patellar instability.

C. Gait

1. Normal gait cycle (walking) has two phases:

a. Swing phase (40%): initial swing, midswing, terminal swing

b. Stance phase (60%): initial contact, loading response, midstance, terminal stance, preswing

2. Three essential actions occur at the knee.

a. Flexion to decrease the impact of initial foot contact

b. Extension for weight-bearing stability

c. Flexion for toe clearance during swing

Bibliography

Amis AA: Current concepts on anatomy and biomechanics of patellar stability. *Sports Med Arthrosc* 2007;15(2):48-56.

Chhabra A, Starman JS, Ferretti M, Vidal AF, Zantop T, Fu FH: Anatomic, radiographic, biomechanical, and kinematic evaluation of the anterior cruciate ligament and its two functional bundles. *J Bone Joint Surg Am* 2006;88(suppl 4):2-10.

Flandry F, Hommel G: Normal anatomy and biomechanics of the knee. *Sports Med Arthrosc* 2011;19(2):82-92.

Fox AJ, Wanivenhaus F, Burge AJ, Warren RF, Rodeo SA: The human meniscus: A review of anatomy, function, injury, and advancements in treatment. *Clin Anat* 2015;28(2):269-287.

LaPrade RF, Engebretsen AH, Ly TV, Johansen S, Wentorf FA, Engebretsen L: The anatomy of the medial part of the knee. *J Bone Joint Surg Am* 2007;89(9):2000-2010.

LaPrade RF, Ly TV, Wentorf FA, Engebretsen L: The posterolateral attachments of the knee: A qualitative and quantitative morphologic analysis of the fibular collateral ligament, popliteus tendon, popliteofibular ligament, and lateral gastrocnemius tendon. *Am J Sports Med* 2003;31(6):854-860.

Musahl V, Herbst E, Burnham JM, Fu FH: The anterolateral complex and anterolateral ligament of the knee. *J Am Acad Orthop Surg* 2018;26:261-267.

Takahashi M, Matsubara T, Doi M, Suzuki D, Nagano A: Anatomical study of the femoral and tibial insertions of the anterolateral and posteromedial bundles of human posterior cruciate ligament. *Knee Surg Sports Traumatol Arthrosc* 2006;14(11):1055-1059.

Chapter 121
Extensor Mechanism Injuries

CHRISTIAN LATTERMANN, MD
ELIZABETH A. ARENDT, MD
JACK ANDRISH, MD
MORGAN H. JONES, MD, MPH

I. LATERAL PATELLAR DISLOCATION

A. Overview/epidemiology

1. Terminology and definitions

   a. Dislocation—A traumatic episode during which the patella loses its confinement in the trochlear groove.

   b. Subluxation—An active event during which the patella is partially translated outside the confines of its groove.

   c. Translation (lateral/medial)—The passive position of a patella in relation to the groove. The term is used to describe the position of the patella on radiographs or its passive position during physical examination.

   d. Tilt—The position of the patella in the horizontal, or axial, plane. The term is used to describe the position of the patella on radiographs or during physical examination.

   e. Limb alignment—A reflection of the three-dimensional geometry of the lower limb. The forces acting on the patellofemoral (PF) joint depend on limb alignment, which includes knee varus/valgus, flexion/extension, and tibial and femoral version or rotation.

2. Epidemiology

   a. Epidemiologic studies are scarce, but lateral PF dislocation appears to occur most frequently in the second and third decades of life.

   b. First-time lateral PF dislocations occur equally in males and females.

   c. Recurrent PF dislocations occur more frequently in females; the reasons for this are speculative.

3. Risk factors

   a. Patella alta

   b. Trochlear dysplasia

   c. Excessive lateral patellar tilt (measured in full extension)

   d. Excessive distance between the tibial tuberosity and the center of the femoral sulcus (measured in full extension), also measured as tibial tuberosity–trochlear groove (TT-TG) distance

B. Pathoanatomy

1. The mechanism of injury is typically a noncontact pivoting force, with the knee near extension and the foot/lower leg externally rotated. The patient may feel the patella move out of place and may contract the quadriceps muscles instinctively, which often will reduce the patella back into the groove.

2. In the absence of previous patellar surgery or substantial dysplastic features of the extensor mechanism, the direction of the dislocation is lateral.

Dr. Lattermann or an immediate family member is a member of a speakers' bureau or has made paid presentations on behalf of Sanofi/Genzyme; serves as a paid consultant to or is an employee of Sanofi/Genzyme room; has received research or institutional support from Smith & Nephew; and serves as a board member, owner, officer, or committee member of the International Cartilage Repair Society. Dr. Arendt or an immediate family member serves as a paid consultant to or is an employee of Tornier and serves as a board member, owner, officer, or committee member of the American Academy of Orthopaedic Surgeons and the International Society of Arthroscopy, Knee Surgery and Orthopaedic Sports Medicine Knee Committee. Dr. Andrish or an immediate family member serves as a board member, owner, officer, or committee member of the International Society of Arthroscopy, Knee Surgery and Orthopaedic Sports Medicine. Dr. Jones or an immediate family member serves as a paid consultant to or is an employee of Allergan.

3. A large hemarthrosis is common, with tearing of the medial retinacular restraints.
4. The medial PF ligament (MPFL) is the main passive restraint to lateral translation of the patella; it is torn in lateral PF dislocations.

C. Evaluation

1. Physical examination
   a. First-time traumatic PF dislocations present with a large effusion and medial-side tenderness along the torn medial retinacular structures. Lateral-side tenderness is often variable.
   b. The absence of swelling after a PF dislocation implies that the medial retinacular structures are so lax that the patella can translate laterally outside of the groove without tearing any structures. This can occur with recurrent PF dislocations or with excessive tissue laxity (eg, Ehlers-Danlos syndrome).
   c. Inhibition of the quadriceps is very common in both acute and recurrent PF dislocations. The patient often resists or performs poorly when asked to perform a straight leg raise test.
   d. Passive patellar translation in the medial and lateral directions is an important maneuver.
      - Patellar motion is measured in quadrants of translation, with the midline on the patella being zero. Lateral translation of the medial border of the patella to the lateral edge of the trochlear groove represents two quadrants of passive lateral translation.
      - Normal motion is less than two quadrants of medial and lateral translation; however, it must be compared with the opposite side, particularly in the absence of current or previous injury to the contralateral limb.
      - During this maneuver, passive lateral translation is often painful or is resisted by the patient. This is known as lateral patellar apprehension.
      - Excessive lateral translation does not confirm the presence of a dislocation because it may be normal for the patient. A PF dislocation cannot occur in the absence of excessive lateral translation, however, making this a powerful physical examination feature.
   e. Lateral patellar tilt—The lateral border of the patella cannot be lifted to the level of the horizon. This is a qualitative test and is difficult to quantify on physical examination. Lateral patellar tilt suggests lateral retinacular tightness.
   f. Quadriceps angle (Q angle)
      - The Q angle is formed by the intersection of a line drawn from the anterosuperior iliac crest to the center of the patella and a line drawn from the center of the patella to the tibial tuberosity.
      - Intraobserver and interobserver variability in the measurement of the Q angle is considerable, and debate exists in the literature as to the limits of the normal value. Using the Q angle as a diagnostic variable is therefore difficult.
      - On average, the Q angle is greater in females (15° ± 5°) than in males (10° ± 5°).
   g. The tuberosity-sulcus angle represents the relationship of the center of the sulcus to the tibial tuberosity.
      - At 90° of flexion, the tubercle-sulcus angle should be zero degrees; that is, the tibial tuberosity should lie directly under the center of the femur. This may be a more reliable way to look for excessive lateral tibial tuberosity placement on physical examination than at zero degrees of flexion.
      - Although quantification schemes have been reported, use of the tubercle-sulcus angle to quantify excessive lateral tibial tuberosity placement has not been widely accepted.
   h. Limb version should be evaluated in all nonacute injuries of the PF joint.
      - Femoral version is best examined with the patient in the prone position; internal rotation in excess of external rotation suggests femoral anteversion.
      - Tibial version can be measured as an angle between the bicondylar femoral axis and the bicondylar tibial axis.
   i. J-tracking—Excessive lateral patellar translation in terminal extension
      - In active flexion, the patella "hops" into the groove.
      - J-tracking is often associated with patella alta.
2. Imaging—The PF joint can be evaluated in three planes: coronal (from the front), sagittal (from the side), and axial (cross-section).
   a. Coronal plane views are helpful in evaluating knee alignment and limb alignment.
      - Knee varus/valgus is most commonly measured on a weight-bearing radiograph of the knee.

- Limb alignment in the coronal plane is best reflected in a weight-bearing radiograph in which the hip, knee, and ankle are visualized.

b. Sagittal plane views are helpful in measuring patellar height and trochlear geometry.

- Patellar height usually is measured on a lateral plain radiograph. Measurements vary depending on whether a quadriceps contracture is present. Most often, a weight-bearing radiograph is used, which presumes a quadriceps-relaxed mode.
- More than a dozen methods of measuring patellar height are described. Currently, the Insall-Salvati (**Figure 1**) and Caton-Deschamps (**Figure 2**) methods are used. These methods have been criticized, however, because they do not take into consideration the relationship between the patella and the trochlear groove, which better defines the degree of functional engagement in early flexion between the patella and the trochlea. No traditional plain radiographic method of measuring the relationship between the patella and the trochlear groove has been clinically accepted with wide use. On CT scans or magnetic resonance images, however, the relationship can be described as the TT-TG distance.
- A positive correlation exists between patella alta and PF instability, PF arthritis, and PF pain.
- Trochlear shape can be determined on a true lateral weight-bearing radiograph, on which the posterior aspects of the medial and lateral condyles are superimposed perfectly. Three contour lines can be seen anteriorly; these represent the anterior curves of the medial and lateral condyles and the floor of

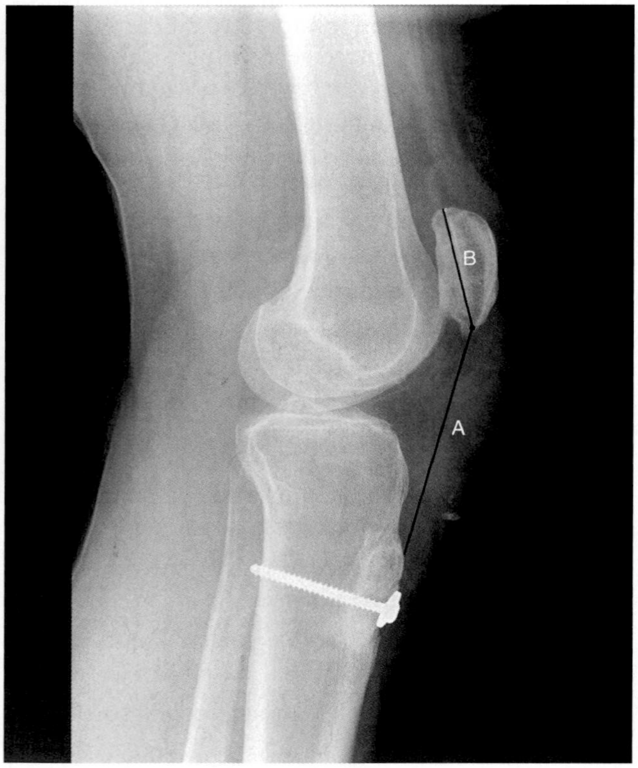

Figure 1 Lateral radiograph shows the Insall-Salvati method of measuring patellar height. This method uses the ratio of AB, where A is the length of the posterior surface of the patellar tendon from the inferior pole of the patella to the tibial tuberosity and B is the greatest diagonal length of the patella. The normal value is 1.0 ± 0.2. This measurement does not take the tibiofemoral joint line into consideration. (Courtesy of Elizabeth Arendt, MD, Minneapolis, MN.)

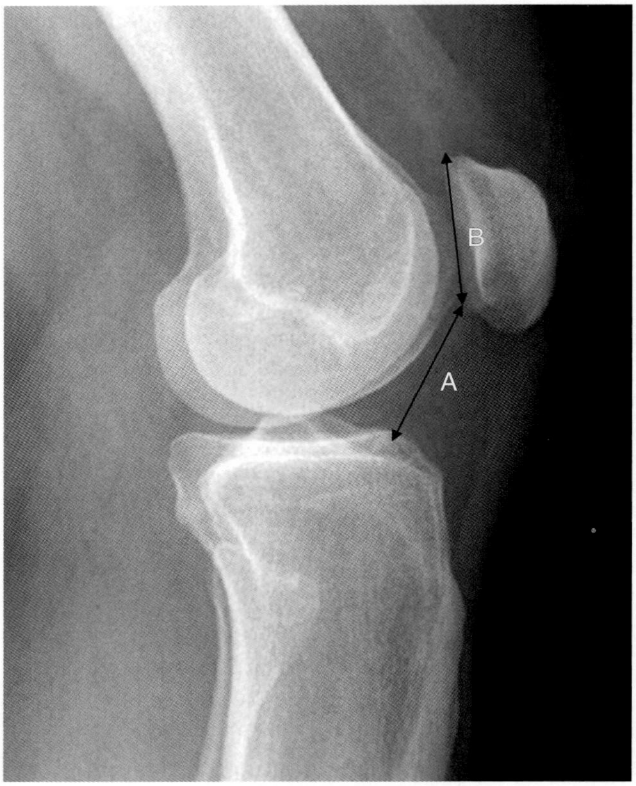

Figure 2 Lateral radiograph shows the Caton-Deschamps method of measuring patellar height. This method creates a ratio of the distance from the inferior articular margin of the patella to the upper edge of the tibial plateau (A) against the length of the patellar articular surface (B) (CD ratio = A/B). The normal value is 0.8 to 1.3. A ratio greater than 1.3 indicates patella alta. This method provides a relative height of the patella to the tibia and is independent from the fixation point of the patellar tendon on the tibia.

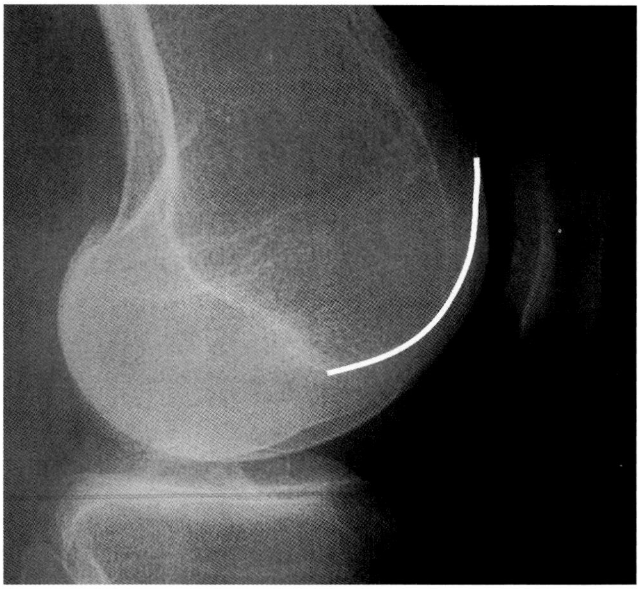

Figure 3 True lateral weight-bearing radiograph of the knee shows the posterior femoral condyles perfectly overlapped. The white line outlines the trochlea, which crosses the anterior cortex, representing a femoral sulcus that is both shortened and shallow (trochlear dysplasia). (Courtesy of David DeJour, MD, Lyon, France.)

the sulcus. These lines are used to define the trochlear depth; the crossing sign (a crossing of the trochlear line over the femoral contour in a perfect lateral radiograph) helps characterize the length and depth of the trochlea and the trochlear boss, or bump.

- Trochlear dysplasia (**Figure 3**) is seen most often in the region of the proximal trochlea, an area that is not visualized well on the axial views obtained in deeper flexion.

c. Axial views help evaluate limb version and patellar position (translation and tilt).

- Patellar tilt can be viewed best on an axial plain radiograph. It is best appreciated at low degrees (~30°) of knee flexion, before the patella is deeply engaged in the groove.
- CT and MRI measurements of patellar tilt are performed on the axial cuts in relation to the posterior condylar line (**Figure 4**). A value greater than 20° is considered excessive lateral patellar tilt.
- Limb version is most often visualized by comparing CT slices at several levels: the femur at the level of the greater trochanter, the distal femur, and the proximal and distal tibia. Femoral anteversion of 15° is normal in adults; anteversion more than 10° greater than normal is believed to warrant surgical correction if determined by symptoms. The value of external tibial torsion that warrants surgical correction is not well defined.
- CT is often used to measure the TT-TG distance. More than 20 mm of lateral displacement is considered excessive and may warrant correction.

D. Treatment

1. First-time (primary) patellar dislocation

a. Physical therapy emphasizing core stability and hip strength is the cornerstone of treatment.

- Aspiration should be performed only if a tense effusion is present. Presence of positive fat globules in the serosanguinous effusion indicates fracture.

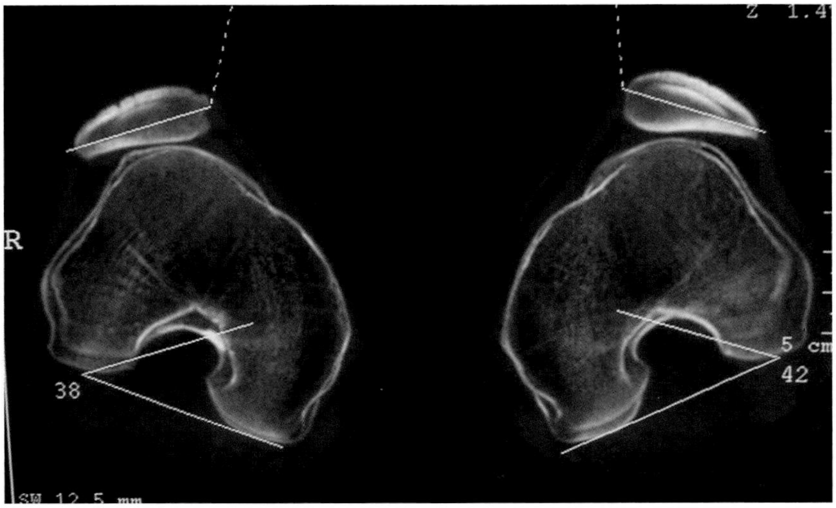

Figure 4 Axial CT of the knees demonstrates how to measure patellar tilt. A line is drawn along the posterior femoral condyles, which shows the "Roman arch" of the notch. A line is then drawn along the long axis of the patella. If the angle between the two lines is greater than 20°, excessive lateral tilting is present. (Courtesy of David DeJour, MD, Lyon, France.)

- Osteochondral fractures can occur as the laterally dislocated patella relocates. In this mechanism, the medial patellar facet contacts the lateral femoral condyle. This is the location where bony fragmentation should be sought; it is recognized most easily on an axial radiograph. Small osteochondral and chondral fractures are identified most readily on MRI.
- MRI should be ordered for every traumatic patellar dislocation with substantial effusion.

b. Immobilization of primary patellar dislocations is controversial, with no best practice established. Ambulation should be modified until a functional gait pattern with appropriate quadriceps activation returns. The emphasis has been on achieving range of motion early and protecting ambulation using crutches or immobilization in extension only as long as quadriceps function limits safe ambulation.

c. Surgical treatment

- If free bony fragments are evident on imaging, arthroscopic examination is the next appropriate step. Depending on the size and location of the fragment, débridement or reduction with fixation is recommended.
- The MPFL is the major structure torn in lateral PF dislocations. Although acute repair of this ligament is gaining popularity, no clinical studies currently support acute repair versus nonsurgical management for first-time dislocations. There is some evidence that primary repair of the MPFL in femoral avulsion may result in a higher failure rate.

2. Recurrent patellar dislocation

a. Surgery is recommended for recurrent dislocations when appropriate rehabilitation has failed.

b. Evidence-based medicine guidance for making decisions regarding surgical treatment choices is sparse in the current literature.

c. Reconstruction of the MPFL using allograft or autograft tissue is commonly used to treat recurrent PF instability.

- The most common graft choice is the gracilis or semitendinosus tendon, which represents a stronger and stiffer graft than the native MPFL.
- Outcomes studies and long-term results of this procedure are sparse.

d. Risk factors and the appropriate surgical correction

- Patella alta: distal tibial tuberosity transfer
- Excessively lateral tibial tuberosity: medial tibial tuberosity transfer
- Severe trochlear dysplasia: trochleoplasty
- Excessive limb rotation: femoral/tibial derotation osteotomy
- Medial patellar dislocation and medial PF arthritis are major complications of the overcorrection of lateral patellar dislocation.

e. Medial patellar dislocation is almost exclusively a result of prior surgery.

E. Physical therapy/rehabilitation

1. When acute injury is associated with joint effusion, rest, ice, compression, and elevation are advised to regain joint motion.
2. Immobilization is advised only when quadriceps function limits safe ambulation.
3. Dysplasia of the vastus medialis oblique (VMO) muscle is associated with PF instability.

   a. This physical examination feature is a product of the bulk of the VMO muscle and its position in relation to the patella.

   b. The usefulness of selective VMO strengthening practices is not supported in the current literature.

4. Strengthening of the knee and limb musculature for improvement of PF function has been shown in the literature to be successful; therefore, its use as a first-line treatment of PF disorders continues to be advocated.
5. Control of the limb under the pelvis is currently the most successful strengthening scheme for the treatment of PF disorders, including PF instability. This includes strengthening of the core musculature (the gluteal and abdominal muscles) as well as the muscles used in extension and abduction of the hip.
6. Using a patellar stabilizing sleeve to help control patellar position and joint effusion is recommended.
7. Restoration of proprioception and balance is recommended.
8. Orthotic control should be considered for the flexible pronated foot.

II. ANTERIOR KNEE PAIN (PATELLOFEMORAL PAIN)

A. Overview/epidemiology

1. Pain is an unpleasant sensory and emotional experience; it occurs as a result of actual or impending tissue damage.
2. Types of pain
   a. Pain can be transmitted rapidly. Rapidly transmitted pain is characterized as sharp and acute and is elicited by mechanical or thermal stimulation, or both. This type of pain sensation is carried on the A fibers.
   b. Pain also can be transmitted slowly. This type is characterized as burning or aching, or patients may report "suffering." It is elicited by mechanical, thermal, and/or chemical stimulation. This type of pain sensation is carried on the C fibers and is transmitted at a lower velocity than rapidly felt pain.
   c. Type IVa free nerve endings constitute the articular nociceptive system. The highest concentration of these free nerve endings in the knee is found in the quadriceps tendon, with the retinacula and the patellar tendon having the second highest concentrations.
3. Epidemiology
   a. Anterior knee pain (AKP; PF pain) is the most common knee condition in adolescents and young adults.
   b. Approximately one-third of knee pain symptoms are related to the PF joint.

B. Pathoanatomy

1. To describe the pathoanatomy of AKP is to suggest that variations in anatomy cause AKP. This is neither completely true nor completely false. AKP has many possible biologic, mechanical, and emotional causes.
   a. Biologic factors associated with AKP include chemical factors, neuroanatomic and intraosseous vascular abnormalities, and degenerative conditions of the articular cartilage (eg, chondromalacia).
      - Chemical factors include substances that stimulate pain, such as histamine, serotonin, and bradykinin, as well as substances that enhance nociceptive stimulation, such as prostaglandins and substance P. Substance P is found in periarticular tissues affected by degenerative changes.
      - Neuroanatomic abnormalities include retinacular neuromata, as well as peripheral nerve entrapment syndromes (eg, saphenous nerve entrapment).
      - Intraosseous vascular abnormalities cause elevated intraosseous pressures (intraosseous hypertension).
      - Degenerative conditions of the articular cartilage, including chondromalacia, are characterized by softening and fibrillation and, at times, fragmentation and erosion.
   b. Mechanical factors that may be associated with AKP are those that produce PF malalignment, characterized as lower extremity alignment resulting from a combination of excessive femoral anteversion (medial femoral torsion), external tibial torsion, and/or excessive foot pronation. PF malalignment also may be characterized by lateral subluxation of the patella, lateral tilt of the patella, or a patella that is positioned more proximally (alta) or distally (baja) than normal.
      - This malalignment can result in excessive medial rotation of the knee during the stance phase, which, in turn, produces an increased lateral patellar force. Increased lateral patellar force can increase retinacular tension and/or cause lateral patellar subluxation.
      - Patellar tilt is thought to be caused by a tight lateral retinaculum, but it also is seen with VMO dysplasia and/or insufficiency of the medial retinacular restraints.
   c. Emotional contributions to AKP—Studies have shown that depression frequently accompanies chronic pain and that patients with AKP often have more stress-related symptoms and elevated levels of hostility and aggression.

C. Evaluation

1. Evaluation of the patient with AKP includes a physical examination and plain radiographs. MRI, CT, and bone scanning also can be helpful, but they are not routinely required.
2. Physical examination—The physical examination includes a behavioral assessment as well as observational assessments of the patient walking, sitting, and lying supine.
   a. A behavioral assessment can help detect emotional factors that may elevate the patient's stress level and enhance the perception of pain.

b. Observation of gait can help detect abnormal adduction moments and rotations that may contribute to increased PF stress. This should include an assessment of foot pronation.

c. Observation of the patient in a sitting position can help detect patella alta, patella baja, and subluxation.

- Active knee extension and flexion can elicit PF crepitus.
- Abnormal lateralization of the tibial tuberosity can be identified by observing lateral positioning of the tuberosity in relation to a plumb line dropped from the midpoint of the patella.

d. Examination of the patient in the supine position can help detect patellar mobility and regions of tenderness.

- Passive medial or lateral patellar glide of less than one quadrant signifies abnormal tightness; medial or lateral glide of three quadrants signifies subluxation and that of four quadrants signifies dislocation.
- Retinacular tenderness may indicate a tight lateral retinaculum or an area of neuromata.
- Quadriceps or PF tenderness may signal inflammation or tendinosis.
- The Q angle is considered excessive if it measures greater than 20° in females and greater than 15° in males; however, as stated earlier, the importance of this measurement continues to be debated.
- Although better assessed with the patient in the prone position, the extent of passive internal and external rotation of the hips observed in a patient in the supine position can reveal excessive femoral version: Internal hip rotation greater than external hip rotation suggests femoral anteversion (or medial femoral torsion). Tibial torsion can be assessed by recording the transmalleolar axis (normal being 15° to 25° of external rotation).
- Joint effusion suggests intra-articular chondral or osteochondral injury.

3. Imaging

a. Plain radiography can detect abnormalities in PF alignment as well as osseous lesions.

- A true lateral view of the knee can detect most PF alignment abnormalities, including tilt, subluxation, patella alta, and patella baja. In addition, trochlear dysplasia can be assessed accurately.
- The Merchant view of the knee is often used to detect PF subluxation and tilt. This view requires precise positioning of the patient and the radiograph beam. The 30° flexion view is used most often.

b. CT is best for detailing bony anatomy and the TT-TG distance (as a measure of detecting abnormal lateral positioning of the tuberosity). Normal TT-TG distance with the knee in extension is 10 to 14 mm. A TT-TG distance greater than 20 mm is abnormal. The limitation of CT imaging is that the contour of the articular surface does not always parallel the contour of the subchondral bone; therefore, the assessment of patellar alignment can be misleading.

c. MRI offers the advantages of detecting abnormalities of articular cartilage and providing a more accurate assessment of joint congruity. Tilt and TT-TG measurements assessed using MRI are similar to CT techniques, even though they tend to underestimate the TT-TG distance by 2 to 4 mm.

D. Classification—AKP can be acute or chronic.

1. Acute AKP is characteristic of acute extensor mechanism overload or traumatic injury. The evaluation should detect the cause.

a. Tenderness may imply patellar or quadriceps tendinitis.

b. The detection of joint effusion suggests intra-articular chondral or osteochondral injury.

c. Peripatellar synovitis is thought to be a common cause of acute and chronic AKP and is classified as a synovial impingement syndrome.

2. Chronic AKP (chronic PF pain)

a. AKP that has lasted longer than 6 months is considered chronic.

b. Although all pain is accompanied by an emotional component, the patient with chronic AKP (chronic PF pain) may have a substantial psychologic history (including childhood emotional trauma).

E. Treatment

1. Nonsurgical treatment—Most often, AKP is managed successfully with nonsurgical treatment.

a. The general principle of nonsurgical treatment is stress management. This includes reducing mechanical stress to the PF joint and reducing emotional stress.

b. Mechanical stress can be reduced by a combination of physical therapy and activity modification.

c. Physical therapy should include assessments of myofascial tightness and muscular weakness and assessments of spine, hip, knee, and foot mechanics.

- VMO strengthening has been overemphasized. A more current understanding of the important role that pelvic stabilizers play in relation to gait has resulted in programs that emphasize core stability.
- Painful exercises reinforce the hypersensitization of the nociceptive system; therefore, all exercises should be performed in a nonpainful manner.
- Knee orthoses and/or taping techniques may reduce PF stress by improving alignment and increasing PF contact area.
- Activity modifications should include an emphasis on low-impact aerobic activities and aquatic exercise.

d. Nutritional counseling should be provided.

e. Emotional stress can be managed most often by reassuring the patient that AKP is nondestructive. Patients with chronic AKP (chronic PF pain) may benefit from psychologic counseling, however.

2. Surgical treatment

a. Surgical treatment of AKP is a slippery slope.

b. Surgery is indicated for patellar instability and pain. Patients with patellar instability and pain in whom instability is the primary symptom and pain is secondary to the instability often have the most consistent surgical results.

c. The relationship between PF malalignment and pain is inconsistent. It cannot be assumed that malalignment is the cause of the AKP. Just as chondromalacia of the patella may or may not be associated with AKP, PF malalignment may or may not be associated with pain.

d. Surgical procedures

- Lateral retinacular release is indicated for the relief of AKP when the lateral retinaculum is tight. Lateral retinaculum tightness can be determined during the physical examination.
- Tibial tuberosity transfer results in load transfer, not necessarily load reduction. Understanding where the patellar chondral injury is located is important. If chondrosis is suspected to be the source of pain, a tibial tuberosity osteotomy may be considered. Medialization of the tibial tuberosity shifts the load to the medial facet. Anteriorization of the tibial tuberosity shifts the PF loading proximally on the patella, whereas anteromedialization shifts patellar load proximally and medially.
- Restoration of the articular cartilage of the PF joint traditionally has produced inconsistent results but may be indicated in cases of central or medial chondral lesions in patients with an abnormal TT-TG distance.
- Resection of inflamed peripatellar synovial tissue (plica syndrome, synovial impingement syndrome, fat pad syndrome) may do no harm.

III. RUPTURE OF THE PATELLAR TENDON OR QUADRICEPS TENDON

A. Overview/epidemiology

1. Rupture of the patellar tendon or quadriceps tendon generally occurs with eccentric loading of the knee extensor mechanism, often when the foot is planted and the knee is slightly bent.
2. Less commonly, these injuries can occur with a direct blow to the tendon when the extensor mechanism is under tension.
3. Rupture of the patellar tendon is most common in patients younger than 40 years.
4. Rupture of the quadriceps tendon is most common in patients older than 40 years.
5. Patients who sustain quadriceps tendon ruptures may have underlying conditions that predispose them to injury, such as obesity, diabetes mellitus, hyperparathyroidism, rheumatoid arthritis, systemic lupus erythematosus, hyperbetalipoproteinemia, hemangioendothelioma, chronic renal failure, or gout.
6. Anabolic steroid use and local corticosteroid injection into the tendon also are associated with both types of tendon ruptures.

B. Pathoanatomy

1. Both patellar tendon and quadriceps tendon ruptures typically occur at the tendon attachment to the patella.
2. Underlying chronic degeneration often is present and is characterized by angiofibroblastic tendinosis, mucoid degeneration, and pseudocyst formation at the attachment of tendon to bone.

3. The quadriceps tendon has been described as having two to four distinct layers. This is important when distinguishing between partial versus complete ruptures and when repairing the tendon.

C. Evaluation

1. History

a. Patients with a rupture of the patellar tendon or quadriceps tendon often report a history of pain, which is consistent with the presence of underlying tendon degeneration.

b. Patellar tendon rupture also has been reported after midthird tendon harvest for knee ligament reconstruction.

c. The rupture typically occurs during an eccentric load on a flexed knee, such as landing from a jump or taking a forceful step while descending stairs. Less commonly, a rupture can occur during a forceful quadriceps contraction when taking off for a jump.

2. Physical examination

a. Physical examination for a complete rupture of either the patellar tendon or the quadriceps tendon demonstrates tenderness at the site of the injury, hematoma, and a palpable defect in the tendon.

b. Patients with a complete rupture of either tendon cannot extend the knee against resistance or perform a straight leg raise. In incomplete ruptures or in patients with a complete rupture of the quadriceps tendon but an intact retinaculum, the ability to perform a straight leg raise against gravity may be uncompromised.

3. Imaging

a. Radiographs

- Radiographs of the knee after patellar tendon rupture demonstrate patella alta, particularly with the knee flexed.
- Radiographs obtained after quadriceps tendon rupture demonstrate patella baja and sometimes show bony fragments in the region of the rupture.

b. MRI can be helpful when the diagnosis is uncertain, particularly when the surgeon is trying to differentiate between a partial and a complete rupture of a tendon.

D. Classification—A rupture is classified according to its severity (partial or complete) and its location (patellar tendon or quadriceps).

E. Nonsurgical treatment

1. Nonsurgical treatment is indicated for partial rupture of the patellar or quadriceps tendon when no disruption of the extensor mechanism is present. It also is indicated for patients who are unable to tolerate surgery because of poor overall medical condition.

2. Nonsurgical treatment consists of an initial period of immobilization in a knee brace followed by progressive range-of-motion and strengthening exercises beginning approximately 6 weeks after injury.

F. Surgical treatment

1. Surgery is indicated for a complete rupture of the patellar or quadriceps tendon.

2. Early surgery (within the first 2 weeks after injury) is recommended.

G. Surgical procedures

1. Patellar tendon rupture repair

a. A midline incision is used.

b. Nonabsorbable sutures are placed in the tendon using a running locking stitch and passed through longitudinal drill holes in the patella.

c. The retinaculum is repaired with a heavy absorbable suture. The paratenon is repaired if possible.

d. Ideally, the knee should flex to 90° after repair.

2. Quadriceps tendon repair

a. Quadriceps tendon repair also is performed via a midline incision.

b. Longitudinal drill holes are placed in the patella, and the tendon is sutured using a heavy nonabsorbable suture in a running locking pattern.

c. The retinaculum is sutured using a heavy absorbable suture.

d. If necessary, reinforcement is performed using a quadriceps turndown, a pull-out wire, or a fascia lata or hamstrings autograft.

e. Ideally, the knee should flex to 90° after repair.

H. Complications

1. Patellar tendon rupture repair—Repair of chronic patellar tendon rupture can be complicated by proximal retraction of the patella and by insufficient tissue for repair. Retraction can be addressed by surgical dissection and mobilization of the quadriceps tendon.

a. Tendon augmentation can be performed with a hamstring autograft passed through tibial and patellar drill holes, a central quadriceps tendon–patellar bone autograft, a contralateral bone–patellar tendon–bone autograft, or an allograft.

b. Augmentation with wire, nonabsorbable tape, or heavy suture also can be considered.

2. Quadriceps tendon rupture repair—Chronic quadriceps tendon ruptures also can be complicated by proximal migration of the tendon stump, which requires débridement and mobilization of the tendon. Following this, the tendon can be augmented with autograft or allograft tissue and secured to bone.

I. Physical therapy/rehabilitation

1. Patellar tendon rupture repair—Postoperatively, the patient may bear weight, but the limb should be protected initially in a cylinder cast or a brace.

2. Quadriceps tendon rupture repair (acute or chronic)—Postoperative care involves a period of immobilization in a cylinder cast or splint followed by progressive flexibility and strengthening exercises.

IV. PATELLAR OR QUADRICEPS TENDINOPATHY

A. Overview/epidemiology

1. Patellar or quadriceps tendinopathy occurs in active individuals who engage in activities that involve forceful, eccentric contraction of the knee extensor mechanism, particularly jumping sports.

2. Harder playing surfaces and increased frequency of practices have been associated with increased rates of tendinopathy.

3. Patellar tendinopathy, or jumper's knee, occurs most frequently in adolescents and young adults, whereas quadriceps tendinopathy occurs in middle-aged and older adults.

B. Pathoanatomy

1. Patellar tendinopathy tends to occur at the deep fibers of the patellar attachment of the tendon.

a. This area has a tenuous blood supply, and affected tissue may demonstrate fibrinoid necrosis, angiofibroblastic change, or mucoid degeneration and disorganized collagen structure.

b. In addition, metaplasia of adjacent fibrocartilage may be present.

c. The medial portion of the patellar tendon often demonstrates thickening compared with the rest of the tendon.

2. The pathoanatomy of quadriceps tendinopathy is similar to that of patellar tendinopathy.

C. Evaluation

1. History

a. Patients with patellar or quadriceps tendinopathy describe an insidious onset of pain and swelling of the affected tendon.

b. These symptoms initially develop after activity, gradually start to bother the individual both during and after activity, and eventually limit athletic performance during the activity.

c. Patients also may report buckling of the knee, which represents reflex quadriceps inhibition due to pain.

2. Physical examination

a. Physical examination reveals tenderness and soft-tissue swelling, usually in the area where the tendon attaches to the patellar bone.

b. Patients often have discomfort with resisted extension of the knee.

3. Imaging

a. Plain radiographs of the knee may demonstrate degenerative spurring where the affected tendon attaches to bone.

b. MRI usually shows thickening in the affected portion of the tendon and also may demonstrate intrasubstance signal abnormalities, but thickening is much more diagnostic than signal changes when identifying abnormal tendon on MRI.

D. Classification—The three stages of tendinopathy, according to Blazina, are listed in **Table 1**.

E. Nonsurgical treatment—Nonsurgical intervention is the mainstay of treatment.

1. Initial treatment consists of activity modification.

2. Progressive flexibility and eccentric strengthening exercises follow.

TABLE 1

Blazina Classification of Patellar or Quadriceps Tendinopathy

Stage	Characteristics
1	Pain after activity
2	Pain during and after activity
3	Pain that limits function during an activity

3. Taping to aid proprioception and patellar tracking or using an infrapatellar strap can be helpful.
4. NSAIDs can be beneficial.
5. Corticosteroid injection is contraindicated because of the increased risk of tendon rupture.
6. No recommendation can be made currently regarding either prolotherapy injections using a local irritant to elicit an inflammatory healing response or platelet-rich plasma injection.

F. Surgical treatment—Surgery is reserved for patients who continue to have pain and swelling of the tendon after a nonsurgical treatment regimen has been attempted.

1. Surgical procedures are performed according to the surgeon's preference.
    a. Options include various methods of débriding diseased tissue and stimulating a vigorous healing response.
        - This can be achieved by simple longitudinal excision of the diseased portion of tendon, followed by abrasion of the bone to provide a bleeding surface for tendon healing, and finishing with the application of side-to-side sutures or suture anchors as needed.
        - Variations of this procedure include drilling of the bone to stimulate a healing response or multiple tendon perforations ("pie crusting") to stimulate healing of the tendon tissue.
    b. All procedures can be performed using a standard anterior midline incision to expose the diseased tendon and its attachment to the patella.

TOP TESTING FACTS

Lateral Patellar Dislocation

1. The MPFL is the main passive restraint to lateral translation of the patella; it is torn in lateral patellar dislocations.
2. Nonsurgical management including physical therapy is the cornerstone of treatment of first-time patellar dislocation.
3. Osteochondral loose bodies and recurrent dislocation after physical therapy are indications for surgical treatment of lateral patellar dislocation.
4. Medial dislocation of the patella is almost exclusively a result of prior surgery—in particular, an overzealous lateral retinacular release.

Anterior Knee Pain (Patellofemoral Pain)

1. The detection of joint effusion in conjunction with AKP suggests intra-articular chondral or osteochondral injury.
2. AKP is usually managed successfully with nonsurgical treatment. Physical therapy includes assessments of spine, hip, knee, and foot mechanics.
3. Lateral retinacular release may be indicated for relief of AKP when the lateral retinaculum is tight.

Rupture of the Patellar Tendon or Quadriceps Tendon

1. Rupture of the patellar tendon is most common in patients younger than 40 years; rupture of the quadriceps tendon is most common in those older than 40 years.
2. Patellar or quadriceps tendon rupture occurs during eccentric loading of the knee extensor mechanism and usually is associated with predisposing factors.
3. Nonsurgical treatment is indicated for partial rupture of the patellar or quadriceps tendon when no disruption of the quadriceps mechanism is present.
4. Surgery is generally indicated for a complete tendon rupture.

Patellar or Quadriceps Tendinopathy

1. Patellar or quadriceps tendinopathy is characterized by disorganized collagen structure visualized on MRI by thickening of the tendon and signal intensity changes.
2. Nonsurgical intervention is the mainstay of treatment. Corticosteroid injection is not recommended because it increases the risk of tendon rupture.

Bibliography

Feller JA, Amis AA, Andrish JT, Arendt EA, Erasmus PJ, Powers CM: Surgical biomechanics of the patellofemoral joint. *Arthroscopy* 2007;23(5):542-553.

Kaar SG, Stuart MJ, Levy BA: Soft-tissue injuries about the knee, in Flynn JM, ed: *Orthopaedic Knowledge Update*, ed 11. Rosemont, IL, American Academy of Orthopaedic Surgeons, 2011.

Lattermann C, Drake GN, Spellman J, Bach BR Jr: Lateral retinacular release for anterior knee pain: A systematic review of the literature. *J Knee Surg* 2006;19(4):278-284.

Lattermann C, Toth J, Bach BR Jr: The role of lateral retinacular release in the treatment of patellar instability. *Sports Med Arthrosc* 2007;15(2):57-60.

Miller MD, Thompson SR: *DeLee & Drez's Orthopaedic Sports Medicine: Principles and Practice*, ed 3. Philadelphia, PA, Saunders, 2009.

Monson J, Arendt EA: Rehabilitative protocols for select patellofemoral procedures and nonoperative management schemes. *Sports Med Arthrosc* 2012;20(3):136-144.

Phillips BB: Recurrent dislocations, in Canale ST, Beaty JH, eds: *Campbell's Operative Orthopaedics*, ed 12. St. Louis, MO, Mosby, 2012, p 2355.

Saggin PR, Saggin JI, Dejour D: Imaging in patellofemoral instability: An abnormality-based approach. *Sports Med Arthrosc* 2012;20(3):145-151.

Shah JN, Howard JS, Flanigan DC, Brophy RH, Carey JL, Lattermann C: A systematic review of complications and failures associated with medial patellofemoral ligament reconstruction for recurrent patellar dislocation. *Am J Sports Med* 2012;40(8):1916-1923.

Smith TO, Davies L, Toms AP, Hing CB, Donell ST: The reliability and validity of radiological assessment for patellar instability: A systematic review and meta-analysis. *Skeletal Radiol* 2011;40(4):399-414.

Tompkins M, Arendt EA: Complications in patellofemoral surgery. *Sports Med Arthrosc* 2012;20(3):187-193.

Chapter 122
LIGAMENTOUS INJURIES OF THE KNEE

CAROLYN M. HETTRICH, MD, MPH
ROBERT G. MARX, MD, MSc, FRCSC
RICHARD D. PARKER, MD
MATTHEW J. MATAVA, MD
JON K. SEKIYA, MD

I. ANTERIOR CRUCIATE LIGAMENT INJURIES

A. Overview and epidemiology

1. The anterior cruciate ligament (ACL) is most commonly injured during sports-related activity, although some ACL injuries occur as a result of high-energy trauma or activities of daily living (ADLs).
2. Approximately 70% of patients hear or feel a "pop" at the time of injury.
3. Almost all patients notice swelling of the knee within 6 to 12 hours of the injury.
4. ACL injuries may be classified as occurring from a contact or noncontact mechanism.
5. Noncontact injuries usually occur during cutting or pivoting.
6. ACL injuries are also commonly sustained during skiing; however, they are less common among snowboarders.
7. Female athletes have a two-fold to eight-fold higher risk of ACL injury than male athletes when level of competition, age, and time exposed are considered.
   a. The reason for the higher rate of injuries among females is not clearly understood but is felt to be due to differences in neuromuscular firing patterns in the quadriceps and hamstrings between males and females.
   b. Potential contributing factors include ACL size and notch width anatomy, biomechanics, alignment, muscle strength, hormonal factors, and training.

B. Pathoanatomy

1. Most ACL injuries are complete disruptions, although disruption of a single anatomic bundle (anteromedial or posterolateral) may occur.
2. In the skeletally mature patient, the femoral insertion or the midsubstance is the most common site of disruption.
3. In the skeletally mature patient, the tibial attachment may be avulsed with or without a piece of bone.

C. Evaluation

1. History
   a. An appropriate and detailed patient history can raise suspicion for an ACL injury.
   b. The patient who sustains a knee injury during sports activity that is followed by knee swelling within 1 to 6 hours should be evaluated carefully for a possible ACL injury.
   c. Patients with a chronic ACL injury may report recurrent episodes of knee instability,

Dr. Hettrich or an immediate family member serves as a board member, owner, officer, or committee member of the American Orthopaedic Society for Sports Medicine. Dr. Marx or an immediate family member has stock or stock options held in Mend and serves as a board member, owner, officer, or committee member of the American Orthopaedic Society for Sports Medicine and the International Society of Arthroscopy, Knee Surgery, and Orthopaedic Sports Medicine. Dr. Parker or an immediate family member has received royalties from Smith & Nephew and serves as a paid consultant to or is an employee of Smith & Nephew. Dr. Matava or an immediate family member serves as a paid consultant to or is an employee of Arthrex, Inc., Breg, Pacira, and Schwartz Biomedical; has received nonincome support (such as equipment or services), commercially derived honoraria, or other non–research-related funding (such as paid travel) from Arthrex, Inc. and Breg; and serves as a board member, owner, officer, or committee member of the Southern Orthopedic Association. Dr. Sekiya or an immediate family member has received royalties from Arthrex, Inc.

mechanical symptoms from a secondary meniscal tear, or pain and swelling.

2. Physical examination
   a. In the setting of acute ACL injury, physical examination can be difficult or limited secondary to pain.
   b. An effusion is related to hemarthrosis secondary to bleeding from the vascular, torn ligament.
   c. The knee should be palpated carefully, with attention focused on the joint lines and the origins/insertions of the medial collateral ligament (MCL) and posterolateral corner (posterior cruciate ligament [PCL]).
   d. Patient apprehension on movement of the patella should be noted because acute patellar dislocations often present with a history that is very similar to ACL injury, and the two injuries can be confused in the acute setting.
   e. The quadriceps and patellar tendons also should be examined in the acute setting because tendon ruptures may be confused with ACL injuries.
   f. The Lachman test is the most useful in diagnosing ACL injuries in the acute setting.
      - The knee is flexed to 30°, and the distal femur is held securely in one hand while the examiner translates the tibia anteriorly with the other hand. A sense of increased movement and lack of a solid end point indicate ACL injury. Grades of injury using the Lachman test are shown in **Table 1**.
   g. The anterior drawer test is performed with the knee at 90° of flexion. Anterior translation of the tibia is assessed in relation to the distal femur. Total amount of translation and the quality of the end point are assessed.

TABLE 1

Anterior Cruciate Ligament Injury Grade[a]

Injury Grade	Increase in Anterior Tibial Translation (mm)
1	3-5
2	5-10
3	10-15

[a]Determined by Lachman test.

   h. The MCL and lateral collateral ligament (LCL) also must be assessed for stability by applying valgus and varus stress, respectively.
   i. The PLC must be examined for posterolateral rotatory laxity as documented by the dial test, reverse pivot shift, and external rotation recurvatum test (see below).
   j. The PCL also must be examined. Ideally, this is performed with the knee at 90° of flexion; however, this maneuver is often difficult in the acute setting because the patient is in pain.
   k. Neurovascular injury must be ruled out by assessing motor and sensory function as well as pedal pulses.
      - In multiligament injuries from higher-energy trauma, vascular injuries can occur. Multiligament disruptions (more than two ligaments disrupted) should raise suspicion for a knee dislocation.
      - With a PLC injury resulting from a varus stress, peroneal nerve injuries also may be detected by loss of ankle dorsiflexion and eversion, and sensory loss in the first web space and lateral aspect of the leg and foot.
   l. The pivot shift test is pathognomonic for ACL injury. This test is best in the chronic setting.
      - The pivot shift test begins with the knee in full extension. The knee is then flexed while the examiner applies a valgus moment.
      - A positive test result occurs when the anterolateral tibial plateau (which is subluxated anteriorly on the femur) reduces with a visible shift at the lateral joint line as the iliotibial band passes posterior to the axis of knee rotation at approximately 15° of knee flexion.
      - There are three grades of pivot shift injury: grade I (pivot glide), grade II ("thud-clunk"), and grade III (impingement).
      - Findings in the injured knee should always be compared with the contralateral side because a physiologic pivot glide occasionally may be present in physiologically lax individuals.
   m. The patient in whom examination for an acute ACL injury is not clearly positive may have a partial ACL injury, despite a positive MRI.
      - Partial ACL injuries require strict physical examination and visualization criteria.

- Partial injuries may not withstand future trauma, allowing the knee to give way.
- If the examiner suspects a partial injury, diagnostic arthroscopy of the affected knee should be performed before graft harvest and/or preparation.

3. Imaging
   a. Radiographs are useful in the acute setting to rule out fracture. The most common fracture pattern is the Segond fracture, which is a small fleck of bone off the lateral tibial plateau that represents an avulsion of the lateral capsule.
   b. In the skeletally immature patient, radiographs should be evaluated for open physes, which can affect surgical options.
   c. In the chronic setting, full-length plain radiographs can be useful to assess the mechanical axis. Unilateral genu varum or genu valgum indicates medial or lateral compartment degeneration, respectively, that may occur from chronic meniscal and/or articular cartilage damage.
   d. MRI is not required for the diagnosis of ACL injury, but it is useful for assessing for other ligamentous injury, meniscal pathology, and subchondral fracture (bone bruise).
      - A characteristic edema pattern on MRI, particularly in the acute setting, is caused by transchondral fractures in the posterolateral tibial plateau and the anterolateral femoral condyle indicating a rotational event that is likely secondary to an ACL injury (**Figure 1**).
      - In sagittal and coronal MRIs, ACL injuries appear as disruptions in the ACL fibers.

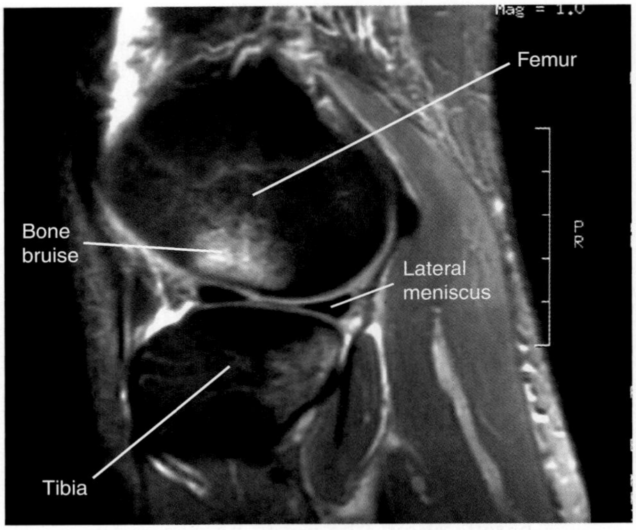

Figure 1 Lateral T2-weighted MRI demonstrates a typical "bone bruise" of the anterolateral femoral condyle and posterolateral tibial plateau. This type of injury is believed to result from an anterolateral rotational event of the tibia in reference to the femur secondary to an anterior cruciate ligament injury.

D. Treatment
1. Nonsurgical
   a. Individualized treatment is appropriate for patients with partial injuries of the ACL, including those with low-energy skiing injuries, who may have a good outcome with nonsurgical treatment.
   b. Nonsurgical treatment involves rehabilitation to strengthen the hamstrings and quadriceps, as well as proprioceptive training.
   c. Activity modification (eg, avoiding cutting and pivoting sports) is also an important part of nonsurgical management, because patients who avoid these activities are at lower risk for knee instability.
   d. ACL sports braces (custom and off-the-shelf) are available, but they have not been shown to prevent abnormal anterior tibial translation. Functional braces and simple knee sleeves improve proprioception, which may give patients a sense of improved knee function and stability.
2. Surgical
   a. In the acute setting, the decision to reconstruct the ACL generally is related to the patient's activity level.
      - Patients who are older or less physically active may elect to modify their activities and proceed with nonsurgical treatment. If nonsurgical treatment fails or knee instability persists, surgery can be performed.
      - Athletes with ACL injuries who perform cutting and pivoting sports, such as basketball, football, soccer, squash, and handball, usually undergo surgery to avoid instability and secondary meniscal and/or articular cartilage damage.
      - The decision about whether ACL surgery is needed for an individual to return to sports activity is not always obvious. Many recreational skiers who do not participate in cutting and pivoting sports can function well without surgery.

- Patients with jobs that may involve physical combat (active military, police officers), risk (firefighters), or activity on unstable surfaces (construction workers) should undergo ACL reconstruction before returning to work.
- Most patients can function well and perform ADLs without instability after a complete ACL injury. Some have difficulty with even simple ADLs, however, because of ACL deficiency–related instability; these patients may require surgery.

b. Contraindications

- Contraindications include lack of quadriceps function, substantial comorbidities, and inability to tolerate the surgery or unwillingness to complete the rehabilitation program.
- After an acute injury, patients should not undergo surgery until the effusion is controlled and they have regained full range of motion (ROM) (especially extension), good quadriceps function, and normal gait. Patients who undergo ACL reconstruction before swelling has been eliminated and full ROM has been reestablished may be at higher risk for postoperative arthrofibrosis.
- Advanced osteoarthritis is a relative contraindication. Patients with osteoarthritis may have substantial pain, swelling, and limited motion following surgery despite a stable knee. Therefore, they may not experience a satisfactory outcome.

c. Surgical procedures

- The most important factor is a well-performed technique, not the type of technique.
- Virtually all ACL reconstructions are performed as an outpatient arthroscopic procedure. Most procedures are done using an endoscopic technique where the femoral tunnel is drilled from inside the joint. Some surgeons still prefer to drill the femoral tunnel from outside-in, which necessitates a second incision. There is no clinical difference between the two techniques.
- There has been an increased conversion to drilling the femoral tunnel through an anteromedial (AM) portal rather than through the tibial tunnel. The transtibial method tends to result in a femoral tunnel that is too vertical resulting in a nonanatomic graft. The AM portal drilling method allows more reliable placement of the femoral tunnel at the native ACL footprint (more obliquely down the intercondylar wall) than is reliably achieved with transtibial drilling. This potentially results in improved rotational stability.
    - Drilling through an AM portal requires knee hyperflexion to avoid posterior femoral wall "blow-out."
    - AM portal drilling can be accomplished with either a low-profile (to avoid damage to the medial femoral condyle) or flexible reamer.
    - AM portal drilling may result in a shorter femoral tunnel than is achieved with transtibial drilling.
- Graft choices for ACL reconstruction include autologous options (bone-patellar tendon-bone, hamstring tendons, and quadriceps tendon) and allograft tissues (bone-patellar tendon-bone, Achilles tendon, and tibialis anterior).
- There has been a renewed interest in ACL repair for selected patients based on limited short-term case series and subsets of long-term clinical cohorts.
    - This procedure may be indicated in younger patients with an acute femoral or tibial avulsion.
    - An internal high-strength suture strut appears to improve histological healing and biomechanical strength.
    - Biological "enhancement" of the repair with platelet-derived growth factors has been shown to improve healing and mechanical strength in animal models.
    - The repaired ACL remains weaker than the native ACL.
- Reconstruction of the anterolateral ligament (ALL) in conjunction with ACL reconstruction has been advocated by several authors in an attempt to confer increased rotational stability to the knee and a higher rate of return to sports above that offered solely by an ACL reconstruction.
    - Suggested indications (level V) for a combined ALL and ACL reconstruction include the following:
        - Revision ACL reconstruction
        - Grade III pivot shift
        - Genu recurvatum or ligamentous laxity

- Anatomically, the ALL originates 4 mm posterior and proximal to the lateral epicondyle and inserts midway between Gerdy tubercle and the fibular head.
- A gracilis autograft or allograft tendon at least 120 mm in length is attached to the femoral socket with an interference screw or suture anchor.
- The graft is brought deep to the iliotibial tract and fixed to the tibia in 20° of extension and neutral tibial rotation using an interference screw or suture anchor.

- Individual reconstruction of both the anteromedial (AM) and posterolateral (PL) bundles (double-bundle reconstruction) have been advocated to improve rotational stability throughout a full ROM above that achieved with a single-bundle reconstruction.
    - A double-bundle procedure is associated with twice as many tunnels, the need for more graft material, and twice as much hardware. This can make a revision reconstruction technically more difficult.
        - Nonaperture fixation is required for the double-bundle technique.
        - The AM bundle should be fixed with the knee at 30° to 45°. The PL bundle should be fixed in full extension.

d. Surgical outcomes

- Reconstruction of the ACL generally results in excellent outcomes; however, most patients have slightly decreased levels of activity.
- Use of the one-incision technique versus the two-incision technique does not appear to affect outcome.
- Rerupture rates vary from 1% to 20% in the literature.
- KT-1000 arthrometer testing shows a 1 to 2 mm difference in side-to-side laxity, which is not clinically significant.
- The risk of future radiographic osteoarthritis after ACL reconstruction is 0% to 13% after an isolated ACL tear and 21% to 48% if the ACL tear is accompanied by a meniscal tear.
- ROM will return to normal.
- Isokinetic strength will be greater than 90% of normal.
- A contralateral ACL tear will occur in 3% to 6% of patients.
- No clinically or statistically relevant differences exist in instrumented laxity, patient-reported outcomes, or quadriceps or hamstring strength between bone-patellar tendon-bone autograft and hamstring tendon autograft. Kneeling pain is more common following use of the bone-patellar tendon-bone autograft. However, return to elite-level sports is also somewhat higher with this graft option.
- During the past few years, allograft use has increased in the United States. A meta-analysis showed that older patients who underwent allograft ACL reconstruction were more likely to experience graft re-rupture and to have greater asymmetry in their hop test (>10% side-to-side difference) than patients who underwent autograft reconstruction. When irradiated and chemically processed grafts were excluded from analysis, no significant differences were found in graft rupture; revision surgery; International Knee Documentation Committee (IKDC) scores, Lachman, pivot shift, or hop test results; patellar crepitus; or return to sport.
    - A level I study found a failure rate of 20% in 18-year-old patients with allograft versus 6% in those with autograft. In 40-year-old patients, a failure rate of 3% occurred with allograft versus 1% with autograft.
    - Based on the growing body of published literature, there is a general perception that allografts should not be used in younger athletes who participate in cutting, twisting, and pivoting sports.
    - If an allograft is used, it should be processed with low-dose irradiation.
    - Allograft tissue carries a risk of HIV disease transmission theorized to be approximately 1 in 1.6 million.
- No clinically significant differences between single-bundle and double-bundle ACL reconstruction have been reported, but the double-bundle procedure is associated with increased cost and longer surgical time. In addition, allograft tissue carries a risk of disease transmission.
- Short-term follow-up of patients undergoing a combined ALL and ACL reconstruction have shown improved measures of knee

stability without improved clinical function. The indications for ALL reconstruction continued to be defined.

E. Complications

1. Anesthesia-related complications (eg, pain related to a spinal or epidural block, spinal headache, femoral nerve palsy following regional block, or major respiratory or allergic problems secondary to general anesthesia) can occur.
2. Deep infection following ACL reconstruction is uncommon (0.8%).
   a. When it does occur, deep infection may require repeat arthroscopy for irrigation and débridement as well as possible hardware removal and graft removal to eradicate the infection.
   b. Deep infections involving the knee are also treated with 6 weeks of intravenous antibiotic therapy.
3. Knee stiffness is generally uncommon and usually can be resolved with physical therapy. It is more common after multiligament reconstructive surgery; in some cases, repeat surgery or manipulation under anesthesia may be required.
4. Thromboembolic disease is uncommon, but patients with a history of deep vein thrombosis, females who use oral contraceptives, and those with a family history of hypercoagulability may be considered for anticoagulation.
5. Lack of full extension occurs in approximately 4% of patients.
   a. It is more common after multiligament reconstructive surgery. In some cases, repeat surgery or manipulation under anesthesia may be required for persistent arthrofibrosis.
   b. Loss of full extension can occur secondary to scarring from the graft or if remaining ACL tissue scars and forms a "cyclops" lesion (nodular scar tissue formed anterior to the ACL graft blocking extension). This can require repeat surgery to remove the tissue that blocks full extension.
6. Painful hardware at the proximal tibia near the tibial tunnel, if it is sufficiently disabling, can result in repeat surgery for hardware removal.

F. Revision surgery

1. When evaluating a failed ACL reconstruction, the surgeon must attempt to determine the etiology of failure.
2. Graft failure is classified as biologic, traumatic, or related to technical failure.
3. Revision surgery is more technically demanding because of the existence of prior tunnels and hardware.
4. Based on the Multicenter ACL Revision Study (MARS) database, outcomes following ACL revision surgery appear to be inferior to outcomes after primary reconstruction.
   a. Combination failure due to more than one cause was most commonly noted.
   b. Femoral tunnel malposition was documented in 80% of patients failing due to "technical error."
   c. Intra-articular pathology in the form of articular cartilage damage of all cartilage surfaces is higher in revision surgery than in primary ACL reconstruction.
   d. Prior partial meniscectomy portends a poor prognosis in terms of articular cartilage damage in revision cases.
   e. Higher rates of primary graft failure have been seen in patients who demonstrate hyperlaxity and undergo an allograft reconstruction.
   f. The surgeon is the most important factor influencing graft choice for revision surgery.

G. Pearls and pitfalls

1. Tunnel placement is the most critical aspect of ACL reconstruction.
2. The most common error in ACL reconstruction is placing the tibial or femoral tunnel too anteriorly, resulting in graft impingement and failure.
3. With a single-incision transtibial technique, the tibial tunnel should begin at the anterior part of the tibial insertion of the MCL to allow the graft to be placed obliquely and arrive at the 10:30 or 1:30 clock position on the intercondylar notch of the femur. If the tibial tunnel is drilled too anteriorly on the tibia, the graft will be vertically placed, which is not desirable. It is important to understand that the direction of the tibial tunnel influences femoral tunnel placement when using a single-incision technique (if the femoral tunnel is drilled through the tibial tunnel). This problem can be avoided by drilling the femoral tunnel through a medial portal or using a two-incision technique.

H. Rehabilitation

1. Studies have shown that a knee immobilizer or continuous passive motion machine is not required postoperatively.

2. Postoperatively, patients are allowed to ambulate as tolerated with crutches until they can walk normally without them, which is generally 1 to 2 weeks after surgery depending on their pain tolerance and lower extremity strength.
   a. Concurrent meniscal or articular cartilage procedures may affect weight-bearing status.
3. Patients are encouraged to emphasize "closed-chain" strengthening. They are allowed to start light running between 3 and 4 months if strengthening has progressed sufficiently.
4. Return to sports depends on the patient's strength and ability to perform specific tasks. For most patients, return to sports is allowed between 6 and 12 months, depending on the rate of progression with rehabilitation, the sport, and the position played.
   a. Psychological factors may affect the timing of return to sports.

II. POSTERIOR CRUCIATE LIGAMENT INJURIES

A. Overview and epidemiology

1. The PCL is the primary restraint to posterior tibial translation in the intact knee.
2. It has been reported that 5% to 20% of all ligamentous injuries to the knee involve the PCL. Many of these injuries are believed to go undiagnosed in the acutely injured knee.
3. Injuries to the PCL may be isolated or combined with other capsuloligamentous injuries in the knee.
4. Although the diagnosis of a combined PCL injury may be obvious in a knee subjected to high-energy trauma, an isolated PCL injury may be less obvious because instability is often subtle or even asymptomatic.

B. Pathoanatomy

1. A direct blow to the proximal aspect of the tibia is the most common cause of PCL injury.
   a. In athletes, the mechanism of injury is usually a fall onto the flexed knee with the foot plantarflexed, which places a posterior force on the tibia and subsequently causes rupture of the PCL.
   b. In high-energy trauma such as motor vehicle accidents, the PCL is often injured with other capsuloligamentous structures.
2. When three or more ligamentous structures are injured, the physician should view the injury as a dislocated knee and should assess the vascular status of the injured limb.
3. The natural history of these injuries is not entirely clear, but evidence shows that certain PCL injuries (especially combined) will progress to instability, pain, and osteoarthritis of the knee—especially of the patellofemoral and medial tibiofemoral compartments.

C. Evaluation

1. History
   a. The history of the injury helps differentiate between high- and low-energy traumas.
   b. Concurrent injuries such as a knee dislocation, neurovascular injury, and any additional injuries (ligamentous or skeletal) may further assist in the evaluation.
2. Physical examination
   a. The physical examination is specific for a PCL injury, which is typically classified based on the degree of injury.
   b. At 90°, there is normally a 1-cm step-off between the tibial plateau and femoral condyle. In a grade I injury, this step-off is < 1 cm but the tibial plateau is still anterior to the femoral condyle. In a grade II injury, the tibial plateau is flush with the femoral condyle. In a grade III injury, the tibial plateau is posterior to the femoral condyle.
   c. The posterior drawer is the primary dynamic test to diagnose a PCL injury and is classified based on the degree of increased posterior tibial translation compared with the uninvolved knee at 90° of flexion: grade I injury: 3 to 5 mm; grade II injury: 6 to 10 mm; and grade III injury: >10 mm. The degree of posterior tibial translation may decrease with internal tibial rotation in partial tears.
   d. The quadriceps-active test is positive when the tibia translates anteriorly at 90° of flexion with resisted knee extension.
   e. A combined PCL and capsuloligamentous injury (PCL injury in conjunction with injury to other structures such as the ACL, posterolateral corner, or medial side) is indicated by more than 15 mm of posterior translation with the knee at 90° and in neutral rotation and more than 10 mm with the knee in internal rotation.
   f. The Lachman test for ACL injury, varus and valgus laxity testing, and determining

differences in external and internal tibial rotation are critical in differentiating between isolated and combined injuries.

3. Imaging
   a. Plain radiographs are important initially to rule out fractures and avulsions.
   b. The key is to recognize that when the knee (intact ACL and PCL) is centered in the sagittal plane, the tibia is anterior to the femoral condyles.
   c. MRI has been shown to have a very high sensitivity and specificity in diagnosing a PCL injury. MRI complements the history and physical examination and helps to determine the site and degree of injury by assessing the continuity of the PCL (**Figure 2**). MRI may also indicate the presence of other meniscal, chondral, or ligamentous injuries, which may influence treatment strategies.

D. Classification
1. PCL injuries occur in isolation or in combination with other injuries.
2. The grades of PCL injuries are based on the physical examination and MRI findings and are listed in **Table 2**.

E. Treatment
1. Nonsurgical
   a. Nonsurgical treatment is reserved for isolated partial PCL injuries with <10 mm of increased posterior tibial translation.
   b. Conservative treatment is also warranted in patients who are unable or unwilling to follow the prescribed rehabilitation regimen.
   c. The PCL can heal with nonsurgical treatment.
      - Nonsurgical treatment consists of bracing treatment with progressive flexion for 4 to 6 weeks.
      - Rehabilitation should emphasize isolated quadriceps strengthening and quadriceps-hamstring isometric cocontractions.
      - Isolated hamstring contraction (especially in a flexed position) should be avoided (**Figure 2**).

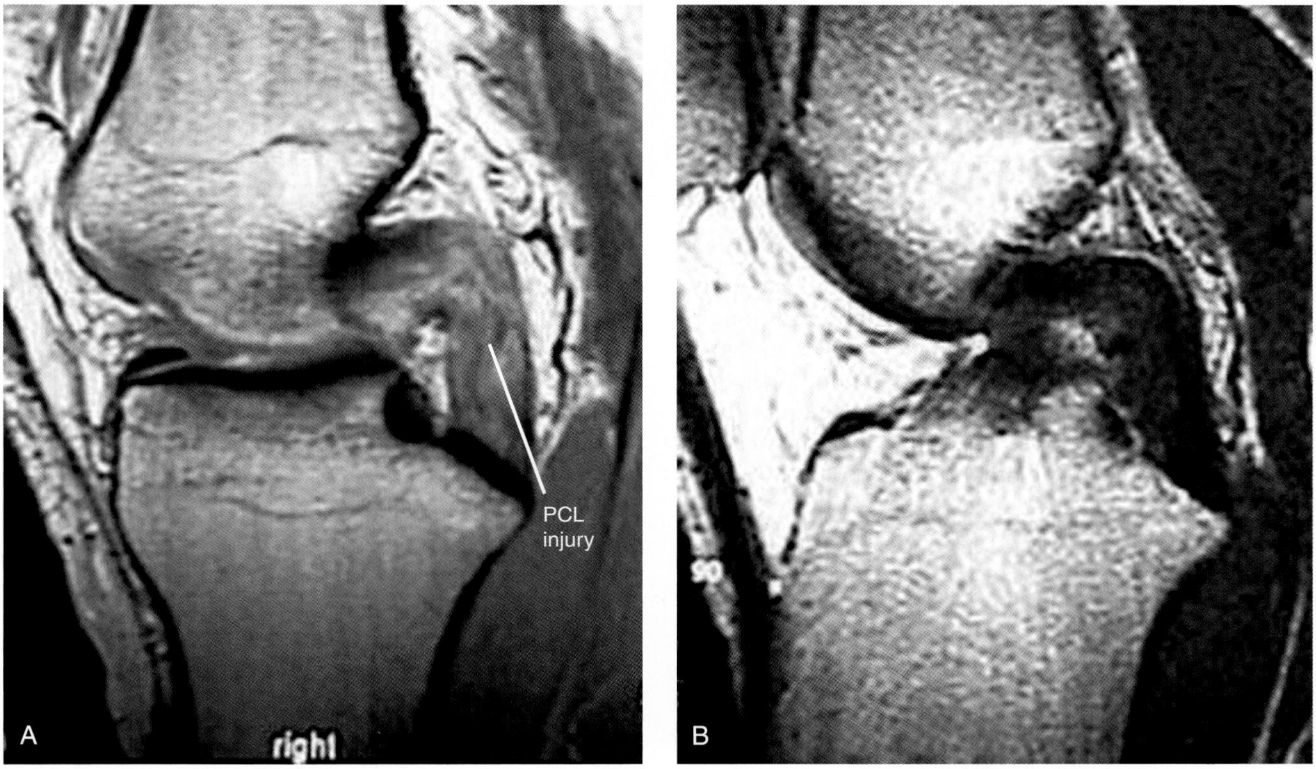

Figure 2 Acute posterior cruciate ligament (PCL) injury. **A**, Initial T1-weighted sagittal MRI demonstrates a PCL injury. **B**, Follow-up T1-weighted sagittal MRI shows healing of the PCL.

TABLE 2

Classification of Posterior Cruciate Ligamentous Injuries

Type of Injury	Characteristics
Partial	Posterior tibial translation <10 mm on posterior drawer test with the knee in neutral rotation End point is present
Complete isolated	Posterior tibial translation of 8-10 mm on posterior drawer test with the knee in neutral rotation and is diminished with the knee in internal rotation
Combined PCL and capsuloligamentous	Posterior tibial translation >10 mm on posterior drawer test with the knee in neutral rotation The PCL is injured in conjunction with other structures such as the ACL, posterolateral corner, or medial side

ACL = anterior cruciate ligament; PCL = posterior cruciate ligament

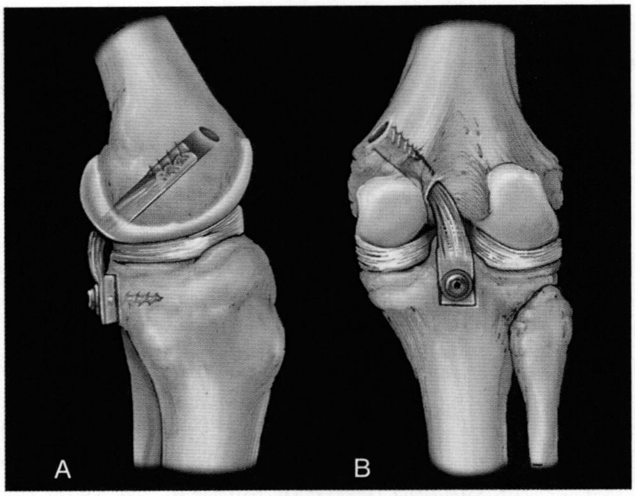

Figure 3 Illustrations depict single femoral tunnel posterior cruciate ligament reconstruction with tibial inlay using bone-patellar tendon-bone graft. **A**, Lateral view. **B**, Posterior view. (Reproduced with permission from the Cleveland Clinic Foundation, Cleveland, OH.)

2. Surgical
   a. Indications for surgery
      - Acute: Isolated PCL injuries with gross laxity to posterior drawer testing and for combined PCL/capsuloligamentous injuries.
      - Chronic: Persistent instability symptoms (particularly during ascending and descending stairs and inclines) and for combined PCL/capsuloligamentous injuries.
   b. Surgical procedures
      - The PCL can be repaired (avulsions), augmented, or reconstructed.
      - PCL reconstruction has been traditionally performed with a single tibial and femoral tunnel. More recently, both open and arthroscopic tibial inlay techniques have been developed in which a blind socket is created at the tibial insertion of the PCL.
         - The inlay technique avoids the so-called "killer curve" that may cause graft abrasion as it exits the tibial tunnel and takes a 90° turn toward the femoral tunnel (**Figures 3** and **4**).
      - Both single-bundle and double-bundle graft techniques have been used. A double-bundle graft most closely reproduces the anatomy of the native PCL by reconstructing both the anterolateral (AL) and posteromedial (PM) bundles and may provide more continuous stability throughout knee ROM. Single-bundle techniques have typically reconstructed on the AL bundle.
      - Graft choices include both autografts (central one-third bone-patellar tendon-bone, hamstring and quadriceps tendon-bone) and allografts (bone-patellar tendon-bone, Achilles tendon-bone, and tibialis anterior tendon).
      - No clinical studies clearly support one technique or graft over another.

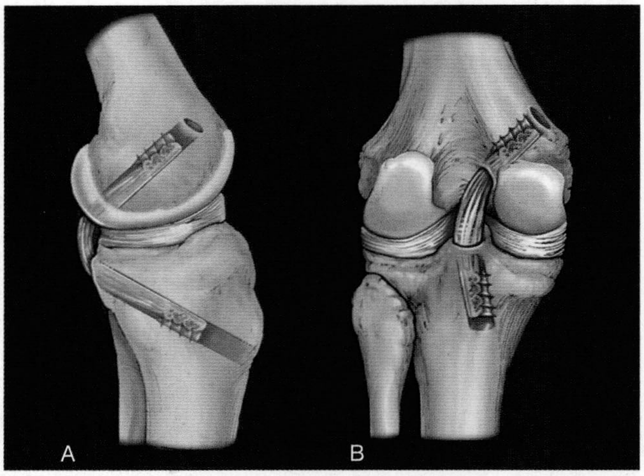

Figure 4 Illustrations show posterior cruciate ligament reconstruction with a single-tunnel technique in the femur and tibia with bone-patellar tendon-bone graft. **A**, Lateral view. **B**, Posterior view. (Reproduced with permission from the Cleveland Clinic Foundation, Cleveland, OH.)

c. Fluoroscopy is recommended during tibial drilling to avoid neurovascular injury of the popliteus structures.

F. Complications

1. Patellofemoral pain and/or arthritis (chronic PCL deficiency) can occur as a result of increased posterior translation and dynamic stabilization by the quadriceps.

2. Neurovascular injury can be a devastating complication and can result from injury to the popliteus neurovascular structures during tibial tunnel drilling.

3. Failure to reference the tibia in relation to the femur can result in misdiagnosis usually due to a false-positive anterior drawer test.

G. Pearls and pitfalls

1. Knee instability occurs less frequently with isolated PCL injuries than it does with ACL injuries.

a. A PCL injury is considered an injury of disability rather than instability.

H. Rehabilitation

1. Rehabilitation goals should focus on quadriceps strengthening.

2. In general, the rehabilitation following a PCL reconstruction is slower than for an ACL reconstruction in terms of advancing knee flexion.

3. Isolated hamstring strengthening should be avoided for 12 weeks following PCL reconstruction.

4. Return to sports usually is possible with 6 to 9 months following PCL reconstruction.

III. MEDIAL COLLATERAL LIGAMENT AND POSTEROMEDIAL CORNER INJURIES

A. Overview and epidemiology

1. The MCL is the most commonly injured ligament of the knee. The true incidence may be underestimated because of underreporting of lower grades of injury.

2. Concomitant ligamentous injuries (95% occur in the ACL) occur in 20% of grade I, 52% of grade II, and 78% of grade III injuries.

3. Concurrent meniscal injuries have been noted in up to 5% of isolated MCL injuries.

B. Anatomy

1. The medial capsuloligamentous complex comprises a three-layered sleeve of static and dynamic stabilizers extending from the midline anteriorly to the midline posteriorly (**Figure 5**).

2. Static stabilizers

a. The superficial MCL

b. The posterior oblique ligament

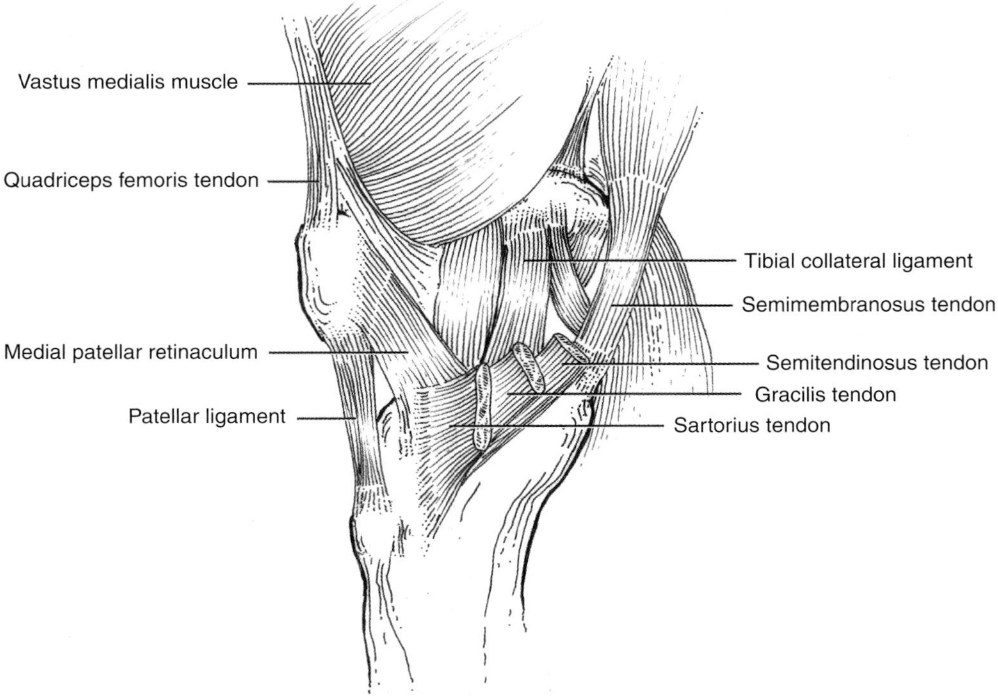

Figure 5 Illustration depicts the static and dynamic stabilizers of the medial and posteromedial aspects of the knee.

c. The deep MCL (also called the deep medial ligament or middle capsular ligament)

3. Dynamic stabilizers—Provide abduction stability under dynamic conditions
   a. The semimembranosus complex (composed of five insertional attachments)
   b. The pes anserinus muscle group (the sartorius, gracilis, and semitendinosus muscles)
   c. The vastus medialis
   d. The medial retinaculum

C. Biomechanics of the medial capsuloligamentous restraints
   1. The main function of this complex is to resist valgus and external rotation loads.
   2. The superficial MCL is the primary restraint to valgus loads at 30° of flexion.
   3. The posterior oblique ligament, the deep MCL, and the cruciate ligaments are secondary restraints to valgus stress.

D. Evaluation
   1. History
      a. Lesser degrees of MCL sprains result from a noncontact valgus, external rotation force. Complete disruption usually results from a direct blow to the lateral aspect of the knee.
      b. Occasionally, a "pop" is noted by the patient.
      c. The ability to ambulate and/or continue to participate in athletic activities depends on the degree of disruption, the player's position, and the presence of any concurrent injuries.
   2. Physical examination
      a. The knee should be inspected for ecchymosis, localized tenderness, and an effusion.
      b. Abduction stress testing should be performed with the knee at 0° and 30° of flexion.
      c. The superficial MCL is isolated with a valgus stress at 30° of flexion.
         - Pathologic laxity is indicated by the amount of increased medial joint space separation compared with the opposite, normal knee
           - Grade I: 1 to 4 mm
           - Grade II: 5 to 9 mm
           - Grade III: ≥10 mm
         - Valgus laxity with the knee at or near full extension implies concurrent injury to the posteromedial capsule and/or cruciate ligaments.
      d. Summary—MCL evaluation
         - Isolated laxity at 30° and stable in 0° of extension; indicates either a grade I or II injury
         - Combined laxity at 0° and 30°; indicates a grade III injury with concurrent injury to the posteromedial capsule (consider ACL or PCL combined injury)
      e. Evaluation of associated and other injuries
         - The Lachman and anterior drawer tests should be performed to rule out an ACL injury.
         - The pivot shift test often has false-negative results in the presence of a grade III MCL sprain.
         - A PCL injury is assessed by palpation of the tibial-condylar step-off and by the posterior drawer test (both performed at 90° of flexion), the quadriceps-active test, and observation of posterior tibial sag.
         - Patellar apprehension and tenderness over the patella and medial retinaculum indicate possible patellar dislocation/subluxation.
         - Diagnosis of an isolated medial meniscal injury is suggested by medial joint line tenderness, the absence of pain to valgus stress, and increased pain on flexion-rotation testing (McMurray test).
           - Injury to the lateral meniscus may occur due to lateral compartment.
   3. Imaging
      a. Plain radiographs
         - Plain radiographs are typically normal but should be inspected for fractures, lateral capsular avulsions (Segond fracture associated with an ACL tear), and Pellegrini-Stieda lesions (indicative of prior MCL injury).
         - Stress radiographs may be indicated in skeletally immature patients to rule out a physeal injury.
      b. MRI has become the imaging modality of choice to evaluate the injured MCL.
         - Advantages: identifies the location and extent of injury; can rule out associated meniscal, chondral, and cruciate ligament injuries
         - Disadvantages: expensive; reader-dependent; may overestimate the degree of injury

c. Contraindications to nonsurgical treatment include complete (grade III) injuries or avulsions of the LCL and combined rotatory instabilities involving the LCL and posterolateral compartment structures.

d. The most common complication of nonsurgical treatment is progressive varus/hyperextension laxity due to unrecognized associated injuries to the posterolateral structures.

e. Return to sports can be expected in 6 to 8 weeks depending on the sport and position played.

2. Surgical

a. Indications

- Complete injuries or avulsions of the LCL
- Rotatory instabilities involving the LCL and arcuate ligament, popliteus tendon, and fabellofibular ligament
- Combined instability patterns involving the LCL/posterolateral corner and cruciate ligaments

b. Surgical procedures: Acute injuries

- Surgical options
    - Primary repair of torn or avulsed structures
    - Reconstruction if the native tissue is of insufficient quality
- Surgery is usually recommended within 2 weeks of injury to prevent the formation of scar tissue and distortion of tissue planes that could hinder a direct repair.
- Arthroscopy is recommended to assist in the diagnosis of all torn structures as well as any meniscal or chondral injuries.
    - Fluid extravasation should be monitored but is rarely an issue.
- Suture anchors can be used to repair avulsed structures.
- Direct suture repair can be used for midsubstance injuries but often results in an unsatisfactory repair.

c. Surgical procedures: Chronic LCL and PLC insufficiency

- Allograft tissue (bone-patellar tendon-bone, Achilles tendon, tibialis anterior) has been used to form a single-stranded graft to reconstruct isolated LCL injuries.
- A bifid or split graft (Achilles tendon or tibialis anterior) can be used to anatomically reconstruct multiple injured structures including the LCL, popliteus, and popliteofibular ligament.
- The "anatomic" reconstruction popularized by LaPrade et al utilizes two separate allograft bundles to reconstruct all ligaments of the PLC:
    - The first bundle goes from the LCL femoral origin through a fibular tunnel (reconstructing the LCL) from an anterolateral to a posteromedial direction to the posterior tibia (reconstructing the popliteofibular ligament) and then anteriorly through a tibial tunnel.
    - The second bundle goes from the popliteus femoral origin posteriorly to the tibial tunnel (reconstructing the popliteus) and then anteriorly through the tibia with the first graft bundle.
- An alternative reconstruction option involves a single allograft bundle from the LCL femoral origin through a fibular tunnel posteriorly and then proximally to the popliteus femoral origin reconstructing the LCL and popliteus.
- The femoral tunnel created for an LCL reconstruction should be drilled with an anterior and proximal trajectory when an ACL reconstruction is performed concurrently to avoid tunnel convergence. Ligamentous reconstruction has a more favorable prognosis than ligament repair.

d. Complications

- Persistent varus or hyperextension laxity often is seen with advancement of attenuated lateral and posterolateral structures in chronic injuries.
- Injury to the peroneal nerve can occur during surgical exposure of the fibular neck or during drilling or graft passage through a transfibular tunnel.
- Loss of knee motion usually occurs with the reconstruction of multiple ligaments, especially the ACL.
- Hardware irritation most commonly occurs at the lateral femoral condyle.

G. Pearls and pitfalls

1. Surgery performed acutely has a more favorable outcome than surgery performed for chronic laxity.

9 | Sports Medicine

2. Ligamentous reconstruction has a more favorable prognosis than ligament repair.
3. All ligamentous deficiencies should be addressed to prevent persistent rotatory instability.
4. Previously described methods of anterior femoral advancement (Hughston procedure) or recession of the attenuated arcuate complex are no longer recommended for chronic instability.
5. Using the biceps femoris as a reconstructive graft in chronic posterolateral instability should be discouraged because it does not prevent external tibial rotation and eliminates the biceps as a dynamic lateral stabilizer of the knee.
6. Ligamentous reconstruction of the LCL should involve placement of graft tissue directly to the fibular head rather than to the lateral tibia to optimize graft isometricity.
7. The peroneal nerve is best identified beginning just posterior to the fibular head and then traced proximally.
    a. In chronic injuries with scarring of the posterolateral structures, the common peroneal nerve is often entrapped in scar tissue and is best identified proximal to the injury and dissected distally.
8. A hinged knee brace with an extended foot piece is recommended for at least the first 4 postoperative weeks to prevent external tibial rotation that may occur with the use of a simple hinged knee brace.
9. Full-length weight-bearing radiographs of both lower extremities should be obtained for all patients with chronic instability to assess for varus mechanical axis. In such cases, a high tibial osteotomy is recommended before ligamentous reconstruction.
    a. In some cases, realignment osteotomy reduces/eliminates the varus thrust associated with chronic ligamentous laxity.

V. MULTILIGAMENT KNEE INJURIES

A. Overview and epidemiology

1. Multiligament knee injuries usually are caused by high-energy trauma and are often considered knee dislocations.
2. Less frequently, low-energy trauma or ultra-low–velocity trauma can result in this injury pattern in obese patients.
3. A bicruciate ligament injury or a multiligament knee injury involving three or more ligaments should be considered a spontaneously reduced knee dislocation.
4. A knee dislocation should be considered a limb-threatening injury, and careful monitoring of vascular status after the injury is imperative.

B. Pathoanatomy

1. Multiligament knee injuries usually involve a partial or complete rupture of both cruciate ligaments.
2. Rare cases of knee dislocation with one cruciate ligament intact have been reported.
3. Most commonly, the medial or lateral side of the knee also will be injured.
4. After high-energy trauma, occasionally both medial- and lateral-side injuries accompany the bicruciate ligament injury.
5. Popliteus artery injury (30%) or peroneal nerve injury (20% to 40%) also can occur.
6. Extensor mechanism injury (quadriceps or patellar tendon) or patellar dislocation also can be encountered in this injury pattern.
7. Associated fractures can complicate management of the multiligament-injured knee, and definitive fixation of unstable fractures should be performed first in a staged fashion or concomitantly with any ligament surgery.

C. Evaluation

1. History
    a. A high index of suspicion for a reduced knee dislocation should accompany any knee injury that involves three or more ligaments.
    b. Mechanism of injury, position of the knee when it was injured, and timing of the injury are all important factors.
    c. A history of previous knee injury and current function are also relevant, as are age, activity level, and previous surgery or other injuries.
2. Physical examination
    a. Vascular examination is critical in an acutely dislocated knee.
        - The pulse and ankle-brachial index (ABI) should be assessed carefully. An ABI less than 0.90, and most certainly an ABI less than 0.80, should be considered abnormal.
        - If any concern exists about an abnormal vascular examination, the surgeon should consider ordering angiography.
        - If pulses are still abnormal or absent following reduction of the dislocation, immediate vascular surgery consultation with intraoperative exploration should be the next step.

- A vascular injury in a knee dislocation is a limb-threatening injury and needs to be corrected within 6 to 8 hours to avoid amputation.

b. Neurologic examination is also critical because peroneal nerve injury can occur with multiligament injuries, particularly in concomitant lateral/posterolateral corner injuries.

c. Swelling should be assessed.

d. A patellar examination should be conducted to assess extensor mechanism integrity and stability.

e. ROM should be evaluated.

f. Stability testing is critical and should include anterior and posterior drawer tests, a posterior sag test, a Lachman test, varus and valgus testing at 0° and 30°, and dial testing at 30° and 90°.

3. Imaging

a. Plain radiographs are essential in the initial evaluation of multiligament knee injuries.

- Associated fractures (ie, fibular head or PCL tibial avulsion) may affect the timing of surgery, and early open reduction and internal fixation of these fractures may improve healing.
- In chronic multiligament-injured knees, weight-bearing long-cassette alignment radiographs should be obtained to evaluate lower limb alignment.
- Radiographs can show posterior tibial subluxation on lateral views or medial or lateral joint space widening on weight-bearing PA views.
- Stress views can be used to document side-to-side differences and to rule out physeal injuries in skeletally immature patients.

b. MRI is required for all patients with a multiligamentous knee injury.

- MRI is useful for determining the site and extent of ligament injuries (ie, distal/proximal/midsubstance collateral ligament injury or cruciate avulsion) in surgical planning (**Figure 7**). This is particularly useful in severe injuries, when physical examination is often difficult because of substantial pain and guarding.

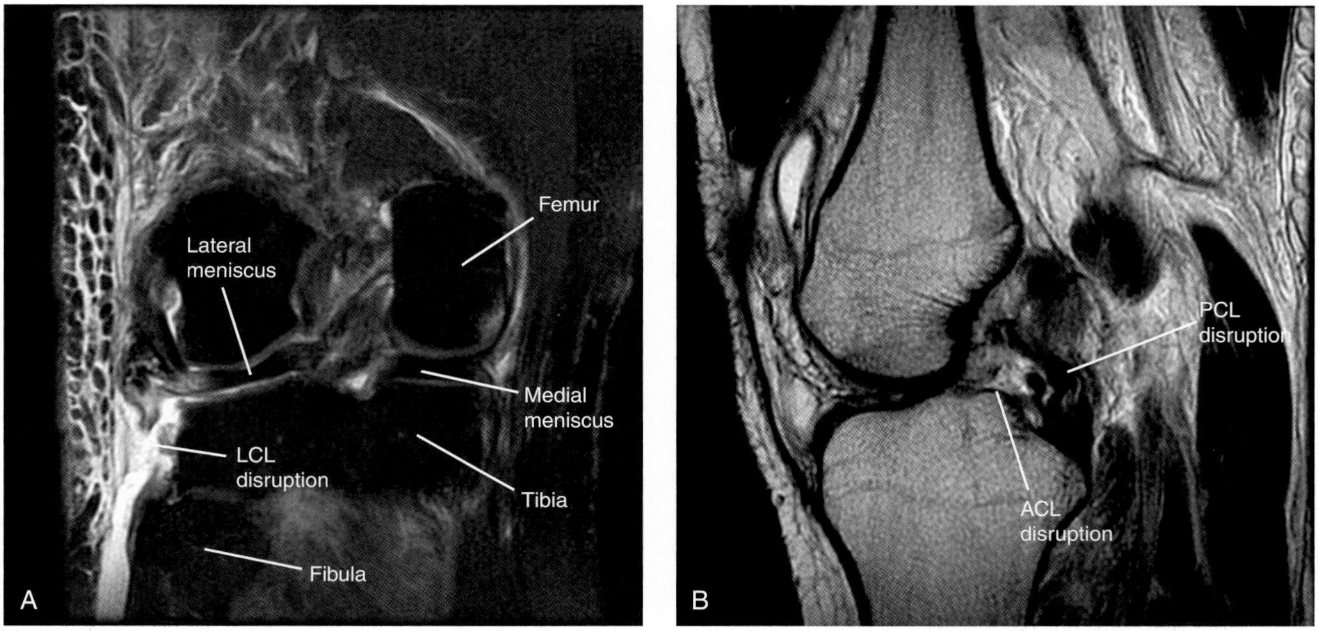

Figure 7 MRI demonstrating a knee dislocation (KDIIIL) in a college football quarterback. **A**, T2-weighted coronal image shows the lateral and posterolateral corner structures avulsed off the posterolateral tibia and fibular head with proximal retraction. **B**, T1-weighted sagittal view shows a bicruciate ligament injury. ACL = anterior cruciate ligament; LCL = lateral collateral ligament; PCL = posterior cruciate ligament.

TABLE 5

Anatomic Classification of Knee Dislocations

Classification	Characteristics
KDI	Single cruciate ligament torn
KDII	Both cruciate ligaments torn, collateral ligaments intact
KDIII	Both cruciate ligaments torn, one collateral ligament torn
KDIIIM	KDIII and MCL torn
KDIIIL	KDIII and LCL torn
KDIV	All four ligaments torn
KDV	Periarticular fracture-dislocation

KD = knee dislocation, LCL = lateral collateral ligament, MCL = medial collateral ligament

D. Classification is based on the direction of dislocation of the tibia and the anatomic area of injury.

1. Direction of dislocation (direction of tibial displacement)

   a. Anterior, posterior, lateral, medial, and posterolateral

   - Posterolateral dislocations often are irreducible as a result of the medial femoral condyle buttonholing through the medial capsule, causing the "dimple" sign.

2. Anatomic classification of knee dislocations is shown in **Table 5**.

E. Treatment

1. In the multiligament-injured knee that presents as a knee dislocation, emergent closed reduction and splinting or bracing treatment should be performed immediately. Postreduction radiographs should be obtained to confirm knee reduction.

2. Repeat radiographs should be obtained in patients with posterior knee dislocations awaiting surgery due to the effect of gravity causing further posterior tibial translation.

3. Nonsurgical

   a. Indications

   - With current reconstructive techniques, nonsurgical management of multiligament injuries usually is reserved for elderly low-demand patients, patients with comorbidities that would increase surgical risks, or patients with concomitant injuries (including vascular or head injuries, compartment syndrome, or associated fractures).
   - Patient preference for nonsurgical management.
   - Partial or incomplete multiligament injuries resulting in reasonable knee stability.
   - Patients unwilling or unable to follow postoperative activity restrictions or rehabilitation.

   b. Contraindications

   - Nonsurgical treatment is contraindicated in the presence of the comorbidities or concomitant injury patterns described above (irreducible dislocations, neurovascular injuries).
   - Surgical stabilization may still be used in a staged fashion after healing of associated fractures or vascular repair or bypass.

   c. Complications

   - Persistent knee instability
   - Knee stiffness or loss of motion (if motion is restricted for extended periods of time as part of nonsurgical management)

   d. Pearls and pitfalls

   - Treatment should include a short period of immobilization in full extension followed by protected ROM, preferably in a hinged knee brace to provide varus/valgus stability.
   - An ankle-foot orthosis should be incorporated into the knee brace in the presence of a footdrop resulting from a peroneal nerve injury.
   - Treatment should include patellar mobilizations to prevent patellar entrapment and the development of arthrofibrosis.
   - Careful monitoring of gait is important to avoid chronic dynamic instability patterns such as a varus thrust.
   - When fractures require skeletal stabilization, this care should be coordinated with the trauma team to ensure appropriate placement of incisions for future planned ligament stabilization.
   - When vascular repair is necessary, consultation with the vascular surgery team about planned incisions, timing of future ligament reconstructions, and motion limitations should be initiated.

   e. Complications, including persistent knee instability, arthrofibrosis, and gait abnormalities, such as a fixed varus deformity or dynamic varus thrust, can occur.

4. Surgical
   a. Indications
      - Injury of two or more ligaments (definition of multiligament injury) that results in an unstable knee
      - Inability to perform ADLs without knee instability
      - Ability to comply with the postoperative rehabilitative protocol
      - Associated fractures requiring stable fixation
      - Emergent surgical indications: irreducible knee dislocation requiring open reduction, open dislocation, vascular injury, or compartment syndrome
   b. Contraindications
      - Urgent concomitant injuries that preclude surgical reconstruction or repair of injured ligaments such as vascular injury, compartment syndrome, certain associated fractures (can sometimes be treated together), open injuries, or head injuries
      - Inability to comply with the postoperative rehabilitative protocol
      - Other medical comorbidities that preclude surgery such as unstable coronary artery disease
   c. Surgical procedures
      - Many approaches to the surgical management of multiligament-injured knees are used.
      - No high level of evidence is currently available on which to base definitive recommendations for surgical management.
      - Current controversies about the optimal surgical management of multiligament injuries include the following:
         - Timing: Acute (restore knee stability early, enabling early protected ROM) versus delayed (regain motion, allow swelling and inflammation to subside)
         - Type of graft: Autograft (improved healing of grafts and "ligamentization") versus allograft (decreased morbidity given the many structures requiring reconstruction but with associated cost and risk of disease transmission)
         - Surgical approach: Open (improved visualization and no risk of arthroscopic fluid-induced compartment syndrome) versus arthroscopic (decreased morbidity)
         - Ligamentous structures addressed: Reconstruct all ligaments (restore knee stability enabling early protected ROM) or reconstruct certain ligaments and perform staged reconstructions (gradual restoration of knee stability while limiting morbidity from each procedure and allowing restoration of motion)
         - Surgical technique: Repair (medial- and lateral-side acute injuries, usually within 2 to 3 weeks) versus reconstruction of torn ligaments (ACL, PCL, and/or delayed reconstruction or augmentation of medial/lateral repairs for added stability)
   d. Complications
      - Arthrofibrosis with loss of motion
      - Recurrent instability
      - Infection
      - Neurovascular injury, including injury to the popliteus artery, or peroneal nerve injury
   e. Pearls and pitfalls
      - The literature suggests that earlier reconstruction may have better outcomes compared with chronically reconstructed knees.
      - With lateral-side injuries, acute repair and/or reconstruction is recommended, preferably within 2 weeks of injury and certainly within 3 weeks. After 3 weeks, the lateral/posterolateral structures are often scarred and retracting, which often necessitates a concomitant reconstruction.
      - In chronic cases, ligament reconstruction should be performed due to the high failure rate of ligament repair in these patients.
      - When performing arthroscopy during multiligament knee surgery, the surgeon should be cognizant of pump pressure and monitor the leg compartments for fluid extravasation and possible compartment syndrome. Waiting 7 to 10 days before attempting surgery is often advised to allow the capsular injury often associated with multiligament knee injuries to heal. Use of gravity flow will reduce the risk of extravasation but may result in compromised visualization.

- Foot/ankle contractures should be suspected in patients with peroneal nerve injuries and can be prevented with the use of an ankle-foot orthosis when peroneal nerve palsy results in a footdrop.
- Missed posterolateral corner injuries have been associated with failed ACL and PCL surgery. Any bicruciate or PCL injury should be examined with a high index of suspicion for such injuries.
- Early protected motion usually is recommended because arthrofibrosis is a common occurrence following surgical reconstruction. This should be monitored carefully because recurrent laxity or instability can complicate an aggressive rehabilitation protocol. Close supervision of the rehabilitation is advised.

TOP TESTING FACTS

1. An effusion after ACL injury is related to hemarthrosis and is secondary to bleeding from the vascular, torn ligament.
2. MRI evidence of a bone bruise pattern in the area of the anterior lateral femoral condyle and the posterior lateral tibial plateau is pathognomonic of ACL injury.
3. The most important surgical factor is a well-performed technique, not the specific type of technique.
4. The most common error in ACL reconstruction is to place the tibial or femoral tunnel too anteriorly, resulting in graft impingement and failure.
5. An increased failure rate is seen when allograft is used in ACL reconstruction in young patients.
6. Primary ACL reconstructions has a better prognosis than revision ACL reconstruction.
7. Grade I and II MCL injuries that are stable in 0° of extension are treated nonsurgically.
8. Valgus laxity with the knee at or near full extension implies concurrent injury to the posteromedial capsule and/or cruciate ligaments.
9. Increased external rotation of the tibia at 30° but not at 90° suggests a posterolateral corner injury.
10. Increased external rotation of the tibia at both 30° and 90° is associated with injury to both the PCL and the posterolateral corner.
11. Neurovascular injuries (eg, common peroneal nerve injuries in the LCL and posterolateral corner and popliteus vascular structure injuries in knee dislocation) are associated multiligament knee injuries.
12. A bicruciate ligament injury or a multiligament knee injury involving three or more ligaments should be considered a spontaneously reduced knee dislocation. Knee dislocation is a limb-threatening injury requiring careful monitoring of vascular status.

Bibliography

Aglietti P, Giron F, Losco M, Cuomo P, Ciardullo A, Mondanelli N: Comparison between single-and double-bundle anterior cruciate ligament reconstruction: A prospective, randomized, single-blinded clinical trial. *Am J Sports Med* 2010;38(1):25-34.

Andersson C, Odensten M, Good L, Gillquist J: Surgical or non-surgical treatment of acute rupture of the anterior cruciate ligament: A randomized study with long-term follow-up. *J Bone Joint Surg Am* 1989;71(7):965-974.

Beynnon BD, Johnson RJ, Abate JA, Fleming BC, Nichols CE: Treatment of anterior cruciate ligament injuries, part I. *Am J Sports Med* 2005;33(10):1579-1602.

Beynnon BD, Johnson RJ, Abate JA, Fleming BC, Nichols CE: Treatment of anterior cruciate ligament injuries, part 2. *Am J Sports Med* 2005;33(11):1751-1767.

Biau DJ, Tournoux C, Katsahian S, Schranz PJ, Nizard RS: Bone-patellar tendon-bone autografts versus hamstring autografts for reconstruction of anterior cruciate ligament: Meta-analysis. *BMJ* 2006;332(7548):995-1001.

Biau DJ, Tournoux C, Katsahian S, Schranz P, Nizard R: ACL reconstruction: A meta-analysis of functional scores. *Clin Orthop Relat Res* 2007;458:180-187.

Boynton MD, Tietjens BR: Long-term follow-up of the untreated isolated posterior cruciate ligament-deficient knee. *Am J Sports Med* 1996;24(3):306-310.

Dunn WR, Lyman S, Lincoln AE, Amoroso PJ, Wickiewicz T, Marx RG: The effect of anterior cruciate ligament reconstruction on the risk of knee reinjury. *Am J Sports Med* 2004;32(8):1906-1914.

George MS, Huston LJ, Spindler KP: Endoscopic versus rear-entry ACL reconstruction: A systematic review. *Clin Orthop Relat Res* 2007;455:158-161.

Halinen J, Lindahl J, Hirvensalo E, Santavirta S: Operative and nonoperative treatments of medial collateral ligament rupture with early anterior cruciate ligament reconstruction: A prospective randomized study. *Am J Sports Med* 2006;34(7):1134-1140.

Harner CD, Waltrip RL, Bennett CH, Francis KA, Cole B, Irrgang JJ: Surgical management of knee dislocations. *J Bone Joint Surg Am* 2004;86(2):262-273.

Hussein M, van Eck CF, Cretnik A, Dinevski D, Fu FH: Prospective randomized clinical evaluation of conventional single-bundle, anatomic single-bundle, and anatomic double-bundle anterior cruciate ligament reconstruction: 281 cases with 3- to 5-year follow-up. *Am J Sports Med* 2012;40(3):512-520.

Indelicato PA: Non-operative treatment of complete tears of the medial collateral ligament of the knee. *J Bone Joint Surg Am* 1983;65(3):323-329.

Kaeding CC, Aros B, Pedroza A, et al: Allograft versus autograft anterior cruciate ligament reconstruction: Predictors of failure from a MOON prospective longitudinal cohort. *Sports Health* 2011;3(1):73-81.

Krych AJ, Jackson JD, Hoskin TL, Dahm DL: A meta-analysis of patellar tendon autograft versus patellar tendon allograft in anterior cruciate ligament reconstruction. *Arthroscopy* 2008;24(3):292-298.

Kurtz CA, Sekiya JK: Treatment of acute and chronic anterior cruciate ligament-posterior cruciate ligament-lateral side knee injuries. *J Knee Surg* 2005;18(3):228-239.

LaPrade RF, Terry GC: Injuries to the posterolateral aspect of the knee: Association of anatomic injury patterns with clinical instability. *Am J Sports Med* 1997;25(4):433-438.

Leys T, Salmon L, Waller A, Linklater J, Pinczewski L: Clinical results and risk factors for reinjury 15 years after anterior cruciate ligament reconstruction: A prospective study of hamstring and patellar tendon grafts. *Am J Sports Med* 2012;40(3):595-605.

Øiestad BE, Engebretsen L, Storheim K, Risberg MA: Knee osteoarthritis after anterior cruciate ligament injury: A systematic review. *Am J Sports Med* 2009;37(7):1434-1443.

Sonnery-Cottet B, Thaunat M, Freychet B, Pupim BH, Murphy CG, Claes S: Outcome of a combined anterior cruciate ligament and anterolateral ligament reconstruction technique with a minimum 2-year follow-up. *Am J Sports Med* 2015;43:1598-1605.

Spindler KP, Kuhn JE, Freedman KB, Matthews CE, Dittus RS, Harrell FE Jr: Anterior cruciate ligament reconstruction autograft choice: Bone-tendon-bone versus hamstring. Does it really matter? A systematic review. *Am J Sports Med* 2004;32(8):1986-1995.

Stannard JP, Brown SL, Farris RC, McGwin G Jr, Volgas DA: The posterolateral corner of the knee: Repair versus reconstruction. *Am J Sports Med* 2005;33(6):881-888.

Taylor SA, Khair MM, Roberts TR, DiFelice GS. Primary repair of the anterior cruciate ligament: A systematic review. *Arthroscopy* 2015;31:2233-2247.

Wright RW, Dunn WR, Amendola A, et al: Risk of tearing the intact anterior cruciate ligament in the contralateral knee and rupturing the anterior cruciate ligament graft during the first 2 years after anterior cruciate ligament reconstruction: A prospective MOON cohort study. *Am J Sports Med* 2007;35(7):1131-1134.

Wright RW, Preston E, Fleming BC, et al: A systematic review of anterior cruciate ligament reconstruction rehabilitation: Part I. Continuous passive motion, early weight bearing, postoperative bracing, and home-based rehabilitation. *J Knee Surg* 2008;21(3):217-224.

Chapter 123
MENISCAL INJURIES

MATTHEW V. SMITH, MD
RICK W. WRIGHT, MD

I. OVERVIEW AND EPIDEMIOLOGY

A. Meniscal function

1. The most important function of the meniscus is load-sharing across the knee joint.
   a. The meniscus increases the contact area between the femur and the tibia.
   b. It also decreases contact stress in the articular cartilage on the femur and tibia.
2. The meniscus also increases articular congruity, provides stability, aids in lubrication, prevents synovial impingement, and limits extremes of flexion and extension.

B. Epidemiology of meniscal injuries

1. Meniscal injuries are among the most common injuries seen in orthopaedic practice.
2. The incidence of acute meniscal tears is 61 cases per 100,000 people per year.
3. Arthroscopic partial meniscectomy is one of the most common orthopaedic procedures.

II. PATHOANATOMY

A. General information

1. The menisci are crescent shaped and have a triangular cross section.
2. The fibers of the menisci have a circumferential orientation, with radial tie fibers presenting longitudinal splits.
3. The medial and lateral menisci have anterior and posterior root attachments to the tibia that prevent meniscal extrusion during load bearing.
4. The lateral meniscus covers 84% of the condylar surface; it is 12 to 13 mm wide and 3 to 5 mm thick.
5. The medial meniscus is wider in diameter than the lateral meniscus; it covers 64% of the condyle surface and is 10 mm wide and 3 to 5 mm thick.
6. The medial meniscus is tethered by the deep medial collateral ligament, making it less mobile than the lateral meniscus.

B. Biochemistry

1. The menisci are 65% to 75% water.
2. Proteoglycans make up 1% of the dry weight.
3. The extracellular matrix is composed predominantly of type I collagen. Types II, III, V, and VI collagen also are identified.

C. Vascularity

1. The meniscal vascular supply arises from the superior medial and lateral, inferior medial and lateral, and middle genicular arteries.
2. Although the percentages are controversial, it appears that 50% of the meniscus is vascularized at birth, whereas only 10% to 25% of the meniscus is vascularized in the adult.
3. The vascularity of the meniscus affects the ability of meniscal repairs to heal.
4. The vascularity has been divided into three regions or zones (**Table 1**).

D. Biomechanics

1. When the knee is in extension, as much as 50% of the load is absorbed by the meniscus, with the percentage of load-sharing increasing to 90% at 90° of knee flexion.

Dr. Smith or an immediate family member has received nonincome support (such as equipment or services), commercially derived honoraria, or other non–research-related funding (such as paid travel) from Breg. Dr. Wright or an immediate family member has received research or institutional support from the National Football League Charities, the National Institutes of Health (NIAMS & NICHD), and Smith & Nephew.

TABLE 1

Vascular Zones of the Meniscus

Zone	Location	Vascular Status
Red-red	Peripheral third of the meniscus	Vascularized
Red-white	Middle third of the meniscus, at the border of the red vascularized zone	Avascular
White-white	Central third of the meniscus	Avascular

2. Beyond 90° of flexion, most of the force is transmitted to the posterior horns of the menisci.
3. The lateral meniscus provides more biomechanical protection to the joint than the medial meniscus.
4. In biomechanical studies, a radial tear of the medial meniscus that extends from the inner rim to the peripheral third (but preserves the peripheral third) has not been found to change maximum contact pressure and contact area in the knee. A radial tear involving 90% of the medial meniscus results in a posterocentral shift in peak-pressure location, however.
5. A vertical tear of the medial meniscus causes increased contact area and maximum contact pressure in both the lateral and medial compartments of the knee.
6. When the meniscus is removed completely, the articular cartilage contact stress increases by two to three times that experienced when the meniscus is intact.
   a. Biomechanical studies of partial meniscectomy have demonstrated increasing contact stresses with increasing loss of meniscal tissue.
   b. Removal of the inner third of the meniscus results in a 10% reduction in contact area and a 65% increase in contact stress on the articular cartilage.
7. Medial meniscus root tears result in peak articular cartilage contact pressure similar to that seen after a complete meniscectomy. Such tears have been associated with the progression of osteoarthritis.

III. EVALUATION

A. History

1. Meniscal tears are unusual in patients younger than 10 years.
2. Most meniscal tears in adolescents and young adults occur with a twisting injury or with a change in direction.
3. Middle-aged and older adults can sustain meniscal tears from squatting or falling.
4. With an acute meniscal tear, an effusion often develops several hours after injury. This differs from an anterior cruciate ligament (ACL) injury, in which swelling develops rapidly within the first few hours.
5. Patients with meniscal injuries localize pain to the joint line or posterior knee and may describe mechanical symptoms of locking or catching.
6. Chronic meniscal tears demonstrate intermittent effusions, often with mechanical symptoms.

B. Physical examination

1. Small joint effusions and joint line tenderness with palpation are common findings with meniscal tears.
2. Manipulative maneuvers, including the McMurray and Apley tests, may produce a palpable or audible click with localized tenderness, but they are not specific for meniscal pathology.
3. In the Thessaly test, the patient flexes the knee to 20° while standing on the affected extremity and twists in internal and external rotation. This maneuver often reproduces pain in patients with a meniscal tear.
4. Range of motion typically is normal.
   a. Longitudinal bucket-handle tears may block full extension of the knee joint.
   b. Patients may report tightness in flexion if an effusion is present.

C. Imaging

1. Standard knee radiographs should be obtained to evaluate for bone injuries or abnormalities.
2. A weight-bearing radiograph is necessary to evaluate for osteoarthritis.
   a. This may include a weight-bearing AP or 45° PA flexion view.
   b. A right-to-left difference of at least 2 mm represents a significant difference that will be verified by articular cartilage chondrosis at the time of arthroscopy.
3. MRI remains the noninvasive diagnostic procedure of choice for confirming meniscal pathology.
   a. In grade III MRI classification of meniscal tears, increased signal intensity reaches the articular surface of the meniscus (**Figure 1**).

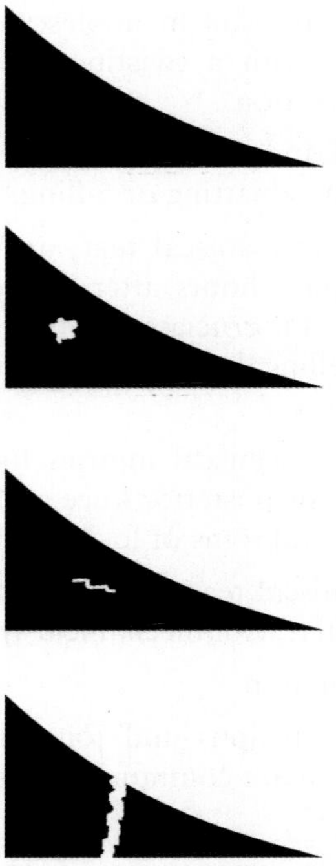

Figure 1 Illustration shows the grading scale for meniscal tears on MRI. Grade 0 is a normal meniscus. Grade I has a globular area of increased signal intensity within the meniscus that does not extend to the surface. Grade II has a linear area of increased signal intensity within the meniscus that does not extend to the surface. Grade III has increased signal intensity that abuts the free edge of the meniscus, indicating a meniscal tear. (Reproduced with permission from Thaete FL, Britton CA: Magnetic resonance imaging, in Fu FH, Harner CD, Vince KG, eds: *Knee Surgery*. Philadelphia, PA, Williams & Wilkins, 1994, pp 325-352.)

b. MRI has demonstrated a high negative predictive value for meniscal tears.

c. A well-performed MRI of a knee with no meniscal pathology will rarely demonstrate a tear.

D. Differential diagnosis

1. Several large studies have also demonstrated the accuracy of the clinical diagnosis of meniscal tears to be 70% to 75%.

2. The differential diagnosis for meniscal tears includes intra-articular and extra-articular diagnoses.

   a. Possible intra-articular diagnoses include osteochondritis dissecans, medial patella plica, patellofemoral pain syndromes, loose bodies, pigmented villonodular synovitis, inflammatory arthropathies, and osteonecrosis.

   b. Possible extra-articular diagnoses include collateral ligament injuries, slipped capital femoral epiphysis, bone or soft-tissue tumors, osteomyelitis, synovial cyst, pes or medial collateral ligament bursitis, injury, complex regional pain syndrome, lumbar radiculopathy, iliotibial band friction, and stress fracture.

IV. CLASSIFICATION

A. **Figure 2** and **Table 2** show classifications of meniscal tears.

B. Discoid meniscus

1. Discoid meniscus is a larger-than-normal meniscus.

2. Discoid meniscus is rare. It more commonly affects the lateral meniscus (1.4% to 15%) (**Figure 3**) than the medial meniscus (<1%).

3. Discoid menisci are classified into three subtypes: type I (incomplete), type II (complete), and type III (Wrisberg variant). Type III lacks posterior attachment to the tibia; it may be repaired.

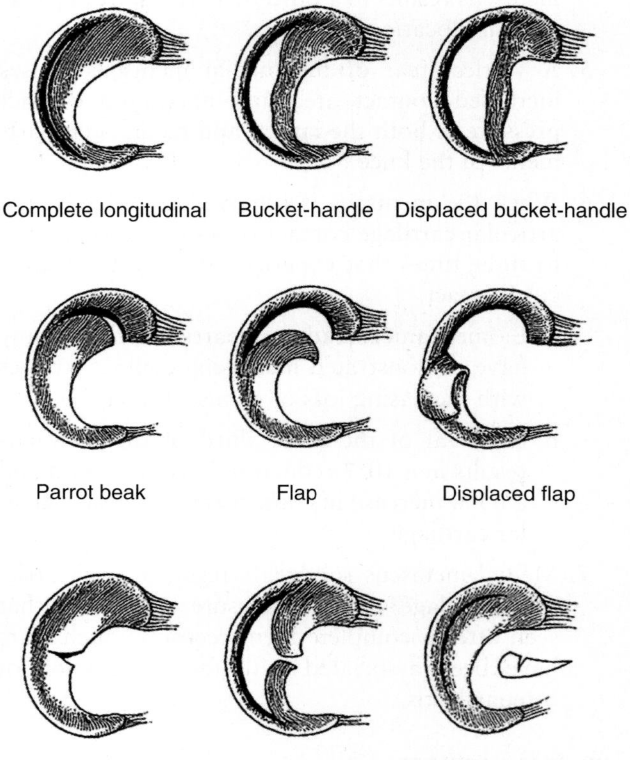

Figure 2 Illustrations depict common meniscal tears. (Adapted with permission from Tria AJ, Klein KS: *An Illustrated Guide to the Knee*. New York, NY, Churchill Livingstone, 1992.)

TABLE 2

Classification of Meniscal Tears

Tear Type	Characteristics
Vertical longitudinal	Common, especially in the setting of anterior cruciate ligament tears; can be repaired if located in the peripheral third of the meniscus
Bucket-handle	A vertical longitudinal tear displaced into the notch
Radial	Starts centrally and proceeds peripherally; not repairable because of loss of circumferential fiber integrity
Flap	Begins as a radial tear and proceeds circumferentially; may cause mechanical locking symptoms
Horizontal cleavage	Occurs more frequently in the older population and may be associated with meniscal cysts
Complex	A combination of tear types; more common in the older population

V. TREATMENT

A. Overview

1. In general, management of meniscal tears is predicated on symptoms.
2. Not all meniscal tears cause symptoms, and many symptomatic tears become asymptomatic.

B. Nonsurgical management

1. Tear types that commonly are managed nonsurgically include:
   a. Stable longitudinal tears less than 10 mm in length with less than 3 to 5 mm of displacement
   b. Degenerative tears associated with significant osteoarthritis
   c. Short (<3 mm in length) radial tears
   d. Stable partial tears
2. Nonsurgical management can include ice, NSAIDs, or physical therapy for range of motion and general strengthening of the lower extremities.

C. Surgical excision

1. Indications—Arthroscopic partial meniscectomy is indicated for radial, oblique, flap, horizontal cleavage, and complex tears, as well as for tears located in the white-white avascular zone.
2. Procedure
   a. Arthroscopic meniscectomy has been demonstrated to reduce surgical morbidity over open meniscectomy and to improve function.
   b. The goal of arthroscopic partial meniscectomy is to débride degenerative or torn meniscal tissue, leaving a stable contoured rim and preserving as much tissue as possible. Peak contact articular cartilage stresses increase proportionally to the amount of meniscus removed.
   c. Studies have demonstrated greater than 80% satisfactory function at minimum 5-year follow-up, despite a 50% finding of Fairbank's changes on radiographs, including osteophytes, flattening of the femoral condyles, and joint space narrowing. Studies also have demonstrated that degenerative changes and a decrease in function occur more quickly in patients who have undergone arthroscopic lateral meniscectomy. This is probably due to the biomechanical protection effect of the lateral meniscus.

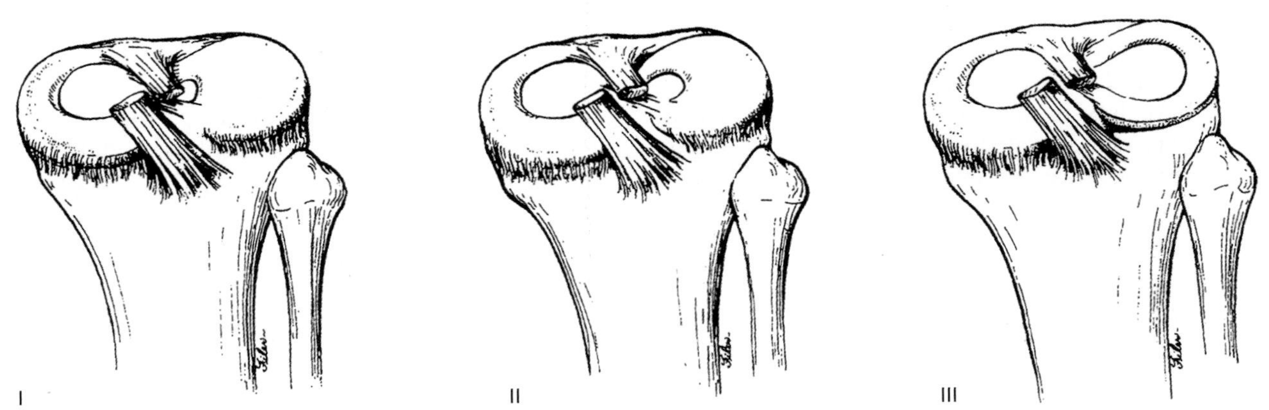

Figure 3 Illustrations show the classification system for lateral discoid menisci: type I (complete), type II (incomplete), and type III (Wrisberg variant). Type III discoid meniscus has no posterior attachment to the tibia. The only posterior attachment is through the ligament of Wrisberg toward the medial femoral condyle. (Reproduced with permission from Neuschwander DS: Discoid lateral meniscus, in Fu FH, Harner CD, Vince KG, eds: *Knee Surgery*. Baltimore, MD, Williams & Wilkins, 1994, p 394.)

9 | Sports Medicine

   d. Factors that seem to predict better long-term function following arthroscopic partial meniscectomy include age younger than 40 years, normal lower extremity alignment, minimal arthritic changes noted at the time of arthroscopy, and a single fragment tear.

D. Surgical repair—Once the function of the meniscus was understood, repair gained importance.

   1. Indications—Tear types appropriate for repair include vertical longitudinal tears in the vascular zone of the meniscus and displaced bucket-handle tears that remain in good condition once they are reduced.
   2. Relative contraindications include advanced degenerative articular cartilage damage, complex tears, poor meniscal tissue quality, and ACL deficiency.
   3. Procedures—The four potential meniscal repair techniques are open, arthroscopic inside-out, arthroscopic outside-in, and arthroscopic all-inside.
      a. Open repair usually is reserved for peripheral tears in the posterior horn approached through a capsular incision.
      b. Arthroscopic inside-out repairs are performed using absorbable or nonabsorbable sutures placed using zone-appropriate cannulas; the sutures are retrieved and tied through a small capsular incision.
      c. The arthroscopic outside-in technique usually is reserved for anterior horn tears. It involves placing a suture through a needle placed across the tear. The suture is retrieved and tied outside the knee through an arthroscopic portal, with the knot pulled into the knee to reduce the tear when tied over the capsule.
      d. Arthroscopic all-inside repairs involve absorbable stents or sutures tied to stents placed through arthroscopic portals. All-inside repairs may offer reduced neurovascular risk. Mechanical studies have investigated many of these devices and have demonstrated reasonable loads to failure, but no device improves on the load to failure of vertically placed inside-out sutures.
   4. Outcomes
      a. Clinical success rates for all meniscal repair techniques in stable knees are reasonable, ranging from 70% to 95%.
      b. Second-look arthroscopy has shown lower rates of success, ranging from 45% to 91%.
      c. Ligamentously unstable knees decrease the success rate of meniscal repair to 30% to 70%.
      d. Several studies have demonstrated meniscal repair success greater than 90% when performed in conjunction with an ACL reconstruction.
      e. Complications include failure to heal the tear, knee stiffness, and potential damage to the articular surface from mechanical devices used to repair the tear.

E. Transplantation

   1. Indications—Typically, meniscal allograft transplantation has been reserved for the patient who remains symptomatic in activities of daily living after partial or total meniscectomy or who develops recurrent pain after partial or total meniscectomy. It usually is reserved for patients who are skeletally mature but younger than 50 years.
   2. Contraindications include uncorrected lower extremity malalignment, uncorrected ligamentous instability, inflammatory arthritis, and significant chondral changes in the treated compartment. Return to strenuous sports generally is not recommended.
   3. Outcomes
      a. Meniscal allograft transplantation has been performed for more than 10 years with varying degrees of reported success.
      b. Subjective improvement in tibiofemoral pain and increased activity levels are seen after meniscal transplant.
      c. A long-term benefit for preventing the progression of osteoarthritis has not been established.
      d. Technically, grafts have performed better when placed with a bone block or plug.
      e. Preservation of at least some peripheral rim is important to prevent peripheral extrusion.
      f. A variety of meniscal scaffold options continue to be investigated, but they have not yet undergone widespread human clinical use or investigation.

Faber KJ, Dill JR, Amendola A, Thain L, Spouge A, Fowler PJ: Occult osteochondral lesions after anterior cruciate ligament rupture: Six-year magnetic resonance imaging follow-up study. *Am J Sports Med* 1999;27(4):489-494.

Frobell RB: Change in cartilage thickness, posttraumatic bone marrow lesions, and joint fluid volumes after acute ACL disruption: A two-year prospective MRI study of sixty-one subjects. *J Bone Joint Surg Am* 2011;93(12):1096-1103.

Gracitelli GC, Moraes VY, Franciozi CE, Luzo MV, Belloti JC. Surgical interventions (microfracture, drilling, mosaicplasty, and allograft transplantation) for treating isolated cartilage defects of the knee in adults. *Cochrane Database Syst Rev* 2016;9:CD010675

Knutsen G, Drogset JO, Engebretsen L, et al: A randomized trial comparing autologous chondrocyte implantation with microfracture: Findings at five years. *J Bone Joint Surg Am* 2007;89(10):2105-2112.

Kocher MS, Tucker R, Ganley TJ, Flynn JM: Management of osteochondritis dissecans of the knee: Current concepts review. *Am J Sports Med* 2006;34(7):1181-1191.

Mandalia V, Fogg AJ, Chari R, Murray J, Beale A, Henson JH: Bone bruising of the knee. *Clin Radiol* 2005;60(6):627-636.

Solheim E, Hegna J, Strand T, Harlem T, Inderhaug E. Randomized study of long-term (15-17 Years) outcome after microfracture versus mosaicplasty in knee articular cartilage defects. *Am J Sports Med* 2018;46(4):826-831.

Wall EJ, Vourazeris J, Myer GD, et al: The healing potential of stable juvenile osteochondritis dissecans knee lesions. *J Bone Joint Surg Am* 2008;90(12):2655-2664.

Wright RW, Phaneuf MA, Limbird TJ, Spindler KP: Clinical outcome of isolated subcortical trabecular fractures (bone bruise) detected on magnetic resonance imaging in knees. *Am J Sports Med* 2000;28(5):663-667.

Yoon KH, Yoo JH, Kim KI: Bone contusion and associated meniscal and medial collateral ligament injury in patients with anterior cruciate ligament rupture. *J Bone Joint Surg Am* 2011;93(16):1510-1518.

Chapter 125
Overuse Injuries

ARMANDO F. VIDAL, MD
ANNUNZIATO AMENDOLA, MD
CHRISTOPHER C. KAEDING, MD
TIMOTHY L. MILLER, MD

I. Stress Fractures

A. Epidemiology

1. Stress fractures are common in highly committed athletes and tend to occur in sports with repetitive, high-impact weight-bearing activity.
2. Stress fractures and stress reactions occur when repetitive microtrauma to a bone exceeds the capacity of the bone to withstand and repair from the microtrauma.
3. Stress fractures are uncommon in the ribs and the upper extremity but occur with upper extremity weight-bearing and repetitive tasks.
4. Most bony stress injuries occur in the lower extremity with the tibia and metatarsals being the most common locations.
5. Stress fractures occur in less than 1% of the general athletic population, but the incidence in running/track athletes can be 10% to 20%. The rate of recurrence may be approximately 10% for all athletes, but as high as 50% in runners.
6. Populations at greatest risk for developing stress fractures include women with the female athlete triad (disordered eating, amenorrhea, and osteoporosis) and those with vitamin D insufficiency. Body mass index (BMI) <19 is a risk factor for stress fracture and extended time to return to sport.

B. Pathophysiology

1. Stress fracture is a fatigue failure of bone that occurs in three stages: *crack initiation, crack propagation,* and *final fracture.*
2. Stress fractures represent a continuum of severity of bone injury (**Table 1**); they occur from accumulation of microdamage that occurs with repetitive loading. The area of initial stress concentration is termed *crack initiation.*
3. If the initial microscopic crack is not repaired and repeated loading of the bone continues, the crack extends and is referred to as *crack propagation,* eventually resulting in a *final fracture.*
4. In vivo, bone responds to crack initiation and propagation with a reparative biologic response that is dependent on age, nutritional status, hormonal status, vascular supply, biomechanical factors, and possibly genetic predisposition.
5. A dynamic balance exists between the accumulation of microdamage and the host repair processes.
   a. When microdamage accumulation exceeds the reparative response, the result is a stress fracture.

Dr. Vidal or an immediate family member is a member of a speakers' bureau or has made paid presentations on behalf of Smith & Nephew; serves as a paid consultant to or is an employee of Smith & Nephew and Stryker; has received nonincome support (such as equipment or services), commercially derived honoraria, or other non–research-related funding (such as paid travel) from Smith & Nephew and Stryker; and serves as a board member, owner, officer, or committee member of the American Orthopaedic Society for Sports Medicine. Dr. Amendola or an immediate family member has received royalties from Arthrex, Inc., arthrosurface, and Smith & Nephew; serves as a paid consultant to or is an employee of Arthrex, Inc.; serves as an unpaid consultant to extremity development corporation, First Ray Inc, and rubber city bracing; has stock or stock options held in First Ray; and serves as a board member, owner, officer, or committee member of the American Orthopaedic Society for Sports Medicine. Dr. Kaeding or an immediate family member serves as a paid consultant to or is an employee of Active Implants and Smith & Nephew; has received research or institutional support from Active Implants, DJ Orthopaedics, and Smith & Nephew; and serves as a board member, owner, officer, or committee member of the American Orthopaedic Society for Sports Medicine and the International Society of Arthroscopy, Knee Surgery, and Orthopaedic Sports Medicine. Neither Dr. Miller nor any immediate family member has received anything of value from or has stock or stock options held in a commercial company or institution related directly or indirectly to the subject of this chapter.

TABLE 1

Locations of High-Risk Stress Fractures

Femoral neck—superolateral
Femoral neck—inferomedial[a]
Patella
Anterior tibial diaphysis
Medial malleolus
Talus
Tarsal navicular
Fifth metatarsal
Sesamoid bones
Olecranon
Scaphoid

Modified from Kaeding CC, Yu JR, Wright R, Amendola A, Spindler KP: Management and return to play of stress fractures. *Clin J Sport Med* 2005;15:442-447.
[a]Less risk of fracture than superolateral location.

b. Any factor that disrupts this dynamic balance can increase the risk of stress fracture.

c. Any factor that increases tensile, compressive, or torsional forces on a bone may cause an increase in microdamage accumulation with each loading episode especially if applied with an abrupt increase in frequency or intensity.

d. Likewise, any factor that impairs the reparative biologic response, such as poor vascularity or an altered hormonal balance, may increase the risk of developing a stress fracture or insufficiency fracture.

C. Evaluation

1. Stress fractures typically present with an insidious onset of pain but may present with an acute onset of pain with or without prodrome pain of weeks to months.

2. A history of a prolonged high-impact activity or a recent abrupt increase in training frequency or intensity is usually present. Alternatively, there may have been a recent change in type of training (eg, introduction of interval training) or equipment (eg, a new brand of shoes).

3. With no history of substantial repetitive loading episodes, an insufficiency fracture or pathologic fracture must be considered, specifically in patients with decreased bone density, inadequate nutrition, or abnormal bone quality.

4. Physical examination may reveal pain with direct palpation or mechanical loading of the affected site with fulcrum testing of long bones and single leg hop testing.

5. Radiography, bone scintigraphy, CT scan, and MRI are the imaging techniques used to evaluate stress fractures. Each has advantages and disadvantages with MRI being the modality of choice due to high sensitivity and specificity.

a. Radiographs are rarely positive unless the injury is severe or chronic. Typically, radiographic findings lag behind clinical symptoms for weeks to months.

b. Bone scans are very sensitive in identifying the presence and location of stress fractures, but they do not reveal macroscopic fracture lines in the bone and may remain positive for up to two years after the injury is clinically healed.

c. MRIs can identify the bony edema associated with early stress concentration or reveal the presence of a fracture line (**Table 2**). MRI is advantageous because it shows the surrounding soft tissues and is most predictive of time to return to athletic activity.

d. Ultrasonography has been described for the imaging of stress fractures but is used much less commonly because of its inability to penetrate the cortex. It is advantageous because no ionizing radiation is used and a focused, real-time evaluation of the fracture can be performed.

e. Identifying the presence of a nonunion and assessing the amount of healing in preparation for possible surgery is best achieved using CT scan, but this carries a significant radiation dose.

TABLE 2

MRI Grading System for Stress Fractures

	Magnetic Resonance Imaging
Grade 1	Positive STIR
Grade 2	Positive STIR and T2WI
Grade 3	Positive T1WI and T2WI but without definite cortical break
Grade 4	Positive T1WI and T2WI with fracture line

Reproduced with permission from Arendt EA, Griffiths HG. The use of mr imaging in the assessment and clinical management of stress reactions of bone in high-performance athletes. *Clin J Sport Med* 1997;16(2):291-306.
STIR, short T1 inversion recovery; T1WI, T1-weighted image; T2WI, T2-weighted image

TABLE 3

Classification of Stress Fractures

	High Risk	Low Risk
Biomechanical environment	Tension	Compression
Natural history	Poor	Good
Management	Aggressive Complete fracture: surgery Incomplete fracture: strict non–weight bearing or surgery	Conservative Symptomatic: activity modification Asymptomatic: no treatment needed, observation

Reproduced with permission from Kaeding CC, Yu JR, Wright R, Amendola A, Spindler KP: Management and return to play of stress fractures. *Clin J Sport Med* 2005;15:442-447.

TABLE 4

Grading System of Fatigue Failure of Bone

Grade	Pain	Imaging*
1	No	Evidence of fatigue failure
2	Yes	Evidence, no fracture line
3	Yes	Fracture line: nondisplaced
4	Yes	Fracture line: displaced
5	Yes	Nonunion

Reproduced from Kaeding CC , Miller TL : The comprehensive description of stress fractures: A new classification system. *J Bone Joint Surg Am* 2013;95:1214-1220.
*Must report imaging modality used.

D. Classification
1. Stress fractures generally are classified as low-risk or high-risk depending on the location; those with a poor natural history are deemed high-risk (**Table 3**) and usually require aggressive management.
2. Delayed recognition or undertreatment of high-risk stress fractures tends to result in fracture progression, nonunion, the need for surgery, refracture, and delayed return to sport.
3. Other fractures have a more benign natural history and are low-risk stress fractures; these fractures tend to heal with activity modification due to compressive forces and adequate vascularity.
4. Recognizing the class of stress fracture is important for optimizing treatment.
   a. Overtreatment of a low-risk stress fracture or undertreatment of a high-risk fracture can result in undue loss of playing time, deconditioning, and prolonged recovery.
5. MRI classification of stress fractures has been correlated with time to return to play (**Table 2**).
6. A recent generalizable clinical and radiologic classification system has been shown to have high intra- and interobserver reliability for grading stress fractures (**Table 4**)

E. Treatment principles
1. Treatment must alter the biomechanical and biologic environment to allow the reparative processes to overcome the accumulation of microdamage at the fracture site. A holistic approach is required to optimize healing potential.
2. The athlete's biologic bone-healing capacity should be evaluated. This includes review of the athlete's nutritional, hormonal, psychological, biomechanical, and medication status.
3. The female athlete triad (amenorrhea, disordered eating, and osteoporosis) must be considered in any female athlete with stress fractures; appropriate evaluation and treatment should be initiated.
4. The fracture site also must be protected from future strain episodes through relative rest, absolute rest, bracing treatment, technique modification, or surgical fixation (**Figure 1**).
   a. Relative rest involves decreasing the frequency or magnitude of strain episodes at the stress fracture site by modifying the athlete's training volume (intensity, duration, and frequency), technique, and equipment, using a brace or orthosis or by cross-training.
   b. Absolute rest removes all strain episodes from the fracture site. This often is achieved by having the athlete bear no weight, use crutches, and undergo immobilization.
5. An assessment of biomechanical risk factors such as malalignment should be performed to assess an athlete's likelihood of recurrence. Video running gait analysis and throwing analysis are ideal for determining form and technique abnormalities.
6. The use of biophysical enhancement technologies in stress fractures such as pulsed ultrasonography and electrical stimulation has not been shown to be a major factor in healing an acute stress injury.
7. Nutritional support with appropriate caloric intake along with calcium and vitamin D supplementation is required to achieve healing and

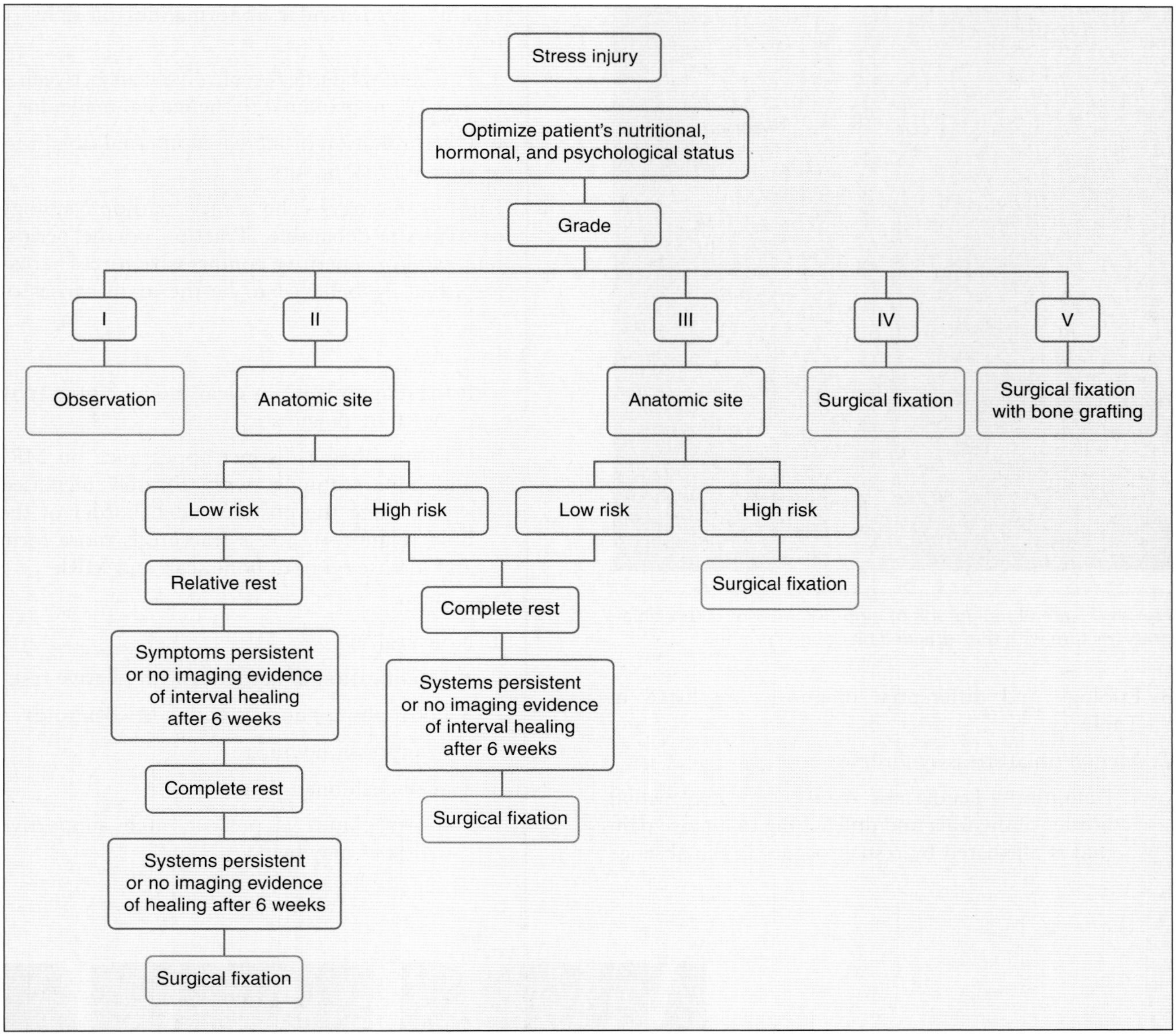

Figure 1 Treatment algorithm for the management of stress fractures based on injury severity on the Kaeding-Miller classification system. (Reproduced with permission from *Rockwood and Green's: Fractures in Adults, ed 9. 2018.)*

prevent recurrence. Nutritional laboratory values may be required in athletes with multiple or recurrent bony stress injuries.

8. With these principles in mind, the management of stress fractures depends on classifying each fracture as either high or low risk (**Figure 1**).
   a. High-risk stress fractures are typically treated with absolute rest or surgery (**Figure 2**).
   b. Level of risk for catastrophic injury must be seriously considered before allowing patients with a high-risk stress fracture to continue to play; however, patients with low-risk stress fractures may do so with activity modification/relative rest (**Figure 3**).

II. EXERCISE-INDUCED LEG PAIN

A. Epidemiology
   1. It is estimated that medial tibial stress syndrome (MTSS) (a nonspecific all-encompassing term) accounts for 10% to 15% of all running injuries.
   2. Shin splints may account for up to 60% of leg pain symptoms in running athletes.

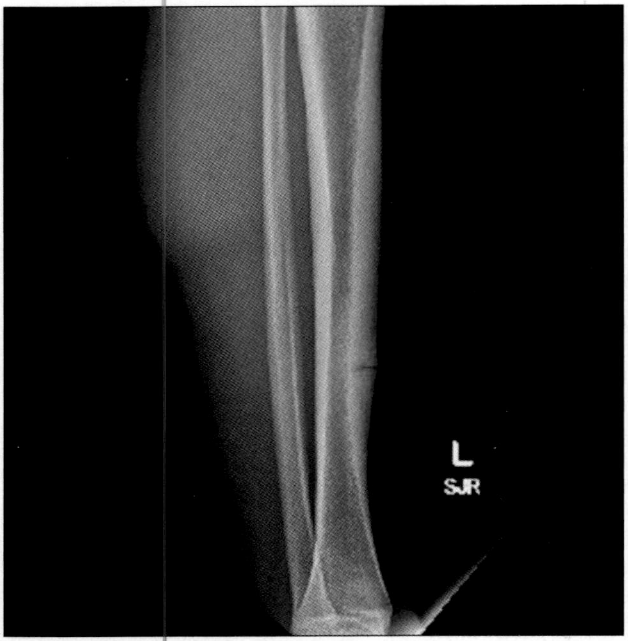

Figure 2 Lateral radiograph of high-risk anterior cortex tibial stress fracture with the "dreaded black line" present.

B. Etiology and differential diagnosis are listed in **Table 5**.

C. Medial tibial stress syndrome

1. Definition—Tenderness over the posteromedial border of the tibia and dull aching to intense pain that is alleviated by rest. It occurs in the absence of any neurovascular abnormalities or signs of fracture.
   a. Pain and tenderness typically occur between 4 and 12 cm proximal to the medial malleolus.
   b. Overpronation or increased internal tibial torsion are risk factors.
2. Pathophysiology—The exact pathophysiology of MTSS is debatable. Traction on the periosteum and/or repetitive compressive forces across the tibia are believed to be the main causes of MTSS.
3. Imaging
   a. If the diagnosis is not clear, bone scintigraphy or MRI are diagnostic.
   b. Periostitis has a distinct appearance on MRI and bone scanning, with diffusely increased signal along the posteromedial border of the tibia (**Figure 4**). Stress fracture is more focal and intense on both bone scan and MRI.
4. Treatment
   a. Nonsurgical
      - Modification of activities with relative rest
      - Local phonophoresis with corticosteroids
      - Compression wraps
      - Well-cushioned shoes
      - If pes planus is present, arch supportive orthotics may help

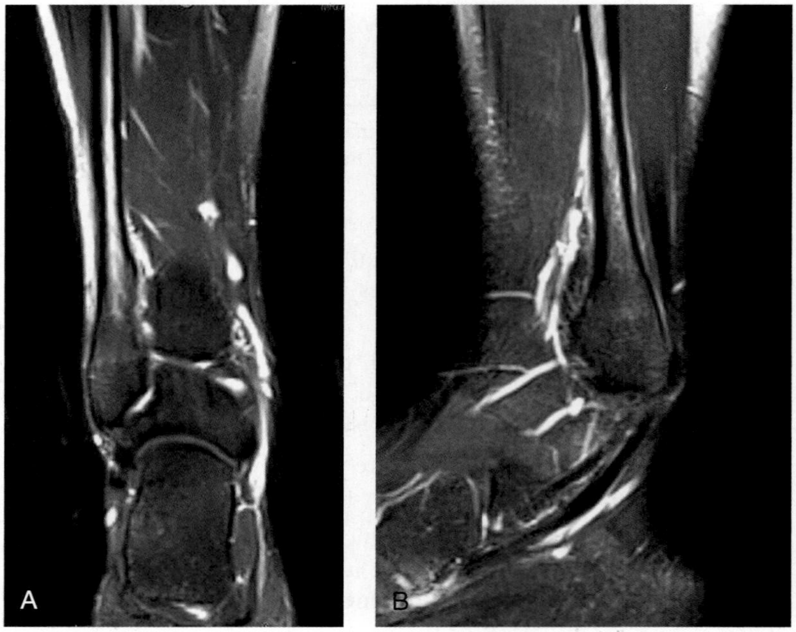

Figure 3 Coronal (**A**) and sagittal (**B**) T2 MRI images demonstrate a Kaeding-Miller grade II fibular stress reaction/fracture.

9 | Sports Medicine

TABLE 5

Etiology and Differential Diagnosis of Exercise-Induced Leg Pain and Compartment Syndrome

Tissue of Origin	Examples of Pathology
Bone	Tibial stress fracture, fibular stress fracture
Periosteum	Periostitis (medial tibial stress syndrome)
Muscle or fascia	Exertional compartment syndrome, fascial herniation
Tendon	Achilles, peroneal, or tibialis posterior tendinopathy
Nerve	Sural or superficial peroneal nerve entrapment
Blood vessel	Popliteus artery entrapment, intermittent claudication, or other insufficiency; venous insufficiency
Distant (referred)	Spinal radiculopathy

- A dedicated program of strengthening of the invertors and evertors of the hindfoot is important in preventing recurrence; recurrence is common after patients resume heavy activity
- A running gait analysis to improve biomechanics may decrease forces on the medial tibia

b. Surgical

- The results of surgery vary given the absence of rigid diagnostic clinical criteria and the variability of potential surgical procedures performed.

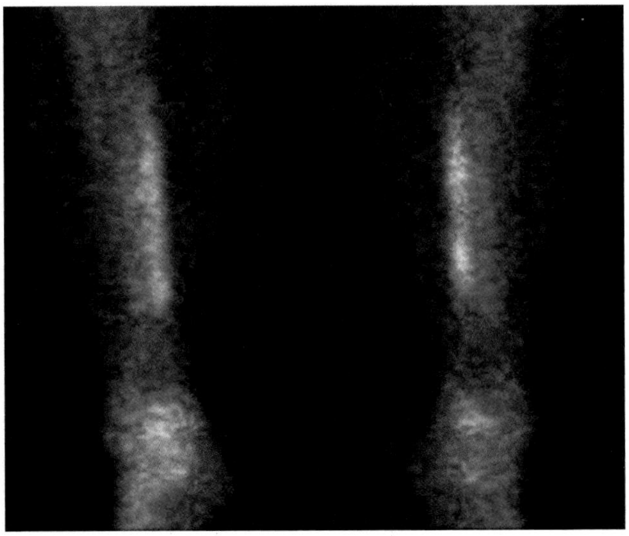

Figure 4 Bone scintigraphy demonstrates medial tibial stress syndrome with diffuse periosteal edema at the medial distal tibial diaphysis.

- If nonsurgical treatment fails and the patient remains symptomatic, fasciotomy of the deep posterior compartment (soleus release) with release of the painful portion of periosteum may be considered.

D. Iliotibial band (ITB) syndrome

1. Definition

a. ITB friction syndrome is a common cause of lateral knee pain in runners, cyclists, and military recruits.

b. It is thought to be caused by repetitive, cyclic friction between the ITB and the lateral femoral epicondyle. Compression of the fat pad and connective tissue deep to the ITB and inflammation of the sub-ITB bursa have also been proposed as causes.

c. Running on chamfered roads is considered a risk factor for increased friction under the ITB.

2. Diagnosis

a. The diagnosis is typically made based on the history and physical examination.

b. Localized tenderness along the ITB between the lateral femoral epicondyle and the Gerdy tubercle is typical.

c. The Ober test helps determine ITB tightness and contracture.

d. Imaging is rarely necessary other than to rule out other causes of pain. MRI typically demonstrates increased signal intensity deep to the ITB in the region of the lateral femoral epicondyle.

3. Treatment

a. Nonsurgical management is the mainstay of treatment.

- Activity modification, rest, and equipment modification (particularly in cyclists) can help alleviate symptoms.
- NSAIDS, localized corticosteroid injections, and physical therapy can be beneficial.
- Physical therapy should consist of specific stretching exercises focusing on the ITB, tensor fascia lata, and gluteus medius.

b. Surgical management

- Surgery is rarely required and is reserved for recalcitrant cases.
- Surgical options include percutaneous or open ITB releases or lengthening. ITB bursectomy performed either open or arthroscopically has been described.

- Favorable results have been published following surgery for recalcitrant cases.

E. Chronic exertional compartment syndrome (CECS)

1. Overview

   a. Definition: A reversible compression within a closed fibro-osseous space that results in decreased tissue perfusion and transient muscle ischemia.

   b. It is most common in the lower leg of athletes in running sports, particularly in distance runners.

   c. Anterior compartment involvement is most common and comprises approximately 70% to 80% of cases.

   d. Posterior compartment involvement is less common and has been associated with less predictable surgical outcomes.

2. Pathophysiology

   a. Muscle volume can increase up to 20% with physical activity.

   b. The combination of muscle enlargement and noncompliant fascia leads to insufficient blood flow to the muscle during the relaxation phase and transient ischemic pain.

3. Diagnosis—The diagnosis of exertional compartment syndrome is made clinically and can often be made using a thorough and detailed history.

   a. The patient characteristically has a normal physical examination and radiographs, no pain at rest, and reproducible exercise-induced leg pain that is completely relieved by stopping the offending activity.

   b. Evaluation—Postexercise intracompartmental pressure measurements, rather than extensive imaging studies, are used to confirm the diagnosis.

   c. Resting pressure, immediate postexercise pressure, and continuous pressure measurements for 30 minutes after exercise are most diagnostic of CECS.

   d. A study is considered positive if the insertional pressure is 15 mm Hg or greater at rest, the immediate postexercise pressure is 30 mm Hg or greater, or the pressure fails to normalize or exceeds 20 mm Hg at 5 minutes post-exercise.

4. Treatment

   a. Nonsurgical

   - Intracompartmental pressure normally rises and falls with activity; therefore, nonsurgical modalities rarely decrease pressure.
   - Physical therapy, NSAIDs, and orthoses have generally been ineffective. Forefoot running, however, has shown some ability to decrease pressure and minimize symptoms for up to 1 year.

   b. Surgical treatment

   - Indicated for patients who have appropriate clinical presentations with confirmatory pressure measurements and are unwilling to modify or give up their sport.
   - Fasciotomy of the affected compartments is the treatment of choice and is >90% effective in appropriately indicated patients.

F. Fascial hernia

1. Pathophysiology—A muscle herniation can become symptomatic because of chronic exertional compartment syndrome, a compressive neuropathy, or ischemia of the herniated muscle tissue.

2. Evaluation—A hernia at the exit of the superficial peroneal nerve or of one of its branches is commonly associated with chronic exertional compartment syndrome.

3. Treatment

   a. Patients with asymptomatic hernias require no treatment.

   b. Symptomatic hernias should be managed initially with education, activity modification, and, possibly, use of a compression stocking.

   c. Failure of these modalities may indicate decompression of the affected compartment with fasciotomy.

   d. Closure of the fascial opening is contraindicated.

G. Peripheral neuropathy

1. Pathophysiology

   a. The superficial peroneal nerve is a branch of the common peroneal nerve.

   b. The nerve is most commonly compressed as it exits the deep fascia at the lateral distal leg to become subcutaneous, a point where localized tenderness may be encountered.

   c. In addition to muscle herniation, the nerve can be compressed by the fascial edge, exertional compartment syndrome, or be subjected to repeated traction by recurrent inversion ankle sprains; 25% of patients report a history of trauma, particularly recurrent ankle sprains.

2. Evaluation
   a. Patients may have activity-related pain and neurologic symptoms in the distal third of the leg or the dorsum of the foot and ankle.
   b. Weakness is not expected because the innervation of the anterior tibialis and peroneal muscles is proximal to the site of compression.
   c. Electromyelogram with nerve conduction velocities may identify site of nerve entrapment if symptoms are not resolved after 6 weeks of observation.
3. Treatment—If the neuropathy is caused by muscle herniation or compression on the fascial edge, fasciotomy with neurolysis may be required to relieve symptoms.

III. SOFT-TISSUE OVERUSE INJURIES

A. Pathophysiology
1. Clinically, tendinosis or tendinopathy is a term that broadly encompasses painful conditions of tendon degeneration that result from overuse and repetitive microtrauma.
2. Histologically, tendinosis is a chronic intratendinous degenerative lesion of the tendon and may involve little to no inflammation.
3. Tendinosis is not a failed healing response; there is no overt acute injury and no inflammatory phase, as is typical for most healing responses.
4. The pathology of tendinosis has been described as *angiofibroblastic hyperplasia*. Microscopically, the pathology of tendinosis demonstrates fibroblasts and vascular, atypical, granulation tissue seen with absence of inflammatory cells.
5. Tendon strain up to 6% is physiologic; strain that ranges from 6% to 8% can result in overuse injuries; and strain greater than 8% can cause complete tendon rupture.
6. In tendinosis, instead of the normal constructive adaptive response of repeated loading, the tendon no longer responds in a positive fashion but starts to accumulate increasing amounts of poorly organized and dysfunctional matrix; this degenerative tissue is the hallmark of tendinosis.
7. Tendinosis occurs most commonly in the rotator cuff, patellar tendon, Achilles tendon, tibialis posterior tendon, and common extensor origin at the elbow (extensor carpi radialis brevis).

B. Classification—The Blazina grading system of tendinitis
1. A grade I lesion is characterized by pain that occurs only after the activity.
2. A grade II tendinitis lesion is characterized by pain that occurs during activity but does not affect performance.
3. A grade III lesion is characterized by pain that occurs during the activity and affects performance, such that the athlete cannot train and perform at the desired level.

C. Treatment
1. Nonsurgical
   a. Initial treatment consists of rest and physical therapy that includes eccentric strengthening.
   b. Many nonsurgical interventions have been advocated, including iontophoresis, hyperbaric oxygen, nitric oxide, sclerotherapy, extracorporeal shockwave therapy, ultrasonography-guided tendon débridement, and platelet-rich plasma injections. Few controlled studies have been conducted that confirm the utility of these options.
   c. Corticosteroid injection is not recommended given the increased risk of tendon rupture.
2. Surgical
   a. If nonsurgical measures fail in a grade III lesion and the tendinosis lesion is well established on MRI, surgery should be considered.
   b. Surgical intervention includes two broad categories:
      - The "excise and stimulate" category includes marginal or wide excision via open or arthroscopic techniques.
      - The "stimulate a healing response" category includes using percutaneous needling or open multiple longitudinal tenotomies.
   c. Both surgical options seek to induce a healing response in the tendon lesion by inflicting an acute traumatic event. This induced acute healing response hopefully results in repair of the degenerative lesion or denervation of the symptomatic tissues.

D. Results
1. Improvement in the patient's ability to perform activities of daily living is typical.
2. Recurrence of symptoms after the athlete returns to aggressive loading activity is not uncommon.
3. A randomized controlled trial has demonstrated that eccentric exercise is as effective as surgery in the treatment of patellar tendinopathy.

TOP TESTING FACTS

1. The tibia and metatarsal bones are the most common sites for the development of stress fractures.
2. Stress fractures occur on a continuum of severity from bony edema to complete fracture with nonunion. They result from crack propagation that exceeds the bone's reparative biologic response.
3. High-risk stress fractures usually involve the tension surfaces of bone or areas of relative avascularity and have a poor natural history requiring aggressive treatment with complete rest or surgery.
4. MTSS is evidenced by diffuse low-intensity increased linear signal on bone scan or MRI as opposed to stress fractures which are of higher intensity and focal.
5. The anterior soft-tissue compartment of the lower leg is the most commonly involved compartment in chronic exertional compartment syndrome.
6. The diagnosis of exertional compartment syndrome can be made if the patient has both reproducible exercise-induced leg pain and an immediate postexercise intracompartmental pressure of 30 mm Hg or greater.
7. Athletes with exertional compartmental syndrome who fail nonsurgical treatment and want to return to sport are treated with surgical fasciotomy of the involved compartments.
8. ITB syndrome is a common overuse injury seen in runners and cyclists and presents with lateral-sided knee pain.
9. Tendinosis, a soft-tissue overuse injury, is considered a failed adaptive response leading to degenerative tearing from repetitive microtrauma and displays angiofibroblastic hyperplasia on histologic evaluation.
10. A randomized controlled trial found eccentric exercise as effective as surgery in treatment of patellar tendinopathy.

Bibliography

Andres BM, Murrell GA: Treatment of tendinopathy: What works, what does not, and what is on the horizon. *Clin Orthop Relat Res* 2008;466(7):1539-1554.

Bahr R, Fossan B, Løken S, Engebretsen L: Surgical treatment compared with eccentric training for patellar tendinopathy (Jumper's Knee): A randomized, controlled trial. *J Bone Joint Surg Am* 2006;88(8):1689-1698.

Dunn JH, Kim JJ, Davis L, Nirschl RP: Ten- to 14-year follow-up of the Nirschl surgical technique for lateral epicondylitis. *Am J Sports Med* 2008;36(2):261-266.

Figueroa D, Figueroa F, Calvo R: Patellar tendinopathy: Diagnosis and treatment. *JAAOS* 2016;24(12):e184–e192.

Kaeding CC, Miller TL: The comprehensive description of stress fractures: A new classification system. *J Bone Joint Surg Am* 2013;95(13):1214-1220.

McInnis KC, Ramey LN: High-risk stress fractures: Diagnosis and management. *PM R* 2016;8(3 suppl):S113-S124.

Miller TL, Best TM: Taking a holistic approach to stress fractures. *J Orthop Surg Res* 2016;11(1):98.

Miller TL, Jamieson M, Everson S, Siegel C: Expected time to return to athletic participation after stress fracture in division I collegiate athletes. *Sports Health* 2018;10(4):340-344.

Pepper M, Akuthota V, McCarty EC: The pathophysiology of stress fractures. *Clin Sports Med* 2006;25(1):1-16, vii.

Reshef N, Guelich DR: Medial tibial stress syndrome. *Clin Sports Med* 2012;31(2):273-290.

Strauss EJ, Kim S, Calcei JG, Park D: Iliotibial band syndrome: Evaluation and management. *J Am Acad Orthop Surg* 2011;19(12):728-736.

Vajapeyajula S, Miller TL: Evaluation, diagnosis and treatment of chronic exertional compartment syndrome. *Phys Sports Med* 2017;45(4):391-398.

Chapter 126

CONCUSSION AND COMMON NEUROLOGIC SPORTS INJURIES

ALLEN K. SILLS, MD, FACS
GARY SOLOMON, PhD
JOHN E. KUHN, MD, MS

I. CONCUSSION

A. Definition

1. A concussion is a transient, trauma-induced alteration in neurologic function.
2. Loss of consciousness (LOC) is not required for a diagnosis of concussion. Only approximately 10% of sport-related concussions include LOC.
3. Other terms for concussion have included mild traumatic brain injury (MTBI), "ding," and "bell-ringer," but these latter two terms are outdated and no longer used.

B. Incidence

1. Between 2 and 4 million MTBIs occur annually in the United States.
2. Concussion comprises 9% of all sports-related injuries at the high-school level, prompting more than 150,000 emergency department visits annually.
3. Sports with the highest incidence of concussion per participant are (in descending order): football, girls' soccer, boys' soccer, girls' basketball, boys' lacrosse, and boys' wrestling.
   a. All sports have a risk of traumatic brain injury.
4. Some data suggest an increasing incidence of concussion ascribed to an increasing size and speed of athletes, a greater risk from the increase in year-round sports, and a greater awareness and more frequent diagnosis.

C. Signs and symptoms of concussion are shown in **Table 1**.

D. Assessment of concussion

1. Numerous scales have been proposed as an attempt to classify concussions based on the severity of the injury.
   a. Each scale is intended to classify the severity of a concussion according to the presenting symptoms, with an historic emphasis on loss of consciousness. Typically, concussions were classified as grade 1 (mild), grade 2 (moderate), and grade 3 (severe); however, the classification scales for concussion have become obsolete.
   b. No standardized definition of concussion has reached universal consensus although common presenting symptoms exist.
   c. No definitive correlation of concussion with outcome exists.
   d. Guidelines for returning to athletic play are based on international consensus opinion.
2. Currently, a concussion is assessed individually on the basis of
   a. The nature and duration of symptoms and signs
   b. The athlete's/player's age
   c. The player's concussion history and medical comorbidities
3. A grading of sports according to type from those with the highest likelihood of concussion to those with the lowest is shown in **Table 2**.

Dr. Sills is a paid employee of the National Football League. Dr. Solomon or an immediate family member serves as a board member, owner, officer, or committee member of the National Football League. Neither Dr. Kuhn nor any immediate family member has received anything of value from or has stock or stock options held in a commercial company or institution related directly or indirectly to the subject of this chapter.

9 | Sports Medicine

TABLE 1

Signs and Symptoms of Concussion

Signs and Symptoms[a]	Physical Symptoms	Cognitive Symptoms	Emotional Symptoms	Sleep Symptoms
Dazed or stunned appearance	Headache	Mental "fogginess"	Irritability	Drowsiness
Forgets plays or assignments	Nausea and/or vomiting	Feeling slow in behavior/reactions	Sadness	Insomnia
Unsure of date of game or opponent	Balance problems	Difficulty in concentrating	Emotional instability	Change in sleep pattern (sleeping more than usual)
Clumsy movement	Dizziness	Difficulty with remembering	Nervousness	
Slow response to questions	Visual problems	Difficulty reading	"Flat" personality	
Behavior or personality change	Fatigue			
Forgets events from before being hit (retrograde amnesia)	Sensitivity to light/noise			
Forgets events after being hit (anterograde amnesia)				

[a]All of these signs and symptoms require honest reporting by the person experiencing them.

4. A more serious neurologic injury requiring transport to a hospital with neurologic services is indicated by
   a. Concussion with spinal cord symptoms
   b. LOC exceeding 1 minute
   c. Seizure (and possibly tonic posturing) in a patient with no history of seizure
   d. A deep scalp laceration with substantial blood loss
   e. Persistent drowsiness
   f. Worsening headache, especially when accompanied by recurrent vomiting
   g. Severe neck pain
   h. Difficulty moving the arms or legs
   i. Any lateralizing neurologic sign such as motor asymmetry, pupil asymmetry, or hemisensory loss

E. Sideline management of suspected concussion
   1. Remove athlete from contest
   2. Obtain a history with a focus on common symptoms
   3. Brief, focused neurologic examination (pupils, extraocular movements)
   4. Motor and sensory screening
   5. Balance and coordination—Single leg balance, tandem walk
   6. Brief cognitive examination—Methods include the Standardized Assessment of Concussion, Sport Concussion Assessment Tool, and ImPACT sideline assessment tool.
   7. The athlete should not be returned to the contest/event if a concussion is diagnosed.
   8. Serial examinations should be performed to determine the duration of symptoms.
   9. An athlete should be accompanied home after the game if symptoms persist.
   10. The athlete should be reassessed on the following day and daily until symptoms resolve.

F. Management of concussion symptoms
   1. Most symptoms will resolve within a few days and not require intensive medical management.
   2. During the acute phase (ie, 24 to 48 hours), physical exertion, loud noise, or bright light may provoke symptoms and should be avoided, and cognitive rest should be encouraged (three-dimensional movies, video games, excessive texting, reading, or computer work should be avoided if symptoms are provoked). Cognitive and physical rest is indicated in this initial time frame.
   3. Acetaminophen or NSAIDs may be used to treat headache (narcotics should be avoided); antiemetics can be used for persistent nausea; and mild sleep aids can be used for persistent sleep problems.

TABLE 2

Risk of Concussion in Different Sports

Collision/ Impact Sports[a,b]	Contact Sports[c]	Limited-Contact Sports[d]	Noncontact Sports
Boxing	Basketball	Baseball	All other sports
Football	Diving	Bicycling	
Ice hockey	Field hockey	Cheerleading	
Rodeo	Lacrosse	Field events	
Rugby	Martial arts	High jump	
	Soccer	Pole vault	
	Wrestling	Gymnastics	
		Horseback riding	
		Skating (ice, inline, roller)	
		Skiing/snow-boarding	
		Softball	
		Surfing	
		Ultimate frisbee	
		Volleyball	

[a]Risk occurs in decreasing order from left to right and in descending order from top to bottom.
[b]Repeated high-energy blows to the head are a common component as part of the game; highest risk of concussion.
[c]Blows to the head are not infrequent but not a primary component of play.
[d]Blows to the head are fairly uncommon but do occur in certain situations.

G. Computerized neurocognitive testing

1. Concussion produces transient alterations in objective measures of visual attention; concentration; visual, verbal, and spatial memory; and reaction time.
2. Measurement of these functions has historically required a written battery of tests administered by a neuropsychologist. This is expensive, time-consuming, and subject to the limited availability of qualified practitioners.
3. Computerized neurocognitive tests can provide a rapid, reproducible assessment of the neurocognitive changes produced by a concussion and eliminates reliance on the accuracy of an athlete's reporting of symptoms.
4. Several products for computerized neurocognitive testing are now commercially available.
5. Ideally, baseline computerized neurocognitive testing of all athletes on a team should be performed before the beginning of the season.
6. Athletes who experience an injury should be retested when their symptoms resolve. These test results should be compared with the baseline results to determine if neurocognitive function has returned to baseline.
7. If no baseline exists, the athlete can be tested in the acute postinjury period, with the test repeated for comparison after symptoms resolve. The neurocognitive test results from the acute postinjury period can also be compared with normative data, although in many cases this may not be as precise as comparison with an individual baseline.

H. Return to play

1. No athlete who has experienced a concussion should return to athletic activity until: (1) all symptoms have resolved both at rest and on exertion, (2) postural stability has returned to normal, and (3) the results of neurocognitive testing have returned to baseline values. Steps in a graduated return to play are as follows:
   a. No activity—Rest until symptoms resolve
   b. Light aerobic exercise (for example, walking, stationary cycling)
   c. More strenuous aerobic activity
   d. Sport-specific training
   e. Noncontact drills
   f. Full-contact drills
   g. Return to play
2. In younger athletes (≤18 years), each step in this progression should last for at least 24 hours.
3. If symptoms develop at any step, rest should be resumed for 24 hours followed by return to the previous step.
4. Game activity is permitted only when all steps have been successfully completed without recurrence of symptoms and full medical clearance.

I. Prognostic aspects of concussion

1. Maximum number of "safe" concussions is unknown.
2. Multiple concussions in a single athletic season should be avoided.
3. A concussion specialist should be consulted when symptoms persist beyond a few weeks or create ongoing academic/cognitive/emotional problems.

4. Any relationship between athletic concussion and (1) chronic neurodegenerative disease or (2) psychiatric disorders is not poorly understood at present.

J. Prevention of concussion
1. Use of a proper fitting, well-maintained helmet.
2. Practice/skill in athletic technique; visualize the target and end result of a football tackle or other objective of play.
3. Maximize safety of play environments.
4. Use age-specific guidelines to determine the allowable extent of contact.
5. Avoid return to play until injuries fully heal.
6. Educate players, families, and athletic staff to recognize signs, symptoms, and the importance of concussion and its reporting.

II. STINGERS

A. Overview and epidemiology
1. Stingers (also called burners) are transient injuries to a single nerve root.
2. In the 1970s, 50% of football players had experienced at least one stinger during their careers; by 1997, this had been reduced to an incidence of 3.7% to 7.7% and prevalence of 15% to 18%, probably through changes in rules and equipment.
3. A single stinger triples the likelihood of experiencing another.

B. Pathoanatomy
1. The most common mechanism of injury in a stinger is downward displacement of the shoulder with lateral flexion of the neck toward the contralateral shoulder, causing traction on the brachial plexus.
2. Lateral turning of the head toward the affected side may cause nerve root compression and may be a source of symptoms.
3. A direct blow to the supraclavicular fossa at the point of Erb may also injure a nerve root and may be equipment related.

C. Evaluation
1. History
   a. A stinger creates a transient, unilateral tingling, burning, or numbing sensation in the distribution of the affected nerve root.
   b. Ipsilateral sensory symptoms and motor weakness are typical in an acute stinger injury.
   c. The distribution of the C6 nerve root is commonly involved, but the upper trunk of the brachial plexus and other cervical roots may also be involved.
   d. Symptoms typically resolve after 1 to 2 minutes.
   e. Neck pain or bilateral complaints should not be present.
2. Physical examination
   a. With chronic or repeated injury, atrophy may be noted.
   b. The physical examination should assess the neck for stiffness, spasm, or pain.
   c. A positive Spurling test result and tenderness on percussion of the supraclavicular fossa may be present.
3. Differential diagnosis and natural history
   a. A player who has stingers in both arms or a leg should be suspected of having a spinal cord injury rather than a simple stinger. The player should be immediately removed from play and undergo a neurologic examination.
   b. Electromyographic (EMG) studies are indicated if symptoms do not resolve after 3 weeks. EMG will demonstrate abnormalities in the spinal cord, nerve roots and trunks, and peripheral nerves.
   c. Other injuries such as a cervical fracture, dislocation, or spinal cord contusion should be ruled out.
   d. The patient should be reexamined frequently.
   e. In 5% to 10% of patients, severe or repeated stingers may cause long-term muscle weakness with persistent paresthesias.
   f. Patients with cervical pain or other symptoms or signs should undergo a thorough workup of the neck.

D. Treatment
1. By definition, stingers are transient injuries and do not require formal treatment.
2. Systemic steroids have not been shown to be beneficial for stingers and may be harmful.
3. Return to play is allowed when the patient is symptom free after rest and rehabilitation. Return to play in a contest may be allowed if symptoms resolve within 10 minutes or less, the neck range of motion is normal, and strength throughout the arms has returned to normal.

4. Players with residual muscle weakness, cervical abnormalities, restricted cervical motion, or abnormal EMG studies should be removed from contact sports.
5. In football, equipment modifications to shoulder pads may reduce the risk of stinger recurrence.

III. LONG THORACIC NERVE INJURY

A. Overview/epidemiology—Injury to the long thoracic nerve is uncommon but has been reported in nearly every sport.

B. Pathoanatomy

1. The long thoracic nerve arises from C5-C7, with a C8 contribution in 8% of individuals. It travels anterior to the scalenus posterior muscle and distally and laterally under the clavicle over the first or second rib and runs along the midaxillary line for 22 to 24 cm.
2. Repetitive stretch injury causes most injuries of the long thoracic nerve, which are typically neurapraxic.
3. Tilting or rotation of the head away from the arm and with the arm in an overhead position put the nerve at risk.
4. A fascial band from the inferior brachial plexus to the proximal serratus anterior muscle may contribute to traction nerve injury.
5. Direct trauma to the thorax may also injure the nerve.
6. Compression of the nerve can occur at many sites.

C. Evaluation

1. History
   a. Patients commonly report pain at the shoulder, neck, or scapula that is exacerbated by activity or tilting of the neck.
   b. Weakness is noted when lifting away from the body or with overhead activity.
   c. Prominent scapular winging may be noted when the patient leans against the back of a chair while sitting.
2. Physical examination
   a. Static and dynamic winging of the scapula is seen, with weakness in shoulder strength testing.
   b. The position of the resting scapula is superior and toward the midline as the trapezius dominates scapula position.
   c. Resisted forward elevation or having the patient perform a push-up will accentuate the winging.
3. Ancillary studies
   a. EMG and nerve conduction velocity (NCV) studies will confirm the diagnosis and delineate the severity of injury.
   b. These studies may also be also helpful to follow recovery.

D. Treatment

1. Most serratus palsies resulting from long thoracic nerve injury recover spontaneously.
2. Physical therapy to strengthen compensatory muscles and braces that help to hold the scapula to the chest may provide some comfort.
3. Recovery typically occurs within 1 year but may take 2 years in some patients.
4. If symptoms warrant and there is no spontaneous recovery, muscle transfers are considered. Transfer of the sternal head of the pectoralis major muscle to the inferior border of the scapula is the most common transfer.

IV. SUPRASCAPULAR NERVE INJURY

A. Overview and epidemiology

1. Suprascapular nerve injury is an uncommon cause of shoulder pain.
2. Infraspinatus muscle impairment is found in 45% of volleyball players, and 1% to 2% of painful shoulder disorders are related to suprascapular nerve compression.

B. Pathoanatomy

1. The suprascapular artery lies above the transverse scapular ligament, and the suprascapular nerve lies below the transverse scapular ligament.
2. The suprascapular nerve is from the upper trunk of the brachial plexus, with roots at C5 and C6 (and occasionally C4).
3. The nerve travels laterally across the posterior cervical triangle, reaching the scapular notch close to the posterior border of the clavicle.
4. Entrapment occurs in three places
   a. The suprascapular notch, by the transverse scapular ligament
   b. The spinoglenoid notch, by the spinoglenoid ligament

c. The spinoglenoid notch, by a ganglion cyst in the notch originating from the shoulder joint (usually associated with a small posterosuperior labral tear)

C. Evaluation

1. History—Patients present with weakness and a poorly localized, dull ache over the lateral shoulder.
2. Physical examination may reveal atrophy of the infraspinatus muscle and sometimes the supraspinatus muscle, with weakness in external rotation of the arm.
3. MRI may demonstrate a ganglion cyst in the spinoglenoid notch or supraspinatus fossa. Patients with MRIs that demonstrate a cyst in the spinoglenoid notch may have compression of the infraspinatus branch of the suprascapular nerve and may present with weakness in external rotation of the arm. The affected muscle is the infraspinatus. In long-standing nerve compression, MRI will also demonstrate fatty infiltration and atrophy of the denervated muscles.
4. An athlete who presents with shoulder pain, weakness in external rotation, and normal MRI findings may have a suprascapular nerve entrapment caused by the transverse scapular ligament or an anterior coracoscapular ligament.
5. EMG and NCV studies will isolate a lesion to the suprascapular notch (affecting the supraspinatus and infraspinatus muscles) or spinoglenoid notch (the supraspinatus muscle is spared).

D. Treatment

1. Nonsurgical treatment can be used for athletes with a suspected microtraumatic injury to the suprascapular nerve if the muscles involved do not show atrophy of fatty infiltration.
2. Symptoms have been reported to resolve within 6 to 12 months following diagnosis.
3. Nonsurgical treatment usually includes rest and stretching of the posterior capsule of the shoulder.
4. Nonsurgical treatment is used for 4 to 6 weeks, followed by a repeat EMG study to assess recovery.
5. Surgery is indicated for masses compressing the suprascapular nerve or when nonsurgical treatment fails, or for patients who are demonstrating early atrophy or fatty infiltration on MRI studies.
6. Surgery entails open or arthroscopic release of the transverse scapular ligament, release of the spinoglenoid ligament, or removal of a ganglion cyst in the spinoglenoid notch.

V. AXILLARY NERVE INJURY

A. Overview and epidemiology

1. Isolated axillary nerve injuries are uncommon and comprise less than 1% of sports-related injuries; however, approximately 48% of patients with an anterior shoulder dislocation will have EMG changes in the axillary nerve. Older patients are at an increased risk for neurologic injury with shoulder dislocation.
2. Quadrilateral space syndrome is very rare, affecting young, active adults from 20 to 40 years of age and is commonly described in baseball players.
   a. The boundaries of the quadrilateral space are the long head of the triceps muscle medially, the humeral shaft laterally, the teres minor muscle superiorly, and the teres major and latissimus dorsi muscles inferiorly.
   b. The quadrilateral space contains the axillary nerve and the posterior circumflex humeral artery.
3. Some patients may exhibit isolated teres minor atrophy from compression of a branch of the axillary artery.

B. Pathoanatomy

1. The axillary nerve originates from C5 and C6 via the posterior cord of the brachial plexus. It travels below the coracoid process obliquely along the anterior surface of the subscapularis muscles; it then descends sharply to the inferior border of the subscapularis. The nerve travels posteriorly adjacent to the inferomedial capsule, then through the quadrilateral space with the posterior circumflex humeral artery.
2. It innervates the teres minor and the deltoid muscles from back to front.
3. The distance from the acromion to the axillary nerve at the middle deltoid muscle is 6 cm.
4. The nerve can be injured by contusion, stretching (as in a dislocation), or entrapment in the quadrilateral space, or iatrogenically (during a deltoid-splitting approach or vigorous retraction during surgery).

C. Evaluation

1. History and physical examination
   a. Patients may be asymptomatic or may describe easy fatigability and weakness.
   b. Physical examination will demonstrate deltoid muscle atrophy. Weakness will also be noted, particularly in abduction, forward punching, and external rotation.

2. A focused cardiovascular examination is important.
   a. Blood pressure must be interpreted on the basis of the patient's age, sex, and height.
   b. In general, blood pressures higher than 140/90 mm Hg merit further evaluation.
3. Symmetric pulses in all four extremities should be noted.
4. Auscultation of the heart should be performed with the patient standing, squatting, and supine. Murmurs that worsen with standing or the Valsalva maneuver, any diastolic murmur, and systolic murmurs greater than or equal to grade 3 of 6 in intensity should be evaluated further before clearance to play.
5. Routine screening with 12-lead electrocardiography and echocardiography is not recommended by the American Heart Association but is recommended by the European Society of Cardiology, the International Olympic Committee, and several professional sports organizations. These tests should be used in assessing athletes thought to be at higher risk for cardiovascular conditions, of either a structural or primary electrical nature, based on history or physical examination.

II. ON-FIELD MANAGEMENT

A. The unconscious athlete
1. Immediate assessment should include an evaluation of the patient's airway, breathing, and circulatory status (ABCs), with spinal immobilization.
2. A cervical spine injury should be assumed in any unconscious athlete.
3. If a player is found lying prone, he or she should be logrolled into the supine position in a controlled effort directed by the person maintaining airway and cervical alignment.
4. Face masks should be removed to allow access to the airway; however, the helmet and shoulder pads should be left in place.
5. The helmet should be removed only if the head and cervical spine are not stabilized with the helmet in place or if the airway cannot be maintained with the helmet in place. If the helmet is removed, the shoulder pads should be removed at the same time to prevent spinal malalignment.
6. The patient should be logrolled or placed on a spine board using the five-man lift and secured in position with straps. The head and neck should be stabilized on either side with blocks or towels.
7. Standard advanced cardiac life support (ACLS) and advanced trauma life support (ATLS) protocols, including rescue breathing, cardiopulmonary resuscitation (CPR), and use of the automated external defibrillator (AED), should be performed in the apneic and pulseless patient.

B. Neck injury
1. Spinal injuries should be assumed in the athlete who is unconscious or has an altered level of consciousness.
2. Spinal injuries should be suspected in the athlete with neck pain, midline bony tenderness on palpation, neurologic signs or symptoms, or a severe distracting injury.
3. On-field assessment should include the ABCs with spinal stabilization and should assume the presence of a spinal injury until proven otherwise.
4. The posterior neck should be palpated for step-offs, deformities, and/or tenderness.
5. Transient quadriplegia is a neurapraxia of the cervical cord that can occur with axial loading of the neck in flexion or extension.
   a. Symptoms include bilateral upper and lower extremity pain, paresthesias, and weakness that, by definition, are transient and typically resolve within minutes to several hours.
   b. Athletes with transient quadriplegia should have the spine stabilized until imaging can be obtained to rule out fractures and spinal cord abnormalities.
6. Criteria for return to play after an episode remain controversial. The use of MRI or CT myelography to rule out functional stenosis has been advocated.

C. Head injury
1. Approximately 300,000 sports-related brain injuries occur in the United States every year.
2. Traumatic head injury is the leading cause of death due to trauma in sports.
3. Severe head injuries in the unconscious or severely impaired athlete, including subdural hematomas (most common), epidural hematomas, subarachnoid hemorrhages, and intracerebral contusions, should be ruled out with a noncontrast CT of the head.
4. The Consensus Statement on Concussion in Sport defines concussion as "a complex pathophysiological process affecting the brain, induced by biomechanical forces."

5. Headache and dizziness are the most common symptoms in concussion; however, the clinical presentation can be extremely varied.
6. Loss of consciousness occurs in less than 10% of concussions.
7. On-field evaluation should include assessment of the ABCs with spinal precautions, the level of consciousness, symptoms, balance, memory (anterograde and retrograde), sensory and motor function, and thought process.
8. Athletes with severe, persistent, or worsening symptoms should be triaged to a medical center for further evaluation.
9. Concussion grading scales and other guidelines for return to play have been published but not validated. Guidelines suggest a stepwise return to physical activity based on recurrence of symptoms.
10. Experts agree that all symptomatic players should be withheld from activity and that return-to-play decisions should be individually based.
11. The use of neurocognitive testing for evaluation of concussion has increased in popularity and may be used as one tool in return-to-play decisions. These tests should not be used as the only means of diagnosis or management of an athlete who may have a concussion.

D. Orthopaedic emergencies—Orthopaedic injuries are the most common injuries encountered in athletes. It is important to evaluate the athlete fully for potentially life-threatening injuries that may be recognized late because of a focus on obvious deformities to the extremities.

1. Fractures
   a. No athlete with a suspected fracture should return to play because a nondisplaced injury could potentially become displaced or open.
   b. Fractures can be splinted in the position in which they are found; however, if vascular compromise exists, reduction of fracture should be performed on the field with gentle traction, and the extremity should be splinted in the position providing best vascular flow.
   c. Open fractures should be suspected when a laceration is seen overlying the deformity.
   d. Open fractures should be covered with moist, sterile dressings and splinted. These injuries require emergent care, including intravenous antibiotics and irrigation and débridement in the operating room.
2. Dislocations
   a. Experienced personnel may attempt to reduce a dislocation on the field; however, the athlete should always be referred for imaging following the reduction to assess for fractures.
   b. A thorough neurovascular examination is imperative before and after the reduction.
   c. Knee dislocations in athletes are rare; however, they should be suspected in the injured knee with multiligamentous instability.
   d. Many dislocations spontaneously reduce before evaluation, requiring a high index of suspicion.
   e. Early on-field reduction with axial traction is imperative.
   f. Rapid transport to a medical facility for orthopaedic and vascular consultation, including vascular studies, is mandatory.

E. Thoracic injuries

1. Pneumothorax
   a. Pneumothorax may be spontaneous or traumatic. Spontaneous pneumothorax occurs more often in sports involving intrathoracic pressure changes, such as weight lifting and scuba diving.
   b. Symptoms of pneumothorax include chest pain, shortness of breath, and diminished breath sounds on auscultation.
   c. Field treatment includes transportation to the emergency department in a position of comfort with supplemental oxygen.
2. Tension pneumothorax
   a. Tension pneumothorax can develop as progressive accumulation of air remains trapped within the pleural space.
   b. This can lead to increased intrathoracic pressure, resulting in a reduced ability to ventilate, and can limit cardiac output.
   c. Patients may present as hypotensive and hypoxic. Tracheal deviation and venous jugular distention also are common.
   d. Unrecognized tension pneumothorax can lead to cardiopulmonary arrest.
   e. Immediate needle decompression should be performed using a 14-gauge angiocatheter placed anteriorly along the midclavicular line in the second intercostal space.
   f. Patients require rapid transport to a medical facility for definitive thoracostomy tube placement.

3. Cardiac contusion
   a. Cardiac contusion can result from blunt anterior chest trauma.
   b. The right ventricle is affected most often because of its anterior position.
   c. Patients present with persistent chest pain and tachycardia.
   d. Patients with suspected cardiac contusion should be referred for electrocardiogram (ECG) and telemetry monitoring because arrhythmias are common.

F. Abdominal injuries
1. Abdominal and pelvic injuries
   a. Abdominal and pelvic injuries typically result from blunt trauma; the liver and spleen are most commonly affected.
   b. The patient may have abdominal pain and potentially referred pain to the shoulder (the Kehr sign).
2. Injuries to the kidney
   a. Kidney injuries may occur with flank or posterior trauma.
   b. Hematuria is present in 90% of cases, but its absence does not exclude injury.
   c. Abdominal pain may not be present because the kidneys are located in the retroperitoneum.
   d. A high index of suspicion based on the mechanism of injury may be required for the diagnosis.
3. Bowel and pancreatic injuries
   a. These injuries can occur with blunt trauma that compresses the organs against the vertebral column.
   b. Presentation may be delayed, and the injury is often missed initially on CT scan.
   c. Laboratory tests and/or serial abdominal examinations may be necessary for diagnosis.
4. On-field examination
   a. A single on-field examination is inadequate to exclude injury. Serial examinations are imperative.
   b. Athletes with a concerning mechanism of injury, persistent or worsening pain, rebound tenderness, or abnormal vital signs should be sent for CT scanning and/or continued observation.

III. MEDICAL CONDITIONS IN SPORTS

A. Sudden death
1. Hypertrophic cardiomyopathy
   a. HCM is the most common cause of sudden cardiac death in athletes.
   b. HCM is characterized by nondilated left ventricular hypertrophy, causing obstruction of the left ventricular outflow tract.
   c. Often asymptomatic, HCM should be considered in athletes with a history of syncope, dyspnea on exertion, chest pain, or a systolic murmur that decreases in intensity upon moving from standing to supine or squatting (or increases in intensity with the Valsalva maneuver) as well as in athletes with a family history of sudden cardiac death.
   d. Death from HCM is believed to be due to fatal arrhythmias.
   e. Diagnosis can be made with echocardiography.
   f. Current recommendations are that athletes with HCM should be excluded from most competitive sports, with few exceptions.
2. Coronary artery abnormality (CAA)
   a. The second most common cause of sudden cardiac death in athletes is CAA.
   b. The most frequent CAA is an anomalous origin of the left main coronary artery; this origin allows for the artery to be compressed between the great vessels under increased cardiac pressure, which restricts circulation to that artery and causes subsequent ischemia to the heart.
   c. Occasionally the athlete may experience chest pain, palpitations, or syncope that is related to exercise, but most often CAAs are asymptomatic and physical examination is normal.
   d. Diagnosis is by CT or MR coronary angiography.
3. Long QT syndrome
   a. Long QT syndrome is a congenital or acquired repolarization abnormality that can lead to sudden cardiac death via the development of ventricular tachycardia and torsades de pointes (a cardiac arrhythmia).
   b. Athletes may be asymptomatic or may have syncope or near-syncope with exercise.
   c. If exercise symptoms exist or the athlete has a family history of sudden cardiac death, an

ECG should be considered to evaluate for long QT syndrome.

d. Diagnosis is based on the corrected QT interval.

e. Sports participation is determined by phenotype, genotype, and the presence of a pacemaker or implanted defibrillator.

4. Commotio cordis

a. Commotio cordis is caused by a blow to the anterior wall of the chest, near the heart, with objects such as a hockey puck or a baseball or with a karate kick; the blow can lead to fatal ventricular fibrillation.

b. Most episodes occur in children and adolescents.

c. Survival rates are often low unless prompt CPR and, more important, early defibrillation can be initiated.

d. Attempts to prevent commotio cordis with chest protectors have not yielded a decline in commotio cordis; however, softer "safety" baseballs may potentially lower the risk.

B. Dermatologic conditions

1. Tinea infections

a. Tinea infections are superficial fungal infections caused by dermatophytes.

b. The infection is named according to the location of the lesion on the body; for example, tinea capitis (head), corporis (body), cruris (groin), and pedis (foot).

c. Direct close contact with dermatophytes, coupled with breaks in the skin, can lead to infection.

d. Diagnosis can be confirmed by scraping the scaly edge of lesions and using microscopic examination with a potassium hydroxide preparation, looking for characteristic hyphae.

e. Tinea corporis, also referred to as ringworm, is common in wrestlers. It must be screened for before competition.

f. Tinea cruris and corporis are often treated with topical antifungals, with systemic antifungals reserved for more severe cases; 72 hours of treatment is recommended before return to competition.

g. Tinea capitis is treated with systemic antifungals; both high school and National Collegiate Athletic Association (NCAA) guidelines recommend 2 weeks of therapy before return to competition.

h. Tinea pedis should be treated but is not considered grounds for disqualification from participation in either high school or collegiate athletics.

2. Methicillin-resistant *Staphylococcus aureus* (MRSA)

a. Community-acquired MRSA is a common problem in sports.

b. MRSA often produces painful boils, pimples, or *spider bite*–type lesions.

c. For small lesions, initial treatment can be with topical mupirocin.

d. Larger lesions often require incision and drainage. Trimethoprim/sulfa, doxycycline, and clindamycin are the usual first-line oral antibiotic agents.

e. More severe infections may require hospitalization, surgical débridement, and intravenous antibiotics.

f. Prevention can be accomplished by avoiding the sharing of personal items (razors, towels, and soaps), by good hygiene, and by protecting compromised skin.

3. Herpes gladiatorum

a. Herpes gladiatorum is caused by the herpes simplex type 1 virus and is transmitted by direct skin-to-skin contact.

b. Infection occurs in 2.6% to 7.6% of wrestlers and primarily affects the head, neck, and shoulders.

c. Treatment includes oral acyclovir or valacyclovir.

d. Lesions close to the eye can progress to the more serious herpetic conjunctivitis.

e. Return to play is often allowed once lesions have scabbed and crusted over.

4. Acne mechanica/folliculitis

a. Acne mechanica is a type of acne seen in athletes that is caused by friction, heat, pressure, and occlusion of the skin.

b. It is frequently seen in sports requiring protective pads (for example, shoulder pads), including lacrosse, hockey, and football.

c. Lesions appear as red papules in the area of occlusion.

d. Treatment is often more difficult than for traditional acne.

e. Washing immediately after exercise can be beneficial, as is wearing moisture-wicking clothing.

f. Treatment can include keratinolytics such as tretinoin, but most cases will resolve after the season is over.

5. Subungual hemorrhage

a. Subungual hemorrhages are common in sports. They result from acute trauma, such as having a toe stepped on, or from repetitive trauma, such as a toe being forced continually into the toe box of a shoe.

b. Acutely, these hemorrhages can be quite painful. Treatment can consist of evacuating the hematoma by creating a hole in the nail with an electrocautery device or a heated, sterile 18-gauge needle.

c. Chronic hemorrhages can lead to nail dystrophy.

C. Exercise-induced bronchospasm (EIB)

1. Definition—EIB occurs during or after exercise and is characterized by coughing, shortness of breath, wheezing, and chest tightness.

2. Factors/conditions contributing to EIB

a. Exercise in cold weather

b. Exercise during viral respiratory illnesses

c. Polluted air environment (eg, in indoor skating rinks, from ice-resurfacing machines; or in heavily chlorinated pool areas)

d. Exercise during allergy seasons

e. Intense exercise

3. Diagnosis

a. EIB often can be suspected from the patient's history and physical examination.

b. Office spirometry can be helpful in diagnosing underlying asthma, especially when the forced expiratory volume (FEV_1) is less than 90%.

c. Exercise challenge testing conducted while observing the patient's symptoms and response to exercising in his or her own sport can be helpful.

d. The International Olympic Committee recommends the eucapnic voluntary hyperventilation test, which is both sensitive and specific for EIB.

e. Testing with a mannitol inhalation challenge is a newer and potentially more sensitive method of diagnosis than the traditional methacholine inhalation challenge used for asthma diagnosis.

4. Treatment

a. Avoidance of environmental and exercise triggers can be effective, but it often is impractical.

b. Adequate warm-up can help reduce symptoms.

c. Pharmacologic treatment often begins with β-2 receptor agonists, such as inhaled albuterol, before exercise.

d. Oral leukotriene modifiers also are effective in controlling symptoms of EIB.

e. For persistent symptoms, the addition of inhaled corticosteroids can be beneficial.

D. Heat illness

1. Heat cramps

a. Heat cramps are characterized by painful muscle cramping, most commonly in the calves, thighs, shoulders, and abdomen.

b. Core temperature typically is not elevated.

c. Treatment includes rest, cooling, oral rehydration and/or intravenous fluids, and the replacement of salt losses.

d. Prevention can include electrolyte sports drinks and, potentially, adding some salt consumption during exercise.

2. Heat exhaustion

a. Heat exhaustion is the most common form of heat illness.

b. Findings include significant fatigue, profuse sweating, core temperatures that may be elevated but are below 40°C (104°F), headache, nausea, vomiting, heat cramps, hypotension, tachycardia, and syncope.

c. Core temperature is best measured rectally.

d. Treatment includes removal from the heat, oral or intravenous rehydration, and rapid cooling.

3. Heatstroke

a. Heatstroke is the most severe of the heat illnesses.

b. Findings include core temperatures above 40°C (104°F) and/or mental status changes.

c. Core temperature is best measured rectally.

d. Heatstroke is a medical emergency, and immediate, rapid, whole-body cooling is a necessity.

e. The most rapid cooling can be achieved by whole-body immersion in an ice bath.

f. Basic life support and ACLS protocols must be followed.

g. Failure to recognize and treat heatstroke can lead to end-organ failure and death.

4. Heat syncope
   a. Heat syncope can occur with a rapid rise from a prolonged seated or lying position in the heat, resulting in orthostatic syncope from inadequate cardiac output and hypotension.
   b. Treatment of heat syncope is accomplished by laying the athlete supine with legs elevated and replacing any fluid deficits from dehydration.

E. Cold exposure
1. Hypothermia
   a. Hypothermia is defined as a core body temperature below 35°C (95°F). Different degrees of hypothermia are defined as shown in **Table 1**.
   b. Athletes with prolonged exposure to the cold, such as cross-country skiers, are more likely to be affected.
   c. Treatment of mild hypothermia includes moving the athlete into a warmer environment, removing wet clothing and replacing it with dry clothing, having the athlete drink hot liquids, and using warmed blankets and rewarming devices.
   d. Moderate to severe hypothermia should be cared for in a controlled medical environment because organ dysfunction and electrolyte imbalances can lead to more serious issues if rewarming is undertaken improperly.
2. Frostbite
   a. Frostbite is a localized freezing of tissues. It can occur in any exposed body part, most commonly the extremities.
   b. Superficial frostbite, also called frostnip, is a milder form of the condition and is characterized by a burning sensation in the affected area that can progress to numbness. Treatment should be initiated as soon as possible by thawing.
   c. Deep frostbite is a more significant problem that is quite painful initially and then progresses to numbness. Thawing and treatment of deeper affected areas should be done in a hospital or emergency department setting.

TABLE 1

Degrees of Hypothermia

Degree	Core Body Temperature
Mild	32°-35°C (89.6°-95°F)
Moderate	28°-32°C (82°-89.6°F)
Severe	20°-28°C (60°-82°F)

3. Prevention of cold illness—Preventing cold exposure–related problems can be achieved by increasing the body's heat production (through eating and increasing muscle activity), proper use of clothing by layering and using wind barriers, and avoiding outdoor activities in extremely cold conditions.

IV. ERGOGENIC AIDS

A. Legal substances
1. Creatine
   a. Creatine is one of the most popular nutritional supplements. It is derived from the amino acids glycine, arginine, and methionine.
   b. Most creatine is stored in muscle. In its phosphorylated form, it contributes to the resynthesis of ATP.
   c. Several studies of the effect of creatine in anaerobic activities have produced conflicting results on its effects on sports performance. No study has shown an improvement in on-the-field performance. Short-term side effects reported include cramping, dehydration, and possible renal dysfunction.
   d. The long-term effects of using creatine supplements are unknown.
2. Caffeine
   a. Consumed daily by athletes and nonathletes alike throughout the world, caffeine can be used to enhance athletic performance.
   b. Doses as low as 2 to 3 mg/kg have been documented to improve performance.
   c. Caffeine is thought to improve performance by reducing fatigue and increasing alertness.
   d. Caffeine is no longer banned by the International Olympic Committee, the World Anti-Doping Agency, or the NCAA, but its use is monitored and restrictions or penalties may be applicable if urine concentrations are found to be greater than 15 mcg/mL.
   e. Athletes must exercise caution in using caffeine. Dietary intake plus the unknown amount of caffeine in supplements because of lack of regulation could lead to an unexpected positive test result.

B. Illegal substances
1. Anabolic steroids
   a. Anabolic steroids are believed to be widely abused in athletes of all ages, with use reported in up to 10% of adolescent athletes.

b. Steroids are synthetically derived to have similar effects to natural testosterone and can be given orally or through an injection.
c. Side effects include the development of atherosclerotic disease, decreased high-density lipoprotein cholesterol, aggression and mood disturbances, testicular atrophy, masculinization in females, gynecomastia in males, acne, and an increased risk for hepatitis and HIV infections in athletes sharing needles to inject steroids.
d. Most side effects are believed to be reversible with cessation of use, but a prolonged period may be required to return to normal.
e. Anabolic steroids are banned by college, Olympic, and most professional sports organizations.
f. Most of these same organizations test for anabolic steroids, looking for a testosterone to epitestosterone ratio greater than 6:1.

2. Erythropoietin (EPO)
   a. EPO acts to stimulate hemoglobin production, which in turn increases the body's oxygen-carrying capacity.
   b. This ability has made EPO widely desirable among elite endurance athletes such as cyclists and cross-country skiers.
   c. Several studies have documented increases in hematocrit and VO_{2max} in time to exhaustion.
   d. Side effects of EPO use include increasing blood viscosity, which can lead to stroke, thromboembolic events, and myocardial infarctions.
   e. EPO is currently illegal in all sports.
   f. Testing does exist, but the substance can still be difficult to detect.
3. Human growth hormone (HGH)
   a. HGH is a peptide secreted by the anterior pituitary gland that stimulates the release of insulin-like growth factors.
   b. Studies in athletes are essentially nonexistent.
   c. Studies that have been conducted were in patients with endocrine dysfunction. They demonstrated increases in muscle size but not in strength.
   d. Resistance with continued use is also thought to occur.
   e. Side effects include water retention and development of myopathy, carpal tunnel syndrome, and insulin resistance.
   f. Newer serologic tests have been developed for detection of HGH.

TOP TESTING FACTS

1. The preparticipation physical examination (PPE) may be normal in athletes with an underlying condition that places them at risk during athletics. A detailed family history and history of exertional symptoms may provide the only clues to a potentially lethal disorder.
2. Cardiac murmurs that increase in intensity with standing or the Valsalva maneuver, any diastolic murmur, and systolic murmurs greater than or equal to grade 3 of 6 in intensity should be evaluated further before clearance to play.
3. A cervical spine injury should be assumed in any unconscious athlete.
4. Face masks should be removed to allow access to the airway in an unstable patient; however, the helmet and shoulder pads should be left in place during transport.
5. Experts agree that all symptomatic players with a concussion should be withheld from activity, and return-to-play decisions should be individually based.
6. Knee dislocations in athletes are rare; however, they should be suspected in the injured knee with multidirectional instability. A vascular study should be performed if this injury is suspected.
7. A single abdominal examination is inadequate to exclude injury. Athletes with a concerning mechanism of injury, persistent or worsening pain, rebound tenderness, or abnormal vital signs should be sent for CT scan and/or continued observation.
8. HCM is the most common cause of sudden cardiac death in athletes.
9. Exercise-induced bronchospasm is frequently managed by limiting environmental aggravators and using β-2 agonists, such as albuterol, before exercise.
10. Heatstroke is a medical emergency, and treatment must be initiated promptly.

Bibliography

AAFP, ACSM, AMSSM, AAP: *PPE Preparticipation Physical Evaluation*, ed 4. Elk Grove Village, IL, American Academy of Pediatrics, 2010, pp 1-168.

Amaral JF: Thoracoabdominal injuries in the athlete. *Clin Sports Med* 1997;16(4):739-753.

Cordoro KM, Ganz JE: Training room management of medical conditions: Sports dermatology. *Clin Sports Med* 2005;24(3):565-598, viii-ix.

DeFranco MJ, Baker CL III, DaSilva JJ, Piasecki DP, Bach BR Jr: Environmental issues for team physicians. *Am J Sports Med* 2008;36(11):2226-2237.

Fitch RW, Cox CL, Hannah GA, Diamond AB, Gregory AJ, Wilson KM: Sideline emergencies: An evidence-based approach. *J Surg Orthop Adv* 2011;20(2):83-101.

Gregory AJ, Fitch RW: Sports medicine: Performance-enhancing drugs. *Pediatr Clin North Am* 2007;54(4):797-806, xii.

Marx RG, Delaney JS: Sideline orthopedic emergencies in the young athlete. *Pediatr Ann* 2002;31(1):60-70.

McCrory P, Meeuwisse W, Johnston K, et al: Consensus statement on concussion in sport: The 3rd International Conference on Concussion in Sport held in Zurich, November 2008. *Br J Sports Med* 2009;43(suppl 1):i76–i90.

Paterick TE, Paterick TJ, Fletcher GF, Maron BJ: Medical and legal issues in the cardiovascular evaluation of competitive athletes. *JAMA* 2005;294(23):3011-3018.

Randolph C: An update on exercise-induced bronchoconstriction with and without asthma. *Curr Allergy Asthma Rep* 2009;9(6):433-438.

Rodriguez NR, Di Marco NM, Langley S; American Dietetic Association; Dietitians of Canada; American College of Sports Medicine: American College of Sports Medicine position stand: Nutrition and athletic performance. *Med Sci Sports Exerc* 2009;41(3):709-731.

Uberoi A, Stein R, Perez MV, et al: Interpretation of the electrocardiogram of young athletes. *Circulation* 2011;124(6):746-757.

Whiteside JW: Management of head and neck injuries by the sideline physician. *Am Fam Physician* 2006;74(8):1357-1362.

Zipes DP, Camm AJ, Borggrefe M, et al: ACC/AHA/ESC 2006 guidelines for management of patients with ventricular arrhythmias and the prevention of sudden cardiac death—executive summary: A report of the American College of Cardiology/American Heart Association Task Force and the European Society of Cardiology Committee for Practice Guidelines (Writing Committee to Develop Guidelines for Management of Patients with Ventricular Arrhythmias and the Prevention of Sudden Cardiac Death) developed in collaboration with the European Heart Rhythm Association and the Heart Rhythm Society. *Eur Heart J* 2006;27(17):2099-2140.

Chapter 128

PREVENTION AND REHABILITATION OF SPORTS INJURIES

TIMOTHY E. HEWETT, PhD
BRUCE BEYNNON, PhD
ROBERT A. MAGNUSSEN, MD
JON DIVINE, MD, MS
GLENN N. WILLIAMS, PT, PhD, ATC

9 | Sports Medicine

I. DEFINITIONS

A. Muscle exercise types

1. Isoinertial exercises

a. Isoinertial exercises, often incorrectly referred to as isotonic exercises, involve applying a muscle contraction throughout a range of motion against a constant resistance or weight. Bench press using free weights is an example of isoinertial exercise.

b. These exercises are beneficial because they strengthen both the primary and synergistic muscles and provide stress to the ligaments and tendons throughout varied ranges of motion.

2. Isotonic exercises

a. Isotonic exercises involve applying a muscle contraction throughout a range of motion against a constant muscle force.

b. These types of muscle contractions rarely occur in the course of normal human activity and require specialized weight devices to ensure isotonic muscle contraction. Most activities commonly referred to as "isotonic" are in fact isoinertial.

3. Isometric exercises

a. Isometric exercise is a process by which a muscle is contracted without appreciable joint motion.

b. These exercises are often used as the first form of strengthening after injury or in persons who are immobilized.

c. Isometric exercises can help improve static strengthening and minimize the extent of muscular atrophy.

4. Isokinetic exercises

a. Isokinetic exercise is a type of strengthening protocol in which the speed of a muscle contraction is fixed but the resistance varies depending on the force exerted throughout a range of motion, with maximum muscle loading postulated to occur throughout the entire range of motion.

b. These exercises are performed using machines that automatically adjust the resistance throughout the range of motion, such as active dynamometers.

c. Isokinetic testing is frequently used to assess the progress of rehabilitation and to objectively determine whether full muscle strength has been regained following an injury.

B. Muscle contraction types

1. Concentric muscle contractions are those in which the individual muscle fibers shorten during

Dr. Magnussen or an immediate family member has received noninicome support (such as equipment or services), commercially derived honoraria, or other non–research-related funding (such as paid travel) from Tornier. Dr. Divine or an immediate family member serves as a board member, owner, officer, or committee member of the American Medical Society for Sports Medicine. Dr. Williams or an immediate family member has received research or institutional support from DJ Orthopaedics. Neither of the following authors nor any immediate family member has received anything of value from or has stock or stock options held in a commercial company or institution related directly or indirectly to the subject of this chapter: Dr. Hewett and Dr. Beynnon.

force production and the origin and insertion of a particular muscle group move closer to one another.

2. Eccentric muscle contractions are those in which the individual muscle fibers lengthen during force production and the origin and insertion of a particular muscle group move apart from one another.

C. Training types

1. Sport specific

a. Sport-specific exercise is characterized by or related to a specific sport.

b. An example of a sport-specific training exercise for hockey is rollerblading, or in-line skating.

2. Periodization

a. Periodization is a planned workout scheme in which the volume and/or the intensity of training is varied over a set period.

b. Periodization of training can generally be divided into phases throughout the year, such as conditioning, precompetition, competition, and rest.

3. Plyometrics

a. Plyometrics is a form of resistance training that involves eccentric loading of a muscle followed by immediate concentric unloading of the muscle to create a fast, forceful movement.

b. Plyometrics trains the muscles, connective tissue, and nervous system to effectively carry out the stretch-shortening cycle.

c. This training modality emphasizes spending as little time as possible in contact with the ground. It may include exercises such as bounding and hopping drills, jumping over hurdles, and depth jumps.

D. Joint motion

1. Active range of motion

a. Active range of motion is the process by which a person moves a joint or muscle group without help from another person or a machine.

b. Active range of motion allows the assessment of a patient's willingness to perform the movement, muscle strength, and joint range.

2. Passive range of motion is the process by which another person or a machine moves a joint or muscle group of an individual.

E. Types of stretching

1. Active stretching

a. Active stretching is also referred to as static active stretching.

b. An active stretch is one in which a position is held with no assistance other than the strength of the agonist muscles.

c. The tension of the agonists in an active stretch helps to relax the muscles being stretched (the antagonists) and is referred to as reciprocal inhibition.

d. Many of the movements (or stretches) in various forms of yoga are active stretches.

e. Active stretches are usually difficult to hold and maintain for more than 10 seconds and rarely are held longer than 15 seconds.

2. Passive stretching

a. Passive stretching is a technique in which the muscle being stretched is relaxed without any active movement on the part of the person to increase the range of motion; instead, an outside agent creates an external force, either manually or mechanically.

b. This position is then held with some other part of the body, with the assistance of a partner, or with some other apparatus.

c. A seated hurdler's stretch for the hamstrings is an example of a passive stretch.

3. Proprioceptive neuromuscular facilitation (PNF)

a. PNF is any type of stretching technique combining passive stretching and isometric stretching.

b. The technique involves a three-step process in which a muscle group is passively stretched, then isometrically contracted against resistance while in the stretched position, and then passively stretched again by postisometric relaxation through the resulting increased range of motion.

c. With PNF stretching, a partner usually provides resistance against the isometric contraction and then later passively moves the joint through its increased range of motion.

F. Open-chain versus closed-chain exercises

1. Open-chain exercises are movements, usually with some type of resistance, in which the hand or foot is not in direct contact with a solid object such as the floor or a wall.

2. In open-chain exercises, the foot, or end of the kinetic chain, is moved freely.

3. Closed-chain exercises are exercises in which the end of the kinetic chain or foot is fixed to the ground or a wall or is otherwise weight bearing and not able to move freely.

4. Open-chain exercises involving the knee, such as leg extensions, are postulated to create greater shear force across the knee and its ligaments, especially the anterior cruciate ligament (ACL); closed-chain exercises, such as leg presses or squats, are postulated to result in greater compression force at the knee and ACL, which is hypothesized to lead to decreased strain on the ACL during the postsurgical rehabilitation process.

G. Modalities

1. Ultrasonography
   a. Ultrasonography is used to apply thermal (deep heat) energy from 2 to 5+ cm below the skin surface, or nonthermal deep massage by using acoustic energy (0.8 to 3.0 MHz) transfer using a round-headed wand or probe that is put in direct contact with the patient's skin.
   b. Sound waves are absorbed by various tissues, causing the production of heat.
   c. The greatest rise in temperature occurs in tissues with high protein content, such as muscle, tendon, and nerve.
   d. Relatively little increase in the temperature of adipose tissue occurs with ultrasonography treatment.
   e. Most ultrasonography treatments last from 3 to 5 minutes.
   f. Contraindications for ultrasonography use include bleeding disorders, cancer, and a cardiac pacemaker.
   g. Ultrasonography should not be used for most acute injuries with edematous or necrotic tissue.
2. Pulsed ultrasonography
   a. Pulsed ultrasonography is used when localized deep tissue massage is desired to reduce edema in an acute injury situation.
   b. Pulsed ultrasonography does not result in increased deep localized heating.
3. Phonophoresis is a noninvasive method of delivering medications to tissues below the skin using ultrasonography.
4. Neuromuscular electrical stimulation (NMES)
   a. NMES is a therapeutic technique that uses a wide variety of electrical stimulators, including burst-modulated AC ("Russian stimulator"), twin-spiked monophasic pulsed current, and biphasic pulsed current stimulators.
   b. NMES has been used for muscle strengthening, the maintenance of muscle mass and strength during prolonged periods of immobilization, selective muscle retraining, and control of edema.
   c. NMES may be beneficial early in the rehabilitation phase when swelling is persistent and reflexively inhibits muscle activation.
   d. The use of NMES is contraindicated in patients with a demand-type pacemaker. NMES also should not be used over the carotid sinus, across the heart, or over the abdomen of a pregnant woman.
5. Transcutaneous electrical nerve stimulation is another form of electrical stimulation that has been used to control a wide variety of acute and chronic pain symptoms.
6. High-voltage stimulation (HVS)
   a. HVS is the delivery of a monophasic pulse of short duration across the skin and into acutely injured, swollen tissue.
   b. HVS works by acting on negatively charged plasma proteins, which leak into the interstitial space and result in edema.
   c. In the setting of an acute injury with edema, a negative electrode is placed over the edematous site and a positive electrode is placed at a distant site.
   d. A monophasic, high-voltage stimulus is applied, creating an electrical potential that disperses the negatively charged proteins away from the edematous site, resulting in reduced swelling.
   e. Acute ankle and knee sprains and postoperative joint effusions are commonly treated with HVS.
   f. HVS is often applied concurrently with the more common methods of acute swelling reduction—ice, elevation, and compression.
   g. Contraindications to the use of HVS are similar to those for electrical stimulation.
7. Ice/cryotherapy
   a. Cryotherapy is the modality used to cool tissue.
   b. Cryotherapy techniques are done at temperatures ranging from 32°F (0°C) to 77°F (25°C).
   c. Depending on the application method and duration, cryotherapy results in decreased local metabolism, vasoconstriction, reduced swelling/edema, decreased hemorrhage, reduced

muscle efficiency, and pain relief secondary to impaired neuromuscular transmission.

8. Heat
   a. Heat is any superficial modality that provides pain relief by using external warming methods with temperatures ranging from 37°C (98.6°F) to 43°C (109.4°F).
   b. The types of heat therapy traditionally are categorized by the method of primary heat transfer. Types include
      - Conduction (hot packs, paraffin baths)
      - Convection (hydrotherapy, moist air)
      - Conversion (sunlight, heat lamp)
   c. Indications for the application of heat may include painful muscle spasms, abdominal muscle cramping, menstrual cramps, and superficial thrombophlebitis.
9. Iontophoresis
   a. Iontophoresis is a transdermal form of medicine delivery in which a charged medication is delivered through the skin and into underlying tissue via DC electrical stimulation.
   b. The charged molecules are placed under an electrode of the same polarity that repels them into the area to be treated.
   c. Many ionic drugs are available, including dexamethasone, lidocaine, and acetate.
   d. Dexamethasone is the medication most commonly used for treating locally inflamed tissues due to tendinitis, bursitis, or arthritis.
   e. Currently, iontophoresis is used in the medical management of inflamed superficial tissues in disorders such as lateral epicondylitis, shoulder tendinitis, and patellar tendinitis.

II. REHABILITATION PHASES OF COMMON SPORTS INJURIES

A. Rehabilitation of the ACL

1. Initial phase after ACL tear or ACL reconstruction
   a. Early rehabilitation regimens after ACL injury and after ACL reconstruction are similar because the goal is to minimize pain and inflammation while obtaining good quadriceps muscle activation and full extension range of motion.
   b. Ice and compression are used to treat pain and inflammation, using a commercially available joint cooling system or crushed ice with a compressive wrap.
   c. Elevation also is important in minimizing swelling because placing the limb in a dependent position leads to edema in the distal leg.
   d. Patients should use an assistive device during ambulation until good quadriceps function and a minimally antalgic gait are achieved.
2. Quadriceps function
   a. Acquiring good control of the quadriceps as soon as possible is critical.
   b. Beginning the day of injury or surgery, the patient should contract the quadriceps muscles as tightly as possible while the knee is in full extension, with a small bolster placed under the Achilles tendon.
   c. Straight-leg raises should begin only after the patient can perform a strong quadriceps contraction in which the heel lifts symmetrically with the opposite side because straight-leg raises can be performed with relatively poor quadriceps function using the hip flexors.
   d. Some patients have severe quadriceps inhibition. For such patients, high-intensity electrical stimulation or assisted eccentric lowering exercises may help improve activation.
3. Range of motion
   a. Efforts should be directed toward obtaining extension range of motion equal to the opposite side as quickly as possible.
   b. Although having a strong quadriceps muscle and early ambulation in full weight bearing are the most effective methods of obtaining full extension, some patients still struggle with gaining full extension.
   c. In these circumstances, low-load, long-duration stretching helps induce tissue creep and gaining motion.
   d. This exercise should not be painful because pain induces counterproductive muscle guarding.
   e. In extremely challenging cases, an extension promotion brace or drop-out casting is helpful.
4. Tailoring rehabilitation
   a. Rehabilitation programs should be tailored to the individual, although general principles apply to all patients.
   b. Aquatic therapy may be helpful.
   c. Strength and control of the entire lower extremity and core are important.

d. Because ACL injury and reconstruction have a particularly severe impact on the quadriceps muscles, this muscle group needs to be treated especially aggressively.

e. The optimal approach includes the combined use of open and closed kinetic chain exercises.

f. Closed kinetic chain exercises should be the primary method of strength training.

g. Rehabilitation exercises need to be performed with an appropriate volume, intensity, and frequency to provide the stimulus for strength improvement.

h. Neuromuscular training, using cushions, disks, balance boards, perturbation training, and/or commercially available devices, is used to progressively improve dynamic joint stability.

i. Cardiovascular training is advised to promote general health and deliver optimal blood supply to healing tissues.

5. Return to play

a. The decision about when it is safe to resume running is case dependent.

b. Running is generally safe 8 to 12 weeks after injury or surgery, as long as the running is in a straight line and progresses gradually.

c. Agility exercises and multidirectional training generally begin about 12 weeks after injury or surgery.

d. Accelerated rehabilitation programs that permit a return to sport at approximately 20 weeks have been shown in some studies to be safe and did not contribute to increased knee laxity or increased injury risk when compared with more traditional nonaccelerated programs that allow a return to sport at approximately 30 weeks. The time to return to sport remains controversial, however, and should be determined through combined decision making that involves the patient, therapist, and surgeon.

e. The return-to-sport decision should be based on a confluence of signs, including patient-based outcomes measures, examination, and indicators of neuromuscular status such as functional tests and strength tests.

f. Thresholds for strength and hop tests should consider the patient's overall status; however, recent evidence suggests that thresholds may need to be higher than previously thought, perhaps as high as 90% relative to the contralateral side.

g. The idea that persistent strength deficits and abnormal kinematics noted at the time of return to sport will normalize quickly through routine sports activity and training is not supported by current evidence. Such abnormalities have been noted to persist for years unless specifically targeted for intervention.

h. Biomechanical screening can detect abnormal kinematics—transverse plane hip kinetics and frontal plane knee kinematics during landing, sagittal plane knee moments at landing, and deficits in postural stability—that have been shown to be independent predictors of a second ACL injury. Further work is needed to determine whether modification of these factors reduces the risk of additional ACL injuries.

B. Ankle ligament injury rehabilitation

1. Lateral ligaments

a. Ankle ligament trauma is the most common sports injury. It can involve sprains of the lateral, medial, and/or syndesmotic ligaments.

b. One of the most well-established treatment modalities for acute injury of the ankle ligaments is RICE (rest, ice cooling, compression, and elevation).

c. Cooling decreases the tissue temperature, which in turn reduces blood flow and metabolism.

d. Cooling also appears to be effective in reducing swelling and limiting pain up to 1 week after the index injury.

e. For minor (grade I) and moderate (grade II) tears of the lateral ankle ligament complex, early mobilization of the injured ankle is recommended, with protection provided by the combination of a brace and an elastic wrap; this approach provides protection from reinjury and compression and has been shown to produce excellent short-term and intermediate-term outcomes in more than 95% of patients.

f. For severe (grade III) sprains of the lateral ligaments, functional treatment produces similar excellent short-term and intermediate-term outcomes.

g. A subgroup of severe sprains does not respond well to functional treatment; patients with these injuries may become candidates for surgical repair if recurrent giving-way episodes of the ankle are experienced.

h. After swelling is controlled, weight-bearing status is restored, and ankle range of motion is reestablished, a rehabilitation program that includes sensory-motor, strength training, and sport-specific exercises is recommended. For minor, moderate, and severe ankle ligament sprains, a 10-week sensory-motor training program that includes balance exercises should be completed. During the sensory-motor training program, muscle strengthening and sport-specific exercises should be implemented and progressed.

i. Loss of strength and its subsequent recovery takes time and depends on the severity of the index injury.

j. Return to play is usually indicated when full ankle range of motion is restored, full muscle strength is regained, sensory-motor control of the ankle is reestablished, and the joint is pain free during activity, with no swelling as a result of activity.

2. Syndesmosis injuries

a. It has been estimated that up to 20% of patients presenting with the more severe lateral ankle ligament sprains have an associated injury to the distal tibiofibular articulation, or syndesmosis (that is, the anterior inferior tibiofibular, interosseous tibiofibular, and/or posterior inferior tibiofibular ligaments).

b. These injuries can range from minor tears of the syndesmosis, which are considered stable, to substantial injuries that involve disruption of the syndesmosis combined with fracture of the fibula, which are unstable.

c. It is important to educate the patient about the longer time interval required for rehabilitation and recovery of injury to the syndesmosis ligament complex in comparison with isolated injury to the lateral ankle ligaments.

d. Treatment of injuries to the syndesmosis without a fracture of the fibula requires particular attention to maintaining anatomic reduction of the ankle mortise and syndesmosis.

e. If the syndesmotic injury is considered stable, the treatment should include RICE combined with a posterior splint, with the ankle in a neutral position and non–weight bearing for at least 4 days.

f. This is followed by partial weight bearing with crutches and the use of a walking boot or ankle stirrup brace and then progression to full weight bearing as tolerated.

g. After obtaining control of swelling, restoration of weight bearing, and reestablishment of ankle range of motion, the same sensory-motor, progressive strength training, and sport-specific exercise program described for the treatment of lateral ankle ligament sprains is recommended.

h. Syndesmotic tears that are considered unstable should be treated within 12 weeks of injury. These injuries may require reduction of the syndesmosis with screw fixation.

i. Rehabilitation of these severe injuries includes protection for 12 weeks followed by the program described for stable syndesmotic injuries.

j. Treatment of chronic (>12 weeks after the index injury) syndesmotic injuries may require reconstruction of the syndesmosis.

C. Shoulder instability rehabilitation

1. Rehabilitation of the patient with shoulder instability is highly dependent on the type of instability (traumatic versus atraumatic or acquired), the direction of instability (anterior, posterior, or multidirectional), the treatment approach (nonsurgical versus surgical), and, in surgical patients, the procedure used (open versus arthroscopic techniques).

2. The goal early after a traumatic instability event or shoulder surgery is to minimize pain and inflammation.

3. Crushed ice or a commercially available joint-cooling system is the primary method of treating pain and inflammation.

4. Minimizing the effects of immobilization is a priority.

a. This is accomplished by performing gentle passive range of motion in the safe range of motion.

b. Range of motion should increase progressively within the safe limits for the specific procedure.

5. Surgeons should clearly determine whether there are any unusual risk factors and what the safe limits are for each patient throughout the rehabilitation process.

6. Rehabilitation programs should be tailored so that they are specific to an individual's unique circumstances.

7. Submaximal isometric exercises are performed within the safe range of motion early in the rehabilitation process to minimize muscle atrophy.

8. Electrical stimulation, biofeedback training, or both can be used as adjunct atrophy-prevention methods.

9. When it is safe, range of motion is progressed using wand exercises, joint mobilization, and low-load, long-duration stretching that promotes gentle creep of the tissues.
10. Developing a stable platform for shoulder movement through scapular stabilization exercise is a prerequisite to aggressive rotator cuff strengthening.
11. Most shoulder strength programs begin with resistance training using exercise bands, cords, and free weights.
12. As strength and control develop, patients are progressed to various resistance-training devices and plyometrics.
13. Neuromuscular control is facilitated by performing reactive training and various exercises that perturb shoulder stability.
14. Care should be taken to promote appropriate responses to perturbations rather than rigid cocontraction because this strategy of joint stabilization is inconsistent with agile movement and skilled performance.
15. The final stages of rehabilitation should involve sport-specific training and the development of skill in sport-specific tasks.
16. Interval training programs, video analysis, and the input of coaches are helpful in obtaining high success rates when treating overhead athletes.
17. Although adjunct measures of patient status such as strength testing can be helpful, the return to sports participation depends on the ability to perform sport-specific tasks in a pain-free manner and on patient-based outcomes.

III. PREVENTION OF COMMON SPORTS INJURIES

A. ACL tear

1. Female athletes have a rate of ACL injury that is two to eight times that of male athletes.
2. Surgical intervention does not change the odds of developing knee osteoarthritis after injury.
3. Researchers have developed ways for clinicians to identify athletes at risk for ACL injury and have begun to use training programs designed for ACL injury prevention.
4. Efforts to prevent ACL injury in female athletes should focus on the factors that make females more susceptible to injury (for example, increased knee dynamic valgus and a tendency to land with less knee flexion) and on developing interventions to aid in the prevention of these injuries.
5. A meta-analysis by Hewett et al attempted to quantitatively combine the results of six independent studies drawn from a systematic review of the published literature on ACL injury interventions in female athletes.
    a. The three studies that incorporated high-intensity plyometrics reported a reduced risk of ACL injury, but the studies that did not incorporate high-intensity plyometrics did not report a reduced ACL injury risk.
    b. This meta-analysis showed that neuromuscular training may assist in the reduction of ACL injuries in female athletes under the following conditions: Plyometrics and technique training are incorporated into a comprehensive training protocol. Balance and strengthening exercise are used as adjuncts, but they may not be effective if used alone. The training sessions are performed more than once per week for a minimum of 6 weeks.

B. Ankle ligament sprains

1. The fundamental premise in ankle ligament injury prevention is that these injuries occur not randomly but in patterns that reflect the process of the underlying causes.
    a. Consequently, it is important to understand the risk factors for these common injuries.
    b. Not only does this facilitate the development of prevention programs, but it also allows the identification of those at increased risk for injury, so an intervention can be targeted.
2. One of the most substantial risk factors for a lateral ankle ligament sprain is a previous ankle injury.
3. In addition, reduced dorsiflexion, poor proprioception, increased postural sway, and strength imbalances of the muscles that span the ankle have been associated with an increased risk of sustaining an inversion ankle ligament injury.
4. Recognizing that one of the most important risk factors for an ankle ligament injury is a prior ankle ligament tear, adequate rehabilitation following an ankle injury before returning to sports participation is an important consideration.
    a. Rehabilitation includes the concept of progressive strength training of the muscles that span the ankle complex and sensory-motor training of the lower extremity.

   b. Sensory-motor training programs that include a minimum of 10 minutes of balance training 5 days a week for at least 10 weeks, with activities such as single-leg stance on an unstable balance pad or balance board training, can have a dramatic effect on improving sensory-motor control.

5. The risk of sustaining an ankle ligament injury (or reinjury) can be minimized with taping or bracing treatment.
   a. Evidence exists that taping is of value in preventing ankle injuries, but a taped ankle loses as much as 40% of the ankle range of restrictiveness following 10 minutes of exercise.
   b. Because of the problems associated with taping, ankle bracing treatment use has increased recently.

TOP TESTING FACTS

1. Isoinertial exercises apply a muscle contraction throughout a range of motion against a constant resistance or weight.
2. Isotonic exercises apply a muscle contraction throughout a range of motion against a constant muscle force.
3. Isometric exercises involve muscle contraction without appreciable joint motion.
4. Isokinetic exercises occur when the speed of a muscle contraction is fixed but the resistance varies depending on the force exerted through the range of motion.
5. Periodization is a planned workout in which the volume and/or intensity of training is varied over time.
6. PNF involves a three-step stretching technique combining passive stretching and isometric stretching.
7. Closed-chain exercises are those in which the foot is fixed to the ground or a wall.
8. The initial treatment of ankle sprain should be RICE.
9. Shoulder rehabilitation for instability is highly dependent on the type and direction of instability and any surgical intervention.
10. Female athletes have a risk of ACL tears that is two to eight times that of their male counterparts.
11. Rehabilitation protocols that include plyometric exercises, such as bounding and hopping, are more effective in preventing ACL injury than programs that do not include such exercises.

Bibliography

Beynnon BD, Johnson RJ, Naud S, et al: Accelerated versus nonaccelerated rehabilitation after anterior cruciate ligament reconstruction: A prospective, randomized, double-blind investigation evaluating knee joint laxity using roentgen stereophotogrammetric analysis. *Am J Sports Med* 2011;39(12):2536-2548.

Beynnon BD, Renström PA, Haugh L, Uh BS, Barker H: A prospective, randomized clinical investigation of the treatment of first-time ankle sprains. *Am J Sports Med* 2006;34(9):1401-1412.

Beynnon BD, Vacek PM, Murphy D, Alosa D, Paller D: First-time inversion ankle ligament trauma: The effects of sex, level of competition, and sport on the incidence of injury. *Am J Sports Med* 2005;33(10):1485-1491.

Di Stasi S, Myer GD, Hewett TE: Neuromuscular training to target deficits associated with second anterior cruciate ligament injury. *J Orthop Sports Phys Ther* 2013;43(11):777-792, A1-A11.

Escamilla RF, Fleisig GS, Zheng N, Barrentine SW, Wilk KE, Andrews JR: Biomechanics of the knee during closed kinetic chain and open kinetic chain exercises. *Med Sci Sports Exerc* 1998;30(4):556-569.

Gaunt BW, Shaffer MA, Sauers EL, et al: The American Society of Shoulder and Elbow Therapists' consensus rehabilitation guideline for arthroscopic anterior capsulolabral repair of the shoulder. *J Orthop Sports Phys Ther* 2010;40(3):155-168.

Hayes K, Callanan M, Walton J, Paxinos A, Murrell GA: Shoulder instability: Management and rehabilitation. *J Orthop Sports Phys Ther* 2002;32(10):497-509.

Hewett TE, Di Stasi SL, Myer GD: Current concepts for injury prevention in athletes after anterior cruciate ligament reconstruction. *Am J Sports Med* 2013;41(1):216-224.

Hewett TE, Ford KR, Myer GD: Anterior cruciate ligament injuries in female athletes: Part 2, a meta-analysis of neuromuscular interventions aimed at injury prevention. *Am J Sports Med* 2006;34(3):490-498.

Hewett TE, Myer GD, Ford KR: Decrease in neuromuscular control about the knee with maturation in female athletes. *J Bone Joint Surg Am* 2004;86-A(8):1601-1608.

Kruse LM, Gray B, Wright RW: Rehabilitation after anterior cruciate ligament reconstruction: A systematic review. *J Bone Joint Surg Am* 2012;94(19):1737-1748.

Nyland J, Nolan MF: Therapeutic modality: Rehabilitation of the injured athlete. *Clin Sports Med* 2004;23(2):299-313, vii.

Paterno MV, Schmitt LC, Ford KR, et al: Biomechanical measures during landing and postural stability predict second anterior cruciate ligament injury after anterior cruciate ligament reconstruction and return to sport. *Am J Sports Med* 2010;38(10):1968-1978.

Prentice WE: *Therapeutic Modalities for Sports Medicine and Athletic Training*, ed 5. Boston, MA, McGraw-Hill, 2002.

Thomeé R, Kaplan Y, Kvist J, et al: Muscle strength and hop performance criteria prior to return to sports after ACL reconstruction. *Knee Surg Sports Traumatol Arthrosc* 2011;19(11):1798-1805.

Thomeé R, Neeter C, Gustaysson A, et al: Variability in leg muscle power and hop performance after anterior cruciate ligament reconstruction. *Knee Surg Sports Traumatol Arthrosc* 2012;20(6):1143-1151.

Verhagen E, van der Beek A, Twisk J, Bouter L, Bahr R, van Mechelen W: The effect of a proprioceptive balance board training program for the prevention of ankle sprains: A prospective controlled trial. *Am J Sports Med* 2004;32(6):1385-1393.

Williams GN, Jones MH, Amendola A: Syndesmotic ankle sprains in athletes. *Am J Sports Med* 2007;35(7):1197-1207.

Section 10

Pediatrics

Section Editors | SCHOENECKER
GOLDSTEIN
MARTUS

Chapter 129

Skeletal Dysplasias and Mucopolysaccharidoses

SAMANTHA A. SPENCER, MD

I. NORMAL GROWTH

A. Anatomy

1. Long bone growth/fracture healing is endochondral.
   a. Vessel invades cartilage in the primary ossification center and growth occurs longitudinally at either end as chondrocytes proliferate, hypertrophy, die, and are replaced by calcified matrix and osteoblasts.
   b. Widening of the bone is achieved by osteoblasts differentiating from stem cells from the ring of LaCroix/node of Ranvier.
2. Flat bone growth/distraction osteogenesis is intramembranous.
   a. The skull is formed by neural crest cells invading a connective tissue scaffold.
   b. The clavicle has both intramembranous and endochondral ossification.
   c. The scapula has seven ossification centers.

B. Physiology

1. An endochondral epiphyseal plate is divided into four main zones.
2. The reserve zone has no diseases associated.
3. Achondroplasia affects the proliferative zone.
4. Fractures occur in the hypertrophic zone.
5. In the zone of calcification, type X collagen is present, but type II collagen is still predominant.
6. Calcifying fracture callus has some type IV collagen.

II. SKELETAL DYSPLASIAS

A. Achondroplasia (**Table 1**)

1. Overview
   a. It is the most common skeletal dysplasia.
   b. It is autosomal dominant, but 90% are new mutations.
   c. Short-limbed dwarfism with abnormal facial features.
2. Pathoanatomy
   a. Mutation affects a single protein in fibroblast growth factor receptor-3 (FGFR-3) gene changing glycine to arginine at position 380.
   b. Result is growth retardation of the proliferative zone of the epiphyseal plate resulting in short limbs.
   c. The growth plates with the most growth (proximal humerus/distal femur) are most affected resulting in rhizomelic (proximal more than distal) short stature.
3. Evaluation
   a. Features include frontal bossing, button nose, trident hands (cannot approximate long and ring fingers), thoracolumbar kyphosis (usually resolves with ambulation), lumbar stenosis with lordosis and short pedicles, posterior radial head dislocation, "champagne glass" pelvic outlet, and genu varum (**Figure 1**).

Dr. Spencer or an immediate family member is a member of a speakers' bureau or has made paid presentations on behalf of AO Trauma and DePuy, A Johnson & Johnson Company and serves as a board member, owner, officer, or committee member of the American Academy of Orthopaedic Surgeons, the Children's Orthopaedic Surgery Foundation, the Massachusetts Orthopaedic Association, the Michigan Medical Alumni Society, the Pediatric Orthopaedic Society of North America, and the Skeletal Dysplasia Meeting Consortium.

TABLE 1

Skeletal Dysplasias: Genetics and Features

Name	Genetics	Features
Achondroplasia	Fibroblast growth factor receptor-3 (FGFR-3); AD; 90% sporadic mutations; affects proliferative zone of physis	Rhizomelic shortening with normal trunk, frontal bossing, button nose, trident hands (cannot approximate long and ring fingers), thoracolumbar kyphosis (usually resolves with sitting), lumbar stenosis and lordosis, radial head subluxations, champagne glass pelvic outlet, genu varum
Hypochondroplasia	FGFR-3 in a different area than achondroplasia; AD	Milder than achondroplasia: short stature, lumbar stenosis, genu varum
Thanatophoric dysplasia	FGFR-3	Rhizomelic shortening, platyspondyly, protuberant abdomen, and a small thoracic cavity. Death by the age of 2 yr
Spondyloepiphyseal dysplasia (SED) congenita	Type II collagen mutation in COL2A1 gene; AD but usually sporadic mutation; affects proliferative zone of physis	Short stature, trunk and limbs, abnormal epiphyses including spine, atlantoaxial instability/odontoid hypoplasia, coxa vara and DDH, genu valgum, early OA, retinal detachment/myopia, sensorineural hearing loss
SED tarda	Unidentified mutation likely in type II collagen, XR	Late-onset at age 8-10 yr, premature OA, associated with DDH but not lower extremity bowing
Kniest dysplasia	Type II collagen mutation in COL2A1 gene, AD	Joint contractures (treat with early PT), kyphosis/scoliosis, dumbbell shaped femurs, respiratory problems, cleft palate, retinal detachment/myopia, otitis media/hearing loss, early OA
Cleidocranial dyplasia	Defect in core-binding factor alpha-1 (CBFA1) a transcription factor that activates osteoblast differentiation. AD. Affects intramembranous ossification	Aplasia/hypoplasia of clavicles (no need to treat), delayed skull suture closure, frontal bossing, coxa vara (osteotomy if neck-shaft angle <100°), delayed ossification pubis, genu valgum, shortened middle phalanges of third-fifth fingers
Nail-patella syndrome (osteoonychodysplasia)	Mutation in Lim homeobox transcription factor 1-β (LMX1β) also expressed in eyes/kidneys; AD	Aplasia/hypoplasia of the patella and condyles, dysplastic nails, iliac horns, posterior dislocation of the radial head, 30% will get renal failure and glaucoma as adults
Diastrophic dysplasia	Mutation in sulfate transporter gene affects proteoglycan sulfate groups in cartilage; AR; 1 in 70 people are carriers of this gene in Finland; very rare elsewhere.	Short stature; rhizomelic shortening, cervical kyphosis, kyphoscoliosis, hitchhiker thumbs, cauliflower ears, rigid clubfeet, skew foot, severe OA, joint contractures
Mucopolysaccharidoses	All defects in enzymes that degrade glycosaminoglycans in lysosomes. The incomplete degradation products accumulate in various organs and cause dysfunction. All AR except Hunter's: XR	Visceromegaly, corneal clouding, cardiac disease, deafness, short stature, mental retardation (except Morquio syndrome—normal intelligence). C1-C2 instability is common as is hip dysplasia and abnormal epiphyses. Hurler syndrome is the most severe; bone marrow transplant improves life expectancy but does not alter orthopaedic manifestations
Metaphyseal dysplasia: Schmid type	Type X collagen mutation in COL10A1 gene. AD. Affects proliferative/hypertrophic zones	Milder; coxa vara, genu varum
Metaphyseal dyplasia: Jansen type	Mutation in parathyroid hormone receptor (affects parathyroid hormone–related protein, PTHRP) which regulates chondrocyte differentiation; affects proliferative/hypertrophic zones; AD	Wide eyes, squatting stance, hypercalcemia, bulbous metaphyseal expansion of long bones and extremity malalignment

TABLE 1

Skeletal Dysplasias: Genetics and Features (Continued)

Name	Genetics	Features
Metaphyseal dysplasia: McKusick type	Mutation in RMRP gene (ribosomal nucleic acid component of mitochondrial ribosomal nucleic acid processing endoribonuclease); affects proliferative/hypertrophic zones	C1-C2 instability, hypoplasia of cartilage, small diameter "fine" hair, intestinal malabsorption and megacolon, increased risk viral infections and malignancies (immune dysfunction), ligamentous laxity, pectus abnormalities, genu varum, and ankle deformities due to fibular overgrowth
Pseudoachondroplasia	Mutation in cartilage oligomeric matrix protein (COMP) on chromosome 19 which is an extracellular matrix glycoprotein in cartilage; AD	C1-C2 instability due to odontoid hypoplasia, normal facial features, metaphyseal flaring, delayed epiphyses, lower extremity malalignment, DDH, scoliosis, early OA
Multiple epiphyseal dysplasia	Mutations in COMP, COL9A2, or COL9A3 genes (collagen IX which is a linker for collagen II in cartilage); AD	Short stature, epiphyseal dysplasia, genu valgum, hip osteonecrosis and dysplasia, early OA. Spine not involved. Short MC/MT, double layer patella
Ellis-van Creveld (EVC) syndrome/chondroectodermal dysplasia	Mutation in the EVC gene; AR	Acromesomelic shortening (distal and middle limb segments), postaxial polydactyly, genu valgum, dysplastic nails/teeth, 60% have congenital heart disease, medial iliac spikes, capitate/hamate fused
Diaphyseal dysplasia aka Camurati-Engelmann syndrome	AD	Symmetric cortical thickening of long bones most commonly seen in tibia, femur, humerus. Treat with NSAIDs, watch for LLD
Leri-Weill dyschondrosteosis	SHOX gene tip of sex chromosome, AD	Mild short stature, mesomelic shortening, Madelung deformity
Menkes syndrome and occipital horn syndrome	Both copper transporter defects; Menkes XR	Menkes syndrome: kinky hair Occipital horn syndrome has bony projections from the occiput

AD = autosomal dominant, AR = autosomal recessive, DDH = developmental dysplasia hip, LLD = leg length discrepancy, MC/MT = metacarpal/metatarsal, OA = osteoarthritis, PT = physical therapy, XD = X-linked dominant, XR = X-linked recessive

b. Foramen magnum stenosis and upper cervical stenosis may be present and cause central apnea and weakness in the first few years of life.

4. Treatment

a. Nonsurgical treatment is usual for the thoracolumbar kyphosis present early on. Avoidance of unsupported sitting may help prevent it.

b. Genu varum is treated with osteotomies if symptomatic.

c. Foramen magnum/upper cervical stenosis may require urgent decompression if cord compression is present; this area does grow bigger in later life.

d. The main issue in adult life is lumbar stenosis requiring decompression and/or fusion.

e. Limb lengthening is controversial and does not treat the other dysmorphic features; if lower limb lengthening is done, humeral lengthening is indicated too.

f. Growth hormone is not effective at increasing stature.

g. Selective FGFR3 inhibitor drug therapies are now in clinical trials: see trials.gov.

B. Pseudoachondroplasia (**Table 1**)

1. Overview

a. Short-limbed rhizomelic dwarfism with normal facial features.

b. Normal development before the age of 2 years.

2. Pathoanatomy

a. Autosomal dominant.

b. Mutation is in Cartilage Oligomeric Matrix Protein (COMP) on chromosome 19.

c. Epiphyses are delayed and abnormal, metaphyseal flaring is present, and early-onset osteoarthritis (OA) is common.

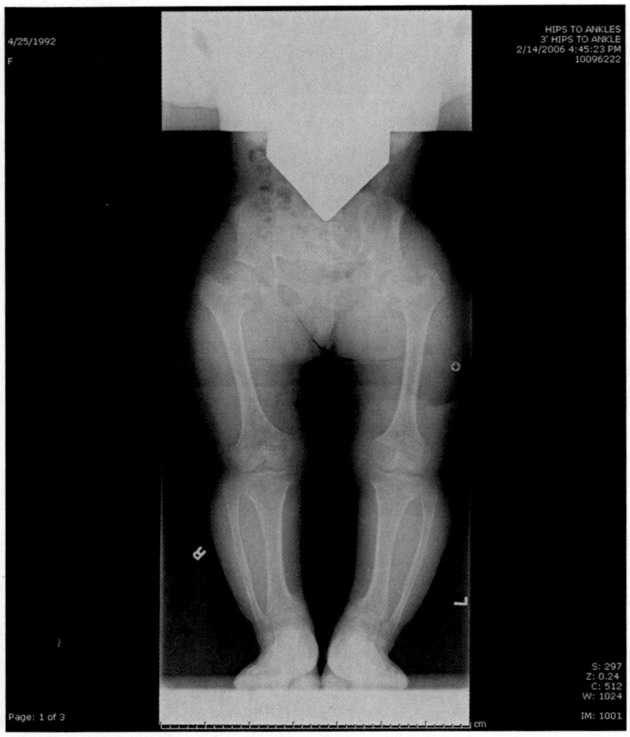

Figure 1 Standing AP hips to ankles radiograph of a child with achondroplasia with classic lower extremity features of a champagne pelvis and genu varum.

3. Evaluation
   a. Cervical instability is common and must be looked for (**Figure 4, A** and **B**).
   b. Lower extremity bowing may be valgus, varus, or windswept.
   c. Joints may be hyperlax in early life, but later on develop flexion contractures and early OA.
   d. Platyspondyly is always present, but spinal stenosis is not present.
4. Treatment
   a. Cervical instability should be stabilized (**Figure 4, C**).
   b. Symptomatic extremity bowing should be surgically corrected, but recurrence is common and OA progressive.

C. Diastrophic dysplasia (**Table 1**)
1. Overview: Short-limbed dwarfism apparent from birth with other common findings including cleft palate and hitchhiker thumbs (**Figures 2, A** and **B, 3**).
2. Pathoanatomy
   a. Autosomal recessive
   b. Mutation in sulfate transport protein that primarily affects cartilage matrix. Present in 1 in 70 Finnish citizens.
3. Evaluation
   a. Cleft palate is present in 60%.
   b. Cauliflower ears are present in 80% and develop after birth from cystic swellings in the ear cartilage (**Figure 2, A** and **B**)
   c. Hitchhiker thumbs are present (**Figure 3**).
   d. Cervical kyphosis and thoracolumbar scoliosis are often present.
   e. Joint contractures (hip flexion, genu valgum with dislocated patellae) and rigid clubfeet or skew feet are often present.
4. Treatment
   a. Surgery for progressive spinal deformity or cord compromise; note that cervical kyphosis often resolves spontaneously.
   b. Surgery for progressive, symptomatic lower extremity deformity; recurrence is common.
   c. The cauliflower ear deformity may be improved by early compressive bandaging (**Figure 2, A** and **B**).

D. Cleidocranial dysostosis (**Table 1**)
1. Overview: Proportionate dwarfism that has mild short stature with a broad forehead and absent clavicles.
2. Pathoanatomy
   a. Autosomal dominant
   b. Defect in core-binding factor alpha-1 (CBFA1) which is a transcription factor for osteocalcin.
   c. Affects intramembranous ossification: skull, clavicles, and pelvis.

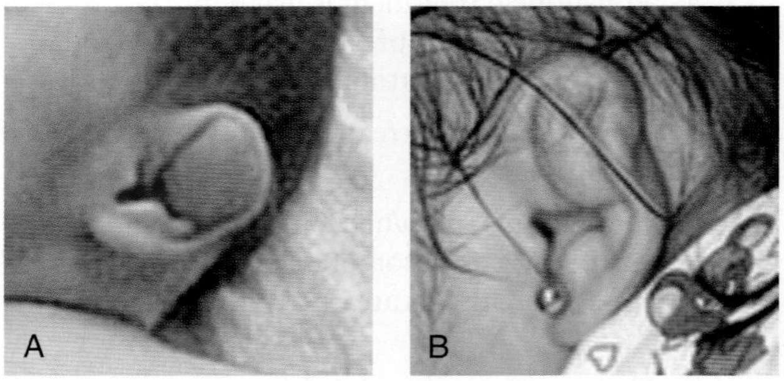

Figure 2 **A**, Photographs showing diastrophic dysplasia's classic cauliflower ear in a neonate. **B**, The same ear several years later after early treatment with compressive bandages. (**A**, Photo courtesy of Ms. Vita Gagne from the 2004 Diastrophic Dysplasia Booklet. **B**, Photo courtesy of Ms. Vita Gagne from the 2004 Diastrophic Dysplasia Booklet.)

Chapter 130

PEDIATRIC MUSCULOSKELETAL DISORDERS AND SYNDROMES

SAMANTHA A. SPENCER, MD

I. CONNECTIVE TISSUE DISEASES

A. Marfan's syndrome (**Table 1**)

1. Overview: Connective tissue disorder affecting elasticity that results in joint laxity, scoliosis, cardiac valve, and aortic dilatation, among other things. Incidence is 1:10,000 with no ethnic or sex predilections.
2. Pathoanatomy
   a. Autosomal dominant (AD); 25% new mutations
   b. Mutation is in fibrillin-1 gene FBN1 on chromosome 15q21; multiple mutations have been identified.
3. Evaluation
   a. Tall and thin with long limbs (dolichostenomelia) and spiderlike fingers (arachnodactyly) and joint hypermobility.
   b. Positive wrist sign (Walker) means the thumb and little finger overlap when used to encircle the opposite wrist.
   c. Positive thumb (Steinberg) sign means when the thumb is adducted across the hand and the fingers are closed in a fist over it, it protrudes out the other side of the hand.
   d. Arm span to height ratio > 1.05 is seen.
   e. Cardiac defects, especially aortic root dilation, and later dissection are common; if Marfan's is suspected, echocardiogram and a cardiology consult are necessary.
   f. Scoliosis is seen in 60% to 70% and is difficult to brace; dural ectasia is common (more than 60%), necessitating MRI before surgery (**Figure 1**).
   g. Pectus excavatum and spontaneous pneumothoraces can occur in the chest (**Figure 2**).
   h. Superior lens dislocation and myopia are common (as opposed to the inferior lens dislocation seen in homocystinuria).
   i. Protrusio acetabuli and severe pes planovalgus are seen in the lower extremity (LE).
4. Classification
   a. Ghent system requires one major criterion in two different organ systems and involvement in a third system
   b. MASS phenotype = Mitral valve prolapse, aortic root diameter at upper limits of normal, stretch marks, skeletal manifestations of Marfan's: these patients do not have ectopia lenis or aortic dissections and have a better prognosis.
5. Treatment
   a. Nonsurgical
      - Beta-blockers for mitral valve prolapse, aortic dilation
      - Bracing treatment for early scoliosis, pes planovalgus
   b. Surgical
      - Long scoliosis fusions due to junctional problems with mandatory preop MRI (to assess dural ectasia) and cardiac workup for progressive scoliosis; high pseudarthrosis rate.
      - Closure of the triradiate cartilage for progressive protrusio acetabuli.
      - Corrective surgery for progressive pes planovalgus.

Dr. Spencer or an immediate family member is a member of a speakers' bureau or has made paid presentations on behalf of AO Trauma and DePuy, A Johnson & Johnson Company and serves as a board member, owner, officer, or committee member of the American Academy of Orthopaedic Surgeons, the Children's Orthopaedic Surgery Foundation, the Massachusetts Orthopaedic Association, the Michigan Medical Alumni Society, the Pediatric Orthopaedic Society of North America, and the Skeletal Dysplasia Meeting Consortium.

TABLE 1

Marfan Syndrome

System	Major Criteria	Minor Criteria
Musculoskeletal[a]	Pectus carinatum; pectus excavatum requiring surgery; dolichostenomelia; wrist and thumb signs; scoliosis greater than 20° or spondylolisthesis; reduced elbow extension; pes planus; protrusio acetabuli	Moderately severe pectus excavatum; joint hypermobility; highly arched palate with crowding of teeth; facial features (dolichocephaly, malar hypoplasia, enophthalmos, retrognathia, down-slanting palpebral fissures)
Ocular[b]	Ectopia lentis	Abnormally flat cornea; increased axial length of globe; hypoplastic iris or hypoplastic ciliary muscle causing decreased miosis
Cardiovascular[c]	Dilatation of ascending aorta ± aortic regurgitation, involving sinuses of Valsalva; dissection of ascending aorta	Mitral valve prolapse ± regurgitation
Family/genetic history[d]	Parent, child, or sibling meets diagnostic criteria; mutation in *FBN1* known to cause Marfan syndrome; inherited haplotype around *FBN1* associated with Marfan syndrome in family	None
Skin and integument[e]	None	Stretch marks not associated with pregnancy, weight gain, or repetitive stress; recurrent incisional hernias
Dura[d]	Lumbosacral dural ectasia	None
Pulmonary[e]	None	Spontaneous pneumothorax or apical blebs

[a]Two or more major or one major plus two minor criteria required for involvement.
[b]At least two minor criteria required for involvement.
[c]One major or minor criterion required for involvement.
[d]One major criterion required for involvement.
[e]One minor criterion required for involvement.
Adapted from Miller NH: Connective tissue disorders, in Koval KJ, ed: *Orthopaedic Knowledge Update*, ed 7. Rosemont, IL, American Academy of Orthopaedic Surgeons, 2002, pp 201-207.

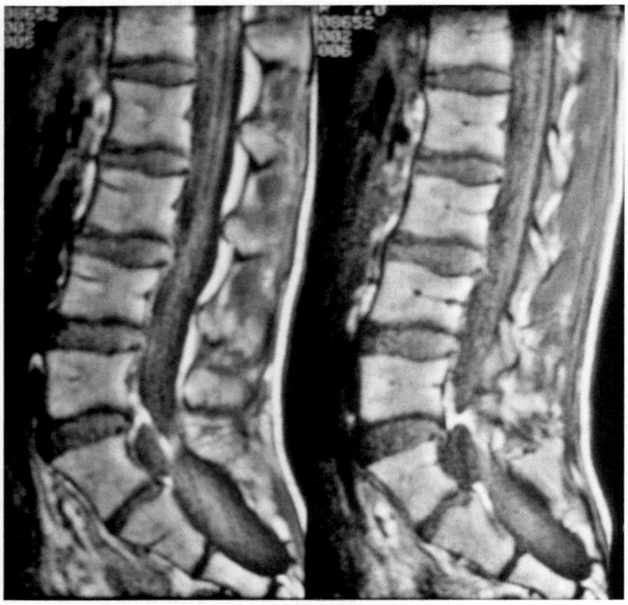

Figure 1 Magnetic resonance image of the lower spine in a Marfan's patient showing dural ectasia of the lumbosacral junction. (Courtesy of Dr. M. Timothy Hresko.)

B. Ehlers-Danlos syndrome (EDS) (**Table 2**)

1. Overview: Connective tissue disorder with skin and joint hypermobility.
2. Pathoanatomy
    a. 40% to 50% of classic form patients have a mutation in COL5A1 or COL5A2, the gene for type V collagen; this classic form is AD.
    b. Type VI is autosomal recessive (AR) and occurs secondary to a mutation in lysyl hydroxylase, an enzyme important in collagen cross-linking. This type particularly has severe kyphoscoliosis.
    c. Type IV is AD and occurs secondary to a mutation in COL3A1, resulting in abnormal collagen III, and arterial, intestinal, and uterine rupture are seen.
    d. Many hypermobility EDS patients do not have an identified mutation.
3. Evaluation
    a. Skin is velvety and fragile. Severe scarring with minor trauma is common.

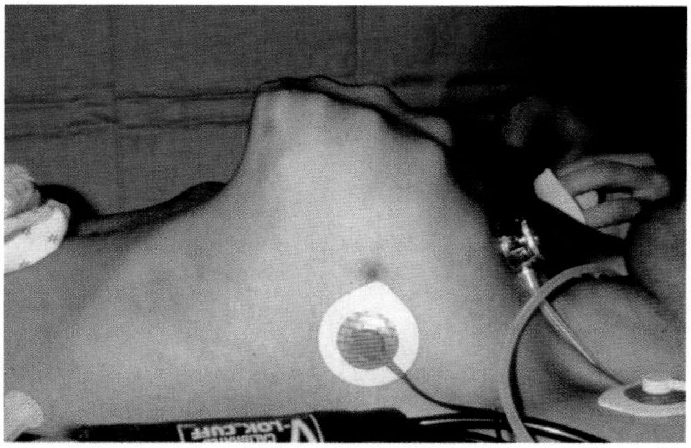

Figure 2 Photograph showing pectus deformity in a Marfan's patient. (Courtesy of Dr. M. Timothy Hresko.)

b. Joints are hypermobile, particularly the shoulders, patellae, and ankles.

c. Up to a third of patients have aortic root dilations; therefore an echo and a cardiac evaluation is mandatory.

d. The vascular subtype can have spontaneous visceral or arterial ruptures.

4. Treatment

a. Avoid surgery for lax joints; soft-tissue procedures are unlikely to work.

b. Scoliosis is most common in type VI and usually progressive. Surgery is indicated for progressive curves, and longer fusions to prevent junctional problems are necessary (**Figure 3, A** and **B**).

c. Chronic musculoskeletal pain is present in over 50%; treat supportively if at all possible.

II. ARTHRITIDES

A. Osteoarthritis (OA) (**Table 3**)

1. Overview: Wear and tear arthritis of older age.

2. Pathoanatomy

a. Mechanical stress due to malalignment (varus or valgus malalignment of >4° to 5° in the knee yields a four times increase in knee OA)

TABLE 2

Ehlers-Danlos Classification

Villefranche Classification (1998)	Berlin Classification (1988)	Genetics	Major Symptomatic Criteria	Biochemical Defects (Minor Criteria)
Classic	Type I (gravis) Type II (mitis)	AD	Hyperextensible skin, atrophic scars, joint hypermobility	*COL5A1, COL5A2* mutations (40%-50% of families); mutations in type V collagen
Hypermobility	Type III (hypermobile)	AD	Velvety soft skin, small and large joint hypermobility; tendency for dislocation, chronic pain, scoliosis	Unknown
Vascular	Type IV (vascular)	AD (rarely AR)	Arterial, intestinal, and uterine fragility; rupture; thin translucent skin; extensive bruising	*COL3A1* mutation, abnormal type III collagen structure of synthesis
Kyphoscoliosis	Type VI (ocular scoliotic)	AR	Severe hypotonia at birth, progressive infantile scoliosis, generalized joint laxity, scleral fragility, globe rupture	Lysyl hydroxylase deficiency, mutations in *PLOD* gene
Arthrochalasis	Type VIIA, VIIB	AD	Congenital bilateral hip dislocation, hypermobility, soft skin	Deletion of type I collagen exons that encode for N-terminal propeptide *(COL1A1, COL1A2)*
Dermatosparaxis	Type VIIIC	AR	Severe sagging or redundant skin	Mutations in type I collagen N peptidase

AD = autosomal dominant, AR = autosomal recessive
Reproduced from D'Astous JL, Carroll KL: Connective tissue disorders, in Vaccaro AR, ed: *Orthopaedic Knowledge Update*, ed 8. Rosemont, IL, American Academy of Orthopaedic Surgeons, 2005, p 246.

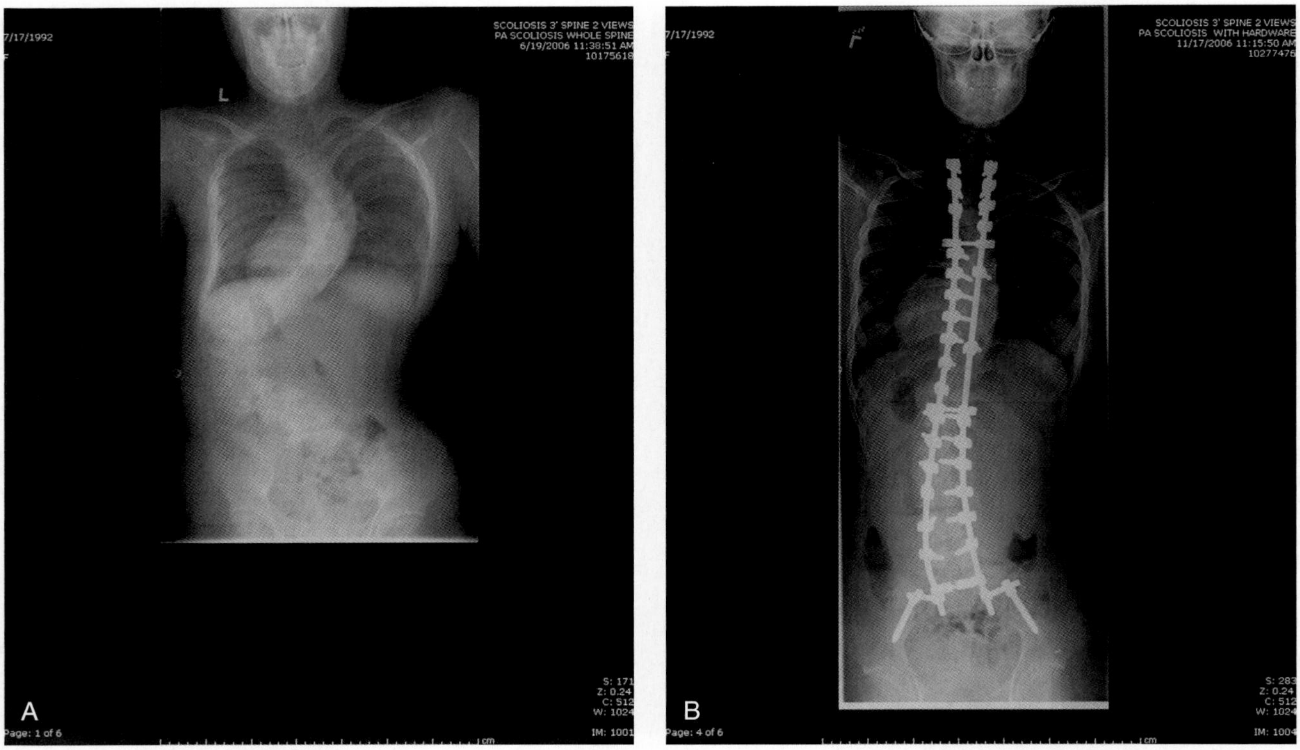

Figure 3 PA spine views of a patient with Ehlers-Danlos type VI. **A**, Preoperative view demonstrates severe scoliosis. **B**, Postoperative view demonstrates the need for long fusion in connective tissue syndromes.

TABLE 3

Osteoarthritis (OA) Versus Rheumatoid Arthritis

	Osteoarthritis	Rheumatoid Arthritis
Age	**Older**	**Younger**
Physical findings	IP joints affected in hands, gradual stiffness/loss of motion in affected joints most common in knees/hips, oligoarticular	MCP joints affected in hands with ulnar deviation, polyarticular, joint effusions, warmth; rheumatoid nodules on extensor surfaces
Pathology	Cartilage fibrillation, increased water content of the cartilage, increased collagen I/II ratio, higher friction and lower elasticity	Thickened synovial pannus that cascades over the joint surface and is filled with numerous T cells and B cells with some plasma cells and macrophages
Radiographic findings	Osteophytes, subchondral sclerosis, subchondral cyst formation; superolateral joint space narrowing in the hip, medial compartment of the knee commonly seen	Symmetric joint space narrowing with osteopenia and periarticular erosions; protrusio in the hip
Pathophysiology	Chondrocytes release matrix metalloproteinases that degrade the extracellular matrix; cytokines such as IL-1 and TNF-alpha are also found in the joint fluid. These cause prostaglandin release which may cause pain.	Autoimmune arthritis in which the joint synovium triggers a T cell–mediated attack leading to release of IL-1 and TNF-alpha, which degrade cartilage.
Associated findings	Obesity is associated with an increased risk of knee (but not hip) and hand OA, particularly in women.	Basilar invagination, eye involvement, entrapment neuropathies, pleural/pericardial effusions

IL = interleukin, IP = interphalangeal, MCP = metacarpophalangeal, TNF = tumor necrosis factor

b. Overuse or joint incongruity or injury damages chondrocytes, leading to cartilage breakdown.

3. Evaluation

a. Physical examination demonstrates joint stiffness most typically in IP joints of hands, hips, and knees without signs of acute systemic inflammation.

b. Radiographs show asymmetric joint space narrowing with osteophytes and subchondral sclerosis

4. Treatment is supportive with PT, NSAIDs/COX-II inhibitors at first, osteotomy and joint replacement for later stages. Cartilage replacement with techniques such as mosaicplasty and ACI is limited at this point. Genetically engineered cartilage regrowth is in the future.

B. Rheumatoid (seropositive) arthritis (RA) (**Table 3**)

1. Overview: Inflammatory autoimmune arthritis that causes joint destruction at a younger age.

2. Pathoanatomy

a. The synovium thickens and fills with B and T cells and macrophages, which erode the cartilage.

b. This is an autoimmune, systemic process.

3. Evaluation

a. Rheumatoid factor is found in only half of RA patients and in 5% of the general population; however, it may help identify more aggressive cases.

b. Prevalence is 1% in the general population; it is higher in aboriginal North Americans. Twin concordance is only 12% to 15% for monozygotic twins.

c. Physical examination demonstrates multiple hot, swollen, stiff joints. Subcutaneous calcified nodules and iridis may be present.

d. Radiographs show symmetric joint space narrowing, periarticular erosions, and osteopenia.

4. Treatment

a. RA treatment is now largely medical with a combination of nonsteroidal anti-inflammatory drugs (NSAIDs) and disease modifying antirheumatic drugs (DMARDs).

b. Most DMARDs are immunosuppressive and must be stopped before orthopaedic procedures with a cell count checked to avoid neutropenia.

c. Surgery involves synovectomy and joint realignment early on and joint replacement in the later stages.

C. Juvenile idiopathic arthritis (JIA) (previously juvenile rheumatoid arthritis or JRA)

1. Overview: Autoimmune inflammatory arthritis of joints in children lasting more than 6 weeks.

2. Pathoanatomy

a. Like that of adult RA, an autoimmune erosion of cartilage occurs.

b. A positive rheumatoid factor and ANA (antinuclear antibody) may indicate a more aggressive course.

3. Evaluation

a. Systemic JIA/JRA (Still's disease)

- Rash, high fever, multiple inflamed joints, acute presentation are typical.
- Anemia and/or a high WBC may occur.
- May have serositis, hepatosplenomegaly, lymphadenopathy, pericarditis.
- Infection must be ruled out.
- It is usually found in ages 5 to 10 and equally affects girls and boys.
- Poorer long-term prognosis
- It is the least common type (20%) of JIA.

b. Oligoarticular JIA/pauciarticular JRA

- It is the most common type (30% to 40%).
- Four or less joints are involved.
- Usually large joints, commonly knees/ankles, are affected.
- Peak age is 2 to 3, and is four times as common in girls as boys.
- A limp which improves during the day is typical.
- 20% have uveitis. Ophthalmology evaluation needed every 4 months if ANA-positive, every 6 months if ANA-negative
- Limb length discrepancy, affected side often longer, is another sequela.
- Best prognosis for long-term remission (70%).

c. Polyarticular JIA/polyarticular JRA

- More than five or more joints are involved and often small joints (hands/wrists) are affected.
- Can have uveitis, but it is less frequent than in oligoarticular JIA.
- It is more common in girls, and prognosis is good (60% remission).

4. Treatment
    a. Leg length discrepancy may need epiphysiodesis; arthroplasty may be needed as an adult
    b. Medical management with NSAIDs or DMARDs by a rheumatologist is generally required.
    c. An arthrocentesis or synovial biopsy for diagnosis may be needed.
    d. Steroid injections and synovectomy may help if medical management fails

D. Seronegative spondyloarthropathies

1. Overview: autoimmune arthropathies that have a negative rheumatoid factor.
2. Pathoanatomy: These are autoimmune in nature.
3. Evaluation
    a. Ankylosing spondylitis
        - Onset age 15 to 35; affects males more commonly than females; characterized by morning stiffness and low back pain.
        - Sacroiliitis and progressive fusion of the spine (bamboo spine) are typical.
        - Peripheral joint arthritis, usually unilateral, is common.
        - Uveitis present in up to 40% of patients; cardiac and pulmonary disease can also occur. Aphthous mouth ulcers and fatigue are common.
        - Aggressive physical therapy and NSAIDs are indicated.
        - Spinal fractures are highly unstable and have high rates of neurologic injury.
        - 95% of whites and 50% of blacks with ankylosing spondylitis are HLA-B27-positive, though <5% of all HLA-B27-positive individuals have ankylosing spondylitis.
    b. Psoriatic arthritis
        - Usually the typical psoriatic skin plaques (extensor surface scaly silvery plaques) precede the arthritis, but in 20% of patients the arthritis is first.
        - A common radiographic finding is "pencil in cup" deformities of the phalanges.
        - Nail pitting and dactylitis commonly found.
    c. Reactive arthritis/Reiter's syndrome
        - An arthritis triggered by diseases such as *Chlamydia*, *Yersinia*, *Salmonella*, *Campylobacter*, *Shigella* infections that lead to an autoimmune complex deposition in the joints (commonly the knee), which leads to painful swelling.
        - Associated with conjunctivitis and dysuria. Mouth ulcers and a rash on the hands and feet can also occur.
        - Treat the underlying condition and manage the arthritis supportively.
    d. Enteropathic arthropathies
        - Arthritis associated with inflammatory bowel disease such as Crohn's or ulcerative colitis, which occurs in 20% of patients with inflammatory bowel disease
        - Managed supportively

III. OTHER CONDITIONS WITH MUSCULOSKELETAL INVOLVEMENT

A. Rickets

1. Overview
    a. Defective mineralization in growing bone due to a variety of causes.
    b. The most common form of rickets in North America is hypophosphatemic rickets.
2. Pathoanatomy
    a. Calcium/phosphate homeostasis is disturbed leading to poor calcification of the cartilage matrix of growing long bones.
    b. Radiographic features include widened osteoid seams, metaphyseal cupping, prominence of the rib heads (osteochondral junction, ie, rachitic rosary), bowing particularly genu varum, and fractures.
    c. Microscopically, the zone of proliferation is disordered and elongated in the epiphyseal plate.
3. Evaluation
    a. Serum calcium, phosphorus, alkaline phosphatase, parathyroid hormone (PTH), 25-hydroxyvitamin D, and 1,25-dihydroxyvitamin D must be checked to assess the cause.
    b. A history of breastfeeding with little sun exposure is the most likely scenario for vitamin D–deficient rickets.
4. Classification/treatment (**Table 4**)
    a. Surgery is indicated for LE bowing that does not resolve after medical treatment of the rickets.

TABLE 4

Rickets

Rickets Type	Genetics	Serum Labs	Associated Features	Treatment
Hypophosphatemic	X-linked dominant, impaired renal phosphate absorption	Decreased phosphate; normal calcium, PTH and vitamin D; increased alkaline phosphatase	Most common type in the United States	High-dose phosphate and vitamin D Burosumab FGF-23 antibody
Vitamin D deficient	Nutritional	Decreased vitamin D, calcium, and phosphate; increased PTH and alkaline phosphatase		Vitamin D replacement
Vitamin D dependent, type 1	Autosomal recessive, defect in renal 25-hydroxyvitamin D 1-α-hydroxylase	Low calcium and phosphate; normal 25-hydroxyvitamin D, very low 1,25-dihydroxyvitamin D; high alkaline phosphatase and PTH		1,25-Dihydroxyvitamin D replacement
Vitamin D dependent, type 2	Defect in the intracellular receptor for 1,25-dihydroxyvitamin D	Low calcium and phosphate; high alkaline phosphatase and PTH; very high 1,25-dihydroxyvitamin D levels	Alopecia	High dose 1,25-dihydroxyvitamin D and calcium
Hypophosphatasia	Autosomal recessive, deficient or nonfunctional alkaline phosphatase	Increased calcium and phosphate levels; very low alkaline phosphatase levels; normal PTH/vitamin D levels	Early loss of teeth	Asfotase alfa

b. Hemiepiphysiodesis or osteotomy may be indicated.

c. Co-management with an endocrinologist is recommended as there are many medical therapeutic options.

B. Trisomy 21 (Down syndrome)

1. Most common chromosomal abnormality with incidence of 1 in 800 to 1 in 1,000 live births; increased incidence with advanced maternal age.

2. Pathoanatomy: usually a duplication of maternal chromosome 21, resulting in three copies of chromosome 21

3. Evaluation

a. Phenotypic features include flattened face, upward slanting eyes with epicanthal folds, single palmar crease, mental retardation (varies), congenital heart disease (endocardial cushion defects 50%), duodenal atresia, hypothyroidism, hearing loss, ligamentous laxity, high incidence of leukemia/lymphoma, diabetes, and Alzheimer's in later adult life.

b. Spine

- Atlantoaxial instability is present in 9% to 22%; it is controversial if flexion-extension cervical spine views are needed before sports participation.
- Scoliosis is present in up to 50%.
- Spondylolisthesis is present in up to 6%

c. Metatarsus primus varus, pes planovalgus, and hallux valgus in the feet are common.

d. Patellar dislocation, pain, and instability are common.

e. Hip instability (often late) is common, sometimes with only mild bony abnormality.

4. Treatment

a. Supportive bracing treatment is indicated for feet and knees, and for reducible hips younger than 6 years old.

b. Treatment of asymptomatic atlanto-dens interval (ADI) of 5 to 10 mm is controversial; many would watch and get a magnetic resonance image.

c. Fusion is always indicated if cord compromise is seen on magnetic resonance image or if there is an ADI > 5 and the patient has symptoms; however, fusion has a high (up to 50%) complication rate.

d. Soft-tissue surgeries fail because of ligamentous laxity and hypotonia; therefore, if surgery is performed, bony realignment is indicated (ie, pelvic osteotomy for hip instability, tibial tubercle osteotomy for lateral patellar dislocation).

C. Osteogenesis imperfecta (OI)

1. Overview

a. Weak organic bone matrix causes frequent fractures and severe bowing and deformity in the more severe types.

b. Normal intelligence

2. Pathoanatomy

a. Types I-IV are a mutation in the COL1A1 and COL1A2 genes, which encode type I collagen, the mainstay of the organic bone matrix.

- The result is bone that has decreased number of trabeculae and decreased cortical thickness, referred to as "wormian" bone.
- Specific mutation is identified by DNA analysis of blood.

b. Types V-VII have no collagen I mutation but have a similar phenotype and abnormal bone on microscopy.

3. Evaluation

a. OI should be considered in children undergoing a nonaccidental trauma workup.

b. Particularly in types II and III, basilar invagination and severe scoliosis may occur.

c. Olecranon apophyseal avulsion fractures are characteristic; children presenting with these should be evaluated for OI.

d. Associated dentinogenesis imperfecta, hearing loss, blue sclera, joint hyperlaxity, and wormian skull bones (puzzle piece appearance to the skull after fontanelle closure) are seen.

4. Treatment

a. Manage fractures with light splints

b. Diphosphonates are used; diphosphonates inhibit osteoclasts yielding increased cortical thickness with decreased fracture rates and pain.

c. For severe bowing of the extremities or recurrent fracture, intramedullary fixation is indicated with or without osteotomy. Newer devices such as telescoping rods allow for growth (**Figure 4**, A and B).

d. Progressive scoliosis/basilar invagination is treated with spinal fusion.

D. Gaucher's disease

1. Overview: An enzymatic defect leads to overaccumulation of glucocerebrosides (lipids) in many organ systems including the bone marrow and the spleen.

2. Pathoanatomy

a. Defect in the gene encoding beta glucocerebrosidase, which breaks down glucocerebrosides. This leads to macrophages stuffed full of glucocerebrosides in many organ systems.

b. Always AR.

3. Evaluation

a. A WBC examination for enzyme activity is diagnostic.

b. Three forms are identified, based on age of onset.

- Type 1 (adult): easy bruising (thrombocytopenia), anemia, enlarged liver/spleen, bone pain/fractures
- Type 2 (infantile): enlarged spleen/liver by age 3 months, brain involved, lethal by age 2
- Type 3 (juvenile): onset in teen years, thrombocytopenia, anemia, enlarged liver/spleen, bone pain/fractures, gradual and mild brain involvement

c. Radiographic findings include Erlenmeyer flask appearance to distal femurs (also seen in osteopetrosis), osteonecrosis of hips/femoral condyles, cortical thinning.

4. Treatment

a. Enzyme replacement therapy is now available and works well for all symptoms except neurologic

b. Bone marrow transplant performed early can be curative.

E. Caffey's disease

1. Overview

a. A cortical hyperostosis of infancy (average age of onset less than 9 weeks old).

b. Self resolving and is a diagnosis of exclusion.

2. Pathoanatomy

a. The ESR and alkaline phosphatase are elevated, but cultures are negative.

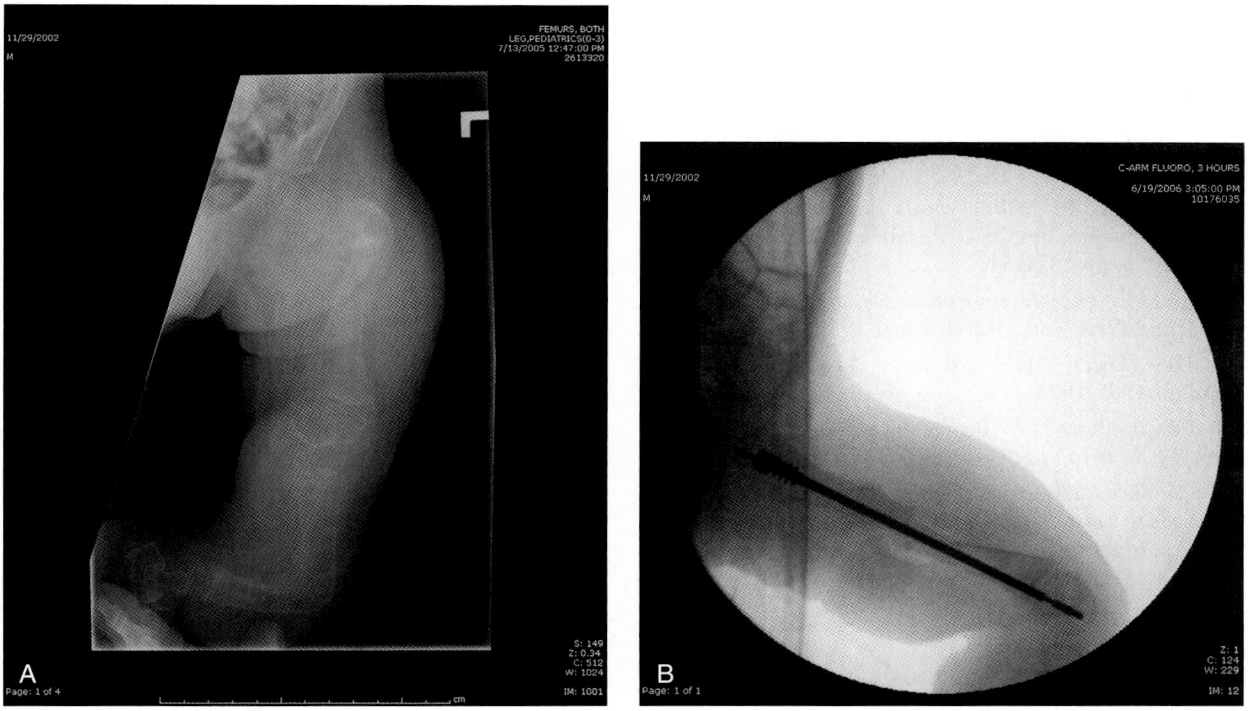

Figure 4 Images of the femur in a patient with type III osteogenesis imperfecta. **A**, Preoperative frog lateral hip to ankle radiograph demonstrates femoral deformity. **B**, Postoperative fluoroscopic radiograph frog lateral of the same hip and femur shows osteotomies and fixation with a telescoping rod.

b. Pathology shows hyperplasia of collagen fibers and fibrinoid degeneration.

3. Evaluation

a. Bones of the jaw (mandible) and forearm (ulna) are most commonly affected with diffuse cortical thickening present, but any bone except the vertebrae and phalanges may be affected.

b. Febrile illness with hyperirritability, swelling of soft tissues, and cortical thickening of the bone is present.

4. Treatment is supportive with occasional glucocorticoid use.

TOP TESTING FACTS

1. Dural ectasia is commonly seen in Marfan's syndrome and may cause back pain and complicate scoliosis surgery; preoperative MRI is mandatory.
2. Marfan's ectopia lentis is a superior dislocation; homocystinuria is an inferior lens dislocation.
3. MASS phenotype Marfan's patients never have ectopia lentis or aortic dissections.
4. Marfan syndrome is caused by a mutation in the fibrillin-1 gene.
5. Juvenile inflammatory arthritis is commonly associated with uveitis, which should be screened for.
6. The most common form of rickets in North America is hypophosphatemic rickets, which is X-linked dominant.
7. The most common chromosomal abnormality is trisomy 21.
8. Olecranon apophysis avulsion fractures are characteristic of OI.
9. Erlenmeyer flask deformities of the femur are seen in Gaucher's disease and osteopetrosis.
10. Juvenile inflammatory arthritis may be associated with a leg length discrepancy.

Bibliography

Aldegheri R, Dall'Oca C: Limb lengthening in short stature patients. *J Pediatr Orthop B* 2001;10:238-247.

D'Astous JL, Carroll KL: *Chapter 22: Connective tissue diseases*, in *Orthopaedic Knowledge Update*, ed 8. Rosemont, AAOS, 2005, pp 245-254.

Fassier F, Hamdy R: *Arthogrypotic syndromes and osteochondrodysplasias*, in *OKU Pediatrics*, ed 3. Rosemont, AAOS, 2006, pp 137-151.

Goldberg MJ: *The Dysmorphic Child an Orthopedic Perspective*. New York, Raven Press, 1987.

Judge DP, Dietz HC: Marfan's syndrome. *Lancet* 2005;366:1965-1976.

Morris CD, Einhorn TA: Bisphosphonates in orthopaedic surgery. *J Bone Joint Surg* 2005;87-A(7):1609-1618.

Nikkel SM: Skeletal dysplasias: What every bone health clinician needs to know. *Curr Osteoporos Rep* 2017;15(5):419-424. http://doi.org/10.1007/s11914-017-0392-x.

Pepe G, Giusti B, Sticchi E, Abbate R, Gensini GF, Nistri S: Marfan syndrome: Current perspectives. *Appl Clin Genet* 2016;9:55-65. http://doi.org/10.2147/TACG.S96233.

Stern CM, Pepin MJ, Stoler JM, Kramer DE, Spencer SA, Stein CJ: Musculoskeletal conditions in a pediatric population with Ehlers-Danlos syndrome. *J Pediatr* 2017;181:261-266. http://doi.org/10.1016/j.jpeds.2016.10.078.

Taybi H, Lachman RS: *Radiology of Syndromes, Metabolic Disorders, and Skeletal Dyplasias*, ed 4. St. Louis, Mosby-Year Book Inc., 1996.

White KK, Bompadre V, Goldberg MJ, et al: Best practices in peri-operative management of patients with skeletal dysplasias. *Am J Med Genet A* 2017;173(10):2584-2595. http://doi.org/10.1002/ajmg.a.38357.

Zeitlin L, Fassier F, Glorieux F: Modern approach to children with osteogenesis imperfecta. *J Pediatr Orthop* 2003;12(2):77-87.

Chapter 131

PEDIATRIC NEUROMUSCULAR DISORDERS

MARGARET SIOBHAN MURPHY-ZANE, MD

I. CEREBRAL PALSY

A. Epidemiology

1. The incidence of cerebral palsy (CP) is from 1 to 3 per 1,000 live births.
2. Prematurity and low birth weight (<1,500 g) increase the incidence to 90 per 1,000 live births.

B. Pathoanatomy

1. CP is a static encephalopathy: a nonprogressive, permanent injury to the brain caused by damage, defectiveness, or illness.
2. CP can affect childhood motor development, speech, cognition, and sensation.
3. Although the brain injury in CP is static, the peripheral manifestations (eg, contractures and bone deformities) of CP are often not static.
4. Ongoing seizures may contribute to loss of function in patients with CP.

C. The risk factors for CP are listed in **Table 1**.

1. CP is not a genetic condition; familial spastic paraparesis, which is manifested by progressive weakness and stiffness of the lower extremities resembling that in CP, is a hereditary condition and should be considered as a diagnostic possibility if there is a family history of CP. Other genetics disorders that may be misdiagnosed as CP include leukodystrophies (eg, Pelizaeus-Merzbacher) or Rett syndrome.

D. Developmental evaluation

1. In normal development, children should
   a. Sit independently by age 6 to 9 months
   b. Cruise, or walk while holding onto furniture, by age 14 months
   c. Walk independently by age 18 months
2. Positive predictive factors for walking include pulling up to a standing position and sitting independently by age 2 years.
3. Poor prognostic indicators for walking are listed in **Table 2**.

E. Classification—Several classification systems are useful in treating CP.

1. Physiologic—The location of the brain injury in CP will cause different types of motor dysfunction.
   a. Patients with spastic-type (pyramidal) CP exhibit increased tone or rigidity with rapid stretching, which can lead to disturbances in gait and limb-muscle contracture. These patients most often benefit from orthopaedic interventions.
   b. Patients with dyskinetic (extrapyramidal) or choreoathetoid CP exhibit involuntary movements, athetosis, and dystonia. This type of CP has been less frequently seen than pyramidal CP with the administration of Rh-immune globulin to pregnant women to prevent Rh incompatibility between mothers and their infants.
   c. Patients with ataxia (cerebellar) exhibit disturbed balance and coordination.
   d. Patients with mixed types of CP show spasticity and dyskinesia.
2. Anatomic (**Table 3**).
3. **Functional—Gross Motor Function Classification System** (**GMFCS**). The patient is assigned a grade from I to V, representing the highest to lowest level of function (**Figure 1**). The GMFCS has been valuable in assessing outcomes across the CP

Dr. Murphy Zane or an immediate family member serves as a board member, owner, officer, or committee member of the American College of Emergency Physicians, the Pediatric Orthopaedic Society of North America, and the Society for Academic Emergency Medicine.

TABLE 1

Risk Factors for Cerebral Palsy

Prematurity
Low birth weight
Multiple births
TORCH (toxoplasmosis, other infections [syphilis and so forth], rubella, cytomegalovirus, herpes) infections
Chorioamnionitis
Placental complications
Third-trimester bleeding
Maternal epilepsy
Toxemia
Low Apgar scores
Anoxia
Intraventricular hemorrhage
Infection
Maternal drug and alcohol use
Teratogens

TABLE 2

Poor Prognostic Indicators for Walking

Not Sitting by 5 yr of age
Not walking by 8 yr of age
Persistence of two or more of the following primitive reflexes at **1** yr of age
Moro: With the child in the supine position, sudden extension of the neck causes arm abduction with finger extension, followed by an embrace
Asymmetric tonic neck: Turning of the head to the side causes a "fencer's pose"
Symmetric tonic neck: Flexion of the neck causes flexion of the arm and extension of the leg
Neck righting: When the child turns his or her head to the side, the trunk and limbs follow
Extensor thrust (abnormal reflex): Touching of the child's feet to the floor causes extension of all joints
Absence of the following postural reflexes at **1** yr of age
Parachute: With the child in the upright position, sudden forward rotation of the child's body causes the arms to extend to break a perceived fall
Foot placement: With support, touching the child's feet to a surface will elicit walking motion

spectrum. Motor function increases in all GMFCS levels until the age of 7 years, remains stable into adulthood in GMFCS I and II, and deteriorates in the teen years in GMFCS III, IV, and V.

TABLE 3

Anatomic Classification of Cerebral Palsy

Type	Area Affected
Quadriplegia	Four limbs
Whole body	Four limbs and bulbar problems (eg, swallowing)
Hemiplegia	One side of the body
Diplegia	Lower extremities, but can have some upper extremity posturing

F. **Gait assessment** is central to the orthopaedic care of patients with CP and myelomeningocele. **Gait motion analysis**, measuring kinematic dynamic joint range of motion, kinetic parameters, electromyography (EMG) muscle activity, foot pressure, and energy expenditure, allows for improved treatment plans and evaluations of the efficacy of surgery and orthotics.

1. Perry/Gage criteria—Five essential factors for normal gait:
    a. Symmetric step length
    b. Stance stability
    c. Swing clearance
    d. Adequate foot position before initial contact
    e. Energy conservation
2. Normal gait (**Figure 2**)
    a. A complete gait cycle is from one foot strike to the next foot strike on the same side of the body.
    b. Stance is the first 62% of the cycle.
    c. Swing is the final 38% of the cycle.
3. The physical examination of gait includes the range of motion (ROM) of the hip, knee, and ankle.
4. Test for spasticity—The "catch" test shows a velocity-dependent difference in muscle tightness, in which a quick passive motion elicits a rapid tightening of the muscles used in walking.
    a. On the Modified Ashworth Scale of tone in response to passive stretching of a limb, grade 1 is resistance to stretch without a catch, grade 2 is a clearly evident catch, and grade 5 is a rigid joint.
5. Tests for contractures and spasticity
    a. Duncan-Ely test (for spasticity of the rectus femoris muscle)—With the child in the prone position, the knee is flexed. If the ipsilateral hip rises, there is spasticity of the rectus femoris.

TABLE 4

Surgical Treatment of Common Gait Disturbances in Cerebral Palsy (Continued)

Gait Disturbance	Problem	Recommended Surgery
Equinovarus foot	Spastic tibialis anterior and/or tibialis posterior overpower the peroneal muscles, with gastrocnemius-soleus equinus	Treat equinus as noted for toe walking Split anterior tendon transfer if anterior tibialis causative Posterior tibialis lengthening or split transfer if posterior tibialis causative Must add calcaneal osteotomy if hindfoot deformity is rigid

AFO = ankle foot orthosis, RF = rectus femoris

5. Selective dorsal rhizotomy (SDR) reduces spasticity by selectively severing dorsal nerve rootlets between L1 and S1.
    a. SDR may be indicated in ambulatory patients between ages 3 and 8 years who have diplegia in the presence of good selective motor control and minimal cognitive delay.
    b. Complications of SDR include scoliosis (44%), spondylolisthesis (19%), risk of bowel/bladder incontinence, dysesthesias, and increasing weakness by adolescence.

I. Scoliosis associated with CP
1. Scoliosis incidence: Hemiplegic and diplegic (20%), quadriplegic (60% to 80%), and bedridden (100%). Neuromuscular scoliosis can lead to thoracic insufficiency syndrome.
2. Hip flexor contractures may cause lumbar increased lordosis, especially in spastic diplegia. Spondylolisthesis up to 21% in spastic diplegia.
3. Progression of scoliosis is common after skeletal maturity in patients with quadriplegia.
4. Bracing treatment and custom seat backs are typically ineffective in treating neuromuscular scoliosis, but it may be used in patients with flexible curves. Bracing treatment may be useful in ambulatory patients with Cobb angles <40.
5. Spinal fusion from the upper thoracic spine to the pelvis in nonambulatory patients may be indicated for large curves that cause pain and/or interfere with sitting.
    a. Prerequisites for surgery include scoliosis >40 to 50, progressive or interfering with sitting, >10yo, hip ROM adequate for seating, and stable medically and nutritionally. Patients who are <fifth percentile weight carry high risk of postoperative complications (fixation failure, infection, pulmonary, GI, neurologic).
    b. Pedicle screw techniques have become widely used over traditional Luque unit rod.
    c. Multilevel pedicle screws, including thoracic screws to T1 or T2, with pelvic fixation if pelvic obliquity >15.
    d. Curves exceeding 90° may require anterior release with a posterior fusion, as a single-step or two-step procedure.
    e. Magnetic growing rods have shown improved Cobb angles and pelvic obliquity, but have a 25% infection rate in CP in some centers, which has improved with process improvement and attention to nutrition pre- and post-op.
    f. Quality of life seems to improve after surgery in regard to sitting balance, cosmesis, caregiver satisfaction, and possibly lifespan. Little evidence to support functional gains.

TABLE 5

Causes of Anterior Knee Pain in Cerebral Palsy

Patella alta
Weak quadriceps
Tight hamstrings
Femoral anteversion
External tibial torsion
Pes valgus
Genu valgum
Patellar instability (may sometimes be asymptomatic)

J. Hip subluxation/dislocation associated with CP (CPHD)
1. Overview
    a. Subluxation is less common in the ambulatory patient, but will develop in 50% of quadriplegic patients with CP.
    b. CPHD is distinct from DDH. Subluxation (usually posterosuperior) results from spasticity of the adductor and iliopsoas muscles and non–weight-bearing status. There are

10 | Pediatrics

rarely soft-tissue obstacles to reduction, unless the migration percentage (MP) is >100%. Subsequent growth in CP, with muscle imbalance, often leads to recurrence.

c. From 50% to 75% of dislocated hips will become painful.

2. Treatment

a. Goals are to prevent subluxation and dislocation of the hip, maintain comfort in seating, and facilitate care and hygiene. Treatment is based on radiologic assessment and use of the Reimer migration percentage index of hip subluxation (MP) (**Figure 4**).

b. Systemic hip surveillance programs have led to early soft-tissue and skeletal hip reconstructions, and decreased hip dislocations and the need for salvage procedures.

c. Systematic hip surveillance programs have shown that hips with MP>30% are at risk. Regardless of treatment, patients at GMFCS levels IV and V have a higher rate of migration than those at GMFCS levels I, II, or III.

d. Botulinum toxin injection to hip adductor and flexor muscles is not effective in preventing progression of subluxation.

e. Surgical management is appropriate when subluxation (MP) progresses to 50%.

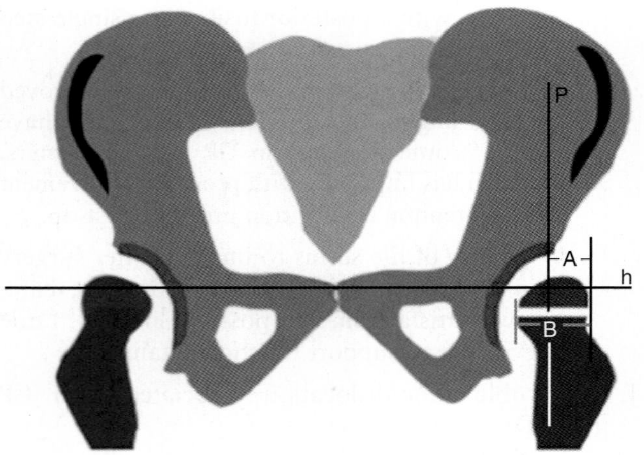

Figure 4 Illustration shows how the Reimer migration percentage is measured using an AP radiograph. The Hilgenreiner (h) and Perkin (P) lines are drawn. Distance A (the distance from P to the lateral border of the femoral epiphysis) is divided by distance B (the width of the femoral epiphysis) and multiplied by 100 to calculate the Reimer migration percentage (A/B × 100). (Reproduced with permission from Miller F: Hip, in Dabney K, Alexander M, eds: *Cerebral Palsy*. New York, NY, Springer, 2005, p 532.)

- Children younger than 8 years and with less than 60% subluxation can be treated with adductor and gracilis tenotomy and with iliopsoas release when hip flexion exceeds 20°. Early soft tissue releases work best in GMFCS II (94% success) and less well in GMFCS V (14% success).
- Children younger than 8 years and with more than 60% subluxation should be treated with a proximal femoral osteotomy (varus derotational osteotomy [VDRO]) and a possible pelvic osteotomy (Dega or Albee type).
- Children older than 8 years and with more than 40% subluxation should be treated with a proximal femoral osteotomy (VDRO) and a possible pelvic osteotomy (Dega or Albee type).
- Older children with closed triradiate cartilage or those with recurrent subluxation may benefit from a Ganz or Chiari pelvic osteotomy or a Staheli shelf with a VDRO.
- Children with a failed hip reconstruction or older children with arthritis, even if they have not undergone previous surgery, may require salvage procedures for pain relief, such as a proximal femoral resection-interposition arthroplasty (Castle procedure), subtrochanteric valgus osteotomy, or proximal femur prosthetic interposition arthroplasty using a humeral prosthesis.

K. Hip adduction contracture

1. Scissoring (caused by adductor tightness) at the hip joint can interfere with gait and hygiene and is treated with proximal release of the adductor muscles.

2. An obturator neurectomy should not be performed.

L. Contracture on hip flexion is treated with intramuscular lengthening of the iliopsoas muscle.

M. Lever-arm dysfunction associated with CP

1. Lever-arm dysfunction results in posterior displacement of the ground-reaction force relative to the knee and often results in crouch and power abnormalities in gait.

2. Intoeing from femoral anteversion can be treated with femoral rotational osteotomies.

3. Intoeing from internal tibial torsion can be treated with supramalleolar tibial osteotomies (a concurrent fibular osteotomy is not needed if correction is less than 25°).

4. Pes planus (pes valgus)—See Section I.P.4.

N. Knee problems specific to CP
  1. Crouched gait
    a. Most common cause is spastic or contracted hamstrings, although crouch may result from excessive dorsiflexion of the ankle or ankle equinus.
    b. Nonsurgical treatment includes physical therapy, bracing treatment (such as the use of knee immobilizers at night), and spasticity management.
    c. Mild crouch—If sustained and complete nonsurgical management fails, surgical treatment can consist of medial (and possibly lateral) lengthening of the hamstring muscles, with concomitant distal transfer of the rectus femoris (DRFT). However, DRFT can result in persistent crouch is not recommended in patients who are GMFCS III and IV. Also, lengthening of the medial and lateral hamstrings in an ambulatory patient carries an increased risk of recurvatum in stance.
    d. Severe crouch or fixed deformity:
      - Guided growth of the distal femur with eight plates or staples is a good option when there is significant growth remaining.
      - Without growth remaining, excellent results have been found with extension distal femoral osteotomy with an anterior closing wedge (fixed with a blade plate, fixed-angle plate, or wires) with shortening or advancement of the patellar tendon. With DFEO, hamstring procedures are not usually necessary.
  2. Stiff-knee gait: Usually from rectus femoris (RF) spasticity, with decreased peak knee flexion and decreased foot clearance in swing, treated with RF transfer or simple transection or intramuscular lengthening. However, DRFT can result in persistent crouch is not recommended in patients who are GMFCS III and IV.
  3. Knee contracture—In a nonambulatory patient, hamstring release may be useful for maintaining leg position in a program to improve standing.

O. Foot and ankle—Abnormal position or ROM at the foot and ankle cause abnormalities of gait and decreased push-off power. Goals of treatment include a painless, plantigrade (stable) foot.
  1. Equinus deformity (the most common foot problem in CP) results from spasticity of the gastrocnemius-soleus muscle complex. It can result in toe-walking or a back-knee (genu recurvatum) gait.
    a. Nonsurgical treatment includes stretching, physical therapy for ROM, the use of AFOs, and spasticity management.
    b. Surgical treatment should be considered only for patients with fixed contractures and is typically deferred until the patient is at least 6 years of age.
      - The Silfverskiöld test (Section I.F.5.c), performed with anesthesia, helps to determine whether a gastrocnemius recession and/or a soleus recession is appropriate. If the ankle rises above neutral with the knee flexed (gastrocnemius relaxed), a gastrocnemius recession should be performed. If the ankle is in equinus with the knee flexed and extended, the soleus is also tight, and a soleus recession should be performed. Lengthening of the Achilles tendon has been used to relieve tightness of the gastrocnemius-soleus complex.
      - Overlengthening of the Achilles tendon may cause a crouched gait and calcaneus foot position, resulting in poor push-off power. This is less of a problem with a gastrocnemius-soleus recession than with a lengthening of the Achilles tendon.
  2. Equinovarus deformity of the foot can cause painful weight bearing over the lateral border of the foot and instability in the stance phase of gait.
    a. Generally, isolated forefoot supination is the result of excessive tension of the tibialis anterior muscle, whereas hindfoot varus comes from excessive tension of the tibialis posterior muscle.
    b. The tibialis anterior and the tibialis posterior muscles (the invertor muscles) overpower the peroneal muscles (the evertor muscles), whereas a tight gastrocnemius-soleus muscle complex causes equinus.
    c. Dynamic EMG is useful in determining whether the anterior tibialis and/or the posterior tibialis is causing a varus deformity of the foot.
    d. Clinically, the tibialis anterior muscle can be assessed using the confusion test.
      - The patient sits on the edge of the examining table and flexes the hip actively.
      - The tibialis anterior muscle will activate and contract.
      - If the forefoot supinates as it dorsiflexes, a varus deformity of the foot is at least partly the result of overactivity of the tibialis anterior muscle.

10 | Pediatrics

e. Clinically, the posterior tibialis muscle is assessed by tightness when the hindfoot is positioned in valgus.

f. Split tendon transfers of the anterior tibialis muscle and/or posterior tibialis muscle are recommended for the correction of varus deformity of the foot in CP, rather than full tendon transfers, because the latter may cause overcorrection.

g. Lengthening of the tibialis posterior muscle is helpful in less severe deformities caused by this muscle.

h. In the case of a rigid varus deformity, both soft-tissue and bony procedures (calcaneal osteotomy) are necessary.

3. Equinovalgus arises from spasticity of the gastrocnemius-soleus muscle complex and peroneus muscle with weakness of the tibialis posterior muscle.

a. Weight-bearing AP radiographs of the ankles must be obtained in cases of equinovalgus because valgus may contribute to ankle deformity.

b. Nonsurgical treatment of equinovalgus includes bracing treatment with a supramalleolar orthosis or AFO, physical therapy for ROM, and may include injection of botulinum toxin.

c. Surgical treatment—Calcaneal osteotomies preserve ROM and are preferred when feasible.

- Moderate deformity—Calcaneal lengthening with lengthening of the peroneus brevis muscle is preferred because it can restore the anatomy of the foot and ankle. Lengthening of the peroneus longus should be avoided because it can increase dorsiflexion of the first ray.
- Severe deformity—A medial calcaneal sliding osteotomy brings the calcaneus into line with the weight-bearing axis of the tibia. It is performed concomitantly with medial closing wedge osteotomy of the cuneiform bone, opening wedge osteotomy of the cuboid bone, and lengthening of the Achilles tendon.
- Arthrodesis should be considered if the patient has poor selective control of the muscles crossing the joint and if deformity is severe.
- Subtalar arthrodesis is sometimes needed but may be necessary in the presence of marked deformity or ligamentous laxity.
- Triple arthrodesis is rarely required.

4. Planovalgus/pes planus

a. Pes planus is common in patients with diplegia and quadriplegia.

b. The foot is externally rotated by spasticity of the gastrocnemius, soleus, and peroneal muscles, with weak function of the tibialis posterior muscle.

c. Patients bear weight on the medial border of the foot, on the talar head.

d. The foot is unstable in push-off.

e. Treatment

- Feet with mild planovalgus can be treated with supramalleolar orthoses or AFOs.
- GMFCS I or II: calcaneal lengthening
- GMFCS III/IV: subtalar fusion
- Moderate to severe deformities can be treated with a calcaneal osteotomy
  - A calcaneal lengthening osteotomy (best undertaken after age 6 years) can restore normal anatomy and is combined with lengthening of the peroneus brevis muscle and tightening of the medial talonavicular joint capsule and/or the posterior tibial tendon. Note that the peroneus longus muscle should be not routinely lengthened because this exacerbates dorsiflexion of the first ray.
  - A medial calcaneal sliding osteotomy with plantar flexion closing-wedge osteotomies of the cuneiform bones and an opening wedge osteotomy of the cuboid bone can also improve foot alignment.
- Severe deformities can be treated with subtalar fusion, although this is usually needed only in very large children and/or those with extreme laxity or poor ambulation (triple arthrodesis is almost never required.)
- Compensatory midfoot supination can be treated with plantar flexion osteotomy of the first ray, often with lengthening of the peroneus brevis muscle.

5. Hallux valgus deformity occurs frequently with pes valgus, equinovalgus, and equinovarus feet.

a. Toe straps added to AFOs or nighttime splinting of hallux valgus may be helpful.

b. Severe hallux valgus should be treated with fusion of the first metatarsophalangeal (MTP) joint.

c. Pes valgus must be simultaneously corrected to avoid recurrence.

d. Pitfalls—At the time of correction of hallux valgus, the patient also will often have valgus interphalangeus, which should be treated with proximal phalanx (Akin) osteotomy.

6. A dorsal bunion is a deformity in which the great toe is flexed in relation to an elevated metatarsal bone, causing a prominence over the uncovered metatarsal head, which can be painful with the wearing of shoes.

   a. Dorsal bunions may be iatrogenic, occurring after surgery to balance the foot. The deformation may be caused either by an overpowering tibialis anterior muscle or an overpowering flexor hallucis longus (FHL) muscle.

   b. Treatment

      - Nonsurgical treatment of a dorsal bunion is done with shoes having soft, deep toe boxes.
      - Surgical treatment is needed in recalcitrant cases. Flexible deformities are treated with lengthening or split transfer of the anterior tibialis muscle and transfer of the FHL muscle to the plantar aspect of the first metatarsal head. Rigid deformities require fusion of the first MTP joint and lengthening or split transfer of the anterior tibialis.

P. Upper extremity problems specific to CP

1. General information—Involvement of the upper extremities is typical in patients with hemiplegia and quadriplegia as effects of CP. Commonly, the hand is in a fist, the thumb is in the palm, the forearm is flexed and pronated, the wrist is flexed, and the shoulder is internally rotated.

2. Nonsurgical treatment

   a. Occupational therapy for patients with upper extremity problems is useful in early childhood for activities of daily living, stretching, and splinting.

   b. Botulinum toxin is useful for treating dynamic deformities.

   c. Constraint-induced therapy (splinting of the uninvolved upper extremity to encourage use of the involved arm) in patients with hemiplegia is becoming common but does not have extensive data.

3. Surgical treatment

   a. Surgical treatment is undertaken primarily for functional concerns, hygiene, and sometimes appearance.

   b. Adduction of the shoulder and contractures on internal rotation may be treated with release of the subscapularis muscle and lengthening of the pectoralis major muscle. A proximal humeral derotational osteotomy is rarely necessary.

   c. Contractures on elbow flexion may be treated with resection of the lacertus fibrosis (bicipital aponeurosis), lengthening of the biceps and brachialis muscles, and release of the brachioradialis muscle at its origin.

   d. Contractures on elbow pronation

      - Release or rerouting of the pronator teres should be considered. Transfer of the pronator teres to an anterolateral position (to act as a supinator) may cause a supination deformity, which is not preferable to pronation.
      - Transfer of the flexor carpi ulnaris (FCU) to the extensor carpi radialis brevis may also ease supination.

   e. Dislocation of the head of the radius is uncommon and, if symptomatic, may be treated with excision of the radial head when the patient reaches maturity.

   f. Wrist deformities usually include flexion contracture with ulnar deviation and are associated with weak wrist extension and a pronated forearm.

      - If finger extension is good and there is little spasticity on flexion of the wrist, the FCU or the flexor carpi radialis (FCR) muscle should be lengthened.
      - Releasing the wrist and finger flexors and the pronator teres from the medial epicondyle of the humerus weakens wrist and finger flexion but is nonselective.
      - In severe spasticity, an FCU transfer is recommended.
         - If grasp is good, release is weak, and the FCU is active in release, it should be transferred to the extensor digitorum communis muscle.
         - If grasp is weak, release is good, and the FCU is active in grasp, it should be transferred to the extensor carpi radialis brevis (ECRB) muscle.

10 | Pediatrics

- A concurrent release of the FCR can excessively weaken flexion of the wrist and should not be done.

4. Hand deformities
   a. Thumb-in-palm deformity can be treated with release of the adductor pollicis muscle, transfer of tendons to improve extension, and stabilization of the metacarpophalangeal (MCP) joint.
   b. Clawing of the fingers, with wrist flexion and hyperextension at the MCP joint, can be treated with transfer of the FCR or FCU muscle to the ECRB.
   c. Contraction on finger flexion is treated with lengthening or tenotomy of the flexor digitorum sublimis (FDS) and flexor digitorum longus (FDL) muscles.
   d. Swan neck deformities of the fingers are a result of intrinsic muscle tightness and extrinsic overpull of the finger extensor muscles. These deformities are sometimes caused by wrist flexion or weak wrist extensors and can sometimes be helped by correcting deformity in wrist flexion.

Q. Fractures specific to CP
1. Nonambulatory patients are at risk for fracture because of low bone-mineral density (BMD), which may be exacerbated by non–weight bearing, poor calcium intake, or antiseizure medications.
2. Intravenous pamidronate should be considered for children with three or more fractures and a dual-energy radiograph absorptiometry Z-score of less than 2 SD.

II. MYELOMENINGOCELE

A. Overview/epidemiology
1. Myelodysplasia/spina bifida disorders comprise a spectrum of congenital malformation of the spinal column and spinal cord resulting from failure of closure of the neural crests (neural tube) at 3 to 4 weeks after fertilization.
2. Spina bifida occulta is the failure of posterior bony spinal elements to fuse but causes no neurologic impairment.
3. In a meningocele, the dura and tissue overlying the spinal cord pouch out through the bony defect, but the spinal cord remains within the spinal canal, frequently causing little neurologic impairment.
4. In a myelomeningocele, overlying tissues and the spinal cord are not contained by the unfused posterior bony spine elements. The neural elements can be found covered in a pouch of skin, or with only dura, or entirely exposed. This can cause major motor and sensory deficits.
5. Myelomeningocele is the most common major birth defect, occurring in 0.9 per 1,000 live births.
6. Prenatal diagnosis made through assay of the a-fetoprotein concentration in maternal serum is 60% to 95% accurate.
7. The diagnosis also can be made with ultrasonography or by amniocentesis.
8. Women of childbearing age should be encouraged to have a diet with adequate folic acid intake. Supplementation with folic acid decreases the risk of spina bifida, but only if done in the first weeks after conception. Supplemental intake of folic acid also has been addressed by adding folic acid to many foods, such as breads and cereals.

B. Risk factors
1. History of a previously affected pregnancy
2. Low folic acid intake
3. Pregestational maternal diabetes
4. In utero exposure to valproic acid or carbamazepine

C. Classification
1. Motor level and functional status are given in **Table 6**.
2. Spinal functional integrity at the L4 level or lower (active quadriceps muscle function) is considered necessary for ambulation in the community.

D. Treatment—The long-term medical and skeletal issues associated with myelomeningocele are often best addressed by multidisciplinary teams.
1. Nonsurgical treatment
   a. Frequent skin checks for pressure sores, and well-fitting braces and wheelchairs, are important in the management of myelomeningocele because those it affects often have substantial sensory deficits.
   b. Urologic and gastrointestinal issues, including detrusor malfunction and abnormal sphincter tone, make early catheterization and bowel regimens important. Kidney reflux and pyelonephritis cause substantial morbidity and mortality in patients with myelomeningocele.
   c. Late issues requiring neurosurgery are common (tethering, syrinx, and shunts), making carefully recorded neurologic examinations important.

TABLE 6

Motor Level and Functional Status for Myelomeningocele

Group	Lesion Level	Muscle Involvement	Function	Ambulation
1	Thoracic/high lumbar	No quadriceps function	Sitter Possible household ambulatory with RGO	Some degree until the age of 13 yr with HKAFO, RGO 95%-99% wheelchair dependent as adults
2	Low lumbar	Quadriceps and medial hamstring function, no gluteus medius or maximus	Household/community ambulator with KAFO or AFO	Require AFO and crutches, 79% community ambulators as adults, wheelchair for long distances; substantial difference between L3 and L4 level, medial hamstring needed for community ambulation
3	Sacral	Quadriceps and gluteus medius function	Community ambulator with AFO, UCBL, or none	94% retain walking ability as adults
	High sacral	No gastrocnemius-soleus strength		Walk without support but require AFO; have gluteus lurch and excessive pelvic obliquity and rotation during gait
	Low sacral	Good gastrocnemius-soleus strength, normal gluteus medius and maximus		Walk without AFO; gait close to normal

AFO = ankle-foot orthosis, HKAFO = hip-knee-ankle-foot orthosis, KAFO = knee-ankle-foot orthosis, RGO = reciprocating gait orthosis, UCBL = University of California/Berkeley Laboratory (orthosis)

Reproduced from Sarwark F, Aminian A, Westberry DE, Davids JR, Karol LA: Neuromuscular disorders in children, in Vaccaro AR, ed: *Orthopaedic Knowledge Update*, ed 8. Rosemont, IL American Academy of Orthopaedic Surgeons, 2005, p 678.

d. Latex allergies are common in patients with myelomeningocele, necessitating precautions against contact with latex for all patients with this condition.

e. Rehabilitation efforts should include early mobilization, physical therapy, bracing treatment, and wheelchair fitting for optimal physical function.

f. Bracing treatment

- Hip-knee-ankle-foot orthoses, KAFOs, or AFOs are frequently used to support stance and/or prevent contracture in patients with myelomeningocele.
- As the child grows, bracing treatment and crutch requirements may decrease with gains in skills or may increase if there is weight gain or development of deformity.

E. The spine

1. Delivery of infants with myelomeningocele is done by cesarean section to avoid further neurologic damage. Neurosurgical closure of myelomeningocele is done within 48 hours after delivery, with a shunt used to treat hydrocephalus. Closure of myelomeningocele also can be done prenatally.
2. Tethering of the spinal cord in a child with myelomeningocele can cause progressive scoliosis, alter the child's functional capabilities, or cause spasticity.
3. Syrinx, shunt problems, or new hydrocephalus can cause new symptoms affecting the upper extremities, such as weakness or increasing spasticity.
4. An Arnold-Chiari malformation is often addressed with shunting in infancy to control hydrocephalus but may later require decompression. Later symptoms may include spasticity or weakness of the lower extremities, problems with swallowing, and absence of the cough reflex.
5. Scoliosis and kyphosis may be progressive in myelomeningocele.

   a. Kyphectomy and posterior fusion may be needed in 90% of patients with thoracic myelomeningocele; surgery may be needed in 10% of patients with myelomeningocele at L4.

   b. Prior to kyphectomy, it is important to check shunt function because shunt failure can result in acute hydrocephalus and death when the spinal cord is tied off during kyphectomy.

F. The hip

1. Flexion contractures are common in patients with myelomeningocele but are often not severe. Contracture exceeding 40° in patients with involvement at the lower lumbar level may require flexor muscle release.
2. Dysplasia and/or dislocation of the hip occurs in 80% of patients with involvement at the midlumbar level.
   a. These patients have medial hamstring and quadriceps muscle function and poor hip extensor and abductor function, causing muscle imbalance that results in hip dysplasia and instability.
   b. Currently, the trend in treatment is not to reduce a dislocated hip in any child with myelomeningocele.
   c. The exception to nontreatment for hip dislocation in children with myelomeningocele may be a unilateral dislocation of the hip in a child with a low-level lesion (ie, a community ambulator). However, the rate of recurrence of dislocation is high, and the procedure is controversial.

G. The knee

1. Flexion contracture of the knee exceeding 20° should be treated with hamstring lengthening, capsular release, growth modulation of the anterior distal femoral physis, and/or distal femoral extension osteotomy. There is, however, a substantial rate of recurrence of flexion contracture after extension osteotomy in growing children.
2. Extension contracture of the knee can be treated with serial casting or V-Y quadriceps lengthening.
3. Knee valgus, often with associated external tibial torsion and femoral anteversion, is common in patients with midlumbar-level involvement by myelomeningocele because they lack functional hip abductors and have a substantial trunk shift when walking with AFOs. This can be addressed with the use of KAFOs or crutches with AFOs.
4. External tibial torsion can be addressed with a distal tibial derotational osteotomy.

H. Myelomeningocele foot

1. About 30% of children with myelomeningocele have a rigid clubfoot.
2. With surgical treatment, portions of the tendons of the foot (eg, Achilles, tibialis posterior, FHL, flexor digitorum communis) may be resected rather than lengthened to decrease the risk of recurrence of clubfoot.
3. Equinus contracture is common in patients with thoracic and high lumbar level involvement by myelomeningocele.
4. Calcaneus foot position can occur with unopposed contraction of the anterior tibialis muscle (myelomeningocele affecting the L3-L4 level of the spine).
5. Equinovarus, equinus, and calcaneal foot deformities are often best treated with a simple tenotomy rather than tendon transfer, achieving a flail but braceable foot.
6. Valgus foot deformities are common in patients with myelomeningocele at the L4-L5 level. If surgery is necessary to achieve a plantigrade foot, fusion should be avoided to maintain foot flexibility and decrease the risk of pressure sores.

I. Fractures in children

1. In children without sensation, fractures often present with erythema, warmth, and swelling.
2. A child with myelomeningocele who presents with a red, hot, and swollen leg should be suspected of having a fracture until proven otherwise.

III. MUSCULAR DYSTROPHIES

A. Overview

1. Muscular dystrophies are muscle diseases of genetic origin that cause progressive weakness (**Table 7**).
2. Although muscular dystrophies are genetically based, new mutations causative of these diseases are frequent; thus, for example, one-third of cases of Duchenne muscular dystrophy (DMD) are the result of new mutations that arise during spermatogenesis on the patient's mother's paternal side.

B. Duchenne muscular dystrophy

1. DMD is an X-linked recessive progressive myopathy involving skeletal and cardiac muscle that has an incidence of 1 in 3,500 males. The involved gene (Xp21.2) encodes dystrophin, a protein that stabilizes the muscle cell membrane. In DMD, dystrophin is absent, whereas its presence in the less severe Becker dystrophy is subnormal.
2. DMD presents between ages 3 and 6 years with toe-walking or flatfootedness, difficulty in running or climbing stairs, and the classic calf pseudohypertrophy, which is seen in 85% of patients (**Figure 5**). Elevated creatine phosphokinase (CPK) levels (100× normal) are usually diagnostic.

TABLE 7

Muscular Dystrophies

Type	Frequency	Inheritance	Gene Defect	Diagnostic Features	EMG/Biopsy	Clinical Course
Duchenne (DMD)	1/3,500 males	X-linked recessive	Xp21 dystrophin, point deletion, nonsense mutation, no dystrophin protein produced	Two of three diagnosed by DNA, CPK 10-200× normal Delayed walking, waddling gait, toe walking, Gowers sign, calf pseudohypertrophy Present deep tendon reflexes, lumbar hyperlordosis, often with static encephalopathy	EMG: Myopathic, decreased amplitude, short duration, polyphasic motor Biopsy: Fibrofatty muscle replacement	Decreasing ambulation by age 6-8 yr, transitions to wheelchair about age 12 yr. Progressive scoliosis and respiratory illness, cardiac failure, death toward end of second decade
Becker	1/30,000 males	X-linked recessive	Xp21 dystrophin in noncoding region with normal reading frame, lesser amounts of truncated dystrophin produced	CPK less elevated than in DMD, similar physical findings but later onset and less progressive	Similar to DMD, but some dystrophin present by biopsy	Onset after age 7 yr, slower progression, walks into teens, Cardiac and pulmonary symptoms present but less severe Equinus frequent
Emery-Dreifuss	Uncommon	X-linked recessive but seen mildly in females	Xq28	Mildly elevated CPK, toe walking Distinctive clinical contractures of Achilles, elbows, and neck extension occur in late childhood	Myopathic	Slowly progressive; walks into sixth decade
Limb girdle	1/14,500	Heterogeneous, mostly AR	AD 5q, AR 15q	CPK mildly elevated, mild DMD symptoms, muscle weakness in the muscles around the shoulder and hip	Dystrophic muscle biopsy	Begins in second or third decade; death before age 40 yr
Adult fascioscapular humeral dystrophy	Rare	AD	4q35	CPK normal Face, shoulder, upper arm affected		Weak shoulder flexion and abduction Normal life expectancy
Infantile fascioscapular humeral dystrophy	Rare	AR	Unknown	Face, shoulder, upper arm affected; weak gluteus maximus muscle leading to substantial lumbar lordosis		Lumbar lordosis leads to wheelchair dependency and fixed hip flexion contractures
Myotonic	13/100,000 adults (most common neuromuscular disease in adults)	AD	C9 near myotin protein kinase gene Severity increases with amplification (number of trinucleotide repeats increases with oogenesis) Mildly affected mothers may have severely affected children	Often severe hypotonia at birth Weakness is worse distally than proximally (unlike DMD)	EMG demonstrates classic "dive bomber" response	75% survive at birth, growing stronger with age, walk by age 5 yr Equinus deformities and distal weakness are common "Drooping face" appearance Cardiomyopathy and conduction problems frequent, very sensitive to anesthesia

AD = autosomal dominant, AR = autosomal recessive, CPK = creatine phosphokinase, DMD = Duchenne muscular dystrophy, EMG = electromyography

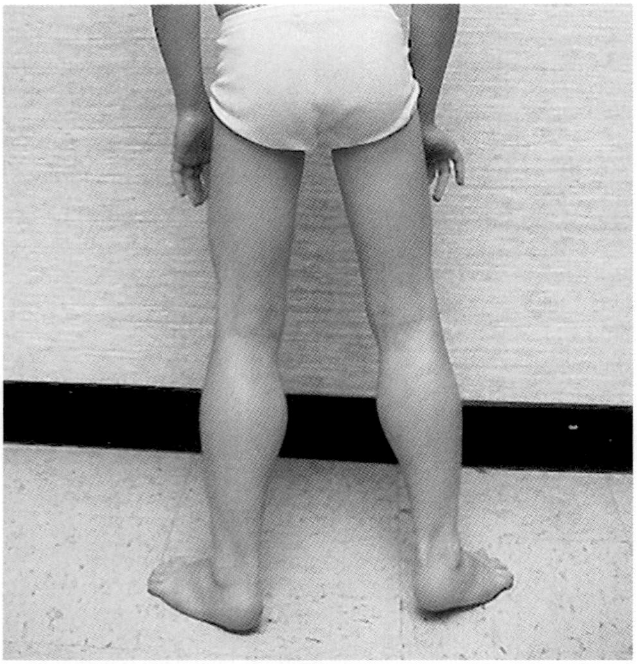

Figure 5 Photograph of a 5-year-old boy with Duchenne muscular dystrophy (DMD). The marked pseudohypertrophy of the calves is a common physical finding in DMD. (Reproduced from Sussman M: Duchenne muscular dystrophy. *J Am Acad Orthop Surg* 2002;10[2]:138-151.)

3. Weakness in DMD presents proximally, first in the gluteus maximus muscle and then in the quadriceps and hip abductors. Gowers sign describes patients' use of their hands to push their legs into extension.
4. With age, DMD in male children continues to worsen, causing shoulder weakness and scoliosis. Ambulation is often limited by the age of 10 years.
5. Nonsurgical management
   a. Corticosteroid therapy: Deflazacort (Emflaza) has been U.S. FDA approved
      - Prolongs ambulation, slows progression of scoliosis, and slows the deterioration of forced vital capacity. With Deflazacort, the rate that boys with DMD develop scoliosis that requires spine fusion has dropped from 92% to 20%.
      - The optimum age for beginning therapy is 5 to 7 years.
      - Treatment is associated with a high risk of complications and side effects, including osteonecrosis, obesity, Cushingoid appearance, gastrointestinal symptoms, mood swings, headaches, short stature, and cataracts.

   b. There is intense interest in gene therapy for DMD, but have as of yet had limited success. For instance, Eteplirsen (Exondys 51, Sarepta Therapeutics) developed to treat DMD, only targets mutations in about 13% of patients.
   c. Nighttime ventilation substantially prolongs survival.
   d. Rehabilitation includes physical therapy for ROM, the use of adaptive equipment and power wheelchairs, and nighttime bracing treatment.
6. Surgical management
   a. Surgery on the lower extremities is controversial in children with DMD.
      - If surgery is performed, the focus should be on early postoperative mobilization and ambulation to prevent deconditioning and deterioration.
      - If surgery is performed, it should include the release of contractures (with lengthening of the hip abductors, hamstrings, Achilles tendon, tibialis posterior muscles) while a child is still ambulatory.

   b. Spine—Scoliosis develops in 95% of patients with DMD after they transition to a wheelchair (usually around age 12 years).
      - Bracing treatment is ineffective and not recommended.
      - Early posterior instrumented fusion (for spinal curvature of 20° or more) is recommended before loss of forced vital capacity from respiratory muscle weakness and progressively decreasing cardiac output.
      - Stiff curves may require anterior and posterior fusion.

   c. Patients with DMD are at risk for malignant hyperthermia and may be pretreated with dantrolene.

IV. SPINAL MUSCULAR ATROPHY

A. Overview

1. Spinal muscular atrophy (SMA) is a genetic disease that is most commonly fatal during childhood. It has an incidence of 1 in 10,000 live births.
2. There are numerous subtypes. The inheritance pattern of SMA is primarily autosomal recessive.

3. Progressive weakness starts proximally and moves distally through the body.

B. Classification:

1. SMA type I (acute Werdnig-Hoffmann disease) onset occurs at birth, with severe involvement of the spinal muscles. Death from respiratory failure occurs by age 2 years.
2. SMA type II (chronic Werdnig-Hoffman disease) onset occurs at age 6 to 18 months and causes diminishing function with time. Weakness is worse in lower extremities.
   a. Hip dislocations (60%), scoliosis, and joint contractures are common.
   b. Life expectancy is 15+ years.
3. SMA type III (Kugelberg-Welander) onset occurs after age 18 months, with physical manifestations similar to those of SMA type II, but patients with type III can stand independently, walking early but progressing to wheelchairs as adults, and have more proximal weakness. Life expectancy is normal.
4. Type IV: Adult onset (after 30 years of age), with moderate proximal muscle weakness.

C. Pathoanatomy

1. Mutations in the survival motor neuron (SMN) gene on chromosome 5q cause deficiency of the SMN protein, resulting in progressive loss of alpha-motor neurons in the anterior horn of the spinal cord and progressive weakness.
2. Two genes, SMN I and SMN II, both at 5q13, are involved in the occurrence of SMA. They both code for the SMN protein, but SMN II codes for a less functional SMN protein.
   a. All patients with SMA lack both copies of SMN I.
   b. The severity of SMA is determined by the number of functional copies of the SMN II gene. Healthy individuals have two SMA II gene copies. In patients with SMA, the mutation in SMN I can functionally convert it to SMN II. Patients with SMA can have up to four functional copies. The more functional copies of SMA II they have, the better they do.

D. Medical treatment:

1. Nusinersen (ISIS-SMN) (SPINRAZA) is an antisense oligonucleotide drug administered intrathecally to treat SMA. Alters the splicing of SMN2 mRNA and increases the amount of functional SMN protein produced. More effective in infantile and childhood onset SMA. Nusinersen is one of the most expensive drugs in the world (>$100,000 per dose), and its cost effectiveness is under review.
   a. Recently, a subcutaneous intrathecal catheter system has been developed to allow repeated outpatient dosing, even in the setting of spine fusion. Spinal fusion can also include a "skip segment" to allow intrathecal access.
2. Scoliosis is very common and progressive in SMA (>90%) Onset can be as early as 8 months of age, average between 6 and 8 years of age. Most type 2 SMA patients develop scoliosis. Progression is faster in patients who have stopped walking, about 10°/yr.
   a. A thoracolumbosacral orthosis improves sitting balance in patients with SMA but does not stop progression of the disease.
   b. Surgery is generally considered for patients >10 years of age with curve >40°
      - A vertical expandable prosthetic titanium rib (VEPTR) for thoracic insufficiency in young patients with SMA II who have spinal curves exceeding 50° has produced good results.
      - Magnetic growing rods (MAGEC) or VEPTR are commonly used in children <5 years of age with severe and/or progressive curves.
      - Posterior spinal fusion with fixation to the pelvis is performed when the spinal curvature exceeds 40° and forced vital capacity is more than 40% of normal. Fusion may cause an ambulatory child to lose the ability to walk (and may cause temporary loss of upper extremity function) because of loss of trunk motion.
3. Hip dislocation
   a. May be unilateral or bilateral
   b. Treatment of hip dysplasia and instability in SMA is controversial, but may become a more viable option as function improves with the use of nusinersen.
   c. The presence of pain should be the main indication for treatment and may require release of the hip adductor and flexor and/or osteotomies to maintain reduction of hip dislocation and minimize symptoms.
4. Contractures of the lower extremities are common in SMA.
   a. Hip and knee contractures exceeding 30° to 40° are not generally treated surgically. Hamstring lengthening may sometimes be considered for contractures smaller than this

in patients who are strong enough and have a strong motivation to walk.

b. Foot deformities such as equinovarus occur commonly in SMA. Rarely, if the patient is ambulatory and retains strength, tenotomy of the gastrocnemius-soleus, posterior tibialis, FDL, and FHL tendons may be done to maintain standing and walking.

V. HEREDITARY MOTOR SENSORY NEUROPATHY (CHARCOT-MARIE-TOOTH DISEASE)

A. Hereditary motor sensory neuropathies (HMSNs) are chronic progressive peripheral neuropathies. They are common causes of cavus feet in children but may not be diagnosed before age 10 years. Presents with cavus feet, claw toes, and sometimes foot drop. Feet are affected first, followed by hands and tongue, with increased incidence of scoliosis and hip dysplasia. Weakness of the proximal muscles is rare in Charcot-Marie-Tooth (CMT) disease, except in the most severe cases. Blood tests currently identify about 90% of known mutations. EMG/nerve conduction studies will also identify demyelinating CMT.

B. Classification

1. HMSN type I (CMT type I)

   a. Is the most common type of HMSN, with an incidence of 1 in 2,500 children.

   b. Peripheral myelin degeneration occurs with decreased motor nerve conduction.

   c. Commonly caused by duplication of the gene at 17p11 affecting peripheral myelin protein 22 (*PMP-22*) and mutations in X-linked connexin 32.

   d. Autosomal dominant inheritance is the most common mode of inheritance of HMSN I, but its inheritance also can be autosomal recessive, X-linked, or sporadic.

   e. The onset of HMSN I occurs in the first to second decade of life.

   f. HMSN I (CMT I) shows slowed nerve conduction velocity (by definition <38 m/s) in upper limbmotor nerves.

2. HMSN type II (CMT type II)

   a. The myelin sheath is intact, but Wallerian axonal degeneration occurs, with decreased motor and sensory conduction.

   b. Autosomal dominant inheritance is the most common mode of inheritance of HMSN II, but it also can be inherited in an autosomal recessive, X-linked, or sporadic manner.

   c. The age at onset of HMSN II is the second decade of life or later.

   d. EMG shows a normal or slightly prolonged duration of the muscle action potential.

3. HMSN type III (Dejerine-Sottas disease)

   a. This type of HMSN is characterized by peripheral-nerve demyelination with severely decreased motor nerve conduction.

   b. An autosomal recessive mode of inheritance is common for HMSN III, with the causative mutation for the disease occurring in the myelin protein zero (*MPZ*) gene.

   c. HMSN III presents in infancy.

   d. HMSN III is characterized by enlarged peripheral nerves, ataxia, and nystagmus. The patient stops walking by maturity.

   e. Other peripheral-nerve abnormalities in HMSN III include polyneuritis and atrophy of the small muscles of the hands.

4. HSMN IV (CMT IV): Severe, early-onset CMT. Multiple subtypes with multiple gene defects.

C. Treatment

1. HMSN commonly presents as distal weakness, affecting intrinsic and extrinsic muscles.

2. Decreased sensation and areflexia also may be present.

3. Hip dysplasia (occurring in 5% to 10% of patients) results from weak hip abductor and extensor muscles.

   a. Hip dysplasia requires treatment, even if not symptomatic.

   b. Acetabular reconstruction is usually performed before VDRO.

4. Cavus foot (**Figure 6**)

   a. Cavus foot in HMSN results from contracted plantar fascia, weak anterior tibialis and peroneal muscles, and tightness of intrinsic muscles of the foot with normal FDL and FHL. The relatively stronger peroneus longus overpowers the tibialis anterior, causing first ray plantarflexion. Weak peroneus brevis allows heel varus.

   b. The peroneus longus muscle is generally somewhat stronger than the peroneus brevis and anterior tibialis muscles.

   c. Initial management includes PT and orthotics

   d. Surgery for cavus feet is performed to balance the muscle forces in the feet and maintain flexibility. Coleman block test assess rigidity of the heel varus.

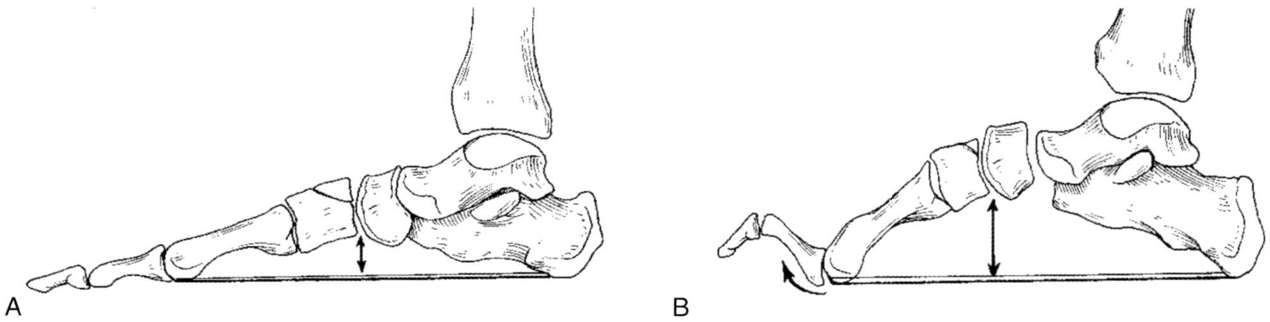

Figure 6 Illustrations show a normal foot and a cavus foot. **A**, Normal foot with normal arch height (double arrow) during standing. **B**, Cavus foot with increased arch height (double arrow) as a result of metatarsophalangeal joint hyperextension (curved arrow), such as occurs at toe-off and as seen in the windlass effect of the plantar fascia. (Reproduced from Schwend RM, Drennan JC: Cavus foot deformity in children. *J Am Acad Orthop Surg* 2003;11[3]:201-211.)

e. Flexible cavovarus foot is typically treated with plantar fascia release, peroneus longus to peroneus brevis transfer, EHL transfer to the first MT head, proximal first MT or medial cuneiform closing wedge osteotomy, tibialis anterior transfer.

f. For fixed hindfoot varus (as determined with the Coleman block test), osteotomies to correct bony deformities in adolescence include a calcaneal osteotomy (Dwyer)

g. Claw toes may become rigid and require treatment, such as interphalangeal fusion, often in conjunction with Jones transfers of the extensor tendons to the metatarsal heads.

5. Scoliosis or kyphoscoliosis is seen in 15% to 37% of children with HMSN and in up to 50% of patients with HMSN who are skeletally mature; it is more common in children with HMSN I and in girls.
   a. Bracing treatment arrests the progression of scoliosis or kyphoscoliosis in a few cases.
   b. Surgery using posterior fusion is effective.
   c. Intraoperative somatosensory cortical evoked potentials may show a lack of signal transmission in patients with HMSN.
6. Intrinsic muscles of the hand and the thenar and hypothenar muscles may show wasting, limiting thumb abduction, and compromising pinch power. Surgically, transfer of the FDS, nerve decompression, release of contractures, and joint arthrodesis may be helpful.

VI. FRIEDREICH ATAXIA

A. Friedreich ataxia (FA) is the most common form of the uncommon spinocerebellar degenerative diseases. It occurs in 1 in 50,000 births. Autosomal recessive; it is a trinucleotide repeat disorder, like Huntington disease and myotonic dystrophy.

1. The onset of FA occurs before the age of 25 years.
2. FA is progressive and affects the heart and nervous system with ataxia, areflexia, a positive extensor plantar response (upgoing Babinski), sensory impairment, and weakness. Often, the gluteus maximus is the first muscle involved, and scoliosis and cavovarus are significant.
3. Associated with hypertrophic cardiomyopathy, diabetes (10%), hearing or vision loss, and dysarthria.
4. Death (from cardiomyopathy) usually occurs by the fourth or fifth decade of life.
5. Nerve conduction velocity is decreased in the upper extremities.

B. Pathoanatomy

1. The genetic mutation responsible for FA is multiple repetition of the base sequence guanine-adenine-adenine (GAA) in the frataxin (*FXN*) gene on chromosome 9q13, causing a lack of the protein frataxin, which is required for normal regulation of cellular iron homeostasis.
2. The age of onset of FA is related to the number of GAA repeats, with a greater number of repeats associated with an earlier age of onset of the disease.

C. Treatment

1. The pes cavovarus in FA is progressive, rigid, and resistant to bracing treatment.
   a. Ambulatory patients may be treated with tendon lengthenings and transfers.
   b. For rigid deformities, arthrodesis is needed to achieve a plantigrade foot.

2. Scoliosis occurs frequently in FA (80%) and will usually progress if the onset of the disease occurred before the age of 10 years, and the scoliosis began before the age of 15 years. Bracing treatment is often ineffective in FA.
3. Posterior instrumented spinal fusion is effective for treating scoliosis in FA if curve is > 50° and does not need to extend to the pelvis. SSEP monitoring is often ineffective with FA.

VII. RETT SYNDROME

A. Overview

1. Rett syndrome (RTT) is a neurodevelopmental disorder affecting the gray matter of the brain. The syndrome has an X-linked dominant pattern of inheritance and is generally caused by a de novo mutation. The affected gene encodes the methyl-CpG-binding protein-2 (*MECP2*), which methylates DNA.
2. Because it is X-linked dominant, RTT is generally lethal in affected male fetuses. Those carried to term frequently die of neonatal encephalopathy by 2 years of age. Males with RTT may result from Klinefelter syndrome, in which the male has an XXY karyotype.
3. The incidence of RTT is 1 in 10,000 births.

B. Clinical presentation

1. Development is normal until 6 to 18 months of age, after which it causes developmental regression.
2. Regression, with signs of mental retardation, autism, and ataxia, is rapid until the age of 3 years, and is followed by a more stable phase until the age of 10 years.
3. Seizures are common (80%).
4. Behavioral abnormalities include hand-wringing and hand-mouthing, lack of purposeful hand function, screaming and crying, loss of speech, and grinding of the teeth.
5. One-half of children with RTT become unable to walk after the age of 10 years as the result of deterioration of motor function. Most have ataxia and spasticity.
6. Gastrointestinal disorders, especially constipation, are common. Swallowing problems are common.

C. Orthopaedic concerns

1. Scoliosis occurs in more than 50% of patients with RTT.
   a. Long, neuromuscular-type thoracolumbar spinal curves develop at about the age of 10 years.
   b. Bracing treatment is ineffective.
   c. Posterior spinal fusion is indicated when curves interfere with sitting or balance.
2. Spasticity frequently causes contractures, particularly equinus, in children with RTT.
3. Coxa valga occurs frequently, with hip instability, and should be treated to optimize function and/or decrease pain.

TOP TESTING FACTS

1. Used in the treatment for CP spasticity, botulinum toxin blocks the presynaptic release of acetylcholine and generally relaxes the muscles into which it is injected for 3 to 6 months.
2. Hip surveillance programs improve rates of successful early soft-tissue releases or pelvic and femoral osteotomies, and decrease the rates of hip dislocation and the need for hip salvage surgeries.
3. Eighty percent of patients with myelomeningocele at the midlumbar level have hip dysplasia or dislocations.
4. In children with myelomeningocele without sensation, fractures often present with erythema, warmth, and swelling.
5. Duchenne muscular dystrophy presents between ages 3 and 6 years with toe walking or flatfootedness, difficulty in running or climbing stairs, and the classic calf pseudohypertrophy (seen in 85% of patients).
6. In Duchenne muscular dystrophy Deflazacort corticosteroid prolongs ambulation, slows progression of scoliosis, and slows the deterioration of forced vital capacity. The optimum age for beginning therapy is 5 to 7 years.
7. In Duchenne muscular dystrophy, early posterior instrumented fusion (for spinal curvature of 20° or more) is recommended before loss of forced vital capacity from respiratory muscle weakness and progressively decreasing cardiac output.
8. In SMA (spinal muscle atrophy), nusinersen is a new antisense oligonucleotide drug used intrathecally; effective in infantile and childhood-onset SMA, but expensive. Progressive scoliosis affects >90% SMA as early as 8 months of age and surgery considered with progressive curves >40°.

9. Charcot-Marie-Tooth disease is the most common type of HMSN (hereditary motor sensory neuropathy), with an incidence of 1 in 2,500, and is the most common cause of bilateral cavus feet.
10. Friedreich ataxia presents by the age of 25 years, with ataxia, areflexia, a positive extensor plantar response, and weakness. Often the gluteus maximus is the first muscle involved. Cardiomyopathy, diabetes, dysarthria, deafness, and vision loss are common. The genetic mutation responsible for FA is multiple repetition of the base sequence GAA in the *FXN* gene on chromosome 9q13, causing a lack of the protein *frataxin*, which is required for normal regulation of cellular iron homeostasis.

Bibliography

Alman BA, Raza SN, Biggar WD: Steroid treatment and the development of scoliosis in males with duchenne muscular dystrophy. *J Bone Joint Surg Am* 2004;86(3):519-524.

Beaty JH, Canale ST: Orthopaedic aspects of myelomeningocele. *J Bone Joint Surg Am* 1990;72(4):626-630.

Boyd RN, Dobson F, Parrott J, et al: The effect of botulinum toxin type A and a variable hip abduction orthosis on gross motor function: A randomized controlled trial. *Eur J Neurol* 2001;8(suppl 5):109-119.

Chambers HG, Sutherland DH: A practical guide to gait analysis. *J Am Acad Orthop Surg* 2002;10(3):222-231.

Chan G, Bowen JR, Kumar SJ: Evaluation and treatment of hip dysplasia in Charcot-Marie-Tooth disease. *Orthop Clin North Am* 2006;37(2):203-209, vii.

Dabney KW, Miller F: Cerebral palsy, in Abel MF, ed: *Orthopaedic Knowledge Update: Pediatrics*, ed 3. Rosemont, IL, American Academy of Orthopaedic Surgeons, 2006, pp 93-109.

Davids JR, Rowan F, Davis RB: Indications for orthoses to improve gait in children with cerebral palsy. *J Am Acad Orthop Surg* 2007;15(3):178-188.

Flynn JM, Miller F: Management of hip disorders in patients with cerebral palsy. *J Am Acad Orthop Surg* 2002;10(3):198-209.

Gabrieli AP, Vankoski SJ, Dias LS, et al: Gait analysis in low lumbar myelomeningocele patients with unilateral hip dislocation or subluxation. *J Pediatr Orthop* 2003;23(3):330-334.

Gage JR, DeLuca PA, Renshaw TS: Gait analysis: Principle and applications with emphasis on its use in cerebral palsy. *Instr Course Lect* 1996;45:491-507.

Karol LA: Surgical management of the lower extremity in ambulatory children with cerebral palsy. *J Am Acad Orthop Surg* 2004;12(3):196-203.

Kerr Graham H, Selber P: Musculoskeletal aspects of cerebral palsy. *J Bone Joint Surg Br* 2003;85(2):157-166.

McCarthy JJ, D'Andrea LP, Betz RR, Clements DH: Scoliosis in the child with cerebral palsy. *J Am Acad Orthop Surg* 2006;14(6):367-375.

Mesfin A, Sponseller PD, Leet AI: Spinal muscular atrophy: Manifestations and management. *J Am Acad Orthop Surg.* 2012;20(6):393-401.

Olafsson Y, Saraste H, Al-Dabbagh Z: Brace treatment in neuromuscular spine deformity. *J Pediatr Orthop* 1999;19:376-379.

Renshaw TS, DeLuca PA: Cerebral palsy, in Morrissey RT, Weinstein WL, eds: *Lovell and Winter's Pediatric Orthopaedics*, ed 6. Philadelphia, PA, Lippincott Williams & Wilkins, 2006, pp 551-604.

Rodda JM, Graham HK, Nattrass GR, Galea MP, Baker R, Wolfe R: Correction of severe crouch gait in patients with spastic diplegia with use of multilevel orthopaedic surgery. *J Bone Joint Surg Am* 2006;88(12):2653-2664.

Saito N, Ebara S, Ohotsuka K, Kumeta H, Takaoka K: Natural history of scoliosis in spastic cerebral palsy. *Lancet* 1998;351:1687-1692.

Sarwark JF, Aminian A, Westberry DE, Davids JR, Karol LA: Neuromuscular disorders in children, in Vaccaro AR, ed: *Orthopaedic Knowledge Update*, ed 8. Rosemont, IL, American Academy of Orthopaedic Surgeons, 2005, pp 677-689.

Scher DM, Mubarak SJ: Surgical prevention of foot deformity in patients with Duchenne muscular dystrophy. *J Pediatr Orthop* 2002;22(3):384-391.

Schwartz MH, Rozumalski A, Steele KM: Dynamic motor control is associated with treatment outcomes for children with cerebral palsy. *Dev Med Child Neurol* 2016;58:1139-1146.

Schwend RM, Drennan JC: Cavus foot deformity in children. *J Am Acad Orthop Surg* 2003;11(3):201-211.

Shore BJ, Yu X, Desai S, Selber P, Wolfe R, Graham HK: Adductor surgery to prevent hip displacement in children with cerebral palsy: The predictive role of the Gross Motor Function Classification System. *J Bone Joint Surg Am* 2012;94:326-334.

Stout JL, Gage JR, Schwartz MH, Novacheck TF: Distal femoral extension osteotomy and patellar tendon advancement to treat persistent crouch gait in cerebral palsy. *J Bone Joint Surg Am* 2008;90(11):2470-2484.

Sussman M: Duchenne muscular dystrophy. *J Am Acad Orthop Surg* 2002;10(2):138-151.

Ward CM, Dolan L, Bennett L, Morcuende J, Cooper R: Long-term results of reconstruction for treatment of a flexible cavovarus foot in Charcot-Marie-Tooth disease. *J Bone Joint Surg Am* 2008;90:2631-2642.

Westberry DE, Davids JR: Cerebral palsy, in Song KM, ed: *Orthopaedic Knowledge Update: Pediatrics*, ed 4. Rosemont IL, American Academy of Orthopaedic Surgeons, 2011, pp 95-104.

Chapter 132

Musculoskeletal Infection of Children and Adolescents

NICOLE MONTGOMERY, MD
HOWARD R. EPPS, MD
SCOTT B. ROSENFELD, MD

10 | Pediatrics

I. OVERVIEW

A. Musculoskeletal infection includes septic arthritis, abscess (intraosseous, subperiosteal, and soft tissue), osteomyelitis, pyomyositis.

1. Infection types may be isolated or occur concurrently.

B. Musculoskeletal infections can cause substantial morbidity and complications in the pediatric population.

C. The annual incidence of osteomyelitis in children is 13 per 100,000 which is twice that of septic arthritis.

D. Pediatric musculoskeletal infection represents a diagnostic challenge due to varying clinical presentation and symptoms which overlap with noninfectious diagnoses.

1. The differential diagnosis includes but is not limited to cellulitis, transient synovitis, fracture/trauma, thrombophlebitis, rheumatic fever, viral illness, chronic recurrent multifocal osteomyelitis (CRMO), juvenile arthritis, bone infarction, Gaucher disease, and malignancy (including leukemia).

E. The evaluation and management of a patient with suspected musculoskeletal infection should be prompt and focused to avoid delay in treatment.

Dr. Epps or an immediate family member is a member of a speakers' bureau or has made paid presentations on behalf of Orthopediatrics; serves as an unpaid consultant to Orthopediatrics; and serves as a board member, owner, officer, or committee member of the Pediatric Orthopaedic Society of North America. Dr. Rosenfeld or an immediate family member serves as a board member, owner, officer, or committee member of the American Orthopaedic Association and the Pediatric Orthopaedic Society of North America. Neither Dr. Montgomery nor any immediate family member has received anything of value from or has stock or stock options held in a commercial company or institution related directly or indirectly to the subject of this chapter.

F. Musculoskeletal infection has been classified into three severity categories which have been shown to be predictive of outcomes as defined in **Table 1**.

1. Inflammation
2. Local infection
3. Disseminated infection

G. Infectious pathogens can take over and upregulate the acute phase response leading to systemic complications.

1. Systemic inflammatory response syndrome (SIRS): criteria are defined in **Table 2**
2. Sepsis: a clinical syndrome characterized by SIRS, immune dysregulation, microcirculatory derangements, and end-organ dysfunction
   a. ≥2 SIRS criteria (**Table 1**) with suspected or proven infection
3. Septic shock: Sepsis with cardiovascular dysfunction
4. Severe sepsis: Dysfunction of ≥2 organ systems

H. Venous thromboembolism (VTE): The rate of VTE in children with musculoskeletal infection is significantly higher than that of hospitalized children in general

II. EVALUATION OF SUSPECTED MUSCULOSKELETAL INFECTION

A. History

1. The focused history of the present illness should cover fever, pain, limp, swelling, skin changes or rashes, refusal to bear weight, duration of symptoms, recent local trauma, recent illness or infections (commonly upper respiratory infections), and recent antibiotic use.

TABLE 1

Musculoskeletal Infection Severity

	Definition
Inflammation	All of the following must be true (if available): • Negative local culture • Negative blood culture • Does not meet any criteria or local or disseminated infection
Local infection	One of the following must be true: • Imaging diagnostic for osteomyelitis or pyomyositis in 1 anatomic site • Local culture positive AND/OR fluid/tissue consistent with infection (grossly purulent, cell count >50,000) • One positive blood culture • Criteria for disseminated infection not met
Disseminated infection	At least one of the following must be true: • Imaging diagnostic for infection in multiple compartments • Two or more positive blood cultures • Two or more positive tissue cultures from multiple anatomic sites • Thromboembolic disease

From Mignemi ME, Benvenuti MA, An TJ, et al: A novel classification system based on dissemination of musculoskeletal infection is predictive of hospital outcomes. *J Pediatr Orthop* 2018;38:279–86.

2. Immunization history must be obtained, particularly with regard to vaccination against *Haemophilus influenzae*.
3. A travel history is useful in including or excluding pathogens endemic to certain areas (eg, Lyme disease associated arthritis in New England or the Midwest).
4. A complete social history including sexual history is obtained as *Neisseria gonorrhoeae* can cause septic arthritis in sexually active adolescents and sexually abused children.
5. In the neonate and infant, a birth and perinatal history is obtained.
6. A past medical history identifies comorbid conditions that may predispose to infection.

B. Physical examination

1. Temperature and vital signs should be measured immediately to rule out toxicity and hemodynamic instability.
2. The patient should specifically be examined for general appearance, the ability to bear weight, point tenderness, range of motion of adjacent joints (including the spine), and localized warmth, edema, and erythema.

TABLE 2

Pediatric SIRS[a] Diagnostic Criteria

Any two of the following must be met, one of which must include abnormal temperature or white blood cell count

1. Abnormal core temperature: >38.5°C or <36.0°F
2. Abnormal heart rate: >2 standard deviations above normal for age or <10th percentile if the child is younger than 1 year
3. Increased respiratory rate: >2 standard deviations above normal for age or mechanical ventilation for acute lung disease
4. Abnormal white blood cell count: above or below normal for age or >10% immature forms

Normal Pediatric Vital Signs and White Blood Cell Counts

	Heart rate (beats/min)				
Age group	**Tachycardia**	**Bradycardia**	**Respiratory rate (breaths/min)**	**WBC[b] (× 10^3/mm^3)**	**Systolic Blood Pressure (mm Hg)**
0-<7 d	>80	<100	>50	>34	<65
≥7 d-<1 mo	>180	<100	>40	>19.5 or <5	<75
≥1 mo-<2 yr	>180	<90	>34	>17.5 or <5	<100
≥2-<6 yr	>140	NA	>22	>15.5 or <6	<94
≥6-<12 yr	>130	NA	>18	>13.5 or <4.5	<105
≥12-<18 yr	>110	NA	>14	>11.5 or <4.5	<117

[a]SIRS = systemic inflammatory response syndrome.
[b]WBC = white blood cell count.
From Mantadakis E, Plessa E, Vouloumanou EK, Michailidis L, Chatzimichael A, Falagas ME. Deep venous thrombosis in children with musculoskeletal infections: the clinical evidence. *Int J Infect Dis* 2012;16:e236-e243.

3. Septic joints have an associated effusion, tenderness, and warmth. Short arc range of motion will illicit pain.
   a. The extremity is typically held in a position that maximizes the volume of the joint.
   b. A septic hip is typically held in flexion, abduction, and external rotation (FABER).

C. Laboratory studies

1. All patients with suspected musculoskeletal infection warrant a workup at presentation to include complete blood count (CBC) with differential, blood chemistries, erythrocyte sedimentation rate (ESR), C-reactive protein (CRP), and blood cultures.
2. CBC with differential: White blood cell (WBC) count is elevated in 25% of patients with osteomyelitis and 30% to 60% of patients with acute septic arthritis. The differential may exhibit a left shift in acute infection.
3. CRP: Elevated with acute musculoskeletal infection and becomes abnormal within 6 hours of infection.
   a. A CRP level of >2.0 mg/dL is an independent risk factor for septic arthritis
4. ESR: Becomes elevated in most patients with musculoskeletal infection and peaks in 3 to 5 days
5. The traditional Kocher criteria (see Section II.e) is commonly used to stratify risk of septic arthritis.
6. Blood cultures: Ideally obtained before initiation of antibiotics. May yield organism in 30% of cases. However, in a patient displaying signs of sepsis, antibiotics should not be held.
7. Synovial fluid analysis
   a. This should be obtained in patients with suspected septic arthritis.
   b. This is performed before initiating antibiotics if the clinical condition of the patient allows.
   c. It is diagnostic and the first step in treatment for septic arthritis as it allows for joint decompression.
   d. Fluid samples should be sent for cell count, Gram stain, aerobic and anaerobic cultures, and *Kingella kingae* polymerase chain reaction (PCR; in patients <5 years).
      - Gram stain may underestimate the presence of gram-negative organisms.
   e. See **Table 3**.

D. Imaging studies

1. Plain radiographs (XR): Always begin with two-view radiographs of the affected area.
   a. Septic arthritis: may see joint effusion, widening of the joint space (compare contralateral side on pelvis XR), lateral displacement of capital femoral epiphysis (hip)
   b. Osteomyelitis: changes visible on radiographs depend on chronicity of infection
      - Early: Normal/loss of soft-tissue planes and soft-tissue edema
      - 5 to 7 days: New periosteal bone formation
      - 10 to 14 days: Osteolysis
      - 1 to 2 weeks: Metaphyseal rarefaction, possible intraosseous abscess

TABLE 3

Synovial Fluid Analysis

Disease	Leukocytes (Cells/mL)	Polymorphonucleocytes (%)
Normal	<200	<25
Traumatic effusion	<5,000, with many erythrocytes	<25
Toxic synovitis	5,000-15,000	<25
Acute rheumatic fever	10,000-15,000	50
Juvenile rheumatoid arthritis	15,000-80,000	75
Lyme arthrtitis	40,000-140,000	> 75
Septic arthritis	>50,000	>75

Adapted with permission from Stans A: Osteomyelitis and septic arthritis, in Morrissy R, Weinstein S, eds: *Lovell and Winters Pediatric Orthopaedics*, ed 6. Philadelphia, PA, Lippincott Williams & Wilkins, 2006, pp 439-492.

10 | Pediatrics

2. Ultrasonography:
   a. Useful in suspected septic arthritis to identify joint effusion
   b. May also identify subperiosteal abscess, soft-tissue swelling, and soft-tissue abscess
3. MRI
   a. Typically performed with and without contrast in the evaluation of possible musculoskeletal infection
   b. Can identify abscesses, myositis, effusions, and osteomyelitis
   c. Judicious use in suspected septic arthritis can identify adjacent or concomitant infection preoperatively (**Figure 1**)
      - A published and validated algorithm includes criteria for MRI in the setting of septic arthritis based on five variables:
         - ≥3 positive variables: Obtain preoperative MRI
         - <3 positive variables: Forgo MRI and take patient to operating room (OR) for irrigation and debridement (I&D) of septic arthritis
            - Age >4 years
            - CRP >13.8 mg/L
            - Duration of symptoms >3 days
            - Platelets <314 × 10^3 cells/µL
            - Absolute neutrophil count (ANC) >8.6 × 10^3 cells/µL
4. CT
   a. Not routinely indicated in acute infection
   b. May demonstrate osseous changes and sequestra in chronic osteomyelitis
5. Technetium-99 bone scan
   a. May demonstrate areas of multifocal infection (in the subacute or chronic setting) or multiple areas of involvement in the setting of CRMO
   b. May be cold in acute infection

E. Differential diagnoses
1. Septic arthritis versus toxic synovitis of the hip
   a. The traditional Kocher criteria: If all four of the following are present, the probability of septic arthritis ranges from 59.0% to 99.6% in various series.
      - Fever with temperature greater than 38.5°C
      - Inability to bear weight
      - ESR greater than 40 mm/hr
      - WBC count greater than 12,000/µL

10 | Pediatrics

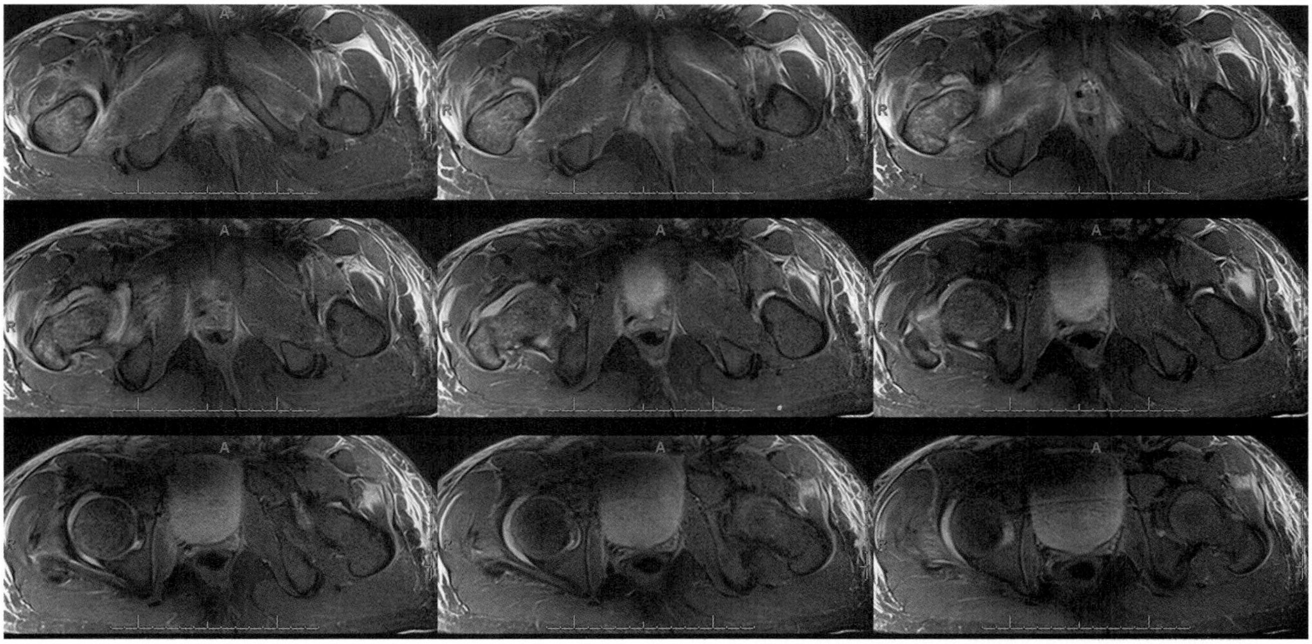

Figure 1 MRI axial T1 FS postcontrast bilateral lower extremities. This series of images is from a 15-year-old male who presented in sepsis with right lower extremity pain. This demonstrates a right hip effusion secondary to septic arthritis, osteomyelitis of the right proximal femur, diffuse bilateral myositis, deep and superficial fascial edema, and subcutaneous edema.

b. Modified Kocher criteria: A CRP level greater than 2.0 mg/dL is an independent risk factor for septic arthritis.

c. The order of importance of predictors is fever with temperature greater than 38.5°C, elevated CRP level, elevated ESR, refusal to bear weight, and elevated WBC count.

2. Neoplasm

a. Acute leukemia: patients may be misdiagnosed as acute osteomyelitis or septic arthritis

- 30% of acute leukemia patients have musculoskeletal symptoms
- Fever, pain, pallor, malaise, increased CRP, ESR
- Anemia, neutropenia, or thrombocytopenia in 80% of patients
- Leukopenia and immature leukocytes on peripheral smear

b. Osteosarcoma

- Aggressive appearing lesion of the metaphysis with mixed lytic and sclerotic components
- Normal laboratory values (but may have elevated alkaline phosphatase) and inflammatory markers

c. Ewing sarcoma

- Aggressive appearing lesion of the metaphysis or diaphysis often with a large soft-tissue mass

d. Chondroblastoma

- Localized tenderness, joint effusion, muscle wasting
- Well-demarcated epiphyseal lytic lesion with sclerotic borders

e. Primary lymphoma of bone

- Poorly defined sclerotic lesion with large, diffuse soft-tissue mass

f. Metastatic neuroblastoma

- Pain, limp, fever
- Metaphyseal lesion
- Elevated homovanillic acid (HVA) or vanillylmandelic acid (VMA) in urine or serum

3. Juvenile idiopathic arthritis

a. An autoimmune-mediated disorder characterized by chronic joint inflammation

b. May have fever, rash, and joint effusion

c. Joint involvement often migratory and polyarticular

d. Diagnostic criteria include a fever for at least 2 weeks and joint effusion for at least 6 weeks

e. Joint aspiration synovial fluid analysis: see **Table 3**

4. CRMO

a. A diagnosis of exclusion after ruling out bacterial osteomyelitis.

b. CRMO is characterized by a prolonged course with periodic exacerbations.

c. CRMO occurs primarily in children and adolescents and is more common in girls; the peak age of onset is 10 years.

d. The metaphyses of long bones are most commonly involved, but CRMO also may involve the medial clavicle and the spine presenting as vertebra plana.

e. The pathophysiology of CRMO is an autoimmune bone inflammatory disorder.

f. Fever of insidious onset, malaise, local pain, tenderness, and swelling.

g. Inflammatory markers may be normal or mildly elevated.

h. Biopsy demonstrates reactive, reparative, and inflammatory changes, and bone cultures are negative.

i. Plain radiography shows eccentric metaphyseal lesions with sclerosis, osteolysis, and new bone formation that is often symmetric.

j. A bone scan or whole body MRI is used in diagnosis to demonstrate other sites of disease.

k. Treatment is successful with scheduled NSAIDs in 79% of patients.

III. ETIOLOGY

A. Acute hematogenous osteomyelitis (AHO)

1. Slow blood flow in the capillaries of the metaphysis allows bacteria to exit the vessel walls.
2. Infection occurs when bacteria lodge in the bone in sufficient numbers to overwhelm local defenses.
3. Osteoblast necrosis, activation of osteoclasts, release of inflammatory mediators, recruitment of inflammatory cells, and blood vessel thrombosis cause a purulent exudate.
4. A subperiosteal abscess forms when the purulent exudate penetrates the porous metaphyseal cortex.
5. Local trauma has been associated with the development of AHO, because it renders the bone more susceptible to bacterial seeding.

B. Primary septic arthritis: hematogenous spread or direct inoculation
   1. Incidence peaks in the first few years of life. One-half of patients with septic arthritis are under the age of 2 years.
C. Secondary septic arthritis: spread of osteomyelitis into the joint (**Figure 1**)
   1. Occurs when the metaphysis is intracapsular: hip, shoulder, elbow, and ankle (not the knee)
D. Overall, *Staphylococcus aureus* continues to be the most common pathogen, but improved awareness and identification techniques has increased diagnosis of other causative organisms
E. Pathogens to consider by age:
   1. <1 year
      a. *S aureus*: nosocomial
      b. Group B streptococcus: community
   2. 1 to 5 years
      a. *S aureus*
      b. *K kingae*
      c. *Streptococcus pneumoniae*
   3. >5 years
      a. *S aureus* is the predominant source of musculoskeletal infection
F. *S aureus*
   1. Methicillin-susceptible *S aureus* (MSSA)
   2. Methicillin-resistant *S aureus* (MRSA): results from mecA gene transfer to *S aureus* resulting in a form of penicillin-binding protein with a low affinity for beta-lactam antibiotics
      a. A 3 to 10 times increase in incidence in the past decade
      b. Associated with more than half of staphylococcal infections in most communities
         - Clindamycin is an appropriate choice for empiric antibiotic therapy
      c. Associated with more severe infection
         - More extensive local soft-tissue destruction, rapid infection spread, higher overall mortality
         - Increased hospital stay, higher risk for need for surgery, and increased intensive care unit (ICU) admissions
         - Increased risk for complications: deep vein thrombosis (DVT), septic pulmonary emboli (PE), persistent bacteremia, and pathologic fracture
      d. Panton-Valentine leukocidin (PVL) is a cytotoxin associated with even greater severity of infections in MRSA
         - Increased cell and tissue necrosis
         - Complex infections, a greater frequency of multifocal infections, prolonged fever, myositis, pyomyositis, intraosseous or subperiosteal abscesses, chronic osteomyelitis, DVT, septic emboli, sepsis, and multisystem organ failure
      e. Most cases are community-acquired MRSA (CA-MRSA)
      f. Hospital-acquired MRSA
G. *K Kingae*
   1. Gram-negative coccobacillus
   2. Typically in children <4 years old
      a. Responsible for up to 50% of septic arthritis in children younger than 2 years
   3. May present as subacute infection
      a. Children appear mildly ill and have normal or mild elevations in ESR and CRP levels
   4. Improved identification due to improved detection techniques
      a. *K kingae*-specific real-time PCR
      b. Oropharyngeal swabs
         - Common in the flora of young children
H. Anaerobic bacteria are a rare cause of pediatric osteomyelitis and usually do this by spreading from infection at a contiguous site, as in conditions such as mastoiditis, otitis media, sinusitis, periodontal abscess, human bites, or decubitus ulcers.
I. *Candida albicans*
   1. A rare fungal infection in the pediatric population
   2. Infection lacks the aggressive inflammatory responses and elevated inflammatory indices of other infections
J. Tuberculosis
   1. The incidence of TB has increased in developed countries in the past 30 years because of immunocompromised patients and the emergence of multidrug-resistant strains.
   2. Bone and/or joint involvement occurs in 2% to 5% of children with TB, most commonly involving the spine (50%), large joints (25%), and long bones (11%). Polyostotic involvement has been reported in 12% of children.
   3. Patients can present with fever, night sweats, weight loss, and pain. Patients with skeletal infections may have more subtle manifestations.

4. In the spine, TB usually involves the anterior one-third of the vertebral body, most often in the region of the thoracolumbar junction; a paravertebral abscess may cause neurologic deficits.
5. Long bone lesions are radiolucent, with poorly defined margins and surrounding osteopenia.
6. The hip and knee are the most commonly affected joints. Involved joints have diffuse osteopenia and subchondral erosions.
7. Laboratory findings—The WBC count is normal, the ESR is usually elevated, and the purified protein derivative test is usually positive.
8. A biopsy with staining and culture showing acid-fast bacilli is diagnostic.
9. Treatment is usually medical and is given for at least 1 year.
10. Surgical débridement of long bone lesions may hasten the resolution of constitutional symptoms, but incisions should be closed to avoid chronic sinus formation.
11. Drainage and stabilization of spinal lesions are indicated for neurologic deficits, spinal instability, progressive kyphosis, or failure of medical therapy.

K. Lyme disease
1. Caused by *Borrelia burgdorferi*, which can induce erythema migrans, intermittent reactive arthritis, neuropathies, cardiac arrhythmias, and acute arthritis.
2. Infection is caused by a bite from the deer tick, which is prevalent in New England and the upper Midwest region of the United States.
3. Patients can present with fever and a swollen, irritable joint but will typically still bear weight.
4. Infection with *B burgdorferi* typically causes erythema migrans, an expanding, red "bulls-eye" rash, although this rash is not always present.
5. Laboratory workup should include an enzyme-linked immunosorbent assay for antibodies to *B burgdorferi* and a confirmatory Western blot assay. The WBC count may be normal or elevated; the ESR and the CRP level are usually elevated.
6. Lyme arthritis is treated with antibiotics, including doxycycline, amoxicillin, and cefuroxime.

L. Gonococcal arthritis
1. Caused by infection with *N gonorrhoeae*, it affects sexually active adolescents, sexually abused children, and neonates of infected mothers.
2. Because of its association with sexual abuse, children with suspected gonococcal arthritis should have cultures of specimens from all mucous membranes.
3. The knee is the most commonly involved joint, but the infection is polyarticular in 80% of cases.
4. Because *N gonorrhoeae* is difficult to culture, synovial aspirates should be cultured on chocolate blood agar.
5. Arthrotomy is required for treating hip infections; other joints can be observed or treated with serial aspiration.
6. Ceftriaxone or cefixime are antibiotics of choice.

M. Coccidioidomycosis
1. Caused by *Coccidioides immitis*, a fungus endemic to the southwestern United States.
2. Manifests as an upper respiratory infection but can progress to disseminated disease resulting in polyostotic osteomyelitis.
3. Both antifungal medical therapy and surgical débridement are usually required for cure.

IV. TREATMENT

A. Once cultures (blood cultures, biopsy, or aspiration) are obtained, empiric treatment with antibiotics should begin (**Table 4**). However, in the setting of sepsis, antibiotic administration should not be delayed.

B. Acute hematogenous osteomyelitis:
1. Aspiration/biopsy—Aspiration or biopsy of the suspected area is critical in both diagnosis and management.
   a. Antibiotic susceptibilities and the incidence of CA-MRSA vary by community, increasing the importance of specimen cultures.
   b. A large-bore needle is used to aspirate both the subperiosteal space and the intraosseous space.
   c. After aspiration, antibiotics may be started according to the guidelines in **Table 4**.
2. Nonsurgical
   a. If no purulent material is aspirated and MRI does not demonstrate subperiosteal abscess, the patient should be admitted for intravenous administration of antibiotics. Because of its frequency, CA-MRSA should be covered in most (if not all) cases.
   b. Intravenous antibiotics can be replaced by oral antibiotics after improvement of clinical and laboratory findings is confirmed.

TABLE 4

Empiric Antibiotic Recommendations for Pediatric Musculoskeletal Infections

Age Group	Antibiotic	Dose (mg/kg)	Route	Frequency
Pediatric and adolescent	Clindamycin	10	IV	Every 6 hr
	Clindamycin	8	Oral	Every 8 hr
	Vancomycin[a]	15	IV	Every 6 hr, initially[b,c]
	Rifampin[d]	10	IV or oral	Every 24 hr
Neonatal 1-3 mo	Vancomycin[e]	15	IV	Every 6 hr, initially[b,c]
	Ceftriaxone[e]	100	IV	Every 24 hr
Neonatal <1 mo	Ampicillin/sulbactam	150	IV	Every 6 hr
	Gentamycin[e]	2	IV	Every 8 hr[b]

[a]Recommended for suspected sepsis/severe infection.
[b]Peak and trough measured after third dose.
[c]Target peak, 45 µg/mL; target trough, 15 µg/mL.
[d]Used in conjunction with vancomycin in cases of osteomyelitis.
[e]Recommended in combination. IV = intravenous.
Reproduced with permission from Copley LA: Pediatric musculoskeletal infection: Trends and antibiotic recommendations. *J Am Acad Orthop Surg* 2009;17(10):618-626.

c. For nonresistant organisms, antibiotics are usually given for at least 3 weeks and/or until the patient's ESR and CRP have normalized.

d. For osteomyelitis caused by MRSA, antibiotics should be given for at least 8 weeks.

3. Surgical

a. Indications for surgical drainage are aspiration of pus, abscess formation seen on imaging studies, and failure to respond adequately to nonsurgical treatment.

b. Hemodynamic instability is a contraindication to emergent surgery; the patient should first be stabilized.

c. Surgical drainage requires evacuation of all purulent material, débridement of devitalized tissue, drilling of the cortex, and débridement of intraosseous collections.

d. Samples should be sent for culture and histology to rule out neoplasm.

e. The wound can be either closed over drains if deemed to be adequately débrided or packed and débrided again after 2 to 3 days before closure over drains.

f. More aggressive débridement may be needed in chronic osteomyelitis, sometimes including excision of a sequestrum.

C. Septic arthritis:

1. Requires urgent surgical treatment

a. Release of proteolytic enzymes from inflammatory cells, synovial cells, cartilage, and bacteria may damage the articular cartilage within 8 hours.

b. Increased joint pressure in the hip may cause osteonecrosis of the femoral head if not promptly relieved.

2. Joint aspiration is necessary for diagnosis and is also the first step in treatment by resulting in decompression of the increased intracapsular pressure

3. Intravenous antibiotics are started after samples are sent for culture and are usually continued for 3 weeks. The patient's immunization status should be checked to determine whether empiric antibiotics should provide coverage of *H influenzae.*

4. Nonsurgical

a. Nonsurgical treatment rarely has a role in septic arthritis, although some authors have advocated intravenous antibiotics and serial aspirations for accessible joints.

b. Recent data support the use of shorter courses of antibiotics, but the treatment plan should be made in concert with an infectious disease specialist familiar with the prevalence and virulence of local strains of pathogens.

5. Surgical
   a. Indications—Surgical drainage by arthrotomy and irrigation is the standard of care for almost all septic joints to remove damaging enzymes. In possible septic arthritis of the hip, it is better to err on the side of surgical drainage, which is associated with a much lower morbidity than a neglected septic hip.
   b. Contraindications—Surgical treatment is contraindicated when the patient's clinical status prevents it.
6. Procedures
   a. Arthrotomy is performed to remove all purulent fluid and irrigate the joint.
   b. In the case of an infected hip, an anterolateral or medial approach is performed to decrease the risk of osteonecrosis.
   c. Drainage of the shoulder, elbow, knee, and ankle can be open or arthroscopic.

V. SPECIFIC INFECTIONS

A. Neonatal infections
1. Overview
   a. Neonates younger than 8 weeks deserve special consideration because their immune systems are immature.
   b. Neonates are more susceptible to infection than older children and often do not show the symptoms and signs that normally assist in the diagnosis of bone or joint infection.
2. Patient groups
   a. Infants in the neonatal intensive care unit
      - Are at risk for infection via sites of phlebotomy, indwelling catheters, invasive monitoring, peripheral alimentation, and intravenous drug administration
      - Those with musculoskeletal infections, which are typically caused by *S aureus* or gram-negative organisms, have multiple sites of infection in 40% of cases
   b. Otherwise healthy infants 2 to 4 weeks of age who develop an infection at home
      - Group B streptococcus is usually the causative organism.
      - Usually, only a single site is involved.
3. Anatomy
   a. Before the secondary center of ossification appears, the metaphyseal vessels also supply the epiphysis, often (76% of cases) causing the spread of osteomyelitis in the metaphysis to the epiphysis and the adjacent joint.

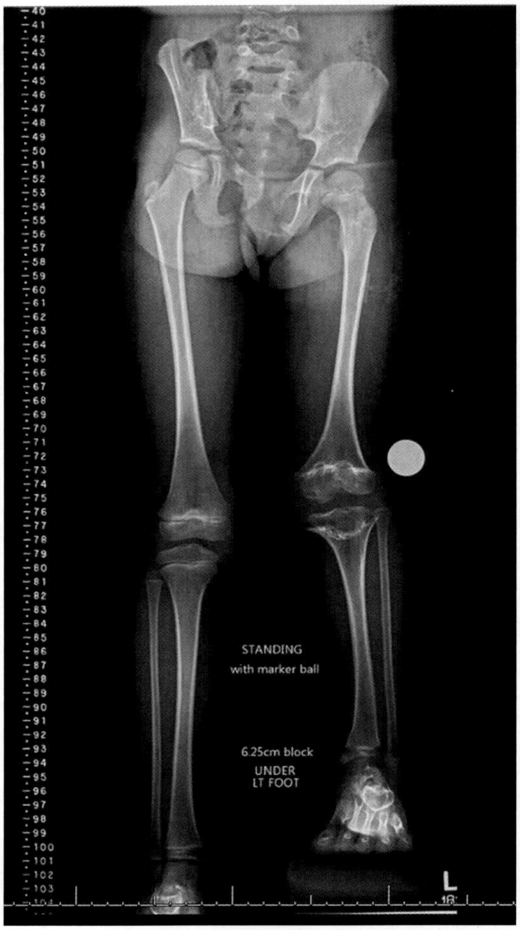

Figure 2 Scanogram radiograph of a 6-year-old female demonstrating a physeal arrest of the proximal tibia and distal femur on the left resulting in a leg length difference. The patient had a history of neonatal osteomyelitis.

   b. Growth disturbance and physeal arrest can occur (**Figure 2**).
4. Diagnosis—Diagnosis of bone or joint infections in the neonate can be difficult.
   a. Fever is usually absent.
   b. Early signs are pain with motion, decreased use of the affected extremity, pseudoparalysis, difficulty in feeding, and temperature instability.
   c. Tenderness, swelling, and erythema occur later.
   d. Laboratory findings
      - The WBC count is usually normal.
      - Blood cultures are positive in 40% of cases, and the ESR may be elevated.

5. Treatment
   a. Neonates with documented sepsis should have aspiration and culture of all suspicious areas.
   b. Areas with sepsis should be surgically drained, with care taken to avoid additional damage to growth centers.

B. Shoe puncture
1. Superficial infections occur in 10% to 15% of children with shoe-puncture wounds, and deep infections occur in approximately 1%.
2. *Pseudomonas* is an organism of concern, although infection by *S aureus* is more common.
3. Tetanus immunization should be documented and provided if not already given.
4. Radiography should be performed to investigate for a retained foreign body.
5. Initial treatment consists of soaks, elevation, rest, and antibiotics that cover both *S aureus* and *Pseudomonas*.
6. Bone scanning or MRI can help identify more complex infections requiring surgical débridement
7. Surgery is indicated for a foreign body, abscess, or septic arthritis or in cases of failure to respond to antibiotics.
8. More than 90% of late, deep infections are caused by *Pseudomonas*.

C. Diskitis
1. Usually occurs in children younger than 5 years.
2. Begins in the vertebral end plates and moves to the disk through vascular channels.
3. *S aureus* is the most common cause.
4. Blood cultures should be performed; local cultures are not routinely needed.
5. Patients present with low-grade fever, a limp, or refusal to bear weight; the child refuses to move the spine.
6. Plain radiographs are normal for the first 2 to 3 weeks but may show loss of normal sagittal spinal contour early; bone scanning or MRI confirms the diagnosis earlier than plain radiography.
7. Antibiotic treatment is effective in most cases; patients who do not respond to antibiotics should have a biopsy.

D. Vertebral osteomyelitis
1. Affects older children.
2. Usually causes more constitutional symptoms than does diskitis and more focal tenderness on examination.
3. MRI or bone scanning is sensitive early in the disease process; plain radiography shows bone destruction later.
4. Treatment with antistaphylococcal agents is typically curative.

E. Sacroiliac infections
1. Infections of the sacroiliac joint cause fever, pain, and a limp.
2. Patients have pain with lateral compression of the pelvis, a positive FABER test, and tenderness over the sacroiliac joint.
3. MRI is the most sensitive diagnostic procedure.
4. Initial antibiotic treatment should cover *S aureus,* which is the most common pathogenic agent.
5. If needed, aspiration or drainage can usually be performed with CT guidance.

F. Sickle cell disease
1. Affected children are at increased risk for both septic arthritis and osteomyelitis.
2. The frequent bone infarcts, sluggish circulation, and decreased opsonization of bacteria in the disease increase the susceptibility to bone or joint infection.
3. Because *S aureus* and *Salmonella* are the most common pathogens, initial antibiotic treatment should cover both.
4. Differentiation between sickle cell crisis and infection can be challenging.
   a. Both entities may cause fever, pain, tenderness, swelling, and warmth.
   b. The WBC count, CRP level, and ESR may be elevated in both conditions.
   c. Bone scanning and MRI are often not specific.
5. Osteoarticular infection is present in only about 2% of children with sickle cell disease who are hospitalized with musculoskeletal pain.
6. A positive blood culture or positive osteoarticular aspirate is diagnostic.

TOP TESTING FACTS

1. A child with bone pain and fever should be assumed to have osteomyelitis until a definitive diagnosis is made.
2. PVL-positive strains of CA-MRSA are associated with complex infections, a greater frequency of multifocal infections, prolonged fever, myositis, pyomyositis, intraosseous or subperiosteal abscesses, chronic osteomyelitis, DVT, septic emboli, sepsis, and multisystem organ failure.
3. Biopsy is required to rule out malignancy in cases of subacute osteomyelitis.
4. Patients with subacute osteomyelitis may present without fever and with a normal WBC count and CRP level.
5. When managing the hip in septic arthritis, drainage should be more strongly considered in equivocal cases; the morbidity of arthrotomy is minimal compared with the sequelae of a neglected septic hip.
6. *Pseudomonas* is responsible for more than 90% of late deep infections following nail puncture through sneakers.
7. In diskitis, the infection begins in the vertebral end plates and moves to the disk through vascular channels.
8. *S aureus* and *Salmonella* are the most common infecting organisms in children with sickle cell anemia and musculoskeletal infection.
9. In children with TB, the most common sites of musculoskeletal infection are the spine (50%), large joints (25%), and long bones (11%). Polyostotic involvement occurs in 12% of children with TB.
10. A fluid specimen collected by arthrocentesis from a joint with suspected sepsis should be placed in a blood culture bottle to evaluate for *K kingae* infection in a young patient and sent for PCR

Bibliography

An TJ, Benvenuti MA, Mignemi ME, Thomsen IP, Schoenecker JG: Pediatric musculoskeletal infection: Hijacking the acute-phase response. *JBJS Rev* 2016;4.

Arkader A, Brusalis C, Warner WC, Jr., Conway JH, Noonan K: Update in pediatric musculoskeletal infections: When it is, when it isn't, and what to do. *J Am Acad Orthop Surg* 2016;24:e112-e121.

Belthur MV, Birchansky SB, Verdugo AA, et al: Pathologic fractures in children with acute Staphylococcus aureus osteomyelitis. *J Bone Joint Surg Am* 2012;94:34-42.

Benvenuti MA, An TJ, Mignemi ME, et al: A clinical prediction algorithm to stratify pediatric musculoskeletal infection by severity. *J Pediatr Orthop* 2019;39(3):153-157.

Boan P, Tan HL, Pearson J, Coombs G, Heath CH, Robinson JO: Epidemiological, clinical, outcome and antibiotic susceptibility differences between PVL positive and PVL negative Staphylococcus aureus infections in Western Australia: A case control study. *BMC Infect Dis* 2015;15:10.

Browne LP, Guillerman RP, Orth RC, Patel J, Mason EO, Kaplan SL: Community-acquired staphylococcal musculoskeletal infection in infants and young children: Necessity of contrast-enhanced MRI for the diagnosis of growth cartilage involvement. *AJR Am J Roentgenol* 2012;198:194-199.

Ceroni D, Cherkaoui A, Ferey S, Kaelin A, Schrenzel J: Kingella kingae osteoarticular infections in young children: Clinical features and contribution of a new specific real-time PCR assay to the diagnosis. *J Pediatr Orthop* 2010;30:301-304.

Copley LA: Pediatric musculoskeletal infection: Trends and antibiotic recommendations. *J Am Acad Orthop Surg* 2009;17:618-626.

Dubnov-Raz G, Ephros M, Garty BZ, et al: Invasive pediatric Kingella kingae infections: A nationwide collaborative study. *Pediatr Infect Dis J* 2010;29:639-643.

Gafur OA, Copley LA, Hollmig ST, Browne RH, Thornton LA, Crawford SE: The impact of the current epidemiology of pediatric musculoskeletal infection on evaluation and treatment guidelines. *J Pediatr Orthop* 2008;28:777-785.

Gamaletsou MN, Kontoyiannis DP, Sipsas NV, et al: Candida osteomyelitis: Analysis of 207 pediatric and adult cases (1970–2011). *Clin Infect Dis* 2012;55:1338-1351.

Goldstein B, Giroir B, Randolph A: International consensus conference on pediatric S. International pediatric sepsis consensus conference: Definitions for sepsis and organ dysfunction in pediatrics. *Pediatr Crit Care Med* 2005;6:2-8.

Hollmig ST, Copley LA, Browne RH, Grande LM, Wilson PL: Deep venous thrombosis associated with osteomyelitis in children. *J Bone Joint Surg Am* 2007;89:1517-1523.

Kocher MS, Zurakowski D, Kasser JR: Differentiating between septic arthritis and transient synovitis of the hip in children: An evidence-based clinical prediction algorithm. *J Bone Joint Surg Am* 1999;81:1662-1670.

Monsalve J, Kan JH, Schallert EK, Bisset GS, Zhang W, Rosenfeld SB: Septic arthritis in children: Frequency of coexisting unsuspected osteomyelitis and implications on imaging work-up and management. *AJR Am J Roentgenol* 2015;204:1289-1295.

Montgomery NI, Rosenfeld S: Pediatric osteoarticular infection update. *J Pediatr Orthop* 2015;35:74-81.

Pendleton A, Kocher MS: Methicillin-resistant staphylococcus aureus bone and joint infections in children. *J Am Acad Orthop Surg* 2015;23:29-37.

Roderick MR, Sen ES, Ramanan AV: Chronic recurrent multifocal osteomyelitis in children and adults: Current understanding and areas for development. *Rheumatology (Oxford)* 2018;57:41-48.

Rosenfeld S, Bernstein DT, Daram S, Dawson J, Zhang W: Predicting the presence of adjacent infections in septic arthritis in children. *J Pediatr Orthop* 2016;36:70-74.

Singhal R, Perry DC, Khan FN, et al: The use of CRP within a clinical prediction algorithm for the differentiation of septic arthritis and transient synovitis in children. *J Bone Joint Surg Br* 2011;93:1556-1561.

Welling BD, Haruno LS, Rosenfeld SB: Validating an algorithm to predict adjacent musculoskeletal infections in pediatric patients with septic arthritis. *Clin Orthop Relat Res* 2018;476:153-159.

Chapter 133
THE PEDIATRIC HIP

TRAVIS H. MATHENEY, MD, MLA
VIDYADHAR V. UPASANI, MD

I. DEVELOPMENTAL DYSPLASIA OF THE HIP

A. Overview

1. Definition

a. Developmental dysplasia of the hip (DDH) refers to the spectrum of pathologic conditions involving the developing hip, ranging from acetabular dysplasia to complete dislocation of the hip.

b. Teratologic dislocation of the hip occurs in utero and is irreducible on neonatal examination. A pseudoacetabulum is usually present. This condition always accompanies other congenital anomalies or neuromuscular conditions, most often arthrogryposis and myelomeningocele.

2. Epidemiology

a. DDH is the most common disorder of the hip in children. One in 1,000 children (0.1%) is born with a dislocated hip; 10 in 1,000 children (1%) are born with hip subluxation or dysplasia.

b. Eighty percent of affected children are female.

c. The left hip is more commonly involved (60%) than the right; bilateral involvement occurs in 20% of cases.

d. The condition is more common in Native Americans and people of northern Finnish descent; DDH is rarely seen in African Americans.

e. The etiology of DDH is unknown but is thought to be multifactorial (genetic, hormonal, and mechanical).

B. Pathoanatomy

1. Risk factors for DDH

a. Female sex, firstborn child, breech presentation

b. Disorders of intrauterine packing phenomenon, such as congenital dislocation of the knee, congenital muscular torticollis, and metatarsus adductus

c. In affected children, 12% to 33% have a family history of DDH. The risk is 6% with one affected sibling, 12% with one affected parent, and 36% with a parent and sibling affected.

C. Evaluation

1. Clinical presentation

a. Clinical presentation varies with age. In the neonatal period, the key clinical finding is instability of the hip.

b. Hip clicks are nonspecific physical findings.

c. Asymmetric skin folds are an unreliable and nonspecific finding.

d. In infants older than 6 months, common findings are asymmetric hip abduction and apparent limb shortening (in unilateral dislocations).

e. In toddlers, restricted motion may be accompanied by a limb-length discrepancy, a limp, or a

Dr. Matheney or an immediate family member is a member of a speakers' bureau or has made paid presentations on behalf of Smith & Nephew; serves as an unpaid consultant to Orthopaediatrics; and serves as a board member, owner, officer, or committee member of the American Academy of Orthopaedic Surgeons and the Pediatric Orthopaedic Society of North America. Dr. Upasani or an immediate family member is a member of a speakers' bureau or has made paid presentations on behalf of BroadWater, DePuy, A Johnson & Johnson Company, Nuvasive, and OrthoPediatrics; serves as a paid consultant to or is an employee of Globus Medical, and OrthoPediatrics; has stock or stock options held in Imagen; has received research or institutional support from EOS Imaging, nView, and Pacira; and serves as a board member, owner, officer, or committee member of the Pediatric Orthopaedic Society of North America and the Scoliosis Research Society.

This chapter is adapted from Choi PD: The pediatric hip, in Boyer MI, ed: *AAOS Comprehensive Orthopaedic Review*, ed 2. Rosemont, IL, American Academy of Orthopaedic Surgeons, 2014, pp 667-683.

TABLE 3

Advantages and Disadvantages of Anterior Versus Medial or Anteromedial Approaches for Developmental Dysplasia of the Hip

Approach	Advantages	Disadvantages
Anterior	Capsulorrhaphy and pelvic osteotomy possible through the same incision Acetabulum (including labrum) directly accessible Lower reported risk of osteonecrosis Shorter duration of spica casting (6 wk) Familiar surgical approach	Postoperative stiffness Potential blood loss Potential injury to the lateral femoral cutaneous nerve
Medial or anteromedial	Allows direct access to medial structures blocking reduction (pulvinar, ligamentum teres, transverse acetabular ligament) Avoids splitting iliac crest apophysis Avoids damage to hip abductors Less invasive, minimal dissection Cosmetically acceptable scar	Capsulorrhaphy and pelvic osteotomy not possible through this incision Poor visualization of acetabulum; labrum not accessible Higher risk of osteonecrosis Longer duration of cast immobilization (3-4 mo)

d. Pelvic osteotomy may be necessary for substantial acetabular dysplasia (typical in children older than 18 to 24 months of age). Osteotomy notably reduces the rate of revision surgery when performed at the time of initial surgery in children in this age group.

4. Residual dysplasia after hip reduction

a. Pelvic osteotomy may be indicated for persistent acetabular dysplasia and hip instability. Clinical practice varies considerably with regard to pelvic osteotomy in children older than 2 years.

b. The two general types of pelvic osteotomy are reconstructive and salvage (**Table 4**).

c. Reconstructive pelvic osteotomies redirect or reshape the roof of the native acetabulum into a more appropriate weight-bearing position. A prerequisite for reconstructive pelvic osteotomy is a hip that can be reduced concentrically and congruently. The hip must also have near-normal ROM.

TABLE 4

Pelvic Osteotomies for the Treatment of Developmental Dysplasia of the Hip

Reconstructive		Salvage
Redirectional	**Reshaping**	
Single innominate (Salter)	Pemberton	Chiari osteotomy
Triple innominate	Dega	Shelf arthroplasty

Adapted from Gillingham BL, Sanchez AA, Wenger DR: Pelvic osteotomies for the treatment of hip dysplasia in children and young adults. *J Am Acad Ortho Surg* 1999;7:325-337.

- Redirectional pelvic osteotomies (**Figure 7**) include the single innominate (Salter), or triple innominate osteotomy.
- The Ganz periacetabular osteotomy or rotational acetabular osteotomies can be used in skeletally mature patients with a closed tri-radiate cartilage and residual acetabular dysplasia.

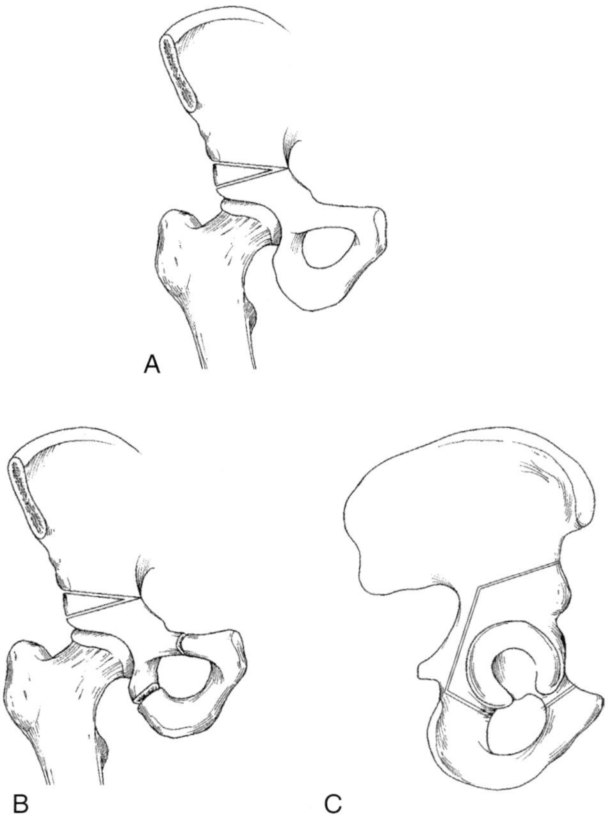

Figure 7 Illustrations show redirectional pelvic osteotomy options. **A**, Single innominate (Salter). **B**, Triple innominate. **C**, Periacetabular.

10 | Pediatrics

- Reshaping pelvic osteotomies (acetabuloplasties) include the Pemberton, Dega, Pembersal, and San Diego osteotomies.

d. Salvage osteotomies increase weight-bearing coverage by using the joint capsule interposed between the femoral head and bone above it. Salvage osteotomies rely on fibrocartilaginous metaplasia of the interposed joint capsule to provide an increased articulating surface. The intent of these osteotomies is to reduce point loading at the edge of the acetabulum.

- Salvage osteotomies are typically indicated for adolescents with severe dysplasia in whom acetabular deficiency precludes a reconstructive osteotomy.
- Salvage osteotomies include the Chiari and shelf osteotomies.

II. LEGG-CALVÉ-PERTHES DISEASE

A. Overview

1. Legg-Calvé-Perthes disease (LCPD) is an idiopathic osteonecrosis of the femoral head in children.
2. Epidemiology
   a. LCPD affects 1 in 1,200 children.
   b. It affects boys between four and five times more commonly than girls.
   c. Bilateral hip involvement is present in 10% to 15% of patients. If both hips are in the same stage of disease, radiographs of the hands, knees and spine could be obtained to evaluate for skeletal dysplasia.
   d. LCPD is more commonly diagnosed in urban than in rural communities.
   e. A predilection appears to exist for certain populations, with an above-average incidence in Asians, the Inuit, and central Europeans. The incidence is below average in native Australians, Native Americans, Polynesians, and African Americans.

B. Etiology

1. The exact etiology of LCPD is unknown, but it is probably caused by a combination of genetic and environmental factors.
2. Historically, the cause was thought to be inflammatory or infectious, with transient synovitis as a possible precursor. Repetitive trauma, exposure to second-hand smoke or carbon monoxide is also believed to be causative.
3. Proposed etiologies include mutations in type II collagen, abnormal insulin-like growth factor-1 action pathways, and various types of thrombophilia.
4. The role of thrombophilia as a cause of LCPD is controversial. Some studies have reported a 50% to 75% association between LCPD and a coagulation abnormality; other studies have not shown any such association.
5. Associated factors
   a. A family history is found in 1.6% to 20.0% of cases.
   b. LCPD is associated with attention deficit hyperactivity disorder in 33%.
   c. Patients are commonly skeletally immature, with delayed bone age in 89%.

C. Pathoanatomy

1. Current theories propose that a disruption of the vascularity of the femoral head serves as the key pathogenic event in LCPD, resulting in ischemic necrosis and subsequent revascularization.
2. The abnormal femoral head (weakened by ischemia) can deform when its mechanical strength is surpassed by loading forces on the hip joint. This deformity may eventually remodel with healing and revascularization.
3. The articular cartilage, capital epiphysis, physis, and metaphysis of the hip joint are histologically abnormal in LCPD, with disorganized cartilaginous areas of hypercellularity and fibrillation.

D. Evaluation

1. LCPD is a diagnosis of exclusion. Other causes of osteonecrosis (eg, septic arthritis, sickle cell disease, corticosteroid therapy) and mimicking conditions (eg, skeletal dysplasias, mucopolysaccharidoses) must be ruled out.
2. Clinical presentation
   a. LCPD occurs most often in children 4 to 8 years of age (range, 2 years to late teens).
   b. The onset is insidious; children with LCPD commonly have a limp and pain in the groin, hip, thigh, or knee regions.
   c. Occasionally, children with LCPD have a history of recent or remote viral illness.
3. Physical examination
   a. Examination may reveal an abnormal gait (antalgic and/or Trendelenburg).

b. Limitation of hip motion depends on the stage of disease. ROM testing often reveals decreased abduction and internal rotation. Hip flexion contractures are seen rarely.

c. Limb-length discrepancy, if present, is mild and a result of femoral head collapse or disruption of the proximal femoral physis. Hip contractures may make the limb-length discrepancy seem greater than it actually is.

E. Diagnostic tests

1. Plain radiographs

a. A standard AP view of the pelvis and lateral view of the proximal femur are critical in making the initial diagnosis and assessing the subsequent clinical course.

b. A perfusion MRI is now often used to assess the extent of femoral head necrosis and has been shown to be a good prognostic tool. However, repeated exposure to IV contrast is concerning for deposition in the brain and other organs and could cause neurocognitive disorders.

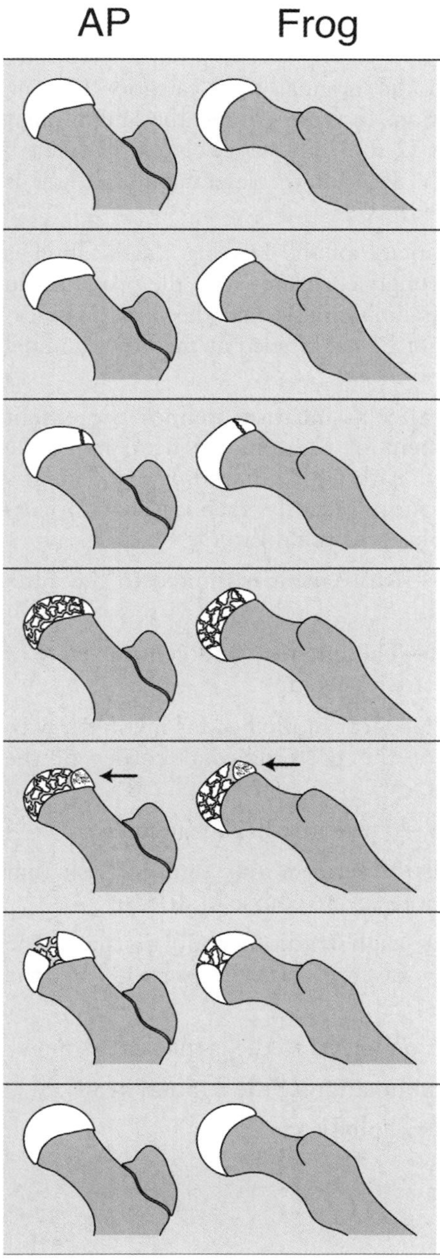

Stage IA
All or part of the epiphysis is sclerotic. There is no loss of height of the epiphysis.

Stage IB
There is sclerosis of the epiphysis. There is loss of epiphyseal height. There is no fragmentation of the epiphysis.

Stage IIA
The epiphysis has just begun to fragment. One or two vertical fissures are present either in the AP view or the frog view.

Stage IIB
Fragmentation is advanced. There is no new bone lateral to the fragmented epiphysis.

Stage IIIA
Early new bone is visible lateral to the fragmented epiphysis (arrows). The texture of the new bone is not normal, it is porotic and covers <1/3 of the width of the epiphysis.

Stage IIIB
New bone of normal texture covers more >1/3 of the width of the epiphysis.

Stage IV
Healing is complete. There no radiographic evidence of avascular bone.

Figure 8 Illustration shows the four stages of the modified Waldenstrom classification system.

2. LCPD typically proceeds through four radiographic stages (The modified Waldenström classification is shown in **Figure 8**).
   a. Initial stage—Early radiographic findings are a sclerotic, smaller proximal femoral ossific nucleus (because of failure of the epiphysis to increase in size) and widened medial clear space (distance between the teardrop and femoral head).
   b. Fragmentation stage (mean duration = 1 year)—Segmental collapse (resorption) of the capital femoral epiphysis, with increased density of the epiphysis.
   c. Reossification or reparative stage (mean duration = 3 to 5 years)—Necrotic bone is resorbed, with subsequent reossification of the capital femoral epiphysis.
   d. Remodeling stage—Remodeling begins when the capital femoral epiphysis is completely reossified.
3. Arthrography is useful for assessing coverage and containment of the femoral head.
   a. Dynamic arthrography is often used at the time of surgery to confirm the degree of correction that femoral and/or pelvic osteotomies need to provide.
   b. Dynamic arthrography may also be used to identify hips with severe deformity and hinged abduction (**Figure 9**).

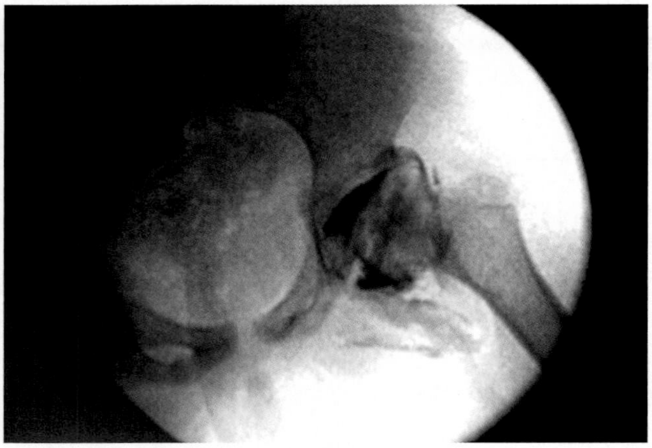

Figure 9 Arthrogram of the left hip shows hinged abduction. With the hip abducted, the lateral edge of the epiphysis hinges on the lateral acetabulum, with concomitant medial dye pooling. (Reproduced from Matheney T: Legg-Calvé Perthes disease, in Song KM, ed: *Orthopaedic Knowledge Update: Pediatrics*, ed 4. Rosemont, IL, American Academy of Orthopaedic Surgeons, 2011, p 183.)

F. Classification
1. The lateral pillar (Herring) classification of LCPD (**Figure 10**) is based on the height of the lateral 15% to 30% of the epiphysis (ie, the lateral pillar) on an AP view of the pelvis. The groups in this classification are described below.
   a. Group A—No involvement of the lateral pillar with no changes in its density and no loss of its height.
   b. Group B—More than 50% of the height of the lateral pillar is maintained.
   c. Group C—Less than 50% of the height of the lateral pillar is maintained.
   d. B/C border groups—These groups were later added to the original three-category Herring classification. In these groups, the lateral pillar is narrow (2 to 3 mm wide) or poorly ossified, or exactly 50% of the lateral pillar height is maintained.
   e. The advantage of the Herring classification is that it strongly correlates with the prognosis in LCPD. Its limitation is that the final classification cannot be determined at the time of initial presentation.
2. The Catterall classification defines the extent of involvement of the femoral head in LCPD (**Figure 11**). Although commonly used in the past, it has more recently been criticized for its poor interobserver reliability.
   a. Group I—Involvement is limited to the anterior head.
   b. Group II—The anterior and central parts of the head are involved.
   c. Group III—Most of the head is involved, with sparing of the posteromedial corner of the epiphysis.
   d. Group IV—The entire head is involved.
3. Catterall also described four signs of risk that indicate a more severe course of disease:
   a. The Gage sign (radiolucency in the shape of a V in the lateral portion of the epiphysis)
   b. Calcification lateral to the epiphysis
   c. Lateral subluxation of the femoral head
   d. A horizontal physis

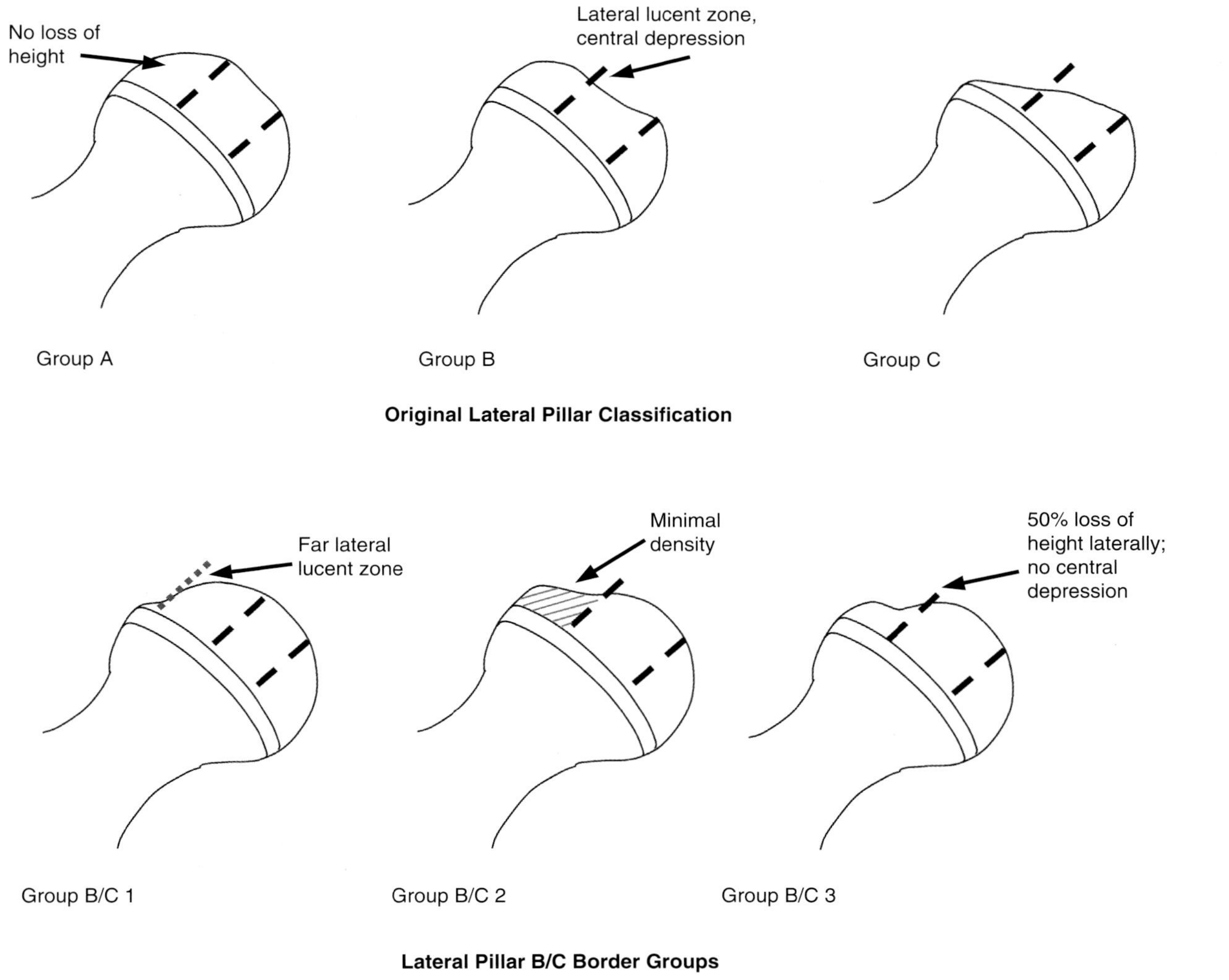

Figure 10 Illustrations show the lateral pillar (Herring) classification for Legg-Calvé-Perthes disease. Group A hips have no loss of height of the lateral pillar (lateral third of the epiphysis). Group B hips have less than 50% loss of lateral pillar height. Group C hips have more than 50% loss of lateral pillar height. In B/C border group hips, the lateral pillar is narrow (2 to 3 mm wide; group B/C 1) or poorly ossified (group B/C 2), or exactly 50% of the height of the lateral pillar is maintained without central depression (group B/C 3). (Reproduced from Matheney T: Legg-Calvé Perthes disease, in Song KM, ed: *Orthopaedic Knowledge Update: Pediatrics*, ed 4. Rosemont, IL, American Academy of Orthopaedic Surgeons, 2011, p 181.)

4. The Stulberg classification is used to evaluate femoral head sphericity and joint congruency at skeletal maturity.
   a. Grade I and II hips are thought to have a good prognosis because of a spherical and congruent hip joint.
   b. Grade III, IV, and V hips have a flat head with poor congruence and are thought to result in hip arthritis.
5. None of the existing classifications of LCPD are sufficiently prospective to provide a prognosis before the onset of deformity.

G. Treatment
1. The treatment of LCPD is highly controversial.
2. Current treatments are largely based on the concept of containing the femoral head in the acetabulum, which optimizes molding of the soft femoral head and minimizes deformity of the head.
3. The aim of treatment is to achieve a spherical femoral head and congruent joint to minimize the risk of osteoarthritis.
4. Treatment is based on the patient's age at disease onset and the severity of involvement of the femoral head (defined by the lateral pillar classification).

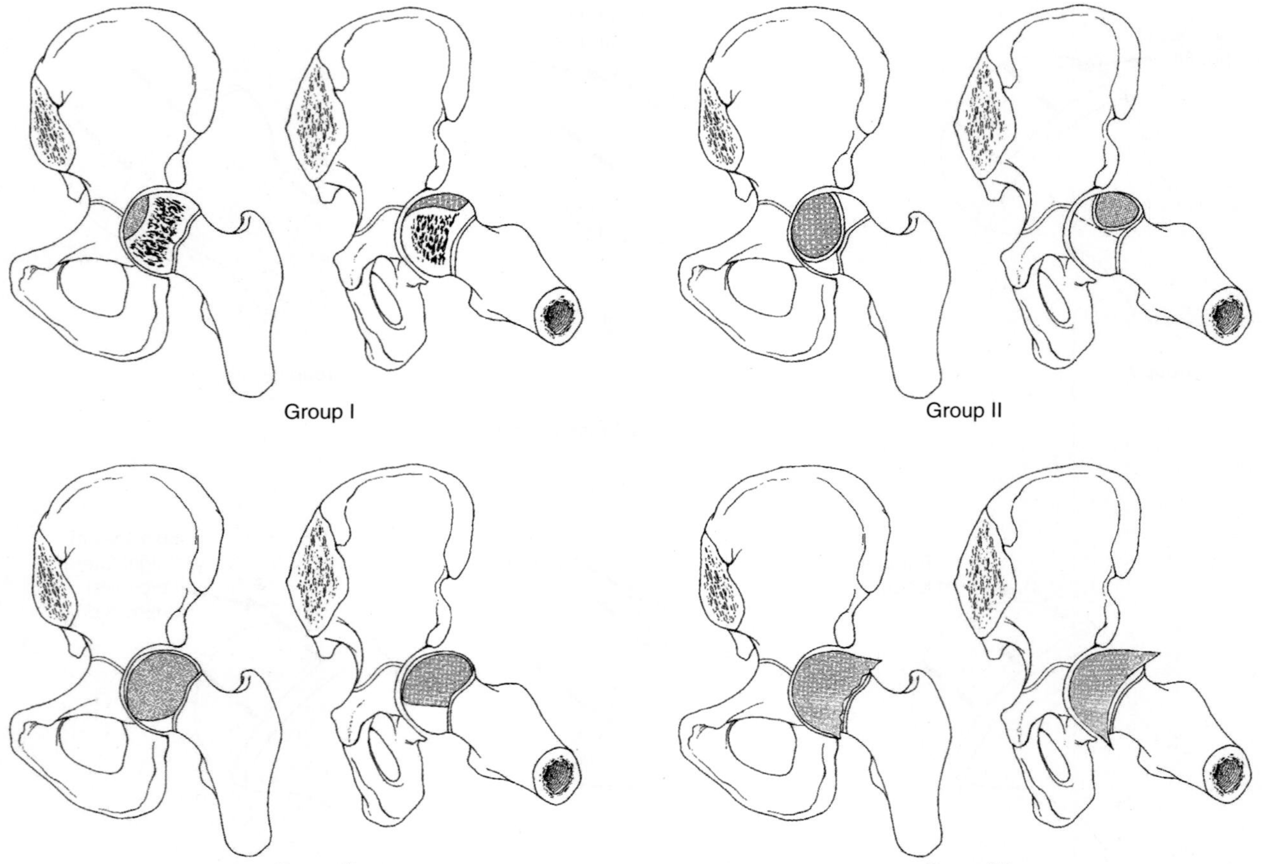

Figure 11 Illustration shows the Catterall classification for Legg-Calvé-Perthes disease.

a. Patients younger than 6 years without complete collapse of the lateral pillar can generally be treated nonsurgically. Most patients achieve Stulberg I or II hips at maturity, with 80% achieving a good outcome.

b. Patients older than 8 years appear to benefit from surgically provided containment of the femoral head. This is particularly true for hips in the lateral pillar B and B/C border groups.

c. Patients with lateral pillar group C hips tend to do poorly regardless of treatment and age at onset.

d. For patients age 6 to 8 years at onset, evidence is not clear regarding potential advantages of a specific surgical procedure in lateral pillar classification.

5. Nonsurgical treatment

a. Containment of the femoral head may be achieved nonsurgically by casting or bracing treatment with the hip in an abducted and internally rotated position.

b. Petrie casts and a variety of abduction orthoses have been used.

c. Protected weight bearing has also been recommended, especially before the reossification stage.

6. Surgical treatment

a. Surgical containment of the femoral head may be approached from the femoral side, the acetabular side, or both, according to the surgeon's preference. These procedures produce comparable outcomes.

b. Containment of the femur is achieved with a proximal femoral varus osteotomy.

c. Containment by the acetabulum is achieved with a redirectional osteotomy (Salter, triple innominate), or acetabular augmentation procedure (shelf arthroplasty).

d. For improved outcomes, the hips must be containable; that is, they must have a relatively full ROM with congruency between the femoral head and the acetabulum.

e. To allow maximal remodeling, the earliest possible initiation of treatment (before or during the early fragmentation stage of LCPD) should be strongly considered.

f. Bracing treatment/casting and physical therapy may be used to improve preoperative joint mobility.

g. Hip arthrodiastasis (via an external fixator) for 4 to 5 months has also been advocated in some centers, but remains controversial.

7. Salvage treatment

a. Salvage is used when the hip has poor congruency or is no longer containable. The goals of treatment are to relieve symptoms and restore stability.

b. Hinged abduction, in which lateral extrusion of the femoral head results in its impinging on the edge of the acetabulum with abduction (**Figure 9**), may be present. Management possibilities are the following:

- An valgus-flexion proximal femoral osteotomy
- Pelvic osteotomy procedures, such as a Chiari osteotomy, shelf arthroplasty, and shelf acetabuloplasty (labral support procedure) may also be beneficial.

8. Residual deformities

a. Deformity of the femoral head may result in femoroacetabular impingement (FAI). FAI in LCPD may be treated with surgical dislocation and proximal femoral osteochondroplasty or the femoral head reduction procedure.

b. An overriding greater trochanter and short femoral neck also may result in FAI. Management options include intertrochanteric valgus osteotomy and surgical dislocation with relative lengthening of the femoral neck.

c. Accommodative acetabular dysplasia that is severe and/or causes instability may require periacetabular osteotomy.

d. The possibility of proximal femoral physeal arrest requires monitoring of leg lengths until skeletal maturity.

e. Osteochondritis dissecans after LCPD may require treatment if it is symptomatic or if the lesion becomes unstable.

H. Outcome

1. Prognosis is related to patient age at disease onset. Patients younger than 6 years old at disease onset typically have a good outcome.

TABLE 5

Stulberg Radiographic Classification of Legg-Calvé-Perthes Disease and Evidence of Osteoarthritis[a]

Class	Descriptive Features	Radiographic Signs of Osteoarthritis (%)	Radiographic Evidence of Joint Space Narrowing (%)
I	Normal hip joint	0	0
II	Spherical head with enlargement, short neck, or steep acetabulum	16	0
III	Nonspherical head (ie, ovoid, mushroom-shaped, umbrella-shaped)	58	47
IV	Flat head	75	53
V	Flat head with incongruent hip joint	78	61

[a]At mean 40-yr follow-up.

2. Deformity of the femoral head also correlates with long-term outcome. The severity of this deformity and the degree of hip joint congruence at maturity (as defined by Stulberg) correlate with the risk of premature osteoarthritis (**Table 5**).

a. The risk of osteoarthritis of the hip is low (0% to 16%) when the femoral head is spherical (classes I and II).

b. The risk of osteoarthritis of the hip is high (58% to 78%) when the femoral head is nonspherical (classes III through V).

3. Longer follow-up (>45 years) reveals substantial deterioration in hip function, with only 40% of patients maintaining good function and the remaining 60% requiring arthroplasty, having severe pain, or having poor function.

III. SLIPPED CAPITAL FEMORAL EPIPHYSIS

A. Overview

1. Definition

a. Slipped capital femoral epiphysis (SCFE) is a disorder of the hip in which the femoral neck displaces anteriorly and superiorly relative to the femoral epiphysis.

b. Displacement occurs through the proximal femoral physis.

c. Uncommonly, the femoral neck displaces posteriorly or medially relative to the femoral epiphysis (*valgus* SCFE).

2. Epidemiology

a. SCFE is the most common disorder of the hip in adolescents.

b. Males are more commonly affected than females (2:1). The cumulative risk in males is 1 per 1,000 to 2,000; the risk in females is 1 per 2,000 to 3,000.

c. Unilateral involvement is more common (80%) than bilateral involvement at the time of presentation. Ultimately, the hips are involved bilaterally in 10% to 60% of cases.

d. SCFE occurs most commonly in Hispanic, Polynesian, and African American populations.

B. Etiology

1. The precise etiology of SCFE is unknown.

2. In general, SCFE is thought to result from an insufficient mechanical ability of the proximal femoral physis to resist loading. This usually results from a combination of abnormally high loads across an abnormally weak physis.

a. Conditions that weaken the physis include endocrinopathies such as hypothyroidism, panhypopituitarism, growth hormone abnormalities, hypogonadism, and hyper- or hypoparathyroidism; systemic diseases such as renal osteodystrophy, hypertension or hyperlipidemia; and prior radiation therapy to the proximal femur.

b. Several mechanical factors that can increase the load across the physis are associated with SCFE, including obesity, relative or absolute femoral retroversion, a decreased femoral neck-shaft angle, and increased physeal obliquity.

C. Pathology—The physis in SCFE is abnormally widened, with irregular organization. The slip occurs through the proliferative and hypertrophic zones of the physis.

D. Evaluation

1. Clinical presentation

a. SCFE is most common in children 10 to 16 years of age.

- In boys, the age at presentation is from age 12 to 16 years (mean, 13.5 years).
- In girls, the age at presentation is from age 10 to 14 years (mean, 11.5 years).

b. Children with SCFE commonly have a limp and localized pain in the groin, hip, thigh, or knee.

c. Symptoms may be present for weeks to months before a diagnosis is made.

2. Physical examination

a. Common physical findings include an abnormal gait (antalgic and/or Trendelenburg), decreased ROM (in particular, decreased hip flexion and decreased internal rotation), and mild limb-length discrepancy.

b. Testing of the ROM of the hip may reveal obligate external rotation (external rotation of the hip as the hip is brought into flexion).

c. The foot and knee progression angles are usually externally rotated.

E. Diagnostic tests

1. Plain radiographs—Standard AP and frog-leg lateral views of the pelvis are recommended. Both hips should be visualized. For patients who cannot be positioned for the frog-leg lateral view, alternate lateral views (eg, cross-table, Dunn lateral) may be warranted.

a. In a normal hip, the Klein line, a line tangential to the superior border of the femoral neck on the AP view, intersects the proximal femoral epiphysis. In a hip with SCFE, the Klein line may fail to intersect the proximal femoral epiphysis, or will be asymmetric between the two hips (**Figure 12**, A).

b. Lateral radiographs are more sensitive than other views in detecting SCFE (**Figure 12**, B).

c. Other radiographic findings in SCFE include a widened, blurred physis and the metaphyseal blanch sign, in which the posteriorly displaced epiphysis is superimposed on the femoral neck on the AP view.

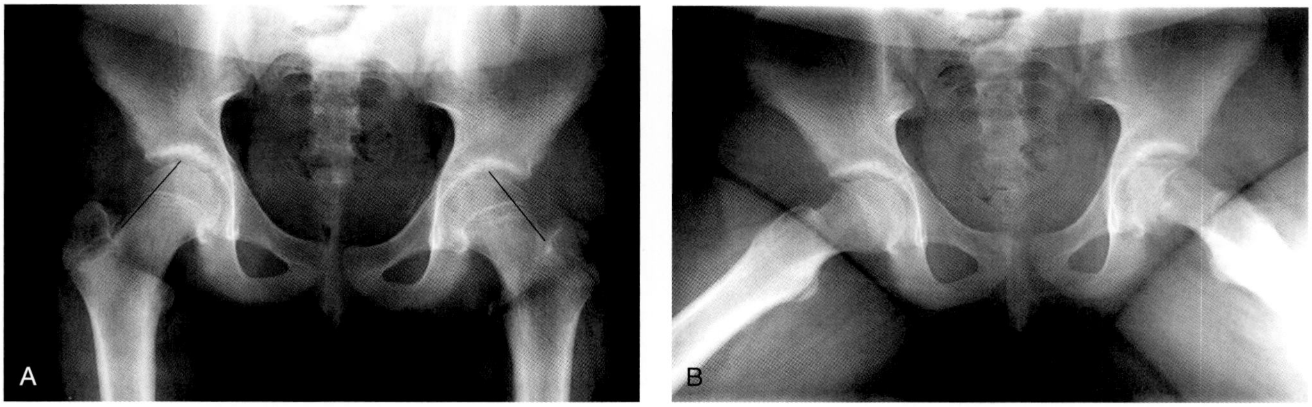

Figure 12 Radiographs of a 10-year-old girl with a stable slipped capital femoral epiphysis (SCFE) on the left. **A**, On the AP view, the Klein line intersects the epiphysis bilaterally. **B**, A frog-leg lateral view of the same patient as in **A** more clearly demonstrates the left SCFE.

2. MRI may be useful in identifying a hip at risk for SCFE before it occurs. An abnormally widened physis with surrounding edematous changes on MRI is suggestive of such a hip.

F. Classification

1. The weight-bearing or Loder classification is the most widely used system. It defines the SCFE as stable or unstable based on the patient's ability to bear weight (**Table 6**).
    a. The SCFE is stable when the patient can bear weight on the involved extremity (with or without crutches).
    b. The SCFE is unstable when the patient cannot bear weight on the involved extremity.
    c. The value of this stability classification is its superior ability to predict osteonecrosis. In a single study, the risk of osteonecrosis in unstable hips was reported as 47% and that in stable hips as zero.
    d. Most cases of SCFE are stable slips (>90%).

TABLE 6

Classification of SCFE

Type of SCFE	Able to Bear Weight?	Risk of Osteonecrosis
Stable	Yes	0%
Unstable	No	47%

Adapted with permission from Loder RT: Unstable slipped capital femoral epiphysis. *J Pediatr Orthop* 2001;21:694-699.

2. The traditional classification was based on duration of symptoms, but it has largely been replaced by the stability classification because of its better prognostic value. This traditional classification used the following categories:
    a. Chronic SCFE: symptoms have been present for more than 3 weeks.
    b. Acute SCFE: symptoms have been present for less than 3 weeks.
    c. Acute-on-chronic SCFE: an acute exacerbation of symptoms follows a prodrome of at least 3 weeks.
3. Radiographic classification
    a. An SCFE is graded according to the percentage of epiphyseal displacement relative to the metaphyseal width of the femoral neck on AP or lateral radiographs. The grades are mild (<33%), moderate (33% to 50%), and severe (>50%).
    b. The Southwick angle (femoral head-shaft angle) is the angle formed by the proximal femoral physis and the femoral shaft on lateral radiographs. An SCFE may also be graded on the basis of the difference in the Southwick angle between the involved and uninvolved hip, with the respective grades of mild (<30° difference), moderate (30° to 50° difference), or severe (>50° difference).

G. Surgical treatment

1. The goal of treatment is to prevent progression of the slip. SCFE should be treated surgically as soon as it is recognized.

2. Stable SCFE—In situ screw fixation is the preferred initial treatment (**Figure 13**).
3. Unstable SCFE—Management is controversial.
   a. The timing of treatment is debated (emergent versus urgent [within 24 hours]).
   b. Decompression of the intracapsular hematoma in SCFE via a capsulotomy (open or percutaneous) may be recommended to decrease the risk of osteonecrosis.
   c. Some centers have moved toward open reduction through a Smith Petersen approach (Parsch procedure), or through a surgical hip dislocation approach (modified Dunn procedure).
   d. Forceful manipulation is never indicated because it is associated with an increased risk of complications, including osteonecrosis.
   e. Serendipitous or gentle reduction does not appear to adversely affect patient outcomes.
4. Technical points of in situ screw fixation
   a. Large (≥6.5 mm), fully threaded, cannulated screw systems are preferred.
   b. A single-screw construct is usually adequate for a stable SCFE. For an unstable SCFE, the use of two screws may be considered for added stability.
   c. The screw or screws are started on the anterolateral femoral neck to allow them to be targeted to the center position of the femoral head and perpendicular to the physis.
   d. Screw heads should be lateral to the intertrochanteric line to minimize the risk of the screw head impinging on the acetabular rim.
5. Indications for prophylactic fixation of the contralateral hip include age younger than 10 years for girls and younger than 12 years for boys, and associated risk factors such as endocrinopathies, renal osteodystrophy, and history of radiation

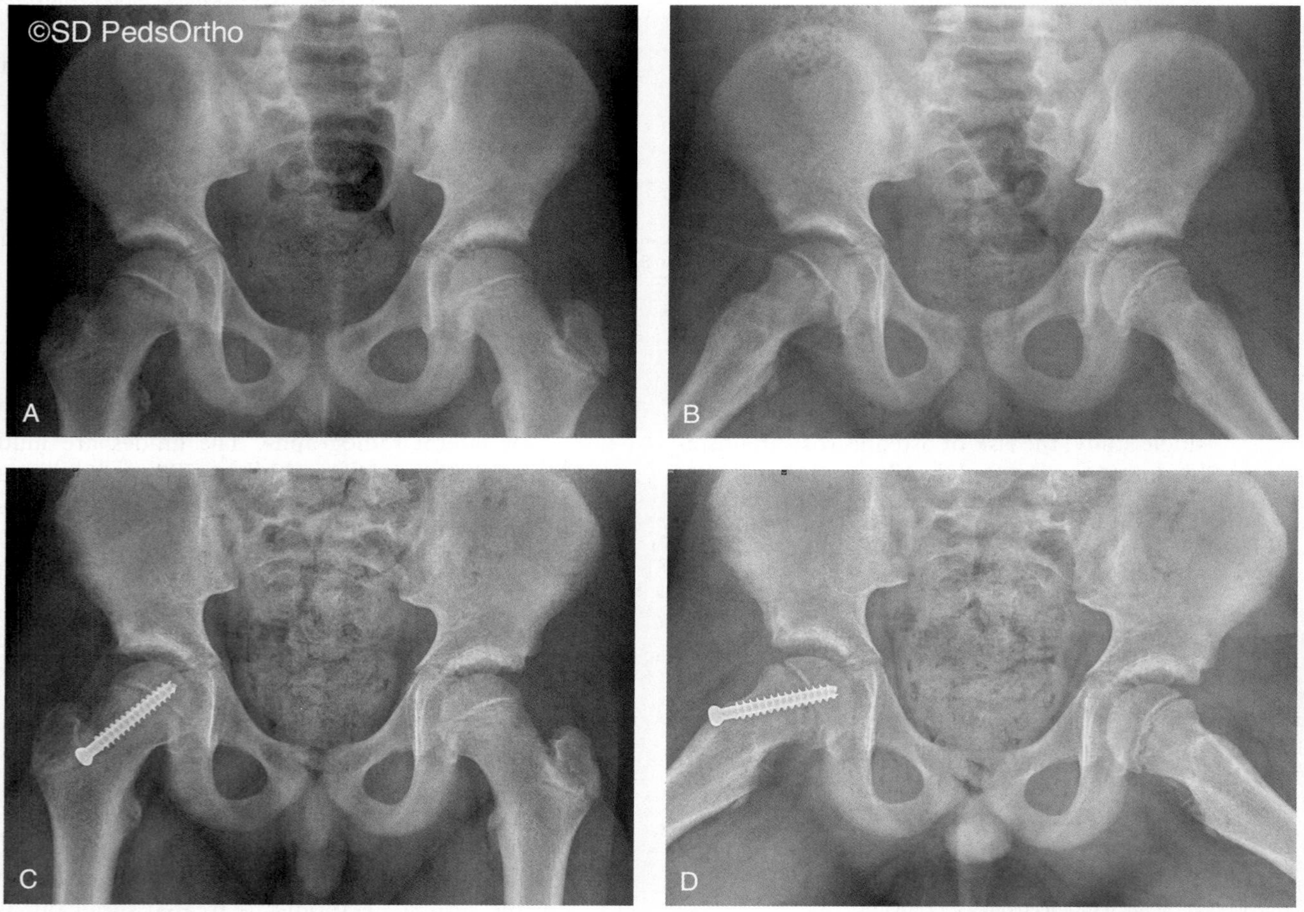

Figure 13 Preoperative AP (**A**) and frog-leg lateral (**B**) and postoperative AP (**C**) and frog-leg **lateral** (**D**) views show in situ screw fixation of a stable slipped capital femoral epiphysis.

therapy. If prophylactic fixation is not performed, the contralateral hip should be monitored radiographically every 6 months.

6. Rehabilitation—Weight bearing is usually protected postoperatively.

H. Management of residual deformity

1. Moderate to severe posteroinferior displacement of the epiphysis relative to the metaphysis can result in substantial proximal femoral deformities, particularly decreased femoral head-neck offset, excessive retroversion of the femoral head, and metaphyseal prominence. These deformities can lead to FAI and pain, stiffness, and premature osteoarthritis of the hip.

2. Moderate to severe SCFE deformities can be corrected to relieve pain and improve function.

a. Hip arthroscopy can be used to improve head-neck offset and address intra-articular pathology.

b. Osteotomy of the proximal femur can be performed at the subcapital, femoral neck, or intertrochanteric (Southwick, Imhäuser) level. Osteotomy at the subcapital level or level of the femoral neck can provide the greatest correction but may be associated with higher rates of complication.

c. Surgical dislocation of the hip with concomitant osteoplasty and/or modified Dunn osteotomy (correction through the physis) has been safely adopted at select centers.

I. Complications

1. Osteonecrosis—Unstable SCFE is the greatest risk factor for osteonecrosis, but hardware placement in the posterior and superior femoral neck can disrupt the interosseous blood supply and also lead to osteonecrosis.

a. Hip arthroplasty is now more commonly performed than hip arthrodesis in young patients with severe osteonecrosis and degenerative joint disease.

2. Chondrolysis—Chondrolysis is usually caused by unrecognized screw penetration of the articular surface. If penetration is recognized and corrected at the time of surgery, chondrolysis does not occur.

3. Slip progression—Progression occurs in 1% to 2% of cases following in situ single-screw fixation.

4. Fracture—The risk of fracture is increased with entry sites through the lateral cortex and those at or distal to the lesser trochanter.

IV. COXA VARA

A. Overview

1. Definition—Coxa vara is an abnormally low femoral neck-shaft angle (<120°).

2. Classification—Coxa vara is classified as congenital, acquired, or developmental.

a. Congenital coxa vara is characterized by a primary cartilaginous defect in the femoral neck. It is commonly associated with a congenitally short femur, a congenitally bowed femur, and proximal femoral focal deficiency (also known as partial longitudinal deficiency of the femur).

b. Acquired coxa vara can result from numerous conditions, including trauma, infection, pathologic bone disorders (eg, osteopetrosis), SCFE, LCPD, and skeletal dysplasias (cleidocranial dysostosis, metaphyseal dysostosis, and some types of spondylometaphyseal dysplasia).

c. Developmental coxa vara occurs in early childhood, with classic radiographic changes (including the inverted Y sign) and no other skeletal manifestations. The remainder of this section focuses on developmental coxa vara.

3. Epidemiology

a. Coxa vara occurs in 1 in 25,000 live births worldwide.

b. Boys and girls are affected equally.

c. Right-side or left-side involvement occurs with equal frequency.

d. Bilateral involvement occurs in 30% to 50% of cases.

e. The incidence does not vary significantly by race.

B. Etiology

1. The precise cause of coxa vara is unclear.

2. A genetic predisposition appears to exist, with an autosomal dominant pattern and incomplete penetrance.

3. Coxa vara may result from a primary defect in endochondral ossification in the medial part of the femoral neck.

a. Bone along the medial inferior aspect of the femoral neck fatigues with weight bearing, resulting in a progressive varus deformity.

b. The vertical orientation of the proximal femoral physis transforms normal compressive forces across the physis into an increasing shear force. Additionally, compressive forces across the medial femoral neck are increased.

C. Evaluation

1. Clinical presentation
   a. The patient usually presents after walking has begun and before 6 years of age.
   b. Pain is uncommon.
   c. An apparent limb shortening or a painless limp may be present in cases of unilateral coxa vara. A waddling gait is more characteristic in cases of bilateral coxa vara.
2. Physical examination
   a. Findings include a prominent greater trochanter, which may also be more proximal than the contralateral greater trochanter.
   b. With unilateral involvement, limb-length discrepancy (usually minor, <3 cm) may be present.
   c. Abductor muscle weakness is common. Consequently, Trendelenburg gait may be present, and the Trendelenburg sign may be positive.
   d. ROM testing may demonstrate a decrease in abduction and internal rotation.
   e. With bilateral involvement, lumbar lordosis may be increased.
3. Plain radiographs—AP and frog-leg lateral views of the pelvis are recommended. Radiographic findings include the following:
   a. A decreased femoral neck-shaft angle (mean femoral neck-shaft angle = 148° at 1 year of age, gradually decreasing to 120° in the adult)
   b. The inverted Y sign (resulting from a triangular metaphyseal fragment in the inferior femoral neck), which is pathognomonic (**Figure 14**)
   c. Vertical orientation of the physis, a shortened femoral neck, and decreased femoral anteversion
   d. An abnormal Hilgenreiner-epiphyseal (H-E) angle (angle formed by a line through the proximal femoral physis and the Hilgenreiner line) (**Figure 15**)

D. Natural history—The H-E angle correlates with the risk of progression of coxa vara.

1. Hips with an H-E angle less than 45° typically remain stable or improve.
2. An H-E angle of 45° to 60° is associated with an indeterminate risk of progression.
3. An H-E angle greater than 60° is associated with a significantly high risk of progression.

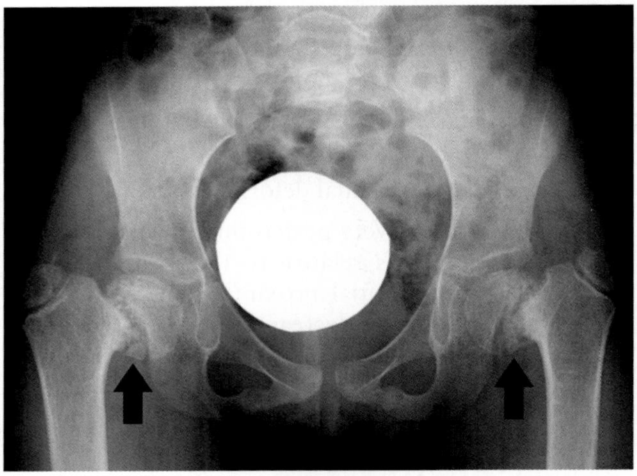

Figure 14 The inverted Y sign (arrows), formed by a triangular metaphyseal fragment in the inferior femoral neck, is pathognomonic for coxa vara

E. Treatment—Recommendations are based on the severity of the H-E angle and the presence of symptoms.

1. Nonsurgical treatment
   a. Asymptomatic patients with an H-E angle less than 45° should be observed.
   b. Asymptomatic patients with an H-E angle between 45° and 59° also can be observed. Serial radiographs are critical to assess for disease progression.
2. Surgical treatment
   a. Indications—Surgery is indicated for the following:
      - Patients with a Trendelenburg gait and/or fatigue pain in the hip abductors and an H-E angle of 45° to 59° or patients with evidence of progression
      - Patients with an H-E angle greater than 60°
      - Patients with a progressive decrease in the femoral neck-shaft angle to 100° or less

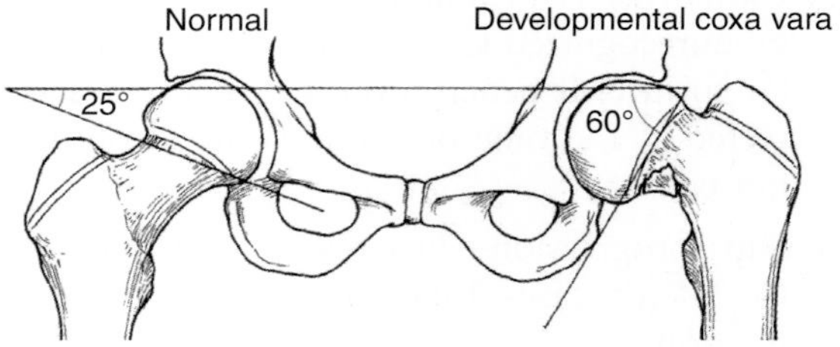

Figure 15 The Hilgenreiner-epiphyseal (H-E) angle is formed by a line through the physis and the Hilgenreiner line. A normal H-E angle is approximately 25°.

b. Before ossification of the navicular at age 3 years, the first metatarsal is used as a proxy for the dorsal alignment of the navicular on the lateral view.

D. Treatment

1. Manipulation and casting (reverse Ponseti method)

a. Entails serial manipulation and casting to reduce the dorsal dislocation of the navicular on the talus and stretch dorsolateral soft tissues

b. Counterpressure is applied to the talar head while the foot is stretched into plantar flexion and inversion.

c. After passive reduction of the talus is achieved and confirmed with a lateral radiograph, surgical release and pinning of the talonavicular joint and percutaneous Achilles tenotomy are performed to complete the correction.

d. More extensive surgical release may be required in cases of incomplete correction.

2. Surgical

a. A traditional pantalar release is usually performed between 12 and 18 months of age.

b. Surgical treatment includes pantalar release with lengthening of the Achilles, toe extensors, and peroneal tendons and pinning of the talonavicular joint. The tibialis anterior is generally transferred to the neck of the talus.

c. The outcome of reconstruction in children older than 3 years is less predictable. Triple arthrodesis is rarely needed as a salvage procedure.

III. OBLIQUE TALUS

A. May have clinical appearance similar to vertical talus

B. The plantar flexion lateral radiograph demonstrates reducible talonavicular subluxation.

C. Treatment is controversial. Many authors propose observation, whereas others advocate for manipulation and/or casting similar to that described for congenital vertical talus.

IV. CALCANEOVALGUS FOOT

A. Overview

1. Calcaneovalgus foot is a positional deformity in infants in which the foot is hyperdorsiflexed secondary to intrauterine positioning (**Figure 2**).

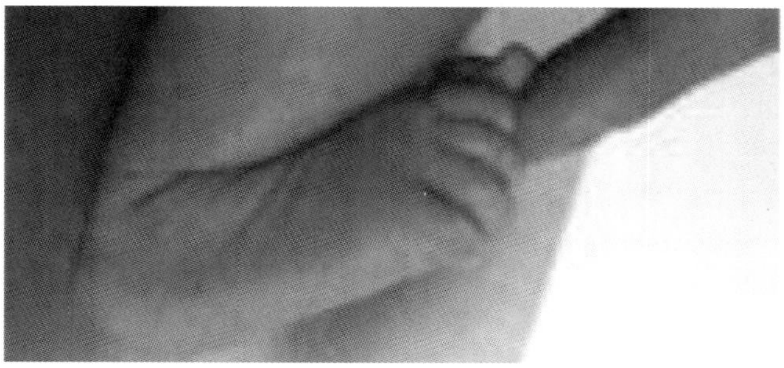

Figure 2 Clinical photograph shows a calcaneovalgus foot in a newborn. Note the characteristic hyperdorsiflexion and hindfoot valgus. (Reproduced from Sullivan JA: Pediatric flatfoot: Evaluation and management. *J Am Acad Orthop Surg* 1999;7[1]:44-53.)

2. It is more common in first-born females.

B. Pathoanatomy

1. A calcaneovalgus foot in newborns is a soft-tissue contracture problem.

2. No dislocation or bony deformity of the foot exists.

C. Evaluation

1. The deformity should be passively correctable to neutral.

2. May be associated with posteromedial bowing of the tibia; however, isolated posteromedial tibial bowing may be misdiagnosed as a calcaneovalgus foot.

D. Treatment

1. The deformity typically resolves without intervention.

2. Stretching may expedite resolution.

V. PES CAVUS

A. Overview

1. A pes cavus (cavus foot) has an elevated medial longitudinal arch secondary to forefoot plantar flexion or, less frequently, as a result of excessive calcaneal dorsiflexion (calcaneus hindfoot).

2. Two-thirds of patients with a cavus foot have an underlying neurologic disorder, most commonly Charcot-Marie-Tooth disease.

B. Pathoanatomy

1. The primary structural problem is forefoot plantar flexion. The first ray is often more markedly plantarflexed, which results in forefoot pronation.

2. For the lateral half of the foot to be in contact with the ground, the hindfoot must deviate into varus (**Figure 3**).

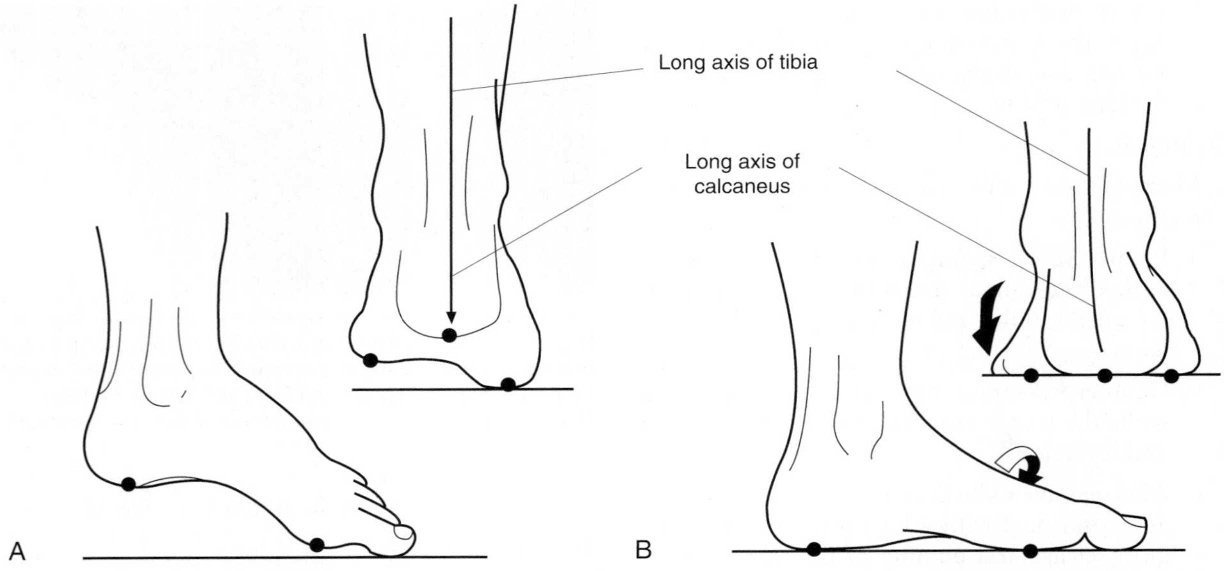

Figure 3 Illustrations show the tripod effect in a cavus foot. **A**, Posterior and lateral views show a cavus foot in the non–weight-bearing position. The long axes of the tibia and the calcaneus are parallel, and the first metatarsal is pronated. Dots indicate the three major weight-bearing plantar areas, the heel and the first and fifth metatarsals. **B**, Posterior and lateral views show a cavus foot in the weight-bearing position. The long axes of the tibia and the calcaneus are not parallel. During weight bearing, a rigid equinus forefoot deformity forces the flexible hindfoot into varus. This is the tripod effect. (Adapted with permission from Paulos L, Coleman SS, Samuelson KM: Pes cavovarus: Review of a surgical approach using selective soft-tissue procedures. *J Bone Joint Surg Am* 1980;62:942-953.)

3. First ray plantar flexion may result from a weak tibialis anterior relative to the peroneus longus, but it is more commonly caused by intrinsic weakness and contracture.
4. Over time, the plantar fascia contracts, and the hindfoot varus deformity becomes more rigid.

C. Evaluation

1. Patients may report instability (ankle sprains).
2. A neurologic examination and a family history are essential.
3. Unilateral involvement suggests a focal diagnosis (for example, spinal cord anomaly or nerve injury).
4. Bilateral involvement and a positive family history are common with Charcot-Marie-Tooth disease. Despite bilateral involvement, asymmetry may be seen in Charcot-Marie-Tooth disease.
5. Hindfoot flexibility is assessed by placing a 1-inch block under the lateral border of the foot (Coleman block test).
6. Radiographs—Weight-bearing views are required.
   a. Increased Meary angle—The long axis of the talus will intersect the long axis of the first metatarsal dorsally on the lateral view of the foot. The normal value is 0° to 5°.
   b. Increased calcaneal pitch—Intersection of a line running along the undersurface of the calcaneus and the floor. Calcaneal pitch greater than 30° indicates a calcaneocavus foot.
7. MRI of the spine is indicated with unilateral involvement.

D. Treatment

1. Joint-sparing procedures are preferred whenever possible.
2. A key to surgical decision making is the flexibility of the hindfoot. Some general guidelines exist (**Table 2**).
3. Percutaneous plantar fascia release is insufficient to correct a cavus foot. At minimum, an open release and soft-tissue rebalancing are needed.
4. Achilles tendon lengthening should not be performed concomitantly with plantar fasciotomy. An intact Achilles tendon provides the resistance necessary to stretch the contracted plantar tissues and correct the cavus deformity.

VI. PES PLANOVALGUS

A. Overview

1. Pes planovalgus (flexible flatfoot) is a physiologic variation of normal.

TABLE 2

Treatment of Pes Cavus

Severity of Deformity	Examination and History	Corrective Treatment
Mild	Flexible, painless	Achilles tendon stretching, eversion/dorsiflexion strengthening program
Mild	Progressive or symptomatic	Plantar release ± peroneus longus to brevis transfer
	Varus because of peroneal weakness	Add tibialis anterior and/or posterior tendon transfer to the peroneal muscles
Moderate	Rigid medial cavus	Dorsiflexion osteotomy of either first metatarsal or cuneiform
	Rigid medial and lateral cavus	Dorsiflexion osteotomies of the cuboid and cuneiforms
	Rigid hindfoot varus	Closing/sliding calcaneal osteotomy
	Clawing of hallux	Add EHL transfer to first metatarsal (Jones)
Severe	Not correctable to plantigrade with other procedures	Triple arthrodesis is rarely needed and should be avoided whenever possible.

EHL = extensor hallucis longus.

2. It is defined by a decreased longitudinal arch and a valgus hindfoot during weight bearing.
3. It is rarely symptomatic, is common in childhood, and resolves spontaneously in most cases.
4. Flexible flatfoot is present in 20% to 25% of adults.

B. Pathoanatomy

1. Generalized ligamentous laxity is common.
2. Approximately one-fourth of flexible flatfeet have a contracture of the gastrocnemius-soleus complex. These cases may be associated with disability.

C. Evaluation

1. An arch should be evident when toe-standing, during dorsiflexion of the hallux, or when not bearing weight.
2. Subtalar motion should be full and painless as evidenced by heel swing from valgus to varus with toe-standing.
3. On a lateral radiograph, the talus is plantarflexed relative to the first metatarsal (decreased Meary angle).
4. Apparent hindfoot valgus may actually be caused by ankle valgus (particularly in children with myelodysplasia). If any suspicion of ankle valgus is present, ankle radiographs should be obtained.
5. The differential of flatfoot includes tarsal coalition, congenital vertical talus, and accessory navicular.

D. Treatment

1. No treatment is indicated for asymptomatic patients.
2. Nonsurgical
   a. Shoes or orthoses do not promote arch development.
   b. Athletic shoes with arch and heel support can help relieve pain.
   c. The University of California Biomechanics Laboratory orthosis is a rigid orthotic insert designed to support the arch and control the hindfoot. A soft molded insert is an alternative but may be inadequate to control hindfoot valgus.
   d. Stretching exercises are recommended if the patient is symptomatic and an Achilles contracture is present.
3. Surgical
   a. Surgery is reserved for rare cases in which pain is recalcitrant to nonsurgical treatment.
   b. A calcaneal neck lengthening with soft-tissue balancing is the treatment of choice. It corrects deformity while preserving motion and growth. Arthrodesis is rarely indicated.

VII. METATARSUS ADDUCTUS

A. Overview

1. Metatarsus adductus is a medial deviation of the forefoot with normal alignment of the hindfoot.
2. It occurs in up to 12% of newborns.

B. Pathoanatomy—Intrauterine positioning of the foot is thought to be one possible cause.

C. Evaluation

1. The foot has a kidney-bean shape (convex lateral border), and the hindfoot is in a neutral position.
2. The amount of active correction is assessed by tickling the foot.
3. The Bleck classification system grades the severity of the deformity based on flexibility. A flexible forefoot is one that could be abducted beyond the midline heel-bisector angle, a partially flexible forefoot could be abducted to the midline, and a rigid forefoot could not be abducted to the midline (**Figure 4**).
4. Must be distinguished from metatarsus primus varus, in which the lateral border of the foot is normal, but a medial crease is present secondary to isolated varus alignment of the first ray. This deformity is typically rigid, requires early casting, and may result in hallux valgus.

D. Prognosis and treatment

1. Nonsurgical
   a. Spontaneous resolution of metatarsus adductus occurs in 90% of children by age 4 years.
   b. Passive stretching is recommended for a flexible deformity but may not improve the final outcome.
   c. Serial casting between 6 and 12 months of age is useful in children with deformity that has a rigid component.
2. Surgical
   a. Surgery is indicated only in children older than 7 years with severe residual deformity that produces problems with shoe wear and pain.
   b. A medial column lengthening (opening wedge osteotomy of cuneiform) combined with lateral column shortening (closing wedge of the cuboid)

VIII. SKEWFOOT

A. Definition—Skewfoot deformity consists of an adducted forefoot and hindfoot valgus with plantar flexion of the talus.

B. Evaluation

1. Patients may become symptomatic at the talar head or the base of the fifth metatarsal.
2. Clinical examination and weight-bearing radiographs confirm the diagnosis.

C. Treatment—Surgery (combined opening wedge medial cuneiform osteotomy and calcaneal osteotomy) is limited to patients who have persistent pain.

IX. IDIOPATHIC TOE WALKING

A. Overview

1. Can occur normally as a child develops the gait pattern; toe walking beyond 2 years of age requires investigation to rule out neuromuscular or developmental abnormalities.
2. The etiology is largely unknown, although proposed causes include defects in sensory processing, abnormalities of underlying muscle fibers, and a possible genetic component.

B. Evaluation

1. A thorough history and physical examination should be performed to rule out neurologic and developmental causes of toe walking.
2. Patients may or may not be able to walk flatfooted, depending on the degree of equinus contracture present.
3. If limited ankle dorsiflexion is present, it is important to determine whether contracture is caused by the gastrocnemius alone or the entire gastrocnemius-soleus complex. Persistent

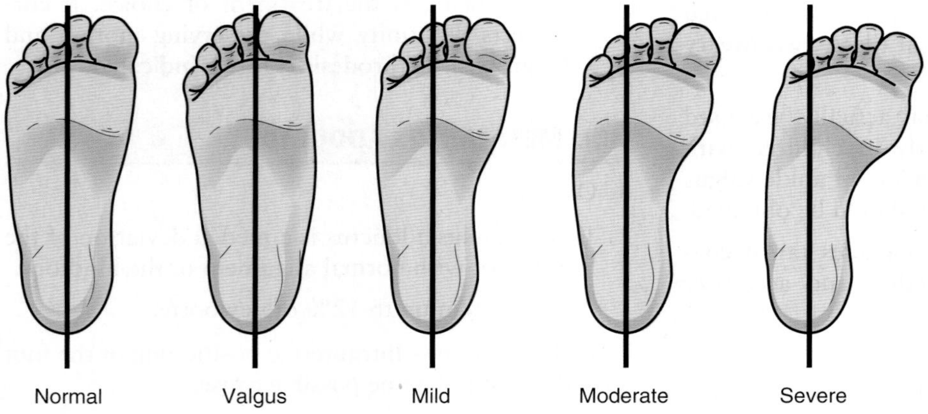

Figure 4 Illustrations depict the heel-bisector line, which defines the relationship of the heel to the forefoot. Normal foot: line bisects the second and third toes; valgus: line bisects the great and second toes; mild metatarsus adductus: line bisects the third toe; moderate metatarsus adductus: line bisects the third and fourth toes; and severe metatarsus adductus: line bisects the fourth and fifth toes.

Chapter 135

Pediatric Lower Extremity Deformities and Limb Deficiencies

ANTHONY A. SCADUTO, MD
NATHAN L. FROST, MD

I. LIMB-LENGTH DISCREPANCY

A. Epidemiology—Small (up to 2 cm) limb-length discrepancies (LLDs) are common, occurring in up to two-thirds of the general population.

B. Secondary problems from LLD

1. The prevalence of back pain may be higher with larger discrepancies (>2 cm).
2. During double-limb stance, the hip on the long side is relatively less covered by the acetabulum. This may predispose patients to hip arthropathy on the long leg side.
3. LLD increases the incidence of structural scoliosis to the short side. In up to one-third of cases, the scoliosis is in a noncompensatory direction.

C. Evaluation

1. The discrepancy is measured by placing blocks under the short leg to level the pelvis.
2. Hip, knee, and ankle contractures will affect the apparent limb length and must be ruled out. A hip adduction contracture causes an apparent shortening of the adducted side.
3. The advantages and disadvantages of various imaging techniques are listed in **Table 1**.
4. Up to 6% of patients with LLD from hemihypertrophy develop embryonal cancers (eg, Wilms tumor). Routine abdominal ultrasonography is recommended until the age of 6 years.

D. Prediction methods

1. Arithmetic or rule-of-thumb method
   a. Assumes growth ends at chronologic age 14 years for girls and 16 years for boys
   b. Estimates the annual contribution to leg length of each physis near skeletal maturity (during the last 4 years of growth)
      - Proximal femoral physis—3 mm
      - Distal femoral physis—9 mm
      - Proximal tibial physis—6 mm
      - Distal tibial physis—3 mm
2. Growth remaining method
   a. LLD prediction based on Green and Anderson tables of extremity length for a given age
   b. Uses skeletal age for predicting discrepancy
3. Moseley straight-line graph method
   a. This method improves the accuracy of the Green and Anderson prediction by reformatting the data in graph form.
   b. It minimizes errors of arithmetic or interpretation by averaging serial measurements.
4. Multiplier method
   a. This method predicts final limb length by multiplying the current discrepancy by a sex-specific and age-specific factor.
   b. It is most accurate for discrepancies that are constantly proportional (eg, congenital).

Dr. Scaduto or an immediate family member serves as a board member, owner, officer, or committee member of the American Academy of Orthopaedic Surgeons, the Pediatric Orthopaedic Society of North America, and the Scoliosis Research Society. Neither Dr. Frost nor any immediate family member has received anything of value from or has stock or stock options held in a commercial company or institution related directly or indirectly to the subject of this chapter.

TABLE 1

Assessment of Limb-Length Discrepancy Using Imaging Techniques

Technique	Description	Advantages	Disadvantages
Teleoradiograph	Single exposure of entire leg on a long cassette	Can assess angular deformity	Magnification error
Orthoradiograph	Three separate exposures (hip, knee, and ankle) on a long cassette	Eliminates magnification error	Cannot assess angular deformity Movement error may occur
Scanogram	Three separate exposures on a small cassette	Eliminates magnification error Small cassette	Cannot assess angular deformity Movement error may occur
CT scanogram	CT scan through hip, knee, and ankle to assess length	Accurate length measurement possible in the presence of joint contractures	Cannot assess angular deformity

E. Classification

1. Causes of LLD include congenital conditions, infection, paralytic conditions, tumors, trauma, and osteonecrosis.
   a. In congenital conditions, the absolute discrepancy increases, but the relative percentage remains constant (eg, a short limb that is 70% of the long side at birth will be 70% of the long side at maturity).
   b. Children with paralysis usually have shortening of the more severely affected side.
2. Static discrepancies (eg, a malunion of the femur in a shortened position) must be differentiated from progressive discrepancies (eg, physeal growth arrest).

F. Treatment (**Table 2**)

1. Surgical correction must address the projected LLD at skeletal maturity.
2. Goals of treatment include a level pelvis and equal limb lengths.
   a. In paralytic conditions or in patients with a stiff knee, it is often best to leave the LLD undercorrected to facilitate foot clearance of the weak leg.
   b. In patients with fixed pelvic obliquity, functional limb-length equality should be the goal of treatment.
3. Nonsurgical management with or without a shoe lift is typically reserved for a projected LLD of less than 2 cm.
4. Shortening techniques
   a. Epiphysiodesis is the treatment of choice for skeletally immature patients with projected discrepancies of 2 to 5 cm because of the low complication rate. If proximal tibial epiphysiodesis is performed, concomitant proximal fibular epiphysiodesis should also be performed if more than 2 to 3 years of growth remain.
   b. Acute osseous shortening, typically of the femur, is used for skeletally mature patients with discrepancies of 2 to 5 cm.
5. Lengthening techniques
   a. Limb lengthening is typically reserved for LLD greater than 5 or 6 cm.
   b. Previous techniques involve osteotomy or corticotomy and incremental distraction using a uniplanar or multiplanar external fixator, often over an intramedullary nail to reduce the time spent in the fixator during the consolidation phase.
   c. Recent technological advances now allow incremental distraction to be carried out with an intramedullary lengthening device. The distraction mechanism is controlled by an externally applied electromagnet while stabilization is provided by the intramedullary device itself.

TABLE 2

Treatment Algorithm for Limb-Length Discrepancy

Discrepancy	Treatment Options
0-2 cm	No treatment if asymptomatic. May use shoe lift if symptomatic
2-5 cm	Shoe lift, epiphysiodesis, shortening, lengthening
5-15 cm	Lengthening(s). May be combined with epiphysiodesis/shortening procedure(s)
>15 cm	Lengthenings plus epiphysiodesis/shortening versus prosthesis

d. Technical considerations for lengthening include making the corticotomy at the metaphyseal level when possible and delaying distraction for 5 to 7 days after the corticotomy.

e. The typical rate of distraction is 1 mm/d (0.25 mm four times daily).

f. Complications of limb lengthening include pin site infection, hardware failure, regenerate deformity or fracture, delayed union, premature union at corticotomy, and joint subluxation/dislocation.

II. ANGULAR DEFORMITIES

A. Overview

1. Normal physiologic knee alignment includes periods of "knock knees" and "bowed legs" (**Figure 1**).

2. Children older than 2 years with bowed legs may require further evaluation.

B. Blount Disease (tibia vara)

1. Overview

a. The most common cause of pathologic genu varum is Blount disease.

b. Progressive tibia vara can occur in infants and adolescents (**Table 3**).

2. Epidemiology

a. Affects less than 1% of US population.

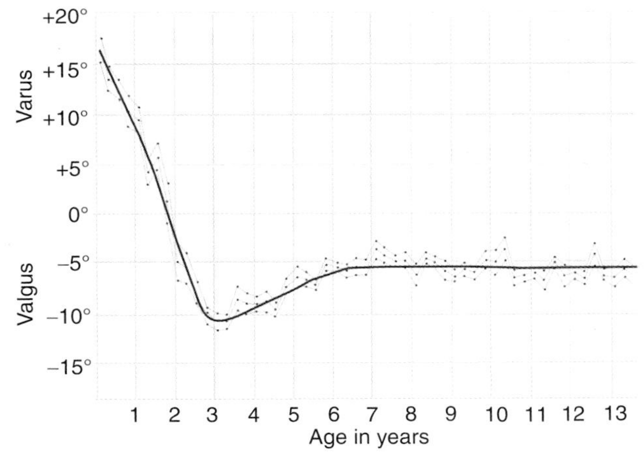

Figure 1 Graph illustrates the development of the tibiofemoral angle in children during growth, based on measurements from 1,480 examinations of 979 children. Of the lighter lines, the middle one represents the mean value at a given point in time, and the other two represent the deviation from the mean. The darker line represents the general trend. (Adapted with permission from Salenius P, Vankka E: The development of the tibiofemoral angle in children. *J Bone Joint Surg Am* 1975;57:259-261.)

b. Higher incidence in African American population and obese individuals as well as those considered to walk early.

3. Pathoanatomy

a. In infantile Blount disease, excess medial pressure (such as obese, early walkers who are in physiologic varus alignment) produces an osteochondrosis of the physis and adjacent epiphysis that can progress to develop a physeal bar.

b. In adolescent Blount disease, a varus moment at the knee during the stance phase of gait further inhibits medial physeal growth according to the Hueter-Volkmann principle (compression = decreased growth of the physis).

4. Evaluation

a. Clinical findings suggestive of pathologic bowing include localized bowing at the proximal tibia, severe deformity, progression, and lateral thrust during gait.

b. Full-length standing radiographs should be performed on children older than 18 months with the aforementioned findings.

c. If the metaphyseal-diaphyseal (MD) angle (**Figure 2**) is less than 10°, there is a 95% chance the bowing will resolve.

d. If the MD angle is greater than 16°, there is a 95% chance the bowing will progress. For MD angles between 11° and 16°, monitoring is required.

5. Classification—Langenskiöld described six radiographic stages that can develop over 4 to 5 years.

a. Early changes include metaphyseal beaking and sloping.

b. Advanced changes include articular depression and medial physeal closure.

6. Nonsurgical treatment of infantile Blount disease

a. The efficacy of bracing treatment is controversial.

b. Bracing treatment with a knee-ankle-foot orthosis may be indicated in patients 2 to 3 years of age with mild disease (stage 1 to 2).

c. Poor results are associated with obesity and bilaterality.

d. Improvement should occur within 1 year, although treatment must be continued until the bony changes resolve, which usually takes 1.5 to 2.0 years.

TABLE 3

Infantile Versus Adolescent Blount Disease

Condition	Age (Years)	Typical History	Location of Deformity	Other Angular Deformities	Laterality	Treatment
Infantile blount	1-3	Early walker, obese	Epiphysis/physis; joint depression in advanced stages	None	Often bilateral	Bracing treatment (limited effectiveness) Proximal tibia/fibula osteotomy
Adolescent blount	9-11	Morbid obesity	Proximal tibia; no joint depression	Distal femur and distal tibia common	Unilateral more common	Bracing treatment not effective Hemiepiphysiodesis if growth remaining Proximal tibia/fibula osteotomy ± femoral and distal tibia osteotomies

7. Surgical treatment of infantile Blount disease
   a. Patients older than 3 years require proximal tibial osteotomy.
   b. To avoid undercorrection, the distal fragment is fixed in slight valgus, lateral translation, and external rotation.

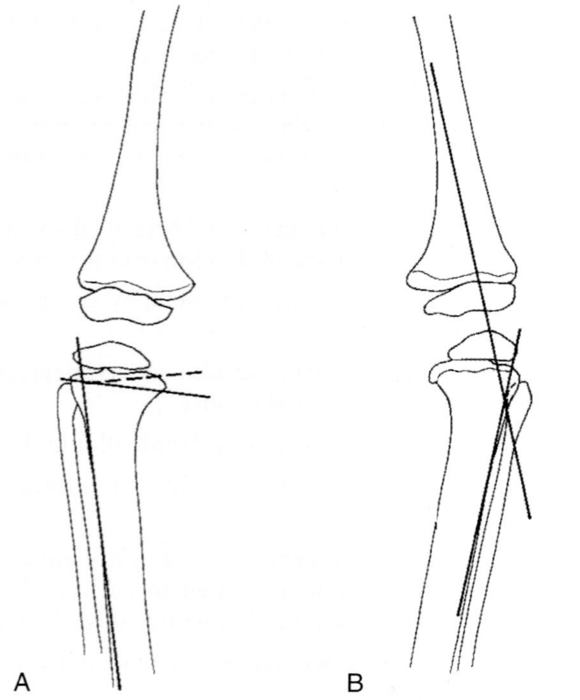

Figure 2 Illustration shows the assessment of the metaphyseal-diaphyseal (**A**) and tibial-femoral (**B**) angles. (Reproduced from Brooks WC, Gross RH: Genu varum in children: Diagnosis and treatment. *J Am Acad Orthop Surg* 1995;3[6]:326-336.)

   c. Performing an anterior compartment fasciotomy at the time of surgery reduces the postoperative risk of compartment syndrome.
   d. The risk of recurrence is much less if the surgery is performed in children younger than 4 years.
   e. If a bony bar is present, a bar resection with interposition of methylmethacrylate (epiphysiolysis) is performed concomitantly.
8. Surgical treatment of adolescent Blount disease
   a. Temporary or permanent hemiepiphysiodesis of the proximal lateral tibia prevents deformity progression and may allow some correction in adolescents with mild to moderate Blount disease in whom at least 15 to 18 months of growth remain.
   b. Severe deformities and/or deformities in skeletally mature patients require proximal tibial osteotomy.
   c. Correction of deformity may be performed acutely or gradually using an external fixator.
   d. Patients should be carefully assessed for distal femoral varus, which can be treated similarly with a hemiepiphysiodesis in immature patients or distal femoral osteotomy in severe cases or in mature patients.

C. Genu valgum
1. Overview
   a. Children aged 3 to 4 years typically have up to 20° of genu valgum.
   b. Genu valgum should not increase after 7 years of age.

TABLE 4

Common Causes of Genu Valgum

Bilateral
Physiologic genu valgum
Rickets
Skeletal dysplasia (eg, chondroctodermal dysplasia, spondyloepiphyseal, morquio syndrome)
Unilateral
Physeal injury (trauma, infection, or vascular)
Proximal tibial metaphyseal (cozen) fracture
Benign tumors (eg, fibrous dysplasia, Ollier disease, osteochondroma)

c. After the age of 7 years, valgus should not exceed 12°, and the intermalleolar distance should be less than 8 cm.

2. Epidemiology
   a. Incidence largely unknown but found to be higher in obese and overweight individuals
3. Pathoanatomy
   a. The deformity is usually in the distal femur but may also arise in the proximal tibia.
   b. The degree of deformity necessary to lead to degenerative changes in the knee is not known.
4. Etiology (**Table 4**)
5. Treatment
   a. There is no role for bracing treatment in genu valgum.
   b. Genu valgum following proximal tibial metaphyseal fractures (Cozen phenomenon) typically remodels spontaneously and should be observed.
   c. Correction is indicated if the mechanical axis (represented by a line drawn from the center of the femoral head to the center of the distal tibial plafond) falls in the outer quadrant of the tibial plateau (or beyond) in children older than 10 years.
   d. In skeletally immature patients, hemiepiphysiodesis or temporary physeal tethering may be performed with staples, transphyseal screws, or plate/screw devices (**Figure 3**).
   e. Varus-producing osteotomies are necessary when insufficient growth remains or the site of the deformity is away from the physis. To reduce the risk of peroneal injury, gradual correction, preemptive peroneal nerve release, or a closing-wedge technique should be considered.

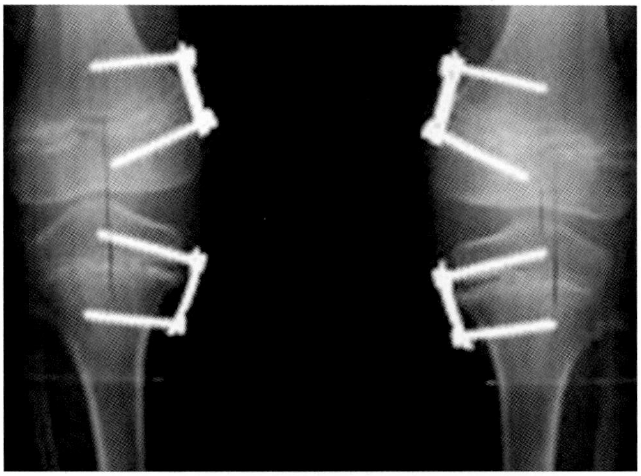

Figure 3 Radiographs demonstrate hemiphyseal tethering with a plate-screw construct. (Courtesy of Orthofix, Lewisville, TX.)

III. ROTATIONAL DEFORMITIES

A. Femoral anteversion

1. Overview
   a. Normal anteversion is 30° to 40° at birth and decreases to 15° by skeletal maturity.
   b. In-toeing from femoral anteversion is most evident between 3 and 6 years of age.
2. Epidemiology
   a. Increased femoral anteversion occurs more commonly in girls than in boys (2:1 ratio) and often is hereditary.
   b. True incidence largely unknown.
3. Pathoanatomy
   a. Rotational variations have not been directly correlated to degenerative changes of the hip or knee.
   b. Patellofemoral pain can arise with increasing femoral anteversion, but a pathologic threshold has not been identified.
4. Evaluation
   a. In-toeing gait with medially rotated patellae is indicative of femoral anteversion.
   b. Rotational profile assessment should include the knee-progression and foot-progression angles during gait, the thigh-foot angle, and the maximum hip internal and external rotation (**Figure 4**). After 10 years of age, internal rotation greater than 70° and external rotation less than 20° suggests excessive femoral anteversion.

10 | Pediatrics

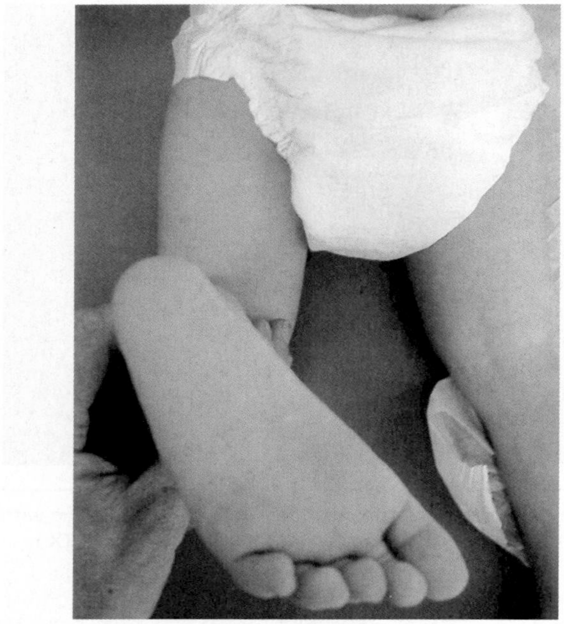

Figure 4 Photograph depicts the measuring of the thigh-foot axis, which is best performed with the child in the prone position. (Reproduced from Lincoln TL, Suen PW: Common rotational variations in children. *J Am Acad Orthop Surg* 2003;11[5]:312-320.)

c. Femoral anteversion is estimated by measuring the degree of internal hip rotation necessary to make the greater trochanter most prominent laterally (trochanteric prominence angle test).

d. CT or MRI can quantify anteversion accurately but are unnecessary in most cases.

e. Differential diagnoses of in-toeing include internal tibial torsion and metatarsus adductus.

5. Treatment

a. Shoes and orthoses are ineffective.

b. Children older than 8 years with unacceptable gait or pain and less than 10° external hip rotation are candidates for a derotational osteotomy.

c. The amount of rotation to correct excessive anteversion = (prone internal rotation – prone external rotation)/2.

B. Internal tibial torsion

1. Epidemiology

a. Most evident between ages 1 and 2 years

b. Usually resolves by age 6 years

2. Evaluation

a. The transmalleolar axis—the angular difference between the bimalleolar axis at the ankle and the bicondylar axis of the knee—is determined; normal is 20° of external rotation.

b. Measurement of the thigh-foot axis in the prone position; by 8 years, normal is 10° of external rotation.

3. Treatment

a. Parent education is the primary treatment.

b. Special shoes and braces do not change outcome.

c. Derotational osteotomy is rarely indicated and should be reserved for children older than 8 years with marked functional and/or esthetic deformity.

IV. TIBIAL BOWING

A. Overview—Three types of tibial bowing exist in children, with considerable differences in prognosis and treatment (**Table 5**).

B. Anterolateral bowing

1. Epidemiology

a. Of patients with anterolateral bowing, 50% have neurofibromatosis.

b. Of patients with neurofibromatosis, 10% have anterolateral bowing.

2. Classification—The presence of sclerosis, cysts, fibular dysplasia, and narrowing are the basis of the Boyd and Crawford classification (**Figure 5**).

3. Natural history

a. Spontaneous resolution is unusual.

b. Good prognostic signs include a duplicated hallux and a delta-shaped osseous segment in the concavity of the bow.

c. Fracture risk decreases at skeletal maturity.

4. Treatment

a. The initial goal of treatment is prevention of pseudarthrosis with a clam-shell total contact brace.

b. Osteotomies to correct bowing are contraindicated because of the risk of pseudarthrosis of the osteotomy site.

c. If pseudarthrosis develops, all treatment options have limited success.

d. Treatment options of pseudarthrosis include

- Intramedullary rod and bone grafting
- Circular fixator with bone transport

TABLE 5

Types of Tibial Bowing

	Anterolateral Bowing	Posteromedial Bowing	Anteromedial Bowing
Associated conditions	Neurofibromatosis	Calcaneal valgus foot	Fibular deficiency
Prognosis	1. Progressive bowing 2. Pseudarthrosis	1. Spontaneous improvement in bowing (rarely complete) 2. Limb-length discrepancy	Varies with severity of shortening and foot function
Treatment	1. Bracing treatment to prevent fracture 2. Osteotomy contraindicated	Observation versus epiphysiodesis for limb-length discrepancy	Osteotomy with lengthening versus amputation

- Vascularized fibular graft
- Adjunctive use of bone morphogenetic proteins is an accepted addition to any of the above treatments

e. Amputation may be considered for persistent pseudarthrosis (usually after two or three failed surgeries).

C. Posteromedial bowing

1. Congenital posteromedial bowing is often associated with a calcaneovalgus foot. The dorsum of the foot may be in contact with the anterior tibia in this condition.
2. The bowing improves in the first years of life, but it rarely resolves completely.

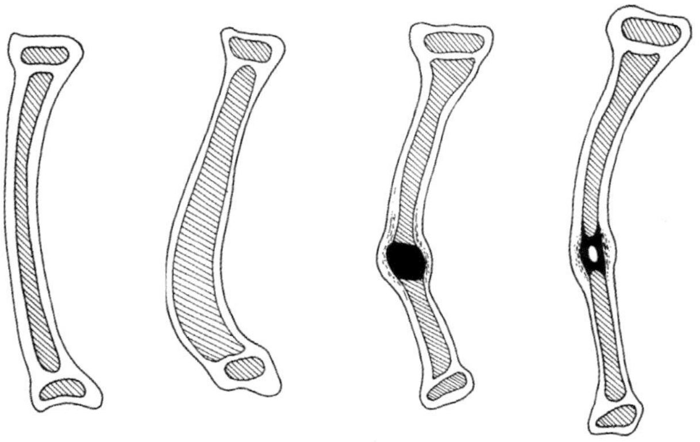

Figure 5 Illustrations show the Boyd and Crawford classification of congenital tibial dysplasia. Type I is characterized by anterior lateral bowing with increased cortical density and a narrow but normal medullary canal; type IIA, by anterior lateral bowing with failure of tubularization and a widened medullary canal; type IIB, by anterior lateral bowing with a cystic lesion before fracture or canal enlargement from a previous fracture; and type IIC, by frank pseudarthrosis and bone atrophy with "sucked candy" narrowing of the ends of the two fragments. (Reproduced from Crawford AH, Schorry EK: Neurofibromatosis in children: The role of the orthopaedist. *J Am Acad Orthop Surg* 1999;7[4]:217-230.)

3. Monitoring for LLD is required—LLDs at maturity are usually in the 3 to 8 cm range (mean, 4 cm) and are treated as described above in Section I.
4. Epidemiology—Incidence largely unknown

D. Anteromedial bowing—See fibular deficiency in Section V.

V. LIMB DEFICIENCIES

A. General principles for amputation, when indicated

1. The optimal age for amputation for limb deficiency is 10 months to 2 years.
2. Early amputation is avoided if severe upper extremity deficiencies require use of the feet for activities of daily living.
3. Syme versus Boyd amputation
   a. The Syme amputation (ankle disarticulation) is simple and accommodates a tapered prosthesis at the ankle for optimal cosmesis.
   b. The Boyd amputation, in which the calcaneus is retained and fused to the distal tibia, prevents heel pad migration, aids prosthesis suspension, and may provide better end bearing. It also may limit prosthetic foot options because of its greater length.

B. Proximal femoral focal deficiency (PFFD) and congenital short femur

1. Overview
   a. The spectrum of femoral hypoplasia ranges from congenital short femur to complete absence of the proximal femur.
   b. Bilateral involvement is seen in 15% of cases. Ipsilateral foot and lower-limb anomalies are present up to 70% of the time.
   c. Fibular deficiency occurs in 50% of patients with PFFD.

TABLE 6

Spectrum of Problems Associated With Proximal Femoral Focal Deficiency

Condition	Acetabulum	Proximal Femur	Knee	Lower Leg
Mild PFFD	Normal	Delayed ossification and varus	AP laxity	Normal
Moderate PFFD	Dysplastic	Pseudarthrosis	Cruciate deficiency	Fibular deficiency
Severe PFFD	Absent	Complete absence	Flexion contracture	Severe fibular and foot deficiency

PFFD = proximal femoral focal deficiency

2. Epidemiology
   a. Incidence of 0.5 to 2 per 100,000 live births
   b. Third most common longitudinal deficiency of the lower limb
3. Pathoanatomy (**Table 6**)
   a. In a congenital short femur, the primary defect is a longitudinal deficiency of the femur.
   b. In PFFD, the Aitken classification outlines the varying deformities of the proximal femur and hip joint, including coxa vara, proximal femoral pseudarthrosis, and acetabular dysplasia (**Figure 6**).
   c. Associated ipsilateral limb anomalies include knee laxity with deficiency of the cruciate ligaments, fibular hemimelia, and absent lateral rays.
4. Evaluation
   a. Patients with a congenitally short femur have an externally rotated limb secondary to femoral retroversion.
   b. In PFFD, the thigh is short, flexed, abducted, and externally rotated (**Figure 7**).
   c. The entire lower extremity should be carefully evaluated for the associated anomalies listed previously.
5. The treatment of congenital short femur consists of treating the associated LLD, as described previously.
6. Treatment of PFFD
   a. Treatment should parallel development; thus initial prosthesis fitting should occur when the patient is pulling to stand.
   b. Surgery is best delayed until the patient is 2.5 to 3.0 years of age.
   c. Proximal femoral deformity (varus, pseudarthrosis) and acetabular dysplasia should be addressed before lengthening.
   d. Lengthening is indicated in the presence of a stable hip, a functional foot, and a projected LLD of less than 20 cm.
   e. Amputation and prosthetic fitting are indicated if the projected LLD is greater than 20 cm.
   f. Van Ness rotationplasty is an option if the projected LLD is greater than 20 cm. This procedure converts the ankle joint into a functional knee joint by rotating the foot 180° (**Figure 8**).

C. Fibular deficiency
1. Overview
   a. Previously termed fibular hemimelia
   b. Most common long-bone deficiency
2. Epidemiology
   a. Most common long bone deficiency
   b. Incidence of 1 to 2 per 100,000 live births
3. Pathoanatomy
   a. The Achterman and Kalamchi classification system describes the spectrum of deficiency ranging from shortened fibula to complete absence of the fibula.
   b. Associated anomalies include femoral deficiency, cruciate ligament deficiency, genu valgum secondary to hypoplasia of the lateral femoral condyle, ball-and-socket ankle joint, tarsal coalition, and absent lateral ray(s) (**Figure 9**).
   c. The tibia also may be shortened with anteromedial bowing.
4. Evaluation
   a. The classic appearance is a short limb with an equinovalgus foot and skin dimpling over the midanterior tibia (**Figure 10**).
   b. Radiographs
      - The fibula is short or absent, and anteromedial bowing of the tibia may be evident.

Tibia Vara (Blount Disease)

1. If the MD angle is greater than 16°, there is a 95% chance the bowing will progress. For MD angles between 11° and 16°, monitoring is required.
2. To avoid undercorrection in infantile Blount disease, the distal fragment should be fixed in slight valgus, lateral translation, and external rotation.
3. The risk of postoperative compartment syndrome is reduced if an anterior compartment fasciotomy is performed at the time of surgery.
4. Recurrence is less common when the osteotomy is performed in children younger than 4 years.

Genu Valgum

1. Children aged 3 to 4 years typically have up to 20° of genu valgum.
2. Unilateral genu valgum following a Cozen fracture almost always resolves spontaneously.
3. When substantial valgus deformity is present in a growing child, treatment through guided growth (temporary hemiepiphysiodesis) is preferred over an osteotomy.

Rotational Deformities

1. Tibial torsion is best evaluated by measuring the thigh-foot axis in the prone position.
2. Internal torsion is physiologic between 1 and 2 years of age, and typically resolves without treatment.
3. Shoes and orthoses are ineffective treatments for in-toeing or out-toeing.

Tibial Bowing

1. Anterolateral bowing is typical of congenital tibial pseudarthrosis, which is often associated with neurofibromatosis.
2. Posteromedial bowing is often associated with development of LLD and a calcaneovalgus foot deformity.
3. Anteromedial bowing is associated with fibular deficiency.

Limb Deficiencies

1. The optimal age range to perform amputation and prosthetic fitting for limb deficiency is 10 months to 2 years.
2. Early amputation should be avoided if severe upper extremity deformities may require the use of the feet for activities of daily living.
3. The Syme amputation is simple and accommodates a tapered prosthesis at the ankle for optimal cosmesis. The medial malleolus does not need to be excised in children as is typically done in adults.
4. The Boyd amputation prevents heel pad migration, aids prosthesis suspension, and may provide better end bearing; however, it also may limit prosthetic foot options because of excessive length.
5. The treatment of fibular deficiency is based on the degree of fibular deficiency and the severity of the foot deformity.
6. In tibial deficiency, a good early radiographic clue to the absence of the proximal tibia is a small, minimally ossified distal femoral epiphysis.
7. The Brown procedure has a high failure rate. In contrast, a tibiofibular synostosis is effective at extending a short proximal tibia segment.

Bibliography

Aitken GT: Proximal femoral focal deficiency – Definition, classification, and management, in Aitken GT, ed: *Proximal Femoral Focal Deficiency: A Congenital Anomaly.* Washington, DC, National Academy of Sciences, 1969, pp 1-22.

Bowen JR, Leahey JL, Zhang ZH, MacEwen GD: Partial epiphysiodesis at the knee to correct angular deformity. *Clin Orthop Relat Res* 1985;198:184-190.

Brooks WC, Gross RH: Genu varum in children: Diagnosis and treatment. *J Am Acad Orthop Surg* 1995;3(6):326-335.

Crawford AH, Schorry EK: Neurofibromatosis in children: The role of the orthopaedist. *J Am Acad Orthop Surg* 1999;7(4):217-230.

Dobbs MB, Purcell DB, Nunley R, Morcuende JA: Early results of a new method of treatment for idiopathic congenital vertical talus. *J Bone Joint Surg Am* 2006;88(6):1192-1200.

Horn J, Hvid I, Huhnstock S, Breen AB, Steen H: Limb lengthening and deformity correction with externally controlled motorized intramedullary nails: Evaluation of 50 consecutive lengthenings. *Acta Orthop* 2018;29:1-11.

Krajbich JI: Lower-limb deficiencies and amputations in children. *J Am Acad Orthop Surg* 1998;6(6):358-367.

Lincoln TL, Suen PW: Common rotational variations in children. *J Am Acad Orthop Surg* 2003;11(5):312-320.

Poloushk JD: Congenital deformities of the knee, in Song KM, ed: *Orthopaedic Knowledge Update: Pediatrics*, ed 4. Rosemont, IL, American Academy of Orthopaedic Surgeons, 2011, pp 195-202.

Richards BS, Anderson TD: rhBMP-2 and intramedullary fixation in congenital pseudarthrosis of the tibia. *J Pediatr Orthop* 2018;38(4):230-238.

Richards BS, Oetgen ME, Johnston CE: The use of rhBMP-2 for the treatment of congenital pseudarthrosis of the tibia: A case series. *J Bone Joint Surg Am* 2010;92(1):177-185.

Spencer SA, Widmann RF: Limb-length discrepancy and limb lengthening, in Song KM, ed: *Orthopaedic Knowledge Update: Pediatrics*, ed 4. Rosemont, IL, American Academy of Orthopaedic Surgeons, 2011, pp 219-232.

Staheli LT: Motor development in orthopaedics, in Abel MF, ed: *Orthopaedic Knowledge Update: Pediatrics*, ed 3. Rosemont, IL, American Academy of Orthopaedic Surgeons, 2006, pp 3-12.

Chapter 136
Limb Deformity Analysis

DAVID W. LOWENBERG, MD
MALCOLM R. DEBAUN, MD

I. GENERAL PRINCIPLES

A. To understand whether a deformity exists, the parameters of a normal limb must be known.

B. If the contralateral limb is unaffected it can be used as a control; with certain conditions (eg, metabolic bone disorders), the contralateral limb is usually abnormal.

C. Many nonunions develop a resultant deformity; malunions, by definition, have a deformity.

D. Limb deformity is more of an issue in the lower extremity than in the upper extremity.

E. Normal lower extremity alignment values have been established and are provided in **Figure 1**.

   1. The mechanical axis of the lower extremity passes from the center of the hip to the center of the talar dome.

   2. Ideal limb alignment occurs when this mechanical axis line passes through the center of the knee.

F. In the pediatric population, a deformity is a dynamic process that can worsen with growth of the limb.

G. Congenital limb-length discrepancy (LLD) may follow five patterns, as defined by Shapiro (**Figure 2**). It is important for the surgeon to realize that not all congenital LLDs follow a linear growth disturbance pattern.

   1. Certain types of deformity and growth impairment characterize one pattern of LLD over another.

   2. Linear progressive pattern (type I) is the most common in congenital LLD, and all predictor methods (Green-Anderson Growth Remaining Method, Moseley Straight Line Graph, Paley Multiplier Method) apply to this linear pattern only.

   3. Growth discrepancy secondary to femoral fracture more commonly follows a type III pattern, whereas type IV is prevalent in Legg-Calvé-Perthes disease.

   4. When growth discrepancy does not follow a linear pattern, treatment must be individualized as to the timing of limb equalization. For this reason, it is sometimes more advantageous to perform definitive limb equalization via lengthening of the affected short limb after skeletal maturity is reached, which ensures that proper limb equality is restored.

H. For treatment of pediatric limb length discrepancies in the growing child, a reproducible method to predict eventual actual leg length at skeletal maturity is required. Many such predictor methods have been described including the White-Menelaus, Anderson-Green, Moseley, and the Paley multiplier method.

   1. The Anderson-Green method uses a graph showing the average growth of the distal femoral and proximal tibia physis from skeletal age of 10 in boys and 8 in girls until maturity ± 2 SD.

   2. The White-Menelaus method uses arithmetic to calculate growth remaining with the premise of on average 3/8 inch/yr in the distal femur and 1/4 inch/yr of growth remains in the proximal tibia until age 16 for males and 14 for females.

   3. The Mosley method uses a logarithmic straight-line graph of limb growth rate to determine the anticipated leg length discrepancy at maturity.

   4. The Paley multiplier method uses age- and sex-specific coefficients to calculate skeletal growth until maturity.

I. The deformities that one encounters in a limb are angulation, translation, length, and rotation; each can exist independent of the other.

Dr. Lowenberg or an immediate family member is a member of a speakers' bureau or has made paid presentations on behalf of Stryker; serves as a paid consultant to or is an employee of Nuvasive; and serves as a board member, owner, officer, or committee member of the Foundation for Orthopaedic Trauma and the Osteosynthesis and Trauma Care Foundation. Dr. DeBaun or an immediate family member has received research or institutional support from Orthofix, Inc. and OsteoCentric.

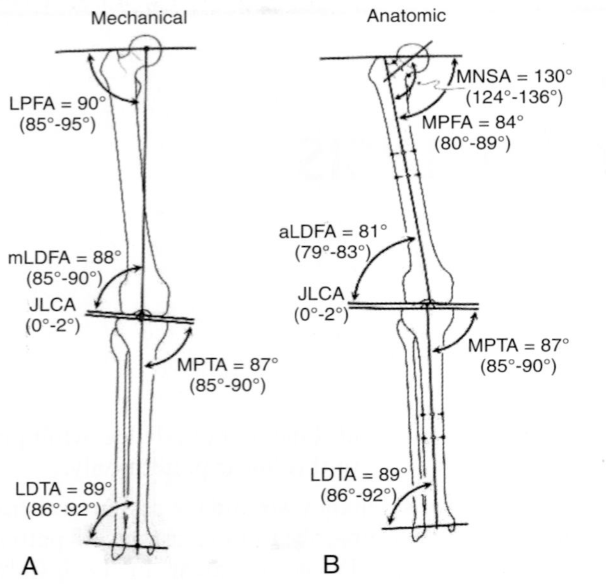

Figure 1 Illustrations show the standard mean values (with ranges) for normal lower extremity limb alignment. **A**, Mechanical alignment values. **B**, Anatomic alignment values. aLDFA = anatomic lateral distal femoral angle; JLCA = joint line convergence angle; LDTA = lateral distal tibial angle; LPFA = lateral proximal femoral angle; mLDFA = mechanical lateral distal femoral angle; MNSA = medial neck-shaft angle; MPFA = medial proximal femoral angle; MPTA = medial proximal tibial angle. (Reproduced with permission from Paley D: *Principles of Deformity Correction*. Berlin, Germany, Springer-Verlag, 2002, pp 1-17.)

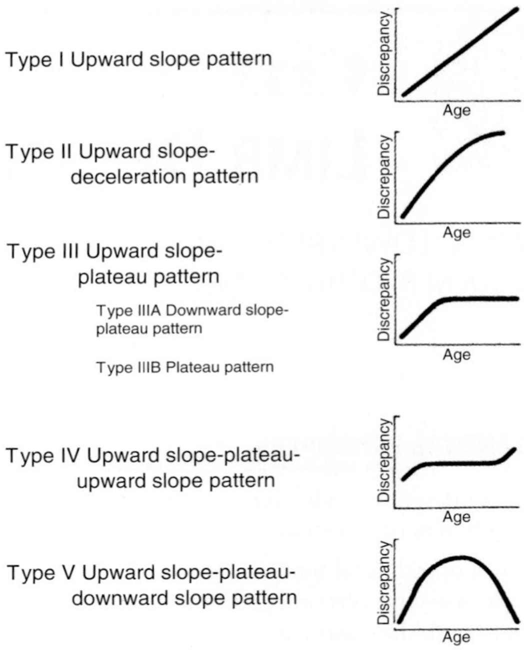

Figure 2 Chart shows the Shapiro classification describing congenital growth disturbance patterns over time. (Adapted with permission from Shapiro F: Developmental patterns in lower extremity length discrepancies. *J Bone Joint Surg Am* 1982;64[5]:639-651.)

II. LIMB DEFORMITY ANALYSIS

A. Mechanical parameters

1. Essential mechanical parameters that must be compared between limbs are the absolute limb segment lengths, the comparative limb segment length, and the total limb rotation.
2. The mechanical axis is defined by a line from the center of the femoral head to the center of the ankle joint.
3. Limb lengths and deformity parameters are independent of each other, as are rotational deformities; all must be measured separately.
4. The nonrotational deformity parameters (**Figure 1, A**) that must be measured and compared with the contralateral limb on appropriate radiographic views include
   a. Lateral proximal femoral angle
   b. Mechanical lateral distal femoral angle
   c. Joint line convergence angle
   d. Medial proximal tibial angle
   e. Lateral distal tibial angle

B. Anatomic parameters

1. Anatomic limb measurement parameters define the alignment of the bones themselves and do not have to mirror the mechanical axis (**Figure 1, B**).
2. The anatomic axis of the lower extremity is represented by the alignment of the intramedullary canals of the femur and tibia.
3. In the normal limb, however, the mechanical and anatomic parameters should yield the same measurements at a level from the knee distally.
4. The unique anatomic parameters of the lower extremity are:
   a. Medial neck-shaft angle
   b. Medial proximal femoral angle
   c. Anatomic lateral distal femoral angle

C. Evaluating lower-limb alignment

1. The benchmark for evaluating lower-limb alignment include a weight-bearing radiograph of both lower extremities from the hips to the ankles with the patellae facing forward and limb length inequality corrected with a block under the short limb, as well as true AP and lateral views of the affected limb segment(s) (**Figure 3**).

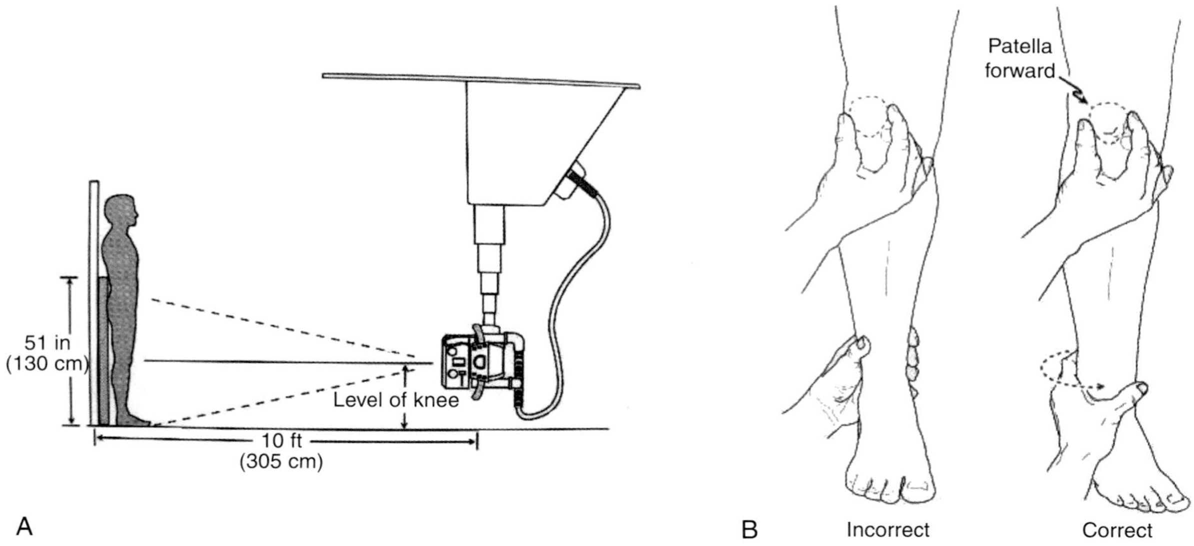

Figure 3 Illustrations show the evaluation of lower-limb alignment. **A**, The correct method of obtaining weight-bearing AP radiographs of both lower extremities. **B**, The correct technique for obtaining consistent, true orthogonal views of the leg. (Reproduced with permission from Paley D: *Principles of Deformity Correction*. Berlin, Germany, Springer-Verlag, 2002, pp 1-17.)

2. The mechanical and anatomic axis angles described previously are measured on the radiographs. This allows determination of the segment level of deformity (whether it is at the level of the femur, tibia, or joint line because of soft-tissue laxity), the degree of deformity, and the type of deformity.
3. To locate the exact site of the deformity, the mechanical axes and often the anatomic axes of each limb segment must be plotted.

D. Mechanical axis deviation (MAD)

1. The MAD is defined as the distance the mechanical axis has deviated from the normal position through the center of the knee (**Figure 4, A**).
2. This measurement is particularly helpful when treating genu varum and genu valgum.
3. The measurement of the MAD combined with the measurement of the accompanying joint orientation angles is particularly useful in the treatment of any juxta-articular deformity about the knee.

E. Diaphyseal deformities

1. These deformities, especially those that are posttraumatic, often are not simply an angulatory problem. An accompanying translational or rotatory deformity usually is present.
2. Translational deformities can contribute at least as much to mechanical axis deformity as can angulatory deformities (**Figure 4, B**).
3. Translational deformities with accompanying angulatory deformities
   a. Compensatory: the translated segment tilts away from the concavity of the deformity.
   b. Additive: the translated distal segment tilts toward the side of the concavity.
   c. A limb with an angulatory deformity and an accompanying compensatory translational component may have none to minimal overall mechanical axis deviation (**Figure 5**).
4. When evaluating posttraumatic deformities, the most common deformity encountered is residual rotational deformity.

F. Center of rotation and angulation (CORA)

1. To determine the true site of deformity, not just the limb segment involved, the CORA must be plotted.
2. The CORA represents both the point in space where the axis of mechanical deformity exists and the virtual point in space where the apex of correction should occur.
3. The CORA is plotted out by drawing the mechanical axes for the limb segments (**Figure 6**).
4. When the affected limb has no translational deformity and no other accompanying juxta-articular deformity or additional site of deformity, then the CORA lies at the site of apparent deformity.

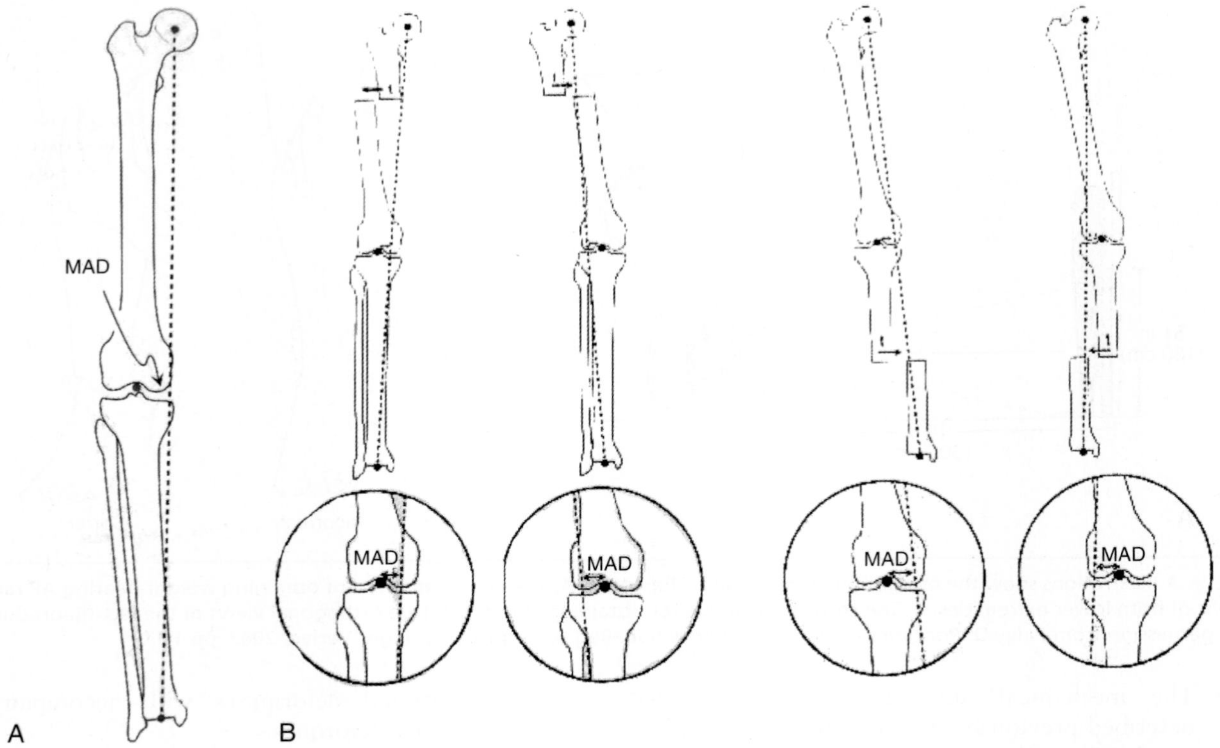

Figure 4 Illustrations depict the mechanical axis deviation (MAD). **A**, The MAD is measured at the level of the knee joint and represents the distance that the mechanical axis is displaced from normal for that limb. "Normal for the limb" is defined as the point that the mechanical axis passes in the contralateral, unaffected limb or a point in a range of 0 to 6 mm medial to the center of the knee, depending on what information is available. **B**, Examples of the effect of femoral and tibial translation on the mechanical axis of the limb. (Reproduced with permission from Paley D: *Principles of Deformity Correction*. Berlin, Germany, Springer-Verlag, 2002, pp 31-60.)

5. If a deformity exists secondary to angulation and translation (eg, malunion), then the CORA will lie at a site other than that of the apparent angulatory deformity. This happens because of the contributory effect (regardless of whether it is a compensatory or additive translational component) of the translated limb segment.

G. Evaluation in the sagittal plane—All the measurements and plotting of limb axes done in the coronal (AP) plane also can be done in the sagittal (lateral) plane, although sagittal plane deformities may be better tolerated in the lower extremity.

H. Upper extremity deformities
   1. The same methods of deformity analysis also can be applied to the upper extremity.
   2. Common sites of posttraumatic deformity:
      a. Elbow: secondary to malreduction of supracondylar humerus fractures
      b. Wrist: secondary to the malreduction of distal radial fractures.

I. The basic rules that can help the surgeon evaluate orthogonal AP and lateral radiographs to characterize limb deformity are listed in **Table 1**.
   1. It is important to understand that radiographs are two-dimensional representations of three-dimensional anatomy.
   2. Limb deformity often is not present in just a true coronal or sagittal plane, but instead somewhere between these two planes. This is why an angulatory deformity is quite often seen on both true AP and true lateral radiographs.
   3. If an AP and/or lateral radiograph show an angulatory deformity, the actual deformity is always greater than or equal to the greater of the two deformities measured.

III. TREATMENT

A. General principles
   1. When external fixation modalities are used, alignment deformities should be corrected in the following order: angulation, translation, length, rotation.

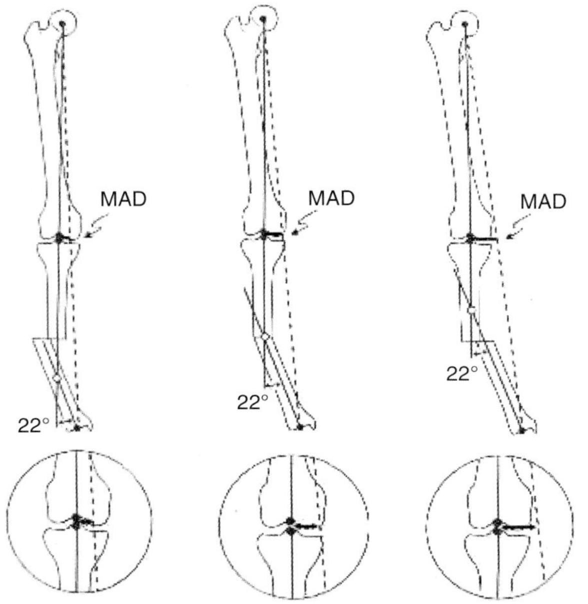

Figure 5 Illustrations show translational limb deformities with accompanying angulatory deformities. Translation of a limb segment can have a compensatory or an additive effect on an angulatory deformity depending on the directional plane of the translation. MAD = mechanical axis deviation. (Reproduced with permission from Paley D: *Principles of Deformity Correction*. Berlin, Germany, Springer-Verlag, 2002, pp 31-60.)

2. Angulatory deformity in skeletally immature patients may be corrected with growth modulation.
   a. In the pediatric population, hemiepiphysiodesis may be performed using tension-band plating, transphyseal screws, or staples.
   b. Growth modulation requires close follow-up to monitor the correction of the deformity and the resultant changes to the mechanical axis.
3. Rotational malalignment
   a. Most common posttraumatic deformity encountered.
   b. Can be imprecise to measure.
   c. It is most often assessed clinically by comparing the affected limb with the contralateral limb.
   d. CT scan may be useful for measuring rotatory malalignment of limbs.
   e. Various values of acceptable lower extremity malalignment have been published, but no definitive value of the maximum acceptable rotatory deformity tolerated in the lower limb has been established. Any rotatory deformity of the leg greater than 10° typically is poorly tolerated.

B. Surgical technique tips for deformity correction
1. Order of correction for external fixation modulated deformity correction.
   a. Alignment deformities should be corrected in the following order: angulation, translation, length, rotation. Following this order of correction results in the most predictable restoration of limb alignment. With the computer modulated external fixation methods using 6-strut technology, these three planar deformities can often be addressed simultaneously.
   b. In correcting the rotation, especially if an external fixator is used, a resultant residual translation can be encountered (**Figure** 7). This translation occurs because of the inevitability of the center of rotational correction not being at the exact center of the bone segment being rotated. This residual translation must be corrected.
2. Simple deformities without clinically substantial limb-length inequality usually can be successfully corrected acutely using locked intramedullary nail or plate and screw osteosynthesis. When possible in the adult population, this is the preferred method of deformity correction. One must factor in ALL deformity parameters choosing the implant.
   a. Improved technology has now allowed for the safe and reproducible utilization of intramedullary lengthening nails for the treatment of primarily pure limb length inequality. Angular and rotational deformities can also be addressed with these nails.
   b. Correction rate should not be hastened when such additional deformity corrections are performed through these osteotomy sites. Distraction rates are variable and can range from 0.5 to 1.25 mm per day depending on a host of local and host variables.
   c. Regardless of the method of fixation, proper preoperative planning and templating remains of paramount importance.
   d. In the adult population, the most common deformity is about the knee. This usually involves a variant of genu varum or genu valgum.
      - In correcting a mechanical axis for genu varum, the ideal correction of the mechanical axis has classically been described as a point at the lateral edge of the tibial spine

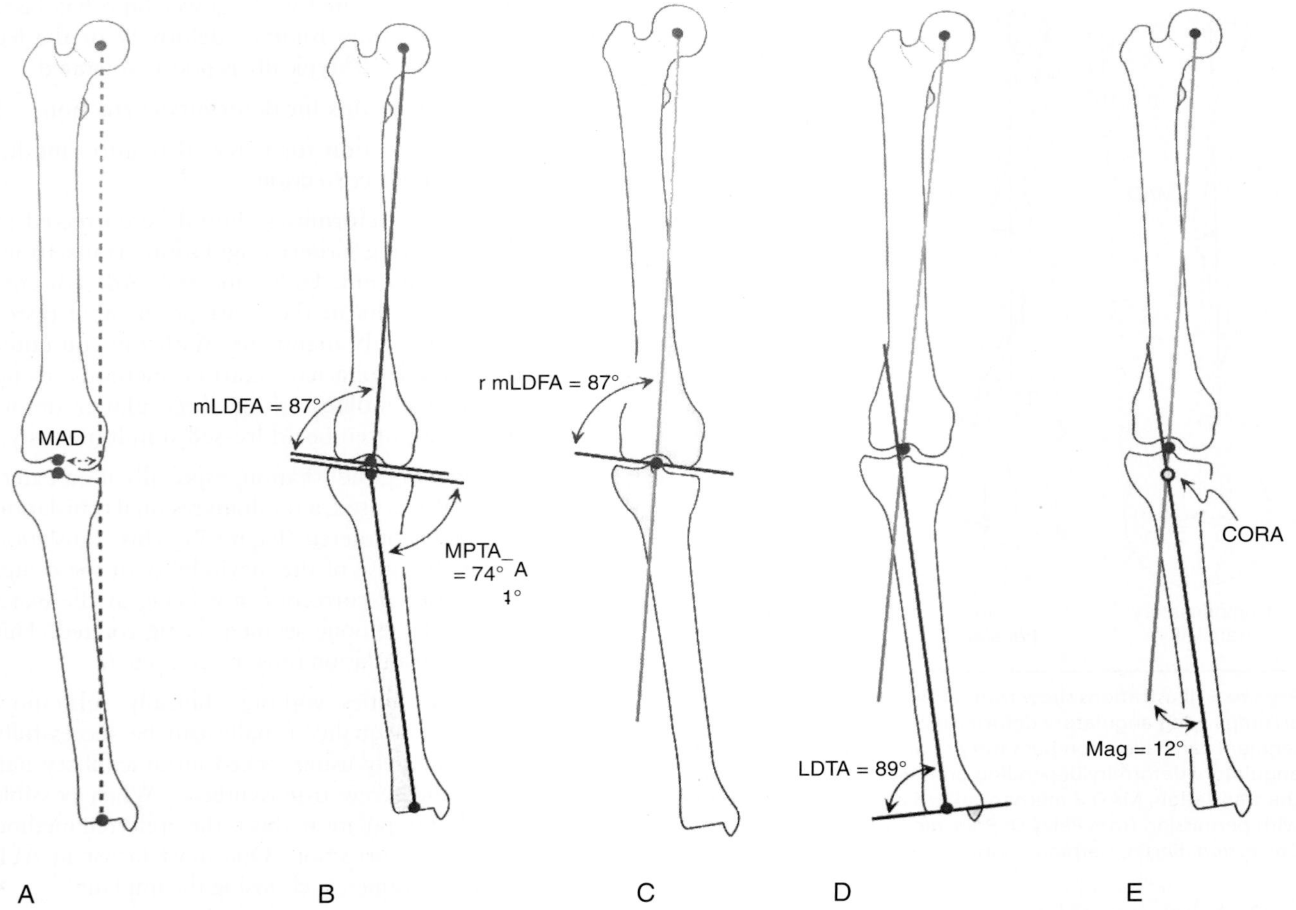

Figure 6 Illustrations depict the determination of the center of rotation of angulation (CORA). **A**, The mechanical axis of the limb is drawn, and the mechanical axis deviation (MAD) is determined. **B**, The mechanical lateral distal femoral angle (mLDFA), joint line convergence angle (JLCA), and medial proximal tibial angle (MPTA) for the limb are determined. Because the mLDFA is in the range of normal, and the JLCA is parallel, then the deformity exists in the tibia, because the MPTA is abnormal at 74°. **C**, Because the mechanical axis of the femur is normal, the mechanical axis line of the femur can then be extended down the limb to represent the mechanical axis of the tibia. **D**, The distal mechanical axis is defined as a line from the center of the ankle and parallel to the shaft of the tibia. The lateral distal tibial angle (LDTA) is found to be normal. **E**, The CORA is now defined as the intersection of the proximal mechanical axis line with the distal mechanical axis line. Imagine translating the distal segment at this level to see how the point of the CORA changes. Mag = magnitude of deformity. (Reproduced with permission from Paley D: *Principles of Deformity Correction*. Berlin, Germany, Springer-Verlag, 2002, pp 195-234.)

known as the Fujisawa point. Correction to this point generally gives an optimal mechanical axis load distribution for symptomatic medial compartment disease.

- The deformity is usually corrected at the level of the proximal tibia, but proper preoperative planning is required to determine the true site of deformity.
- Deformities under 10° of varus can usually be corrected with a supra tibial tubercle opening wedge osteotomy and plating.
- Deformities greater than 10° of varus often require an infra-tibial tubercle corticotomy and correction with ring fixation.
- Opening wedge osteotomies greater than 10° are risk fracture of the lateral cortical hinge and resultant uncontrolled cortical translation deformity.
- In the correction of adult genu valgum, the site of needed correction is usually at the level of the distal femur and is generally treated with a distal femoral osteotomy.

TABLE 1

The Five Rules of Deformity Analysis

1. The true angle of bone deformity is always equal to or greater than the measured angle of deformity on a radiograph.
2. The closer the measured values of deformity on AP and lateral radiographs are to each other, the closer the true plane of deformity is to the 45° axis.
3. Equal angles of deformity on true AP and true lateral radiographs define a true axis of deformity at the 45° axis, with the actual degree of deformity being 1.43 times that measured on the AP or lateral projection.
4. If a measured deformity on an AP view = 0°, then the plane of deformity is 90° to this plane, and the degree of deformity equals that measured on the lateral radiograph; and vice versa.
5. No direct relationship exists between angulation and translation in a deformity, although translation can have an additive or compensatory effect to angulation on limb mechanical axis.

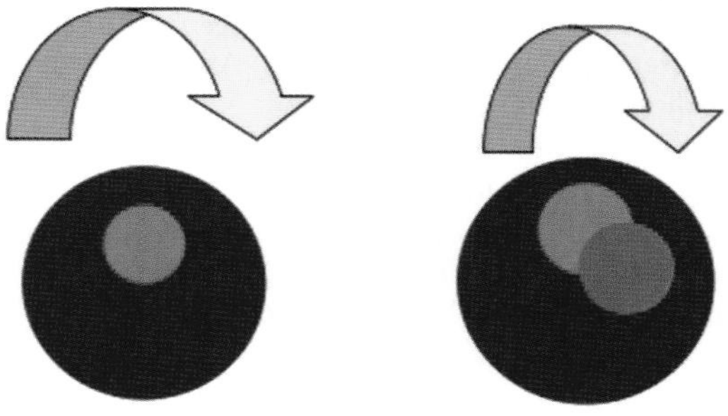

Figure 7 Illustrations depict residual translation. **A,** Initial graphic shows the bone (inner circle) within the soft-tissue envelope (outer circle) before rotational limb correction. **B,** Bone translation following limb rotational correction. Because of the eccentric position of the bone within the rings of the fixator, a resultant translation occurs, which needs subsequent correction.

TOP TESTING FACTS

1. The mechanical axis of the lower extremity passes from the center of the hip to the center of the talar dome. Ideal limb alignment is defined as passage of this mechanical axis line through the center of the knee.
2. If the surgeon suspects a nonlinear congenital growth disturbance, it must be weighed when deciding the timing of definitive limb equalization and deformity correction.
3. The types of deformity that can exist in a limb are angulation, translation, length, and rotation. Rotation is generally measured clinically, whereas the other parameters are measured on appropriate radiographs.
4. It is important to recognize that translation deformities can be compensatory or additive to an angulatory deformity.
5. Because angulation is a phenomenon independent of translation, an apparent site of deformity might not actually be the true CORA. Therefore, this site must be precisely determined by obtaining the measurements on long radiographs.
6. Rotational deformities are the most common posttraumatic deformity encountered.
7. In congenital deformity analysis, limb-length inequality is an important accompanying deformity parameter that must be evaluated and projected over time.
8. The pattern of growth disturbance and resultant deformity is not always linear and can follow certain described growth rate disturbance patterns.
9. Projected leg length discrepancy at maturity less than 2 cm is generally managed with a shoe lift or observation depending on the symptomatology of the patient.
10. Lengthening along the anatomical axis of the femur leads to lateralization of the mechanical axis, whereas shortening leads to medialization.

Bibliography

Aiona M, Do KP, Emara K, Dorociak R, Pierce R: Gait patterns in children with limb length discrepancy. *J Pediatr Orthop* 2015;35:280-284.

Bowen JR, Leahey JL, Zhang ZH, MacEwen GD: Partial epiphysiodesis at the knee to correct angular deformity. *Clin Orthop Relat Res* 1985;198:184-190.

Green SA, Gibbs P: The relationship of angulation to translation in fracture deformities. *J Bone Joint Surg Am* 1994;76(3):390-397.

Green SA, Green HD: The influence of radiographic projection on the appearance of deformities. *Orthop Clin North Am* 1994;25(3):467-475.

Handy RC, McCarthy JJ, eds: *Management of Limb-Length Discrepancies*. Rosemont, IL, American Academy of Orthopaedic Surgeons, 2011.

Herring JA: Limb length discrepancy, in Herring JA, Texas Scottish Rite Hospital for Children, eds: *Tachdjian's Pediatric Orthopaedics: From the Texas Scottish Rite Hospital for Children*, ed 5. Philadelphia, PA, Elsevier Saunders, 2014, vol 2, pp 884-928.

Iobst C: Growth of the musculoskeletal system, in Martus J, ed: *Orthopaedic Knowledge Update Pediatrics*, ed 5. Rosemont, IL, American Academy of Orthopaedic Surgeons, 2016, pp 59-68.

Makarov MR, Jackson TJ, Smith CM, Jo CH, Birch JG: Timing of epiphysiodesis to correct leg-length discrepancy. *J Bone Joint Surg Am* 2018;100(14):1217-1222.

Paley D: *Principles of Deformity Correction*. Berlin, Germany, Springer-Verlag, 2002.

Shapiro F: Developmental patterns in lower-extremity length discrepancies. *J Bone Joint Surg Am* 1982;64(5):639-651.

Stevens PM: Guided growth for angular correction: A preliminary series using a tension band plate. *J Pediatr Orthop* 2007;27(3):253-259.

Chapter 137
Musculoskeletal Conditions and Injuries in the Young Athlete

JAY C. ALBRIGHT, MD
ALEXIA G. GAGLIARDI, BA
STEPHANIE W. MAYER, MD

I. OVERVIEW

A. Child athlete versus adult athlete

1. A child athlete is not a small adult.
2. Because children have open physes growing at variable rates, they are susceptible to injury.
3. Children are less coordinated and have poorer mechanics than adults.
4. Children have less efficient thermoregulatory mechanisms than adults, including a less efficient sweating response, and cannot acclimatize as rapidly.

B. Sex-specific considerations

1. The female athlete triad—amenorrhea, disordered eating, and osteoporosis—places the female athlete at higher risk of insufficiency or stress fractures, overuse injuries, and recurrent injuries.
2. Knee injuries
   a. The female knee becomes more susceptible to injury at puberty.
   b. Differences in anatomy, sex hormone levels, neuromuscular control, and overall strength and coordination have been implicated in the higher incidence of knee injuries in females than in males in the same sport.

II. LITTLE LEAGUER'S SHOULDER

A. Overview and epidemiology

1. Little Leaguer's shoulder is an epiphysiolysis, or stress fracture, through the proximal humeral epiphysis caused by repetitive microtrauma.
2. It occurs most commonly in overhead athletes such as pitchers and tennis players who are skeletally immature.
3. Mechanism of injury—Results from repeated high loads of torque on the physis in a skeletally immature athlete.

B. Evaluation

1. Presentation—Insidious onset of generalized shoulder pain. Pain is usually worst during late cocking or early deceleration phases of throwing.
2. Physical examination—Point tenderness over the physis of the proximal humerus, pain with extremes of range of motion in all directions, pain with resisted elevation of the shoulder. This can be hard to discern from subdeltoid bursitis.
3. Imaging—Radiographs may show a widened proximal humeral physis compared with the opposite side (**Figure 1**). Other findings can include sclerosis, cystic changes, or fragmentation of the physis. MRI is usually not needed for diagnosis.

Dr. Albright or an immediate family member is a member of a speakers' bureau or has made paid presentations on behalf of Arthrex, Inc.; has received research or institutional support from Arthrex, Inc.; and serves as a board member, owner, officer, or committee member of the American Board of Orthopaedic Surgery, Inc., the American Orthopaedic Society for Sports Medicine, the Pediatric Orthopaedic Society of North the America, and PRISM. Dr. Mayer or an immediate family member serves as a paid consultant to or is an employee of Arthrex, Inc. and Stryker. Neither Ms. Gagliardi nor any immediate family member has received anything of value from or has stock or stock options held in a commercial company or institution related directly or indirectly to the subject of this chapter.

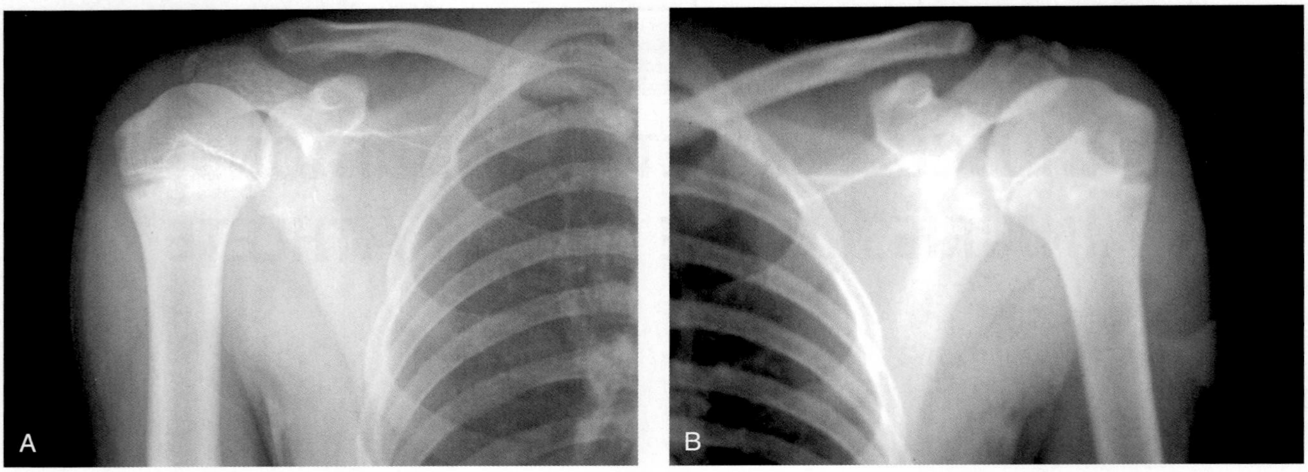

Figure 1 AP radiographs show the shoulders of a 12-year-old child who had right shoulder pain during the deceleration phase of throwing. Compare the physeal widening of the right shoulder (**A**) with the unaffected left shoulder (**B**).

C. Treatment is nonsurgical, with no throwing for at least 2 to 3 months.

D. Rehabilitation

1. When painless full range of motion (ROM) is achieved, physical therapy for scapular stabilizer and rotator cuff strengthening is initiated.
2. Strengthening is followed by a progressive throwing program.
    a. The athlete begins with short tosses at low velocity and gradually progresses to longer tosses and then longer tosses with increasing velocity.
    b. After long tosses at higher velocities have been achieved, the patient can fully return to play.
    c. Time to symptom resolution has been shown to be approximately 2.6 months, and return to sports, 4.2 months.

E. Complications

1. Most common complication is recurrence at a rate of approximately 7%. Low incidence of premature growth arrest with or without angular deformity.
2. Subsequent Salter-Harris fractures also can occur while the physis is healing.

F. Prevention—Little league shoulder (LLS) may be prevented by adherence to guidelines set by multiple entities, including the American Academy of Orthopaedic Surgeons, USA Baseball, and the American Society for Sports Medicine (**Table 1**). Glenohumeral internal rotation deficit (GIRD) has been shown to be a risk factor for recurrence. Therefore, physical therapy for GIRD may also help prevent LLS.

III. LITTLE LEAGUER'S ELBOW

A. Overview and epidemiology—Little Leaguer's elbow is a generic term for any injury to a child's elbow accompanied by pain along the medial aspect of the proximal forearm or elbow. These injuries are commonly related to the excessive stresses experienced by the immature skeleton during overhead athletics. Little Leaguer's elbow is a progressive problem resulting from repetitive microtrauma.

B. Mechanism of injury

1. The valgus-hyperextension overloading of the elbow during throwing causes repetitive microtrauma and shear stresses to the medial elbow at the medial epicondyle physis, ulnar collateral ligament

TABLE 1

Pitching Recommendations for the Young Baseball Player

Age (Years)	Maximum Pitches per Game	Maximum Games per Week
8-10	52 ± 15	2 ± 0.6
11-12	68 ± 18	2 ± 0.6
13-14	76 ± 16	2 ± 0.4
15-16	91 ± 16	2 ± 0.6
17-18	106 ± 16	2 ± 0.6

Reproduced from Pasque CB, McGinnis DW, Griffin LY: Shoulder, in Sullivan JA, Anderson ST, eds: *Care of the Young Athlete*. Rosemont, IL, American Academy of Orthopaedic Surgeons, 2000, p 347.

(UCL), and flexor pronator origin. The symptoms in a child can be more varied than adults. Children often experience pain on the compressed radial side of the joint in addition to the distracted ulnar side.

2. The syndrome is associated with throwing curveballs or with an infielder bent-elbow throw that involves a whipping mechanism used to gain adequate speed.
3. The younger the patient, the more likely the diagnosis is to be an apophysitis or an avulsion injury, rather than a UCL sprain.

C. Evaluation

1. Presentation—Patients often first experience pain after and then during a game. The pain may be mild at first but eventually inhibits throwing. Forces are highest on the medial elbow during late cocking and early acceleration phases of throwing.
2. Less common is acute avulsion of medial epicondyle.
3. Patient may at first report decreased throwing distance or accuracy, and as the injury progresses, a loss of throwing velocity.
4. Physical examination
   a. Chronic conditions may produce an increased carrying angle or a flexion contracture.
   b. Note point tenderness over the medial epicondyle, sublime tubercle, or flexor mass.
   c. Stability testing involves several maneuvers.
      - Moving valgus stress test—Valgus stress is applied, with the arm in varied degrees of flexion and extension.
      - Milking maneuver—Valgus stress with forearm supination and >90° elbow flexion.
5. Imaging
   a. Bilateral AP, lateral, and oblique radiographs of the elbow should be obtained.
   b. Compare with the unaffected side to determine whether an irregular appearance of the physis is evident. This step also may help determine the degree of displacement.
   c. Fragmentation of the medial epicondyle, trochlea, olecranon, or capitellum may be present.
   d. Medial epicondyle hypertrophy or radial head hypertrophy also may be present.
   e. Advanced imaging with MRI is indicated in cases of possible UCL injury or when radiographs and physical examination are inconclusive. Magnetic resonance (MR) arthrogram may be helpful for diagnosis of UCL injury.

D. Treatment

1. Nonsurgical
   a. Medial epicondylitis is managed initially with 4 to 6 weeks of rest.
   b. Management of osteochondritis dissecans (OCD) and Panner disease is discussed in Section V.
   c. Valgus extension overload and posterior stress syndromes typically can be managed with rest or activity and throwing modifications depending on severity of symptoms.
   d. Alterations in the athlete's form, motion, and playing habits as well as adherence to recommended pitch and inning counts are advised when return to throwing is initiated.
   e. Intra-articular steroid injection may be used to control inflammation.
2. Surgical
   a. Indications
      - Failure to respond to nonsurgical treatment.
      - Instability of the elbow with avulsion fracture or fragmentation of the medial epicondyle.
   b. Procedures
      - UCL reconstruction with auto- or allograft when indicated for UCL insufficiency (**Figure 2**).
      - Open reduction and internal fixation (ORIF) for medial epicondyle avulsion fractures displaced more than 5 mm. Consideration for ORIF for less displaced avulsion fractures in competitive throwers, although definitive research is lacking.
      - Arthroscopic débridement of posterolateral synovium and olecranon osteophytes for recalcitrant posterior symptoms of valgus extension overload.
   c. Complications
      - Ulnar nerve neuropathy
      - Loss of motion
      - Infection
      - Continued pain
      - Inability to return to play at same level
      - Aggressive débridement of the olecranon or osteophytes may result in instability

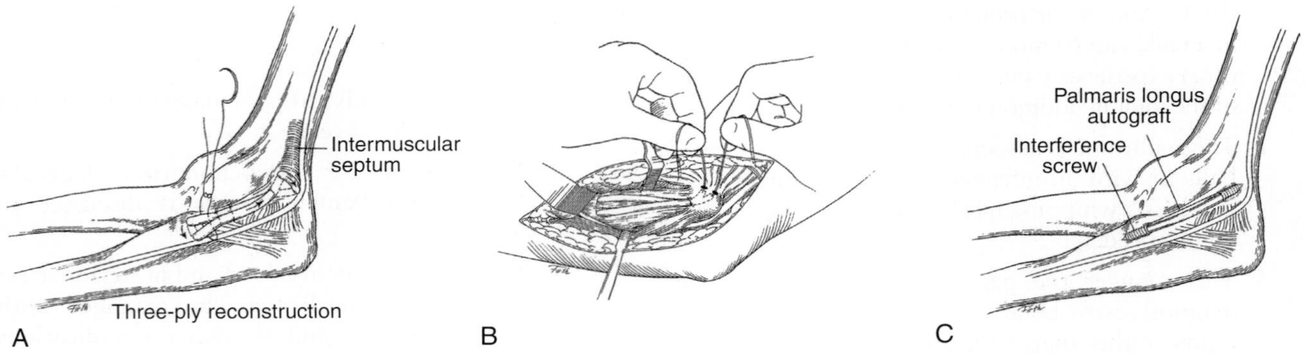

Figure 2 Illustrations show medial ulnar collateral ligament reconstruction techniques. **A**, Tendon graft passed through bone tunnels. **B**, Docking technique. **C**, Anatomic interference technique. (Reproduced with permission from El Attrache NS, Bast SC, David T: Medial collateral ligament reconstruction. *Tech Shoulder Elbow Surg* 2001;2:38-49.)

E. Rehabilitation

1. For surgery not involving ligaments, minimal immobilization with early ROM, strengthening, and pain modalities
2. For ligament reconstructions, a short course of immobilization followed by protected ROM

F. Prevention—Educating coaches, parents, and athletes on pitch counts, proper mechanics of throwing.

IV. DISTAL RADIUS EPIPHYSIOLYSIS/ EPIPHYSITIS

A. Overview and pathoanatomy

1. Injury to the distal radial epiphysis most commonly occurs in adolescent athletes in sports that require weight bearing on the upper extremities, such as gymnastics or cheerleading.
2. Children aged 10 to 14 years at higher skill levels spend more time in intensive training, so these injuries are more likely to occur in this age group.

B. Mechanism of injury—Overloading of the distal radial epiphysis, causing inflammation and/or fracture of the epiphysis.

C. Evaluation

1. History—Painful wrist with weight-bearing activities.
2. Physical examination consistent with pain and swelling at the joint with or without deformity of the wrist.
3. Imaging—Radiographs may show a widened physis, blurred epiphyseal plate, metaphyseal changes, and fragmentation of radial and volar aspects of the plate, as shown in **Figure 3**.

D. Treatment

1. Nonsurgical
   a. The patient should be allowed to participate in choosing treatment.
   b. Relative rest is indicated in mild to moderate cases, complete rest in severe cases. In-season athletes and less severe cases may be managed with relative rest in a splint and physical therapy.
   c. Immobilization is always indicated, a splint in mild to moderate cases, and casting in more severe cases. Aggressive immobilization is encouraged.
   d. For severe cases, bone stimulation can be used.

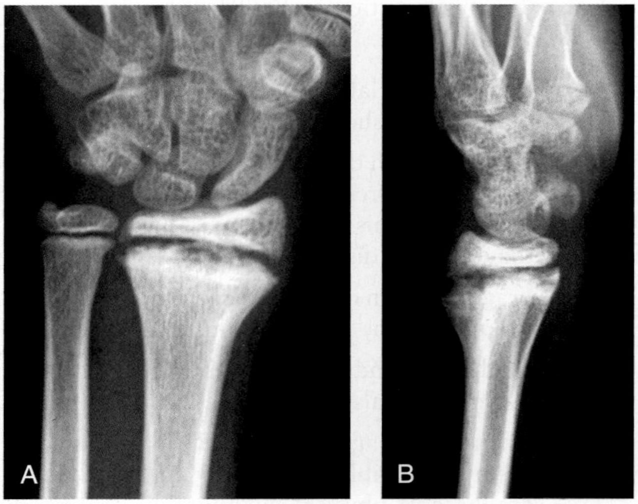

Figure 3 AP (**A**) and lateral (**B**) radiographs of the wrist of a 13-year-old elite-level female gymnast who presented with persistent pain and progressive deformity of the left wrist.

2. Surgical—Typically indicated only for the correction of complications.

E. Rehabilitation—Physical therapy is useful for regaining motion after casting and helps control the return to activity.

F. Complications

1. This injury may recur, even with casting for 6 to 8 weeks, particularly if the athlete returns to full activities immediately.
2. Positive ulnar variance is a common eventual outcome in untreated athletes and may result in triangular fibrocartilage complex pathology or ulnar abutment.

V. OSTEOCHONDRITIS DISSECANS AND PANNER DISEASE

A. Overview

1. OCD occurs in the elbow, knee, and ankle in asymptomatic skeletally immature individuals but may not be detected until early adulthood.
2. No single etiologic theory is uniformly accepted; potential causes include macrotrauma or microtrauma and vascular, hereditary, or constitutional factors.

B. Elbow OCD

1. Epidemiology

    a. Panner disease, or osteonecrosis of the capitellum, is generally thought to be an idiosyncratic loss of blood supply of the majority, if not all, of the capitellum, has a relatively benign course, and typically occurs in the first decade of life.

    b. Capitellar OCD typically occurs after 10 years of age. It frequently causes permanent disability.

2. Pathoanatomy

    a. Panner disease and capitellar OCD result from repetitive overuse or overload compression-type injuries, resulting in insult to the blood supply of the immature capitellum.

    b. Ossification of the capitellum usually is complete by 10 years of age, distinguishing Panner disease from OCD.

3. Staging and classification of OCD—Based on radiographic studies and arthroscopy (**Figure 4**).

    a. Type I lesions—Intact cartilage with or without bony stability underneath

    b. Type II lesions—Cartilage fracture with bony collapse or displacement

    c. Type III lesions—Loose fragments in the joint

4. Evaluation

    a. Presentation—An insidious onset of activity-related pain with or without stiffness in the dominant arm of an overhead throwing or weight-bearing athlete

    b. A history of locking or catching may be present.

    c. Physical examination—Reveals a flexion contracture, point tenderness, and possibly crepitus

    d. Radiographs—AP, lateral, and oblique views

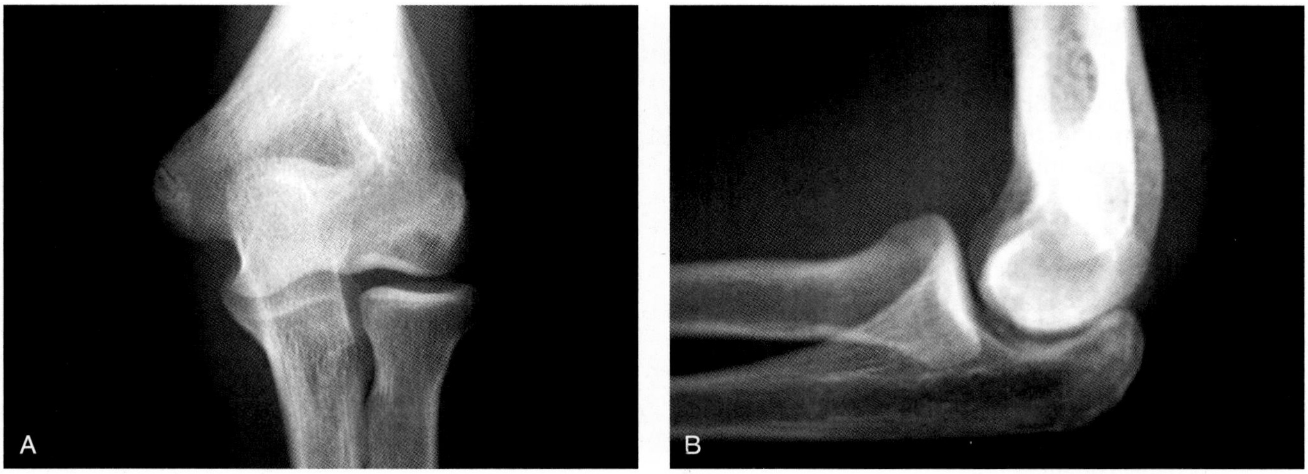

Figure 4 AP (**A**) and lateral (**B**) radiographs show capitellar osteochondritis dissecans in a 14-year-old child who is a gymnast.

5. Nonsurgical treatment
   a. Panner disease and type I OCD lesions are best managed nonsurgically, with a success rate greater than 90%.
   b. Rest with or without immobilization for 3 to 6 weeks, longer for OCD than Panner disease
   c. A slow progression back to activity is allowed over the next 6 to 12 weeks.
6. Surgical treatment
   a. Indications
      - Failure of nonsurgical management
      - Persistent pain
      - Symptomatic loose bodies
      - Displacement of OCD lesions
   b. Contraindications—Stable lesions;, patients younger than 10 years, without loose bodies, chondral fractures, or displacement of the OCD.
   c. Procedures
      - Extra-articular or transarticular drilling of type I lesions without bony stability or type II lesions that are stable arthroscopically has good clinical success.
      - Fixation of OCD lesions of the capitellum has variable success and should be reserved for large lesions with primary intact fragments that sit well or are not completely displaced.
      - Débridement of the base of the lesion with or without drilling of the subchondral bone and loose body excision is frequently required in unstable type II and type III lesions.
      - Cartilage restoration may be necessary if symptoms continue or the lesion is large.
   d. Pearls
      - The posterior portals and anconeus portal are used for most of the work; nearly all of the capitellum can be visualized through this approach.
      - Excessive cartilage débridement should be avoided; only flaps or loose cartilage should be débrided.
      - Extra-articular drilling avoids damaging the cartilage.
      - Large lesions may need cartilage restoration initially or if symptoms do not abate after débridement.
7. Complications—Elbow stiffness, infection, progression of arthritis, continued pain, and an inability to return to sports.
8. Rehabilitation
   a. The rehabilitation protocol depends on the procedure.
      - Débridement or loose body excisions call for early ROM with or without an elbow brace. Progression to strengthening can be initiated when painless ROM is achieved, with avoidance of valgus positions, throwing, and weight bearing for 3 to 4 months.
      - Elbows that undergo fixation or drilling procedures need more prolonged protection, with protected early ROM followed by strengthening at approximately 2 months, then a slow return to valgus position. Throwing and then weight bearing may begin at 4 to 6 months.
   b. Overhead or weight-bearing athletes may not be able to return to the same level of play.
   c. Changes in mechanics, position, or sport may be necessary.

C. Knee OCD
1. Overview and epidemiology
   a. The knee is the most common site of osteochondrosis in growing children.
   b. The actual incidence may be far greater than thought; no studies exist for a general population of asymptomatic children.
   c. Often confused with irregularities of epiphyseal ossification, knee OCD does not always improve with benign neglect.
   d. Age and level of skeletal maturity at onset are considered prognostic. Generally, children with closed or nearly closed growth plates at the onset have a worse prognosis.
2. Classification—Lesions are classified by evaluating radiographs and MRIs and using arthroscopic evaluation; multiple classifications exist in the literature, including the Guhl classification (**Figure 5**).
3. Evaluation
   a. Patients present with generalized, often anterior, knee pain and variable swelling with or without temporally related trauma.
   b. Onset may be associated with an increase or change in activity.

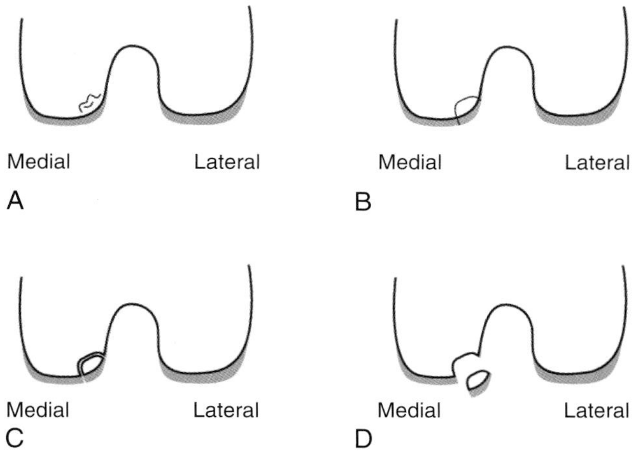

Figure 5 Illustrations show the Guhl classification for osteochondritis dissecans. **A**, Type I: Signal change around the lesion without bright signal. **B**, Type II: High signal intensity surrounding the bone portion of the lesion without signs of cartilage breach. **C**, Type III: High signal intensity around the whole lesion including cartilage (unstable lesion). **D**, Type IV: Empty bed of the lesion with loose body. (Courtesy of Jay Albright, MD, and the Children's Specialists of San Diego, San Diego, CA.)

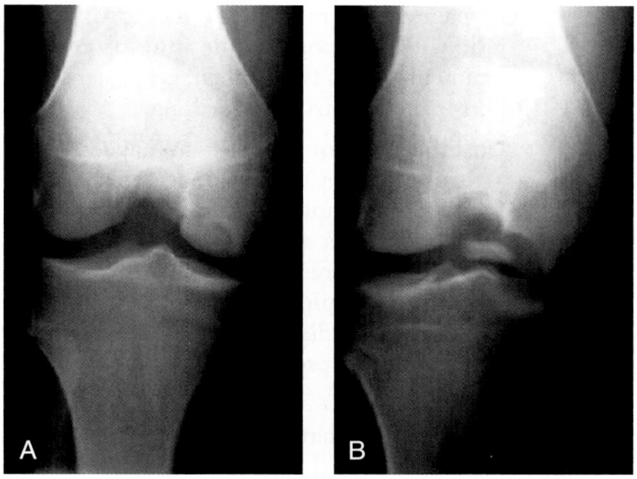

Figure 6 Tunnel radiographic views of the knee demonstrate the classic location of an osteochondritis dissecans lesion on the lateral aspect of the medial femoral condyle, before (**A**) and after (**B**) displacement. (Reproduced from Crawford DC, Safran MR: Osteochondritis dissecans of the knee. *J Am Acad Orthop Surg* 2006;14[2]:90-100.)

c. Careful assessment can clarify whether symptoms include only pain or mechanical popping and locking to determine appropriate treatment.

d. In thin patients, deep pressure over the medial parapatellar area may produce pain when the knee is flexed, but not when it is extended.

e. Application of varus or valgus stress throughout a full ROM may produce reports of pain and popping if a medial or lateral femoral condylar fragment is sufficiently loose.

f. Physical examination—A thorough provocative and ligamentous examination is necessary to identify any comorbid conditions, such as meniscal tears, loose bodies, or instability.

g. Imaging—Standard weight-bearing AP, lateral, tunnel, and Merchant radiographic views should be obtained.
   - An OCD lesion in the classic position on the lateral aspect of the medial femoral condyle may be overlooked on the AP view in extension because of overriding bone.
   - Classic lesions are best visualized on the tunnel view (**Figure 6**).

h. MRIs and bone scans are adjunctive studies that help stage the lesions and predict the prognosis.

4. Nonsurgical treatment
   a. Patients of any age with stable lesions are treated with rest, activity restriction, anti-inflammatory medication, and pain modalities as needed.
   b. If symptoms persist, 6 weeks of protected weight bearing or immobilization may be needed.

5. Surgical treatment
   a. Indications
      - Unstable lesions with or without loose bodies.
      - Older children with persistent pain despite sufficient nonsurgical treatment.
      - Younger patients with continued pain and swelling with or without loss of motion in whom 3 to 6 months of nonsurgical treatment has failed.
   b. Contraindications—Very young patients with inconsistent pain in whom a long course of nonsurgical treatment has been successful.
   c. Procedures
      - Stable lesions are amenable to extra-articular or transarticular arthroscopic drilling. When drilling a stable OCD lesion arthroscopically, care must be taken to avoid slipping across the cartilage or producing excessive heat that creates cartilage

10 | Pediatrics

damage when transarticularly perforating a lesion. Fluoroscopy or an anterior cruciate ligament (ACL) type of drill guide is used to perform extra-articular drilling.

- Unstable lesions are managed with arthroscopic or open débridement with fixation. In young adolescents, fixation of unstable lesions should be attempted; additional procedures may be necessary later. Bioabsorbable pins or screws of appropriate length work well; they must be cut flush so that no excess protrudes from the cartilage surface.
- A loose body that does not fit or is severely damaged should be removed, followed by chondroplasty or a cartilage restoration procedure; the piece should be retained if possible by trimming it and securing it with pins and/or screws.

6. Complications—Stiffness, infection, failure of fixation, continued pain, and arthrofibrosis.
7. Rehabilitation
    a. Crutches and touchdown weight bearing are prescribed for 6 weeks.
    b. Immediate active-assisted and passive motion is begun, along with quadriceps activation and strengthening.
    c. Progression of weight bearing is allowed between 6 and 12 weeks with or without radiographic evidence of healing, as long as no pain or swelling is clinically present.

VI. KNEE LIGAMENT INJURIES

A. Overview and pathoanatomy

1. Posterior cruciate ligament (PCL) and lateral collateral ligament tears are relatively rare. Medial collateral ligament tears are the most common, but ACL tears in adolescents are significantly increasing in frequency.
2. Ligaments fail when loaded at speeds and forces that result in elongation in excess of 10% of the original length of the ligament.
3. The speed at which the load is applied determines whether the ligament fails or the bone or physis fails.
4. Among patients participating in a cutting, jumping, or pivoting sport or activity, approximately 70% of patients will present with a noncontact injury and 30% of patients present with a contact injury.
5. Approximately 70% of patients who present to the emergency department or clinic with a large knee effusion after an injury will have an ACL injury.

B. Classification—Ligament injuries are graded according to the severity of injury of each ligament.

C. Evaluation

1. The history can be traumatic, such as a motor vehicle accident or an injury sustained during contact or noncontact sports, or atraumatic. Patients present with acute pain and swelling, with or without instability. Loss of motion is frequent.
2. Physical examination may be difficult in the acute setting. Instability and point tenderness in this setting can be diagnostic. Examination should be repeated at up to two weeks post-injury to aid in the diagnosis in lieu of an MRI.
3. The physical examination to diagnose a meniscus injury should include Lachman test, McMurray test, and Apley test.
4. Radiographs obtained during the initial examination can rule out physeal or other fractures about the knee. They may demonstrate abnormalities of alignment, such as an anteriorly translated tibia seen on a lateral view, that make diagnosis of a ligament injury possible.
5. MRI is useful for confirming a suspected diagnosis or when an adequate physical examination is not possible.

D. Treatment

1. General principles
    a. When determining treatment, factors including the ligament injured and the patient's age, remaining growth, severity of injury, and planned level of activity should be considered.
    b. For a patient who is not within 2 years of skeletal maturity, treatment is chosen carefully and all factors, particularly the amount of growth remaining, are weighed. When in doubt, other pathology is repaired and rehabilitation is initiated, with or without bracing treatment.
    c. Although uncommon, physeal injury or arrest can occur no matter what procedure is used.
    d. When considering ligament reconstruction, skeletal age should be determined using growth charts, bone age, and Tanner staging.

e. Complete tears
   - Complete PCL injuries seem to cause less instability than ACL tears but probably have the same potential for long-term arthritis, although surgical intervention is more easily avoided until skeletal maturity.
   - Posterolateral corner injuries rarely occur in isolation. When combined with PCL injuries, a more difficult problem is created.

f. When managing any ligament injury, the surgeon must balance the risk of iatrogenic physeal injury from surgical reconstruction with potential long-term disability and/or arthritis resulting from nonsurgical treatments. The younger the patient, the greater the risk of deformity if a growth arrest occurs after a reconstructive procedure.

2. Nonsurgical treatment
   a. Surgical treatment should be considered for complete ACL ruptures to avoid further meniscal and chondral injury.
   b. Partial tears of the ACL, PCL, medial collateral ligament, or lateral collateral ligament without other intra-articular pathology are amenable to nonsurgical treatment.
      - Bracing treatment provides initial stabilization and support for the return to sports.
      - Physical therapy, including strength and gait training and pain modalities, helps achieve full ROM.
      - Anti-inflammatory medications may be used initially, but uncertainty exists about their effect on the soft-tissue healing process.
      - Return to sports is allowed when full motion, strength, and stability have returned with or without a brace.
   c. Activity modification, brief immobilization, physical therapy, and pain modalities are all indicated initially.
   d. Obtaining full motion and relative stability with bracing treatment and muscle control may obviate the need for surgical intervention in a select group of individuals (copers: those who can perform activities without an ACL and not sustain further pivot shift or buckling events) even when skeletally mature.

3. Surgical treatment
   a. Indications
      - Failure to maintain stability despite physical therapy and bracing treatment
      - Unwillingness to modify activities
      - Need to assess other pathology, such as meniscal pathology
   b. Procedures
      - Ligament repair has a high rate of failure in adolescent patients but has the potential to prevent long-term disability or arthritis in skeletally immature or mature patients.
      - Transphyseal tibial tunnel combined with over-the-top graft positioning on the femur, although not commonly performed.
      - Physeal sparing—All-epiphyseal or extra-articular reconstructions (**Figure 7**).
      - Hybrid procedures, ie, all-epiphyseal femoral tunnel with transphyseal tibial tunnel (**Figure 8**).
      - Transphyseal procedures with soft tissue only.

E. Pearls
   1. Spanning the physis with bone or metal must be avoided.
   2. Transphyseal tunnels should be kept to a minimum size in a central location.

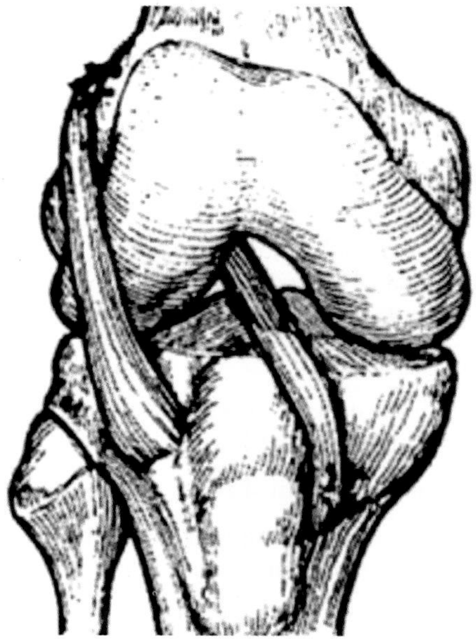

Figure 7 Illustration shows extraphyseal anterior cruciate ligament reconstruction. (Reproduced with permission from Kocher MS, Garg S, Micheli Li: Physeal sparing reconstruction of the anterior cruciate ligament in skeletally immature prepubescent children and adolescents. *J Bone Joint Surg Am* 2005;87:2371-2379.)

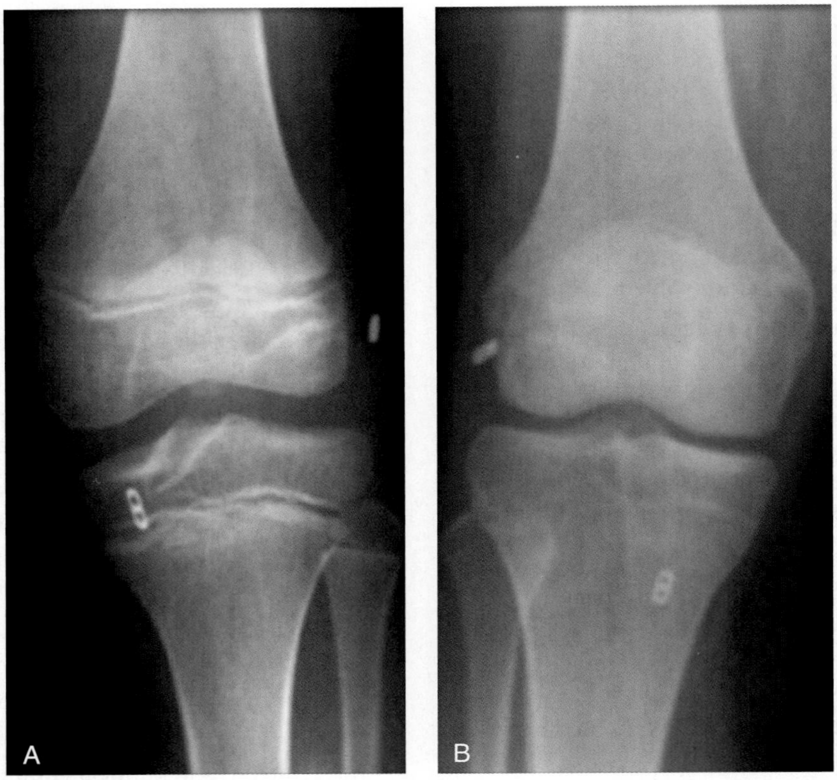

Figure 8 **A**, All-epiphyseal drilling technique in both the tibia and femur for anterior cruciate ligament (ACL) reconstruction in a skeletally immature patient. **B**, All-epiphyseal drilling technique in the femur and transphyseal drilling technique in the tibia. (Courtesy of Jay Albright, and Children's Hospital Colorado, Aurora, CO.)

3. Dissection or damage to the perichondral ring should be avoided (do not dissect subperiosteally) when passing the graft via over-the-top position on the femur.

F. Complications—Partial or complete physeal arrest, arthrofibrosis, infection, short-term or long-term ligament failure, arthritis, and atrophy.

G. Rehabilitation

1. Immediate motion, quadriceps activation, swelling, and pain control
2. Prolonged physical therapy
   a. Slow, steady progress back to straight line activities at approximately six months
   b. No start-stop or cutting action for 8 to 12 months
   c. Return to sports in 1 year with or without a brace

VII. PATELLOFEMORAL INSTABILITY

A. Pathoanatomy

1. More than 90% occur with lateral patellar translation.
2. Common injuries occurring during a patellar instability event.
   a. Torn medial patellofemoral ligament (MPFL) and/or medial retinaculum (femoral-, midsubstance-, or patellar-based)
   b. Avulsion fracture of the medial patella at the insertion of the MPFL
   c. Osteochondral injuries resulting in intra-articular loose bodies
   d. Bone bruising of the patella and lateral femoral condyle

3. Risk Factors
    a. Valgus alignment
    b. Increased quadriceps angle
    c. Excessive femoral anteversion
    d. Excessive external tibial torsion
    e. Trochlear dysplasia
    f. Patella alta
    g. Previous patellar dislocation
    h. Skeletal immaturity
    i. Disorders that affect ligamentous laxity, such as Ehlers-Danlos or Down syndrome

B. Classification—Patellofemoral instability is classified descriptively.
1. Subluxation or dislocation
2. First time dislocation or recurrent

C. Mechanism of injury—Patellofemoral subluxation or dislocation can result from a direct blow forcing the patella out of place or from noncontact mechanisms.

D. Evaluation
1. History
    a. May report noncontact twisting mechanism or contact with direct blow.
    b. With frank dislocation, patella may spontaneously reduce or may require positioning with leg in hip flexion and knee extension for reduction.
2. Physical examination
    a. Point tenderness is maximal at the site of the retinacular or ligament tear along its course from the medial epicondyle to the medial patella.
    b. An effusion may be subtle or large.
    c. Apprehension test is typically positive.
    d. Evaluation of axial and rotational alignment is performed.
    e. The quadriceps angle is assessed.
    f. A J-sign may be appreciated.
3. Imaging
    a. Plain radiographs may appear normal or may show an osteochondral loose body.
    b. Evaluate trochlear morphology and patellar height and tilt on lateral and sunrise views.
    c. After a dislocation, ordering an MRI is controversial but is advised if a tense knee effusion is present without radiographic signs of an osteochondral injury, as this effusion may signify a chondral loose body.
    d. Evaluation of tibial tubercle to trochlear groove (TTTG) distance.
    e. Evaluation of skeletal maturity if surgical intervention is planned.

E. Nonsurgical treatment
1. Initial management includes immobilization for comfort, rest, ice, compression, and elevation.
2. Physical therapy is initiated to strengthen the injured extremity and address core and hip weakness.
3. A patellar stabilizing brace initially for activities of daily living also can be used after the athlete is ready to return to play.

F. Surgical treatment
1. Indications
    a. Osteochondral injury with loose body
    b. Recurrent instability
    c. Failure of nonsurgical treatment with persistent pain or instability
2. Contraindications
    a. Procedures which would compromise an open physis such as tibial tubercle osteotomy or MPFL graft transphyseal tunnel
3. Procedures depend on constellation of symptoms and radiographic abnormalities.
    a. Lateral release
    b. Medial retinacular or MPFL repair
    c. Medial plication of VMO fascia
    d. MPFL reconstruction
    e. Guided growth with hemiepiphysiodesis
    f. Rotational osteotomy of the femur and/or tibia
    g. Removal or fixation of osteochondral fragment
    h. Tibial tubercle osteotomy in skeletally mature patients for increased TTTG distance
4. Pearls
    a. Osteochondral injuries should be addressed.
    b. Evaluation of anatomic abnormalities which are risk factors for dislocation is important, as these should be addressed if possible.

c. Anatomic reconstruction of the MPFL is important for optimal outcome.
   - The tension of the construct is set with the patella centered in the trochlea with the knee in 30° of flexion.
   - The location of the graft attachment sites on the patella and femur should be checked that they produce an isometric graft with the knee in 0° to 60° of flexion.
   - The femoral attachment can be within 1 to 3 mm from the epiphyseal plate. Generally, in younger patients, this site is just distal to the physis, but in older adolescents, it can be at or proximal to the physis. Femoral drill tunnels should be aimed away from the physis. This may mean the drill will be aimed distal and posterior if starting below the physis.

d. Avoid overconstraining the patella. Patella should have one to two quadrants of medial and lateral translation following repair similar to the native patella. Flexion past 90° will be difficult after overtensioning of the repair or reconstruction.

e. Excessive lateral release can result in iatrogenic medial instability or dislocation.

f. Tibial tubercle osteotomy should be avoided in skeletally immature patients to prevent angular deformity.

g. Quadriceps/femoral nerve stimulation intraoperatively may be helpful to fine-tune the amount of medialization during tibial tubercle osteotomy.

5. Complications
   a. Arthrofibrosis
   b. Recurrent dislocations
   c. Premature growth arrest
   d. Overcorrection of axial or rotational alignment
   e. Iatrogenic medial dislocation

6. Rehabilitation
   a. Immediate weight bearing locked in extension is allowed.
   b. Range of motion should be restricted to 0° to 90° for 4 to 6 weeks.
   c. Early physical therapy is important for quadriceps activation and ROM.
   d. Return to sports or activities may occur when strength and neuromuscular control has returned. Generally, this will be around 6 month postoperatively.
   e. A patellar stabilizing brace may be used for return to play.

VIII. MENISCAL INJURIES AND DISCOID MENISCUS

A. Pathoanatomy

1. Injuries to the meniscus result from twisting events during loading of the knee.
2. Meniscus functions as shock absorber between femur and tibia and relies on intact circumferentially oriented fibers to absorb force and hoop stresses.
3. Vascular supply is from the periphery. Outer third of the meniscus is termed red-red zone due to abundant blood supply, middle third is red-white zone, and inner third is white-white zone due to lack of vascularity.
4. Tear location and pattern have implications for the success of repair or nonsurgical treatment attempts; tears occurring close to the vascular zone have the highest rates of success.
5. Discoid meniscus refers to an abnormally large meniscus which does not have the usual contour. They are classified as partial, complete, or Wrisberg variant (**Figure 9**).

B. Classification

1. Meniscal tears are classified descriptively.
   a. Location of tear—Red-red zone, vascular, outer third; red-white zone, middle third; white zone, avascular, inner third.
   b. Size
   c. Pattern—Horizontal, vertical, radial, bucket-handle, parrot beak, complex, or combination (**Figure 10**).

C. Evaluation

1. History
   a. Meniscal tears can follow a traumatic or atraumatic event. Generally, there is an axial load with flexion or twisting at the knee simultaneously.
   b. Young children may present with insidious onset.

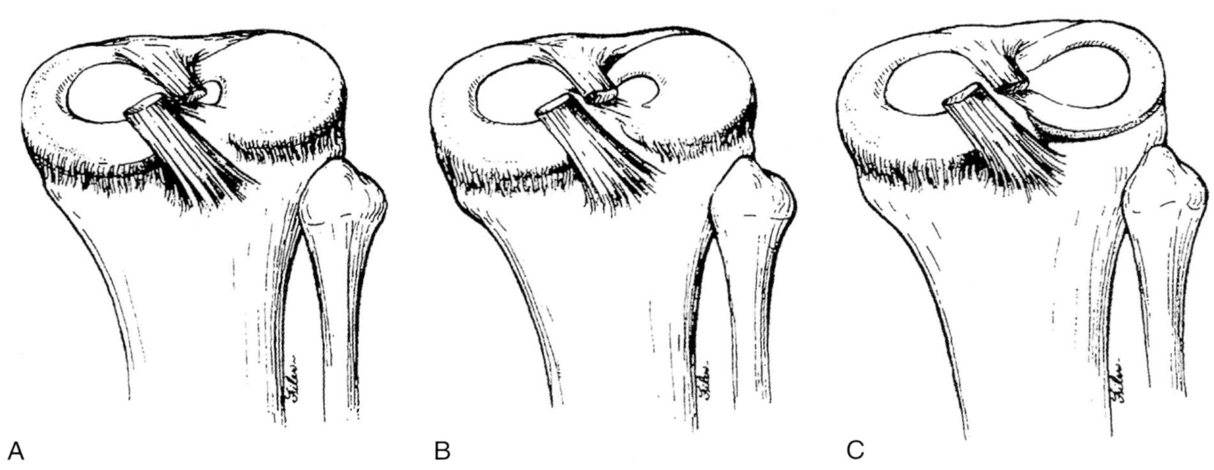

Figure 9 Illustrations show the classification system for lateral discoid menisci. **A**, Type I (complete); **B**, Type II (incomplete); and **C**, Type III (Wrisberg ligament). Type III discoid menisci have no posterior attachment to the tibia. The only posterior attachment is through the ligament of Wrisberg toward the medial femoral condyle. (Reproduced with permission from Neuschwander DC: Discoid lateral meniscus, in Fu FH, Harner CD, Vince KG, eds: *Knee Surgery*. Baltimore, MD, Williams and Wilkins, 1994, p 394.)

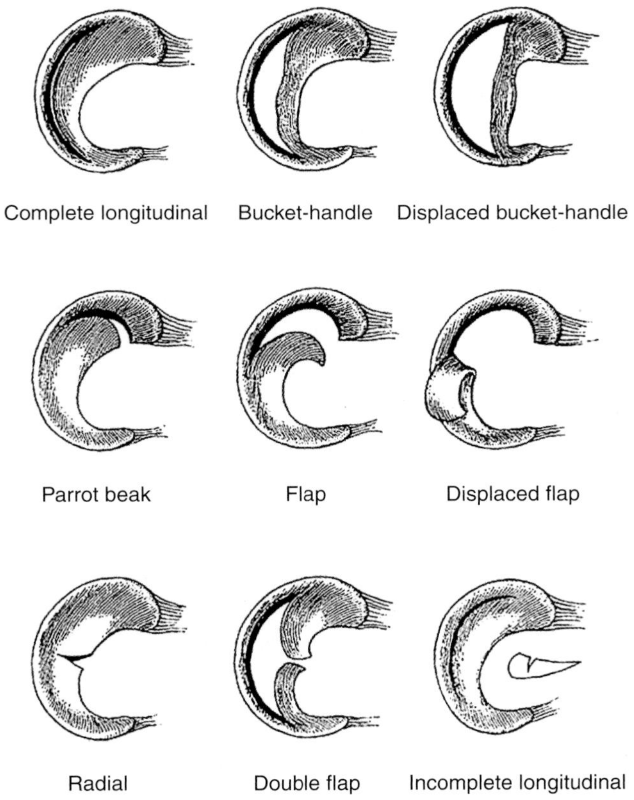

Figure 10 Illustrations show common meniscal tear morphology. (Reproduced with permission from Tria AJ, Klein KS: *An Illustrated Guide to the Knee*. New York, NY, Churchill Livingstone, 1992.)

c. Patients may report a pop followed by pain and swelling.

2. Physical examination
   a. Effusion may be present.
   b. Range of motion may be limited due to effusion, pain, or mechanical block.
   c. Point tenderness at the joint line.
   d. Provocative testing including hyperflexion, McMurray test, Apley test, and Thessaly test which may produce pain and a pop.
   e. Examination of ligaments is important due to the potential for concomitant injury.
3. Imaging
   a. Radiographs may appear normal; however, they can indicate a discoid lateral meniscus with a widened lateral joint line or lateral femoral condyle flattening.
   b. MRI is indicated to rule out a discoid meniscus, meniscal tears, and other intra-articular diagnoses.
   c. MRI has a high false-positive rate in children younger than 10 years because of the abundant vascularity of the meniscus in this age group which can appear similar to a tear.

D. Nonsurgical treatment
   1. The management of incidentally noted, asymptomatic discoid menisci is observation.

2. Small peripheral tears (in the red-red zone) may heal or become asymptomatic with nonsurgical treatment.
   a. Rest with or without bracing treatment to limit range of motion past 90° for 4 to 6 weeks, followed by physical therapy to regain strength and range of motion.

E. Surgical treatment
1. Indications
   a. Mechanical symptoms, bucket-handle tears, meniscal root tears, meniscal tears causing extrusion of the meniscus or loss of circumferential fiber integrity, tears of a discoid meniscus, and associated ligament injury.
   b. Failure of nonsurgical treatment with persistent pain.
2. Procedures
   a. Fixation methods
      - Inside-out repair technique is the benchmark.
      - All-inside devices are increasingly common given their ease of use. More recent studies cite similar outcomes to inside-out repairs.
      - Outside-in technique may be useful for anterior horn repair.
   b. Partial meniscectomy is reserved for irreparable tears or small tears of the white-white zone.
   c. Saucerization of a torn discoid meniscus with repair of remaining torn meniscal tissue.
3. Pearls
   a. A vertical mattress suture pattern has been shown to be the strongest.
   b. Partial meniscectomy is reserved only for tears that are irreparable. Given the potential for healing is higher in the pediatric patient, a more aggressive attempt at repair should be undertaken.

F. Complications
1. Arthrofibrosis
2. Retear or propagation of new tear from repair site
3. Iatrogenic cartilage damage during repair

G. Rehabilitation
1. Early physical therapy for range of motion, quadriceps activation, swelling, and pain control
2. For a repaired meniscus, 4 to 6 weeks of touch-down weight bearing and range of motion from 0° to 90°, depending on the size and location of tear

For meniscectomy, weight bearing as tolerated and no range of motion restrictions.

IX. PLICA SYNDROME

A. Epidemiology
1. Painful plica is a diagnosis of exclusion; its true incidence is difficult to discern.
2. Plicae are medially based parapatellar bands in approximately 90% of symptomatic patients.

B. Pathoanatomy
1. A plica is a remnant of embryologic development; it consists of normal synovial tissue that causes mechanically based synovitis from repetitive motion.
2. Plicae may even cause arthroscopically visible evidence of chondromalacia of the edge of the femoral condyle.

C. Evaluation
1. Plica syndrome is diagnosed by excluding other pathologies.
2. Patients report activity-related anteromedial to medial knee pain, sometimes with catching or partial giving way.
3. Physical examination reveals a painful, palpable band of tissue along the medial parapatellar area.
   a. The knee is palpated while the patient performs active motion. If patellar compression is not painful in 45° of knee flexion, but is painful in the parapatellar soft tissue, then plicae may be present.
   b. Examining for an accompanying, highly sensitive lateral suprapatellar soft-tissue mass lying under the vastus lateralis is helpful.
   c. The parapatellar bands also can be palpated lateral and even inferior to the patella.
   d. MRI may not reveal a plica, which is easier to see when knee effusion is present, but usually is difficult to visualize. A high index of suspicion is warranted.

D. Treatment
1. Nonsurgical
   a. Anti-inflammatory medications, ice, activity modification, immobilization

b. Physical therapy modalities, such as ultrasonography and iontophoresis of cortisone solution

c. Cortisone injections

2. Surgical

a. Indications

- Pain not resolved by nonsurgical methods
- An erroneous diagnosis explained only by an irritated plica

b. Contraindications—Reflex sympathetic dystrophy, chronic regional pain syndrome, or saphenous neuritis, which can be ruled out before surgery.

c. Procedure

- Arthroscopic resection of the plica is performed using a standard two-portal or three-portal approach.
- The inferomedial parapatellar portal or the medial/lateral suprapatellar portals are sufficient for excision using the shaver, biter, or heat probe of choice.

d. Pearls

- The most worrisome pitfall is an overaggressive resection of the plica that includes the retinaculum and not just the abnormal band of synovium.
- Denudement, irritation, or deformation of the medial condylar articular surface under the contact area of the plica is an indication that the plica should be resected.
- An arthroscopic punch or heat device can create a working resection edge in the thickened yet smooth plicae that are difficult to treat using a shaver.

E. Complications—Same as those that occur after routine arthroscopy: arthrofibrosis, infection, nerve or vessel injury, patellar instability, unresolved pain.

F. Rehabilitation

1. Immediate motion and quadriceps activation, with quick return to weight bearing as tolerated
2. At 3 to 4 weeks, the patient may be ready to return to full participation, depending on any other pathology present at the time of surgery.

TOP TESTING FACTS

1. Little Leaguer's shoulder is an epiphysiolysis, or a fracture through the proximal humeral physis, that causes pain during the late cocking or deceleration phases of pitching.
2. Little Leaguer's elbow (medial epicondylitis) occurs secondary to valgus loading of the elbow during throwing/pitching. Initial management of this epicondylitis is nonsurgical.
3. The radiographic diagnosis of a capitellar lesion in a child younger than 10 years is Panner disease; in a child older than 10 years, it is OCD.
4. OCD of the knee classically involves the lateral aspect of the medial femoral condyle and is best visualized on a tunnel radiograph. Treatment is determined based on the stability of the lesion.
5. Initial management of OCD of the knee includes activity modification and/or rest with or without immobilization, unless locking symptoms or a loose body is present.
6. Partial ACL tears can be managed nonsurgically with physical therapy, with or without bracing treatment. Surgical management is recommended for complete ACL rupture to prevent subsequent meniscal damage.
7. Partial or complete physeal arrest in the skeletally immature patient is a potential complication of ACL reconstruction. Growth arrest may lead to leg length discrepancy or valgus or varus deformity.
8. MPFL graft should be placed and tensioned to produce an isometric graft from 0° to 60° of flexion.
9. If a femoral socket is placed to secure an MPFL graft, care should be taken to determine the location of the physis and the socket may need to be directed distal and posterior to avoid the physis.
10. Surgery should be performed for tears of the meniscus in the outer, vascular zone only if locking symptoms exist or if no improvement occurs after prolonged nonsurgical treatment.

Bibliography

Andrish JT: Meniscal injuries in children and adolescents: Diagnosis and management. *J Am Acad Orthop Surg* 1996;4(5):231-237.

Crebs DT, Anthony CA, McCunniff PT, Nieto MJ, Beckert MW, Albright JP: Effectiveness of Fulkerson osteotomy with femoral nerve stimulation for patients with severe femoral trochlear dysplasia. *Iowa Orthop J* 2015;35:34-41.

Heyworth BE, Kramer DE, Martin DJ, Micheli LJ, Kocher MS, Bae DS: Trends in the presentation, management, and outcomes of little league shoulder. *Am J Sports Med* 2016;44(6):1431-1438.

Kocher MS, Saxon HS, Hovis WD, Hawkins RJ: Management and complications of anterior cruciate ligament injuries in skeletally immature patients: Survey of the Herodicus Society and the ACL Study Group. *J Pediatr Orthop* 2002;22(4):452-457.

Lawrence JT, Argawal N, Ganley TJ: Degeneration of the knee joint in skeletally immature patients with a diagnosis of an anterior cruciate ligament tear: Is there harm in delay of treatment? *Am J Sports Med* 2011;39(12):2582-2587.

Leahy I, Schorpion M, Ganley T: Elbow OCD vs Panner's disease. *J Hand Ther* 2015;28(2):201-210.

Lin KM, James EW, Spitzer E, Fabricant PD: Pediatric and adolescent anterior shoulder instability: Clinical management of first-time dislocators. *Curr Opin Pediatr* 2018;30(1):49-56.

Murray MM, Fleming BC: Use of a bioactive scaffold to stimulate anterior cruciate ligament healing also minimizes posttraumatic osteoarthritis after surgery. *Am J Sports Med* 2013;41(8):1762-1770.

Nepple JJ, Milewski MD, Shea KG: Research in osteochondritis dissecans of the knee: 2016 update. *J Knee Surg* 2016;29(8):696.

Newman JT, Carry PM, Terhune EB, et al: Factors predictive of concomitant injuries among children and adolescents undergoing anterior cruciate ligament surgery. *Am J Sports Med* 2015;43(2):282-288.

Noyes FR, Albright JC: Reconstruction of the medial patellofemoral ligament with autologous quadriceps tendon. *Arthroscopy* 2006;22(8):e1–e7.

Shea KG, Martinson WD, Cannamela PC, et al: Variation in the medial patellofemoral ligament origin in the skeletally immature knee: An anatomic study. *Am J Sports Med* 2018;46(2):363-369.

Chapter 138
PEDIATRIC POLYTRAUMA AND UPPER EXTREMITY FRACTURES

ERIN MEISEL, MD
ROBERT M. KAY, MD

I. SKELETAL DIFFERENCES BETWEEN CHILDREN AND ADULTS

A. Pediatric bone is more elastic, leading to unique fracture patterns, including torus (buckle) fractures and greenstick fractures.

B. The thicker periosteum generally remains intact on the side of the bone toward which the distal fragment is displaced.

   1. This periosteal hinge facilitates reduction.
   2. Aggressive reduction attempts can disrupt the hinge, making a satisfactory reduction more difficult.

C. Open physes (epiphyseal plates) can allow remodeling and straightening of a malunited fracture; however, with growth disturbance, ongoing growth can result in angular deformity, limb-length discrepancy, or both.

   1. Remodeling occurs more rapidly and fully in the plane of joint motion (eg, sagittal malalignment at the wrist remodels more successfully than a coronal plane deformity).
   2. In the upper extremity, the fastest growth occurs at the upper and lower ends of the extremity (ie, at the proximal humerus and distal radius and ulna), whereas in the lower extremity, most growth occurs in the middle (ie, at the distal femur and proximal tibia and fibula).
   3. Fractures most commonly occur through the hypertrophic zone.

Dr. Meisel or an immediate family member has stock or stock options held in Joint Development LLC. Dr. Kay or an immediate family member serves as a paid consultant to or is an employee of Intrinsic Therapeutics; has stock or stock options held in Biomet, Johnson & Johnson, Medtronic, Pfizer, and Zimmer; and serves as a board member, owner, officer, or committee member of the Commission for Motion Lab Accreditation.

II. EPIPHYSEAL PLATE (PHYSEAL) FRACTURES

A. Classification—Most commonly used is the Salter-Harris classification (**Figure 1**).

   1. Advantages—Ease of use and prognostic value.
   2. Disadvantage—Salter-Harris V fractures, which are rare, cannot be distinguished from Salter-Harris I fractures at initial presentation; the differentiation cannot be made until a growth arrest has occurred.

B. Growth arrest following physeal fracture

   1. Recognition—Following fracture healing, Park-Harris lines should be moving away from the physis while remaining parallel to the physis (**Figure 2**). If the lines are not moving away from or are not parallel to the physis, then a growth arrest (partial or whole) has occurred (**Figure 3**).
   2. Imaging—Advanced imaging, particularly MRI, facilitates the determination of physeal bar size and location. CT is now used less frequently because of radiation exposure.
   3. Management—Depends on physeal bar size and location and the amount of growth remaining in the affected bone.
      a. Upper extremity growth arrests result in fewer functional problems than do lower extremity arrests and less commonly require intervention.
      b. Physeal bar excision—Attempts at excision (with interposition of an inert material such as autogenous fat) may be considered for bars less than 33% to 50% of the cross-sectional area of the physis in a physis with more than 2 years of remaining growth. Results of physeal bar excision are best with small bars in younger children.

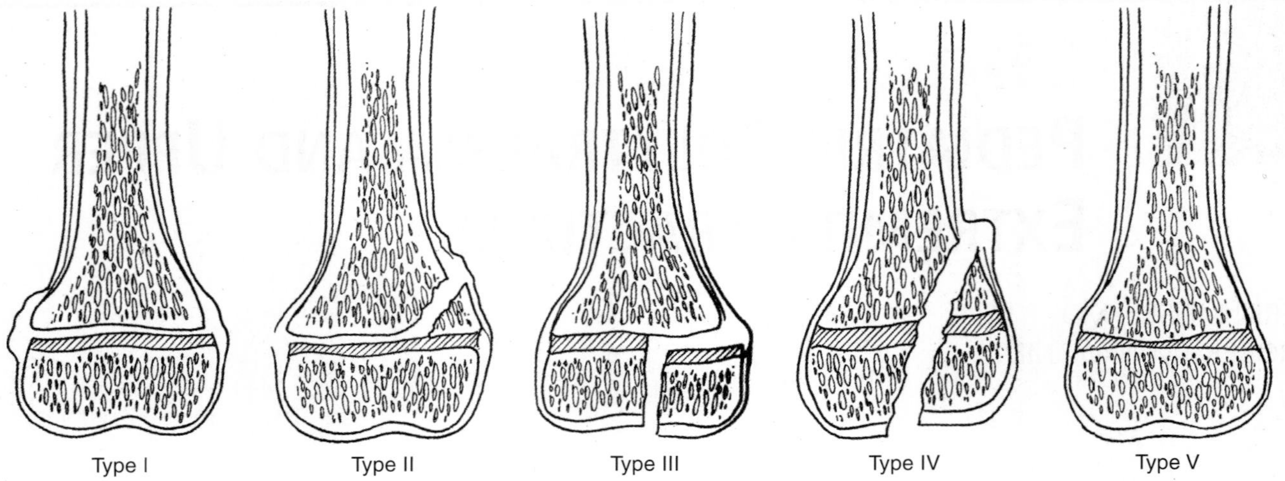

Figure 1 Illustrations show the Salter-Harris classification of physeal fractures. Type I is characterized by a physeal separation; type II by a fracture that traverses the physis and exits through the metaphysis; type III by a fracture that traverses the physis before exiting through the epiphysis; type IV by a fracture that passes through the epiphysis, physis, and metaphysis; and type V by a crush injury to the physis. (Reproduced from Kay RM, Matthys GA: Pediatric ankle fractures: Evaluation and treatment. *J Am Acad Orthop Surg* 2001;9[4]:268-278.)

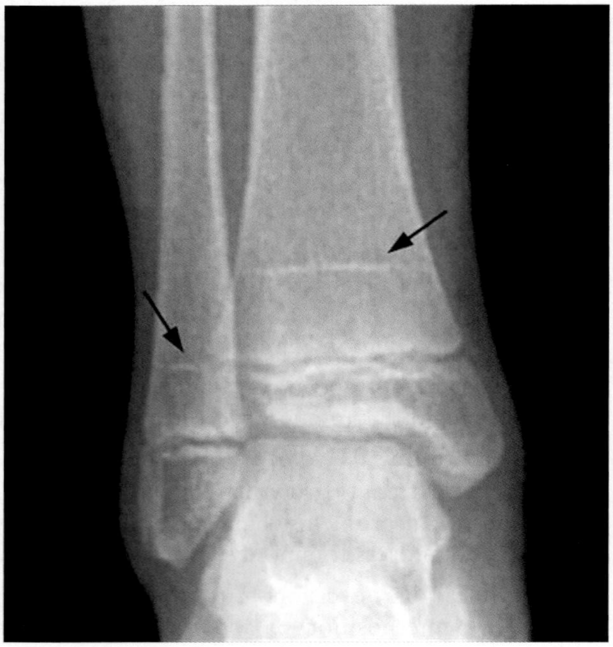

Figure 2 AP radiograph demonstrates growth arrest lines (arrows) following ankle fracture in a pediatric patient. These lines lie parallel to the adjacent physes and thus do not represent asymmetrical growth. (Reproduced from Wuerz TH, Gurd DP: Pediatric physeal ankle fracture. *J Am Acad Orthop Surg* 2013;21[4]:234-244.)

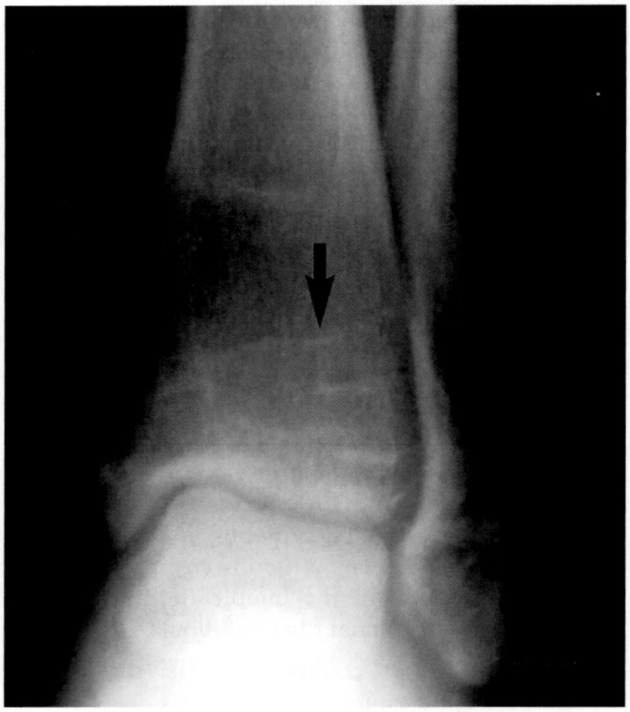

Figure 3 AP radiograph of a 14-year-old girl obtained 4 years after a distal tibial fracture complicated by medial growth arrest shows a 1.7-cm leg-length disparity and a 15° varus deformity of the ankle. Growth-disturbance lines (arrow) converge medially because of the medial growth arrest. (Reproduced from Kay RM, Matthys GA: Pediatric ankle fractures: Evaluation and treatment. *J Am Acad Orthop Surg* 2001;9[4]:268-278.)

4. Epiphysiodesis
   a. Ipsilateral extremity—The functioning part of the affected physis may be ablated if angular deformity is developing.
   b. Contralateral epiphysiodesis is considered if the physeal arrest will result in unacceptable limb-length discrepancy, typically 2 cm or larger, in the lower extremities

III. POLYTRAUMA

A. Epidemiology
1. Trauma is the most common cause of death in children older than 1 year.
2. The most common causes are falls and motor vehicle accidents.
   a. Many injuries and deaths could be avoided by appropriate use of child seats and restraints.
   b. Cervical spine injuries following a motor vehicle accident are more common in children younger than 8 years. Two contributing elements are restraints that do not fit young children well, and the disproportionately large size of the head relative to the trunk. Deceleration mechanisms lead to distraction injuries.

B. Initial evaluation, resuscitation, and transport
1. Hypotension (systolic blood pressure [SBP] ≤ 100) and low Glasgow Coma Scale (GCS) score upon initial evaluation are strongly associated with increased risk of in-hospital mortality after trauma.
2. Fluid resuscitation
   a. If venous access is difficult, intraosseous infusion with a large-bore needle may be necessary.
   b. Unlike adults, children often remain hemodynamically stable for extended periods of time following substantial blood loss. Hypovolemic shock eventually ensues if fluid resuscitation is inadequate.
   - Blood volume—70 mL/kg
   - Children develop hypotension with loss of 25% of blood volume
3. Because young children have a large head size, a special transport board with an occipital cutout or a mattress pad to elevate the body is necessary when transporting children younger than 6 years to the hospital, to prevent cervical spine flexion and potential iatrogenic cervical spinal cord injury.

C. Systemic response to trauma
1. Timing of multiorgan failure in children differs from adults, occurring almost immediately after injury and simultaneously rather than in a stepwise fashion.
   a. Rate of acute lung injury in children is 1/6 as frequent in children as it is in adults.
2. Children mount a strong local inflammatory response to facilitate healing as compared with adults (**Table 1**).

D. Secondary evaluation
1. The Glasgow Coma Scale (GCS, **Table 2**), scored on a scale of 3 to 15 points, is most commonly used for evaluating head injury.
   a. A GCS score less than 8 at presentation in verbal children indicates a higher risk of mortality.
   b. The GCS motor score at 72 hours post injury predicts permanent disability following traumatic brain injury.
2. Abdominal bruising (lap belt sign) often indicates abdominal visceral injuries and spine fractures.
   a. Greater likelihood of multiple organ injuries given their close proximity.

TABLE 1

Comparison of Adult and Pediatric Physiologic Response to Polytrauma Trauma

Factor	Adults	Children
Timing of organ failure	48-72 hr after injury	Immediate
Organ failure sequence	Sequential	Simultaneous
Acute lung injury	High risk	Low risk
Systemic inflammatory response	Robust	Dampened
Local inflammatory response	Dampened	Robust
Death due to pelvic fracture	High risk	Low risk
Morbidity	Associated with pelvic fracture	Associated with organ injuries
Neurologic injury	Low recovery rate	High recovery rate

TABLE 2

Pediatric Glasgow Coma Scale

Score	Age 5 yr and Older	Age 1-5 yr	Age 1 yr and Younger
Best Motor Response			
6	Obeys commands	Obeys commands	
5	Localizes pain	Localizes pain	Localizes pain
4	Withdrawal	Withdrawal	Abnormal withdrawal
3	Flexion to pain	Abnormal flexion	Abnormal flexion
2	Extensor rigidity	Extensor rigidity	Abnormal extension
1	None	None	None
Best Verbal Response			
5	Oriented	Appropriate words	Smiles/cries appropriately
4	Confused	Inappropriate words	Cries
3	Inappropriate words	Cries/screams	Cries inappropriately
2	Incomprehensible	Grunts	Grunts
1	None	None	None
Eye Opening			
4	Spontaneous	Spontaneous	Spontaneous
3	To speech	To speech	To shout
2	To pain	To pain	To pain
1	None	None	None

Reproduced from Sponseller PD, Paidas C: Management of the pediatric trauma patient, in Sponseller PD, ed: *Orthopaedic Knowledge Update: Pediatrics*, ed 2. Rosemont, IL, American Academy of Orthopaedic Surgeons, 2002, pp 73-79.

3. Up to 10% of injuries are initially missed by the treating team because of head injury and/or severe pain in other locations.

E. CT—Only approximately one half of pelvic fractures identified on CT scans are identified on AP pelvic radiographs.

F. Head and neck injuries
   1. Children can make remarkable recoveries following severe traumatic brain injury and should be treated as if such a recovery will occur.
   2. Intracranial pressure should be controlled to minimize ongoing brain damage.
   3. Musculoskeletal manifestations of head injuries
      a. Spasticity begins within days to weeks; splinting helps prevent contractures.
         - Part-time positioning of the hip and knee in flexion can reduce the plantar flexor tone to help prevent equinus contracture.
         - Pharmacologic intervention with botulinum toxin A may help acutely control spasticity and facilitate rehabilitation.
      b. Heterotopic ossification (HO), especially around the elbow, is common following traumatic brain injury.
         - An increase in serum alkaline phosphatase may herald the onset of HO.
         - Treatment is either observation or excision if heterotopic bone interferes with rehabilitation.
         - The use of NSAIDs, salicylates, and low-dose radiation for postexcision prophylaxis is controversial.
      c. Fractures heal more rapidly following traumatic brain injury, but the mechanism is not yet understood.
      d. The timing of surgical intervention for fractures in patients with head injuries should be decided in concert with trauma surgeons and neurosurgeons to minimize secondary injuries to the brain.

G. Treatment of the patient with multiple injuries
   1. Surgical fracture treatment is much more common in multiple-trauma patients because

TABLE 3

Antibiotics Used in the Treatment of Pediatric Open Fractures

Antibiotic	Dose	Interval	Maximum Dose	Indications
Cefazolin	100 mg/kg/d	Q8 hr	6 g/d	All open fractures
Gentamicin	5-7.5 mg/kg/d	Q8 hr	None specified	Severe grade II and III injuries
Penicillin	150,000 units/kg/d	Q6 hr	24 million units/d	Farm-type or vascular injuries
Clindamycin	15-40 units/kg/d	Q6-8 hr	2.7 g/d	Patients with allergies to cefazolin or penicillin

it facilitates patient care and mobilization and reduces the risk of pressure sores from immobilization.

a. Decreased risk of multiorgan failure in the first 48 hours after injury.

2. Open fractures are discussed in Section IV.

H. Complications in multiply injured patients

1. Mortality rates can be as high as 20% following pediatric multiple trauma.

2. Long-term morbidity is present in one-third to one-half of children following multiple trauma. Most long-term morbidity results from head injuries and orthopaedic injuries.

a. GCS score at 6 weeks after injury is the best predictor of long-term disability.

b. Spine fractures have highest morbidity and mortality of the musculoskeletal injuries.

3. Fat embolism syndrome in children is a rare, but life-threatening, complication.

I. Rehabilitation

1. Pediatric patients often improve for 1 year or more following injury; many make dramatic neurologic and functional gains; orthopaedic care should be based on the assumption of full recovery.

2. Splinting and bracing treatment prevent contractures and enhance function.

IV. OPEN FRACTURES

A. Epidemiology

1. Open fractures are often high-energy injuries; associated injuries are common.

2. Lawnmower injuries are a common cause of open fractures in children. They are devastating, with high rates of amputation, infection, and growth disturbance.

B. Initial evaluation and management

1. Thorough evaluation for other injuries is essential; up to 50% of children with open fractures have injuries to the head, abdomen, chest, or multiple extremities.

2. Significantly lower infection rates seen in children with open fractures as compared with adults.

3. Tetanus status should be confirmed and updated; children with an unknown vaccination history or who have not had a booster within 5 years should receive a dose of tetanus toxoid.

4. Prompt administration of intravenous antibiotics is essential to minimize the risk of infection (**Table 3**).

C. Classification—As in adults, the Gustilo-Anderson classification is used to grade open fractures (**Table 4**).

D. Treatment

1. Prompt administration of intravenous antibiotics is the most important factor in preventing infection following open fractures.

2. Irrigation and débridement should be performed in all open fractures.

a. Type I fractures generally need only one instance of irrigation and débridement, whereas grade II and III injuries often need repeat irrigation and débridement every 48 to 72 hours until all remaining tissue appears clean and viable.

b. The risk of infection following open fractures is no higher if irrigation and débridement is performed 6 to 24 hours post injury than if performed within 6 hours.

c. Because of the better soft-tissue envelope and vascularity in children, tissue of apparently marginal viability may be left behind at initial débridement. Tissue viability often declares itself by re-exploration time, 2 to 3 days later.

TABLE 4

Gustilo-Anderson Classification of Open Fractures

Grade	Contamination	Wound Length	Defining Feature
I	Clean	<1 cm	
II	Moderate	1-10 cm	
III	Severe	>10 cm	
IIIA	Severe	>10 cm	Adequate soft-tissue coverage
IIIB	Severe	>10 cm	Bone exposure without adequate soft-tissue coverage; soft-tissue coverage often required
IIIC	Severe	Any length	Major vascular injury in injured segment

d. Because of enhanced periosteal new bone formation in children, some bone defects may fill in spontaneously, particularly in young children.

3. Wound cultures

a. Wound cultures are not indicated in the absence of clinical signs of infection.

b. The correlation of predébridement and postdébridement cultures with the development of infection is low; such cultures should not be performed routinely.

4. Fracture fixation (internal or external) is almost universally indicated to stabilize the soft tissues, allow wound access, and maintain alignment.

E. Complications

1. Compartment syndrome (discussed below in Section V) is a substantial risk, particularly in children with a head injury or other distracting injuries.

2. Infection risk is minimized with the prompt administration of intravenous antibiotics and appropriate irrigation and débridement.

3. Chronic pain and psychological sequelae are common manifestations following severe trauma.

V. COMPARTMENT SYNDROME

A. Epidemiology

1. May occur in any location where skeletal muscle is contained within a confined fascial compartment.

B. Pathophysiology

1. Elevated pressure within the fascial space compromises nerve and muscle perfusion leading to ischemia and irreversible damage if not corrected.

2. Etiology

a. Trauma

- Most commonly in the setting of displaced fractures of the tibia (most common) or of forearm, particularly in conjunction with an elbow fracture (so-called floating elbow injuries).

b. Tight circumferential cast, bandage

c. Bleeding diatheses

d. Swelling due to reperfusion

C. Anatomy

1. Lower leg

a. Four compartments: anterior, lateral, superficial, and deep posterior

- Associated with pediatric tibial tubercle fractures due to injury to anterior tibial recurrent artery

2. Forearm

a. Three compartments: volar (most commonly affected by compartment syndrome), dorsal and mobile wad

3. Hand (10 compartments)

4. Foot (nine compartments)

D. Evaluation

1. Primarily a clinical diagnosis

a. Pain out of proportion to the injury and pain with passive stretch (most common) are early signs, but are often unreliable in children.

b. The 3 "A's"—anxiety, agitation, and increased analgesic requirements—are better applied to pediatric population.

2. Compartment pressure measurements may aid in diagnosis, particularly in nonverbal, polytrauma, and/or comatose patients.

a. Intracompartmental pressure >30 mm Hg or within 30 mm Hg of the diastolic pressure (ΔP) is considered diagnostic.

E. Treatment
  1. Nonsurgical
    a. Bivalve cast, loosen bandage and repeat evaluation
  2. Surgical
    a. Emergent fasciotomies: release all potentially involved compartments
      - Lower leg: whether using single- or dual-incisions, must take care to protect common peroneal nerve proximally

F. Neonatal forearm compartment syndrome
  1. Rare and commonly missed diagnosis
  2. Sentinel skin lesions: bullae, desquamation
  3. No role for intracompartmental pressure measurements since no norms have been established for neonates
  4. Best prognosis with emergent fasciotomies

VI. CHILD ABUSE (NONACCIDENTAL TRAUMA)

A. Evaluation
  1. Nonaccidental trauma (NAT) should be suspected in the following circumstances.
    a. Any fracture before walking age
    b. Femur fractures
      - Most femur fractures before walking age result from abuse.
      - Femur fractures up to age 3 years are sometimes related to abuse.
    c. Multiple injuries in a child without a witnessed and reasonable explanation
    d. Multiple injuries in a child younger than 2 years
    e. A child with long bone and head injuries
  2. Corner fractures (seen at the junction of the metaphysis and physis) and posterior rib fractures are essentially pathognomonic for NAT, but isolated, transverse long bone fractures are actually more common following NAT. Corner fractures result from shear forces associated with pulling and twisting an extremity.
  3. A skeletal survey must be obtained in all children in whom child abuse is suspected to rule out additional fractures (including skull and rib fractures). Repeat imaging may be necessary in these children because periosteal new bone formation, which often does not appear for 1 week or more after injury, may be the first evidence of fracture.
  4. Thorough examination of the child by nonorthopaedists is necessary to rule out other evidence of abuse, including skin bruising (especially bruises of different ages) or scarring, retinal hemorrhages, intracranial bleeds, or evidence of sexual abuse.
  5. Skin lesions, including bruising and scarring, are the most common signs of nonaccidental trauma.

B. Treatment
  1. Reporting of suspected child abuse is mandatory.
    a. The orthopaedic surgeon is protected from litigation when reporting cases of suspected abuse.
    b. Failure to report suspected abuse puts the abused child at a 30 to 50% risk of repeat abuse and up to a 5 to 10% risk of death.
  2. Many fractures are sufficiently healed at the time of presentation that they do not require treatment.

VII. PATHOLOGIC FRACTURES

A. General—A pathologic fracture occurs when a low-energy mechanism (not usually sufficient to cause fracture) results in a fracture through a weakened bone (see Chapter 45). Common causes in children include neoplasm, metabolic bone disease, infection, and disuse osteoporosis (especially in children with neuromuscular diseases).

B. Evaluation
  1. A high index of suspicion is necessary for a fracture resulting from a low-energy mechanism.
  2. Plain radiographs are evaluated for the appearance of bone quality, the presence of osseous lesions, and any evidence (eg, periosteal new bone) of preexisting osseous injury.
  3. Lesions are staged before intervention.

C. Treatment
  1. Children with potentially malignant lesions are referred to tertiary musculoskeletal oncology centers.
  2. For benign lesions, the tumor is treated appropriately; the fracture can typically be treated concomitantly.

VIII. FRACTURES OF THE SHOULDER AND HUMERAL SHAFT

A. Clavicle fractures
  1. Overview
    a. Common in all pediatric age groups; account for 90% of obstetric fractures; often associated with brachial plexus palsy.

b. Clavicle fractures may be confused with congenital pseudarthrosis of the clavicle.
   - Congenital pseudarthrosis results from a congenital failure of fusion of the medial and lateral ossification centers of the clavicle; may be related to external compression by the subclavian artery against the developing clavicle.
   - Typical findings include (1) presence at birth, although prominence of a "bump" often increases with age, (2) right-sidedness, (3) no pain, and (4) radiographs showing convexity of the ends of the nonfused portions of the clavicle.

2. Fracture location
   a. Medial clavicle fracture
      - The medial clavicular physis is the last physis in the body to close, at 23 to 25 years of age.
      - Many medial clavicle fractures are physeal fractures; sternoclavicular joint dislocations also can occur.
      - Posteriorly displaced fractures or dislocations may impinge on the mediastinum, including the great vessels, esophagus, and trachea.
   b. Clavicle shaft fracture—Displaced fractures rarely cause problems, although compression of the subclavian vessels and/or brachial plexus can occur.
   c. Lateral clavicle fracture—May be confused with an acromioclavicular joint dislocation, which is rare in children.

3. Treatment
   a. Medial clavicle fractures and sternoclavicular dislocations
      - Nonsurgical treatment, with a sling for 3 to 4 weeks as needed.
      - Percutaneous reduction with a towel clip may be indicated for posteriorly displaced fractures or dislocations impinging on the mediastinum. Some authors recommend a vascular surgeon be present because of potential vascular complications.
      - Open reduction may be needed for open fractures or if percutaneous reduction fails. Suture fixation generally suffices in such cases.
   b. Clavicle shaft fractures
      - Nonsurgical treatment with a figure-of-8 harness or sling for 4 to 6 weeks is appropriate. A swathe may be used in infants.
      - Open reduction and internal fixation (ORIF); indications may include floating shoulder injuries, open fractures, and multiple trauma; some authors recommend ORIF for substantially displaced and/or shortened fractures (>2 cm) in adolescents.
   c. Lateral clavicle fractures
      - Most are treated symptomatically with a sling.
      - For markedly displaced fractures, surgical treatment is controversial.

4. Complications
   a. Medial fractures and dislocations—Compression of the mediastinal structures may occur with posterior displacement.
   b. Shaft fractures
      - Complications are rare with closed treatment; prominence at the fracture site is expected.
      - Compression of the subclavian vessels and brachial plexus is rare.
      - Surgical treatment increases the risks of infection and delayed union, and hardware prominence is very common.
   c. Lateral fractures—Complications are rare with closed treatment.

B. Proximal humerus fractures

1. General—because 80% of humeral growth is proximal, these are very forgiving fractures.
2. Evaluation
   a. Plain radiographs are almost universally sufficient for evaluating fracture configuration and to rule out associated shoulder dislocation.
   b. Thorough neurologic examination is necessary because of the proximity of the brachial plexus.
3. Classification—The Neer and Horwitz classification is used to define the amount of fracture displacement. Grade I fractures are displaced 5 mm or less, grade II fractures one-third of the humeral diameter or less, grade III fractures two-thirds of the humeral diameter or less, and grade IV fractures greater than two-thirds of the humeral diameter.
4. Nonsurgical treatment
   a. Most can be treated nonsurgically with a sling and swathe, shoulder immobilizer, or coaptation splint.

b. Reduction may be performed for grade III and IV fractures.
   - Reduction is generally obtained by shoulder abduction, flexion to 90°, and external rotation.
   - Impediments to reduction may include the long head of the biceps or the periosteum.

c. Gentle shoulder range of motion (ROM) exercises should begin 1 to 3 weeks after injury.

5. Surgical treatment
   a. Surgical treatment is indicated for adolescents with grade III and IV injuries and for open fractures.
   b. Closed reduction and percutaneous pinning is used in most surgical cases.
      - Risks include iatrogenic damage to the axillary nerve, unrecognized joint penetration, and soft-tissue complications and infection.
   c. Open reduction and pinning is necessary if interposed structures (biceps tendon, periosteum) prevent closed reduction in adolescents with grade III or IV injuries.

6. Complications
   a. Malunion, growth arrest, and other complications are rare.
   b. Brachial plexus injuries are almost always stretch injuries, which resolve spontaneously.

C. Humeral shaft fractures
   1. Evaluation—Radial nerve palsy occurs in less than 5% of humeral shaft fractures and is almost always a neurapraxia following middle or distal third fractures.
   2. Nonsurgical treatment
      a. Nonsurgical therapy (with sling and swathe, coaptation splint, or fracture brace) is the mainstay of treatment.
      b. Substantial displacement and angulation up to 30° are acceptable because range of shoulder motion is generally excellent.
      c. ROM exercises are started by 2 to 4 weeks post injury.
   3. Surgical treatment
      a. Indications for surgical treatment include open fractures, multiple trauma, and floating elbow or shoulder injuries.
      b. Procedures
         - Intramedullary rod fixation (flexible titanium nails) is preferred for many shaft fractures requiring fixation.
         - Plate fixation involves more surgical dissection and puts the radial nerve at risk during surgery.
   4. Complications
      a. Malunion rarely has functional consequences because normal shoulder ROM can compensate for the humeral malalignment.
      b. Radial nerve palsy—primary radial nerve palsies (present at the time of injury) are almost always caused by neurapraxia, resolve spontaneously, and should be observed.
         - If they do not resolve spontaneously by 3 to 5 months, electrophysiologic studies are indicated, and surgical exploration may be needed.
         - Secondary nerve palsies (present after intervention) are more complete injuries and typically require exploration acutely.
      c. Stiffness is rare; early ROM minimizes this risk.
      d. Limb-length discrepancy is common but generally mild and of no functional consequence.

IX. SUPRACONDYLAR HUMERUS FRACTURES

A. Epidemiology
   1. Supracondylar humerus (SCH) fractures account for more than one half of pediatric elbow fractures.
   2. Extension-type injures account for 95% to 98% of SCH fractures.

B. Relevant anatomy
   1. Distal humeral anatomy is shown in **Figure 4**.
   2. The Baumann angle may be measured on AP radiographs of the distal humerus to assess the coronal plane fracture alignment but is used less commonly now because of variability in measurement.

C. Associated injuries
   1. Vascular injuries occur in approximately 1% of SCH fractures. Because of the rich collateral flow at the elbow, distal perfusion may remain good despite a vascular injury (**Table 5**).
   2. Nerve injuries—Described in **Table 6**.

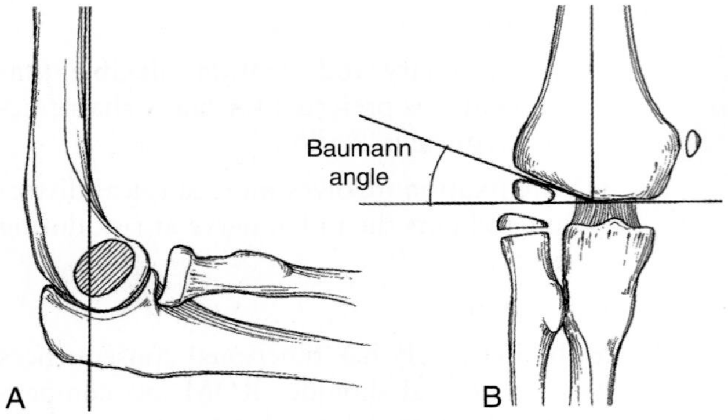

Figure 4 Illustrations show the typical anatomic relationships in the elbow. **A**, The anterior humeral line, shown as would be drawn on a lateral radiograph, should bisect the capitellum. In extension-type supracondylar fractures, the capitellum moves posterior to the anterior humeral line. **B**, The Baumann angle, shown as would be measured on an AP view, is the angle subtended by a line perpendicular to the long axis of the humerus and a line along the lateral condylar physis. The Baumann angle may be used to assess the adequacy of the reduction in the coronal plane and may be compared with the contralateral elbow. (Reproduced from Skaggs DL: Elbow fractures in children: Diagnosis and management. *J Am Acad Orthop Surg* 1997;5[6]:303-312.)

D. Classification—The modified Gartland classification is used to classify SCH fractures (**Figure 5**).

E. Nonsurgical treatment

1. Type I fractures are treated closed with a long arm cast in approximately 90° of elbow flexion.
2. Type II fractures may be treated closed only if the following criteria are met.
   a. No substantial swelling is present.
   b. The anterior humeral line intersects the capitellum.
   c. No medial cortical impaction of the distal humerus and/or varus malalignment is present.
3. The casts are removed after fracture healing at 3 weeks.

TABLE 5

Treatment for Vascular Injuries With Supracondylar Humerus Fractures

Vascular Status	Treatment
Pulse lost after reduction and pinning	Explore brachial artery and treat
Pulseless, well-perfused hand	Observe for 24-72 hr
Pulseless, cool hand	Explore brachial artery and treat

TABLE 6

Nerve Injuries With Supracondylar Humerus Fractures

Nerve Injury	Association
Anterior interosseous nerve	Most common nerve injury with supracondylar humerus fracture
Median nerve	Associated with posterolateral fracture displacement
Radial nerve	Seen with posteromedial fracture displacement, second most common
Ulnar nerve	Seen with flexion type fractures; also may be iatrogenic in 3%-8% of pinnings (due to medial pin)

F. Surgical treatment

1. Indications—Most type II and all type III and IV fractures are treated with reduction and pinning.
2. Pin configuration (**Figure 6** and **Table 7**)
   a. Crossed pins
      - Crossed pins are more stable biomechanically in laboratory studies than lateral-entry pins.
      - Using a medial pin results in a substantial (3% to 8%) risk of iatrogenic ulnar nerve injury, especially if the medial pin is inserted with the elbow fully flexed.

   b. Lateral-entry pins
      - Lateral-entry pins should be separated sufficiently to engage the medial and lateral columns of the distal humerus at the level of the fracture.
      - When inserted with appropriate technique, lateral-entry pins are comparable in maintaining reduction of SCH fractures.
         - Three pins are biomechanically stronger than two pins in bending and torsion.
      - Iatrogenic ulnar nerve injury does not occur with lateral-entry pins.

G. Complications

1. Volkmann ischemic contracture is a devastating complication that more commonly results from compression of the brachial artery with casting in greater than 90° of flexion than from arterial injury at the time of fracture.
2. Cubitus varus (gunstock deformity) is a cosmetic deformity with few functional sequelae in childhood, although it may increase the risk

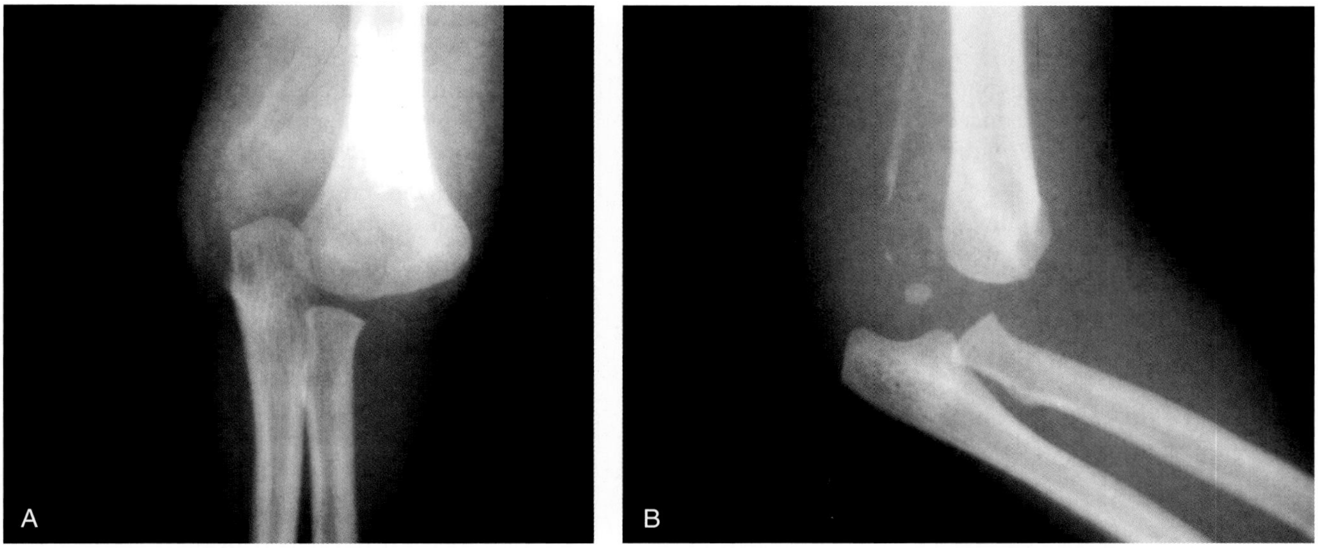

Figure 11 AP (A) and lateral (B) radiographs of the elbow of an 18-month-old infant show the typical alignment of the elbow following a physeal fracture of the distal humerus. Although the appearance resembles an elbow dislocation, the age of the child is younger than the age at which dislocation typically occurs, and the radius is directed at the capitellum in these radiographs. Most of these injuries are displaced posteromedially. Periosteal new bone is evident in this 2-week-old fracture. (Reproduced from Sponseller PD: Injuries of the arm and elbow, in Sponseller PD, ed: *Orthopaedic Knowledge Update: Pediatrics*, ed 2. Rosemont, IL, American Academy of Orthopaedic Surgeons, 2002, pp 93-107.)

G. Proximal radius fractures

1. Overview
   a. Most fractures are radial neck and/or physeal fractures.
   b. Most are associated with extension and valgus loading of the elbow or elbow dislocation.
2. Classification—Based on the location of the fracture (neck or head) and the angulation and/or displacement.
3. Nonsurgical treatment
   a. Most of these fractures are treated closed.
   b. Manipulative techniques
      - Patterson maneuver—The elbow is held in extension and supination, distal traction is applied pulling the forearm into varus while direct pressure is applied to the radial head.
      - Israeli technique—Direct pressure is applied over the radial head with the elbow flexed 90° while the forearm is taken from supination to pronation.
      - Elastic bandage—Spontaneous reduction may occur with tight application of an elastic bandage around the forearm and elbow.
   c. Early mobilization (within 3 to 7 days) minimizes stiffness.
4. Surgical treatment
   a. Indications following attempted closed reduction
      - More than 30° of residual angulation
      - More than 3 to 4 mm of translation
      - Less than 45° of pronation and supination
   b. Procedures
      - Percutaneous manipulation is attempted using a K-wire, awl, elevator, or other metallic device.
      - In the Metaizeau technique, a flexible rod or nail is inserted retrograde, passed across the fracture site, rotated to reduce the fracture, and advanced into the proximal fragment.
      - Open reduction via a lateral approach is rarely necessary but may be required for severely displaced fractures.
      - Internal fixation is used only for fractures that are unstable following reduction.
5. Complications
   a. Elbow stiffness is extremely common, even after nondisplaced fractures.
   b. Overgrowth of the radial head also is common.

H. Olecranon fractures

1. Evaluation—Palpation over the radial head is necessary to rule out a Monteggia fracture. Tenderness over a reduced radial head indicates a Monteggia fracture with spontaneous reduction of the radial head.
2. Classification—Apophyseal fractures may be the first indication of osteogenesis imperfecta and must be differentiated from the more common metaphyseal fractures.
3. Nonsurgical treatment—Most are treated nonsurgically, with casting in relative extension (usually 10° to 45° of flexion) for 3 weeks.
4. Surgical treatment
   a. Indications—Fractures with intra-articular displacement greater than 2 to 3 mm benefit from surgery.
   b. Fixation—Stabilized using tension-band fixation, often with an absorbable suture as the tension band.
5. Complications are rare and rarely of clinical significance, although failure to diagnose associated injuries (such as radial head dislocation) may result in substantial morbidity.

I. Nursemaid elbow

1. Epidemiology—Occurs with longitudinal traction on the outstretched arm of a child younger than 5 years as the orbicular ligament subluxates over the radial head.
2. Evaluation
   a. The history and physical examination are classic, with the child holding the elbow extended and the forearm pronated.
   b. Radiographs are not needed unless the classic history and arm positioning are absent. If radiographs are obtained, they are normal.
3. Treatment—With one thumb held over the affected radial head (to feel for a "snap" as the orbicular ligament reduces), the forearm is supinated and the elbow is flexed past 90°.
4. Complications—Recurrent nursemaid elbow is relatively common in children younger than 5 years.

XI. FRACTURES OF THE FOREARM, WRIST, AND HAND

A. Diaphyseal forearm fractures

1. Evaluation—Open wounds are often punctate and are commonly missed when not evaluated by an orthopaedic surgeon.
2. Classification
   a. Greenstick fractures are incomplete fractures common in children. They should be described as apex volar or apex dorsal to guide reduction.
   b. Complete fractures are categorized as in adults, by fracture location, pattern, angulation, and displacement.
3. Nonsurgical treatment
   a. Most pediatric forearm fractures can be treated nonsurgically.
   b. Greenstick fractures are generally rotational injuries. Apex volar fractures (supination injuries) may be treated by forearm pronation; apex dorsal injuries (pronation injuries) by forearm supination.
   c. Casting for 6 weeks is typical.
4. Surgical treatment
   a. Indications
      - Persistent malalignment following closed reduction (angulation >15° in children younger than 10 years and >10° in children 10 years or older, and bayonet apposition in children 10 years or older) may necessitate open reduction.
      - Substantially displaced fractures in adolescents are at high risk for redisplacement and are a relative indication for surgery.
      - Open fractures are commonly treated surgically.
   b. Technique
      - Internal fixation with intramedullary devices or plates has high rates of success in children.
      - Fixation of one bone is often sufficient to stabilize an unstable forearm, particularly in children younger than 10 years.
5. Complications
   a. Refracture occurs in 5% to 10% of children following forearm fractures.
   b. Malunion is unusual if serial radiographs are obtained in the first 3 weeks following fracture.
   c. Compartment syndrome may occur, particularly in high-energy injuries. The rate after intramedullary fixation is high, especially with multiple attempts at reduction and rod passage.
   d. Loss of pronation and supination is common, although generally mild.

TABLE 9

Bado Classification of Monteggia Fractures

Bado Type	Apex of Ulnar Fracture	Radial Head Pathology
I	Anterior	Anterior dislocation
II	Posterior	Posterior dislocation
III	Lateral	Lateral dislocation
IV	Any direction (typically anterior)	Proximal radius dislocation and fracture

B. Monteggia fractures

1. Evaluation

a. Palpation over the radial head must be performed for all children with ulnar fractures to rule out Monteggia injuries.

b. Isolated radial head dislocations almost never occur in children. Presumed "isolated" injuries almost universally result from plastic deformation of the ulna with concomitant radial head dislocation.

2. Classification

a. The Bado classification (**Table 9**) is most commonly used.

b. Fractures may be classified as acute or chronic (>2 to 3 weeks since injury).

3. Nonsurgical treatment

a. Much more common (and successful) in children with Monteggia fractures than in adults.

b. Reestablishment of ulnar length is necessary to maintain reduction of the radial head.

c. For Bado I fractures, the elbow should be immobilized in hyperflexion >110° and supination.

4. Surgical treatment

a. Acute fractures

- Indications for surgery include open and/or unstable fractures.
- Fixation
    - An intramedullary nail is often sufficient to maintain ulnar length (**Figure 12**) in transverse fractures.
    - Plate fixation is needed for comminuted fractures.
- Annular ligament reconstruction is rarely needed for acute fractures.

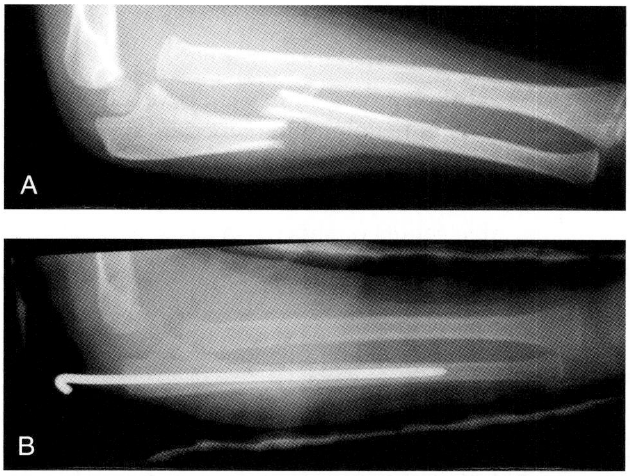

Figure 12 Radiographs show a Bado I Monteggia fracture-dislocation. **A**, Preoperative radiograph shows the injury. **B**, Postoperative radiograph shows the fracture after treatment by closed reduction and intramedullary nail fixation. (Reproduced from Waters PM: Injuries of the shoulder, elbow, and forearm, in Abel MF, ed: *Orthopaedic Knowledge Update: Pediatrics*, ed 3. Rosemont, IL, American Academy of Orthopaedic Surgeons, 2006, pp 303-314.)

b. Chronic fractures

- Most should be reduced surgically if symptomatic (preferably within 6 to 12 months following injury).
- Technique—These complex reconstructions require ulnar osteotomy with internal fixation, radial head reduction, and annular ligament reconstruction.

5. Complications

a. Posterior interosseous nerve palsy occurs in up to 10% of acute injuries but almost always resolves spontaneously.

b. Delayed or missed diagnosis of a Monteggia fracture is common when the child is not evaluated by an orthopaedic surgeon.

c. Complication rates and severity are much greater if the diagnosis is delayed more than 2 to 3 weeks.

C. Distal forearm fractures

1. Classification

a. Physeal fractures are categorized using the Salter-Harris classification.

b. For metaphyseal fractures, distinction is made between buckle fractures and complete fractures.

2. Nonsurgical treatment
   a. Most are treated by closed means.
      - Short arm casts are as effective as long arm casts in maintaining reduction for displaced fractures.
      - Buckle fractures may be treated with removable splints or short arm casts.
   b. Healing times
      - Physeal fractures heal in 3 to 4 weeks.
      - Metaphyseal fractures heal in 4 to 6 weeks.
      - Buckle fractures heal in 3 weeks.
3. Surgical treatment
   a. Indications
      - Open fractures are treated surgically with ORIF following irrigation and débridement.
      - Unacceptable closed reduction
        - Complete metaphyseal fractures—Quoted unacceptable alignment is greater than 20° of angulation in a child of any age and bayonet apposition in children older than 10 years, although the growth potential in this area allows such fractures to remodel successfully.
        - Physeal fractures—Residual displacement greater than 50% is unacceptable. Attempting reduction of a physeal fracture more than 5 to 7 days post injury is discouraged because of the increased risk of iatrogenic physeal injury.
        - Floating elbow injuries—Percutaneous pinning of the distal radius results in much lower rates of fracture reduction loss and malunion.
   b. Procedures
      - Closed reduction successfully reduces most of these fractures.
      - Percutaneous pinning (avoiding the superficial radial nerve) is generally sufficient to maintain reduction for very unstable fractures or those with associated injuries.
4. Complications
   a. Malunion generally results in cosmetic deformity rather than functional deficits and often remodels spontaneously.
   b. Growth arrest occurs in <1% to 2% of distal radius physeal fractures and <1% of metaphyseal fractures.
   c. Compartment syndrome is a substantial risk in children with floating elbow injuries (ipsilateral forearm and humeral fractures).

D. Carpal injuries
1. Nonsurgical treatment
   a. Scaphoid fractures are most commonly treated with a short arm or long arm thumb spica cast.
      - Distal pole fractures routinely heal with closed treatment.
      - Waist fractures have worse results (especially in adolescents) and may result in osteonecrosis and/or nonunion.
   b. Triangular fibrocartilage complex (TFCC) tears may accompany distal radial and/or ulnar styloid fractures and are treated closed.
2. Surgical treatment
   a. Scaphoid fractures may be treated with ORIF for displaced waist fractures or with ORIF and bone grafting for established nonunions.
   b. If ongoing wrist pain occurs following closed treatment of a wrist fracture, TFCC tears may be repaired arthroscopically.
3. Complications
   a. Scaphoid waist fractures—Osteonecrosis and nonunion.
   b. TFCC tears—Chronic wrist pain.

E. Metacarpal fractures
1. Classification
   a. For physeal injuries, the Salter-Harris classification is used.
   b. For nonphyseal fractures, classification is based on fracture location, configuration, angulation, and displacement, as in adults.
   c. Some of these fractures are "open" injuries ("fight bites" or "clenched-fist" injuries); lacerations over the knuckles should be sought to rule out such an injury.
2. Nonsurgical treatment
   a. Most of these fractures are treated closed.
      - Rotational alignment must be good for acceptable closed treatment.
      - Acceptable sagittal angulation increases from radial to ulnar as in adults, according to these guidelines: Second metacarpal, 10° to 20°; third metacarpal, 20° to 30°; fourth metacarpal, 30° to 40°; and fifth metacarpal, 40° to 50°.

b. Closed treatment is successful for diaphyseal and metaphyseal fractures of the thumb metacarpal.

3. Surgical treatment

a. Indications—Unacceptable rotational, sagittal, and/or coronal alignment.

b. Physeal fractures of the base of the thumb metacarpal often require surgery because of instability and/or intra-articular step-off.

4. Complications—Most common is malalignment (including rotational deformity, which results in overlapping fingers), requiring late osteotomy.

F. Phalangeal fractures

1. Classification

a. Physeal fractures are described using the Salter-Harris classification.

b. Shaft and neck fractures are categorized by fracture type and displacement.

c. Seymour fracture—displaced distal phalanx physeal fracture with associated nail bed injury.

- Most commonly treated surgically with removal of interposed tissue, reduction across distal interphalangeal joint, and nail bed repair.
- Antibiotics required for open injuries.
- Complications—nail deformity most common; osteomyelitis, nonunion, and malunion rare with appropriate diagnosis and treatment.

2. Nonsurgical treatment suffices for most fractures, with healing in approximately 3 weeks.

3. Surgical treatment

a. Indications—Most intra-articular phalangeal fractures.

b. Procedures

- Closed reduction and pinning is indicated for most minimally displaced intra-articular fractures.
- Open reduction and pinning is often needed for more displaced unicondylar and bicondylar fractures.

4. Complications—Stiffness, fixation loss, growth disturbance, and malunion are relatively uncommon.

TOP TESTING FACTS

1. The surgeon should assume that complete recovery from other injuries (including head injuries) will occur; many children make excellent recoveries from such injuries.
2. Prompt administration of intravenous antibiotics is the most important factor in reducing the rate of infection following open fractures.
3. A pulseless, well-perfused hand may need only careful observation following SCH fracture because of the excellent collateral circulation around the elbow.
4. Injury to the anterior interosseous nerve is the most common nerve injury associated with SCH fractures.
5. Ulnar nerve injury with extension-type SCH fractures is almost always iatrogenic from medial pin insertion, particularly if the medial pin is inserted with the elbow in a fully flexed position.
6. The internal oblique radiograph is the most sensitive for detecting maximal displacement of lateral condyle fractures and is required when contemplating closed treatment.
7. Elbow dislocations in children younger than 3 to 6 years are very rare, so transphyseal fractures should be suspected in young patients with displacement of the proximal radius and ulna relative to the humerus.
8. Isolated radial head dislocations almost never occur in children. These presumed "isolated" injuries almost always result from plastic deformation of the ulna with concomitant radial head dislocation (Monteggia fracture).
9. Buckle fractures of the distal radius can be treated with removable wrist splints.
10. Floating elbow injuries have high complication rates, including loss of forearm fracture reduction when internal fixation has not been used and increased risk of compartment syndrome.

Bibliography

Abzug JM, Dua K, Bauer AS, Cornwall R, Wyrick TO: Pediatric phalanx fractures. *J Am Acad Orthop Surg* 2016;24(11):e174-e183.

Heggeness MH, Sanders JO, Murray J, Pezold R, Sevarino KS: Management of pediatric supracondylar humerus fractures. *J Am Acad Orthop Surg* 2015;23(10):e49-e51.

Kay RM, Skaggs DL: Pediatric polytrauma management. *J Pediatr Orthop* 2006;26(2):268-277.

Livingston KS, Glotzbecker MP, Shore BJ: Pediatric acute compartment syndrome. *J Am Acad Orthop Surg* 2017;25(5):358-364.

Pandya NK, Upasani VV, Kulkarni VA: The pediatric polytrauma patient: Current concepts. *J Am Acad Orthop Surg* 2013;21(3):170-179.

Popkin CA, Levine WN, Ahmad CS: Evaluation and management of pediatric proximal humerus fractures. *J Am Acad Orthop Surg* 2015;23(2):77-86.

Price CT: Surgical management of forearm and distal radius fractures in children and adolescents. *Instr Course Lect* 2008;57:509-514.

Ring D: Monteggia fractures. *Orthop Clin North Am* 2013;44(1):59-66.

Ring D, Jupiter JB, Waters PM: Monteggia fractures in children and adults. *J Am Acad Orthop Surg* 1998;6(4):215-224.

Sink EL, Hyman JE, Matheny T, Georgopoulos G, Kleinman P: Child abuse: The role of the orthopaedic surgeon in nonaccidental trauma. *Clin Orthop Relat Res* 2011;469(3):790-797.

Skaggs DL, Cluck MW, Mostofi A, Flynn JM, Kay RM: Lateral-entry pin fixation in the management of supracondylar fractures in children. *J Bone Joint Surg Am* 2004;86(4):702-707.

Skaggs DL, Friend L, Alman B, et al: The effect of surgical delay on acute infection following 554 open fractures in children. *J Bone Joint Surg Am* 2005;87(1):8-12.

Stewart DG Jr, Kay RM, Skaggs DL: Open fractures in children: Principles of evaluation and management. *J Bone Joint Surg Am* 2005;87(12):2784-2798.

Tejwani N, Phillips D, Goldstein RY: Management of lateral humeral condylar fracture in children. *J Am Acad Orthop Surg* 2011;19(6):350-358.

Weiss JM, Graves S, Yang S, Mendelsohn E, Kay RM, Skaggs DL: A new classification system predictive of complications in surgically treated pediatric humeral lateral condyle fractures. *J Pediatr Orthop* 2009;29(6):602-605.

Wood JN, Henry MK, Berger RP, et al: Use and utility of skeletal surveys to evaluate for occult fractures in young injured children. *Acad Pediatr*. 2018. pii:S1876-2859(18)30536-9.

Chapter 139

PEDIATRIC PELVIC AND LOWER EXTREMITY FRACTURES

OUSSAMA ABOUSAMRA, MD
ROBERT M. KAY, MD

I. PELVIC FRACTURES

A. Epidemiology: pelvic fractures are rare in children with an incidence of 1 per 100,000 children. These injuries are seen in 5% of all pediatric trauma patients. The mean age in population studies is around 9 to 11 years.

Half of pelvic fractures identified on CT are not identified on plain AP pelvis radiographs.

B. Classification

1. The most common systems are the Tile classification system and the Torode and Zieg classification system.
   a. Tile classification
      - Type A—Stable fractures
      - Type B—Rotationally unstable but vertically stable
      - Type C—Rotationally and vertically unstable
   b. Torode and Zieg classification
      - Type I—Avulsion fractures
      - Type II—Iliac wing fractures
      - Type III—Ring fractures without segmental instability
        - Type IIIA—Simple anterior ring fractures
        - Type IIIB—Have anterior and posterior ring disruptions, but are stable
      - Type IV—Ring disruptions with segmental instability
2. Regardless of the classification system, it is essential to determine whether the pelvic fracture is stable.

C. Treatment

1. Nonsurgical—Most pelvic fractures in children are treated nonsurgically with good results. Management includes bed rest and bed-to-chair transfers for 3 to 4 weeks, followed by progressive weight bearing. Some may need protection and immobilization by a spica cast.
2. Surgical indications
   a. In general, the indications for surgical fixation are:
      - Bleeding control. External fixation may be applied rapidly and is occasionally indicated to stabilize the pelvic ring and/or decrease the volume of the pelvis in open book injuries.
      - Prevention of deformity and subsequent osteoarthritis in severely displaced fractures: Open reduction and internal fixation (ORIF) is most commonly indicated in adolescents with vertically unstable injuries or displaced acetabular fractures of more than 2 mm. To prevent limb length discrepancy (LLD), ring fractures displaced more than 2 cm need reduction and fixation.
      - To encourage mobility in some situations such as polytrauma.

D. Complications

1. Malunion and nonunion are uncommon.
2. LLD may occur in vertically unstable fractures.
3. Fractures involving the triradiate cartilage in young children might result in growth

Dr. Kay or an immediate family member serves as a paid consultant to or is an employee of Intrinsic Therapeutics; has stock or stock options held in Biomet, Johnson & Johnson, Medtronic, Pfizer, and Zimmer; and serves as a board member, owner, officer, or committee member of the Commission for Motion Lab Accreditation. Neither Dr. Abousamra nor any immediate family member has received anything of value from or has stock or stock options held in a commercial company or institution related directly or indirectly to the subject of this chapter.

disturbance and possible hip dysplasia and hip joint incongruity.

4. Systemic complications such as thrombosis, acute respiratory distress syndrome, or multiorgan failure are significantly lower in children compared with adults.

II. AVULSION FRACTURES OF THE PELVIS

A. Epidemiology

1. Typically occur in adolescent athletes involved in explosive-type activities, such as sprinting, jumping, and/or kicking.
2. The most common avulsion sites (and the causative muscles) are shown in **Table 1**.

B. Treatment

1. Nonsurgical—Local measures, including rest, ice, and anti-inflammatory medication for 2 to 3 weeks, followed by gradual resumption of activities.
2. Surgical—Almost never indicated for these injuries; surgery may be considered for symptomatic nonunions.

C. Complications—Few, if any, long-term sequelae.

III. HIP FRACTURES

A. Epidemiology: Hip fractures are <1% of all pediatric fractures. Most are caused by high-energy mechanisms, although pathologic fractures are also seen with low-energy trauma.

B. Classification—The Delbet classification is used for proximal femur fractures (**Figure 1**).

C. Treatment

1. Nonsurgical—Rarely indicated because of the increased risks of coxa vara and nonunion with closed treatment.

TABLE 1

Pelvic Avulsion Fracture Sites and Causative Muscles

Avulsion Site	Causative Muscles
Ischium	Hamstrings/adductors
Anterior-superior iliac spine	Sartorius
Anterior-inferior iliac spine	Rectus femoris
Iliac crest	Abdominals
Lesser trochanter	Iliopsoas

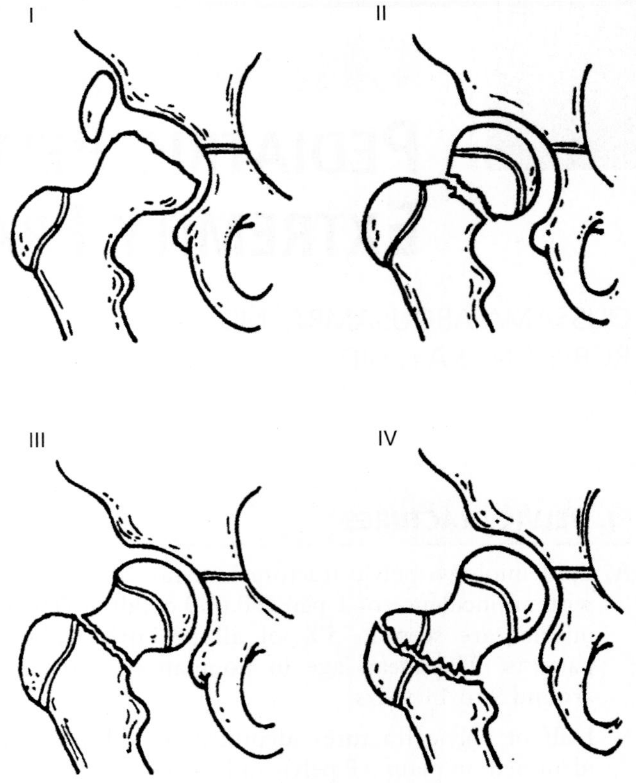

Figure 1 Illustrations depict the Delbet classification of pediatric hip fractures. Type I fractures are physeal; type II, transcervical; type III, cervicotrochanteric; and type IV, intertrochanteric. (Reproduced with permission from Hughes LO, Beaty JH: Fractures of the head and neck of the femur in children. *J Bone Joint Surg Am* 1994;76:283-292.)

2. Surgical
   a. When feasible, gentle, closed reduction and internal fixation is preferred.
   b. Fixation
      - Fixation is performed with Kirschner wires (K-wires) or cannulated screws for Delbet type I fractures, cannulated screws for type II and III fractures, and a pediatric hip screw, dynamic hip screw, or proximal femoral locking plate for type IV fractures.
      - Stability of fixation is paramount to reduce the chance of nonunion or malunion; fixation should extend across the physis if needed for stability.

D. Complications

1. Osteonecrosis is the most common, and severe, complication and is related to fracture level. The risk of osteonecrosis is 90% to 100% for type I fractures, 50% for type II, 25% for type III, and 10% for type IV. Femoral head collapse often

leads to joint penetration of the previously placed hardware, which may result in chondrolysis and exacerbation of pain.

2. Coxa vara and nonunion are much more common after nonsurgically treated fractures, particularly Delbet type II and III fractures.
3. LLD is common after hip fractures in young children because the proximal femoral physis accounts for about 15% of total leg length.
4. After closed reduction of traumatic hip dislocations, imaging is needed to rule out structural injury to the hip, especially the posterior labrum/chondrolabral junction. MRI has been shown as superior to CT scan in detecting such injuries.

IV. FEMORAL SHAFT FRACTURES

A. Epidemiology
1. The femur is a common orthopaedic injury in children.
2. Most femur fractures in children are caused by accidental trauma.
3. However, children with diaphyseal femur fractures less than 3 years old, and any child with a femur fracture less than 1 year old, should be evaluated for possible child abuse.
4. Pathologic fractures are also seen in children due to local pathology (bone cyst, benign or malignant tumors, etc) or systemic conditions (osteogenesis imperfecta, cerebral palsy, etc).
5. In younger children, femur fractures are most likely due to falls, whereas in older children, motor vehicle collisions are more common. The mechanism and energy of the trauma would impact the complexity of the fracture pattern and further need for surgery. Rotational forces usually result in long spiral fractures, while direct impact injuries result in transverse and short oblique fractures.

B. Treatment
1. Nonsurgical
   a. Indication—Spica casting is routine in children younger than 6 years. Two prospective studies indicate equivalence in outcomes of single leg compared with both leg spica casting with great parent satisfaction.
   b. Contraindications to immediate spica casting
      - Shortening greater than 2.5 to 3.0 cm is a relative contraindication.
      - Multiple trauma is a relative contraindication.
   c. Complications
      - LLD
         - Ipsilateral overgrowth of 7 to 10 mm occurs in children aged 2 to 10 years who sustain a femur fracture.
         - LLD may result from excessive overgrowth or excessive shortening at the time of fracture healing following cast treatment.
      - Malunion
         - Angular malunion (usually varus and/or procurvatum) can be minimized with careful technique and cast molding.
         - Torsional malunion is common but mild and rarely of clinical consequence.
2. Surgical treatment
   a. Indications—Most children older than 6 years are treated surgically, as are many younger multiple-trauma patients.
   b. Procedures
      - Flexible intramedullary (IM) rodding
         - Indications—Most pediatric femoral shaft fractures in children aged 6 to 10 years.
         - Relative contraindications—Comminuted or very distal or proximal fractures are harder to control with flexible IM rods.
         - Complication rates (particularly loss of reduction) are higher in children older than 10 years and in those who weigh more than 50 kg.
      - Antegrade rigid femoral nails
      - Generally, a trochanteric entry nails are used in children.
         - This technique is often used in children older than 8 to 10 years, in those weighing more than 50 kg, or in extremely comminuted fractures.
         - Complications—(1) Rarely, may cause abnormalities of proximal femoral growth resulting in a narrow femoral neck. (2) The risk of iatrogenic osteonecrosis and/or coxa valga appear to be low.
      - Submuscular bridge plating
         - Indications—Submuscular plating may be considered especially for comminuted and length-unstable femoral shaft fractures.

10 | Pediatrics

- Complications—(1) Fracture following hardware removal may occur because of numerous stress risers in the femoral shaft following hardware removal. (2) Distal femoral valgus is relatively common following healing due to possible vascular compromise of the distal femoral physis; therefore, the distal end of the plate should be at least 20 mm from the physis. (3) Complications, including malunion, may occur more commonly until the surgeon gains experience with this technique because a substantial learning curve exists.

- Open femoral plating
  - Indications—Rarely used currently but may be used for comminuted fractures, particularly in those with osteoporotic bone.
  - Complications—Numerous stress risers increase the risk of fracture after hardware removal.
- External fixation
  - Indications—For comminuted or segmental fractures or in "damage control" situations requiring rapid application (sometimes at the bedside). External fixation is also helpful in contaminated open fractures when the risk of infection is high with internal fixation.
  - Complications—(1) Delayed union and refracture are more frequent than with other forms of fixation. (2) Pin tract infections (usually superficial) are frequent.

V. DISTAL FEMUR FRACTURES

A. Distal femoral metaphyseal fractures: Non physeal supracondylar distal femoral fractures account for ~ 12% of all pediatric femur fractures.

1. Nonsurgical treatment—Casting suffices for most low-energy insufficiency fractures in children with neuromuscular disease.
2. Surgical treatment
   a. Indications—Displaced fractures require surgical treatment with closed reduction and fixation.
   b. Technique—Hardware should not cross the physis, if possible.
3. Complications—Malunion is the most common complication following displaced fractures because accurate assessment of coronal plane alignment is difficult following casting.

B. Distal femoral physeal fractures: Physeal fractures of the distal femur are rare injuries and account for <2% of all physeal fractures.

1. Classification—The Salter-Harris classification.
2. Nonsurgical treatment is indicated for nondisplaced Salter-Harris type I and II fractures.
3. Surgical treatment
   a. Indications—Displaced fractures of the distal femoral physis.
   b. Procedures
      - Closed reduction and internal fixation if anatomic reduction is obtainable closed.
      - ORIF if closed reduction is not satisfactory.
      - Fixation avoids the physis when possible. When fixation must cross the physis, smooth K-wires are used and should be removed by 3 to 4 weeks after surgery.
      - Some surgeons prefer antegrade pin placement to avoid intra-articular pins and reduce the chance of septic arthritis, which may be associated with pin tract sepsis.
4. Complications: Distal femur physeal fractures tend to have a worse prognosis than physeal fractures in other locations.
   a. Popliteal artery injury and compartment syndrome are rare but more likely when the epiphysis displaces anteriorly. Initial treatment of any indication of vascular compromise is immediate reduction of the fracture.
   b. Growth arrest occurs in 30% to 50% of distal femoral physeal injuries.
      - Sequelae of distal femoral physeal fractures include LLD and angular deformity.
      - These sequelae are often severe because the distal femur accounts for 70% of femoral growth.
      - A higher incidence of growth arrest has been noted with displaced fractures Salter-Harris type IV. A higher incidence was also found when fixation implants cross the physis, although this might be needed to achieve stable fixation in certain fracture patterns.
      - Timely contralateral epiphysiodesis should be performed in cases of complete physeal arrest with significant growth remaining.

VI. PATELLAR FRACTURES

A. Epidemiology: Patellar fractures in children are rare with an incidence of around 0.44%.

1. Evaluation—Patellar fractures need to be differentiated from bipartite patella, which is a normal variant (in ≤5% of knees) and differs from a patellar fracture in two ways.
   a. Bipartite patella has rounded borders.
   b. Bipartite patella is located superolaterally.
2. A history of trauma, knee effusion, inability to actively extend the knee, high riding patella, and sometimes a palpable gap would help raising suspicion of a patellar fracture.

B. Classification

1. Categorized based on location, fracture configuration, and amount of displacement
2. Patellar sleeve fractures are the most common type of patellar fractures in children, and occur when a chondral sleeve of the patella separates from the main portion of the patella and ossific nucleus.
   a. These fractures are usually seen between 8 and 12 years of age.
   b. The only finding on plain radiographs may be apparent patella alta for distal fractures (**Figure 2**) or patella baja for proximal fractures, so these fractures are often missed on initial presentation.
   c. Patellar sleeve fractures should be considered when the examination is concerning for patellar tendon rupture. Ultrasonography is helpful when plain radiographs are not conclusive, and MRI can show the extent of cartilaginous injury and displacement of the fracture fragments.

C. Treatment

1. Nonsurgical—Indicated for nondisplaced and minimally displaced fractures in children without an extensor lag.
2. Surgical
   a. Indications
      - Patellar fractures displaced greater than 2 mm at the articular surface should be fixed surgically. The indication for surgery is confirmed by an extensor lag or the inability to actively extend the knee.
      - Patellar sleeve fractures require surgery.

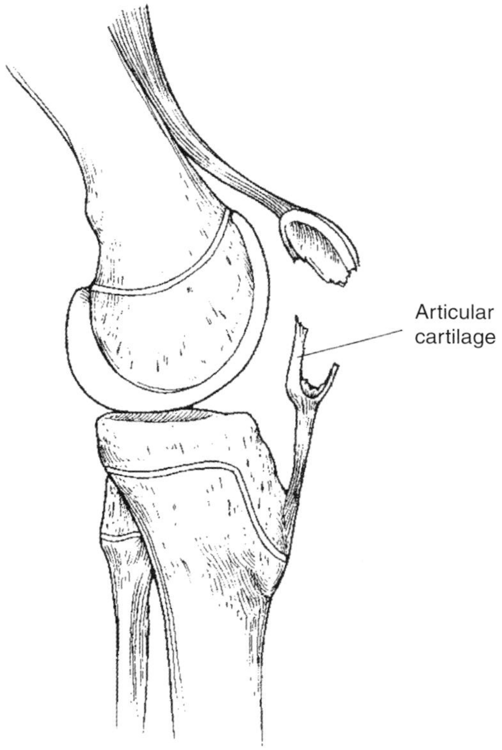

Figure 2 Illustration shows a lateral view of a patellar sleeve fracture. The only sign on plain radiographs may be patella alta. (Adapted with permission from Tolo VT: Fractures and dislocations around the knee, in Green NE, Swiontkowski MF, eds: *Skeletal Trauma in Children*. Philadelphia, PA, WB Saunders, 1994, vol 3, pp 369-395.)

   b. Procedures
      - For osseous fractures, fixation (as in adults) with tension banding; a cerclage wire may be needed for extensively comminuted fractures.
      - For patellar sleeve fractures, repair of the torn medial and lateral retinaculum along with sutures through the cartilaginous and osseous portions of the patella

VII. TIBIA AND FIBULA FRACTURES

A. Tibial spine (eminence) fractures1

1. Epidemiology: Tibial spine fractures occur in around 3 per 100,000 children annually. They account for 2% to 5% of pediatric knee injuries with effusion. These fractures are more common in skeletally immature patients between 8 and 14 years of age.
2. Evaluation
   a. Children with fractures of the tibial spine present with a mechanism consistent with an

anterior cruciate ligament (ACL) tear and an acutely unstable knee. Because ligaments are typically stronger than bones in children, pediatric tibial spine fractures occur more frequently than ACL tears in children with open physes.

b. The physical examination is comparable to that following a ligamentous ACL tear.

c. Plain radiographs, especially lateral view of the knee, help identify the injury. MRI would be helpful in identifying associated injuries, such as injuries to the medial meniscus or the fibers of ACL.

3. Classification—The Meyers and McKeever classification (**Figure 3**) is used. Type I are minimally displaced; type II are hinged with displacement of the anterior portion; and type III are completely displaced.

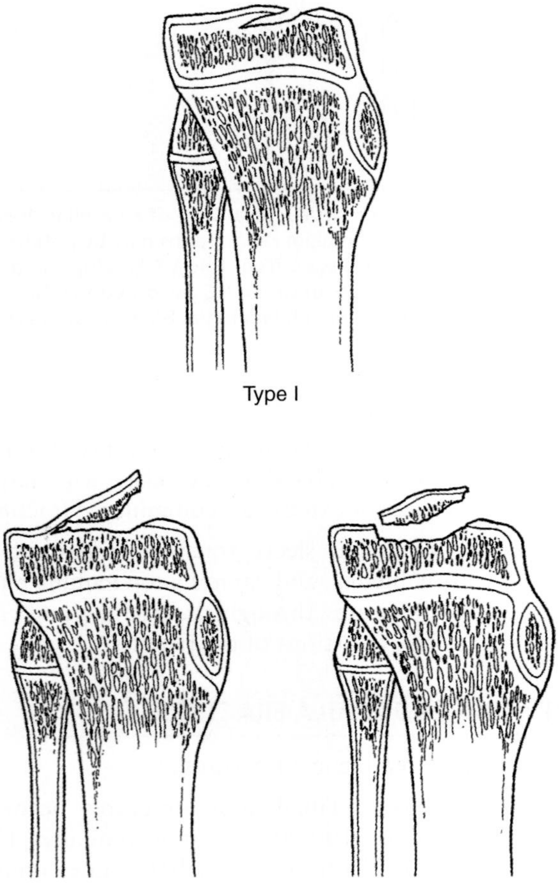

Figure 3 Illustrations depict the Meyers and McKeever classification of tibial spine fractures. (Adapted with permission from Tolo VT: Fractures and dislocations around the knee, in Green NE, Swiontkowski MF, eds: *Skeletal Trauma in Children*. Philadelphia, PA, WB Saunders, 1994, pp 369-395.)

4. Nonsurgical treatment
   a. Indications—Closed reduction and casting suffices for type I and some type II fractures. For type II fractures, the reduction must be within a few millimeters of anatomic to accept closed treatment.
   b. Procedure
      - Arthrocentesis before casting if a large hemarthrosis is present.
      - The optimal amount of knee flexion for reduction is controversial but generally recommended to be 0° to 20°.
5. Surgical treatment
   a. Indications—Type II fractures that do not reduce with casting and type III fractures.
   b. Procedures
      - ORIF and arthroscopic reduction and internal fixation are both effective.
      - Type of fixation used (sutures versus suture anchors versus screws) is often determined by fracture configuration; comminuted fractures with small fracture fragments typically require suture fixation. Fixation should avoid the physis.
      - The anterior horn of the medial meniscus is often entrapped and must be moved to allow reduction.
6. Complications
   a. Arthrofibrosis is common after surgically and nonsurgically treated tibial spine fractures. Early mobilization following surgical fixation seems to reduce the rate.
   b. ACL laxity is common but generally not clinically significant.
   c. Malunion with persistent elevation of the fracture fragment may result in impingement in the notch.

B. Tibial tubercle fractures

1. Epidemiology: Tibial tubercle fractures account for less than 1% of physeal fractures. The mean age at injury is around 14 years (13-16 years).
2. Classification—The classification has evolved since Watson-Jones first described three types of fractures (**Figure 6**).
3. Nonsurgical treatment is rarely indicated but may be used in children with minimally displaced fractures (<2 mm) and no extensor lag.

4. Surgical treatment
   a. Indications—Recommended for children with fractures having greater than 2 mm of displacement and/or an extensor lag.
   b. Procedures
      - ORIF with screws for fracture types I through IV. For type III fractures, the joint must be visualized to accurately reduce the joint surface and to assess for meniscal injury.
      - Suture reattachment (which may be supplemented with small screws) of the periosteal sleeve is the technique of choice for type V fractures.
5. Complications—Compartment syndrome and genu recurvatum are rare. Disruption of branches of the anterior recurrent tibial artery could result in compartment syndrome.

C. Proximal tibial physeal fractures

1. Epidemiology: proximal tibial physeal fractures are relatively infrequent injuries. Salter-Harris type I and II fractures occur commonly ~ 12 years of age, and Salter-Harris type III and IV fractures occur ~ 14 years of age.
2. Classification—The Salter-Harris classification is used (**Figure 4**).
3. Nonsurgical treatment indications—Nondisplaced fractures (which include 30% to 50% of Salter-Harris type I and II fractures) may be treated with cast immobilization.
4. Surgical treatment
   a. Indications—Displaced fractures are treated with closed (or open) reduction and internal fixation.
   b. Procedures
      - Closed reduction typically suffices. If unsuccessful, open reduction is required.
      - Fixation devices
         - Crossed smooth K-wires for most Salter-Harris type I and II fractures; they are removed by 3 to 4 weeks after surgery.
         - Cannulated screws (inserted parallel to the physis) for Salter-Harris type III and IV fractures (and type II fractures with large metaphyseal fragments).
5. Complications
   a. Neurovascular complications include popliteal artery injuries (5%), compartment syndrome (3% to 4%), and peroneal nerve injury (5%). Vascular complications are particularly common with hyperextension injuries (**Figure 5**).
   b. Redisplacement of the fracture is common in displaced fractures treated without internal fixation.
   c. Growth arrest occurs in 25% of patients and can result in LLD and/or angular deformity.

D. Proximal tibial metaphyseal fractures

1. Epidemiology: proximal tibial fractures through the metaphysis occur usually in younger children, typically between ages of 3 and 6 years.
2. Classification—No specific classification is used.
3. Nonsurgical treatment with a long leg cast is the mainstay treatment of low-energy injuries in children younger than 10 years.
4. Surgical treatment—Generally necessary for high-energy proximal tibial fractures in older children because these fractures are often substantially displaced and unstable.

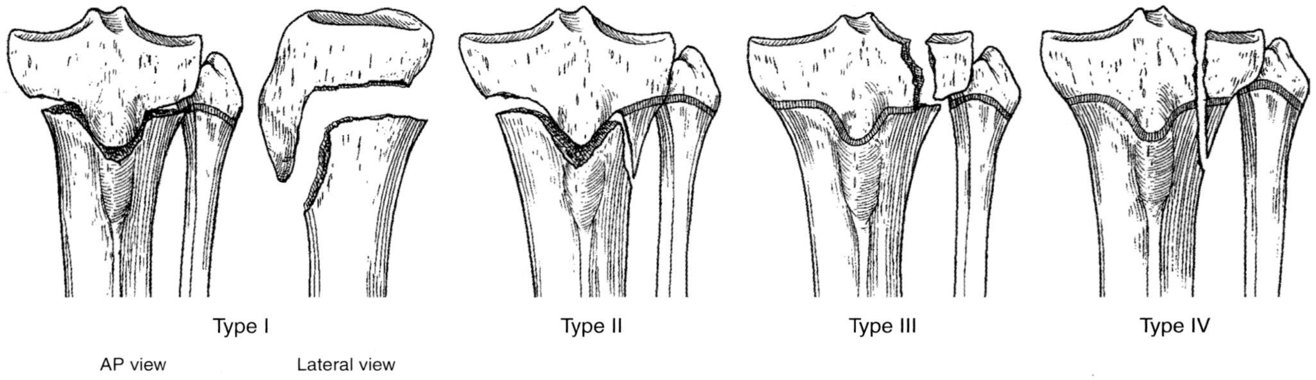

Figure 4 Illustrations show Salter-Harris fractures of the proximal tibial physis. (Adapted from Hensinger RN, ed: *Operative Management of Lower Extremity Fractures in Children*. Park Ridge, IL, American Academy of Orthopaedic Surgeons, 1992, p 49.)

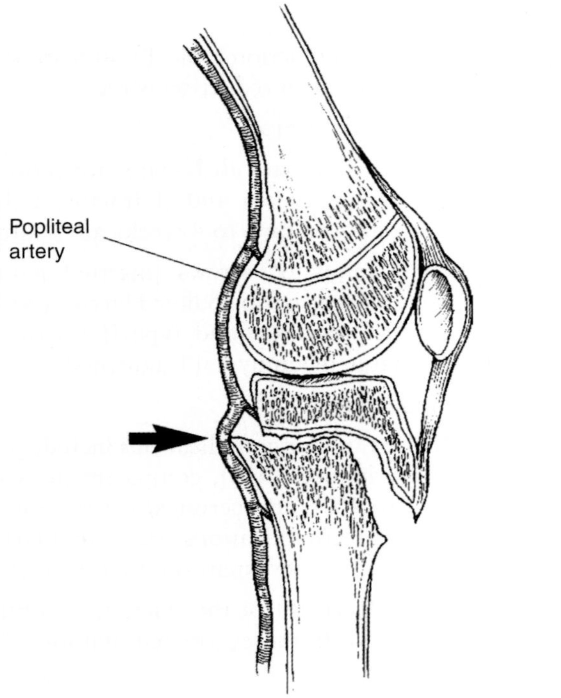

Figure 5 Lateral illustration of the knee depicts the potential for popliteal artery injury from proximal tibial physeal fracture. Arrow indicates the point at which the fractured bone can injure the artery. (Adapted with permission from Tolo VT: Fractures and dislocations around the knee, in Green NE, Swiontkowski MF, eds: *Skeletal Trauma in Children*. Philadelphia, PA, WB Saunders, 1994, pp 369-395.)

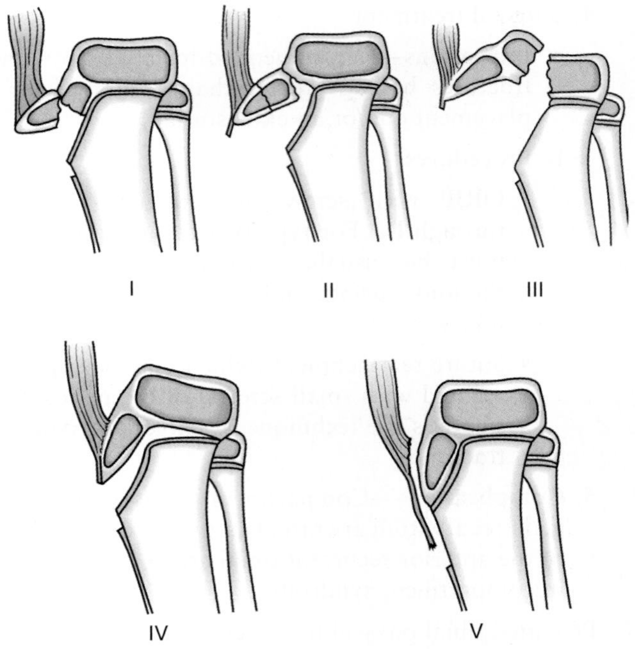

Figure 6 Illustrations show the classification of tibial tubercle injuries. Types I through IV are true fractures, whereas type V is actually a soft-tissue injury with detachment of the periosteal sleeve.

5. Complications
   a. Genu valgum is common following low-energy injuries (Cozen phenomenon). No treatment is needed acutely because these deformities often remodel and improve spontaneously.
   b. Neurovascular damage, compartment syndrome, and malunion may occur after high-energy fractures.

E. Tibial shaft fractures

1. Epidemiology: Tibial shaft fractures are considered among the most common pediatric fractures. The average age is ~ 8 years.
2. Nonsurgical treatment
   a. Most tibial fractures in children can be treated with reduction and casting.
   b. Healing takes 3 to 4 weeks for toddler fractures and 6 to 8 weeks for other tibial fractures.
3. Surgical treatment
   a. Indications include open fractures, marked soft-tissue injury, unstable fractures, multiple trauma, more than 1 cm of shortening, and unacceptable closed reduction (>10° of angulation).
   b. Fixation options include IM rod fixation, external fixation, or percutaneous pins or plates.
4. Complications
   a. When closed reduction is lost, isolated tibial fractures typically drift into varus, and combined tibia and fibula fractures drift into valgus.
   b. Delayed union and nonunion are almost never seen in closed fractures but are more common following external fixation.
   c. Compartment syndrome can occur with open or closed fractures.

VIII. ANKLE FRACTURES

A. Epidemiology: Ankle fractures represent around 5% of all pediatric fractures and 15% to 20% of all physeal injuries. These fractures are considered the most common physeal fracturs of the lower extremity.

B. Classification

1. An anatomic classification system is typically used for ankle fractures. The Salter-Harris classification is commonly used for physeal fractures.

2. A mechanistic classification system such as the Dias-Tachdjian classification may be used. This classification is patterned after the Lauge-Hansen categorization of adult fractures and describes four main mechanisms: supination-inversion, supination–plantar flexion, supination–external rotation, and pronation/eversion–external rotation.

C. Special considerations

1. Inversion ankle injuries in children typically result in distal fibular physeal fractures (almost exclusively Salter-Harris type I or II).

a. These fractures are believed to be more common than ankle sprains following an ankle inversion injury in a child, but MRI studies do not show physeal injuries of the distal fibula and question this dogma.

b. Salter type I fractures are diagnosed clinically by tenderness at the level of the physis and radiographs that show no malalignment of the physis and soft-tissue swelling over the distal fibula.

2. Transitional fractures occur as the distal tibial physis is closing.

a. These fractures involve the anterolateral distal tibial epiphysis because the distal tibial physis closes centrally first, then medially, and finally laterally.

b. Tillaux fractures (**Figure** 7) are Salter-Harris type III fractures of the anterolateral tibial epiphysis that occur with supination–external rotation injuries.

c. Triplane fractures (**Figures** 8 and 9) are Salter-Harris type IV fractures that include an anterolateral fragment of the distal tibial epiphysis (as in a Tillaux fracture) in conjunction with a metaphyseal fracture. They may be 2, 3, 4, or even 5-part fractures. The most common pattern in the metaphysis is medial-lateral in the posterior metaphysis. In the epiphysis, anteroposterior pattern is common.

D. Nonsurgical treatment

1. Distal tibial physeal fracture indications

a. Most distal tibial Salter-Harris type I, II, and III fractures; closed reduction is acceptable if postreduction radiographs show less than 2 to 3 mm of displacement and up to 10° of angulation for Salter-Harris type I and II fractures and postreduction CT shows less than 2 to 3 mm of displacement (fracture diastasis or articular step-off) for type III fractures.

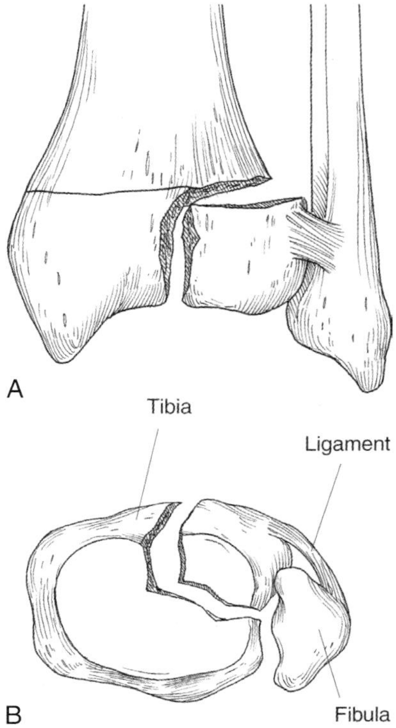

Figure 7 Illustrations depict a Tillaux fracture as seen from the anterior (**A**) and inferior (**B**) views. The anterolateral fragment is avulsed by the anterior-inferior tibiofibular ligament. (Part A adapted with permission from Weber BG, Sussenbach F: Malleolar fractures, in Weber BG, Brunner C, Freuler F, eds: *Treatment of Fractures in Children and Adolescents*. New York, NY, Springer-Verlag, 1980.)

b. Nondisplaced or minimally displaced Salter-Harris type IV fractures (medial malleolus or triplane) can be treated closed. CT should be obtained after casting for triplane fractures to confirm that reduction is satisfactory (<2 to 3 mm of fracture diastasis and articular step-off).

2. Distal fibular fractures

a. Isolated injuries—Almost always Salter-Harris type I and II fractures; typically treated closed with a short leg walking cast or fracture boot for 3 weeks.

b. Closed treatment suffices for almost all distal fibula fractures associated with distal tibia fractures, unless the fibula fracture is "high" and/or comminuted in a child nearing skeletal maturity.

E. Surgical treatment

1. Distal tibial physeal fracture indications

a. Salter-Harris type I and II fractures with greater than 2 to 3 mm of displacement or greater than 10° of angulation

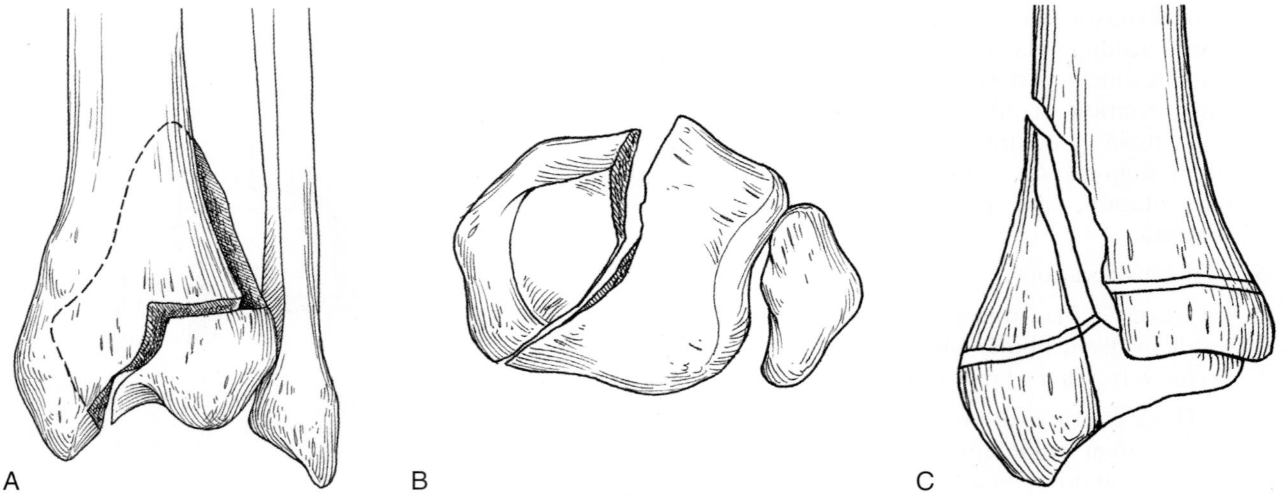

Figure 8 Illustrations show a two-part lateral triplane fracture as seen from the anterior (**A**) and inferior (**B**) aspects of the ankle. **C**, A two-part medial triplane fracture. (Panels A and B adapted with permission from Jarvis JG: Tibial triplane fractures, in Letts RM, ed: *Management of Pediatric Fractures*. Philadelphia, PA, Churchill Livingstone, 1994, p 739 and Panel C adapted with permission from Rockwood CA Jr, Wilkins KE, King RE: *Fractures in Children*. Philadelphia, PA, JB Lippincott, 1984, p 933.)

b. Salter-Harris type III fractures with greater than 2 to 3 mm articular displacement (diastasis or step-off) on postreduction CT

c. Salter-Harris type IV fractures with greater than 2 to 3 mm of displacement postreduction

2. Distal fibular fractures

a. Isolated injuries—Surgery may be necessary for the unusual Salter-Harris type III or IV fracture that is displaced.

b. Distal fibula fractures associated with distal tibia fractures—ORIF may be needed for a "high" and/or comminuted fibula fracture in a child nearing skeletal maturity.

F. Complications

1. Growth arrest with angular deformity and/or LLD is minimized by reduction within 2 mm of anatomic. Medial malleolar Salter-Harris type IV shear ankle fractures have the highest risk of growth arrest.

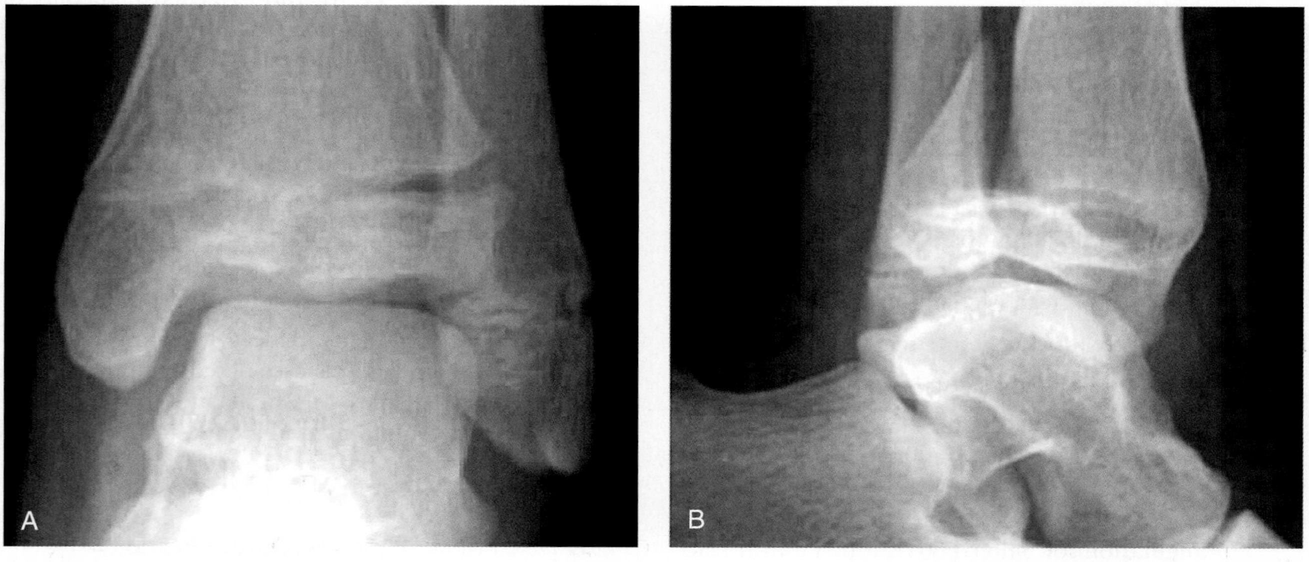

Figure 9 AP (**A**) and lateral (**B**) radiographs show a classic triplane fracture. (Reproduced from Schnetzler KA, Hoernschemeyer D: The pediatric triplane ankle fracture. *J Am Acad Orthop Surg* 2007;15[12]:738-747.)

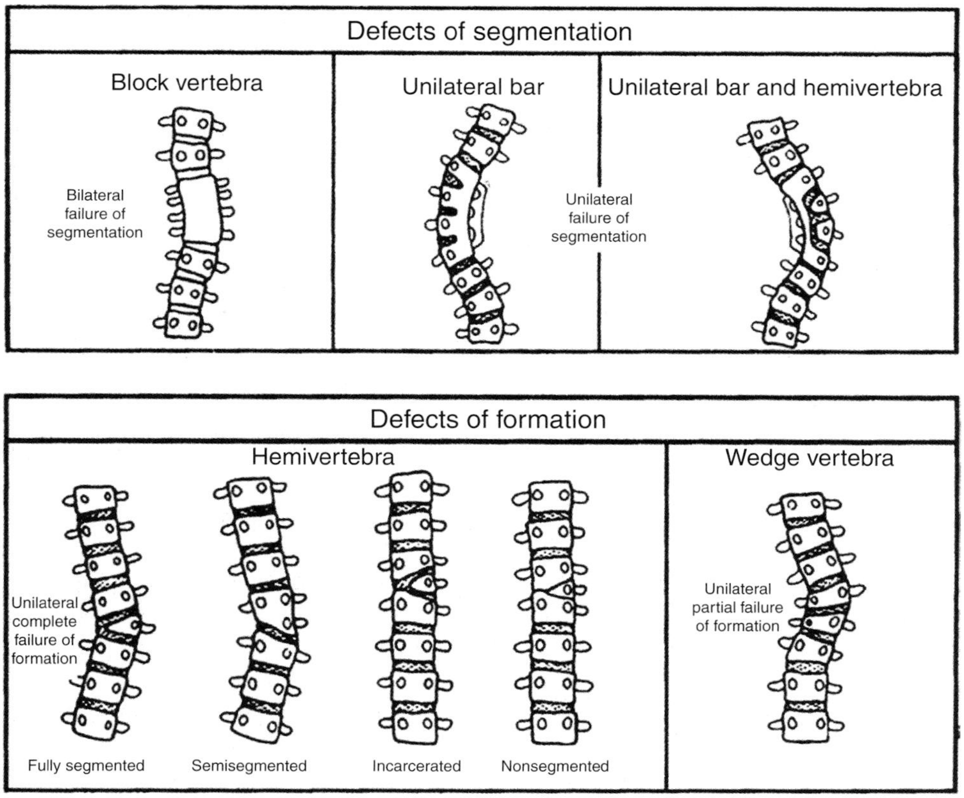

Figure 5 Illustrations showing the classification of congenital vertebral anomalies resulting in scoliosis. (Reproduced with permission from McMaster MJ: Congenital scoliosis, in Weinstein SL, ed: *The Pediatric Spine: Principles and Practices*. New York, NY, Raven Press, 1994, pp 227-244.)

- A unilateral unsegmented bar associated with a contralateral hemivertebra has the poorest prognosis for development of scoliosis, and patients with this abnormality are most often candidates for early surgery.
- A block vertebra (bilateral failure of segmentation) has the best prognosis.

c. A congenital vertebral anomaly in the thoracolumbar region with fused ribs is associated with a high risk of progression.

TABLE 2

Rates of Progression for Specific Anomalies

Type of Anomaly	Progression (per year)
Block vertebra	<2°
Wedge vertebra	<2°
Hemivertebra	2°-5°
Unilateral bar	5°-6°
Unilateral bar with contralateral hemivertebra	5°-10°

Data obtained from McMaster MJ, Ohtsuka K: The natural history of congenital scoliosis: A study of two hundred and fifty-one patients. *J Bone Joint Surg Am* 1982;64:1128-1147.

d. Incarcerated hemivertebrae do not cause scoliosis because deficiencies above and below the hemivertebrae compensate.

2. Thoracic insufficiency syndrome (TIS)
   a. TIS is defined as the inability of the thorax to support normal respiration or lung growth.
   b. TIS is usually associated with substantial scoliosis (idiopathic or congenital), a shortened thorax, rib fusions or rib aplasia, or poor rib growth (Jeune syndrome).
   c. Jarco-Levin syndrome (extensive congenital fusions of the thoracic spine) is a common cause of TIS, with two important subtypes.
      - Spondylothoracic dysplasia (primarily vertebral involvement)
      - Spondylocostal dysplasia (fused or missing ribs)
   d. Without treatment, TIS can cause substantial cardiopulmonary insufficiency or early mortality.
3. Progression of deformity in congenital scoliosis correlates with growth, which is rapid during the first 3 years of life.

C. Evaluation

1. Associated systemic abnormalities are present in up to 61% of patients with vertebral anomalies.
   a. Congenital heart defects (26%)
   b. Congenital urogenital defects (21%)
   c. Limb abnormalities (hip dysplasia, limb hypoplasia, Sprengel deformity)
   d. Anal atresia
   e. Hearing deficits
   f. Facial asymmetry
2. Approximately 38% to 55% of patients with vertebral anomalies present with a constellation of defects that constitute a syndrome, such as the vertebral, anal, cardiac, tracheal, esophageal, renal, and limb defects (VACTERL) syndrome and Goldenhar syndrome (dysplastic or aplastic ears, eye growths or an absent eye, and asymmetry of the mouth/chin, usually affecting one side of the face).
3. Workup of patients with congenital scoliosis includes renal (MRI or ultrasonography) and cardiac evaluation.
4. Pulmonary function should also be evaluated, with attention given to TIS.
5. MRI should be considered for patients with congenital spinal deformity because 20% to 40% will have a neural axis abnormality (Chiari type 1 malformation, diastematomyelia, tethered spinal cord, syringomyelia, low conus, and intradural lipoma).
6. MRI in young children (who would require general anesthesia) may be delayed if the curve is not progressive or does not require surgery.
7. Dysplasia of the chest (fused or absent ribs) may affect treatment options for congenital scoliosis.

D. Treatment

1. Nonsurgical—Bracing has no effect on congenital scoliosis.
2. Surgical
   a. Indications
      - Substantial progression of scoliosis
      - Known high risk of future progression, such as in the case of a unilateral bar opposite a hemivertebra
      - Declining pulmonary function
      - Neurologic deficit
   b. Contraindications
      - Poor skin at the surgical site
      - Minimal soft-tissue coverage of the spine
      - Substantial medical comorbidities
   c. Procedures
      - Unilateral unsegmented bars with minimal deformity, after progression has been demonstrated, are best treated with early in situ arthrodesis, either anterior and posterior or posterior alone.
      - Progressive, fully segmented hemivertebrae in children younger than 5 years with a spinal curve of less than 40° and without notable spinal imbalance have traditionally been treated with an in situ anterior and/or posterior contralateral hemiepiphysiodesis with hemiarthrodesis when progression has been documented.
      - Hemivertebra excision is recommended for patients with progressive spinal curve with marked trunk imbalance caused by a hemivertebra. This technique has best results for patients younger than 6 years who have flexible curves of less than 40°.
      - Anterior and/or posterior osteotomy/vertebrectomy is recommended for more severe, rigid deformities, fixed pelvic obliquity, or decompensated deformities that present late.
      - Growing rod constructs may be attached to the spine and/or ribs to control deformity and encourage spinal growth. Improved results have been reported with lengthening of the construct at intervals of approximately 6 to 12 months, or often more frequently with magnetically controlled growing rods which can be lengthened noninvasively.
      - TIS—A shortened hemithorax with fused ribs may benefit from an opening wedge thoracostomy, expansion of the hemithorax, and growth implants across the hemithorax, although the benefit of thoracotomy remains unproved.
   d. Rehabilitation is usually not needed.

E. Complications

1. Iatrogenic shortening of the spinal column due to fusion.
   a. Surgery at an earlier age and a greater number of fused spinal levels have a greater effect on growth and long-term pulmonary function.
   b. The goal of growth constructs is to optimize spinal growth.

2. Neurologic deficit—Can occur secondary to overdistraction or overcorrection, harvesting of segmental vessels, or spinal implant intrusion into the spinal canal.
3. Soft-tissue problems over spinal implants.
   a. Children with congenital scoliosis, especially those with pulmonary compromise, often have an insufficient volume of subcutaneous tissue to safely pad an implant.
   b. Optimization of preoperative nutrition is vital.
4. Continued progression of a scoliotic curve and crankshaft deformity requiring additional surgery.

III. NEUROMUSCULAR SCOLIOSIS

A. Overview (epidemiology)
1. Scoliosis can result from a variety of conditions that alter muscular forces acting on the spine (eg, cerebral palsy, spinal muscular atrophy, muscular dystrophy, spinal cord injury, etc...).
2. Scoliosis can develop in up to 90% of patients with neuromuscular disease, with Gross Motor Function Classification System (GMFCS) level and nonambulatory status being significant predictors of development and severity of spinal involvement.

B. Pathoanatomy
1. Impaired muscle function acting on the spine leads to progressive truncal imbalance.
2. Can result from hypotonia, spasticity, or dystonia.
3. Curves often involve the entire spine with a long, sweeping, C-shaped deformity with the apex at the thoracolumbar junction, leading to progressive pelvic obliquity, and difficulty with sitting due to pain and/or body alignment.

C. Evaluation
1. History
   a. Progressive deformity and difficulty sitting.
   b. Pelvic obliquity can be associated with increased pressure over the trochanters and decubitus ulcers.
   c. There may be progressive pain with sitting as the more cephalad pelvis pushes into the lower ribs. In severe cases this can cause skin problems.
   d. Patients frequently present with multiple medical comorbidities, including seizure disorders, malnutrition requiring gastrostomy tubes, and respiratory issues, in addition to other orthopaedic concerns such as hip dysplasia, joint contractures, and foot deformities.
2. Physical examination focuses on gait, sitting or standing balance and truncal shift, kyphosis, and pelvic obliquity. Detailed neurologic examination is often difficult in this population.
3. Imaging studies
   a. Plain radiography—ideally upright PA and lateral radiographs, whether in a standing or seated position, are obtained. Supine coronal bending or traction and sagittal radiographs can be obtained to determine curve flexibility for preoperative planning.
   b. CT—Can be useful in surgical planning and determining pelvic anatomy, though not commonly indicated.
   c. MRI—not routinely obtained.

D. Classification
1. Based on underlying neuromuscular disorder (cerebral palsy, myelomeningocele, Duchenne muscular dystrophy [DMD], etc)
2. Age
   a. Early-onset (age 10 years or younger) versus late-onset (older than 10 years)
3. Location
   a. Cervical (C2 through C6), cervicothoracic (C7 through T1), thoracic (T2 through T11-12 disk), thoracolumbar (T12 through L1), lumbar (L1-2 disk through L4)

E. Treatment
1. Nonsurgical
   a. Bracing treatment—rigid thoracolumbosacral orthoses (TLSOs) generally do not alter the natural history of neuromuscular scoliosis and can increase the risk of skin, respiratory, or gastrointestinal problems. Soft orthoses and custom wheelchair modifications can be used to improve sitting balance, especially in patients with hypotonia.
   b. Glucocorticoid treatment in DMD has been shown to alter the progression of scoliosis in this disease and decrease the need for surgery.
2. Surgical
   a. Indications
      - The decision for surgery is individualized for each patient based on the severity and progression of the deformity, caregiver wishes,

and medical comorbidities. In ambulatory patients, curves greater than 50° could be considered for surgery, while it is reasonable to delay surgery until deformity impacts care or sitting balance in nonambulatory patients.

- Surgical intervention in DMD is typically early (Cobb angle of 20° to 30°) before significant pulmonary disease develops. Forced vital capacity (FVC) <35% puts patients at risk for prolonged mechanical ventilation postoperatively.
- Thorough preoperative evaluation is mandatory in these complex patients. Malnutrition is common in this population.

b. Procedures

- In nonambulatory patients, fusions typically are performed from the upper thoracic spine to the pelvis and to the lower lumbar spine in ambulatory patients.
- Low bone density, hyperkyphosis, hyperlordosis, and significant rotation can make placement of implants challenging.
- Intraoperative traction can be useful in patients with pelvic obliquity.

3. Complications

a. Complications are common, with pulmonary issues, implant complications, and infection being the most common.

b. Reliable neuromonitoring data can be more difficult to obtain than the IS population but important if patient uses the upper extremities functionally, can weightbear (ambulate with assistance or standing frame) or is bowel or bladder continent.

IV. KYPHOSIS

A. Overview (epidemiology)

1. The most common types are postural, Scheuermann (**Figure 6**), and congenital (**Figures 7 and 8**) kyphosis.
2. Less commonly, kyphosis is secondary to trauma, infection, or spinal instrumentation.
3. The incidence of Scheuermann kyphosis ranges from 1% to 8%, with a male-to-female ratio that ranges from 2:1 to 7:1.
4. Scheuermann kyphosis is traditionally defined as thoracic hyperkyphosis caused by three consecutive vertebrae with more than 5° of anterior wedging (Sorensen criteria). Increased kyphosis with gibbus deformity on clinical examination may be considered diagnostic of Scheuermann kyphosis if congenital kyphosis has been ruled out.

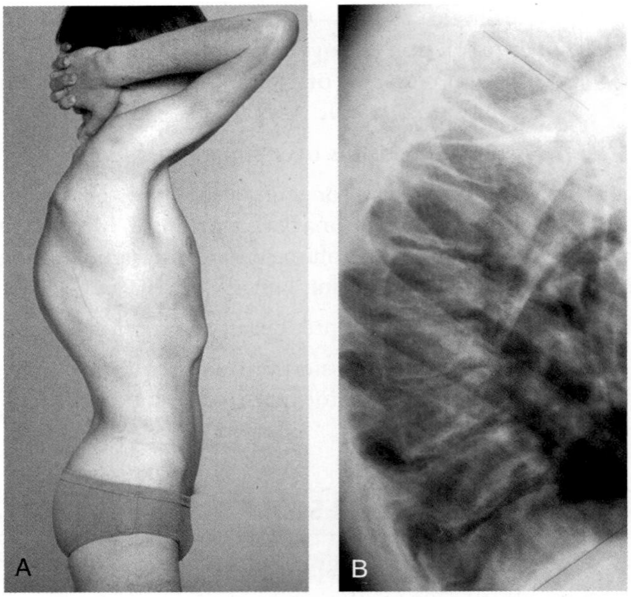

Figure 6 Patient with Scheuermann kyphosis. **A**, Clinical photograph shows sharp angulation typical of Scheuermann kyphosis. **B**, Lateral radiograph shows wedging of vertebrae and irregularity of end plates. (Reproduced with permission from Arlet V, Schlenzka D: Scheuermann kyphosis: Surgical management. *Eur Spine J* 2005;14[9]:817-827.)

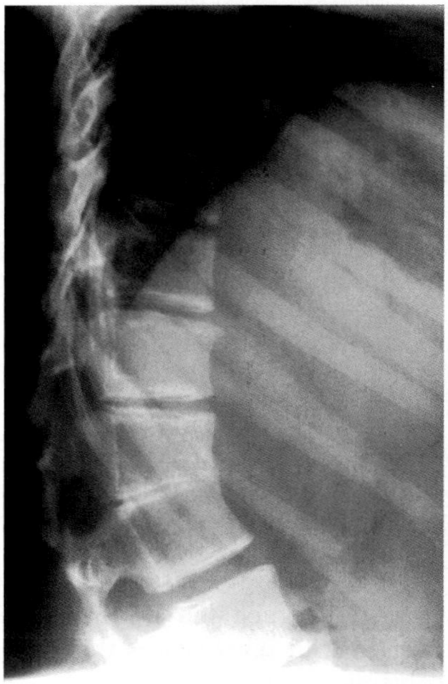

Figure 7 Lateral radiograph demonstrates congenital kyphosis with failure of segmentation.

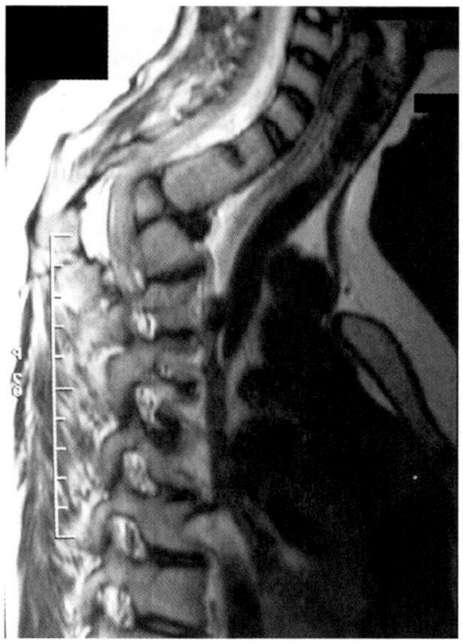

Figure 8 Sagittal MRI demonstrates congenital kyphosis, primarily resulting from a posterior hemivertebra, with a block vertebra immediately cephalad.

B. Pathoanatomy

1. Scheuermann kyphosis

a. Etiology is not well established. May be related to a developmental error in collagen aggregation resulting in disturbance of endochondral ossification of the vertebral end plates; this results in wedge-shaped vertebra and increased kyphosis.

b. It is most common in the thoracic spine; less common in the lumbar spine

c. The natural history of Scheuermann kyphosis in adults with mild forms of the disease (mean curvature, 71°) is back pain that only rarely interferes with ADLs or professional careers.

d. More severe deformities (curvature >75°) are more likely to cause thoracic pain.

e. Pulmonary compromise is not generally a concern unless the curvature exceeds 100°.

2. **Congenital kyphosis—divided into four types (types I and III associated with the greatest risk of neurologic injury; Figure 9)**

a. Type I—Failure of vertebral formation (posterior hemivertebrae). Rate of progression in this type of kyphosis is 7° to 9° per year.

b. Type II—Failure of segmentation (anterior bar). Rate of progression is 5° to 7° per year.

c. Type III (mixed)—Has the poorest prognosis for any types of the four types of congenital

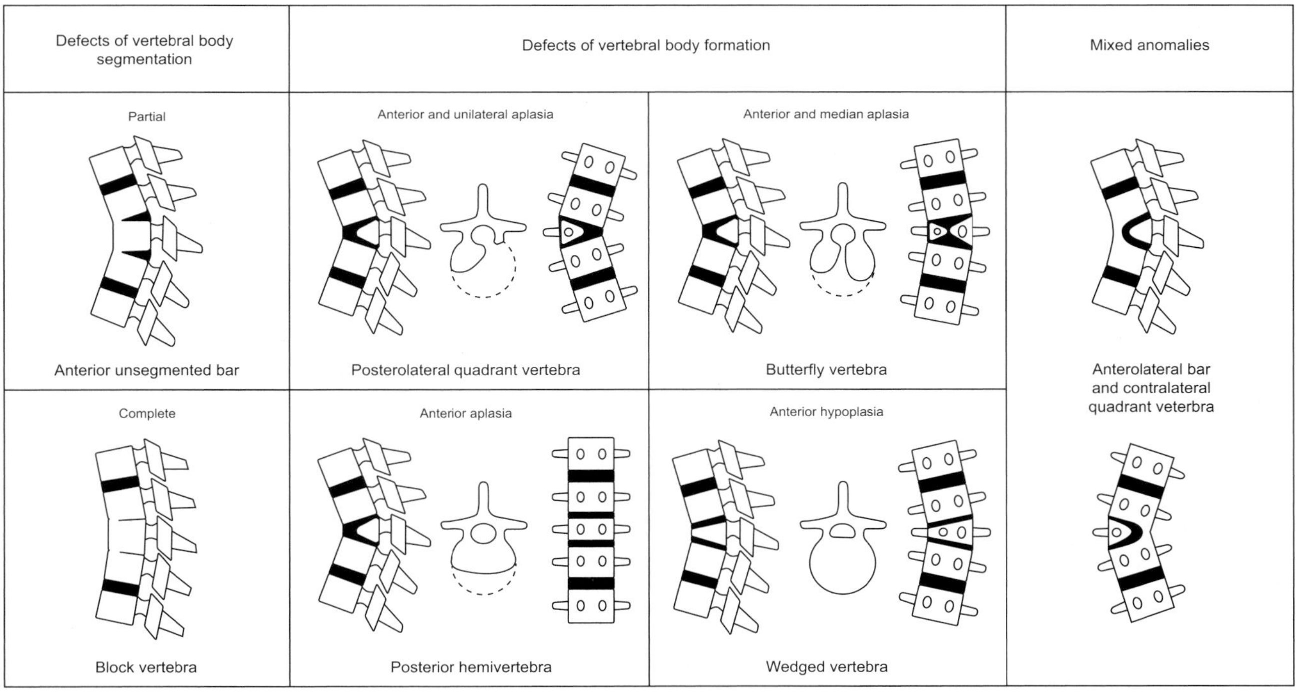

Figure 9 Illustration showing the classification of congenital vertebral anomalies resulting in kyphosis. (Reproduced with permission from McMaster MJ, Singh H: Natural History of Congenital Kyphosis and Kyphoscoliosis. *J Bone Joint Surg Am* 1999;81[10]:1367-1383.)

kyphosis for spinal deformity in the sagittal plane.

d. Type IV—Rotatory/congenital dislocation of the spine.

C. Evaluation

1. Normal thoracic kyphosis is 20° to 45° with no kyphosis at the thoracolumbar junction.
2. The patient usually presents because of cosmetic concerns or pain, which can be in the thoracic region or in the hyperlordotic lumbar spine.
   a. Thoracolumbar kyphosis is typically painful, whereas thoracic kyphosis is typically not painful.
   b. Patients with congenital and Scheuermann kyphosis often demonstrate an acute gibbus deformity at the site of spinal pathology.
3. Postural kyphosis presents a gentler, rounded contour (without gibbus deformity) of the back, with up to 60° of kyphosis.
4. Classic plain radiographic findings in Scheuermann kyphosis are vertebral end plate abnormalities, loss of disk height, Schmorls nodes, and wedge vertebra. The lumbar spine should be evaluated to rule out concomitant spondylolisthesis.
5. MRI
   a. MRI is indicated for all patients with congenital kyphosis, which has a 56% incidence of intraspinal anomalies.

D. Treatment

1. Nonsurgical
   a. Congenital kyphosis—Bracing is ineffective.
   b. Scheuermann kyphosis
      - Bracing treatment can be effective if more than 1 year of growth remains and kyphosis is between 50° and 70° with the apex of the spinal deformity at or below T7.
      - Bracing treatment is continued for a minimum of 18 months.
      - Pain can respond to physical therapy and NSAIDs.
      - Patient noncompliance with bracing treatment is common.
      - Hyperextension stretching may be of benefit.
2. Surgical
   a. Indications—Congenital kyphosis
      - Surgery is indicated for most patients with type II (failure of segmentation) or type III (mixed) congenital kyphosis, especially those with neurologic deficits.
      - For patients with type I (failure of formation) congenital kyphosis, progressive local kyphosis exceeding 40° or neurologic symptoms are an indication for surgery.
   b. Scheuermann kyphosis—Relative indications for surgery
      - Kyphosis exceeding 75°
      - Deformity progression
      - Cosmesis
      - Neurologic deficits
      - Substantial pain unresponsive to nonsurgical management
   c. Contraindications—Asymptomatic Scheuermann kyphosis in a child without cosmetic concerns
   d. Procedures
      - Congenital kyphosis—For children with failure of segmentation who are younger than 5 years and have less than 55° of kyphosis, posterior fusion is recommended to stabilize the kyphosis and permit some correction. For progressive congenital kyphosis exceeding 55°, a vertebral resection may be necessary, which has an extremely high risk for causing a neurologic deficit.
      - Scheuermann kyphosis—Posterior spinal fusion with instrumentation. Anterior release has been recommended for deformities that do not correct to more than 50° on hyperextension on a lateral radiograph over an apical bolster. Newer thoracic pedicle screw constructs with multiple posterior osteotomies may obviate the need for anterior releases, and the two techniques have similar radiographic outcomes and complication rates. Traditional recommendations are to limit correction to less than 50% of a deformity to prevent proximal or distal junctional kyphosis or implant pullout. Upper instrumented vertebra is generally the upper end vertebra or one level above the end vertebra. The fusion should include the sagittal stable vertebra as the lower instrumented vertebrae.
   e. Rehabilitation—generally not needed

E. Complications

1. Neurologic deficits (paralysis, nerve root deficit) can result from vascular compromise in a corrected spinal position, mechanical impingement,

or stretching of the spinal cord by implants in the spine or bony/soft-tissue structure. This is most common in the correction of kyphosis and kyphoscoliosis and least common in adolescent IS.

2. Anterior approaches to the thoracic spine can injure the artery of Adamkiewicz, the main blood supply to the spinal cord from T4 through T9, and generally arises variably from T8 to L2 on the left.
3. Junctional kyphosis occurs in 20% to 30% of patients, although this is usually not clinically significant.

V. SPONDYLOLYSIS/SPONDYLOLISTHESIS

A. Overview (epidemiology)

1. The incidence of spondylolysis is 5% (occurring in males more than females). Its incidence is 53% in Eskimos.
2. Of patients with spondylolysis, 25% have associated spondylolisthesis.
3. Of patients with isthmic spondylolisthesis, males are affected more commonly than females, but females are four times more likely to develop high-grade slip.
4. Primarily affects L5 (87% to 95% of patients); less frequently L4 (≤10%) and L3 (≤3%).

B. Pathoanatomy

1. Spondylolysis is an acquired condition presumed to be a stress fracture through the pars interarticularis.
2. Spondylolisthesis is anterior slippage of one vertebra relative to another, and is most common in the lumbar spine.
3. Progression is associated with the adolescent growth spurt, lumbosacral kyphosis (slip angle >40°), a higher Meyerding grade (>grade II or >50% translation), younger age, female sex, dysplastic posterior elements, and a dome-shaped sacrum.
4. Dysplastic spondylolistheses have an intact posterior arch, increasing the risk of neurologic symptoms due to entrapment of the cauda equina and the exiting nerve roots (**Figure 10**).

C. Evaluation

1. Back pain is usually localized to the lumbosacral area but may radiate down the legs.
2. Pain is exacerbated by activities involving lumbar extension and is improved with rest.

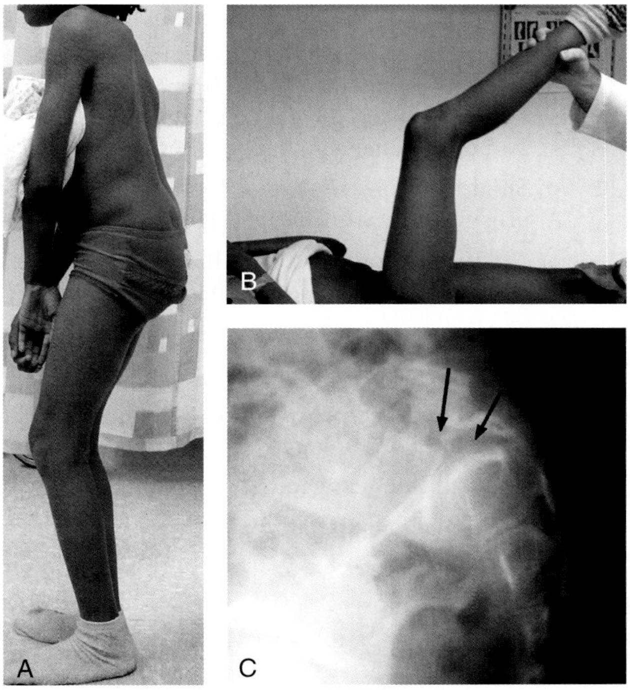

Figure 10 Grade IV dysplastic (Wiltse type I) spondylolisthesis of L5-S1 in a 9-year-old girl. **A**, Clinical photograph. Note the position of flexion of the patient's hips and knees. **B**, Clinical photograph of popliteal angle measurement of 55° caused by contracture of the hamstring muscles. **C**, Lateral weight-bearing radiograph of the lumbosacral spine illustrates high-grade dysplastic spondylolisthesis with severe lumbosacral kyphosis (arrows). (Reproduced from Cavalier R, Herman MJ, Cheung EV, Pizzutillo PD: Spondylolysis and spondylolisthesis in children and adolescents: I. Diagnosis, natural history, and nonsurgical management. *J Am Acad Orthop Surg* 2006;14[7]:417-424.)

3. Physical examination findings include paraspinal muscle spasms, tight hamstrings, and limited lumbar mobility.
   a. High-grade spondylolisthesis can produce a waddling gait (Phalen-Dickson syndrome) and hyperlordosis of the lumbar spine.
   b. The nerve root most commonly affected by an isthmic spondylolisthesis at L5-S1 is L5 because of foraminal stenosis caused by fracture callus.
4. Imaging
   a. Often can be visualized on lateral plain radiographs.
   b. CT is the best option for visualizing a pars defect, but radiation exposure must be considered. Oblique radiographs have traditionally been utilized (Scotty dog sign), but do not substantially improve sensitivity of diagnosis and

add significantly to radiation exposure and cost.

c. In high-grade vertebral slips with substantial angulation of the cephalad vertebra, a Napoleon's hat sign may be seen on AP views.

d. Single-photon emission CT (SPECT) is highly sensitive for pars defects (**Figure 11**).

e. MRI is suboptimal for evaluating pars defects but has a role in assessing nerve entrapment.

D. Classification

1. Wiltse system

a. Describes six types of spondylolisthesis on the basis of their etiology

- Dysplastic (congenital, type 1)
- Isthmic (acquired, type 2)
- Degenerative
- Traumatic
- Pathologic
- Iatrogenic

b. Isthmic (type 2) spondylolisthesis has an 85% to 95% occurrence at L5 and a 5% to 15% occurrence at L4 and is most common in adolescents.

2. Meyerding classification (**Figure 12**)

a. Based on the amount of forward slip of a superior vertebra on an inferior vertebra and is graded in quadrants according to the degree of slip.

b. Grade V in this system is spondyloptosis or 100% anterior translation of the superior vertebra.

E. Treatment

1. Nonsurgical

a. Asymptomatic patients with spondylolysis and grade I or II spondylolisthesis do not require treatment or activity restrictions.

b. Symptomatic patients (spondylolysis and grade I or II spondylolisthesis) may be treated with lumbosacral orthoses (antilordotic) for up to 4 to 6 months, as well as core strengthening and/or electromagnetic bone stimulation.

2. Surgical

a. Indications for surgery

- Uncontrolled pain (with nonsurgical management)
- Neurologic symptoms (radicular symptoms or cauda equina syndrome)
- Grade III or higher slip or progressive slip to 50%

b. Procedures

- Spondylolysis can be treated with pars repair, although this is not always successful. If disk desiccation is present (dark disk), an L5-S1 fusion should be performed.
- Posterolateral fusion (with or without instrumentation) may be performed for spondylolysis and spondylolisthesis. With noninstrumented fusions, the deformity may progress over many years. Pedicle screw constructs may increase fusion rates and decrease the postoperative slip progression.

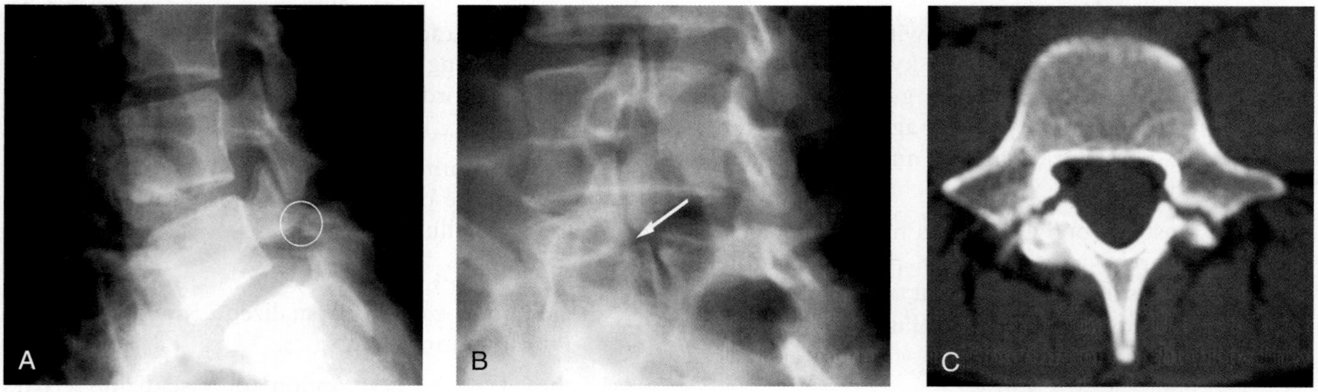

Figure 11 Patient with spondylolytic defect of the pars interarticularis of L5. Lateral weight-bearing (**A**) and supine oblique (**B**) radiographs demonstrate the defect (circle **[A]**, arrow **[B]**). **C**, Axial CT scan through the L5 vertebra demonstrates the bilateral spondylolytic defects. (Reproduced from Cavalier R, Herman MJ, Cheung EV, Pizzutillo PD: Spondylolysis and spondylolisthesis in children and adolescents: I. Diagnosis, natural history, and nonsurgical management. *J Am Acad Orthop Surg* 2006;14[7]:417-424.)

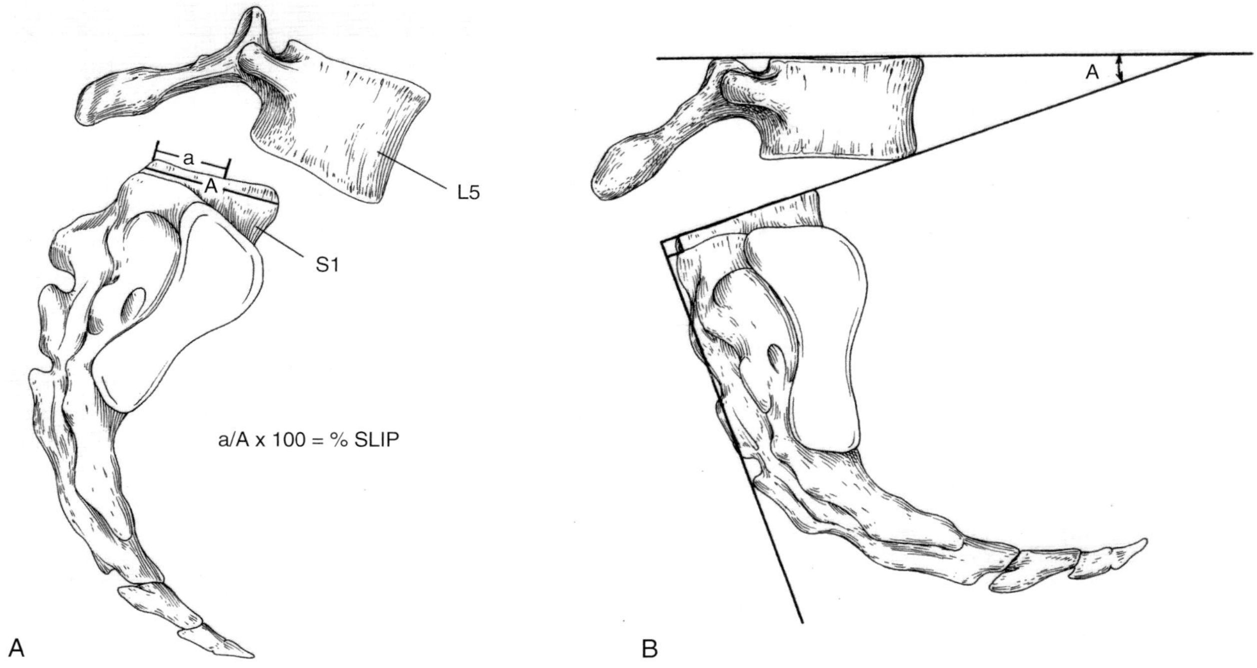

Figure 12 Diagrams illustrate the measurements used in the Meyerding classification. **A**, The Meyerding classification is used to quantify the degree of spondylolisthesis. Grade I is a slip of 0%-25%, grade II is a slip of 26%-50%, grade III is a slip of 51%-75%, and grade IV is a slip of 75%-99%. A = width of the superior end plate of S1, a = distance between the posterior edge of the inferior end plate of L5 and the posterior edge of the superior end plate of S1. **B**, Slip angle A quantifies the degree of lumbosacral kyphosis. A value that exceeds 50° correlates with a substantially increased risk of progression of spondylolisthesis. (Adapted with permission from Herman MJ, Pizzutillo PD, Cavalier R: Spondylolysis and spondylolisthesis in the child and adolescent athlete. *Orthop Clin North Am* 2003;34:461-467.)

- In the presence of a neurologic deficit, nerve root decompression is generally recommended, although neurologic improvement has been demonstrated with in situ fusion alone.
- Indications for reduction are controversial, with no universally accepted guidelines. The reduction of spondylolistheses that exceeds 50% is associated with stretching of the L5 nerve root and neurologic injury.
- Concomitant anterior fusion (transforaminal lumbar interbody fusion) is likely to increase the probability of fusion.

F. Complications

1. Cauda equina syndrome (rare) is most likely to occur in type 1 (dysplastic/congenital) slip, with the intact posterior neural arch trapping the sacral nerve roots against the posterosuperior corner of the sacrum. This may occur without surgery.
2. Implant failure (rare)
3. Pseudarthrosis (occurs in ≤45% of high-grade fusions without implants and ≤30% of high-grade slips treated with posterior instrumentation, but is rare in high-grade slips treated with circumferential fusion)
4. Postoperative slip progression
5. Pain (occurs in approximately 14% of patients at 21 years postoperatively)

VI. CERVICAL SPINE ABNORMALITIES

A. Overview (epidemiology)

1. In Down syndrome, 61% of patients have atlanto-occipital hypermobility and 21% have atlantoaxial instability; the subaxial cervical spine is not affected.
2. Klippel-Feil syndrome is characterized by failure of segmentation in the cervical spine, with a short, broad neck, torticollis, scoliosis, a low hairline posteriorly, a high scapula, and jaw anomalies. Sprengel deformity is seen in 33% of patients with Klippel-Feil syndrome.
3. Intervertebral disk calcification is most common in the cervical spine.

B. Pathoanatomy of os odontoideum

1. The odontoid develops from two ossification centers that coalesce before 3 months of age.
2. The tip of the dens is not ossified at birth but appears at 3 years of age and fuses to the dens by 12 years of age.
3. Os odontoideum is usually a result of nonunion and may result in instability of the atlantoaxial joint. The odontoid process is separated from the body of the axis by a synchondrosis (which has a "cork in a bottle" appearance), which usually fuses by age 6 to 7 years.

C. Evaluation

1. Physical examination findings in patients with basilar invagination include loss of upper/lower extremity strength, spasticity, and hyperreflexia. Patients with intervertebral disk calcification present with neck pain but have normal neurologic examination results.
2. Radiographic imaging of the cervical spine includes primarily plain AP, lateral, and odontoid views.
   a. Basilar invagination is evaluated on the lateral view and defined by protrusion of the dens above the McRae line or 5 mm above the McGregor line.
   b. Atlantoaxial instability is present when the atlanto-dens interval (ADI) exceeds 5 mm (**Figure 13**). Normal ADI in adults is 2 to 3 mm, but up to 5 mm can occur in children younger than 8 years with an intact transverse ligament.
   c. Atlantoaxial instability is also evaluated using the Powers ratio (**Figure 13**), which is the ratio of the length of the line from the basion to the posterior margin of the atlas, divided by the distance from the opisthion to the anterior arch of the atlas. A normal Powers ratio is less than 1.0.

D. Classification

1. Basilar invagination
   a. Commonly associated with Klippel-Feil syndrome, hypoplasia of the atlas, bifid posterior arch of the atlas, and occipitocervical synostosis.
   b. Also commonly found in systemic disorders such as achondroplasia, osteogenesis imperfecta, Morquio syndrome, and spondyloepiphyseal dysplasia.
   c. Motor and sensory disturbances occur in 85% of individuals with basilar invagination. Patients may present with headache, neck ache, and neurologic compromise.
2. In occipitocervical synostosis, clinical findings are a short neck, low posterior hairline, and limited neck range of motion. Atlantoaxial instability is present in 50%.
3. Odontoid anomalies range from aplasia to varied degrees of hypoplasia, which secondarily causes atlantoaxial instability.
4. Congenital muscular torticollis is associated with developmental hip dysplasia (5%). Its etiology is presumed to be secondary to compartment syndrome.
5. The etiology of torticollis also includes ophthalmologic, vestibular, congenital, and traumatic causes, as well as tumors. If a tight sternocleidomastoid muscle is not present, other causes of torticollis should be sought.
6. Atlantoaxial rotatory displacement (AARD)
   a. Ranges from mild displacement to a fixed subluxation of C1 on C2. It is most often caused by upper respiratory infection (Grisel syndrome) or trauma.
   b. CT can be used to confirm the diagnosis and rule out AARD grades III and IV, which are associated with neurologic injury and sudden death. In patients who present acutely and without significant trauma, limited cuts of C1 and C2 in a neutral position can confirm the diagnosis with much less radiation than a CT of entire cervical spine or with repeating scans with dynamic views. MRI can be useful to evaluate the C1-2 ligamentous complex or if other underlying causes (infection, tumor) are suspected, without the risk of ionizing radiation.
7. Patients with Morquio syndrome commonly have atlantoaxial instability resulting from odontoid hypoplasia.

E. Treatment

1. Nonsurgical
   a. Intervertebral disk calcification is treated with analgesics.
      - Biopsy and antibiotics are not needed.
      - Calcifications usually resolve over a period of 6 months.
   b. Congenital muscular torticollis—Initial treatment is passive stretching.

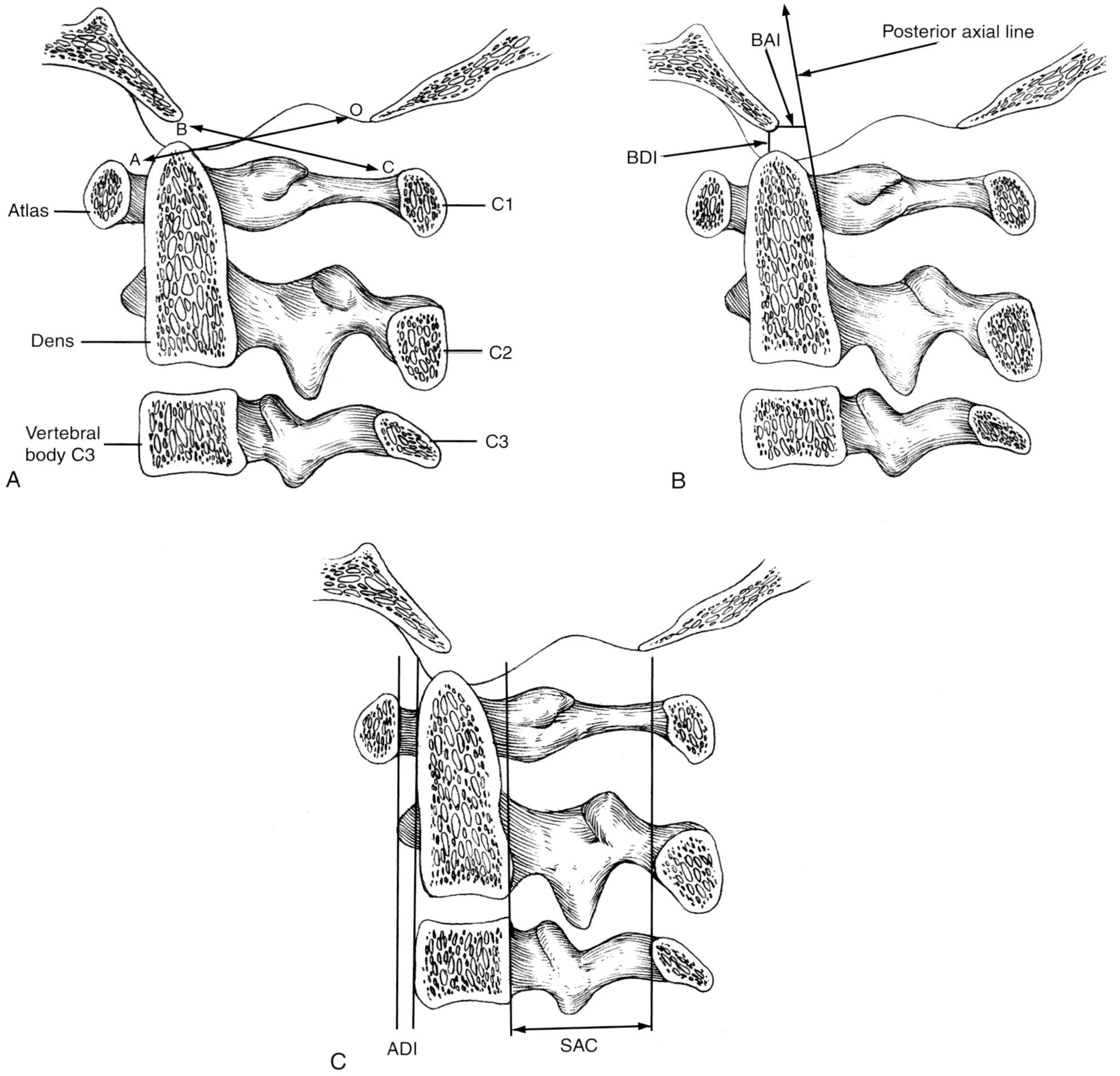

Figure 13 Illustration showing upper cervical spine and occiput (C1 through C3). **A**, Powers ratio = BC/AO. A = anterior arch of the atlas, B = basion, C = posterior arch of the atlas, O = opisthion. **B**, The basion-dental interval (BDI) and basion-axial interval (BAI) should each measure less than 12 mm. **C**, Atlanto-dens interval (ADI) and space available for the spinal cord. Atlantoaxial instability should be suspected with an ADI exceeding 5 mm. If the ADI is greater than 10-12 mm, the space available for the cord (SAC) becomes negligible and cord compression occurs. (Reproduced from Eubanks JD, Gilmore A, Bess S, Cooperman DR: Clearing the pediatric cervical spine following injury. *J Am Acad Orthop Surg* 2006;14[9]:552-564.)

c. AARD is initially managed with NSAIDs, rest, and a soft collar.

d. Patients with Down syndrome who have an ADI exceeding 5 mm without symptoms should not engage in stressful weight bearing on the head, such as in gymnastics and diving.

2. Surgical
   a. Indications
      - Basilar invagination
      - Occipitocervical synostosis with atlantoaxial instability

- Odontoid anomalies—neurologic involvement, instability exceeding 10 mm on flexion-extension radiographs, or persistent neck symptoms
- Congenital muscular torticollis if limitation exceeds 30° or condition persists longer than 1 year
- Klippel-Feil syndrome—Indications for surgery are not clearly defined
- In patients with Down syndrome, surgery should be performed when the ADI exceeds 5 mm with neurologic symptoms or exceeds 10 mm without symptoms
- Morquio syndrome and spondyloepiphyseal dysplasia—More than 5 mm of instability (regardless of symptoms)

b. Procedures

- Basilar invagination is treated with decompression and fusion of the occiput to C2 or C3.
- Occipitoaxial synostosis requires atlantoaxial reduction with fusion of the occiput-C1 complex to C2. If neural impairment exists, decompression should be considered in combination with this fusion.
- Odontoid anomalies with instability undergo C1-C2 fusion.
- Congenital muscular torticollis has been effectively treated with bipolar (proximal and distal) release of the sternocleidomastoid muscle.
- If atlantoaxial rotatory displacement persists for more than 1 week and is reducible, it should be treated with head halter traction (at home or in the hospital). If symptoms persist for more than 1 month, use of a halo or rigid brace should be considered. Fusion of C1 to C2 may be indicated if neurologic involvement or persistent deformity is present.

F. Complications

1. Complications are common with halo bracing treatment.

   a. Anterior pins most commonly injure the supraorbital nerve.

   b. More pins (6 to 12) with less insertional torque (≤5 inch-pounds) are used in young children.

   c. The sixth cranial (abducens) nerve is the nerve most commonly injured with halo traction, which is seen as a loss of lateral gaze. If neurologic injury is noted with halo traction, the traction should be removed.

2. Nonunion and a mortality rate of up to 25% are reported with C1-C2 fusion in patients with Down syndrome.

3. Posterior cervical fusions have a high rate of union with iliac crest bone grafting, but the rate of union is reported to be much lower with allograft bone.

VII. SPINE TRAUMA

A. Overview (epidemiology)

1. Injuries to the cervical spine comprise 60% of pediatric spinal injuries.
2. Mortality from cervical injury in pediatric trauma victims ranges from 16% to 17%.
3. The most common mechanisms of injury across all pediatric age groups occur in motor vehicle accidents. Toddlers and school-age children are injured most commonly in falls, and adolescents experience many sports-related injuries.
4. Nonaccidental trauma (NAT) should also be considered. Up to 40% of spinal injuries in children younger than 2 years are a result of NAT. Upper cervical spine injuries predominate, and many injuries are purely ligamentous. Multilevel injuries and other associated trauma are common.

B. Pathoanatomy

1. Children younger than 8 years have an increased risk of injury to the cervical spine because of their larger head-to-body ratio, greater ligamentous laxity, and relatively horizontal facet joints.
2. Among children with cervical spine injuries, 87% of those younger than 8 years have injuries at C3 or higher. These children also have a higher mortality than do older children, ranging from 17.0% with injury at C1 to 3.7% with injury at C4.
3. The immature spinal column can stretch up to 5 cm without rupture; the spinal cord ruptures at 5 to 6 mm of traction.
4. In children with cervical spine injuries, 33% show evidence of neurologic deficit.
5. Injuries to other organ systems occur in 42% of children with spinal injuries.

C. Evaluation

1. Initial management—Patients should be transported on a backboard with a cut-out for the occiput or on a mattress to elevate the body, to

prevent inadvertent flexion of the cervical spine resulting from the child's disproportionately large head.

2. Physical examination
   a. A detailed neurologic examination should be conducted (absence of anal wink indicates spinal shock).
   b. Upper cervical spine injuries should be suspected in young children with facial fractures and head trauma.
3. Imaging
   a. Initial imaging should consist of plain radiography of the injured region (**Table 3; Figure 14**).
      - Atlantoaxial instability is evaluated using the ADI, which should be less than 5 mm in children. When the ADI exceeds 10 mm, all ligaments have failed, creating cord compression from the negligible space available for the spinal cord.
      - On a lateral radiograph, the retropharyngeal space should be less than 6 mm at C2 and less than 22 mm at C6. However, this space at these locations may be enlarged because of crying and its enlargement is therefore not necessarily a sign of underlying injury in children.
      - Instability of the subaxial cervical spine should be suspected when intervertebral angulation exceeds 11° or translation exceeds 3.5 mm.
      - It is crucial to always visualize the C7-T1 junction on the lateral view.

TABLE 3

Normal Radiographic Findings Unique to the Pediatric Cervical Spine

Increased atlanto-dens interval	>5 mm abnormal
Pseudosubluxation C2 on C3	>4 mm abnormal
Loss of cervical lordosis	
Widened retropharyngeal space	>6 mm at C2; >22 mm at C6
Wedging of cervical vertebral bodies	
Neurocentral synchondroses	Closure by 7 yr of age

Reproduced from Hedequist D: Pediatric spine trauma, in Abel MF, ed: *Orthopaedic Knowledge Update: Pediatrics*, ed 3. Rosemont, IL, American Academy of Orthopaedic Surgeons, 2006, p 324.

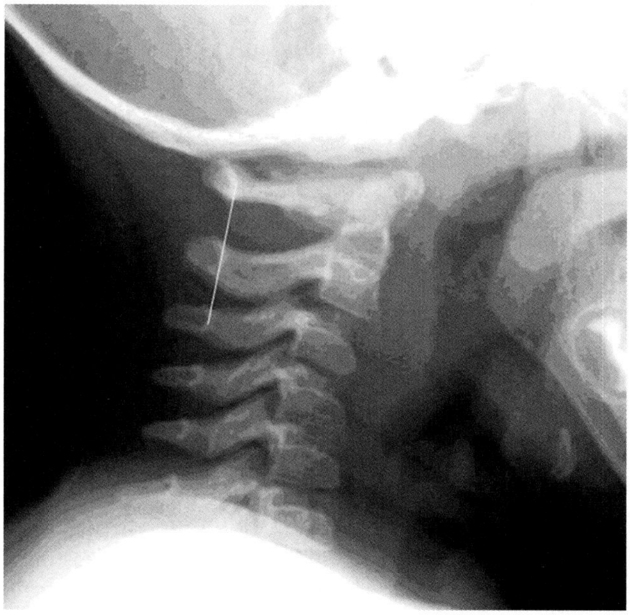

Figure 14 Lateral radiograph demonstrates pseudosubluxation of C2-C3. The Swischuk line (white line) connects the spinolaminar junction of C1 to C3. When the spinolaminar junction of C2 is no more than 1 mm anterior to this line, the subluxation is physiologic.

   b. Three-dimensional imaging—CT and MRI help assess injury and the extent of spinal canal encroachment.
   c. Atlanto-occipital junction injuries are assessed with the Powers ratio, the C1-C2:C2-C3 ratio, and the basion-axial interval (BAI) (**Figure 13**). The BAI is the distance from the basion to the tip of the odontoid and should be less than 12 mm in all children.
      - The Powers ratio is the ratio of the length of the line from the basion to the posterior arch of the atlas to that of a second line from the opisthion to the anterior arch of the atlas. A Powers ratio exceeding 1.0 or less than 0.55 represents a disruption of the atlanto-occipital joint.
      - The C1-C2:C2-C3 ratio is less than 2.5 in healthy children.

D. Classification
1. Cervical
   a. Atlanto-occipital junction injuries are highly unstable ligamentous injuries that are rare but commonly fatal. Common mechanisms are motor vehicle accidents and pedestrian-vehicle collisions.

b. Atlas fractures (also known as Jefferson fractures) are uncommon injuries usually caused by axial loading.
   - Neurologic dysfunction is atypical.
   - Widening of the lateral masses of C2 to more than 7 mm beyond the borders of the axis on an AP view indicates injury to the transverse ligament.

c. Atlantoaxial injuries are usually ligamentous injuries to the main stabilizing structures of this joint (transverse ligament) or to secondary stabilizers (apical and alar ligaments).

d. Odontoid fractures usually occur through a synchondrosis, as the result of a flexion moment causing anterior displacement.

e. Hangman's fractures (fractures through the pars articularis of C2) are usually the result of hyperextension, causing angulation and anterior subluxation of C2 on C3 (**Figure 15**).
   - Subluxation does not usually exceed 1.5 mm

f. Lower cervical spine (C3 through C7) injuries are more common in adolescents.

g. Pseudosubluxation is a common (40%) incidental finding.
   - Most common at C2-C3, followed by C3-C4
   - Reduces on extension radiographs

2. Thoracolumbar

a. Flexion injuries result in compression or burst fractures.
   - Compression fractures rarely exceed more than 20% of the vertebral body.
   - With more than 50% loss of vertical height, a burst fracture should be considered and a CT scan should be obtained.

b. Distraction and shear injuries are highly unstable and usually associated with spinal cord injury.

c. Chance fractures are caused by hyperflexion over automobile lap belts and are frequently associated with intra-abdominal injuries.

d. Spinal cord injury without radiographic abnormality (SCIWORA).
   - MRI is the study of choice, which may show ligamentous and spinal cord injury in the absence of findings on plain radiographs.
   - SCIWORA is the cause of paralysis in approximately 20% to 30% of children with injuries of the spinal cord.
   - Approximately 20% to 50% of patients with SCIWORA have a delayed onset of

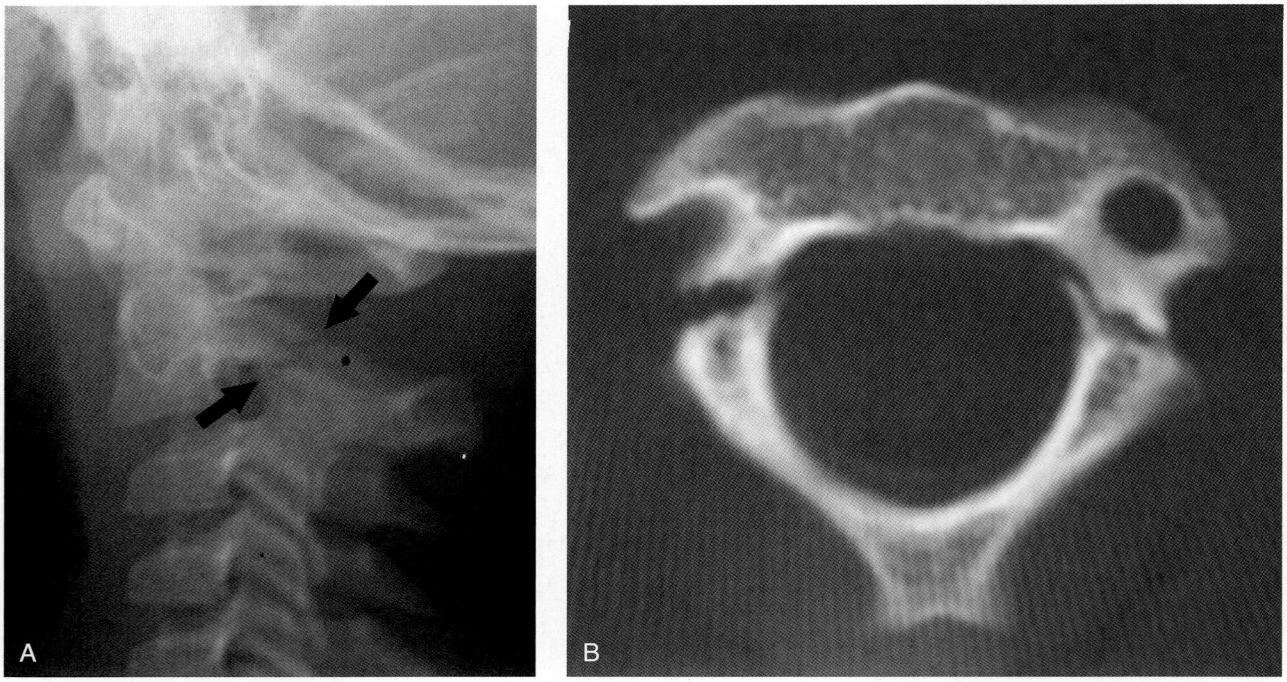

Figure 15 Lateral radiograph (**A**) and axial CT scan (**B**) of a 5-year-old boy who sustained a hangman's fracture (arrows) in a motor vehicle accident. (Reproduced with permission from Children's Orthopaedic Center, Los Angeles, CA.)

neurologic symptoms or late neurologic deterioration.

- Children younger than 10 years are more likely than older children to have permanent paralysis.

E. Treatment

1. Nonsurgical

a. Cervical

- Intervertebral disk calcification—Treated with rest and NSAIDs
- Atlas fractures—Treated with a cervical collar or halo

b. Thoracolumbar

- Compression fractures—Bracing for 6 weeks
- Burst fractures—Bracing if the fracture is stable
- Chance fractures with less than 20° of segmental kyphosis—Treated in a hyperextension cast
- SCIWORA—Immobilization for 6 weeks to prevent further spinal cord injury

2. Surgical

a. Indications

- Craniocervical instability
- Atlantoaxial instability with an ADI that exceeds 5 mm
- Displaced odontoid fracture
- Displaced and angulated hangman's fracture
- Thoracolumbar burst fractures with neurologic injury and canal compromise
- Distraction and shear injuries with displacement
- Chance fractures that are purely ligamentous injuries and bony injuries with more than 20° of kyphosis

b. Procedures

- Craniocervical instability is treated with an occiput-to-C2 fusion with halo stabilization, preferably with internal fixation.
- Atlantoaxial instability requires a C1-C2 posterior fusion, with multiple options available:
  - Transarticular C1-C2 screws.
  - Brooks-type wiring construct.
  - C1 lateral mass screws with C2 pars, pedicle, or translaminar screws, or at times hooks if screws cannot be placed safely.
- Odontoid—reduction of the displacement, with extension or hyperextension if necessary and with halo immobilization for 8 weeks.
- Hangman's fractures with minimal angulation and translation can be treated with closed reduction in extension, with immobilization in a Minerva cast or halo device for 8 weeks. Fractures with substantial angulation or translation require a posterior fusion or anterior C2-C3 fusion.
- Halo placement—in toddlers and children younger than 8 years, more pins (8 to 12) are used for halo fixation and tightened only to finger tightness (2 to 4 inch-pounds).
- Unstable thoracolumbar burst fractures are treated with fusion. Indirect canal decompression is accomplished by surgical distraction of the injured level. Direct decompression may be indicated for neurologic deficits.
- Distraction and shear injuries are treated with reduction and fusion.
- Chance injuries that are purely ligamentous should be surgically stabilized with instrumentation and arthrodesis. Bony injuries with more than 20° kyphosis or inadequate reduction are treated with posterior compression instrumentation and arthrodesis.

F. Complications

1. Os odontoideum

a. Caused by nonunion of an odontoid fracture that may cause episodic or transient neurologic symptoms.

b. Instability occurs with more than 8 mm of motion; requires C1-C2 fusion.

2. Posttraumatic kyphosis usually does not remodel and may worsen

3. Pseudarthrosis

4. Implant failure

VIII. OTHER CONDITIONS

A. Diskitis

1. Pathoanatomy—presumed infection appears to begin by seeding of the vascular vertebral end plate with extension into the disk space.

2. Evaluation

a. Symptoms

- Fever
- Back pain

- Abdominal pain
- Refusal to ambulate
- Painful limp
- Lower extremity discomfort

b. Is febrile in 25% of cases.

c. Laboratory studies show the erythrocyte sedimentation rate (ESR) and C-reactive protein (CRP) level are elevated.

d. Radiographs can demonstrate disk space narrowing with vertebral end plate irregularities (**Figure 16**). Further imaging is generally not needed if typical changes are encountered. MRI can be useful to identify earlier stages of infection than would be seen on plain radiograph such as inflammatory changes of the disk and adjacent end plate.

3. Classification

a. The typically causative organism is *Staphylococcus aureus*.

b. Langerhans cell histiocytosis (the "great imitator") must be considered in the differential diagnosis.

4. Treatment

a. Nonsurgical

- Typically consists of parenteral antibiotics (to cover *S aureus*) for 7 to 10 days, followed by oral antibiotics for several more weeks
- If the diskitis does not respond to antibiotics, a biopsy should be performed and sent for cultures and pathologic tissue evaluation.

b. Surgical

- Indications—Paraspinal abscess in the presence of a neurologic deficit; unresponsive to nonsurgical care
- Contraindications—Standard diskitis
- Procedures—Culture, irrigation, and débridement

5. Complications

a. Long-term disk space narrowing

b. Intervertebral fusions

c. Back pain

6. Pearls and pitfalls—*Salmonella* infection should be considered in the setting of sickle cell anemia because it is unique to patients with sickle cell disease.

B. Cervical disk calcification

1. Presents with neck pain universally
2. Radiographs show calcification of the cervical disk (**Figure 17**)
3. May be accompanied by fever and elevated ESR and CRP concentration

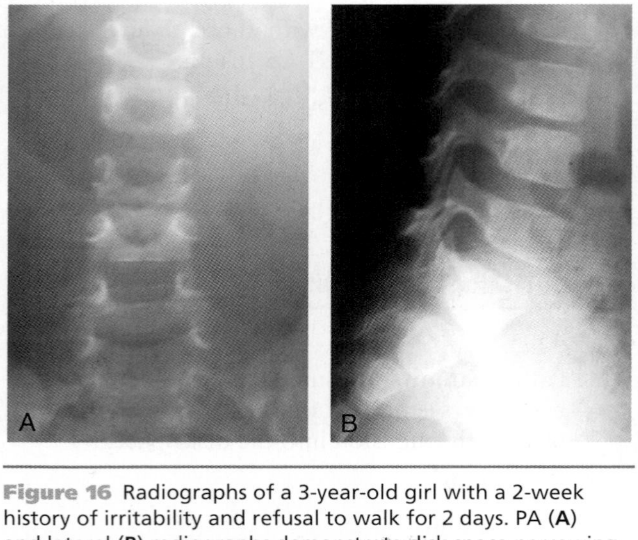

Figure 16 Radiographs of a 3-year-old girl with a 2-week history of irritability and refusal to walk for 2 days. PA (**A**) and lateral (**B**) radiographs demonstrate disk space narrowing at L3-4 consistent with diskitis. (Reproduced from Early SD, Kay RM, Tolo VT: Childhood diskitis. *J Am Aced Orthop Surg* 2003;11[6]:413-420.)

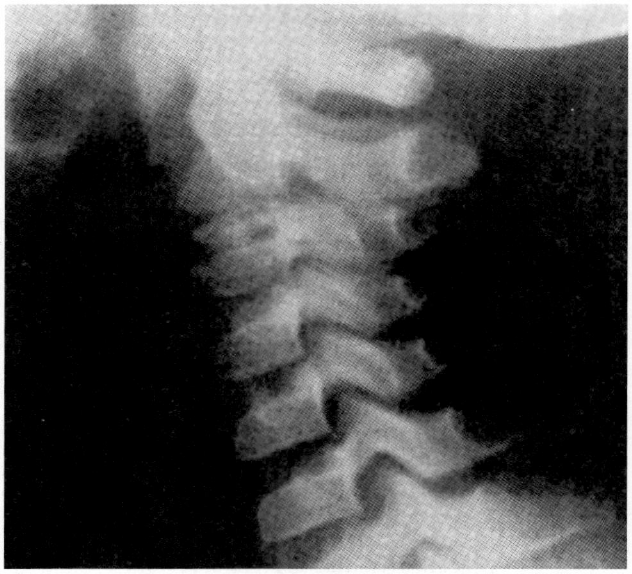

Figure 17 A 7-year-old boy was admitted with pain and a stiff neck. Lateral radiograph shows calcification of the C2-C3 disk space. (Reproduced with permission from Dai LY, Ye H, Qian QR: The natural history of cervical disk calcification in children. *J Bone Joint Surg Am* 2004;86:1467-1472.)

4. Treatment
   a. Observation—Biopsy and surgery are not indicated.
   b. Mean time to resolution is just over 1 month.

C. Septic arthritis of the sacroiliac joint
1. Epidemiology—More common in children older than 10 years
2. Pathoanatomy
   a. *S aureus* is the most common
3. Evaluation
   a. Tenderness is usually present directly over the sacroiliac joint; testing the hip in the flexed, abducted, and externally rotated position reproduces pain.
   b. MRI or bone scanning confirms the diagnosis; CT-guided needle biopsy is technically possible but not necessary for treatment.

IX. BACK PAIN

A. Overview (epidemiology)
1. More than 50% of children experience back pain by the age of 15 years. In 80% to 90%, the pain resolves within 6 weeks.
2. The differential diagnosis of back pain is shown in **Table 4**.

B. Pathoanatomy
1. In children younger than 10 years, serious underlying pathology should be considered, although conventional mechanical back pain is still most common.
2. Older children and adolescents commonly suffer "adult" low back pain.
3. Spinal deformities (scoliosis and kyphosis) can cause pain.
4. Intra-abdominal pathology such as pyelonephritis, pancreatitis, and appendicitis should be considered.
5. Studies suggest that more weight in a backpack is associated with a higher incidence of back pain.
6. Apophyseal ring fractures occur at the junction of the vertebral body and the cartilaginous ring apophysis, with the posteroinferior portion displaced into the canal.

C. Evaluation
1. History
   a. Pain at night is traditionally associated with tumors.

TABLE 4

Differential Diagnosis of Back Pain in Children

Common
Muscular strain/apophysitis/overuse
Spondylolysis
Spondylolisthesis
Trauma: microfracture
Less common
Infection (diskitis/osteomyelitis)
Scheuermann disease
Trauma: fracture
Uncommon
Herniated nucleus pulposus
Ankylosing spondylitis
Juvenile rheumatoid arthritis
Bone tumor
Spinal cord tumor
Psychogenic

Reproduced from Garg S, Dorman JP: Tumors and tumor-like conditions of the spine in children. *J Am Acad Orthop Surg* 2005;13[6]:372-381.

   b. Visceral pain is not relieved by rest or exacerbated by activity.
2. A detailed musculoskeletal, abdominal, and neurologic examination is necessary.
3. Imaging studies
   a. Plain radiography should be obtained first.
   b. Technetium Tc-99m bone scanning helps localize tumor, infection, or fracture.
   c. CT is best for identifying bone-related abnormalities (spondylolysis, apophyseal ring fracture).
   d. MRI is recommended for any neurologic signs or symptoms. MRI has been shown to be a sensitive initial advanced imaging modality for identifying structural causes of back pain when there are concerning findings on history or physical examination, with the advantage of avoiding radiation exposure associated with CT or bone scan.
4. Laboratory studies such as complete blood count with a peripheral smear, CRP, and ESR are indicated for patients with back pain and constitutional symptoms.

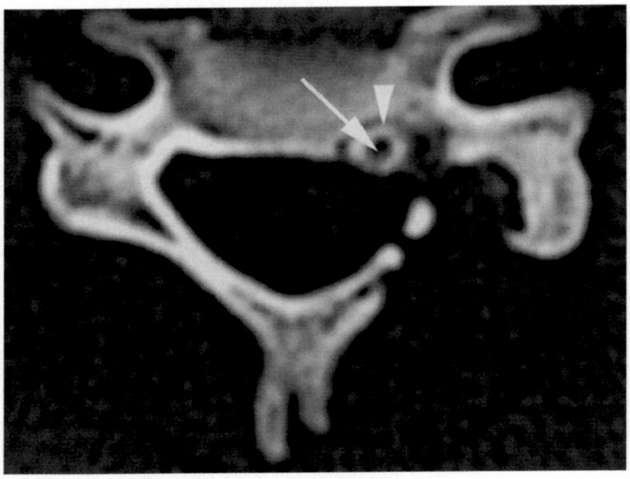

Figure 18 Axial CT scan shows C5 in a 12-year-old girl with an osteoid osteoma of the left pedicle. The arrow indicates the center of the lesion (nidus). The nonlesional, reactive sclerotic bony rim around the nidus (arrowhead) is characteristic of osteoid osteoma seen on CT. (Reproduced from Garg S, Dormans JP: Tumors and tumor-like conditions of the spine in children. *J Am Acad Orthop Surg* 2005;13[6]:372-381.)

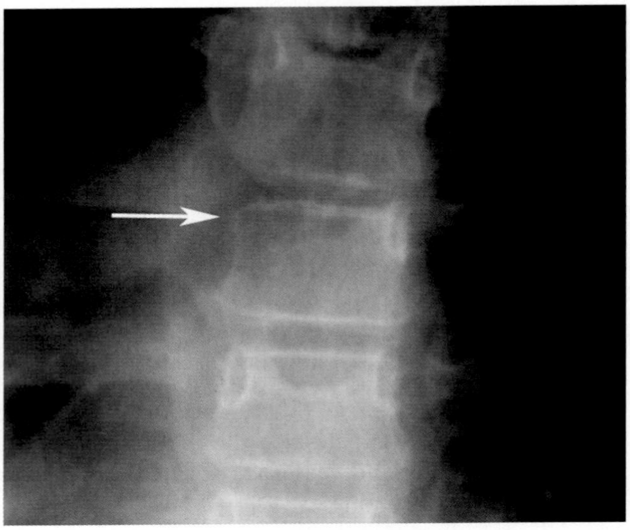

Figure 19 AP radiograph of the thoracic spine of an 8-year-old girl with an aneurysmal bone cyst at T5 demonstrates the "winking owl" sign. The left pedicle of T5 is missing (arrow). (Reproduced from Garg S, Dormans JP: Tumors and tumor-like conditions of the spine in children. *J Am Acad Orthop Surg* 2005;13[6]:372-381.)

D. Classification

1. Possible specific causes include diskitis, spinal deformity (scoliosis and kyphosis), neoplasia, spondylolysis/spondylolisthesis, disk herniation, and vertebral apophyseal end plate fracture.
2. Posteriorly, common tumors include osteoid osteoma (**Figure 18**), osteoblastoma, and aneurysmal bone cyst (**Figure 19**). Anteriorly, Langerhans cell histiocytosis has a predilection for the vertebral body, causing vertebrae plana (**Figure 20**).
3. The most common malignant cause of back pain is leukemia.

E. Treatment

1. Nonsurgical
   a. Osteoid osteomas are initially treated with NSAIDs and observation.
   b. Steroid injections, epidural (ESI), and selective nerve root (SNRI) can be performed safely in the pediatric population and are an option in children and adolescents with symptomatic disk herniations, although outcomes studies are lacking in this population.
2. Surgical
   a. Indications
      - Lumbar disk herniation—If unresponsive to nonsurgical management for a minimum of 6 weeks or if neurologic symptoms are present. Approximately ¼ of patients with a lumbar disk herniation also have evidence of an apophyseal ring fracture, and more frequently require surgical management.
      - Osteoid osteomas—If nonsurgical pain management is unsuccessful. Radioablation is not commonly used in the spine because of the risk of neurologic injury.

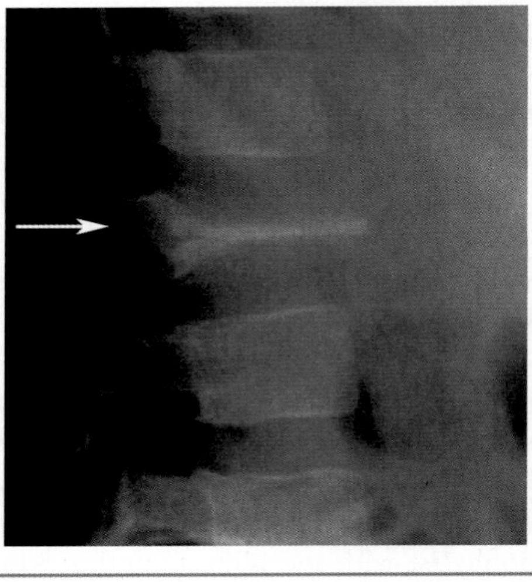

Figure 20 Lateral radiograph of the spine of a 5-year-old girl with Langerhans cell histiocytosis shows vertebra plana at L2. The collapse of the vertebral body of L2 (arrow) without soft-tissue extension or loss of disk-space height is characteristic of Langerhans cell histiocytosis. (Reproduced from Garg S, Dormans JP: Tumors and tumor-like conditions of the spine in children. *J Am Acad Orthop Surg* 2005;13[6]:372-381.)

- Osteoblastomas—Surgical treatment is always indicated because these tumors do not respond to nonsurgical interventions.

b. Procedures—Benign bone lesions can be marginally excised.

F. Red flags for pathologic back pain

1. History

a. Pain that is well localized; a positive finger test result can be used, in which the patient points to pain in one location with one finger.

b. Pain that progressively worsens over time

c. Pain that is not associated with activities and is present at rest or at night

d. Bowel or bladder incontinence

2. Physical examination

a. Tight hamstrings—Popliteal angle exceeding 50°

b. Localized bony tenderness

c. Neurologic abnormalities

TOP TESTING FACTS

1. In IS curves that are not standard, such as a left primary thoracic curve, MRI is indicated because intraspinal anomalies are common in this population.
2. The general indication for surgical treatment of patients with adolescent IS is a curve of more than 45° to 50°.
3. Maximal curve progression in IS occurs at peak growth velocity, which precedes menarche in females.
4. Congenital scoliosis is associated with a substantial risk of cardiac and renal anomalies; therefore, a cardiac workup and renal ultrasonographic examination are generally indicated.
5. Congenital scoliosis also is associated with intraspinal pathology in up to 40% of patients, so evaluation with MRI is indicated.
6. The most progressive type of congenital scoliosis is a unilateral unsegmented bar with a contralateral hemivertebra.
7. Scheuermann kyphosis is defined as thoracic hyperkyphosis caused by three consecutive vertebrae with more than 5° of anterior wedging.
8. The lower end of the instrumentation for Scheuermann kyphosis should include the first lumbar vertebrae touched by the posterior sacral line or the risk of junctional kyphosis is increased.
9. Spondylolysis or spondylolisthesis occurs in 5% of the population, most of whom are asymptomatic.
10. The end point of treatment for spondylolysis is the absence of pain and not necessarily a radiographic demonstration of healing.
11. Children younger than 8 years tend to have cervical injuries at C3 and above; children older than 8 years tend to have injuries below C3.
12. In children, the ADI should be less than 5 mm on radiographs, and the retropharyngeal space should be less than 6 mm at C2 and less than 22 mm at C6.

Bibliography

Agabegi SS, Kazemi N, Sturm PF, Mehlman CT: Natural history of adolescent idiopathic scoliosis in skeletally mature patients: A critical review. *J Am Acad Orthop Surg* 2015;23(12):714-723.

Copley LA, Dormans JP: Cervical spine disorders in infants and children. *J Am Acad Orthop Surg* 1998;6(4):204-214.

Hardesty CK, Huang RP, El-Hawary R, et al: Early-onset scoliosis: Updated treatment techniques and results. *Spine Deform* 2018;6(4):467-472.

Lenke LG, Betz RR, Harms J, et al: Adolescent idiopathic scoliosis: A new classification to determine extent of spinal arthrodesis. *J Bone Joint Surg Am* 2001;83-A(8):1169-1181.

Pahys JM, Guille JT: What's new in congenital scoliosis? *J Pediatr Orthop* 2018;38(3)e172-e179.

Shah SA, Saller J: Evaluation and diagnosis of back pain in children and adolescents. *J Am Acad Orthop Surg* 2016;24(1):37-45.

Weinstein SL, Dolan LA, Spratt KF, Peterson KK, Spoonamore MJ, Ponseti IV: Health and function of patients with untreated idiopathic scoliosis: A 50-year natural history study. *JAMA* 2003;289(5):559-567.

Weinstein SL, Dolan LA, Wright JG, Dobbs MB: Effects of bracing in adolescents with idiopathic scoliosis. *N Engl J Med* 2013;369(16):1512-1521.

Section 11

Oncology

Section Editors | KRISTY WEBER, MD
PETER ROSE, MD

Chapter 141
Overview of Orthopaedic Oncology and Systemic Disease

FRANK J. FRASSICA, MD

I. GENERAL INFORMATION AND TERMINOLOGY

A. Overview

1. Approximately 3,260 new bone and joint sarcomas and 12,390 new soft-tissue sarcomas are diagnosed annually in the United States.
2. Most of these sarcomas are high-grade malignancies with a high propensity to metastasize to the lungs.
   a. Well-differentiated sarcomas have a risk of metastasis less than 10%.
   b. Moderately differentiated sarcomas have a risk of metastasis between 10% and 30%.
   c. High-grade undifferentiated sarcomas have a risk of metastasis greater than 30%.

B. Benign bone conditions

1. Developmental processes
2. Reactive processes (osteomyelitis, stress fractures, bone cysts)
3. Benign tumors (giant cell tumor, chondroblastoma)

C. Malignant bone conditions

1. Malignancies that arise from mesenchymal derivatives are called sarcomas.
2. Primary bone sarcomas include osteosarcoma, Ewing tumor, and chondrosarcoma.
3. Bone malignancies that are not sarcomas include metastatic bone disease, multiple myeloma, and lymphoma.

D. Soft-tissue masses

1. Most common soft-tissue tumors
   a. Benign: lipoma
   b. Malignant: undifferentiated pleomorphic sarcoma (previously called malignant fibrous histiocytoma), liposarcoma, synovial sarcoma
2. Nonneoplastic reactive conditions include hematomas and heterotopic ossification.

II. BONE TUMORS

A. Classification/staging systems

1. Lichtenstein system—Modified by Dahlin to group conditions together based on the type of proliferating cell and whether the lesion is benign or malignant (**Table 1**).
2. Bone tumors can be classified according to whether the process involves the intramedullary area or the surface of the bone.
   a. Common intramedullary tumors
      - Enchondroma
      - Nonossifying fibroma
      - Osteosarcoma
      - Chondrosarcoma
      - Undifferentiated pleomorphic sarcoma of bone
   b. Common surface tumors
      - Osteochondroma
      - Periosteal chondroma
      - Parosteal osteosarcoma
3. Bone sarcomas can also be characterized as primary or secondary.
   a. Common primary bone sarcomas
      - Osteosarcoma
      - Ewing sarcoma
      - Chondrosarcoma

Neither Dr. Frassica nor any immediate family member has received anything of value from or has stock or stock options held in a commercial company or institution related directly or indirectly to the subject of this chapter.

TABLE 1

Dahlin Modification of the Lichtenstein Classification System

Cell Type	Benign	Malignant
Bone	Osteoid osteoma	Osteosarcoma
	Osteoblastoma	Parosteal osteosarcoma
		Periosteal osteosarcoma
		High-grade surface osteosarcoma
Cartilage	Enchondroma	Chondrosarcoma
	Periosteal chondroma	Dedifferentiated chondrosarcoma
	Osteochondroma	Periosteal chondrosarcoma
	Chondroblastoma	Mesenchymal chondrosarcoma
	Chondromyxoid fibroma	Clear cell chondrosarcoma
Fibrous	Nonossifying fibroma	Fibrosarcoma
		Undifferentiated pleomorphic sarcoma
Vascular	Hemangioma	Hemangioendothelioma
		Hemangiopericytoma
Hematopoietic		Myeloma
		Lymphoma
Nerve	Neurilemmoma	Malignant peripheral nerve sheath tumor
Lipogenic	Lipoma	Liposarcoma
Notochordal	Notochordal rest	Chordoma
Unknown	Giant cell tumor	Ewing sarcoma
		Adamantinoma

b. Common secondary bone sarcomas
- Chondrosarcoma arising in an osteochondroma
- Undifferentiated pleomorphic sarcoma arising in a bone infarct
- Osteosarcoma occurring in a focus of Paget disease
- Sarcoma following external beam irradiation (PIS)

4. Bone tumor grade (**Table 2**)

TABLE 2

Bone Tumor Grades

Grade	Characteristic	Examples
G1	Low grade (well differentiated)	Parosteal osteosarcoma
		Low-grade intramedullary osteosarcoma (rare)
		Adamantinoma
		Intramedullary grade 1 chondrosarcoma (represent two-thirds of chondrosarcomas)
		Chordoma
G2	Intermediate grade (moderately differentiated)	Periosteal osteosarcoma
		Grade 2 chondrosarcoma of bone
G3, G4	High grade (poorly differentiated or undifferentiated)	Osteosarcoma
		Ewing sarcoma
		Undifferentiated pleomorphic sarcoma of bone

5. Enneking system—Staging system for benign and malignant bone tumors.
   a. Benign lesions—See **Table 3**.
   b. Malignant bone tumors—See **Table 4**.
   c. Most high-grade osteosarcoma present at an Enneking stage IIB lesion
6. American Joint Committee on Cancer (AJCC) classification system for bone tumors (**Table 5**)
   a. Based on the tumor grade, size, and presence or absence of discontinuous tumor or regional/systemic metastases. The staging system is different now that the eighth edition has come out and divides the staging for sarcomas into extremity, retroperitoneum, and head/neck.
   b. In this system, the order of importance of prognostic factors is:
      - Presence of metastasis (stage IV)
      - Discontinuous tumor (stage III)
      - Grade (I—low, II—high)
      - Size
        - T1 ≤ 8 cm
        - T2 > 8 cm

TABLE 3

Enneking Classification of Benign Bone Tumors

Stage	Description	Tumor Examples
1	Inactive (latent)	Nonossifying fibroma
		Enchondroma
2	Active	Giant cell tumor[a]
		Aneurysmal bone cyst[a]
		Chondroblastoma
		Chondromyxoid fibroma
		Unicameral bone cyst
3	Aggressive	Giant cell tumor[a]
		Aneurysmal bone cyst[a]

[a]Giant cell tumor and aneurysmal bone cyst can be either stage 2 (active) or stage 3 (aggressive) lesions, depending on the amount of bone destruction, soft-tissue masses, and joint involvement.

TABLE 4

Enneking Classification of Malignant Bone Tumors

Stage	Description
IA	Low grade, intracompartmental
IB	Low grade, extracompartmental
IIA	High grade, intracompartmental
IIB	High grade, extracompartmental
III	Metastatic disease

Suffix A = intracompartmental (confined to bone, no soft-tissue involvement); suffix B = extracompartmental (penetration of the cortex with a soft-tissue mass)

TABLE 5

Definitions of TNM Stage I Through Stage IV

Stage	Tumor Grade	Tumor Size
IA	Low	<8 cm
IB	Low	>8 cm
IIA	High	<8 cm
IIB	High	>8 cm
III	Any tumor grade, skip metastases[a]	
IV	Any tumor grade, any tumor size, distant metastases	

Reproduced with permission from Amin MB, Edge SB, Greene FL: *AJCC Cancer Staging Manual*, 8 ed. Springer International, 2017.
[a]Skip metastases: discontinuous tumors in the primary bone site. This designation is only appropriate for intermediate- and high-grade lesions.
TNM = tumor, nodes, metastasis

c. The staging system has been divided into the appendicular skeleton, pelvis, and spine. The individual stage of the tumor has not changed. Location in the spine and pelvis has a worse prognosis than the appendicular skeleton.

- For the spine:
  - T1—one or two adjacent vertebral segments
  - T2—three adjacent vertebral segments
  - T3—four or more or nonadjacent segments
  - T4—tumors that have invaded the great vessels or spinal canal
- For the pelvis:
  - T1—one pelvic segment without extraosseous extension
  - T2—one pelvic segment with extraosseous extension or two pelvic segments without extraosseous extension
  - T3—two pelvic segments with extraosseous extension
  - T4—tumors that occupy three pelvic segments, or extend across the sacroiliac joint, or encase the external iliac vessels, or display tumor within the vessels
- Pelvic segments: sacrum, iliac wing, pubic rami. symphysis, acetabulum/periacetabulum

III. SOFT-TISSUE TUMORS

A. Classification

1. Soft-tissue tumors are classified histologically, according to the predominant cell type.
2. Staging systems can include benign and malignant tumors and reactive conditions.
3. There are hundreds of different soft-tissue tumors; some of the most significant are listed in **Table 6**.

B. Staging—The most common system is the AJCC system (**Table 7**). The order of importance of prognostic factors is:

1. Presence of metastasis (stage IV)
2. Grade
   a. Low—stage I
   b. High—stage II
3. Size (>5 cm)
   a. T1 ≤ 5 cm
   b. T2 > 5 cm
4. Location (superficial or deep)

TABLE 6

Histologic Classification of Soft-Tissue Tumors

Type	Benign	Malignant
Fibrous	Nodular fasciitis	Fibrosarcoma
	Proliferative fasciitis	Infantile fibrosarcoma
	Elastofibroma	
	Infantile fibromatosis	
	Adult fibromatosis	
Fibrohistiocytic	Fibrous histiocytoma	DFSP
		Undifferentiated pleomorphic sarcoma
Lipomatous	Lipoma	Well-differentiated liposarcoma
	Angiolipoma	Myxoid round cell liposarcoma
	Hibernoma	Pleomorphic liposarcoma
	Atypical lipoma	Dedifferentiated liposarcoma
Smooth muscle	Leiomyoma	Leiomyosarcoma
Skeletal muscle	Rhabdomyoma	Rhabdomyo-sarcoma
Blood vessels	Hemangioma	Angiosarcoma
	Lymphangioma	Kaposi sarcoma
Perivascular	Glomus tumor	Hemangio-pericytoma
Synovial	Focal PVNS	Malignant PVNS
	Diffuse PVNS	
Nerve sheath	Neuroma	MPNST
	Neurofibroma	
	Neurofibromatosis	
	Schwannoma	
Neuroectodermal	Ganglioneuroma	Neuroblastoma
		Ewing sarcoma
		PNET
Cartilage	Chondroma	Extraskeletal chondrosarcoma
	Synovial chondromatosis	
Bone	FOP	Extraskeletal osteosarcoma
Miscellaneous	Tumoral calcinosis	Synovial sarcoma
	Myxoma	Alveolar soft-part sarcoma
		Epithelioid sarcoma

DFSP = dermatofibrosarcoma protuberans, FOP = fibrodysplasia ossificans progressiva, MPNST = malignant peripheral nerve sheath tumor, PNET = primitive neuroectodermal tumor, PVNS = pigmented villonodular synovitis

TABLE 7

AJCC Version 8 Staging for Soft-Tissue Sarcomas

Primary Tumor (T)				
TX	Primary tumor cannot be assessed			
T1	Tumor 5 cm or less			
T2	Tumor more than 5 cm but equal or less than 10 cm			
T3	Tumor more than 10 cm but equal or less than 15 cm			
T4	Tumor greater than 15 cm			
Note: Superficial tumor is located exclusively above the superficial fascia without invasion of the fascia; deep tumor is located either exclusively beneath the superficial fascia, superficial to the fascia with invasion of or through the fascia, or both superficial yet beneath the fascia.				
Regional Lymph Nodes (N)				
	Regional lymph nodes cannot be assessed			
N0	No regional lymph node metastasis			
N1	Regional lymph node metastasis			
Distant Metastasis (M)				
M0	No distant metastasis			
M1	Distant metastasis			
Staging of Soft-Tissue Sarcomas of the Trunk and Extremities				
Stage IA	T1	N0	M0	G1, GX
Stage IB	T2,3,4	N0	M0	G1, GX
State II	T1	N0	M0	G3, G3
Stage IIIA	T2	N0	M0	G2,G3
Stage IIIB	T3,4	N0	M0	G2,G3
Stage IV	Any T	N1	M0	Any G
Stage IV	Any T	Any N	M1	Any G

Reproduced with permission from Amin MB, Edge SB, Greene FL: *AJCC Cancer Staging Manual*, 8 ed. Springer International, 2017.
AJCC = American Joint Committee on Cancer

C. This system now uses the anatomic site of the tumor: trunk and extremity, abdomen and thoracic visceral organisms, gastrointestinal stromal tumor, retroperitoneum, unusual histologies, and sites.

IV. PATIENT EVALUATION

A. History

1. Current symptoms (pain, rate of growth, skin changes, presence of mass)

a. Pain
- Destructive bone tumors
  - Pain is intermittent and progresses to constant pain that does not respond to NSAIDs or weak narcotic medications.
  - A common presentation is severe pain that occurs at rest and with activity.
  - Night pain often present (must be carefully elicited, especially if the patient is a child)
    - Pain that wakes the patient up at night
    - Any requirement for analgesic medication at night (aspirin, nonsteroidal anti-inflammatories Tylenol, etc)
- Malignant soft-tissue tumors—Patients with these tumors often present without pain unless there is rapid growth or impingement on neural structures.

b. Rate of growth—A rapidly growing soft-tissue mass may suggest malignancy. Some malignant soft-tissue tumors grow slowly (synovial sarcoma, epithelioid sarcoma).

c. Presence of a mass—Assess when noticed in relation to other symptoms and rate of growth. A soft-tissue mass may also develop from a bone tumor.

2. Relevant history/family history

a. History of cancer or family history of cancer/masses (neurofibromatosis)

b. Exposure (eg, toxic chemicals, cats—cat scratch disease causes enlarged lymph nodes)

c. History of infection or trauma (myositis ossificans)

B. Physical examination

1. Mass—With bone tumors, patients present with a hard, fixed mass adjacent to the bone lesion that is often tender on deep palpation. Soft-tissue masses can be compressible (lipoma) or firm (sarcoma, desmoid).

2. Range of motion—Range of motion of the joint adjacent to a bone or soft-tissue tumor is often diminished.

3. Muscle atrophy—Common, adjacent to painful lesion.

4. Lymphadenopathy—Lymph nodes can be enlarged as a result of infection or metastasis.

5. Pathologic fractures

a. Fractures through a bone lesion occur in 5% to 10% of patients.

b. A history of antecedent pain is common.

c. Pathologic fractures generally occur with minor trauma or following activities of daily living.

C. Imaging

1. Plain radiographs

a. Primary bone lesion
- Plain radiographs alone (two planes) are often sufficient for benign bone lesions.
- Cortices should be inspected for bone destruction.
- Lesion should be assessed for mineralization.
  - Rings/stipples suggest a cartilage lesion.
  - Cloud-like lesions suggest bone formation.
- Periosteal reaction should be checked for.

b. Primary soft-tissue lesions
- Synovial sarcomas: Scattered calcifications are noted in 30%.
- Myositis ossificans: Peripheral mineralization is present.
- Hemangiomas: Phleboliths present in soft tissue.
- Lipomas: Radiolucent on plain radiographs.

2. Technetium Tc-99m bone scan

a. Technetium Tc-99m forms chemical adducts to sites of new bone formation.

b. Detects multiple sites of bone involvement or skip metastases

c. Very sensitive but not specific

d. High false-negative rate in multiple myeloma and occasionally in very osteolytic bone metastasis such as renal cell carcinoma

3. CT

a. Determines the mineral distribution in normal and abnormal bone

b. Helpful in evaluating pelvic and spine lesions

c. Thin-cut CT should be ordered if osteoid osteoma is suspected.

4. MRI

a. Sensitive and specific for detecting bone marrow involvement

b. Defines anatomic features (T1-weighted sequences)

c. Helpful in evaluating pelvic and spine bone lesions

d. Key study for evaluation of soft-tissue tumors

- Determinate masses—If nature of lesion can definitively be determined by analysis of MRI (lipoma, ganglion cyst, hemangioma, muscle injury). These can be definitively treated without a biopsy.
- Indeterminate masses—If nature of lesion cannot be determined by analysis of MRI. These require a biopsy before definitive treatment.

5. Pulmonary staging

a. CT is used as a baseline to detect pulmonary metastases and for future comparison.

b. Chest radiographs (or repeated CT scans) are used for future follow-up if initial CT of the chest is negative.

c. PET scanning is very controversial (the cost is about $5,000); when this modality is allowed by the insurance company, patients often have PET scans to look for pulmonary and other sites of metastasis. PET scanning is not routinely done in patients with sarcomas (as opposed to lymphomas where it is an integral part of staging).

V. BIOPSY

A. General

1. Biopsy is a key step in the evaluation and treatment of patients with bone or soft-tissue lesions.

2. Significant problems can occur when a biopsy is not done correctly.

a. Altered treatment

b. Major errors in diagnosis

c. Complications (eg, infection, nerve injury)

d. Nonrepresentative tissue

e. Adverse outcome (local recurrence)

f. Unnecessary amputation

B. Major types of biopsy

1. Needle biopsy—Most common method of establishing a diagnosis, but requires an experienced cytopathologist and surgical pathologist.

a. Fine-needle aspiration—Needle aspiration of cells from the tumor.

b. Core needle biopsy—A larger bore needle is placed into the tumor and a core of tissue is extracted.

2. Open incisional biopsy—Surgical procedure to obtain tissue.

a. The biopsy tract should be designed to be excised at the time of the definitive resection if the tumor is malignant.

- The incision should be small and usually is oriented longitudinally.
- The following nonlongitudinal incisions are used occasionally:
  - A transverse incision for the clavicle
  - An oblique incision for the scapular body

b. Soft-tissue flaps are not elevated; the biopsy is performed directly onto the tumor mass.

c. Hemostasis is critical; usually, no indwelling drains are used.

d. A frozen section analysis is often performed to ensure that diagnostic tissue has been obtained.

3. Excisional biopsy

a. Indicated only when the surgeon is sure that the lesion is benign or when the tumor can be removed with a wide margin (eg, if the radiographic appearance suggests a superficial, small soft-tissue malignancy).

b. Two low-grade malignancies for which an excisional biopsy is sometimes performed are parosteal osteosarcoma and low-grade chondrosarcoma.

VI. MOLECULAR MARKERS/GENETIC CONSIDERATIONS

A. Tumor suppressor genes and associated conditions are listed in **Table 8**.

B. Chromosomal alterations

1. Chromosomal alterations in malignant tumors are generally translocations (**Table 9**).

2. Alterations often produce unique gene products that may affect the prognosis.

TABLE 8

Tumor Suppressor Genes

Gene	Syndrome	Tumor Examples
RB	Hereditary neuroblastoma	Retinoblastoma, osteosarcoma
P53	Li-Fraumeni syndrome	Sarcomas, breast cancer
P16INK4a	Familial melanoma	Chondrosarcoma, osteosarcoma, melanoma
APC	Familial adenomatous polyposis	Colon adenomas, desmoids
NF1	Neurofibromatosis	Neurofibroma, sarcomas
EXT1/ EXT2	Hereditary multiple exostosis	Osteochondromas, chondrosarcomas

Note: *EXT1* has a greater burden of disease and increased risk for secondary chondrosarcoma

TABLE 9

Chromosomal Alterations in Malignant Tumors

Tumor	Translocation	Genes
Ewing sarcoma, PNET	t(11;22)(q24;q12)	*EWS, FLI1*
Synovial sarcoma	t(X;18)(p11;q11)	*SYT, SSX*
Clear cell sarcoma	t(12;22)(q13;a12)	*EWS, ATF1*
Alveolar rhab-domyosar-coma	t(2;13)(q35;q14)	*PAX3, FKHR*
Myxoid liposarcoma	t(12;16)(q13;p11)	*CHOP, TLS*

PNET = primitive neuroectodermal tumor

TOP TESTING FACTS

1. The most common site of metastases from bone and soft-tissue sarcomas is the lungs.
2. The most common low-grade bone sarcomas are chondrosarcoma, parosteal osteosarcoma, adamantinoma, and chordoma.
3. The most common high-grade sarcomas are osteosarcoma, Ewing sarcoma, and undifferentiated pleomorphic sarcoma.
4. The order of importance of prognostic factors in bone tumor staging is presence of metastases, discontinuous tumor, grade, and size. The most common stage of osteosarcoma is stage IIB (Enneking) and stage II (AJCC).
5. A high rate of false-negative results occurs with technetium Tc-99m bone scanning in multiple myeloma.
6. The order of importance of prognostic factors in soft-tissue tumor staging is presence of metastases, grade, and size.
7. The *RB* gene is the tumor suppressor gene associated with osteosarcoma and is located on chromosome 15.
8. *EXT1/EXT2* are the tumor suppressor genes associated with hereditary multiple exostoses. *EXT1* has a greater burden of disease and a greater risk of secondary chondrosarcoma.
9. Ewing sarcoma and primitive neuroectodermal tumor have a characteristic chromosomal translocation t(11;22).
10. Synovial sarcoma has a characteristic chromosomal translocation t(X;18).

Bibliography

Amin MB, Edge SB, Greene FL: *AJCC Cancer Staging Manual*, ed 8. Springer International, 2017, pp 471-545.

Enneking WF: A system of staging musculoskeletal neoplasms. *Clin Orthop Relat Res* 1986;204:9-24.

Enneking WF, Spanier SS, Goodman MA: A system for the surgical staging of musculoskeletal sarcoma. *Clin Orthop Relat Res* 1980;153:106-120.

Goldblum JR, Folpe AL, Weiss SW: General considerations, in Weiss SW, Goldblum JR, eds: *Enzinger and Weiss's Soft Tissue Tumors*, ed 6. Elesevier, 2014, pp 1-10.

11 | Oncology

Hopyan S, Wunder JS, Randall RL: Molecular biology in musculoskeletal neoplasia, in Schwartz HSS, ed: *Orthopaedic Knowledge Update: Musculoskeletal Tumors*, ed 2. Rosemont, IL, American Academy of Orthopaedic Surgeons, 2007, pp 13-21.

Mankin HJ, Lange TA, Spanier SS: The classic: The hazards of biopsy in patients with malignant primary bone and soft-tissue tumors. The Journal of Bone and Joint Surgery, 1982;64:1121-1127. *Clin Orthop Relat Res* 2006;450:4-10.

Mankin HJ, Mankin CJ, Simon MA: Members of the musculoskeletal tumor society: The hazards of the biopsy, revisited. *J Bone Joint Surg Am* 1996;78(5):656-663.

Papp DF, Khanna AJ, McCarthy EF, Carrino JA, Farber AJ, Frassica FJ: Magnetic resonance imaging of soft-tissue tumors: Determinate and indeterminate lesions. *J Bone Joint Surg Am* 2007;89(suppl 3):103-115.

Siegel R, Miller KD, Jemal A: Cancer statistics, 2017. *CA Cancer J Clin* 2017;67:7-30.

Unni KK: Introduction and scope of study, in Unni KK, ed: *Dahlin's Bone Tumors: General Aspects and Data on 11,087 Cases*, ed 5. Philadelphia, PA, Lipppincott-Raven, 1996.

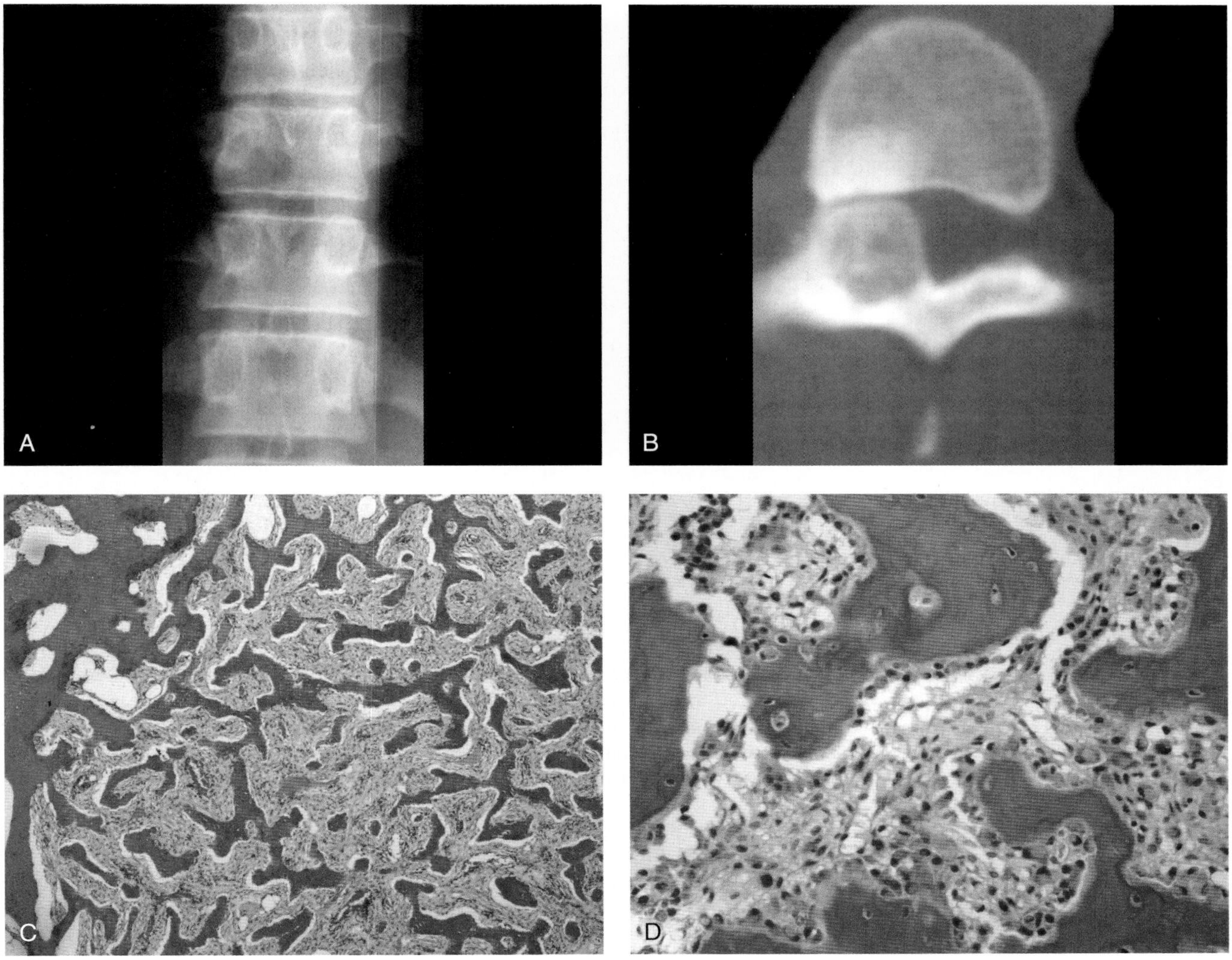

Figure 2 Osteoblastomas. **A**, AP radiograph of the lower portion of the thoracic spine of a 17-year-old boy shows a possible lesion on the right side of T10. **B**, A CT scan of the same patient shown in **A** better shows the location of the osteoblastoma in the pedicle of T10. **C**, The histologic appearance of an osteoblastoma shows interlacing trabeculae surrounded by fibrovascular connective tissue. The tumor merges into the normal bone at the periphery of the lesion. **D**, Higher power magnification shows osteoblastic rimming around the trabecular bone. The osteoblasts can appear plasmacytoid. (Reproduced from Weber KL, Heck RK Jr: Cystic and benign lesions, in Schwartz HS, ed: *Orthopaedic Knowledge Update: Musculoskeletal Tumors*, ed 2. Rosemont, IL, American Academy of Orthopaedic Surgeons, 2007, pp 87-102.)

5. Imaging appearance
    a. Uniform radiodense lesion attached to the outer bone cortex with a broad base ranging from 1 to 8 cm in size (**Figure 3, A**).
    b. Well-defined, with smooth, lobulated borders.
    c. No cortical or medullary invasion; this is best noted on CT scan (**Figure 3, B**).
    d. Radiographic differential diagnosis includes parosteal osteosarcoma, healed stress fracture, and osteoid osteoma.
6. Pathology
    a. Histologic appearance is of mature, hypocellular lamellar bone with intact haversian systems.
    b. No atypical cells are present.
7. Treatment/outcome
    a. Nonsurgical treatment is preferred for incidental or minimally symptomatic lesions.
    b. Biopsy should be performed if the diagnosis is unclear.

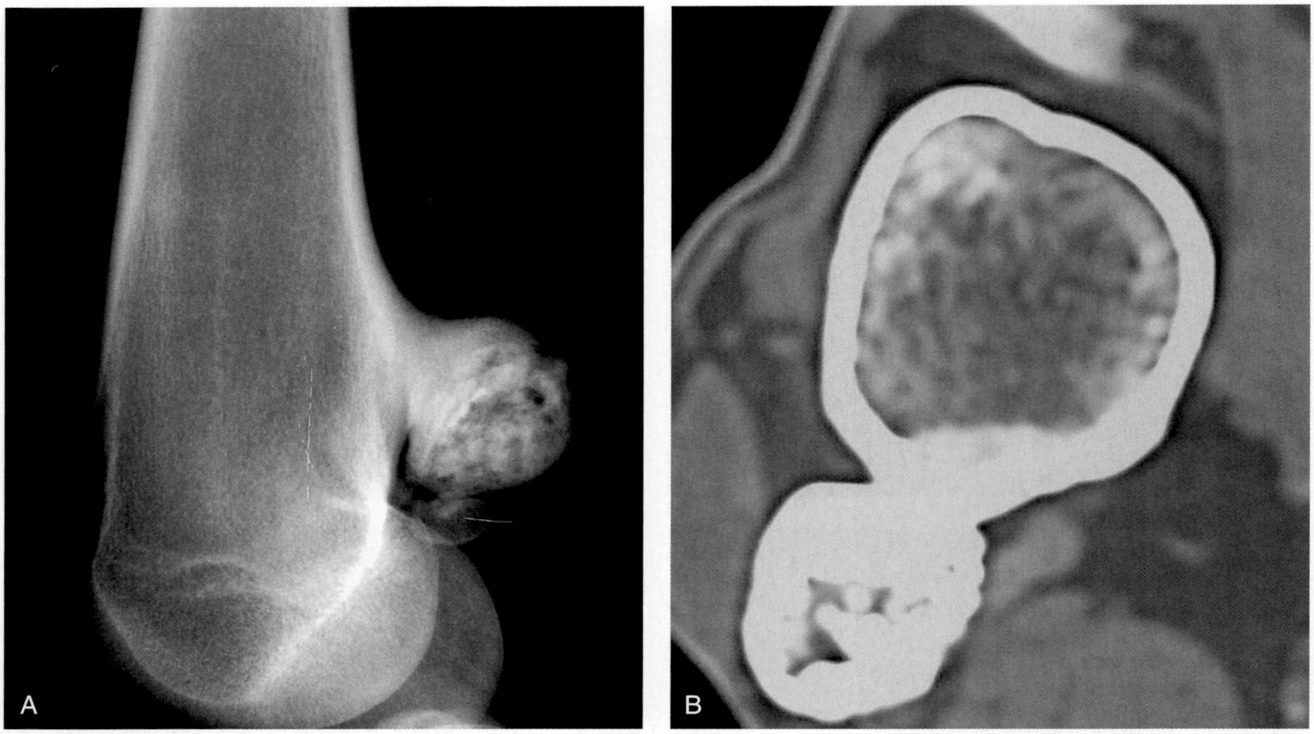

Figure 3 Parosteal osteoma. **A**, Lateral radiograph of the distal femur in a 37-year-old man reveals a heavily ossified surface lesion attached to the posterior femoral cortex. **B**, CT scan of the same patient reveals the relationship of the lesion to the cortex and differentiates it from myositis ossificans. An excisional biopsy revealed a parosteal osteoma.

c. Local recurrence of the lesion suggests it was initially not recognized as a parosteal osteosarcoma.

D. Bone island (enostosis)—A usually small (but occasionally large) deposit of dense, compact bone within the medullary cavity. Bone islands are nontumorous lesions.

1. Demographics—Bone islands occur frequently in adults, but their true incidence is unknown because they are usually found incidentally.
2. Genetics/etiology—Possible arrested resorption of mature bone during endochondral ossification.
3. Clinical presentation
   a. Bone islands are asymptomatic and are found incidentally.
   b. Any bone can be involved, but the pelvis and femur are most common.
   c. Osteopoikilosis is a hereditary syndrome that manifests as hundreds of bone islands throughout the skeleton, usually centered about joints.
4. Radiographic appearance
   a. Well-defined, round focus of dense bone within the medullary cavity, usually 2 to 20 mm in diameter (**Figure 4**)
   b. Occasionally, radiating spicules of bone are present around the lesion that blend with the surrounding medullary cavity.
   c. Approximately one-third of lesions show increased activity on bone scan.
   d. No surrounding bony reaction or edema on T2-weighted MRI.
   e. Low signal intensity on T1- and T2-weighted MRI.
   f. Radiographic differential diagnosis includes well-differentiated or parosteal osteosarcoma, osteoblastic metastasis, and bone infarct.
5. Pathology
   a. Bone islands appear histologically as cortical bone with a well-defined lamellar structure and haversian systems.
   b. The border between the lesion and surrounding medullary bone shows no endochondral ossification.
6. Treatment/outcome—No treatment is required, but follow-up radiographs should be taken if any question about the diagnosis exists.

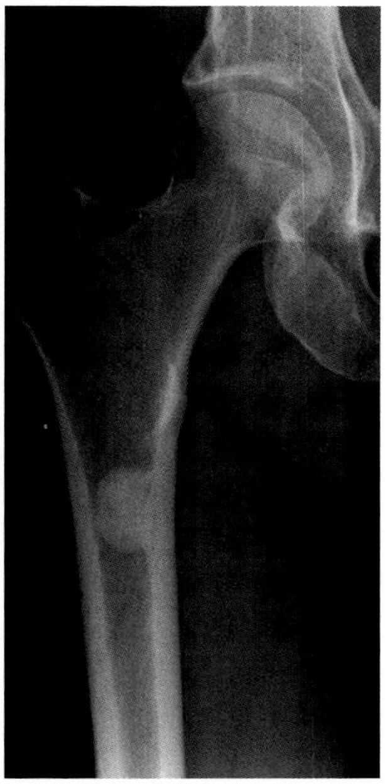

Figure 4 AP radiograph of the hip in an asymptomatic 45-year-old woman with a benign-appearing lesion in the proximal femur consistent with a bone island. (Reproduced from Weber KL, Heck RJ Jr: Cystic and benign bone lesions, in Schwartz HS, ed: *Orthopaedic Knowledge Update: Musculoskeletal Tumors*, ed 2. Rosemont, IL, American Academy of Orthopaedic Surgeons, 2007, p 98.)

II. CARTILAGE

A. Enchondroma—A benign tumor composed of mature hyaline cartilage and located in the medullary cavity.

1. Demographics
   a. Enchondromas can occur at any age, but they are most common in patients 20 to 50 years of age.
   b. The incidence is unclear because most lesions are found incidentally.
2. Genetics/etiology
   a. Thought to be related to incomplete endochondral ossification, in which fragments of epiphyseal cartilage displace into the metaphysis during skeletal growth.
   b. *IDH1* and *IDH2* somatic mutations are reported in most enchondromas.
3. Clinical presentation
   a. Most enchondromas are asymptomatic and are noted incidentally on radiographs.
   b. Lesions in the small bones of the hands and feet can be painful, especially after a pathologic fracture.
   c. In a patient with an enchondroma and pain localized to the adjacent joint, the pain often has a cause that is unrelated to the tumor.
   d. If a patient has pain and the radiographic appearance is concerning, low-grade chondrosarcoma must be considered.
   e. One-half of all enchondromas occur in the small tubular bones, with most in the hands. Enchondroma is the most common bone tumor in the hand.
   f. Other common locations include the metaphysis or diaphysis of long bones (proximal humerus, distal femur, proximal tibia); enchondromas are rare in the spine, pelvis, and chest wall.
   g. Enchondromas are classified by Enneking as inactive or latent bone lesions.
   h. The incidence of high-grade malignant transformation is less than 1%. Rarely, a dedifferentiated chondrosarcoma develops from an enchondroma.
4. Imaging appearance
   a. Enchondromas begin as well-defined, lucent, central medullary lesions that calcify over time
   b. The classic radiographic appearance involves rings and stippled calcifications within the lesion (**Figure 5, A**).
   c. Lesions can be 1 to 10 cm in size.
   d. Minimal endosteal erosion (<50% of the width of the cortex) or cortical expansion may be present.
   e. In hand enchondromas, the cortices may be thinned and expanded (**Figure 5, B**).
   f. Cortical thickening or moderate to extensive cortical destruction suggests a chondrosarcoma.
   g. The radiographic differential diagnosis includes a bone infarct and low-grade chondrosarcoma.
   h. The radiographic appearance is more important than the pathologic appearance in differentiating an enchondroma from a low-grade chondrosarcoma.
   i. Enchondromas frequently have mild increased uptake on bone scans due to continual remodeling of the endochondral bone within the lesion.
   j. MRI is not necessary for diagnosis, but it will show the lesion as lobular and bright on T2-weighted images with no surrounding bone marrow edema or periosteal reaction.

11 | Oncology

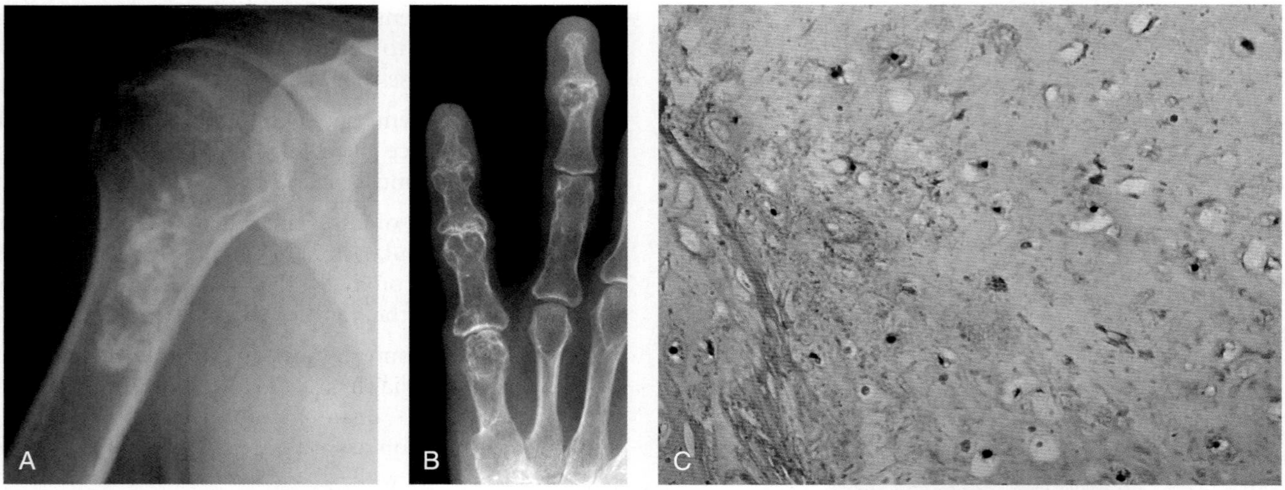

Figure 5 Enchondromas. **A**, AP radiograph of the right proximal humerus in a 49-year-old woman with shoulder pain reveals a calcified lesion in the metaphysis that is centrally located within the bone. The ring-like or stippled calcifications are consistent with an enchondroma. There is no endosteal erosion or cortical thickening. **B**, Radiograph demonstrates enchondromas in the hand of a patient with Ollier disease. Note the multiple expansile lytic lesions affecting the metacarpals and phalanges. Areas of calcified cartilage are evident within the lucent areas. **C**, Histologic appearance of an enchondroma. Note the normal chondrocytes in lacunar spaces with no mitotic figures. (Part C reproduced from Weber KL, O'Connor MI: Benign cartilage lesions, in Schwartz HS, ed: *Orthopaedic Knowledge Update: Musculoskeletal Tumors*, ed 2. Rosemont, IL, American Academy of Orthopaedic Surgeons, 2007, p 111.)

5. Pathology
   a. Gross: blue-gray, lobulated hyaline cartilage with a variable amount of calcification within the tumor.
   b. The low-power histologic appearance is of mature hyaline cartilage lobules separated by normal marrow, which is key to differentiating an enchondroma from a chondrosarcoma.
   c. Endochondral ossification encases the cartilage lobules with lamellar bone.
   d. Lesions in the small tubular bones and proximal fibula are more hypercellular than lesions in other locations.
   e. Enchondromas in long bones have abundant extracellular matrix but no myxoid component.
   f. The cells are bland, with uniform, dark-stained nuclei; they have no pleomorphism, necrosis, mitoses, or multinucleate cells (**Figure 5, C**).
6. Treatment/outcome
   a. Asymptomatic lesions require no treatment and can be followed with serial radiographs to ensure inactivity for a period of time.
   b. Rarely, when pain due to other causes is excluded, symptomatic enchondromas can be treated with curettage and bone grafting.
   c. Pathologic fractures through enchondromas in small, tubular bones can be allowed to heal before consideration of curettage and bone grafting.
   d. Surgery is necessary when clinical presentation and radiographic findings are suspicious for a chondrosarcoma.
   e. A needle biopsy is not reliable to differentiate enchondroma from low-grade chondrosarcoma and should be performed only if confirmation of cartilage tissue type is needed.
7. Related conditions: Ollier disease; Maffucci syndrome
   a. Ollier disease is characterized by multiple enchondromas with a tendency toward unilateral involvement of the skeleton (sporadic inheritance).
   b. Multiple enchondromas are thought to indicate a skeletal dysplasia with failure of normal endochondral ossification throughout the metaphyses of the affected bones.
   c. *IDH1* and *IDH2* mutations are present in patients with Ollier disease and Maffucci syndrome.
   d. Patients with multiple enchondromas have growth abnormalities causing shortening and bowing deformities.

e. Maffucci syndrome involves multiple enchondromas and soft-tissue angiomas.

f. Radiographically, the enchondromas in Ollier disease and Maffucci syndrome have variable mineralization and often expand the bone markedly.

g. The angiomas in Maffucci syndrome can be identified on radiographs because of the presence of phleboliths (small, round, calcified bodies).

h. The histologic appearance of lesions in a patient with multiple enchondromas is similar to solitary lesions in small tubular bones (hypercellular with mild chondrocytic atypia).

i. Patients with multiple enchondromas may require surgical correction of skeletal deformities at a young age.

j. Patients with Ollier disease have an increased risk of malignant transformation of an enchondroma to a low-grade chondrosarcoma (25% to 30%).

k. Patients with Maffucci syndrome have an increased risk of malignant transformation of an enchondroma to a low-grade chondrosarcoma (23% to 100%), as well as a high risk of developing a fatal visceral malignancy.

l. Patients with Ollier disease or Maffucci syndrome should be followed long-term because of the increased chance of malignancy.

B. Periosteal chondroma—A benign hyaline cartilage tumor located on the surface of the bone.

1. Demographics—Periosteal chondromas occur in patients from 10 to 30 years of age.

2. Genetics/etiology—Periosteal chondromas are rare lesions thought to arise from pluripotential cells deep in the periosteum that differentiate into chondroblasts instead of osteoblasts.

3. Clinical presentation

a. Patients usually present with pain; sometimes the lesions are found incidentally in asymptomatic patients.

b. Any bone can be involved, but the proximal humerus, the femur, and the small bones of the hand are the most common locations.

c. The lesions can grow slowly after patients reach skeletal maturity, but they have no malignant potential.

4. Imaging appearance

a. The classic appearance is a well-defined surface lesion that creates a saucerized defect in the underlying cortex (**Figure 6**).

b. The lesion ranges from 1 to 5 cm in size and is metaphyseal or diaphyseal.

c. A rim of sclerosis is seen in the underlying bone.

d. The edges of the lesion often have a mature buttress of bone.

e. The amount of calcification is variable. Soft-tissue swelling may be present because of the surface location.

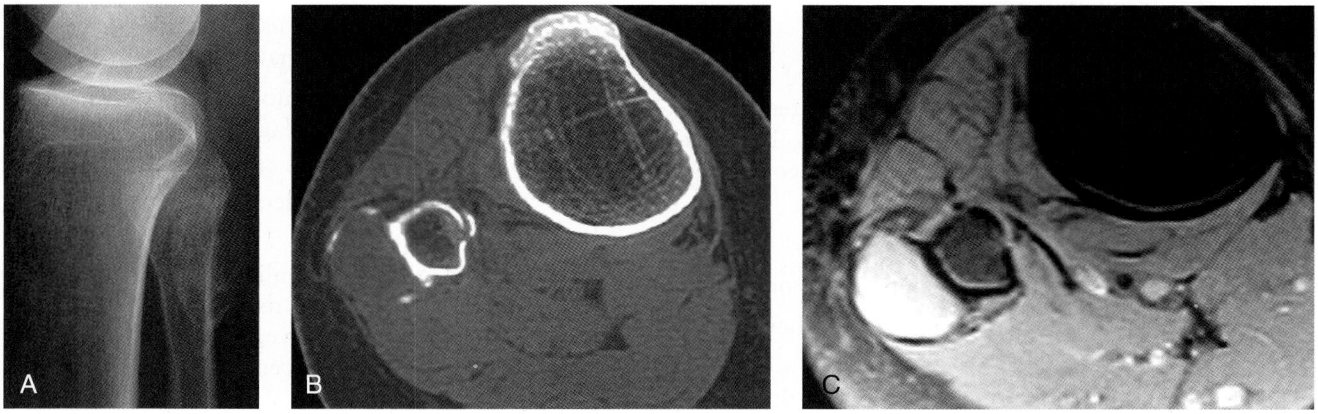

Figure 6 Periosteal chondroma. **A**, Lateral view of the right knee in a 28-year-old woman with lateral calf pain. Extraosseous calcification is seen around the proximal fibula. **B**, Axial CT reveals a surface lesion with a calcified rim and nondisplaced pathologic fracture in the fibula. **C**, T2-weighted MRI reveals bright signal intensity and defines this as a surface lesion without medullary involvement. A biopsy revealed a periosteal chondroma.

f. The radiographic differential diagnosis includes periosteal chondrosarcoma and periosteal osteosarcoma.

5. Pathology
   a. The low-power appearance is of well-circumscribed hyaline cartilage lobules.
   b. The histologic appearance is similar to that of an enchondroma, with mildly increased cellularity, binucleated cells, and occasional mild pleomorphism.

6. Treatment/outcome
   a. No treatment is needed for asymptomatic patients.
   b. Symptomatic patients are treated with excision with an intralesional or marginal margin.
   c. Local recurrence is rare.

C. Osteochondroma—A benign osteocartilaginous tumor arising from the surface of the bone.

1. Demographics
   a. Osteochondromas are the most common benign bone tumor.
   b. The true incidence of osteochondromas is unknown because most lesions are asymptomatic.
   c. Most lesions are identified in the first 2 decades of life.

2. Genetics/etiology
   a. Osteochondromas are hamartomatous proliferations of both bone and cartilage.
   b. They are thought to arise from trapped growth-plate cartilage that herniates through the cortex and grows via endochondral ossification beneath the periosteum.
   c. A defect in the perichondrial node of Ranvier may allow the physeal growth to extend from the surface; as the cartilage ossifies, it forms cortical and cancellous bone that comprises the stalk of the lesion.

3. Clinical presentation
   a. Most lesions are solitary and asymptomatic.
   b. Most are less than 3 cm in size, but they can be as large as 15 cm.
   c. Depending on size and location, patients can have pain from an inflamed overlying bursa, fracture of the stalk, or nerve compression.
   d. When close to the skin surface, osteochondromas can be palpated as firm, immobile masses.
   e. Osteochondromas continue to grow until the patient reaches skeletal maturity.
   f. The lesions most commonly occur around the knee (distal femur, proximal tibia), proximal humerus, and pelvis; spinal lesions (posterior elements) are rare.
   g. A subungual exostosis that arises from beneath the nail in the distal phalanx is a posttraumatic lesion and not a true osteochondroma.
   h. When multiple lesions are present, the condition is called multiple hereditary exostoses.
   i. The risk of malignant degeneration of a solitary osteochondroma to a chondrosarcoma is less than 1%.
   j. Rarely, a dedifferentiated chondrosarcoma can develop from a solitary osteochondroma.

4. Imaging appearance
   a. Osteochondromas can be sessile or pedunculated on the bone surface (**Figure 7, A**).
   b. Sessile lesions are associated with a higher risk of malignant degeneration.
   c. Lesions arise near the epiphyseal plate and appear to become more diaphyseal with time.
   d. Pedunculated lesions grow away from the adjacent joint (**Figure 7, B** and **C**).
   e. The medullary cavity of the bone is continuous with the stalk of the lesion.
   f. The cortex of the underlying bone is continuous with the cortex of the stalk.
   g. The affected bony metaphysis is often flared or widened.
   h. The cartilage cap is usually radiolucent and involutes at skeletal maturity.
   i. Metaplastic cartilage nodules can occur within a bursa over the cartilage cap.
   j. The radiographic differential diagnosis includes parosteal osteosarcoma and myositis ossificans.
   k. CT and MRI can evaluate the cartilage cap and surrounding soft tissues better than plain radiographs and are useful when malignant degeneration is a concern.

5. Pathology
   a. The gross appearance of a pedunculated lesion is similar to that of a cauliflower, with cancellous bone beneath the cartilage cap.

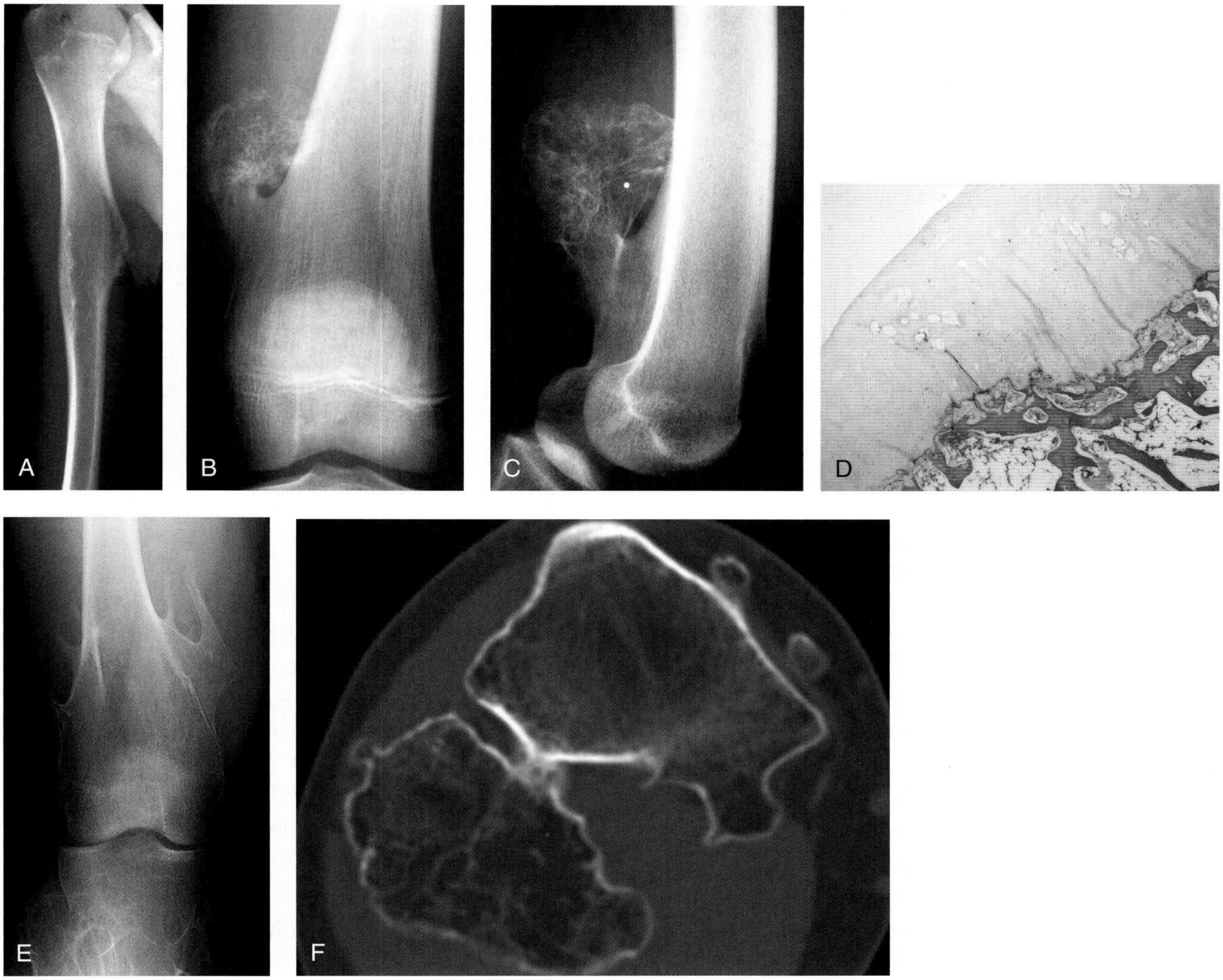

Figure 7 Osteochondromas. **A**, Sessile osteochondroma noted on an AP radiograph of the right humerus in a 14-year-old boy. AP (**B**) and lateral (**C**) radiographs of the distal femur in an 11-year-old boy reveal a pedunculated osteochondroma of the medial distal femur. The medullary portion of the lesional stalk is continuous with the medullary cavity of the distal femur. Note the cortical sharing. **D**, At low-power magnification, the histologic appearance of an osteochondroma shows the cartilage cap with the cartilage cells arranged in columns similar to an epiphyseal plate. **E**, AP radiograph of the right knee in an 18-year-old man with multiple hereditary exostosis. Note the multiple small lesions and the widened metaphysis. **F**, Axial CT scan of the same patient shown in **E** shows the posteromedial extension of a lesion in the proximal fibula. (Part F reproduced from Weber KL, O'Connor MI: Benign cartilage lesions, in Schwartz HS, ed: *Orthopaedic Knowledge Update: Musculoskeletal Tumors*, ed 2. Rosemont, IL, American Academy of Orthopaedic Surgeons, 2007, p 106.)

b. Histologically, the cartilage cap consists of hyaline cartilage and is organized like an epiphyseal plate with maturation to bony trabeculae (**Figure** 7, **D**).

c. A well-defined perichondrium surrounds the cartilage cap.

d. The stalk consists of cortical and trabecular bone, with spaces between the bone filled with marrow.

e. The chondrocytes within the lesion are uniform, without pleomorphism or multiple nuclei.

f. A thick cartilage cap implies growth but is not a reliable indicator of malignant degeneration.

6. Treatment/outcome

a. Nonsurgical treatment is preferred in asymptomatic or minimally symptomatic patients who are still growing.

b. Relative indications for surgical excision of an osteochondroma (performed by excision at the base of the stalk).
   - Symptoms secondary to inflammation of surrounding soft tissues (bursae, muscles, joint capsule, tendons) not controlled by NSAIDs or activity modification
   - Symptoms secondary to frequent traumatic injury
   - Significant aesthetic deformity
   - Symptoms secondary to nerve or vascular compression
   - Concern for malignant transformation

c. The perichondrium over the cartilage cap must be removed to decrease the likelihood of local recurrence.

d. Delaying surgical excision until skeletal maturity increases the chance of local control.

e. The surgeon should be aware that a patient with an osteochondroma extending into the popliteus fossa can have a pseudoaneurysm and is at risk for vascular injury during excision.

7. Related condition: multiple hereditary exostoses

a. Multiple hereditary exostoses is a skeletal dysplasia that is inherited with an autosomal dominant pattern.

b. Patients may have up to 30 osteochondromas throughout the skeleton.

c. *EXT1* and *EXT2* are genetic loci associated with this disorder. Loss of function mutations in these genes are found in most patients affected with the disorder; they are considered tumor-suppressor genes.

d. *EXT1* and *EXT2* proteins function in the biosynthesis of heparan sulfate proteoglycans, which are involved in growth factor signaling in normal epiphyseal plate. Mutations in *EXT1* or *EXT2* result in systemic heparan sulfate deficiency. Osteochondroma development requires a somatic "second hit" that adds to the germline EXT mutation to further decrease heparan sulfate production at perichondrial sites of osteochondroma formation.

e. Clinically, patients with the disorder have skeletal deformities and short stature.

f. The lesions are similar radiographically and histologically to solitary osteochondromas.

g. Radiographs reveal primarily sessile lesions that may grow to be very large.

h. Metaphyseal widening is present in affected patients (**Figure 7, E** and **F**).

i. Deformities occur as a result of disorganized endochondral ossification in the epiphyseal plate and may require surgical correction, especially in the paired bones (radius/ulna, tibia/fibula).

j. The risk of malignant transformation is higher (~5% to 10%) in patients with this condition than in patients with solitary lesions.

k. The most common location of a secondary chondrosarcoma is the pelvis. The malignant tumors are usually low grade and grow slowly.

D. Chondroblastoma—A rare, benign bone tumor differentiated from giant cell tumor by its chondroid matrix.

1. Demographics

a. Male-to-female ratio = 2:1.

b. 80% of patients are younger than 25 years.

2. Genetics/etiology

a. Chondroblastoma has been categorized as a cartilage tumor because of its areas of chondroid matrix, but type II collagen is not expressed by the tumor cells.

b. It is thought to arise from the cartilaginous epiphyseal plate.

3. Clinical presentation

a. Patients present with pain that is progressive at the site of the tumor.

b. Because these tumors often occur adjacent to a joint, decreased range of motion, a limp, muscle atrophy, and tenderness over the affected bone may be present.

c. Most chondroblastomas are found in the distal femur and proximal tibia, followed by proximal humerus, proximal femur, calcaneus, and flat bones.

d. Benign pulmonary metastasis develops from chondroblastoma in less than 1% of patients.

4. Imaging appearance

a. Chondroblastomas are small, round tumors that occur in the epiphysis or apophysis; they can extend into the metaphysis (**Figure 8, A** and **B**).

b. Most are 1 to 4 cm in size, have a sclerotic rim, and are centrally located in the epiphysis.

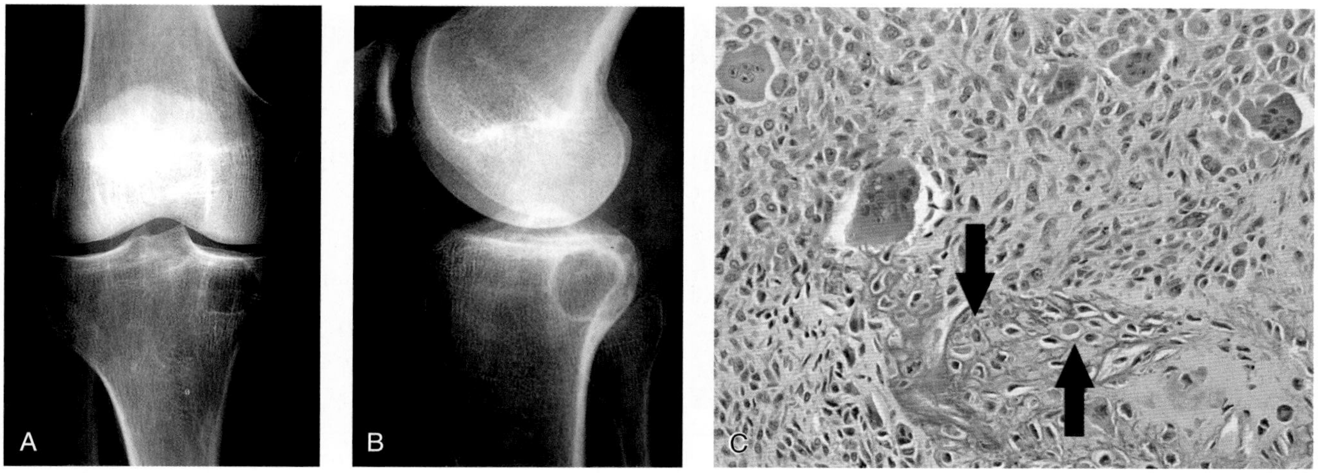

Figure 8 Chondroblastoma. AP (**A**) and lateral (**B**) views of the right knee in a 19-year-old man show a well-circumscribed round lesion in the proximal tibial epiphysis extending slightly into the metaphysis. Note the sclerotic rim. **C**, Histologic appearance of a chondroblastoma. Note the round or oval chondroblasts (arrows). On higher power magnification, areas of dystrophic calcification are visible around the individual cells in a "chicken-wire" pattern. (Part C reproduced from Weber KL, O'Connor MI: Benign cartilage lesions, in Schwartz HS, ed: *Orthopaedic Knowledge Update: Musculoskeletal Tumors*, ed 2. Rosemont, IL, American Academy of Orthopaedic Surgeons, 2007, p 116.)

c. Cortical expansion of the bone may be present, but soft-tissue extension is rare.

d. A small subset has a more aggressive appearance due to secondary ABC formation.

e. Stippled calcifications are seen within the lesion in 25% to 40% of chondroblastomas.

f. The differential diagnosis includes giant cell tumor, osteomyelitis, ganglion cyst, and clear cell chondrosarcoma.

g. Three-dimensional imaging is not required, but a CT scan will define the bony extent of the lesion.

h. MRI shows extensive edema surrounding the lesion.

5. Pathology

a. The tumor consists of a background of mononuclear cells, scattered multinucleate giant cells, and focal areas of chondroid matrix.

b. The mononuclear stromal cells are distinct, round, S100+ cells with large, central nuclei that can appear similar to histiocytes; the nuclei have a longitudinal groove resembling a coffee bean (**Figure 8, C**).

c. Chicken-wire calcifications are present in a lace-like pattern throughout the tumor.

d. Mitotic figures are present but not atypical.

e. One-third of chondroblastomas have areas of secondary ABC.

6. Treatment/outcome

a. Curettage and bone grafting is indicated for the treatment of chondroblastoma.

b. Surgical adjuvants such as phenol, liquid nitrogen, or argon beam coagulation can be used to decrease local recurrence.

c. The local recurrence rate is 10% to 15%.

d. Surgical resection is indicated for the rare cases of benign pulmonary metastasis.

E. Chondromyxoid fibroma (CMF)—A rare, benign cartilage tumor containing chondroid, fibrous, and myxoid tissue.

1. Demographics

a. Most CMFs occur in the second and third decades of life, but they may be seen in patients up to 75 years of age.

b. Slight male predominance.

2. Genetics/etiology—CMF is thought to arise from remnants of the epiphyseal plate.

3. Clinical presentation

a. Most patients present with pain and mild swelling of the affected area.

b. Occasionally, the lesions are noted incidentally on radiographic examination.

c. The most common locations are the long bones of the lower extremities (proximal tibia) and pelvis. Small bones in the hands and feet are also affected.

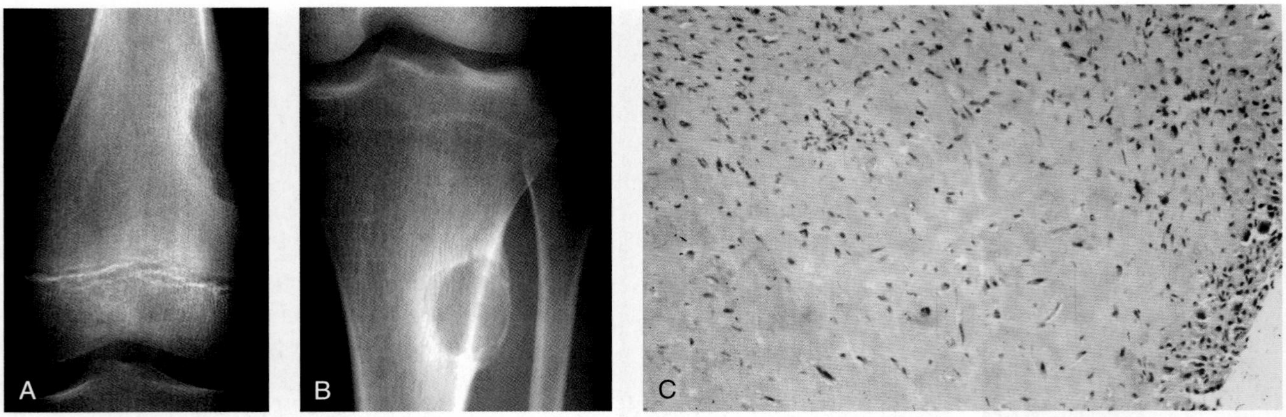

Figure 9 Chondromyxoid fibromas. **A**, AP radiograph of the right distal femur in a 12-year-old boy with knee pain shows an eccentric lytic lesion with a well-defined intramedullary border. A periosteal shell that is not easily seen is consistent with a chondromyxoid fibroma. **B**, AP radiograph of the proximal tibia in a 22-year-old woman with an eccentric lesion expanding the cortex with a visible rim. **C**, The histologic appearance of a chondromyxoid fibroma shows hypercellular regions at the periphery of the lobules. Note the spindled, stellate cells and myxoid stroma.

4. Imaging appearance
   a. CMF is a lucent, eccentric lesion found in the metaphysis of long bones (**Figure 9, A**).
   b. It can cause thinning and expansion of the adjacent cortical bone (**Figure 9, B**).
   c. It often has a sharp, scalloped sclerotic rim.
   d. Radiographic calcifications within the lesion are rare.
   e. CMFs range in size from 2 to 10 cm.
   f. The radiographic differential diagnosis includes ABC, chondroblastoma, and nonossifying fibroma.
   g. Increased tracer uptake is seen within the lesion on bone scan.
5. Pathology
   a. On low-power magnification, the lesion is lobulated, with peripheral hypercellularity.
   b. Within the lobules, the cells are spindled or stellate, with hyperchromatic nuclei.
   c. Multinucleated giant cells and fibrovascular tissue are seen between the lobules.
   d. Areas of myxoid stroma are present, but hyaline cartilage is rare (**Figure 9, C**).
   e. The cellular areas may resemble chondroblastoma.
   f. Areas with pleomorphic cells with bizarre nuclei are common.
   g. The histologic differential diagnosis includes chondroblastoma, enchondroma, and chondrosarcoma.
6. Treatment/outcome
   a. CMF is treated with curettage and bone grafting.
   b. The local recurrence rate is 10% to 20%.

III. FIBROUS/HISTIOCYTIC

A. Nonossifying fibroma (NOF)—A developmental abnormality related to faulty ossification; not a true neoplasm.
1. Demographics
   a. Very common skeletal lesions.
   b. Occur in children and adolescents (age 5 to 15 years).
   c. NOFs are found in 30% of children with open physes.
   d. Also frequently called fibrous cortical defect or metaphyseal fibrous defect.
2. Genetics/etiology—Possibly caused by abnormal subperiosteal osteoclastic resorption during remodeling of the metaphysis.
3. Clinical presentation
   a. Usually an incidental finding
   b. May be multifocal. Types include
      - Familial multifocal
      - Neurofibromatosis
      - Jaffe-Campanacci syndrome (congenital, with cafe-au-lait pigmentation, mental retardation, and nonskeletal abnormalities involving the heart, eyes, and gonads)

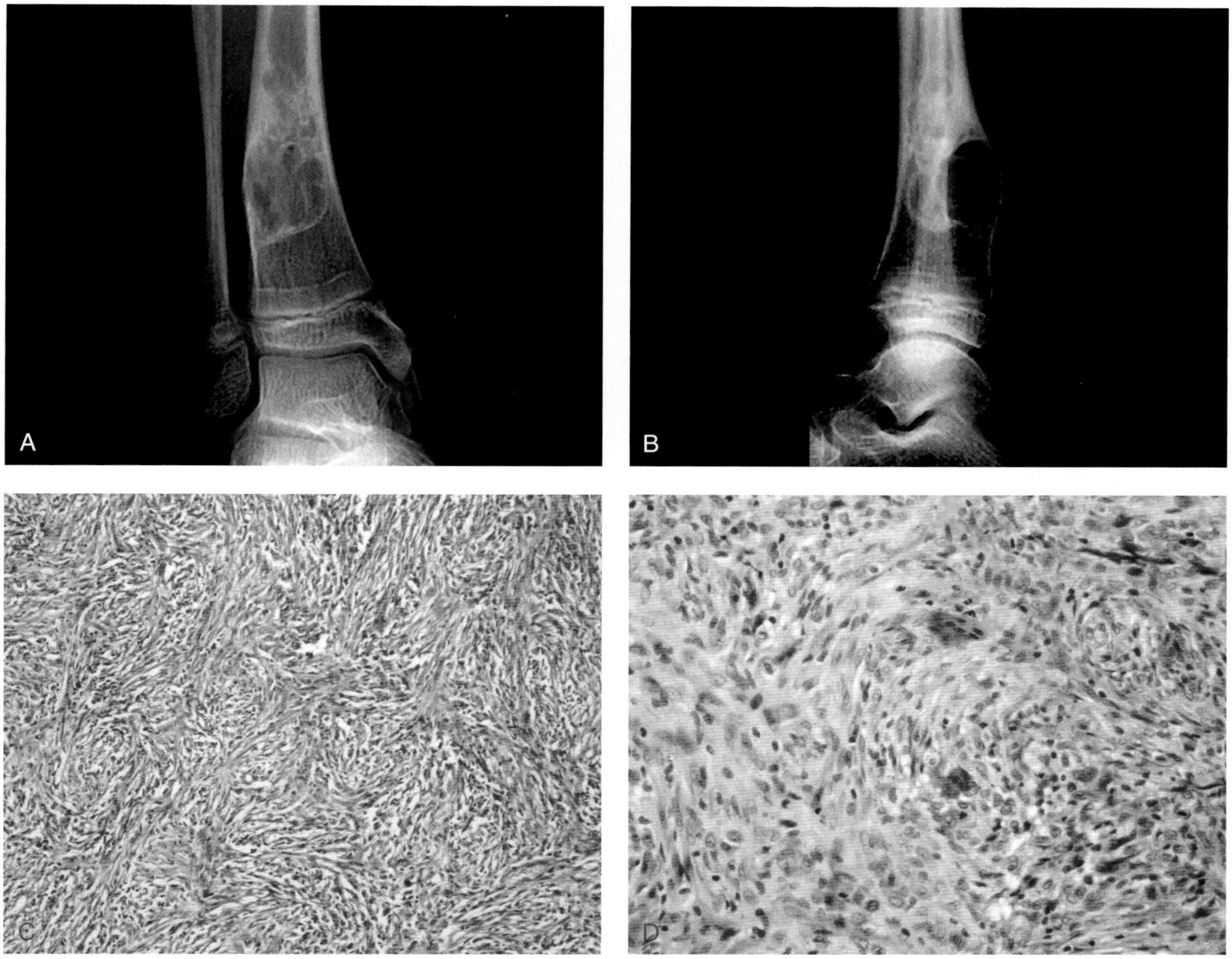

Figure 10 Nonossifying fibromas (NOFs). AP (**A**) and lateral (**B**) radiographs of the distal tibia in an 11-year-old boy reveal an NOF that has healed after a minimally displaced pathologic fracture. It is an eccentric, scalloped lesion with a sclerotic rim. Anteriorly, the lesion is filling in with bone. **C**, Histologic appearance of an NOF. Bands of collagen fibers and fibroblasts can be seen coursing throughout the lesion. **D**, High-power magnification of the same specimen shown in **C** reveals multinucleated giant cells and hemosiderin-laden histiocytes that are characteristic of an NOF. (Parts C and D reproduced from Pitcher JD Jr, Weber KL: Benign fibrous and histiocytic lesions, in Schwartz HS, ed: *Orthopaedic Knowledge Update: Musculoskeletal Tumors*, ed 2. Rosemont, IL, American Academy of Orthopaedic Surgeons, 2007, p 122.)

c. Most common in long bones of lower extremity (80%)

d. Patients occasionally present with a pathologic fracture (more common in the distal tibia)

4. Radiographic appearance

a. Eccentric, lytic, cortically based lesions with a sclerotic rim (**Figure 10, A** and **B**).

b. Occur in the metaphysis and appear to migrate to the diaphysis as bone grows.

c. May thin the overlying cortex with expansion of the bone.

d. Lesions enlarge (1 to 7 cm) as the patient grows.

e. As the patient reaches skeletal maturity, the lesions ossify and become sclerotic.

f. Occasionally associated with secondary ABC.

g. Plain radiographs are diagnostic.

h. An avulsive cortical irregularity is the result of an avulsion injury at the insertion of the adductor magnus muscle on the posteromedial aspect of the distal femur and can be similar in appearance to an NOF.

5. Pathology
   a. Prominent storiform pattern of fibrohistiocytic cells (**Figure 10, C and D**).
   b. Variable numbers of giant cells.
   c. Areas of xanthomatous reaction with foamy histiocytes may be present.
   d. Prominent hemosiderin.
   e. Occasional secondary ABC component.
6. Treatment/outcome
   a. Most are managed with observation; spontaneous regression usually occurs.
   b. Large lesions can be monitored along with skeletal growth.
   c. Curettage and bone grafting may be indicated for symptomatic and large lesions.
   d. Pathologic fractures are often allowed to heal and then are observed or treated with curettage and grafting.
   e. Internal fixation is rarely needed; depends on anatomic location.

B. Fibrous dysplasia—A common developmental abnormality characterized by hamartomatous proliferation of fibro-osseous tissue within the bone.

1. Demographics
   a. Can be seen in patients of any age, but approximately 75% are seen in patients younger than 30 years
   b. Females affected more commonly than males
2. Genetics/etiology
   a. Solitary focal or generalized multifocal inability to produce mature lamellar bone.
   b. Areas of the skeleton remain indefinitely as immature, poorly mineralized trabeculae.
   c. Not inherited.
   d. Monostotic and polyostotic forms are caused by the dominant activating mutations of GSα on chromosome 20q13, which produce a sustained adenylate cyclase–cyclic adenosine monophosphate activation (**Table 2**).
   e. Fibrous dysplasia tissue has high expression of fibroblast growth factor-23, thought to be the cause of hypophosphatemia in patients with McCune-Albright syndrome or oncogenic osteomalacia.
3. Clinical presentation
   a. Usually asymptomatic and found incidentally.
   b. Can be monostotic or polyostotic.

TABLE 2

Characteristic Cytogenetic and Molecular Events of Benign Bone and Soft-Tissue Tumors

Histologic Type	Cytogenetic Events	Molecular Events
Aneurysmal bone cyst	t(16;17)(q22;p13)	*CDH11-USP6* fusion
Nodular fasciitis	t(17;22)(p13;q13)	*MYH9-USP6*
Fibrous dysplasia		*GNAS mutation (α subunit)*
Tenosynovial giant cell tumor	t(1;2)(p13;q35-37)	*COL6A3-CSF1*

Reproduced with permission from *JBJS Reviews* (Wustrack R, Cooper K, Weber K: Molecular markers in bone and soft tissue tumors. *JBJS Rev* 2016;4:1-11).

   c. Can affect any bone but has a predilection for the proximal femur, rib, maxilla, and tibia.
   d. Fatigue fractures through the lesion can cause pain.
   e. Swelling may be present around the lesion.
   f. Severe cranial deformities and blindness with craniofacial involvement may be present.
   g. Patients occasionally present with pathologic fractures.
   h. McCune-Albright syndrome—Triad of polyostotic fibrous dysplasia, precocious puberty, and pigmented skin lesions (with irregular borders likened to the coast of Maine).
      - Unilateral bone lesions
      - Skin lesions usually on the same side as bone lesions
      - The syndrome is present in 3% of patients with polyostotic fibrous dysplasia.
   i. Myriad endocrine abnormalities are associated with polyostotic forms.
   j. Most common entity causing oncogenic osteomalacia (renal phosphate wasting due to fibroblast growth factor-23).
   k. Mazabraud syndrome—Fibrous dysplasia (usually polyostotic) associated with multiple intramuscular myxomas.
      - Females affected more commonly than males
      - Lower limbs more frequently affected

4. Radiographic appearance
   a. Central lytic lesions within the medullary canal, usually diaphysis/metaphysis
   b. Sclerotic rim
   c. May be expansile with cortical thinning
   d. Ground glass or shower-door glass appearance (**Figure 11, A**)
   e. Bowing deformity in proximal femur (shepherd's crook) or tibia
   f. Vertebral collapse and kyphoscoliosis may be seen
   g. Long lesion in a long bone (**Figure 11, B**)
   h. Plain radiographs usually diagnostic
5. Bone scan—Increased activity is seen, but bone scan is not required.
6. Pathology
   a. Gross: yellow-white gritty tissue
   b. Histology: poorly mineralized immature fibrous tissue surrounding islands of irregular, often poorly mineralized trabeculae of woven bone (**Figure 11, C**)
   c. "Chinese letters" or "alphabet soup" appearance
   d. Metaplastic bone arises from fibrous tissue without osteoblastic rimming
   e. Common mitoses
   f. Metaplastic cartilage or areas of cystic degeneration may be present
   g. Can be associated with secondary ABC
   h. Differential diagnosis includes low-grade intramedullary osteosarcoma
7. Treatment/outcome
   a. Asymptomatic patients may be observed.
   b. Surgical indications include painful lesions, impending/actual pathologic fracture, severe deformity, and neurologic compromise (spine).
   c. Surgical treatment: curettage and bone grafting of the lesion. (It is important to use cortical allograft, not cancellous autograft, because cancellous autograft is replaced by dysplastic bone.)
   d. Internal fixation (intramedullary device more effective than plate) usually required to achieve pain control in the lower extremity
   e. Osteotomies for deformity

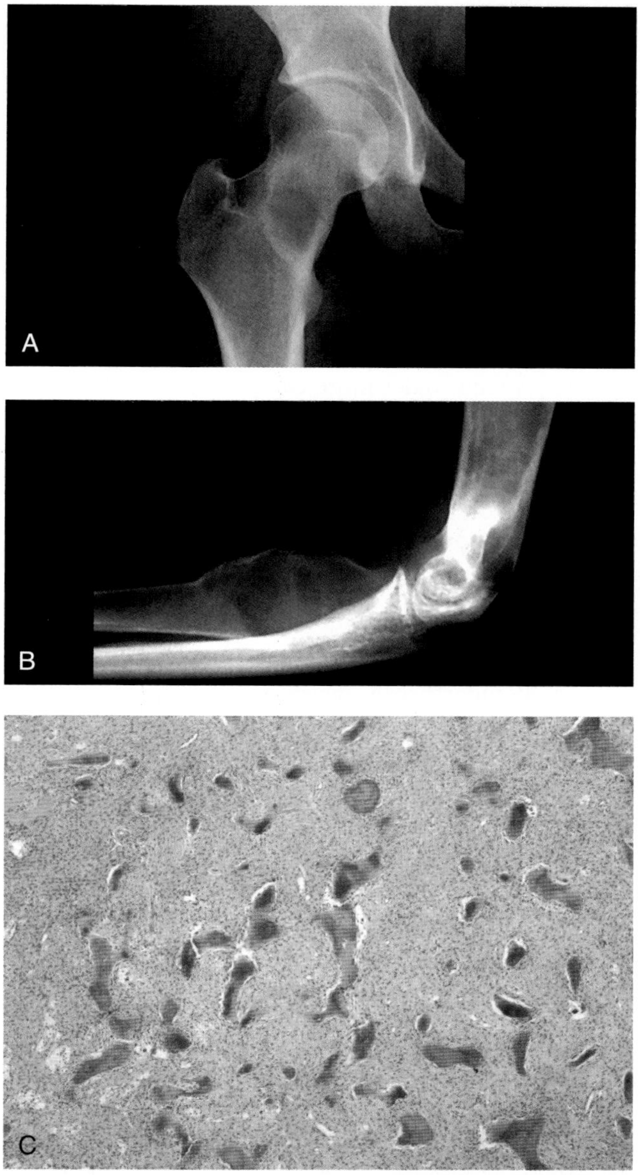

Figure 11 Fibrous dysplasia. **A**, AP radiograph of the right proximal femur in an 18-year-old woman with groin pain. A central, lytic bone lesion with a ground glass appearance fills the femoral neck, consistent with fibrous dysplasia. **B**, A lateral radiograph of an elbow reveals an expansile lesion in the proximal radius with a ground glass appearance. There is no evidence of cortical destruction. **C**, Histologic appearance on intermediate magnification. Metaplastic bone spicules can be seen scattered haphazardly; this pattern produces the characteristic radiographic ground glass appearance of fibrous dysplasia. (Part B reproduced from Prichard DJ, ed: *Musculoskeletal Tumors and Diseases Self-Assessment Examination.* Rosemont, IL, American Academy of Orthopaedic Surgeons, 1999. Part C reproduced from Pitcher JD Jr, Weber KL: Benign fibrous and histiocytic lesions, in Schwartz HS, ed: *Orthopaedic Knowledge Update: Musculoskeletal Tumors*, ed 2. Rosemont, IL, American Academy of Orthopaedic Surgeons, 2007, p 125.)

f. Beneficial long-term outcomes of long-term diphosphonate therapy in most patients with fibrous dysplasia. In approximately 1% of lesions, malignant transformation to osteosarcoma, fibrosarcoma, or undifferentiated pleomorphic sarcoma occurs, with extremely poor prognosis.

C. Osteofibrous dysplasia—A nonneoplastic fibro-osseous lesion affecting the long bones of young children.

1. Demographics
   a. Affects males more commonly than females
   b. Usually noted in the first decade of life
2. Genetics/etiology: Trisomies 7, 8, 12, and 22 have been reported.
3. Clinical presentation
   a. Unique predilection for the tibia.
   b. Anterior or anterolateral bowing deformity may be present.
   c. Pseudarthrosis develops in 10% to 30% of patients.
   d. Patients usually present with painless swelling over the anterior border of the tibia.
4. Radiographic appearance
   a. Eccentric, well-defined anterior tibial lytic lesions (**Figure 12, A**)
   b. Usually diaphyseal
   c. Single or multiple lucent areas surrounded by dense sclerosis
   d. Confined to the anterior cortex; may expand
   e. No periosteal reaction
   f. Differential diagnosis: adamantinoma (radiographic appearance can be identical)
5. Pathology
   a. Moderately cellular fibroblastic stroma
   b. Islands of woven bone with prominent osteoblastic rimming (**Figure 12, B**)
   c. No cellular atypia
   d. May have giant cells
   e. Differential diagnosis: fibrous dysplasia
6. Treatment/outcome
   a. Surgery should be avoided if possible; bracing treatment may be used when necessary.
   b. Lesions may spontaneously regress or stabilize at skeletal maturity.
   c. Deformity correction may be required.
   d. Controversy: whether a continuum exists from osteofibrous dysplasia to adamantinoma; most authors suggest not.

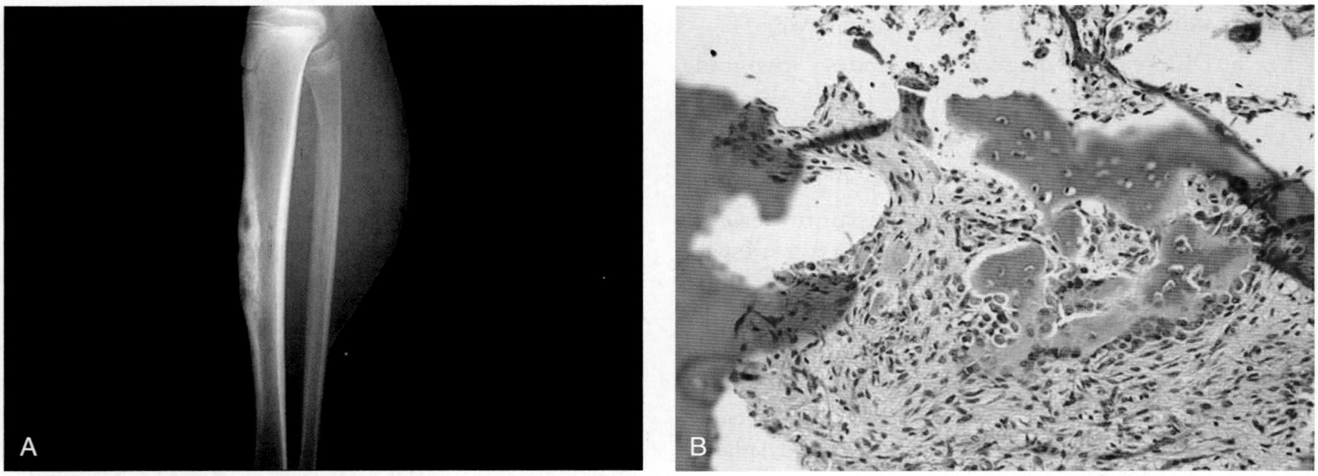

Figure 12 Osteofibrous dysplasia. **A**, Lateral radiograph of the tibia in a skeletally immature patient reveals a cortically based lytic lesion. There are multiple lucencies surrounded by dense sclerosis, consistent with osteofibrous dysplasia. There is no periosteal reaction. **B**, A high-power histologic section reveals woven bone arising from a fibrous stroma. The new bone is prominently rimmed by osteoblasts, thereby differentiating this from fibrous dysplasia. (Reproduced from Scarborough MT, ed: *Musculoskeletal Tumors and Diseases Self-Assessment Examination*. Rosemont, IL, American Academy of Orthopaedic Surgeons, 2005.)

D. Desmoplastic fibroma—An extremely rare benign bone tumor composed of dense bundles of fibrous connective tissue.

1. Demographics—Most common in patients aged 10 to 30 years.
2. Genetics/etiology
   a. Bone counterpart of the aggressive fibromatosis (desmoid) in soft tissue; may originate from myofibroblasts.
   b. Gene loss and rearrangements have been reported.
3. Clinical presentation
   a. Can occur in any bone
   b. Intermittent pain unrelated to activity
   c. Palpable mass/swelling
4. Imaging appearance
   a. Lytic lesion centrally located in metaphysis
   b. Honeycomb/trabeculated appearance (**Figure 13**)
   c. Usually no periosteal reaction unless a fracture is present (12%)
   d. May appear aggressive with cortical destruction and soft-tissue extension
   e. No calcification within lesion
   f. Increased activity on bone scan
5. Pathology
   a. Gross: dense, white, scarlike tissue
   b. Histology: abundant collagen fibrils with intermixed spindle cells

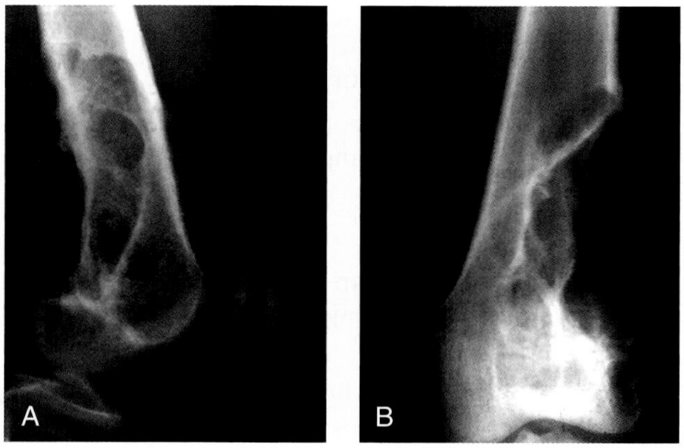

Figure 13 Desmoplastic fibroma. Lateral (**A**) and AP (**B**) radiographs of the distal femur reveal a lytic lesion expanding the posterolateral cortex and having an internal honeycomb appearance. This is consistent with the aggressive behavior of a desmoplastic fibroma.

   c. Appearance is hypocellular and similar to scar tissue
   d. Monotonous, with uniform nuclei
   e. Infiltrative growth pattern, trapping native trabeculae
   f. Differential diagnosis includes low-grade fibrosarcoma
6. Treatment/outcome
   a. Surgical treatment is the standard of care.
   b. Thorough curettage allows good results.
   c. Wide resection is used for expendable bones, extensive cortical destruction or locally recurrent lesions.
   d. Tumors do not metastasize but often recur locally.

E. Langerhans cell histiocytosis (LCH)—A rare clonal disease characterized by the proliferation of CD1a-positive immature dendritic cells; can have varied clinical presentations.

1. Demographics
   a. Most common in children (80% younger than 20 years)
   b. Male-to-female ratio = 2:1
2. Genetics/etiology: Presence of oncogenic BRAF mutations and proinflammatory cytokines and chemokines
3. Clinical presentation
   a. Previously categorized as eosinophilic granuloma, Hand-Schüller-Christian disease (chronic, disseminated), and Letterer-Siwe disease (infantile, acute).
   b. Now believed to be three types.
      - Solitary disease (eosinophilic granuloma)
      - Multiple bony sites
      - Multiple bony sites with visceral involvement (lungs, liver, spleen, skin, lymph nodes)
   c. Rarely, bone lesions are asymptomatic; usually, they cause localized pain/swelling/limp.
   d. Can occur in any bone; most commonly, the skull, ribs, clavicle, scapula, vertebrae (thoracic > lumbar > cervical), long bones, and pelvis.
4. Radiographic appearance
   a. Classic appearance: "punched-out" lytic lesion (**Figure 14, A**)
   b. May have thick periosteal reaction

11 | Oncology

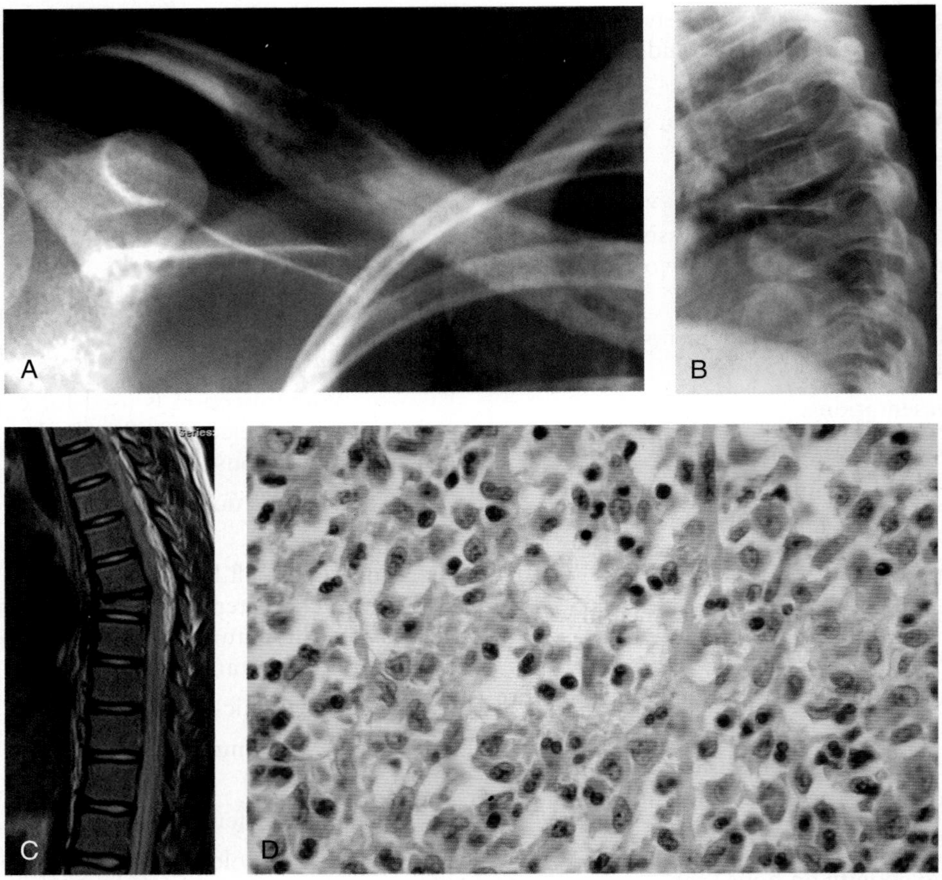

Figure 14 Eosinophilic granulomas/Langerhans cell histiocytosis. **A**, AP radiograph of a lytic lesion in the right clavicle of a child demonstrates cortical expansion, periosteal reaction, and no sclerotic edges. This is an eosinophilic granuloma, but the radiographic appearance can also be consistent with osteomyelitis or Ewing sarcoma. **B**, A lateral radiograph of the thoracic spine shows the classic appearance of vertebra plana in a patient with eosinophilic granuloma. **C**, MRI appearance of a patient with thoracic vertebra plana which improves with bracing treatment in most patients. **D**, Histologic appearance of an eosinophilic granuloma shows a mixed inflammatory infiltrate with Langerhans histiocytes having large indented nuclei, lymphocytes, and eosinophils.

   c. Can appear well-demarcated or permeative (**Figure 14, B**)
   d. Commonly causes vertebral collapse (vertebra plana) when affecting the spine (**Figure 14, C**)
   e. Great mimicker of other lesions (osteomyelitis, Ewing sarcoma, leukemia)

5. Pathology
   a. The characteristic tumor cell is the Langerhans cell or histiocyte (**Figure 14, D**).
   b. Histiocytes have indented nuclei (“coffee bean” appearance) and eosinophilic cytoplasm.
   c. Histiocytes stain with CD1a.
   d. Giant cells are present.
   e. Eosinophils are variable in number.
   f. Mixed inflammatory cell infiltrate.
   g. Birbeck granules (“tennis racket” appearance) seen in Langerhans cells on electron microscopy.

6. Treatment/outcome
   a. Solitary lesions can be treated effectively with an intralesional injection of methylprednisolone acetate.
   b. Curettage and bone grafting is reasonable if open biopsy is being performed for diagnosis.
   c. In 90% of patients with vertebra plana caused by Langerhans cell histiocytosis, bracing treatment alone will correct the deformity; 10% will need corrective surgery.

TABLE 1

Characteristic Cytogenetic and Molecular Events of Primary Bone Sarcomas

Histologic Type	Cytogenetic Events	Molecular Events
Chondrosarcoma of bone	Complex	*IDH1* and *IDH2* mutations
Ewing sarcoma	t(11;22)(q24;q12) t(21;22)(q22;q12) t(2;22)(q35;q12) t(7;22)(p22;q12) t(17:22)(q21;q12) inv((22)(p36;q12)) t(16;21)(p11;q22) t(2:16)(q35;p11) t(20;22)(q13;q12) t(6;22)(p21;q12) t(4;22)(q31;q12) t(2;22)(q31:q12) t(4;19)(q35:q13)	*EWSR1-FLI1* fusion *EWSR1-ERG* fusion *EWSR1-FEV* fusion *EWSR1-ETV1* fusion *EWSR1-E1AF* fusion *EWSR1-ZSG* *FUS-ERG* *FUS-FEV* *EWSR1-NFATC2* *EWSR1-POU5F1* *EWSR1-SMARCA5* *EWSR1-SP3* *CIC-DUX4*
Ewing-like sarcoma	t(X;X)(p11;p11)	*BCOR-CCNB3*
Mesenchymal chondrosarcoma	t(8;8)(q13;q21)	*HEY1-NCOA2*
Osteosarcoma:		
Low-grade central	Simple	*MDMD2* and *CDK4* amplification
Parosteal	Ring chromosomes	12q13-15 amplification
High grade	Complex	*MDMD2* and *CDK4* amplification

Reproduced with permission from JBJS Reviews (Wustrack R, Cooper K, Weber K: Molecular markers in bone and soft tissue tumors. *JBJS Rev* 2016;4:1-11).

d. Osteosarcoma is defined by the presence of malignant osteoid.

e. Extensive pleomorphism and numerous mitotic figures are present.

f. Areas of necrosis, cartilage, or giant cells may be present within the lesion.

g. The histologic differential diagnosis includes fibrous dysplasia.

6. Treatment/outcome

a. The standard treatment of osteosarcoma is neoadjuvant chemotherapy followed by surgical resection (limb-sparing or amputation), followed by additional adjuvant chemotherapy.

b. The most common chemotherapy agents include adriamycin (doxorubicin), cisplatinum, methotrexate, and ifosfamide (**Table 2**).

c. Radiation plays no role in the standard treatment of osteosarcoma, although it is used for palliative control in inoperable primary tumors or metastatic sites.

d. Limb-sparing surgery is performed in 90% of cases.

e. Patients who present with a pathologic fracture can be treated with limb-salvage surgery but have a higher risk of local recurrence if the fracture is widely displaced.

f. Local recurrence after surgical resection is approximately 5%; these patients have a dismal prognosis.

g. Good histologic response and wide surgical margins are associated with a low risk of local recurrence.

h. The most common reconstructive options depend on patient age and tumor location and include metal prostheses, intercalary allografts, allograft-prosthetic composites, expandable prostheses, and vascularized fibular autografts.

i. Tumor stage is the most important prognostic indicator.

j. The percentage of necrosis within the tumor after neoadjuvant chemotherapy is related to overall survival (>90% necrosis is associated with significantly increased survival).

k. Elevated lactate dehydrogenase (LDH) and alkaline phosphatase have been reported to

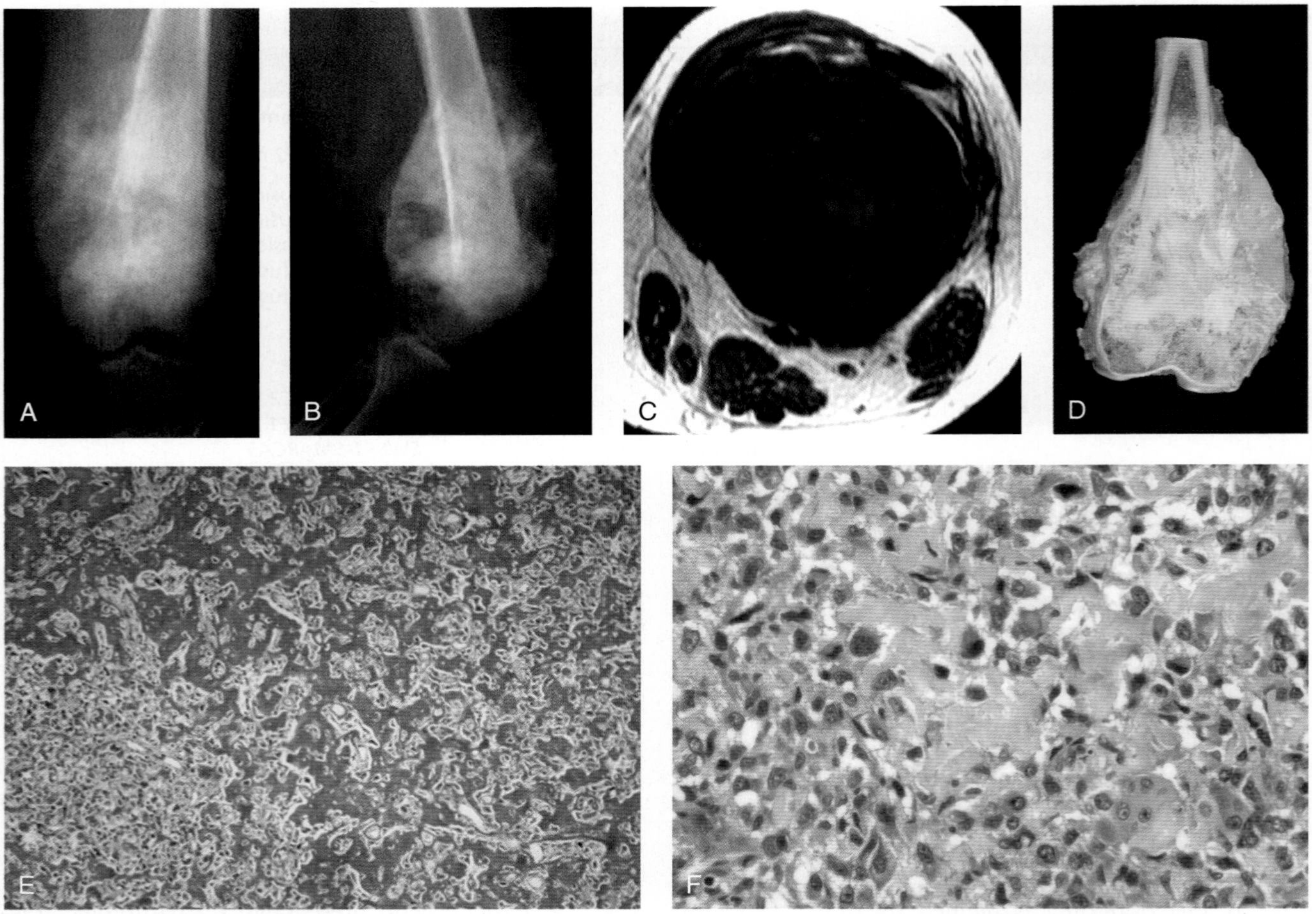

Figure 1 Osteosarcoma of the left distal femur in a 15-year-old boy. AP (**A**) and lateral (**B**) radiographs demonstrate extensive bone formation and an ossified soft-tissue mass after several cycles of chemotherapy. **C**, Axial T1-weighted MRI reveals an extensive circumferential soft-tissue mass abutting the neurovascular bundle posteriorly. **D**, Gross specimen after distal femoral resection shows a clear proximal margin and tumor extending into the epiphysis. **E**, Low-power histologic image shows the classic osteoid formed by malignant stromal cells. Note the lacelike pattern. **F**, High-power histologic image reveals the pleomorphic cells producing the new bone. (Panel E reproduced from Scarborough MT, ed: *2005 Musculoskeletal Tumors and Diseases Self-Assessment Examination*. Rosemont, IL, American Academy of Orthopaedic Surgeons, 2005.)

be poor prognostic factors, as is overexpression of vascular endothelial growth factor (VEGF).

l. Survival
- The 5-year survival of patients with localized osteosarcoma in an extremity is 70%.
- The 5-year survival of patients with localized pelvic osteosarcoma is 25%.
- The 10-year overall survival of patients with metastatic disease is 25%.
- Intensifying treatment in response to poor prognostic variables allows no improvement in outcome.
- Overall survival has remained constant for several decades.

m. The most common site of metastasis is the lungs (61%), followed by the bones (16%).
- Aggressive treatment of late (>1 year) pulmonary metastasis with thoracotomy allows 5-year survival of approximately 30%.
- Patients with bone metastasis usually die of the disease.

n. Skip lesions occur in 10% of patients; the prognosis in these patients is similar to that of patients with lung metastasis.

B. Osteosarcoma subtypes

1. Parosteal osteosarcoma

a. Definition and demographics
- Low-grade surface osteosarcoma composed of dense bone

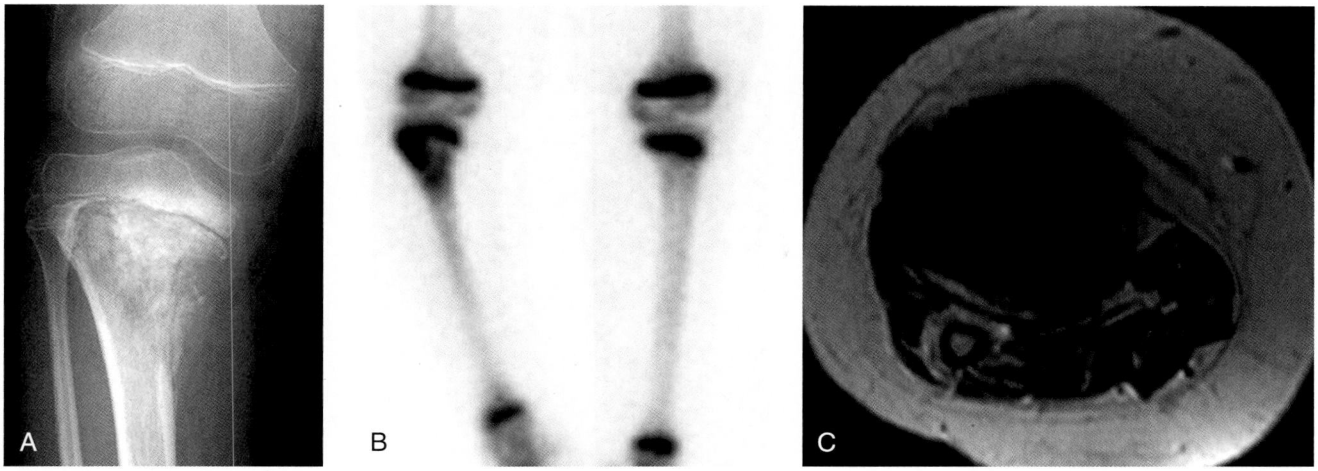

Figure 2 Osteosarcoma of the right proximal tibia in an 8-year-old boy. **A**, AP radiograph demonstrates collapse of the medial cortex with a minimally displaced fracture. Both bone destruction and formation are seen. **B**, Technetium Tc-99m bone scan reveals avid uptake in the area of the tumor. **C**, Axial T1-weighted MRI reveals a small, medial soft-tissue mass.

- Female-to-male ratio = 2:1
- Accounts for 5% of all osteosarcomas
- Most patients are 20 to 45 years of age

b. Clinical presentation

- Classic presentation is swelling of long duration (often, years).
- Pain, limited joint range of motion, and limp all vary.
- The most common location is the posterior aspect of the distal femur (75%), followed by the proximal tibia and the proximal humerus.

TABLE 2

Chemotherapy Drugs Used in the Treatment of Osteosarcoma

Drug	Mechanism of Action	Major Toxicities
Adriamycin/ doxorubicin	Blocks DNA/RNA synthesis Inhibits topoisomerase II	Cardiotoxicity
Cisplatinum	DNA disruption by covalent binding	Hearing loss Neuropathy Renal failure
Methotrexate	Inhibits dihydrofolate reductase (inhibits DNA synthesis)	Mucositis
Ifosfamide	DNA-alkylating agent	Renal failure Encephalopathy

c. Imaging

- Dense, lobulated lesion on the surface of the bone (**Figure 3**, A).
- Underlying cortical thickening may be seen.
- Attachment to the cortex may be broad.
- Minor intramedullary involvement is occasionally seen.
- The tumor is most dense in the center and least ossified peripherally.
- Radiographic differential diagnosis includes myositis ossificans and osteochondroma.
- MRI or CT is helpful in defining the lesional extent before surgery (**Figure 3**, B).
- Dedifferentiated parosteal osteosarcoma has ill-defined areas on the surface of the lesion and hypervascularity on angiographic studies.

d. Pathology

- Regular, ordered osseous trabeculae (**Figure 3**, D and E).
- Bland, fibrous stroma with occasional slightly atypical cells (grade 1).
- Dedifferentiated parosteal osteosarcoma contains a high-grade sarcoma juxtaposed to the underlying low-grade lesion.

e. Treatment/outcome

- Wide surgical resection is the treatment of choice (**Figure 4**).
- High risk of local recurrence with inadequate resection.

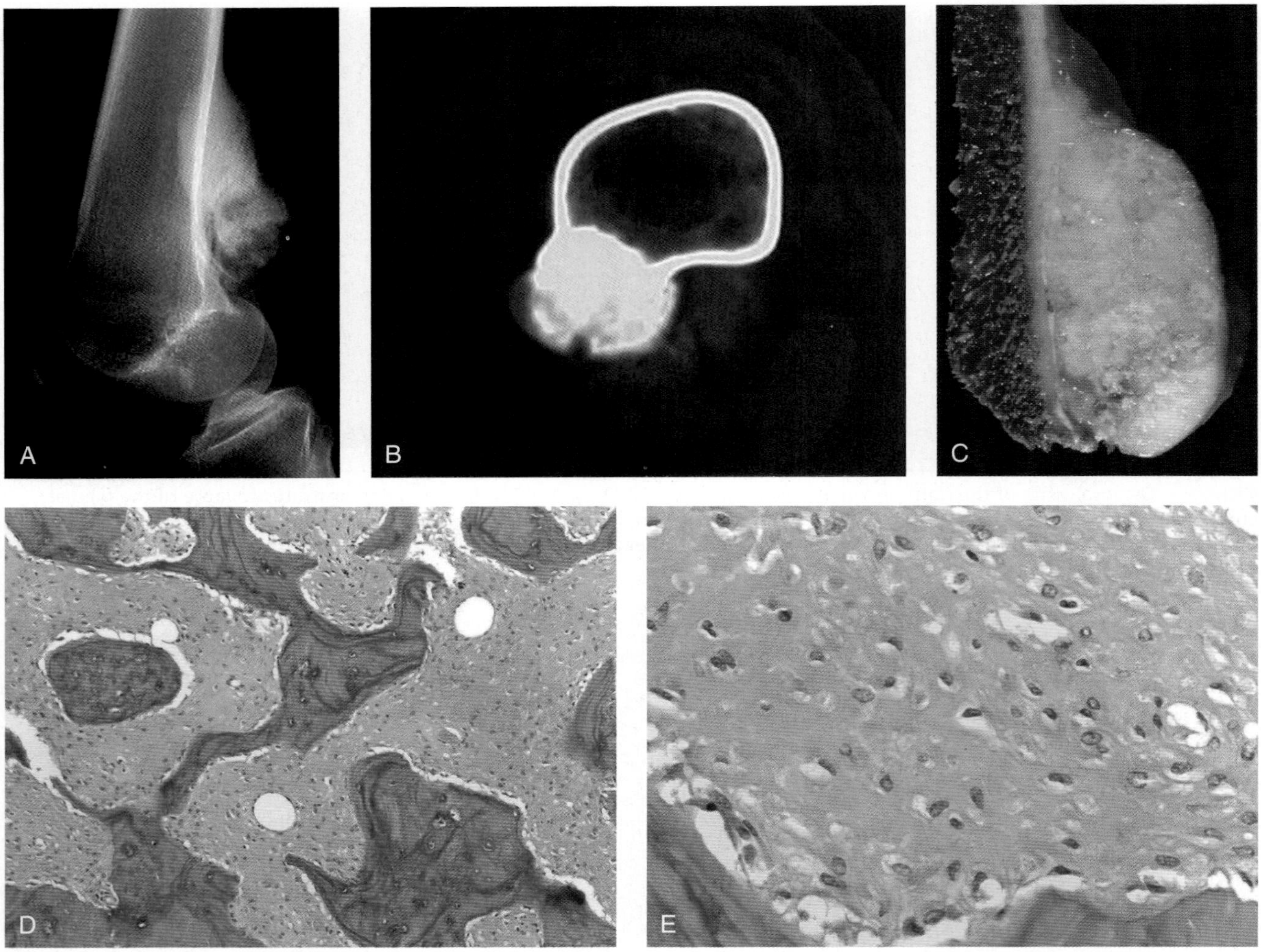

Figure 3 Parosteal osteosarcoma of the distal femur. **A**, Lateral radiograph of the knee reveals a densely ossified surface lesion on the posterior distal femur that is consistent with a parosteal osteosarcoma. **B**, CT scan demonstrates the relationship between the tumor and the femoral cortex. **C**, Gross specimen confirms that it is truly a surface osteosarcoma. **D**, Low-power histologic image reveals a bland appearance with regular, ordered, dense trabeculae and interspersed fibrous stroma. **E**, Higher power histologic image reveals minimal cellular atypia. (Panel A reproduced from Scarborough MT, ed: *2005 Musculoskeletal Tumors and Diseases Self-Assessment Examination*. Rosemont, IL, American Academy of Orthopaedic Surgeons, 2005.)

- Often, the knee joint can be maintained after resection of the lesion and posterior cortex of the femur.
- Survival is 95% if wide resection is achieved.
- Dedifferentiated variants occur in 25% of patients and are more common after multiple low-grade recurrences; survival is 50%.

2. Periosteal osteosarcoma
   a. Definition and demographics
      - Intermediate-grade surface osteosarcoma.
      - Occurs in patients 15 to 25 years of age.
      - Extremely rare.
   b. Clinical presentation
      - Pain is the most common presenting symptom.
      - Most commonly occurs in the femoral or tibial diaphysis.
   c. Imaging
      - Lesion has a sunburst periosteal elevation in the diaphysis of long bones (**Figure 5**, A).
      - The underlying cortex may be saucerized.
      - No involvement of the medullary canal.
   d. Pathology
      - Gross appearance is lobular and cartilaginous (**Figure 5**, B).

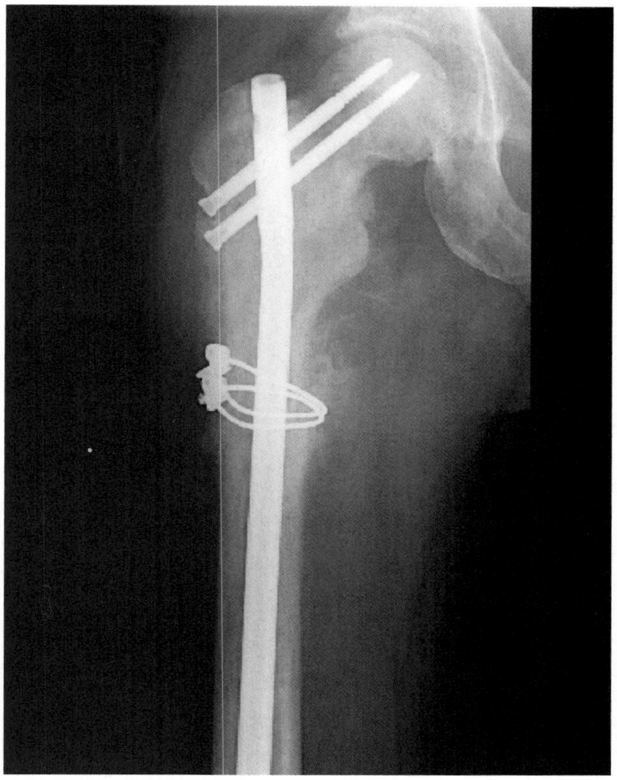

Figure 4 Radiograph shows the proximal femur of a 43-year-old man who was assumed to have metastatic disease; an intramedullary rod was placed in the right femur. Note the osteoblastic appearance of the proximal femur. A later biopsy obtained after continued pain revealed an osteosarcoma. The patient required a hindquarter amputation. This case highlights the importance of a preoperative biopsy.

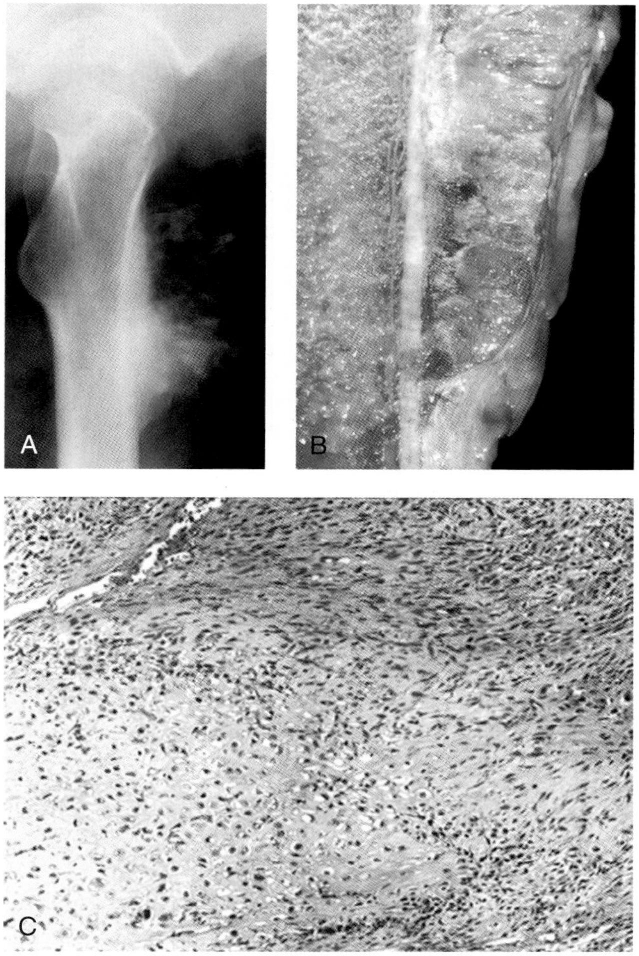

Figure 5 Periosteal osteosarcoma. **A**, Radiograph demonstrates a lesion in the proximal femur. **B**, Gross pathology. **C**, The histologic image reveals a lobular cartilaginous lesion with moderate cellularity. From this appearance, a malignant cartilage lesion would be suspected. One area reveals osteoid production confirming the diagnosis of periosteal osteosarcoma, which is typically chondroblastic in appearance. (Reproduced from Hornicek FJ: Osteosarcoma of bone, in Schwartz HS, ed: *Orthopaedic Knowledge Update: Musculoskeletal Tumors*, ed 2. Rosemont, IL, American Academy of Orthopaedic Surgeons, 2007, p 167.)

- Histology reveals extensive areas of chondroblastic matrix, but the tumor produces osteoid (**Figure 5**, C).
- Without any osteoid production, the lesion would be a chondrosarcoma.
- Cellular appearance is grade 2 to 3.

e. Treatment/outcome

- Controversial whether to use chemotherapy; the more common current treatment is neoadjuvant chemotherapy followed by wide surgical resection followed by additional chemotherapy.
- Ten-year survival of 77% with surgical resection with or without chemotherapy.
- Metastasis develops in 25% of patients.

3. High-grade surface osteosarcoma

a. Definition—Rare, high-grade variant of osteosarcoma that occurs on the bone surface.

b. Demographics, genetics, etiology, clinical presentation, and pathology are the same as for classic osteosarcoma (see Section I.A).

c. Radiographic appearance

- Similar to the appearance of a classic osteosarcoma except that high-grade surface osteosarcoma occurs solely on the cortical surface.
- No intramedullary involvement.

4. Telangiectatic osteosarcoma

a. Definition—Rare histologic variant of osteosarcoma containing large, blood-filled spaces.

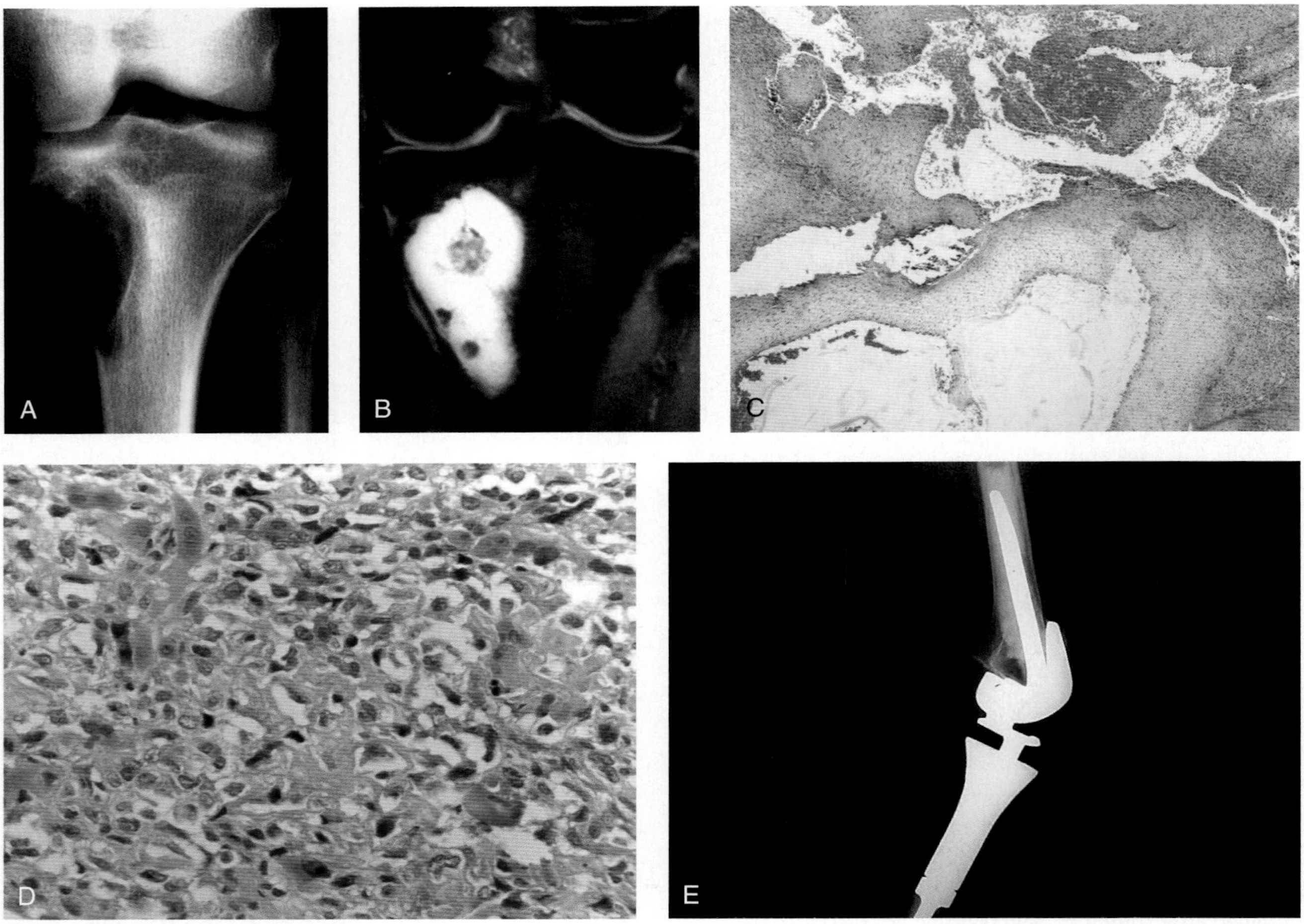

Figure 6 Telangiectatic osteosarcoma. **A**, AP radiograph of the knee of a 14-year-old girl reveals an osteolytic lesion in the medial aspect of the left proximal tibia. The differential diagnosis includes telangiectatic osteosarcoma and aneurysmal bone cyst. **B**, Coronal T2-weighted MRI reveals a lesion of high signal intensity, but no fluid levels are seen. **C**, Low-power histologic image reveals large blood-filled spaces with intervening fibrous septa. **D**, High-power histologic image is required to determine that this is a telangiectatic osteosarcoma with pleomorphic osteoblasts producing osteoid. **E**, Postoperative lateral radiograph obtained after wide resection of the proximal tibia and reconstruction with a modular proximal tibial endoprosthesis. (Panels A and B reproduced from Scarborough MT, ed: *2005 Musculoskeletal Tumors and Diseases Self-Assessment Examination*. Rosemont, IL, American Academy of Orthopaedic Surgeons, 2005.)

b. Demographics, genetics/etiology, clinical presentation
   - Similar to classic osteosarcoma.
   - Rare (only 4% of all osteosarcomas).
   - Twenty-five percent of patients present with pathologic fracture.

c. Imaging
   - Purely lytic lesion that occasionally obliterates entire cortex (**Figure 6**).
   - Differential diagnosis primarily includes aneurysmal bone cyst (ABC).
   - Osteosarcoma has more intense uptake than ABC on bone scan.
   - MRI may show fluid-fluid levels and extensive surrounding edema.

d. Pathology
   - Grossly, the tumor is described as a “bag of blood.”
   - Histology shows large blood-filled spaces (**Figure 6**, C).
   - Intervening septa contain areas of high-grade sarcoma with atypical mitoses (**Figure 6**, D).
   - May produce only minimal osteoid.

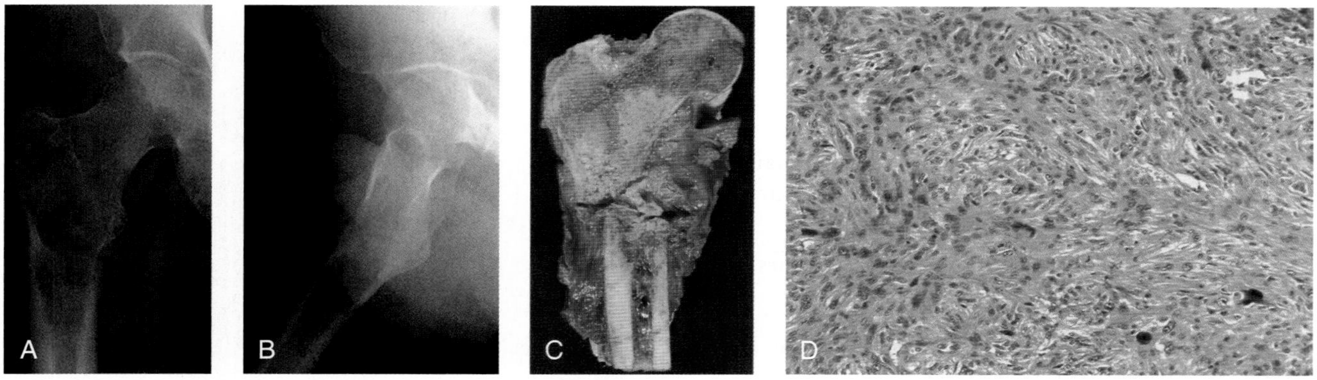

Figure 7 Undifferentiated pleomorphic sarcoma (UPS). AP (**A**) and lateral (**B**) radiographs of the hip of a 43-year-old man with a destructive lesion in the intertrochanteric region of the right femur. A needle biopsy revealed UPS of bone. The patient sustained a pathologic fracture during preoperative chemotherapy. **C**, Gross specimen after proximal femoral resection and reconstruction with a modular endoprosthesis. **D**, Histologic image reveals a storiform pattern with marked pleomorphism and a few multinucleated cells.

- Occasionally contains benign giant cells.
- Differential diagnosis: primarily ABC.

e. Treatment/outcome—Same as classic osteosarcoma (see Section I.A.6).

II. FIBROUS/HISTIOCYTIC TUMORS

A. Undifferentiated pleomorphic sarcoma

1. Definition and demographics
    a. Primary malignant bone tumor similar to osteosarcoma but with histiocytic differentiation and no osteoid (**Figure** 7).
    b. Occurs in patients 20 to 80 years of age (most older than 40 years).
    c. Slight male predominance.
2. Genetics/etiology—25% of cases occur as secondary lesions in the setting of a bone infarct, Paget disease, or prior radiation.
3. Clinical presentation
    a. Pain is the primary symptom, followed by swelling, limp, decreased range of motion, and pathologic fracture.
    b. Undifferentiated pleomorphic sarcoma of bone most commonly occurs in the metaphyses of long bones, primarily the distal femur, proximal tibia, and proximal humerus.
4. Imaging
    a. Lytic, destructive lesion with variable periosteal reaction (**Figure** 7, A and B).
    b. No bone production.
    c. Cortical destruction with a soft-tissue mass is often seen.
    d. Appearance is often nonspecific; the differential diagnosis includes any malignant bone tumor or metastasis.
5. Pathology
    a. Storiform appearance with marked pleomorphism and mitotic figures (**Figure** 7, D)
    b. Fibrous fascicles radiate from focal hypocellular areas
    c. Multinucleated tumor cells with histiocytic nuclei (grooved)
    d. Areas of chronic inflammatory cells
    e. Variable collagen production
6. Treatment/outcome
    a. Undifferentiated pleomorphic sarcoma of bone is treated similarly to osteosarcoma, with neoadjuvant chemotherapy, wide surgical resection, and postoperative chemotherapy.
    b. As with osteosarcoma, reconstructive options depend on patient age and tumor location but include metal prostheses, intercalary allografts, allograft-prosthetic composites, expandable prostheses, and vascularized fibular autografts.
    c. Survival is slightly worse than for osteosarcoma, with metastasis primarily to the lung and bones.
    d. Secondary undifferentiated pleomorphic sarcoma in a preexisting lesion has a worse prognosis than primary undifferentiated pleomorphic sarcoma.

11 | Oncology

III. CARTILAGE TUMORS

A. Chondrosarcoma

1. Definition and demographics
   a. Classic chondrosarcoma is a malignant cartilage-producing bone tumor that arises de novo or secondary to other lesions.
   b. Occurs in adult patients (40 to 75 years).
   c. Slight male predominance.
   d. Central (intramedullary) and surface lesions occur with equal frequency.
   e. Incidence
      - Grade 1 = 60%
      - Grade 2 = 25%
      - Grade 3 = 5%
      - Dedifferentiated = 10%
2. Genetics/etiology—mutations of isocitrate dehydrogenase 1 and 2 (IDH1 and IDH2) identified in primary and secondary central chondrosarcomas and enchondromas
3. Clinical presentation
   a. Pain of prolonged duration (lesional pain can differentiate low-grade chondrosarcoma from benign enchondroma).
   b. Slow-growing firm mass (surface lesion).
   c. Bowel/bladder symptoms may develop with large pelvic lesions.
   d. Most common locations, in order of occurrence, include pelvis, proximal femur, scapula.
   e. Location is important for diagnosis (scapula usually malignant, hand usually benign).
   f. Wide range of aggressiveness, depending on grade
   g. Secondary chondrosarcomas occur in the setting of a solitary osteochondroma (<1%), multiple hereditary osteochondromas (5% to 10%), Ollier disease (25% to 30%), or Maffucci disease (23% to 100%).
4. Imaging
   a. Radiographic appearance varies by grade of tumor.
   b. Low-grade intramedullary lesions are similar to enchondromas, but they have cortical thickening/expansion, extensive endosteal erosion, and occasional soft-tissue extension (**Figure 8**).

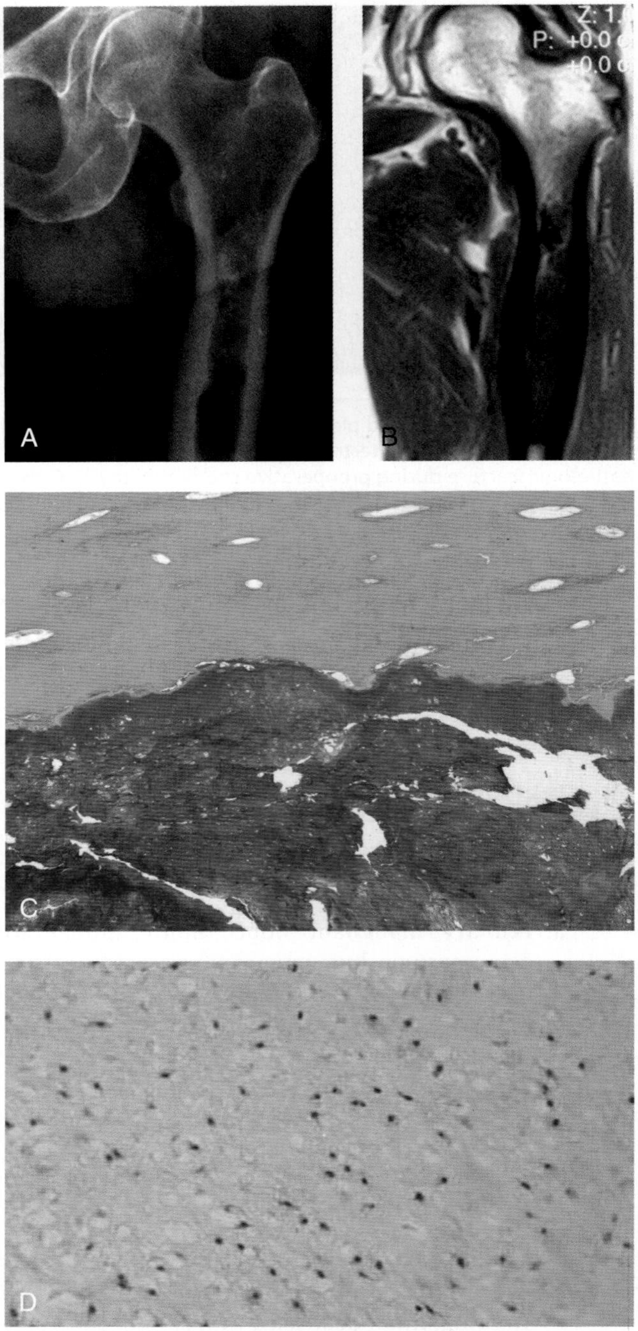

Figure 8 Low-grade chondrosarcoma in a 65-year-old woman who presented with constant thigh pain. **A**, AP radiograph of the left proximal femur shows thickened cortices and proximal intramedullary calcification within the lesion. These findings are consistent with a low-grade chondrosarcoma. **B**, Coronal T1-weighted MRI reveals the intramedullary extent of the lesion. No soft-tissue mass is evident. **C**, Low-power histologic image reveals the interface between the bone and a relatively hypocellular cartilage lesion. **D**, Higher power histologic image reveals a grade 1 chondrosarcoma with a bland cellular appearance, extensive basophilic cytoplasm, and no mitotic figures.

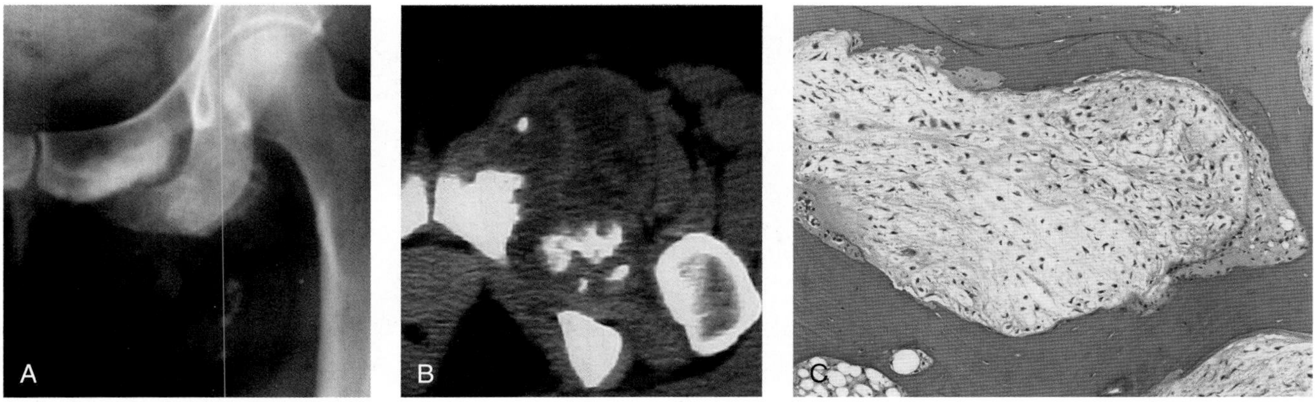

Figure 9 High-grade chondrosarcoma in a 42-year-old woman. **A**, AP radiograph of the left pelvis reveals a destructive lesion of the inferior pubic ramus with a soft-tissue mass. **B**, CT scan defines the mass. Evidence of intralesional calcium within the mass is seen. This radiographic appearance is consistent with a chondrosarcoma. **C**, Histologic image reveals a hypercellular lesion with atypical cells and permeation of the trabecular spaces consistent with a high-grade lesion. (Panels A and B reproduced from Scarborough MT, ed: *2005 Musculoskeletal Tumors and Diseases Self-Assessment Examination*. Rosemont, IL, American Academy of Orthopaedic Surgeons, 2005.)

c. Low-grade lesions have rings, arcs, and stipples and are usually mineralized.

d. Low-grade chondrosarcomas in the long bones are usually larger than 8 cm.

e. Low-grade pelvic chondrosarcomas can grow to large size (>10 cm) with extensive soft-tissue extension toward surrounding viscera.

f. Intermediate- or high-grade chondrosarcoma is less well defined, involves frank cortical destruction, and often has an associated soft-tissue mass (**Figures 9** through **11**).

g. Dedifferentiated chondrosarcoma is a high-grade sarcoma juxtaposed to a benign or low-grade malignant cartilage lesion, noted radiographically by a calcified intramedullary lesion with an adjacent destructive lytic lesion (**Figure 12**).

h. Secondary chondrosarcomas appear with ill-defined edges or rapid thickening of cartilage caps next to an enchondroma or osteochondroma, respectively (**Figure 13**).

i. Bone scan shows increased uptake in all variants and grades of chondrosarcoma.

j. CT or MRI is helpful in defining cortical destruction and marrow involvement, respectively.

5. Pathology

a. Low-grade tumors are grossly lobular; higher grade tumors may be myxoid.

b. Needle biopsy is not helpful in determining the grade of a cartilage tumor (especially differentiating an enchondroma from a low-grade chondrosarcoma).

c. Low-grade chondrosarcomas have a bland histologic appearance, but permeation and entrapment of the existing trabeculae are present (**Figure 8**, C and D).

d. Mitotic figures are rare.

e. Higher grade chondrosarcomas have a hypercellular pattern with binucleate forms and occasional myxoid change (**Figure 9**, C).

f. Dedifferentiated chondrosarcomas reveal a high-grade sarcoma (undifferentiated pleomorphic sarcoma, fibrosarcoma, osteosarcoma) adjacent to a low-grade or benign cartilage tumor (**Figure 12**, D).

6. Treatment/outcome

a. Grade 1 chondrosarcomas in the extremities can be treated with thorough intralesional curettage or wide resection.

b. All pelvic chondrosarcomas should be resected with an adequate margin (may require amputation).

c. Local recurrence rate at 10 years is approximately 20%.

d. Recurrent lesions have a 10% chance of increasing in grade.

e. Grade 2 or 3 or dedifferentiated chondrosarcomas require wide surgical resection regardless of location.

f. Metastasis to the lungs is treated with thoracotomy.

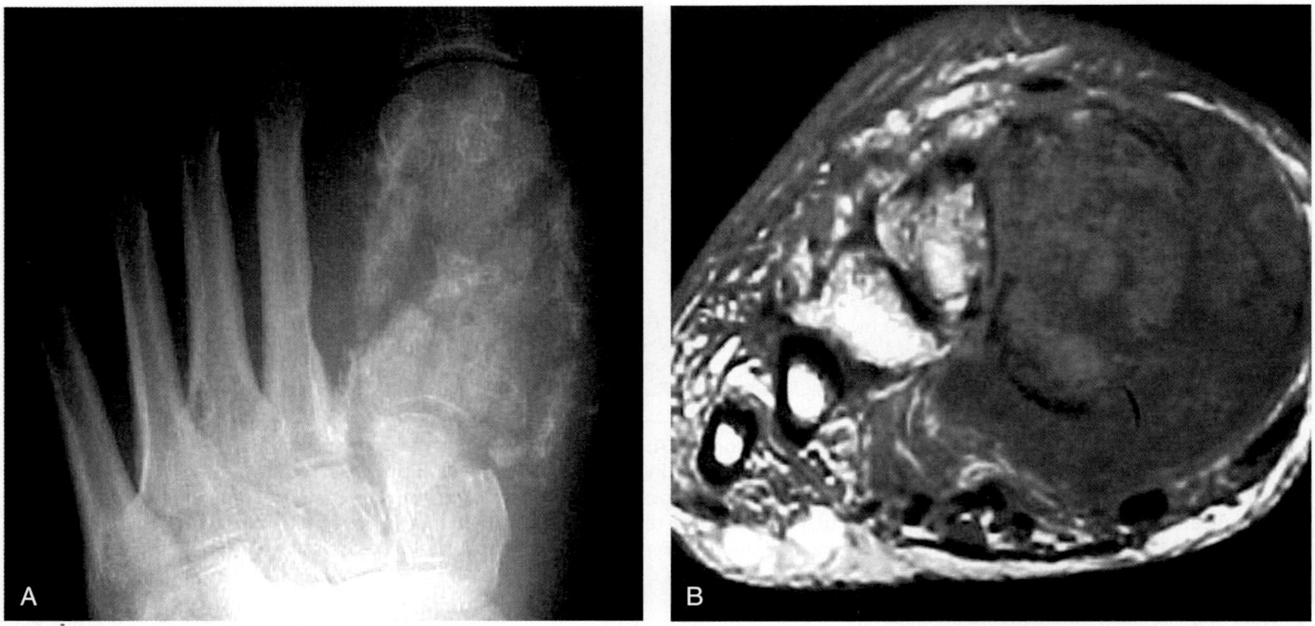

Figure 10 Grade 2 chondrosarcoma of the left foot in a 68-year-old man. **A**, AP radiograph reveals a destructive lesion in the metatarsal. **B**, Axial T1-weighted MRI reveals an extensive soft-tissue mass; the tissue diagnosis was a grade 2 chondrosarcoma. The patient required a transtibial amputation.

g. Slow progression of disease requires long-term follow-up (approximately 20 years).

h. Overall survival depends on the grade of the tumor.

- Grade 1 > 90%
- Grade 2 = 60% to 70%
- Grade 3 = 30% to 50%
- Dedifferentiated = 10%

i. No current role for chemotherapy or radiation except in dedifferentiated chondrosarcoma (chemotherapy may be used for high-grade sarcomas, depending on patient age/condition)

B. Chondrosarcoma subtypes

1. Clear cell chondrosarcoma

a. Definition—Rare malignant cartilage tumor with immature cartilaginous histogenesis.

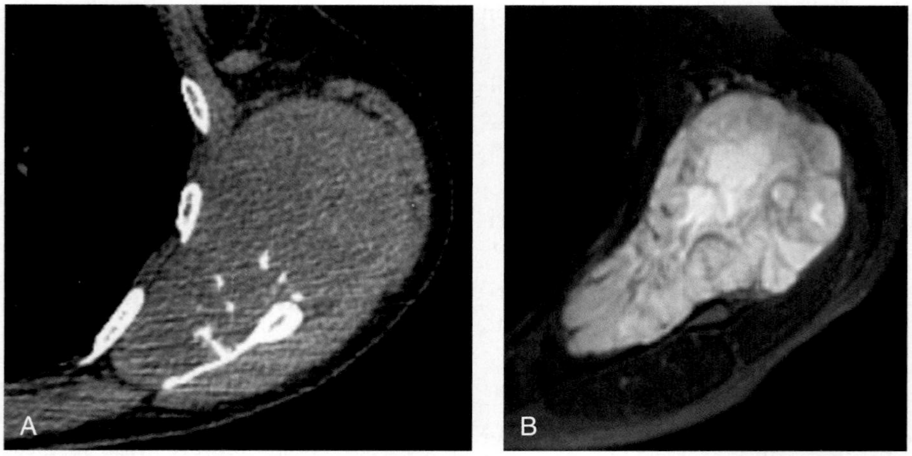

Figure 11 **A**, CT scan of the scapula reveals a large soft-tissue mass with tissue consistent with a grade 3 chondrosarcoma. Note the intralesional calcifications. **B**, Axial T2-weighted MRI reveals the extent of the soft-tissue mass emanating from the scapular body. The scapula is a common location for this tumor.

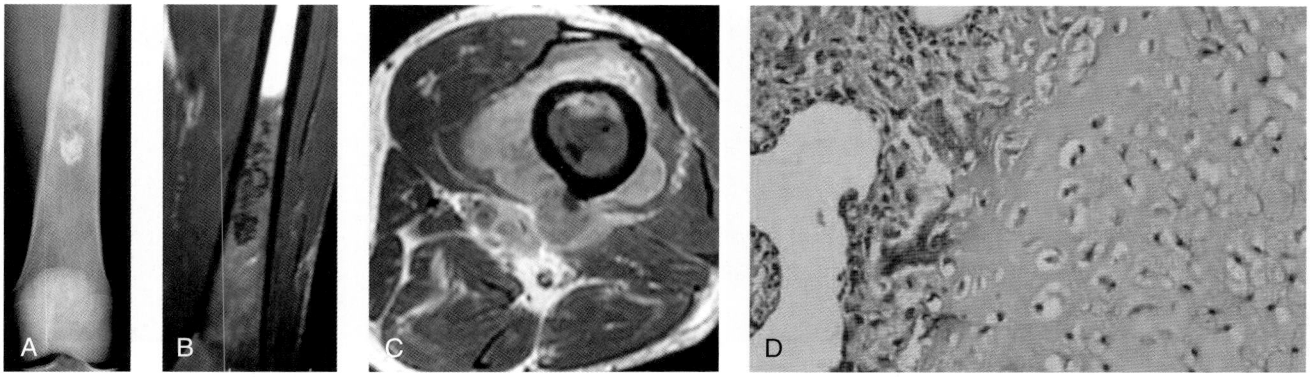

Figure 12 Dedifferentiated chondrosarcoma of the femur in a 73-year-old man. **A**, AP radiograph reveals a lesion similar to an enchondroma within the medullary canal, but there is an ill-defined lucency distal to the lesion. **B**, Coronal T1-weighted MRI reveals the intramedullary extent of the lesion, which is much different from an enchondroma and raises the concern for a dedifferentiated chondrosarcoma. **C**, Axial T1-weighted MRI demonstrates a circumferential soft-tissue mass consistent with a high-grade lesion. **D**, A high-power histologic view shows low-grade cartilage juxtaposed to a high-grade sarcomatous lesion, indicating a dedifferentiated chondrosarcoma. (Panels A and B reproduced from Scarborough MT, ed: *2005 Musculoskeletal Tumors and Diseases Self-Assessment Examination*. Rosemont, IL, American Academy of Orthopaedic Surgeons, 2005.)

b. Demographics, genetics/etiology, and clinical presentation are the same as for classic chondrosarcoma (see Section I.A.1-3).

c. Radiographic appearance

- Clear cell chondrosarcoma occurs in the epiphysis of long bones, most commonly in the proximal femur or proximal humerus (**Figure 14**).
- Lytic, round, expansile well-defined lesion. No periosteal reaction.
- Mineralization may be evident within the lesion.
- Most often confused with a benign chondroblastoma.

d. Pathology

- Intermediate- to high-grade lesion formed of immature cartilage cells (**Figure 14**, C)

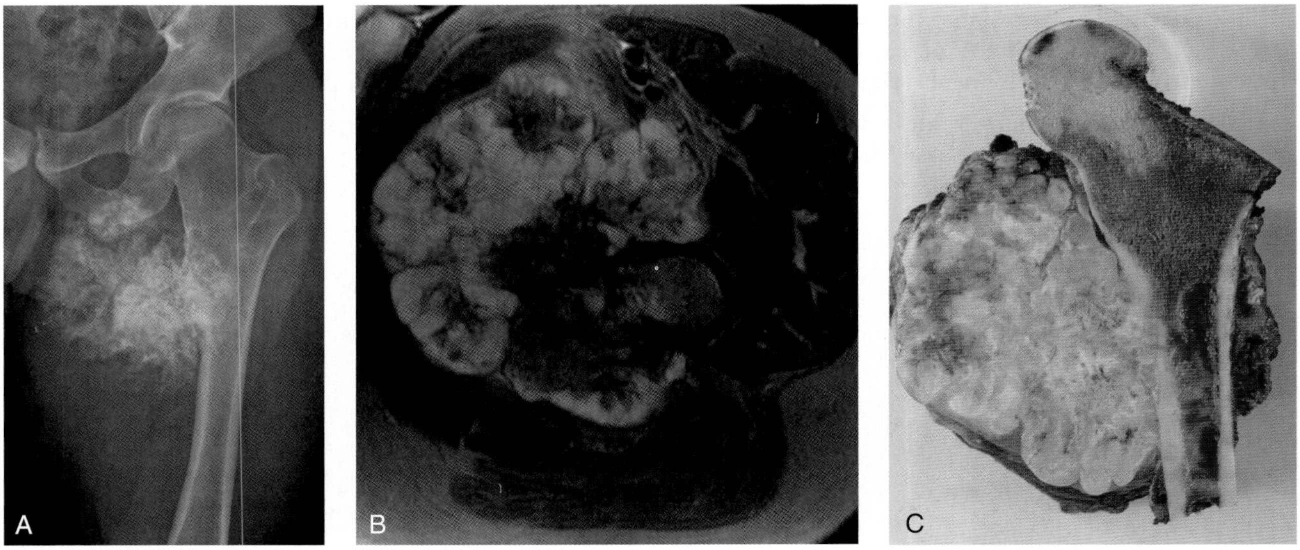

Figure 13 Chondrosarcoma in a 24-year-old man with multiple hereditary osteochondromas who presented with 6 months of increasing left hip pain. **A**, AP radiograph of the left proximal femoral osteochondroma with large associated soft-tissue mass with internal calcifications. **B**, Axial T2-weighted MRI reveals the secondary chondrosarcoma emanating from the posteromedial osteochondroma. **C**, Gross appearance of the lesion after resection of the proximal femur. The histology revealed a grade 2 chondrosarcoma.

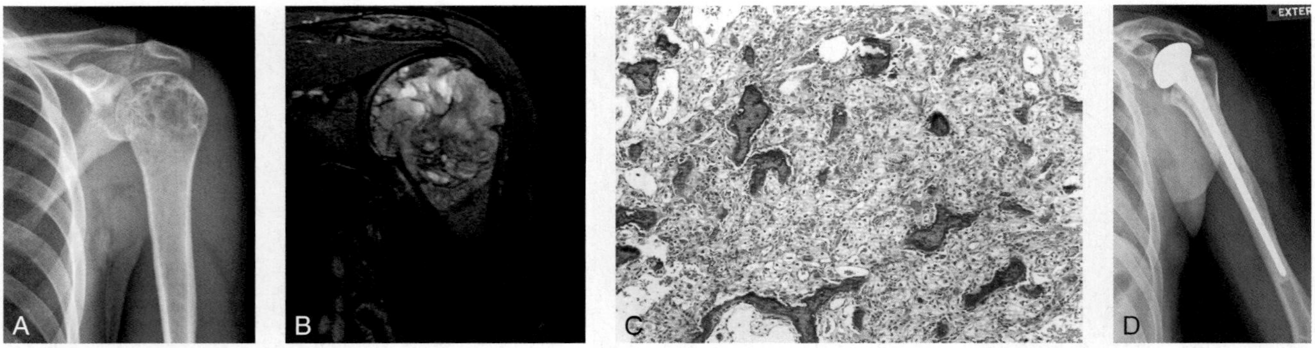

Figure 14 **A**, AP radiograph in an 18-year-old man with a clear cell chondrosarcoma in the left proximal humerus. **B**, Coronal MRI revealing the discrete epiphyseal location of this low-grade malignancy. **C**, Low-power histologic image of a clear cell chondrosarcoma reveals a cellular lesion with minimal matrix. The cartilage cells have clear cytoplasm. Additional benign giant cells are within the lesion. **D**, AP radiograph 4 years after wide resection and allograft-prosthetic composite reconstruction.

- Lobular growth pattern
- Benign giant cells throughout the tumor
- Extensive clear cytoplasm with minimal matrix

e. Treatment/outcome

- Wide surgical resection required for cure
- Chemotherapy and radiation not effective
- Metastasis to bones and lungs
- Good prognosis (5-year survival is 80%)

2. Mesenchymal chondrosarcoma

a. Definition and demographics

- Rare primary bone tumor composed of a biphasic pattern of cartilage and small round cell components (**Figure 15**).
- Occurs in younger individuals (10 to 40 years of age) than classic chondrosarcoma.
- A novel fusion protein, NEY1-NCOA2, is identified (absent in other chondrosarcomas).

b. Clinical presentation

- Most common in the flat bones (ilium, ribs, skull) but can occur in the long bones.
- Thirty percent of cases involve only soft tissue.
- May involve multiple skeletal sites at presentation.
- Pain and swelling of long duration are the most common symptoms.

c. Radiographic appearance

- Lytic destructive tumors with stippled calcification within the lesion (**Figure 15**, A).
- Expansion of bone with cortical thickening and poor margination.

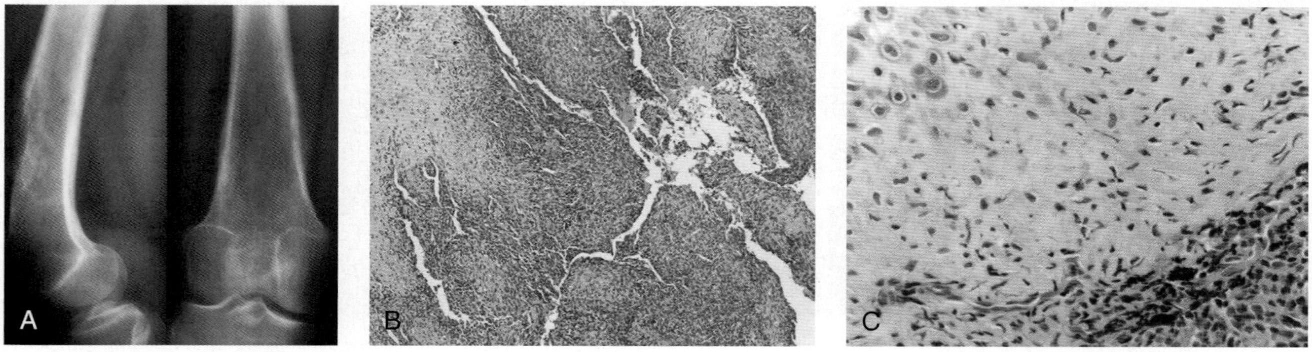

Figure 15 Chondrosarcoma of the distal femur in a 28-year-old woman. **A**, Composite lateral and AP radiographs reveal a poorly defined lytic lesion with destruction of the anterior cortex. **B**, Low-power histologic image reveals a biphasic appearance to the lesion with cartilage as well as small round cells consistent with a mesenchymal chondrosarcoma. **C**, Higher power histologic image shows the junction between the low-grade cartilage and the sheets of small cells.

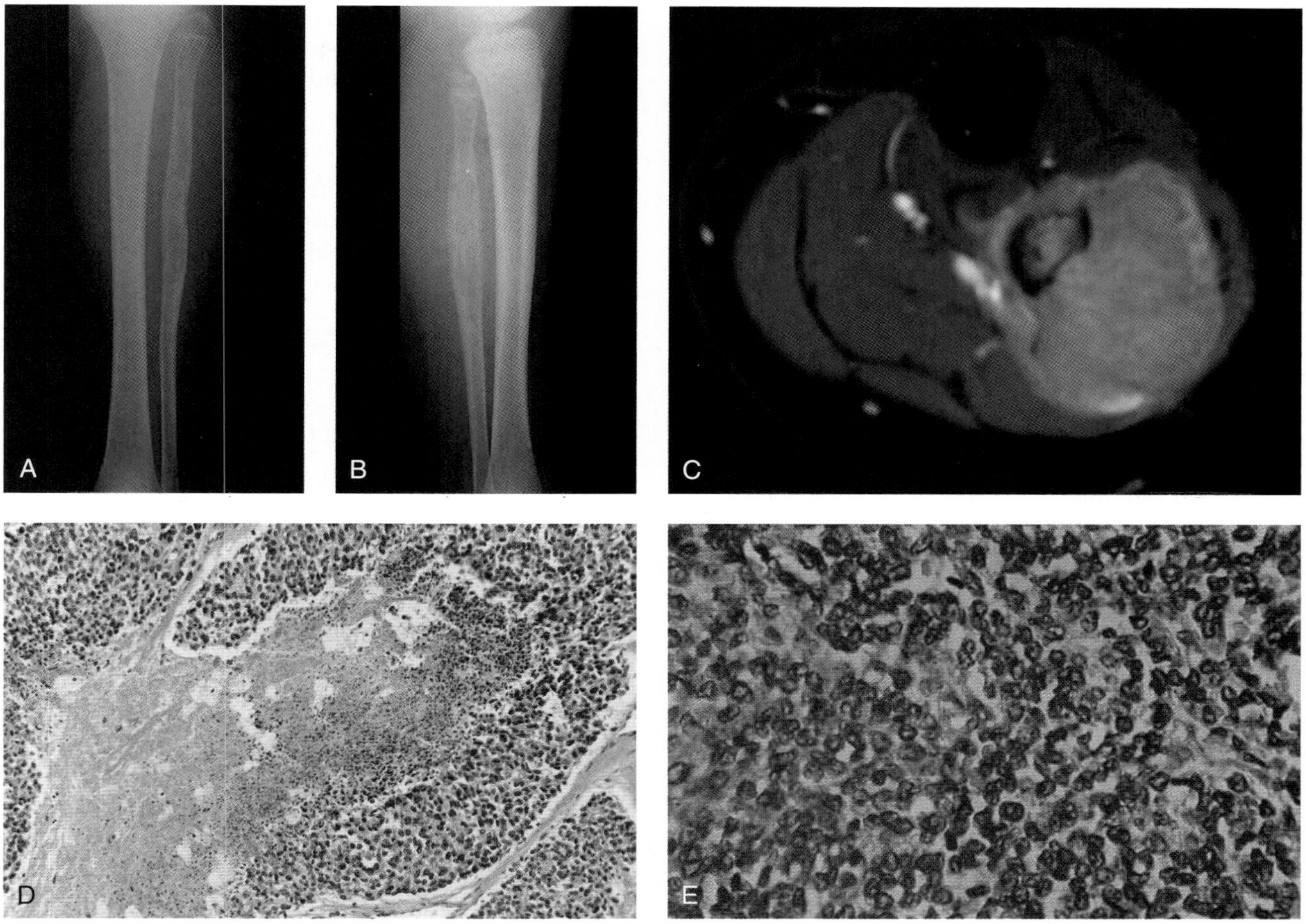

Figure 16 Ewing sarcoma/primitive neuroectodermal tumor (PNET) in an 11-year-old boy. AP (**A**) and lateral (**B**) radiographs of the left tibia/fibula reveal a lesion in the fibular diaphysis. Needle biopsy was consistent with Ewing sarcoma. The initial periosteal reaction ossified slightly after two cycles of neoadjuvant chemotherapy. **C**, Axial T2-weighted fat-saturated MRI obtained at diagnosis reveals an extensive soft-tissue mass at diagnosis consistent with a small round cell lesion. **D**, Low-power histologic image reveals a small round blue cell lesion with large sheets of necrosis. **E**, Higher power image reveals the monotonous small cells with prominent nuclei and scant cytoplasm characteristic of Ewing sarcoma/PNET.

- Nonspecific appearance can be included in a differential of any malignant or metastatic lesion.

d. Pathology—Biphasic histologic pattern of low-grade islands of cartilage alternating with sheets of small anaplastic round cells (**Figure 15**, B and C).

e. Treatment/outcome

- Treatment is chemotherapy (controversial) and wide surgical resection.
- The 5-year survival is 30% to 60%.
- Few series in the literature.

IV. ROUND CELL LESIONS

A. Ewing sarcoma/primitive neuroectodermal tumor (PNET)

1. Definition and demographics

a. Malignant bone tumor composed of small round blue cells.

b. Male-to-female ratio = 3:2.

c. Uncommon in African Americans and Chinese.

d. Second most common primary malignant bone tumor in children (1 case/million persons/year; 80% younger than 20 years).

e. Can also be a soft-tissue sarcoma.

2. Genetics/etiology
   a. Cell of origin unknown.
   b. Hypothesized to be of neuroectodermal differentiation. PNET is thought to be the differentiated neural tumor, and Ewing sarcoma the undifferentiated variant.
   c. Possible mesenchymal stem cell derivation.
   d. Classic 11:22 chromosomal translocation (*EWS/FLI1* is the fusion gene) in 85% of cases.
3. Clinical presentation
   a. Pain is the most common symptom.
   b. Swelling, limp, and decreased range of motion are variable.
   c. Frequent fever and occasional erythema (mistaken for infection).
   d. Elevated erythrocyte sedimentation rate, LDH, and white blood cell count (**Figure 17**).
   e. The most common locations are the pelvis, diaphysis of long bones, and scapula.
   f. Twenty-five percent of patients present with metastatic disease.
   g. Staging workup includes a bone marrow biopsy in addition to the standard studies (CT chest, radiograph/MRI of primary lesion, PET scan).
4. Imaging
   a. Purely lytic bone destruction.
   b. Periosteal reaction in multiple layers (the classic reaction, called "onion skin") or sunburst pattern (**Figure 16**, A and B).
   c. Poorly marginated and permeative.
   d. Extensive soft-tissue mass often present despite more subtle bone destruction (**Figures 16**, C and **18**, C).
   e. MRI necessary to identify soft-tissue extension and marrow involvement (**Figure 16**, C).
   f. Radiographic differential diagnosis includes osteomyelitis, osteosarcoma, eosinophilic granuloma, osteoid osteoma, lymphoma.
5. Pathology
   a. Gross appearance may be a liquid consistency, mimicking pus.
   b. Small round blue cells with round/oval nuclei (**Figure 16**, D and E).
   c. Indistinct cell outlines.
   d. Prominent nuclei and minimal cytoplasm.
   e. Reactive osseous or fibroblastic tissue may be present.
   f. Can be broad sheets of necrosis and widely separated fibrous strands.
   g. Differential diagnosis includes lymphoma, osteomyelitis, neuroblastoma, rhabdomyosarcoma, eosinophilic granuloma, and leukemia.
   h. Immunohistochemical stains are helpful; CD99+ (013 antibody).
   i. 11:22 chromosomal translocation produces *EWS/FLI1*, which can be identified by polymerase chain reaction in 85% of cases and differentiates Ewing sarcoma from other round cell lesions.
   j. Additional features seen only in PNET include a more lobular pattern and arrangement of the cells in poorly formed rosettes around an eosinophilic material (**Figure 19**).

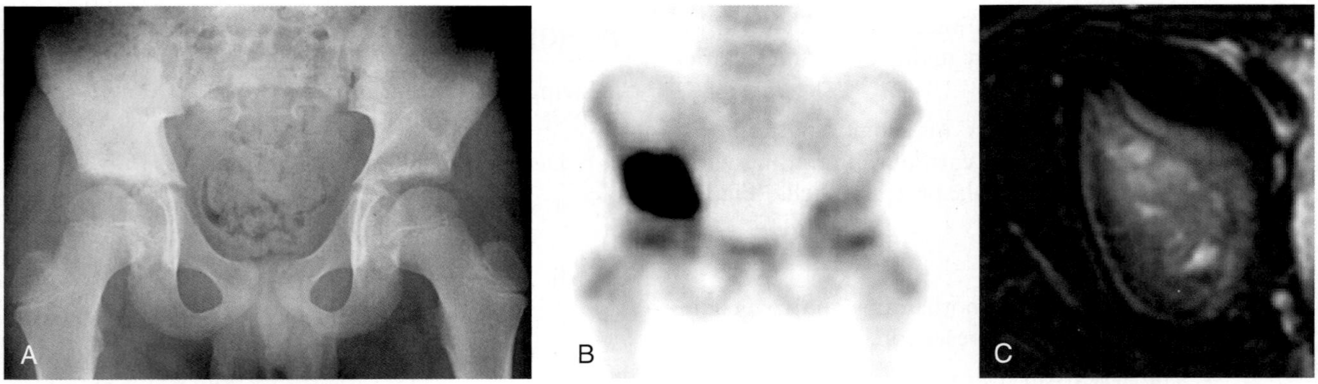

Figure 17 Ewing sarcoma of the pelvis. **A**, AP radiograph reveals an indistinct abnormality in the right supra-acetabular region. **B**, Technetium Tc-99m bone scan reveals avid uptake in this area. **C**, Axial MRI of the acetabular region reveals an elevated periosteum. A biopsy was consistent with Ewing sarcoma.

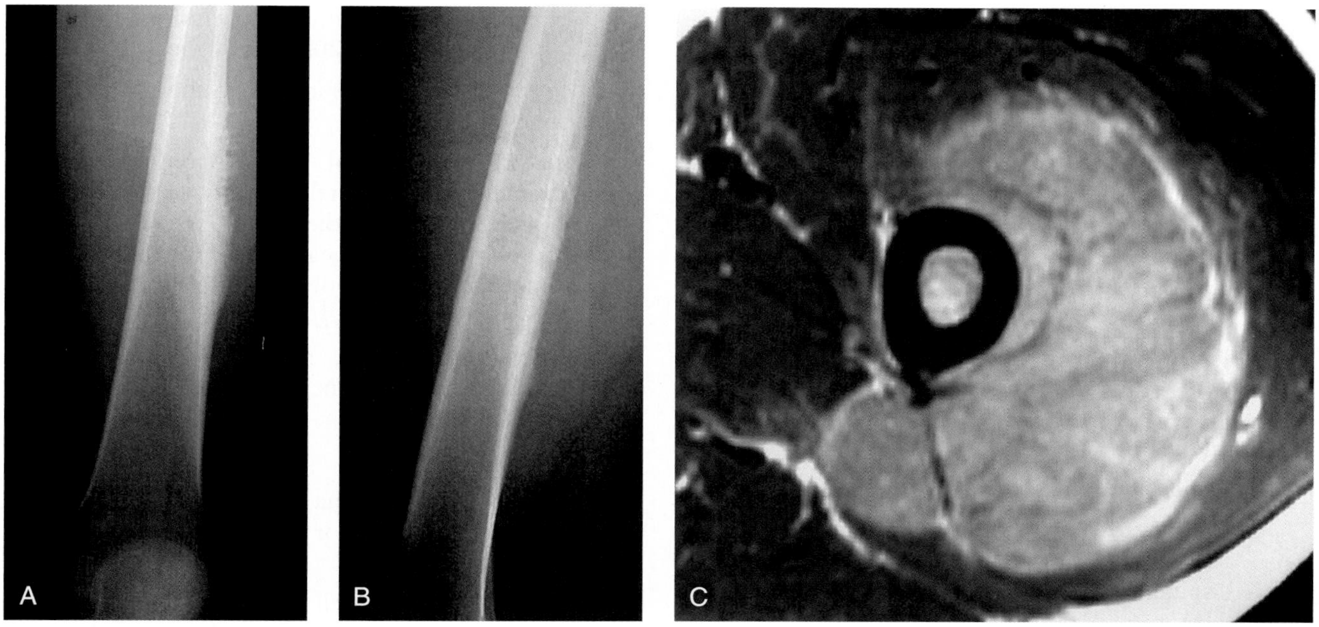

Figure 18 Ewing sarcoma in the femur of a 14-year-old boy. AP (**A**) and lateral (**B**) radiographs of the femur reveal a diaphyseal lesion with a sunburst pattern of periosteal reaction. **C**, Axial MRI reveals an extensive soft-tissue mass. A biopsy revealed Ewing sarcoma.

6. Treatment/outcome
   a. Standard treatment of Ewing sarcoma is neoadjuvant chemotherapy.
   b. Most common chemotherapy drugs include vincristine, Adriamycin (doxorubicin), ifosfamide, etoposide, Cytoxan, and actinomycin D.
   c. Local control of the primary tumor can be achieved by either wide surgical resection or external beam radiation.

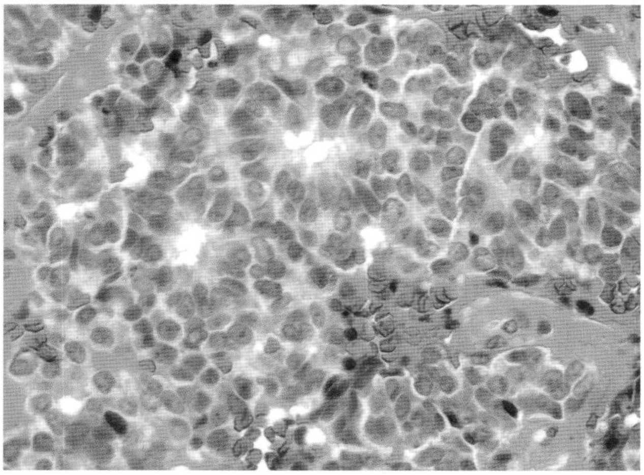

Figure 19 High-power histologic image of a primitive neuroectodermal tumor. Note that the cells are arranged in a rosette pattern around a central eosinophilic substance.

   d. Most isolated extremity lesions are treated with surgical resection rather than radiation because of short-term and long-term side effects of radiation and better potential local control with surgery.
   e. Radiation is often used for the primary lesion in patients who have inoperable tumors or present with metastatic disease.
   f. Local control is controversial for localized pelvic Ewing sarcoma: surgery or radiation or both are used.
   g. Complications of radiation in skeletally immature patients include joint contractures, fibrosis, growth arrest, fracture, and secondary malignancy (usually 10 to 20 years later).
   h. Response to chemotherapy (percent necrosis) is used as a prognostic indicator for overall survival (>99% necrosis associated with improved survival).
   i. Patients with localized extremity Ewing sarcoma have a 5-year event-free survival of 73%.
   j. Patients who present with metastatic disease have a poor prognosis (5-year survival < 20%).
   k. Metastases occur primarily in the lungs (60%) but also in the bone (43%) and bone marrow

(19%). With recurrent disease, the event-free survival is less than 10% at 3 years.

l. Adverse prognostic factors include nonpulmonary metastasis, less than 90% necrosis, large tumor volume, and pelvic lesions.

m. Different *EWS-FLI* fusion protein subtypes do not predict different outcomes.

n. PNET is thought to have a slightly worse prognosis than Ewing sarcoma.

V. NOTOCHORDAL AND MISCELLANEOUS TUMORS

A. Chordoma

1. Definition and demographics
   a. Slow-growing malignant bone tumor arising from notochordal rests and occurring in the spinal axis.
   b. Male-to-female ratio = 3:1 (most apparent in sacral lesions).
   c. Occurs in adult patients (>40 years).
   d. Lesions at base of skull present earlier than sacral lesions.
2. Genetics/etiology
   a. Chordoma is thought to develop from residual notochordal cells that eventually undergo neoplastic change.
   b. Brachyury gene duplication is a major susceptibility mutation in familial chordoma. No clear marker for sporadic forms is known.
3. Clinical presentation
   a. Insidious onset of low-back or sacral pain.
   b. Frequently misdiagnosed as osteoarthritis, nerve impingement, or disk herniation.
   c. Infrequent distal motor/sensory loss because most lesions occur below S1.
   d. Bowel/bladder symptoms are common.
   e. Fifty percent can be identified on a careful rectal examination. (Transrectal biopsy should not be performed.)
   f. Fifty percent occur in the sacrococcygeal region, 35% in the spheno-occipital region, and 15% in the mobile spine.
4. Imaging
   a. Chordomas occur in the midline, consistent with prior notochord location.
   b. Findings on plain radiographs of sacrum are subtle because of overlying bowel gas.
   c. Cross-sectional imaging with CT or MRI required (**Figure 20**, A through C).
   d. CT reveals areas of calcification within the lesion.
   e. MRI (low signal intensity on T1-weighted images, high signal intensity on T2-weighted images) defines the extent of the frequently anterior soft-tissue mass and the bony involvement (usually involves multiple sacral levels).
   f. Radiographic differential diagnosis includes chondrosarcoma, multiple myeloma, metastatic disease, giant cell tumor, and lymphoma (**Table 3**).
5. Pathology
   a. Grossly, chordoma appears lobulated and jellylike, with tumor tracking along the nerve roots.
   b. The signature cell is the physaliferous cell, which contains intracellular vacuoles and appears bubbly (cytoplasmic mucous droplets) (**Figure 20**, D and E).
   c. Lobules of the tumor are separated by fibrous septa.
   d. Physaliferous cells are keratin positive, which differentiates this tumor from chondrosarcoma.
   e. Weakly S100 positive.
   f. Differential diagnosis includes chondrosarcoma and metastatic carcinoma.
6. Treatment/outcome
   a. The main treatment is wide surgical resection.
   b. Local recurrence is common (50%) and is directly related to the surgical margin achieved.
   c. To achieve a satisfactory wide margin, the surgeon must be willing to sacrifice involved nerve roots, viscera, and so forth.
   d. Radiation (protons preferred) can be used as an adjunct for locally recurrent disease, as positive margins, or as primary treatment of inoperable tumors (protons or photons).
   e. High-dose proton radiation alone (70 Gy) has reasonable short-term local control.
   f. Chemotherapy is not effective and is currently not indicated.
   g. Chordoma metastasizes late to the lungs and, occasionally, bone and requires long-term follow-up (20 years).
   h. Long-term survival is 25% to 50%, due in part to local progression.

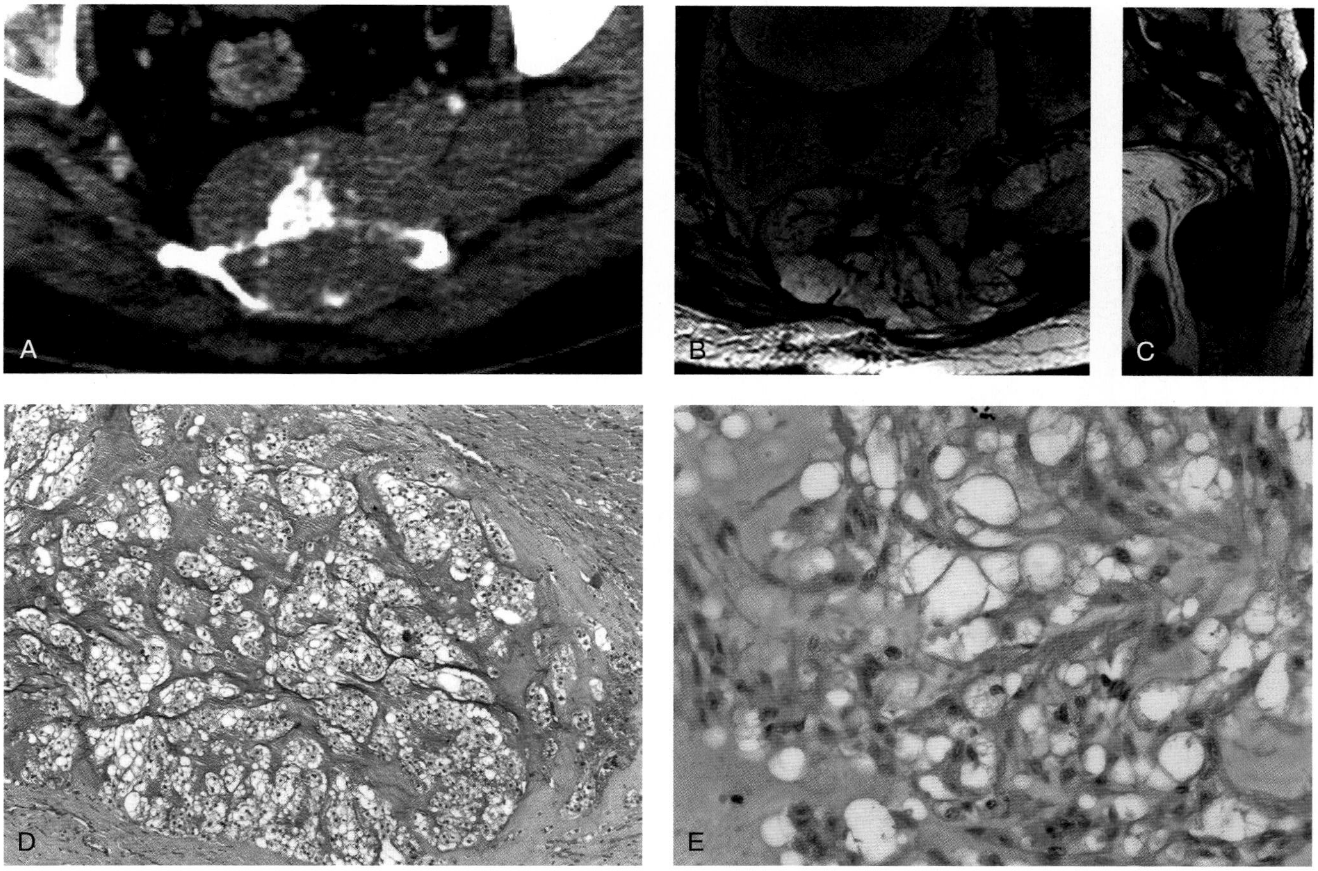

Figure 20 Chordoma of the sacrum in a 66-year-old man. **A**, CT scan reveals a destructive lesion with an anterior soft-tissue mass containing calcifications. **B**, Axial MRI further defines the soft-tissue extension anteriorly and toward the left pelvic sidewall. **C**, Sagittal T1-weighted MRI shows the lesion at S3 and below. Note that the anterior extension abuts the rectum. **D**, Low-power histologic image of this lesion reveals a tumor lobule surrounded by fibrous tissue. **E**, Higher power histologic image reveals the physaliferous cells of a chordoma with a bubbly appearance to the cytoplasm.

TABLE 3

Tumors Occurring in the Vertebrae

Anterior (Vertebral Body)
Giant cell tumor
Eosinophilic granuloma Metastatic disease
Multiple myeloma
Ependymoma
Chordoma
Lymphoma
Primary bone tumors (chondrosarcoma, osteosarcoma)
Posterior Elements
Osteoid osteoma
Osteoblastoma
Aneurysmal bone cyst

B. Adamantinoma
1. Definition and demographics
   a. Unusual, rare, slow-growing malignant bone tumor with a predilection for the tibia (**Figure 21**).
   b. Male slightly more common than female.
   c. Patients are generally 20 to 40 years of age.
   d. Fewer than 300 cases in the literature.
2. Genetics/etiology—Controversial whether adamantinoma evolves from osteofibrous dysplasia; most believe it does not.
3. Clinical presentation
   a. Pain of variable duration and intensity is the major symptom.
   b. Occasional tibial deformity or a mass.

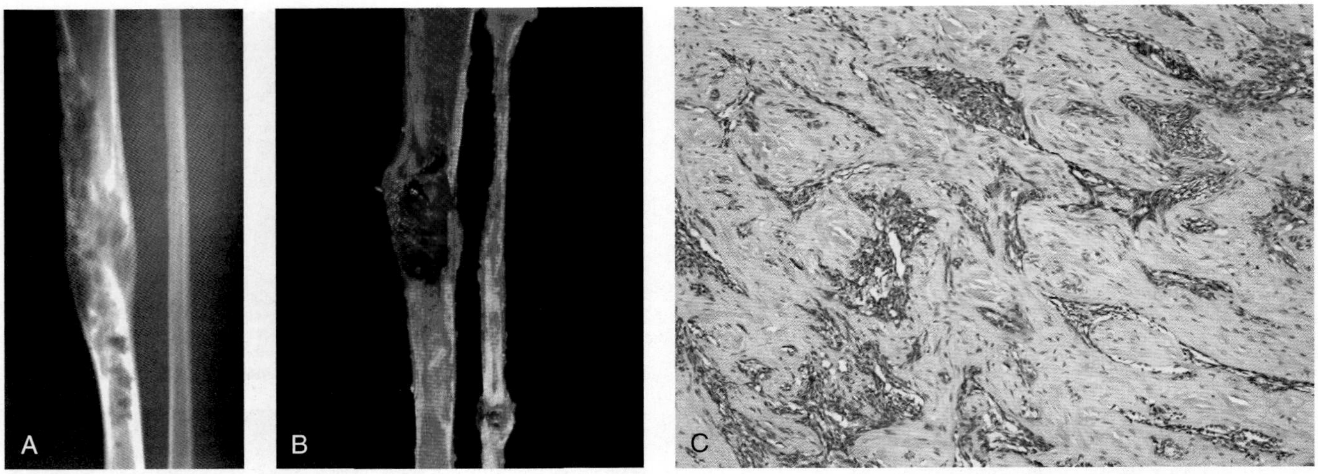

Figure 21 Adamantinoma of the tibia in a 38-year-old woman. **A,** AP radiograph reveals multiple diaphyseal lucent lesions separated by sclerotic bone. They have a bubbly appearance consistent with adamantinoma. **B,** A gross specimen from a different patient reveals lesions in both the tibia and fibula that expand the bone. **C,** The histologic appearance is nests of epithelial cells in a fibrous stroma.

c. Tenderness over the subcutaneous tibial border.

d. History of preceding trauma is common (30% to 60%).

e. About80% to 90% of lesions occur in the tibial diaphysis.

f. Synchronous involvement of the ipsilateral fibula in 10% to 50% of cases.

4. Imaging

a. Classic radiographic appearance is multiple well-circumscribed lucent defects, usually with one dominant defect that may expand the bone locally (**Figure 21**, A).

b. Sclerotic bone between defects.

c. "Soap bubble" appearance.

d. Lesions may be intracortical or intramedullary, with occasional (10%) soft-tissue mass.

e. No periosteal reaction.

5. Pathology

a. Nests of epithelial cells in a benign fibrous stroma (**Figure 21**, C).

b. Epithelial cells are columnar in appearance and keratin positive.

c. Epithelial cells are bland without mitosis.

6. Treatment/outcome

a. Standard of care is wide surgical resection.

b. Chemotherapy and radiation are not indicated.

c. Local recurrence is more common when adequate margins are not achieved.

d. Given diaphyseal location, common reconstruction is intercalary allograft.

e. Late metastasis to lungs, bones, and lymph nodes in 10% to 30% of patients.

f. Requires long-term follow-up.

g. Case series from 2000 described 87% survival at 10 years.

VI. SYSTEMIC DISEASE

A. Multiple myeloma

1. Definition and demographics

a. Neoplastic proliferation of plasma cells producing a monoclonal protein.

b. Considered the most common primary malignant bone tumor (30,000 persons/year) in the United States.

c. Affects patients older than 40 years.

d. Twice as common in African Americans as in Caucasians.

e. Affects males more commonly than females.

2. Genetics/etiology

a. Immunoglobulins (Igs) are composed of two heavy chains and two light chains.

- Heavy chains = IgG, IgA, IgM, IgD, and IgE (IgG and IgA are common in myeloma)
- Light chains = κ and λ (Bence Jones proteins)

b. In myeloma, both heavy and light chains are produced.

c. Major mediators of osteoclastogenesis in myeloma include receptor activator of nuclear factor-κ B ligand (RANKL), interleukin-6, and macrophage inflammatory protein-1α.

d. Osteoblastic bone formation is suppressed by tumor necrosis factor and Dickkopf-related protein 1 (Dkk-1).

3. Clinical presentation

a. Common symptoms include bone pain, pathologic fractures, cord compression, and recurrent infections.

b. Lesions occur throughout the skeleton but are common in bones that contain hematopoietic marrow, including the skull, spine, and long bones (**Figure 22**).

c. Laboratory findings: normochromic, normocytic anemia; hypercalcemia; renal insufficiency; amyloidosis; and elevated erythrocyte sedimentation rate.

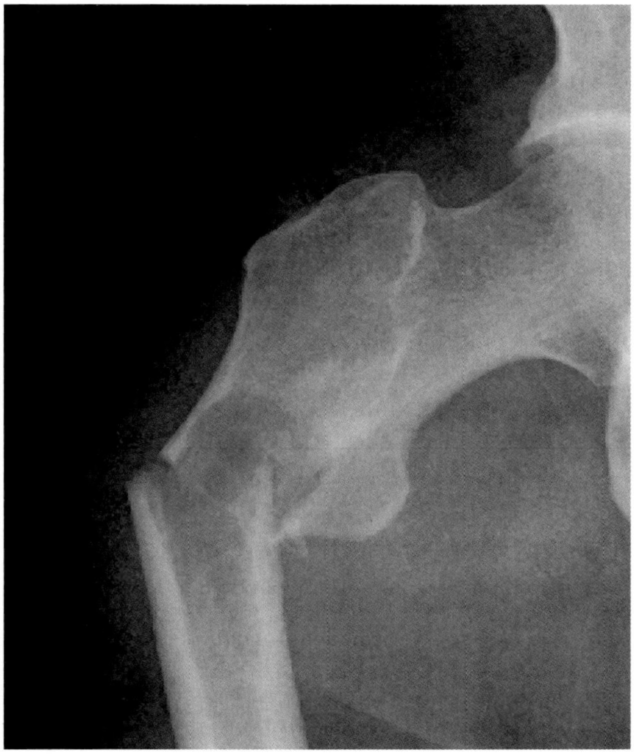

Figure 22 AP radiograph of the hip of a 47-year-old woman who presented with a pathologic fracture of the proximal femur through a lytic lesion. Open biopsy at the time of surgery showed a plasma cell lesion consistent with multiple myeloma.

d. Electrophoresis: 99% of patients have a spike in serum or urine or both.

- Serum: identifies types of proteins present
- Urine: identifies Bence Jones proteins

e. 24-hour urine collection quantifies protein in urine.

f. β_2-microglobulin (>5.5) and serum albumin—tumor markers with prognostic ability (increased β_2-microglobulin and decreased serum albumin = poor prognosis).

g. Diagnosis—One major and one minor (or three minor) diagnostic criteria must be present.

- Major criteria
  - Plasmacytoma: tissue diagnosis on biopsy
  - More than 30% plasma cells in bone marrow
  - Serum IgG greater than 3.5 g/dL, IgA greater than 2 g/dL or urine greater than 1 g/24 hours, or Bence Jones protein
- Minor criteria
  - 10% to 30% plasma cells in bone marrow
  - Serum/urine protein levels lower than listed for major criteria
  - Lytic bone lesions on skeletal survey
  - Lower-than-normal IgG levels

4. Imaging

a. Classic appearance is multiple "punched-out" lytic lesions throughout the skeleton (**Figures 23, A, B,** and **24**, A).

b. No surrounding sclerosis.

c. Skull lesions and vertebral compression fractures are common (**Figures 23, A** and **24**, A).

d. Diffuse osteopenia (**Figure 24**, A).

e. Bone scan is usually negative because there is minimal osteoblastic response in myeloma.

f. PET-CT is now the screening tool of choice. Skeletal survey is still helpful in determining fracture risk.

g. MRI is helpful in defining vertebral lesions (**Figure 24**, B).

5. Pathology

a. The lesion consists of sheets of plasma cells with eccentric nuclei; little intercellular material is present (**Figure 23**, C)

b. Nuclear chromatin arranged in a "clock face" pattern

11 | Oncology

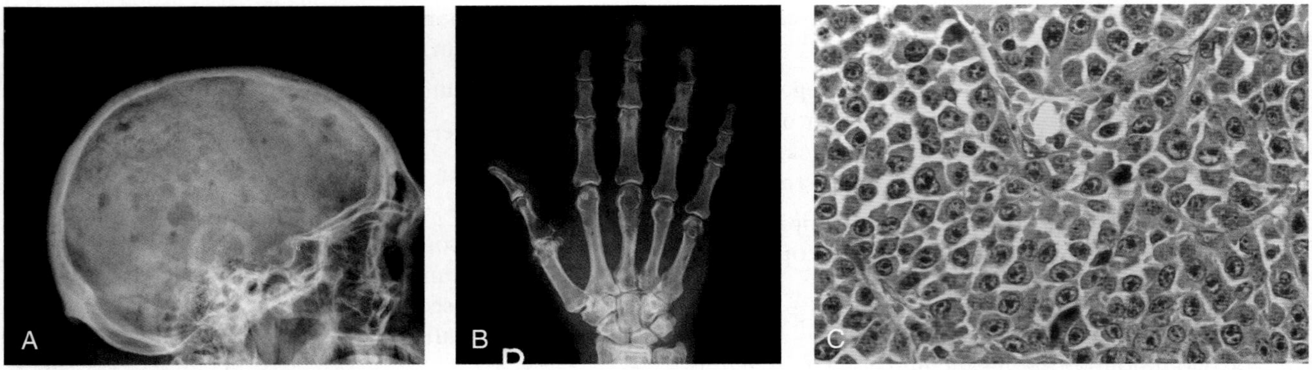

Figure 23 **A** and **B**, Examples radiographs of multiple myeloma in the skull and hand showing typical round, punched-out lesions. **C**, A high-power histologic image reveals numerous plasma cells with eccentric nuclei and extensive vascularity.

c. Abundant eosinophilic cytoplasm
d. Rare mitotic figures
e. Extremely vascular, with an extensive capillary system
f. Immunohistochemistry stains: CD38+

6. Treatment/outcome
   a. Dramatic improvement in survival over the past 10 years
   b. Standard of care is high-dose chemotherapy with autologous stem cell support
   c. Risk stratification of patients allows for individualized treatment
   d. Six sets of active agents in myeloma
      - Alkylating agents (melphalan, cyclophosphamide)
      - Anthracyclines (doxorubicin, liposomal doxorubicin)
      - Corticosteroids (dexamethasone, prednisone)
      - Immunomodulatory drugs (thalidomide, lenalidomide)
      - Proteosome inhibitors (bortezomib, carfilzomib)
      - Monoclonal antibodies (daratumumab, elotuzumab)
   e. Bisphosphonates or RANKL inhibitors help decrease number of lesions, bone pain, and serum calcium
   f. Same improved survival for early or late autologous stem cell transplant
   g. Radiation effective to decrease pain, avoid surgery
   h. Surgical stabilization of pathologic fractures or impending fractures (principles similar to those used in metastatic disease)
   i. Kyphoplasty/vertebroplasty common to treat vertebral compression fractures
   j. Survival worse with renal failure
   k. Median survival is 8 years (prognosis and treatment more individualized)

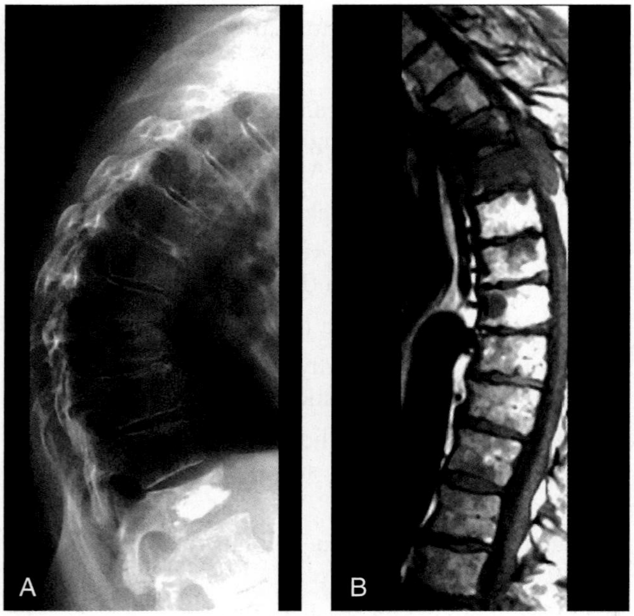

Figure 24 Multiple myeloma. **A**, A lateral radiograph of the thoracic spine demonstrates the severe osteopenia present in multiple myeloma contributing to compression fractures. Note the prior injection of cement to stabilize a vertebral body in the lower part of the figure. **B**, Sagittal MRI of the thoracic spine in a patient with long-standing multiple myeloma shows multiple vertebral lesions with an area of epidural extension.

B. Solitary plasmacytoma
   1. Plasma cell tumor in a single skeletal site

2. Represents 5% of patients with plasma cell lesions
3. Can have positive or negative serum/urine protein electrophoresis
4. Negative bone marrow biopsy/aspirate
5. Treated with radiation alone (4,500 to 5,000 cGy)
6. Progresses to myeloma in approximately 55% of patients

C. Osteosclerotic myeloma

1. Accounts for 3% of myeloma cases
2. POEMS syndrome = *p*olyneuropathy, *o*rganomegaly, *e*ndocrinopathy, *M*-spike, and *s*kin changes
3. Elevated serum VEGF is a marker

D. B cell lymphoma

1. Definition and demographics
   a. Clonal proliferation of B cells commonly presenting as nodal disease and occasionally affecting the skeleton.
   b. Can occur at any age; most common in patients 35 to 55 years of age.
   c. Affects males more commonly than females.
   d. Non-Hodgkin lymphoma most commonly affects the bone (B cell much more common than T cell variants).
   e. Of patients with non-Hodgkin lymphoma, 10% to 35% have extranodal disease.
   f. Primary lymphoma of bone can occur but is quite rare (2% to 5%).
2. Genetics/etiology—Risk factors for B cell lymphoma include immunodeficiency (HIV, hepatitis), benzene exposure, and viral/bacterial infection (Epstein-Barr).
3. Clinical presentation
   a. Constant pain unrelieved by rest.
   b. A large soft-tissue mass that is tender or warm is common.
   c. Lymphoma affects bones with persistent red marrow (femur, spine, pelvis).
   d. Neurologic symptoms from spinal lesions
   e. Twenty-five percent of patients present with pathologic fracture.
   f. B-symptoms = fever, weight loss, and night sweats.
   g. Primary lymphoma of bone is rare; occurs when there are no extraskeletal sites of disease (other than a single node) for 6 months after diagnosis.
4. Imaging appearance
   a. Lytic, permeative lesions that can show subtle bone destruction (**Figure 25**, A)
   b. Generally involves the diaphysis in long bones
   c. Can involve multiple sites in the skeleton
   d. Intensely positive on bone scan but used less frequently due to PET scan
   e. Extensive marrow involvement noted on MRI
   f. Large soft-tissue mass (**Figure 25**, B and C) is common

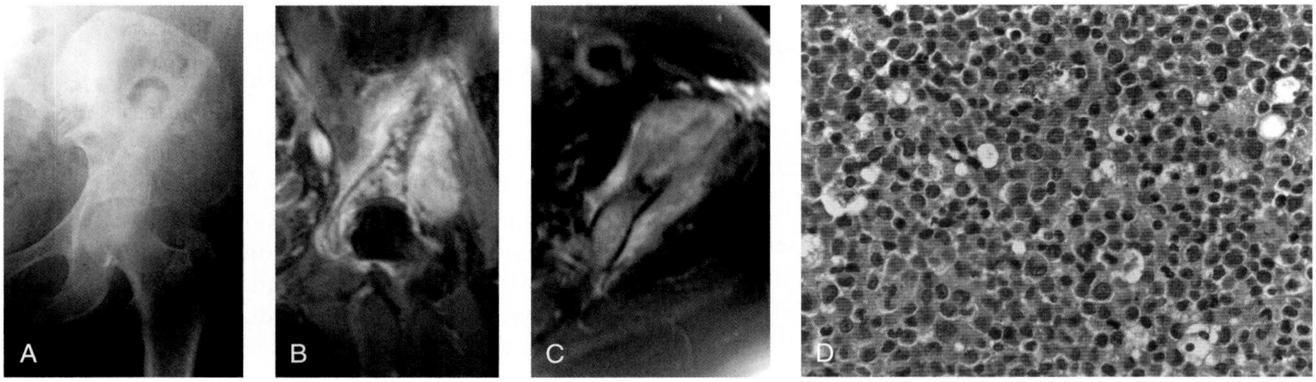

Figure 25 Lymphoma in a 72-year-old woman who presented with lateral hip pain. **A**, AP radiograph of the left pelvis reveals an extensive lytic lesion of the ilium and a resultant pathologic fracture. Coronal (**B**) and axial (**C**) MRIs reveal the extent of the surrounding soft-tissue mass. **D**, A high-power histologic image reveals a small round blue cell lesion (larger than lymphocytes). A CD20 stain was positive for a B cell lymphoma.

g. PET is standard imaging modality for staging and follow-up to assess disease viability

h. Radiographic differential diagnosis includes metastatic disease, myeloma, and osteomyelitis

5. Pathology

a. Can be difficult to diagnose on needle biopsy because the tissue is often crushed

b. Diffuse infiltrative rather than nodular pattern

c. Lesion comprised small round blue cells (2× size of lymphocytes; can be variable) (**Figure 25**, D)

d. Immunohistochemistry stains

- B cell (CD20+, CD79a+, CD10+), BCL2, BCL6, MYC
- Atypical/large cells (CD15+, CD30+, CD45+)

e. Increased percentage of cleaved cells improves prognosis in primary lymphoma of bone

6. Treatment/outcome

a. Bone marrow biopsy and PET-CT are required as part of staging/workup.

b. Chemotherapy is the primary treatment. Chemotherapeutic agents include cyclophosphamide, doxorubicin, prednisone, and vincristine for large B cell lymphoma.

c. Radiation of the primary site (bone) is used in some individuals for persistent disease after chemotherapy.

d. Surgical treatment is necessary only for pathologic fractures as chemotherapy alone or +/− radiation is effective for most lesions.

e. Reported 5-year survival is as high as 70% when chemotherapy and radiation are used for disseminated disease.

f. Secondary involvement of bone in lymphoma has a worse prognosis than primary lymphoma of bone.

VII. SECONDARY LESIONS

A. Overview (**Table 4** and **Figures 26** and **27**)

1. Secondary lesions can be benign (secondary ABC), but most commonly they are malignant (postradiation sarcoma, Paget sarcoma, sarcomas emanating from infarct or fibrous dysplasia, secondary chondrosarcomas from benign cartilage tumors, squamous carcinomas from osteomyelitis/draining sinus).

2. Secondary chondrosarcomas are described in Section III.A.

TABLE 4

Secondary Lesions

Type	Histology
Benign	Aneurysmal bone cyst
Postradiation (for ewing sarcoma, carcinoma, giant cell tumor)	Osteosarcoma Undifferentiated pleomorphic sarcoma Fibrosarcoma Chondrosarcoma
Paget sarcoma	Osteosarcoma Undifferentiated pleomorphic sarcoma Fibrosarcoma
Secondary to bone infarction	Undifferentiated pleomorphic sarcoma
Secondary to fibrous dysplasia	Osteosarcoma Undifferentiated pleomorphic sarcoma Fibrosarcoma
Secondary to benign cartilage lesion (enchondroma/osteochondroma)	Chondrosarcoma
Secondary to chronic osteomyelitis/draining sinus	Squamous cell carcinoma

3. These lesions develop from a preexisting tumor, process, or treatment.

B. Postradiation sarcoma

1. Definition and demographics

a. A postradiation sarcoma develops after a latent period when radiation has been used to treat a benign or malignant bone, soft-tissue, or visceral tumor.

b. These lesions can occur at any age after radiation of a prior tumor (Ewing sarcoma, cervical/breast/prostate cancer, giant cell tumor, soft-tissue sarcoma, retinoblastoma).

c. More common in children exposed to radiation than in adults

d. Latent period is variable (range, 4 to 40 years; median, approximately 10 years)

e. Literature suggests children with Ewing sarcoma treated with radiation have a 5% to 10% risk of postradiation malignancy at 20 years (7% for a postradiation sarcoma).

2. Genetics/etiology

a. Ionizing radiation causes DNA damage and creates free radicals.

b. Incidence depends on dose, type, and rate of radiation treatment. In survivors of atomic

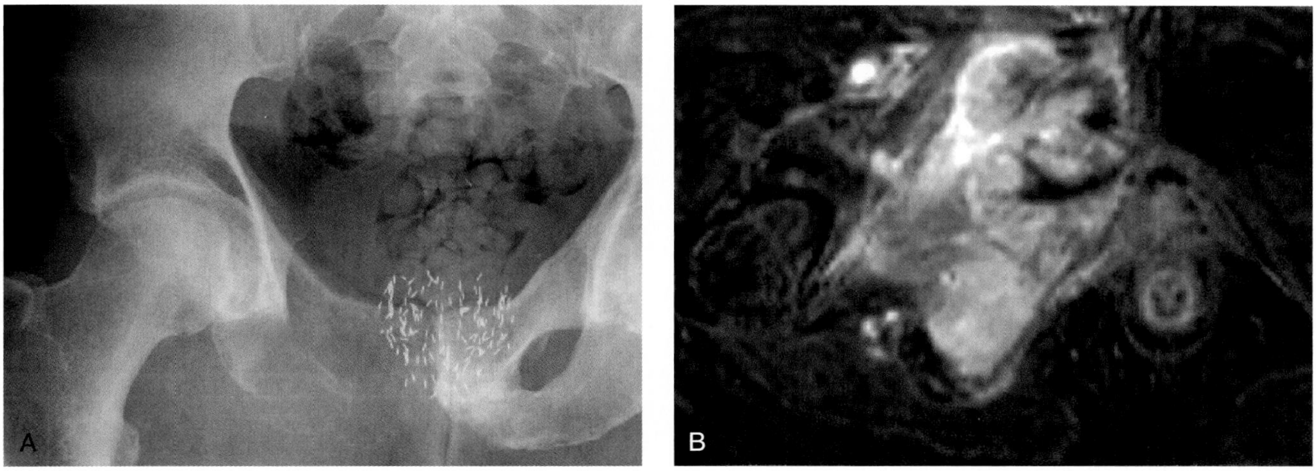

Figure 26 Secondary sarcoma in a 68-year-old man with a history of treatment for prostate cancer. **A**, AP radiograph of the right pelvis shows a destructive lesion in the right pubic rami. Note the radiation seeds. **B**, Axial MRI shows the extent of the surrounding soft-tissue mass. The biopsy revealed a high-grade sarcoma that was presumably radiation induced.

bombs, dose threshold is 0.85 Gy (lower than previously thought to be associated with secondary development of sarcoma).

c. May be affected by the use of chemotherapy (especially alkylating agents).

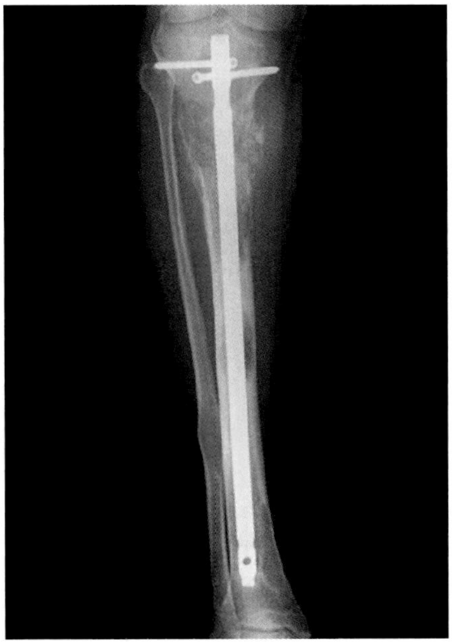

Figure 27 AP radiograph of the right lower extremity of a 64-year-old man with a diagnosis of polyostotic fibrous dysplasia. He sustained a pathologic fracture of the right proximal tibia through a lytic lesion, and an intramedullary device was placed without a preoperative biopsy. The eventual biopsy revealed a high-grade osteosarcoma developing from an area of fibrous dysplasia. The patient required a transfemoral amputation.

3. Clinical presentation
   a. Gradual onset of intermittent, then constant, pain in a previously radiated site
   b. Can affect any skeletal site
4. Imaging appearance
   a. Lytic, aggressive, destructive bone lesion (**Figure 26**, A)
   b. Possible soft-tissue mass (**Figure 26**, B)
   c. MRI used to define the extent of the lesion
5. Pathology
   a. Histology shows high-grade sarcoma (osteosarcoma, undifferentiated pleomorphic sarcoma, fibrosarcoma, chondrosarcoma)
   b. May be histologic evidence of prior irradiation in the surrounding tissues
6. Treatment/outcome
   a. Treatment is chemotherapy and surgical resection
   b. Occasionally neoadjuvant radiation is used when the margin is adjacent to critical structures
   c. Poor prognosis, with 25% to 50% 5-year survival (worse in sites not amenable to surgical resection)
   d. Metastasis primarily to the lung

C. Paget sarcoma
1. Definition and demographics
   a. Sarcoma that arises from a skeletal area affected by Paget disease

b. Occurs in older patients (older than 50 years)

c. Occurs in approximately 1% of patients with Paget disease

2. Clinical presentation

a. New onset of pain in an area affected by Paget disease

b. Possible swelling or pathologic fracture

c. Commonly affects pelvis and proximal femur

3. Imaging appearance

a. Marked bone destruction and possible soft-tissue mass in a skeletal site affected by Paget disease

b. Helpful to have prior documentation of the radiographic appearance

c. MRI is helpful to define the extent of the sarcoma within the abnormal bone

4. Pathology—Histology shows a high-grade sarcoma (osteosarcoma, undifferentiated pleomorphic sarcoma, fibrosarcoma, chondrosarcoma) within an area of pagetoid bone.

5. Treatment/outcome

a. Poor prognosis; survival is less than 10% at 5 years.

b. Treat as a primary bone sarcoma, with chemotherapy and surgical resection.

c. Radiation is palliative only.

d. High rate of metastasis to the lung.

TOP TESTING FACTS

Osteosarcoma and Undifferentiated Pleomorphic Sarcoma

1. Osteosarcoma is the most common malignant bone tumor in children.
2. Osteosarcoma classically occurs in the metaphysis of long bones and presents with progressive pain.
3. Osteosarcoma has a radiographic appearance of bone destruction and bone formation starting in the medullary canal.
4. The osteoblastic stromal cells are malignant in osteosarcoma.
5. Osteosarcoma is a genetically complex tumor with a high level of chromosomal instability.
6. The 5-year survival of patients with localized osteosarcoma in an extremity is 70%.
7. Parosteal and periosteal osteosarcomas occur on the surface of the bone.
8. Parosteal osteosarcoma is a low-grade lesion that appears fibrous histologically and is treated with wide surgical resection alone.
9. Telangiectatic osteosarcoma can be confused with an ABC.
10. Undifferentiated pleomorphic sarcoma of bone (previously called malignant fibrous histiocytoma) presents and is treated like osteosarcoma, but no osteoid is noted histologically.

Chondrosarcoma

1. Chondrosarcoma occurs de novo or secondary to an enchondroma or osteochondroma.
2. Chondrosarcoma occurs in adults, whereas osteosarcoma and Ewing sarcoma occur primarily in children.
3. The pelvis is the most common location for chondrosarcoma.
4. Secondary chondrosarcomas can occur in prior enchondromas or osteochondromas (more commonly in patients with Ollier disease, Maffucci syndrome, or multiple hereditary osteochondromas).
5. Pelvic chondrosarcomas require wide resection regardless of grade.
6. Tumor grade is a major prognostic factor for chondrosarcoma.
7. Grade 1 chondrosarcomas rarely metastasize and have a >90% survival.
8. The survival for patients with dedifferentiated chondrosarcoma is the lowest of all bone sarcomas (10%).
9. Clear cell chondrosarcoma has a radiographic appearance similar to chondroblastoma.
10. Chemotherapy is not effective in conventional chondrosarcoma (occasionally used in dedifferentiated and mesenchymal chondrosarcoma variants).
11. Radiation is not used in the treatment of chondrosarcoma.

Ewing Sarcoma/Primitive Neuroectodermal Tumor

1. Ewing sarcoma is one of a group of small round blue cell tumors not distinguishable based on histology alone.
2. Ewing sarcoma is the second most common primary malignant bone tumor in children.
3. Ewing sarcoma is found most commonly in the diaphysis of long bones as well as in the pelvis.
4. No matrix is produced by the tumor cells, so the radiographs are purely lytic.
5. There may be extensive periosteal reaction and a large soft-tissue mass.
6. Ewing sarcoma is CD99 positive and has an 11:22 chromosomal translocation.
7. Ewing sarcoma is radiation sensitive, but surgery is used more commonly for local control unless the patient has metastatic disease or cannot undergo surgery.
8. Ewing sarcoma requires multiagent chemotherapy.
9. Ewing sarcoma can metastasize to the lungs, bone, and bone marrow.
10. The 5-year survival rate of patients with isolated extremity Ewing sarcoma is 73%.

Chordoma and Adamantinoma

1. Chordoma occurs exclusively in the spinal axis, although many lesions should be considered in the differential of a destructive sacral lesion.
2. Sacral chordoma occurs in adults and has a prolonged course; misdiagnosis is common.
3. Chordoma of the skull base presents more quickly with symptoms.
4. Plain radiographs often do not identify sacral destruction from chordoma—cross-sectional imaging is required.
5. CT scan of a chordoma shows calcified areas within the tumor.
6. Chordoma consists of physaliferous cells on histologic examination.
7. Surgical cure of chordoma requires a wide resection, possibly removing nerve roots, bowel, bladder, and so forth.
8. Radiation (protons preferable) can be used in an adjunct or primary fashion for chordoma, but chemotherapy has no role.
9. Adamantinoma occurs primarily in the tibial diaphysis and has a soap bubble radiographic appearance.
10. Adamantinoma consists of nests of epithelial cells in a fibrous stroma and is keratin positive.
11. Adamantinoma requires a wide surgical resection for cure.

Multiple Myeloma and Lymphoma

1. Multiple myeloma is the most common primary malignant bone tumor.
2. Myeloma often presents with normochromic, normocytic anemia.
3. Myeloma presents radiographically with multiple punched-out lytic lesions.
4. Bone scan is typically negative with myeloma.
5. Myeloma lesions are composed of sheets of plasma cells.
6. Myeloma is treated with systemic therapy, osteoclast inhibitors, and often autologous stem cell transplant.
7. Lymphoma affecting bone is usually non-Hodgkin B cell subtype.
8. Subtle radiographic bone destruction with extensive marrow and soft-tissue involvement in lymphoma is typical.
9. Lymphoma B cells are CD20+ on immunohistochemistry staining.
10. B cell lymphoma is treated with chemotherapy and radiation; it rarely requires surgery.

Secondary Lesions

1. Secondary lesions can be benign (secondary ABC) but are most commonly sarcomas.
2. Secondary sarcomas arise in areas of Paget disease, prior radiation, or previous lesions (bone infarcts, fibrous dysplasia).
3. New-onset pain in the site of a previous lesion or site of radiation is suspicious for a secondary lesion.

4. Radiographic appearance of a secondary sarcoma is an aggressive, destructive bone tumor.
5. Histologic appearance is of a high-grade sarcoma (osteosarcoma, undifferentiated pleomorphic sarcoma, fibrosarcoma, chondrosarcoma).
6. Secondary sarcomas have a uniformly poor prognosis; treatment is with chemotherapy and surgery.
7. Undifferentiated pleomorphic sarcoma of bone can arise in a prior infarct and has a poor prognosis.
8. Fewer than 1% of fibrous dysplasia lesions undergo malignant change to undifferentiated pleomorphic sarcoma or osteosarcoma.
9. Secondary squamous cell carcinoma can arise in long-standing osteomyelitis with a draining sinus tract (Marjolin ulcer).

Bibliography

Bacci G, Longhi A, Versari M, Mercuri M, Briccoli A, Picci P: Prognostic factors for osteosarcoma of the extremity treated with neoadjuvant chemotherapy: 15-year experience in 789 patients treated at a single institution. *Cancer* 2006;106(5):1154-1161.

Cesari M, Alberghini M, Vanel D, et al: Periosteal osteosarcoma: A single-institution experience. *Cancer* 2011;117(8):1731-1735.

Chou AJ, Malek F: Osteosarcoma of bone, in Biermann JS, ed: *Orthopaedic Knowledge Update: Musculoskeletal Tumors*, ed 3. Rosemont, IL, American Academy of Orthopaedic Surgeons, 2014, pp 159-170.

Douis H, Saifuddin A: The imaging of cartilaginous bone tumours: II. Chondrosarcoma. *Skeletal Radiol* 2013;42(5):611-626.

Fuchs B, Dickey ID, Yaszemski MJ, Inwards CY, Sim FH: Operative management of sacral chordoma. *J Bone Joint Surg Am* 2005;87(10):2211-2216.

Harrison DJ, Geller DS, Gill JD, Lewis VO, Gorlick R: Current and future therapeutic approaches for osteosarcoma. *Expert Rev Anticancer Ther* 2018;18:39-50.

Hickey M, Farrokhyar F, Deheshi B, Turcotte R, Ghert M: A systematic review and meta-analysis of intralesional versus wide resection for intramedullary grade I chondrosarcoma of the extremities. *Ann Surg Oncol* 2011;18(6):1705-1709.

Kabolizadeh P, Chen YL, Liebsch N et al: Updated outcome and analysis of tumor response in mobile spine and sacral chordoma treated with definitive high-dose photon/proton radiation therapy. *Int J Rad Oncol Biol Phys* 2017; 97:254-262.

Kim HJ, McLawhorn AS, Goldstein MJ, Boland PJ: Malignant osseous tumors of the pediatric spine. *J Am Acad Orthop Surg* 2012;20(10):646-656.

Kuttesch JF Jr, Wexler LH, Marcus RB, et al: Second malignancies after Ewing's sarcoma: Radiation dose-dependency of secondary sarcomas. *J Clin Oncol* 1996;14(10):2818-2825.

Levin AS, Arkader A, Morris CD: Reconstruction following tumor resections in skeletally immature patients. *J Am Acad Orthop Surg* 2017;25:204-213.

Maheshwari AV, Cheng EY: Ewing sarcoma family of tumors. *J Am Acad Orthop Surg* 2010;18(2):94-107.

Mavrogenis AF, Ruggieri P, Mercuri M, Papagelopoulos PJ: Dedifferentiated chondrosarcoma revisited. *J Surg Orthop Adv* 2011;20(2):106-111.

McGough RL III: Chondrosarcoma of bone, in Biermann JS, ed: *Orthopaedic Knowledge Update: Musculoskeletal Tumors*, ed 3. Rosemont, IL, American Academy of Orthopaedic Surgeons, 2014, pp 1818-2194.

Most MJ, Sim FH, Inwards CY: Osteofibrous dysplasia and adamantinoma. *J Am Acad Orthop Surg* 2010;18:358-366.

Ostrowski ML, Unni KK, Banks PM, et al: Malignant lymphoma of bone. *Cancer* 1986;58(12):2646-2655.

Palumbo A, Avet-Loiseau H, Oliva S, et al: Revised international staging system for multiple myeloma: A report from international myeloma working group. *J Clin Oncol* 2015;33:2863-2869.

Rajkumar SV, Kumar S: Multiple myeloma: Diagnosis and treatment. *Mayo Clin Proc* 2016;91:101-119.

Schwab JH, Springfield DS, Raskin KA, Mankin HJ, Hornicek FJ: What's new in primary bone tumors. *J Bone Joint Surg Am* 2012;94(20):1913-1919.

Steensma M: Ewing sarcoma, in Biermann JS, ed: *Orthopaedic Knowledge Update: Musculoskeletal Tumors*, ed 3. Rosemont, IL, American Academy of Orthopaedic Surgeons, 2014, pp 171-180.

Unni KK, Inwards CY: *Dahlin's Bone Tumors*, ed 6. Philadelphia, PA, Lippincott-Raven, 2012.

Wustrack R, Cooper K, Weber K: Molecular markers in bone and soft tissue tumors. *JBJS Rev* 2016;4:1-11.

Wold LE, Unni KK, Sim FH, Sundaram M: *Atlas of Orthopedic Pathology*, ed 3. Philadelphia, PA, WB Saunders, 2008.

Chapter 145
Benign Soft-Tissue Tumors and Reactive Lesions

KRISTY L. WEBER, MD

I. LIPOMA

A. Definition and demographics
   1. Lipoma—A benign tumor of adipose tissue.
   2. Slightly more common in men than in women.
   3. Occurs primarily in patients 40 to 60 years of age.
   4. Superficial/subcutaneous lesions are common; deep lesions are uncommon.
   5. Hibernomas are tumors of brown fat; they occur in slightly younger patients (20 to 40 years).

B. Genetics/etiology
   1. Lipomas (white fat) are common.
   2. Lipomas occur when white fat accumulates in inactive people.
   3. Chromosomal abnormalities have been described.
   4. Brown fat usually occurs in hibernating animals or human infants.

C. Clinical presentation
   1. A soft, painless, mobile mass characterizes the common superficial variety.
   2. Of patients with superficial lipomas, 5% to 8% have multiple lesions.
   3. Superficial lipomas are common in the upper back, the shoulders, the arms, the buttocks, and the proximal thighs.
   4. Deep lipomas are usually intramuscular, fixed, and painless and can be large.
   5. Deep lesions are found frequently in the thigh, shoulder, and calf.
   6. Most are stable after an initial period of growth.

Dr. Weber or an immediate family member serves as a board member, owner, officer, or committee member of the American Academy of Orthopaedic Surgeons .

D. Imaging appearance
   1. Plain radiographs—Not helpful for diagnosing lipomas; in deep lipomas, a radiolucency may be seen.
   2. CT—Appearance of subcutaneous fat.
   3. MRI
      a. Bright on T1-weighted images, moderate on T2-weighted images (**Figure 1**, A and B).
      b. Lipomas image exactly as fat on all sequences (suppress with fat-suppressed images); hibernomas have increased signal intensity on T1-weighted images but not always the same appearance as fat.
      c. Homogeneous, although minor linear streaking may occur.
      d. Appearance is usually classic on MRI; biopsy not required.
   4. Occasionally, lipomas contain calcific deposits or bone.

E. Pathology
   1. Gross appearance
      a. Lipoma: soft, lobular, white, or yellow, with a capsule.
      b. Hibernoma: red-brown in color because of profusion of mitochondria and more extensive vascularity than lipoma.
   2. Histology
      a. Mature fat cells with moderate vascularity (**Figure 1**, C).
      b. Occasionally, focal calcium deposits, cartilage, or bone.
      c. Histologic variants include spindle cell lipoma, pleomorphic lipoma, angiolipoma. (All are benign but can be confused histologically with malignant lesions.)

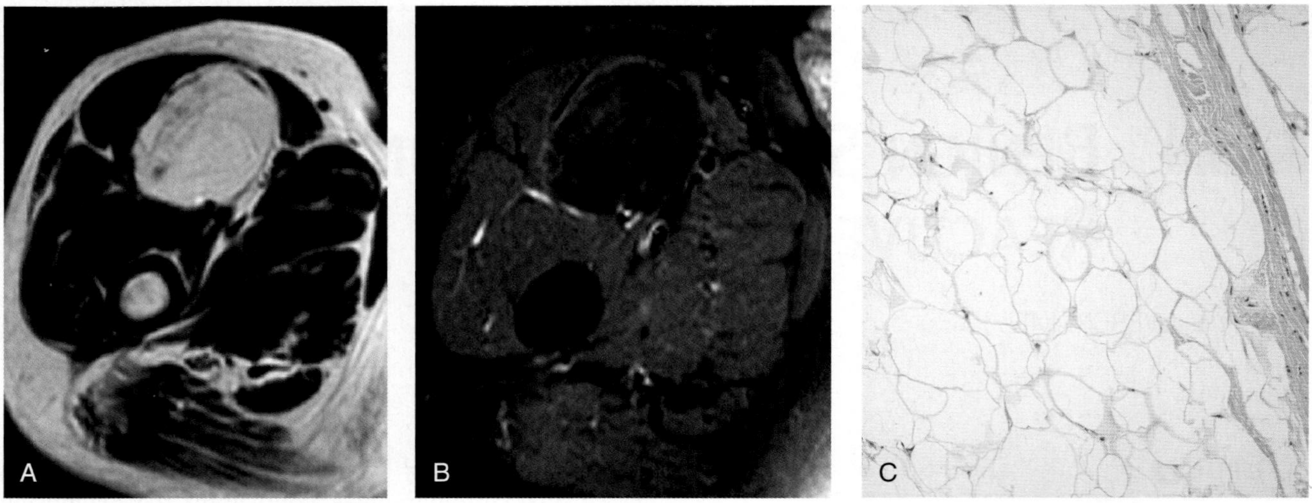

Figure 1 Intramuscular lipoma. Axial T1-weighted fat-suppressed (**A**) and T2-weighted fat-suppressed (**B**) MRIs of the right thigh reveal a well-circumscribed lesion with the same signal as the subcutaneous fat. Note that the lesion is suppressed on the fat-suppressed images, as is classic for an intramuscular lipoma. **C**, The histologic appearance is of mature fat cells without atypia (hematoxylin and eosin). A loose fibrous capsule is visible.

F. Treatment/outcome
   1. Treatment is observation or local excision (excisional biopsy with marginal margin can be performed if imaging studies clearly document a lipoma).
   2. Local recurrence is less than 5% if removed.
   3. Malignant transformation is not clinically relevant; few cases have been reported.

G. Atypical lipoma/well-differentiated liposarcoma
   1. Called atypical lipoma in the extremities and well-differentiated liposarcoma in the retroperitoneum due to different levels of aggressiveness
   2. Usually very large, deep tumors
   3. May look identical to classic lipomas or may have increased stranding on MRI (**Figure 2**, A)

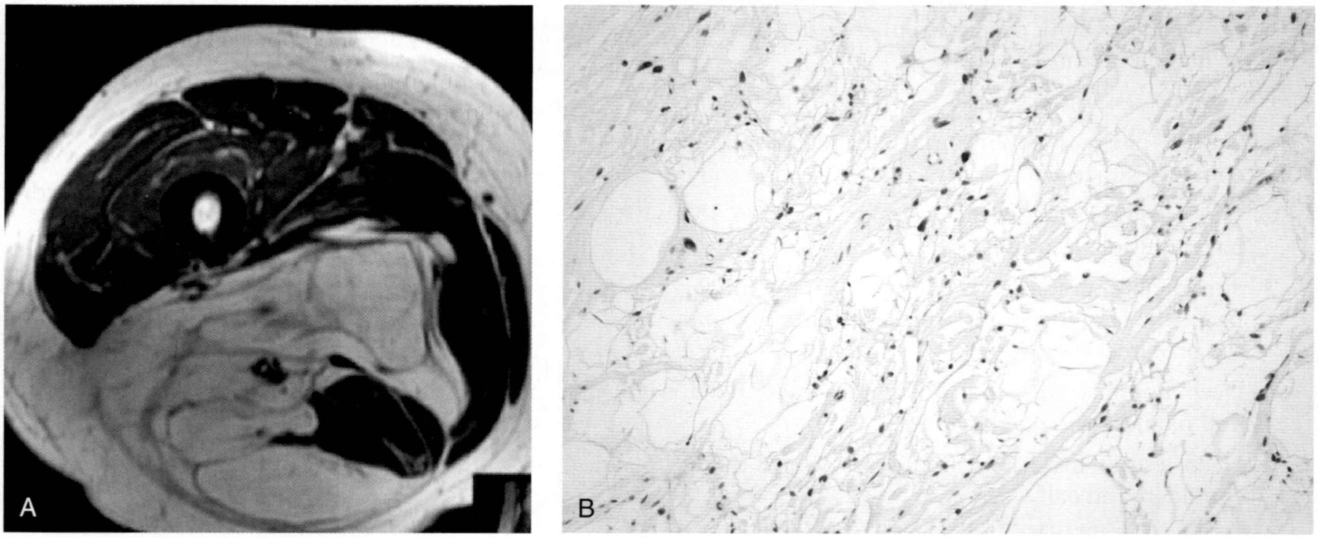

Figure 2 Atypical lipoma. **A**, Axial MRI reveals an extensive intramuscular lipomatous lesion infiltrating the posterior thigh musculature. Note the extensive stranding within the lesion. From this appearance, an intramuscular lipoma cannot be differentiated from an atypical lipoma. **B**, The histologic appearance of this atypical lipoma is more cellular than a classic lipoma (hematoxylin and eosin) and is positive for MDM2 overexpression.

4. Histology shows greater cellularity than classic lipoma (**Figure 2**, B)
5. Atypical lipoma has overexpression of MDM2 (diagnostic)
6. Treatment is marginal excision; often not differentiated from classic lipoma until after excision (based on histology)
7. Higher chance of local recurrence (50% at 10 years) compared with lipoma, but does not metastasize
8. Higher chance of dedifferentiation in the retroperitoneal well-differentiated liposarcoma (20%) than in extremity atypical lipoma (2%)

II. VASCULAR MALFORMATIONS

A. Definition and demographics
1. International Society for the Study of Vascular Anomalies (ISSVA) system
   a. Two biologic categories: Vascular neoplasms and vascular malformations
   b. Vascular neoplasms—subdivided on presence (infantile hemangiomas) or absence (congenital hemangiomas) of glucose transporter 1 (GLUT1) isoform protein
   c. Vascular malformations—subdivided into slow-/low-flow (venous, capillary, lymphatic) versus fast-/high-flow (arterial) malformations
2. Final diagnosis of vascular anomalies determined by the pathologist
3. Infantile hemangioma—most common tumor of infancy
   a. Presents between 2 weeks and 2 months
   b. Noted on skin in the head, neck, trunk, and extremities
   c. Rapid proliferative phase in first year of life to gradual regression by puberty
4. Congenital hemangioma
   a. Present at birth
   b. Observation only—usually regress spontaneously
5. Vascular malformations
   a. Most common situation in orthopaedic surgery is low-flow intramuscular vascular malformation (not a neoplasm)—previously called "hemangioma."
   b. Both low- and high-flow lesions grow during childhood and can present at any age.
   c. Males and females are affected equally.

B. Genetics/etiology—Vascular malformations
1. Low-flow malformations are congenital (venous, lymphatic, or both)
2. High-flow malformations are congenital (single, multiple, or part of a genetic disorder)

C. Clinical presentation
1. Low-flow vascular malformation
   a. Usually present before 2 years of age
   b. Common sites include neck/face, limbs, trunk, bones, muscle
2. High-flow vascular malformation
   a. Common sites in the cranium, bone, muscle, subcutaneous fat
3. Growth is variable and often fluctuates with activity.
4. Pain is variable and can increase with activity.

D. Imaging appearance
1. Plain radiographs
   a. Low-flow vascular malformation—May reveal phleboliths or calcifications within the lesion (**Figure 3**, C).
   b. Adjacent bone erosion may be seen.
2. Ultrasonography
   a. Can help differentiate high- and low-flow vascular malformation based on flow.
   b. Low-flow vascular malformations—color Doppler reveals partially solid multicystic mass.
3. MRI
   a. Low-flow vascular malformation
      - Partially solid, partially cystic lesion with fluid-fluid levels and phleboliths. They enhance with gadolinium contrast.
      - Focal areas of low signal intensity are due to blood flow or calcifications.
      - Lesions are often ill-defined or described as a "bag of worms"; they can appear infiltrative within the muscle.
   b. Helps determine the extent of the lesion in high-flow vascular malformations
   c. Increased signal intensity on T1- and T2-weighted images for both types (**Figure 3**, A and B)
   d. Frequently mistaken for a malignant soft-tissue tumor

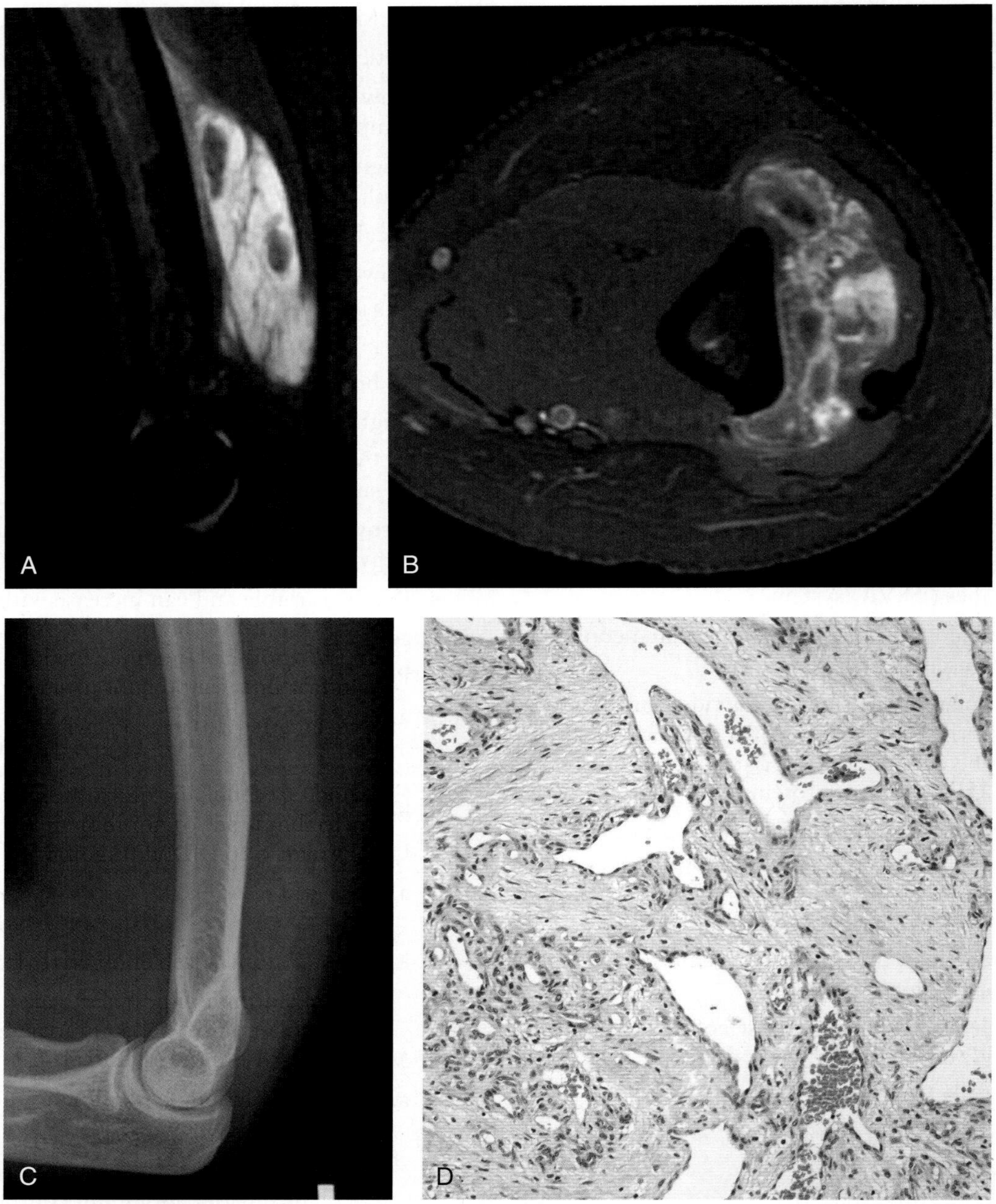

Figure 3 Vascular malformation. **A**, Sagittal and **B**, axial T2-weighted MRI of a vascular malformation in the distal triceps in a 19-year-old woman. Note the poorly circumscribed soft-tissue lesion with both fatty and vascular features within the muscle. **C**, Phleboliths seen in the posterior arm on this plain radiograph are intralesional calcifications. **D**, Histologic image of this venous or capillary low-flow lesion shows large blood-filled spaces but no cellular atypia (hematoxylin and eosin).

E. Pathology

1. Gross appearance
   a. Varies, depending on whether the lesion is the venous (more common) or arterial type.
   b. Color varies from red to tan to yellow with obvious blood vessels visible.
2. Histology
   a. Capillary-sized vessels with large nuclei (**Figure 3**, D)
   b. Well-developed vascular lumens, infiltration of muscle fibers
   c. No significant cellular pleomorphism or mitoses
3. Differential diagnosis includes angiosarcoma.

F. Treatment/outcome

1. Most vascular malformations can be symptomatically managed with observation, anti-inflammatory medications, and compression sleeves.
2. Many are amenable to interventional radiology techniques of embolization (high flow) or sclerotherapy (low flow) to decrease the size of the lesion or relieve symptoms.
3. Surgical excision carries a high risk of local recurrence—can be helpful for solid lesions.
4. No incidence of malignant transformation.

III. NEURILEMOMA (SCHWANNOMA)

A. Definition and demographics

1. Neurilemoma (schwannoma)—An encapsulated benign soft-tissue tumor composed of Schwann cells.
2. Commonly discovered in patients 20 to 50 years of age (may also occur in older patients)
3. Affects males and females equally
4. Can affect any motor or sensory nerve
5. More common than neurofibroma

B. Genetics/etiology

1. *NF2* tumor suppressor gene encodes schwannomin.
2. Inactivating *NF2* mutations are linked to neurofibromatosis type 2 (NF2; hallmark is schwannomas).

C. Clinical presentation

1. Usually asymptomatic; sometimes causes pain with stretch or activity.
2. Occurs frequently on the flexor surfaces of the extremities as well as the head/neck.
3. Pelvic lesions can become quite large.
4. May change in size given frequent occurrence of cystic degeneration.
5. Multiple lesions occur rarely.
6. Positive Tinel sign may be elicited.

D. Appearance on MRI

1. Low signal intensity on T1-weighted MRI; high signal intensity on T2-weighted MRI (**Figure 4**, A and B).
2. Diffusely enhanced signal with gadolinium administration.
3. On sagittal or coronal images, the lesion may appear in continuity with the affected nerve (**Figure 5**).
4. Difficult to differentiate neurilemoma and neurofibroma.

E. Pathology

1. Gross appearance
   a. Well-encapsulated lesion, gray-tan in color (**Figure 6**)
   b. Grows eccentrically from the nerve
2. Histology
   a. Alternating areas of compact spindle cells (Antoni A) (**Figure 4**, C) and loosely arranged cells with large vessels (Antoni B) (**Figure 4**, D)
   b. The appearance of Verocay bodies (two rows of aligned nuclei in a palisading formation) is pathognomonic.
   c. Strongly uniform positive staining for S100 antibody

F. Treatment/outcome

1. Treatment is observation or marginal/intralesional excision with nerve fiber preservation as symptoms dictate.
2. Small risk of sensory deficits or long-standing palsies after dissection.
3. Extremely rare risk of malignant degeneration.

IV. NEUROFIBROMA

A. Definition and demographics

1. Neurofibroma—A benign neural tumor involving multiple cell types.
2. Occurs in patients 20 to 40 years of age (or younger when associated with neurofibromatosis).
3. Affects males and females equally.

B. Genetics/etiology

1. Most neurofibromas arise sporadically.
2. Neurofibromatosis type 1 (NF1) is an autosomal dominant syndrome characterized by multiple neurofibromas.
   a. NF1: abnormal chromosome 17 (1 in 3000 births)
   b. NF2: abnormal chromosome 22 (1 in 33,000 births)

C. Clinical presentation

1. Can affect any nerve; may be cutaneous or plexiform (infiltrative).

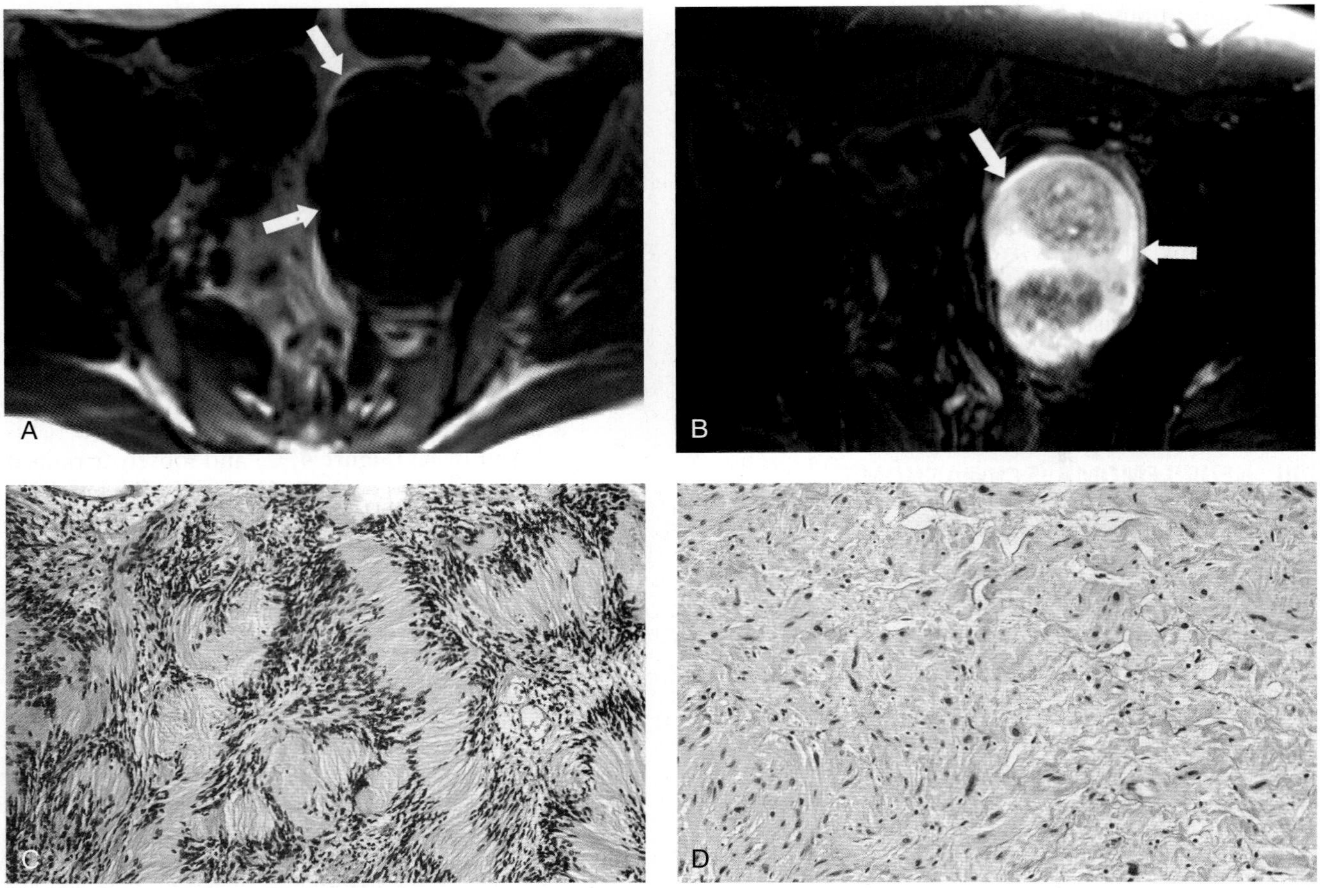

Figure 4 Neurilemoma of the pelvis. Axial T1-weighted (**A**) and T2-weighted (**B**) MRIs reveal a large soft-tissue mass (arrows) that has low signal intensity on T1 sequences and high signal intensity on T2 sequences. It would enhance after gadolinium administration. **C**, Low-power histologic image reveals the compact spindle cell areas (Antoni A) of a neurilemoma (hematoxylin and eosin). Note the palisading nuclei and Verocay bodies. **D**, Another histologic image from within the same tumor reveals areas of loosely arranged cells within a haphazard collagenous stroma (Antoni B; hematoxylin and eosin). Antoni B areas contain numerous blood vessels.

2. Most are asymptomatic, but sometimes neurologic symptoms are present.
3. Tumors are slow growing.
4. Positive Tinel sign may be elicited.
5. National Institutes of Health criteria for NF1 (requires two of the following):
   a. Six or more café-au-lait spots (size/age dependent)
   b. Two or more Lisch nodules (melanocyte hamartoma affecting the iris)
   c. Axillary or inguinal freckling
   d. Two neurofibromas (any type) or one plexiform neurofibroma
   e. Optic glioma
   f. Definitive bone lesion
   g. First-degree relative with NF1
6. Rapid enlargement of a neurofibroma suggests malignant transformation.

D. Imaging appearance
   1. Varies in size; usually a fusiform expansion of the nerve
   2. MRI
      a. Low signal intensity on T1-weighted sequences, high on T2-weighted sequences (**Figure 7**, A and B).
      b. Dumbbell-shaped lesion that can expand a neural foramen.
      c. More likely than neurilemoma to have "target sign" (peripheral high signal intensity and center of low signal intensity on T2-weighted sequences).
      d. Plexiform neurofibroma has extensive signal on MRI; infiltrative.

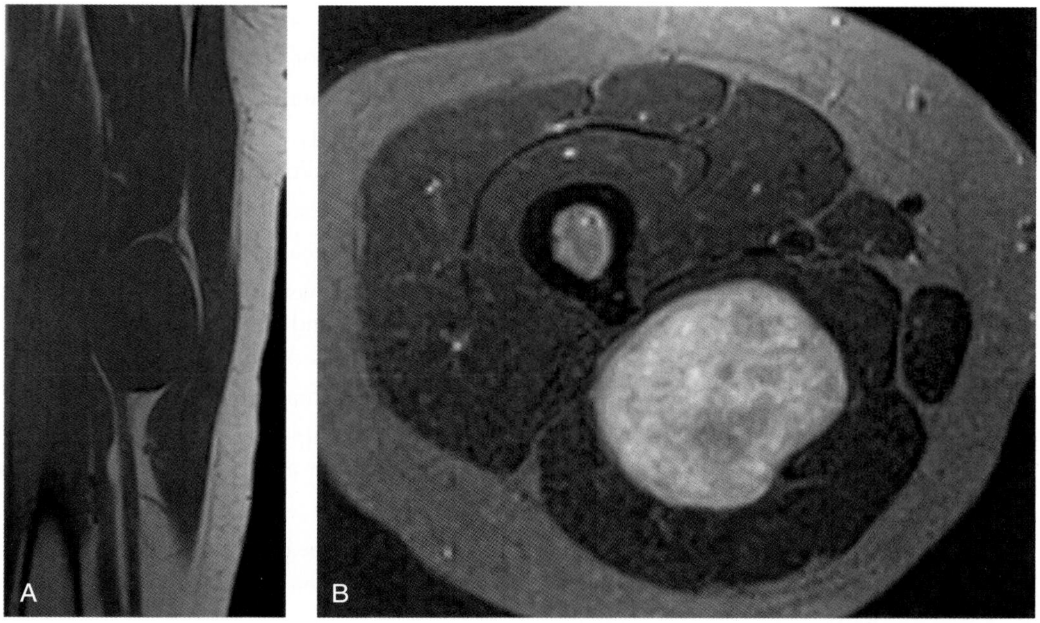

Figure 5 **A**, Sagittal T1-weighted and **B**, axial T2-weighted MRI of the right thigh reveals a well-circumscribed soft-tissue mass that is low signal on T1 and bright signal on T2 consistent with a benign nerve tumor. On the sagittal view, the lesion is in continuity with the sciatic nerve. This lesion was histologically a schwannoma.

3. Radiographs—Orthopaedic manifestations of NF1 include penciling of the ribs, sharp vertebral end plates, tibial congenital pseudarthrosis, non-ossifying fibromas, osteopenia, and scoliosis.

E. Pathology
   1. Gross appearance
      a. Fusiform expansion of the nerve
      b. Usually unencapsulated
   2. Histology
      a. Interlacing bundles of elongated cells with wavy, dark nuclei (**Figure** 7, C and D).
      b. Cells are associated with wirelike collagen fibrils.

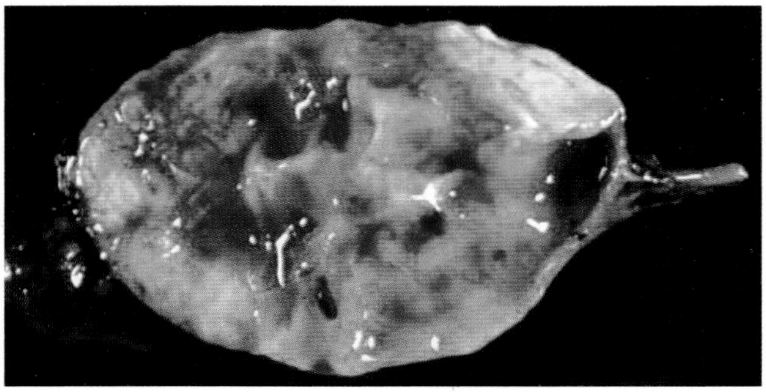

Figure 6 Photograph shows gross appearance of a bisected neurilemoma (schwannoma). Note the cystic degeneration of the well-encapsulated lesion.

      c. Cells are sometimes arranged in fascicles or a storiform pattern.
      d. Mixed cell population of Schwann cells, mast cells, and lymphocytes.
      e. Stroma may have a myxoid appearance.
      f. S100 staining is variable.

F. Treatment/outcome
   1. If asymptomatic, treatment is observation.
   2. Surgical excision; can leave significant nerve deficit and may require grafting.
   3. In 8% to 13% of patients with neurofibromatosis, malignant transformation of a lesion develops (often a plexiform neurofibroma).
   4. Malignant transformation of a solitary lesion is rare.

V. NODULAR FASCIITIS

A. Definition and demographics
   1. Nodular fasciitis—A self-limited process induced by genomic rearrangement of USP6 locus
   2. Most common in adults 20 to 40 years of age
   3. Males and females affected equally
   4. Most common fibrous soft-tissue lesion

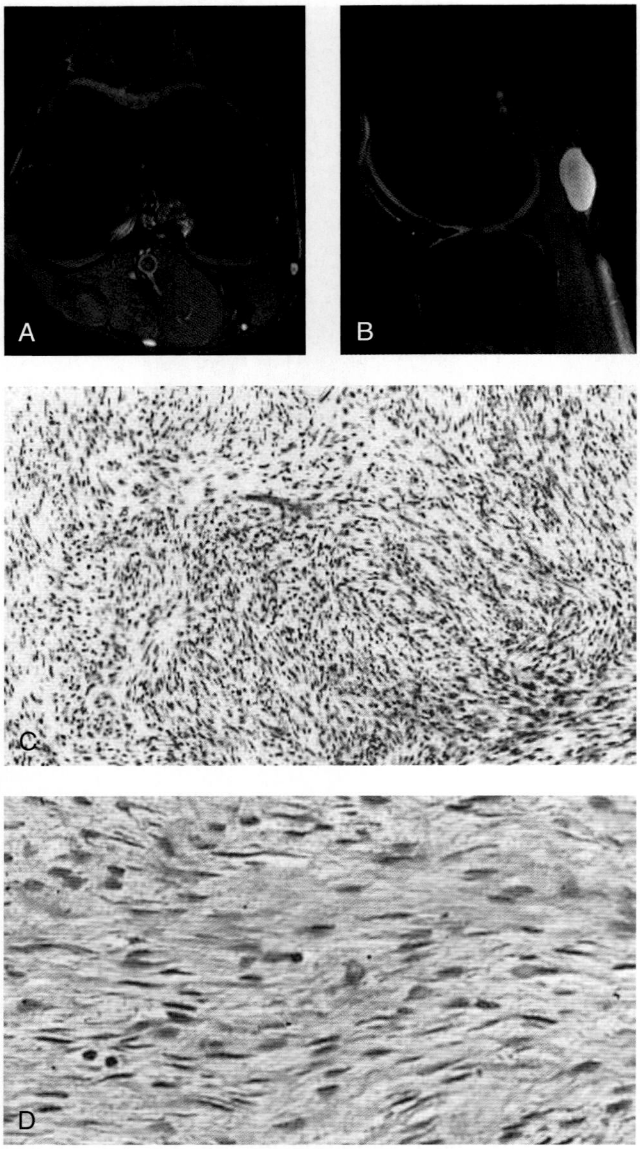

Figure 7 Neurofibroma around the knee. **A**, Axial T1-weighted and **B**, sagittal T2-weighted MRI of the right knee of a 30-year-old man reveals an area of low signal intensity on T1 imaging and high signal on T2 imaging consistent with a neurofibroma in the posterolateral subcutaneous tissues. **C**, Low-power histologic image reveals a cellular lesion with a wavy or storiform appearance (hematoxylin and eosin). **D**, Higher power histologic image reveals elongated cells with dark nuclei and no atypia (hematoxylin and eosin).

B. Genetics/etiology
   1. USP6 genomic rearrangement confirms clonal, neoplastic nature of lesion
   2. Rearrangement of USP6 locus in 90% of nodular fasciitis lesions

C. Clinical presentation
   1. Rapid growth of a nodule over 2 to 4 weeks
   2. Common h/o preceding trauma
   3. Pain and/or tenderness in 50% of patients
   4. Lesion usually 2 to 4 cm
   5. Commonly occurs on volar forearm, back, chest wall, head/neck
   6. Solitary lesion

D. Imaging appearance
   1. MRI shows nodularity, extension along fascial planes, and avid enhancement with gadolinium (**Figure 8**, A)
   2. Usually small
   3. Occurs superficially (most common), intramuscularly, or along the superficial fascial planes

E. Pathology
   1. Gross appearance—Nodular without a surrounding capsule.
   2. Histology
      a. Cellular with numerous mitotic figures (**Figure 8**, B).
      b. Cells are plump, regular fibroblasts arranged in short bundles or fascicles (**Figure 8**, C).
      c. Additional cells include lymphoid cells, erythrocytes, giant cells, and lipid macrophages.
      d. Can have an infiltrative growth pattern.
   3. Often misdiagnosed as a sarcoma
   4. USP6 rearrangement (by fluorescence in situ hybridization [FISH]) is diagnostic

F. Treatment/outcome
   1. Treatment is marginal or intralesional excision; has a low risk of local recurrence.
   2. Can observe if asymptomatic—can resolve spontaneously
   3. No risk of malignant transformation
   4. Reports of resolution of lesion after needle biopsy

VI. INTRAMUSCULAR MYXOMA

A. Definition and demographics
   1. Intramuscular myxoma—A benign, nonaggressive myxomatous soft-tissue tumor.
   2. Occurs in adults 40 to 70 years of age
   3. Male-to-female ratio = 1:2

B. Clinical presentation
   1. Usually presents as a painless mass
   2. Pain/tenderness in approximately 20% of patients

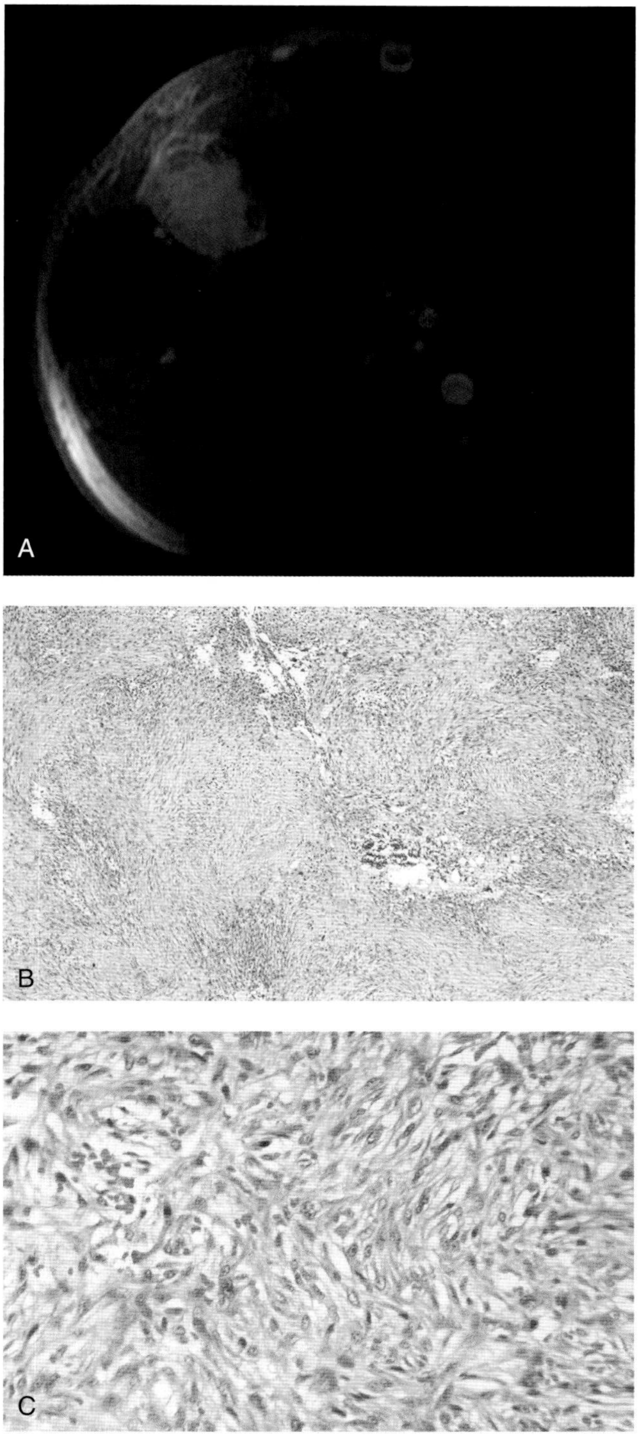

Figure 8 Nodular fasciitis. **A**, Axial T2-weighted MRI of the right upper arm reveals a bright lesion along the anterolateral fascial plane that developed after a prior history of trauma. The area is tender on examination. **B**, Low-power histologic image reveals a highly cellular lesion with a nodular pattern (hematoxylin and eosin). **C**, Higher power histologic image shows regular, plump fibroblasts with vessels, erythrocytes, and lipid macrophages consistent with nodular fasciitis (hematoxylin and eosin). The lesion was positive for a USP6 gene rearrangement.

3. Possible numbness or paresthesias in patients with large lesions
4. Usually solitary
5. Most commonly located in the thigh, buttocks, shoulder, and upper arm
6. Often close to neurovascular structures
7. The presence of multiple intramuscular myxomas is associated with fibrous dysplasia (Mazabraud syndrome). In Mazabraud syndrome, fibrous dysplasia develops at a young age and the myxomas occur later in the same general anatomic area.

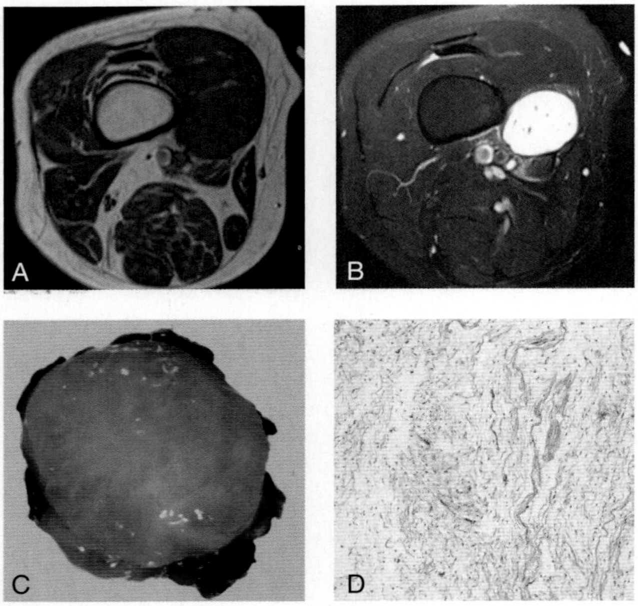

Figure 9 Intramuscular myxoma. Axial T1-weighted (**A**) and T2-weighted (**B**) MRIs of the right knee in a 58-year-old woman show a soft-tissue mass along the posteromedial aspect of the vastus medialis consistent with an intramuscular myxoma. It has lower signal intensity than muscle on the T1-weighted image and is bright on the T2-weighted image. **C**, Photograph shows the gross appearance of a bisected intramuscular myxoma; note the white, gelatinous surface. **D**, The histologic appearance reveals a paucicellular lesion with extensive reticulin fibers and a mucoid stroma (hematoxylin and eosin).

C. Imaging appearance
1. MRI appearance is homogeneous.
2. Low signal intensity (lower than muscle) on T1-weighted sequences, high on T2-weighted sequences (**Figure 9**, A and B).
3. Located within the muscle groups; usually 5 to 10 cm in size.

D. Pathology
1. Gross appearance—Lobular and gelatinous with cyst-like spaces (**Figure 9**, C)
2. Histology
   a. Minimal cellularity with cells suspended in abundant mucoid material (**Figure 9**, D).
   b. Loose network of reticulin fibers.
   c. No atypia, and only sparse vascularity.
   d. "Cellular myxoma" has increased cellularity and can be mistaken for a malignant myxoid neoplasm.

E. Treatment/outcome
1. Marginal excision is the preferred treatment.
2. Can observe if asymptomatic.
3. Very rarely recurs locally and does not metastasize.

VII. DESMOID TUMOR (EXTRA-ABDOMINAL FIBROMATOSIS)

A. Definition and demographics
1. Desmoid tumor—A benign, locally aggressive fibrous neoplasm with a high risk of local recurrence.
2. Approximately 900 cases annually in the United States.
3. Occurs in young persons (15 to 40 years).
4. Slight female predominance.
5. Desmoid tumors occur within a family of fibromatoses that also includes superficial lesions in the palmar and plantar fascia (Dupuytren disease, Ledderhose disease).

B. Genetics/etiology
1. Most spontaneous desmoid tumors are associated with mutations of the β-catenin gene (85% of cases), which results in decreased activation of Wnt/β-catenin signaling.
2. A minority of desmoid tumors are associated with Gardner syndrome and have mutations in the adenomatous polyposis coli (APC) gene.
3. Cytogenetic abnormalities include trisomy of chromosomes 8 or 20.

C. Clinical presentation
1. Usually a painless mass
2. Rock hard, fixed, and deep on examination
3. Most commonly occurs in the shoulder, chest wall/back, thigh
4. More than 50% are extra-abdominal; the rest are intra-abdominal (pelvis, mesentery)
5. Occasionally multicentric; usually a subsequent lesion occurs more proximal in the same limb

D. Imaging appearance
1. Typical MRI appearance: low signal intensity on T1-weighted sequences, low to medium signal intensity on T2-weighted sequences (**Figure 10**, A and B)
2. Enhanced appearance with gadolinium administration
3. Infiltrative within the muscles; usually 5 to 10 cm in size
4. Adjacent osseous changes (erosion) may be seen.

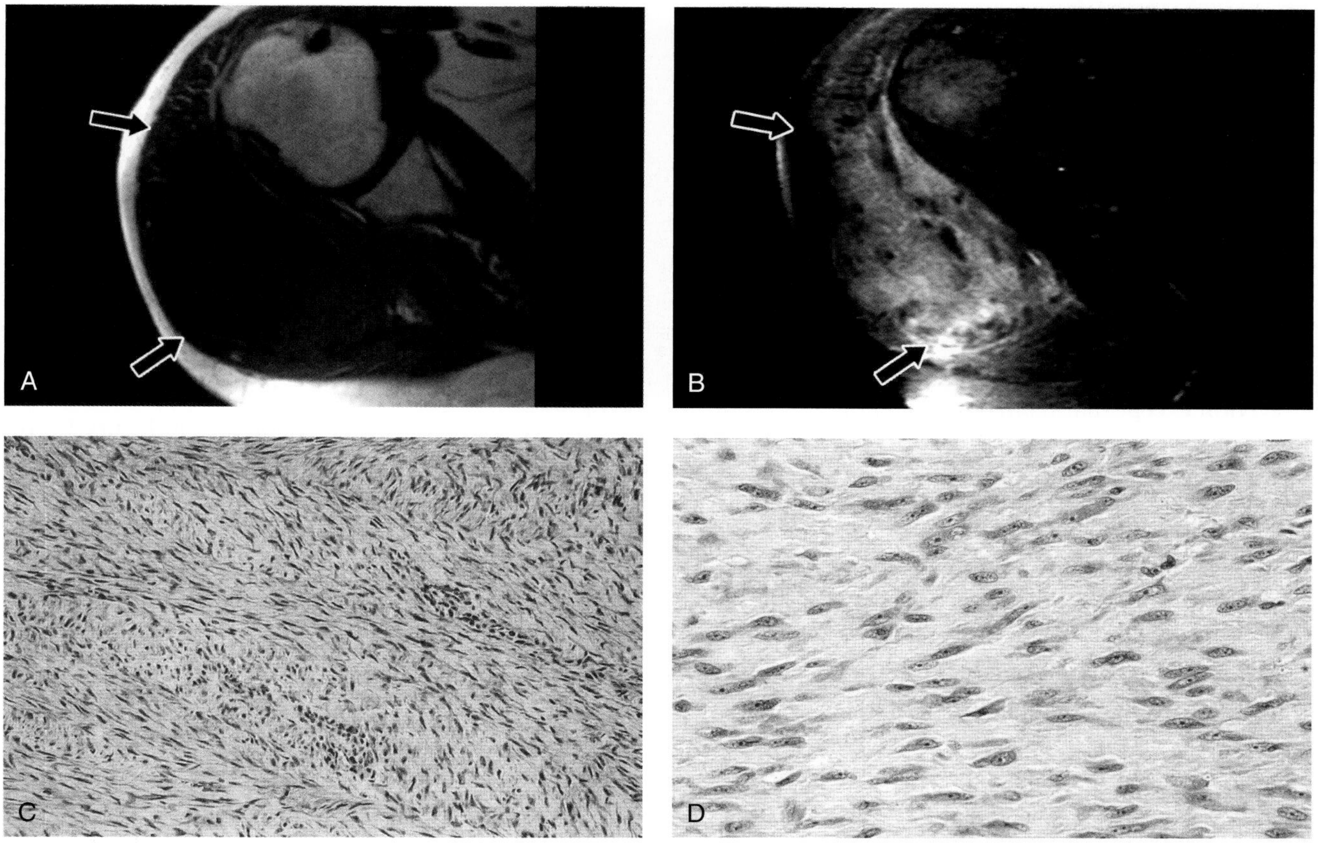

Figure 10 Desmoid tumors. Axial T1-weighted (**A**) and short tau inversion recovery (STIR) (**B**) MRIs of the right shoulder of a 58-year-old woman reveal a desmoid tumor (arrows). The STIR sequence is fluid sensitive and reveals findings similar to those found on a fat-sensitive T2-weighted image. Low signal intensity is seen on both images. **C**, Low-power histologic image reveals sweeping bundles of collagen (hematoxylin and eosin). **D**, Higher power histologic image demonstrates bland, elongated, fibrous cells without atypia (hematoxylin and eosin). The lesion stained positive for β-catenin.

E. Pathology

1. Gross appearance: gritty, white, poorly encapsulated
2. Histology
    a. Bland fibroblasts with abundant collagen (**Figure 10**, C and D)
    b. Uniform spindle cells with elongated nuclei and only occasional mitoses
    c. Moderate vascularity
    d. Sweeping bundles of collagen; less defined than in fibrosarcoma
    e. Often infiltrates into adjacent tissues and has no tumor capsule
    f. Nuclear staining for β-catenin helps differentiate from other fibrous lesions
    g. Positive staining for estrogen receptor β
3. Differential diagnosis includes fibrosarcoma, nodular fasciitis, and hypertrophic scar

F. Treatment/outcome

1. Overall treatment should be determined by a multidisciplinary team.
    a. Medical treatment of most desmoid tumors (especially large or those where wide margins are not achievable) is the current standard.
        - Tyrosine kinase inhibitors (sorafenib) is first-line treatment followed by (in no order) antihormonal drugs (tamoxifen), NSAIDs (cyclo-oxygenase [COX]-2 inhibitors), or classic chemotherapy.
    b. Observation for asymptomatic stable lesions.
    c. Surgery if symptomatic after failed medical therapy or resectable with wide margin.
    d. Radiation (up to 60 Gy) as an adjuvant or definitive therapy (although risk exists for secondary sarcoma).
    e. Results are highly variable regardless of treatment option.

2. If surgery is performed, treatment is similar to that for sarcoma, requiring wide resection.
3. High risk of local recurrence after surgery given infiltrative pattern.
4. Difficult to differentiate recurrent tumor from scar tissue (use gadolinium with MRI).
5. Unusual natural history: hard-to-predict behavior, occasional spontaneous regression.
6. Treatment should not be worse than the disease; avoid amputation.
7. No risk of metastasis or malignant transformation except that related to radiation.

VIII. ELASTOFIBROMA

A. Definition and demographics
1. Elastofibroma—An unusual, tumorlike reactive process that frequently occurs between the scapula and chest wall
2. Occurs in patients aged 60 to 80 years
3. More common in females than in males

B. Genetics/etiology
1. High familial incidence
2. Often occurs after repeated trauma

C. Clinical presentation
1. Usually asymptomatic; found in approximately 17% of elderly people at autopsy
2. Snapping scapula on examination
3. Firm, deep lesion
4. Occurs almost exclusively in the soft tissues between the tip of the scapula and the chest wall
5. Bilateral in 10% of cases (can be noted incidentally on chest CT scans)

D. Imaging appearance
1. CT—Ill-defined lesion with appearance of muscle.
2. MRI—Mixed low and high signal intensity on T1- and T2-weighted sequences (**Figure 11**, A).

E. Pathology
1. Gross appearance: gray with cystic degeneration, 5 to 10 cm in length.
2. Histology
   a. Elastic fibers having a beaded appearance with characteristic staining for elastin (**Figure 11**, B).
   b. Equal proportion of intertwined collagen fibers.

F. Treatment/outcome
1. Treatment for asymptomatic lesions is observation.
2. Simple excision is curative.
3. No risk of malignant transformation

IX. GLOMUS TUMOR

A. Definition and demographics
1. Glomus tumor—A benign tumor of the normal glomus body usually occurring in the subungual region.
2. Extremely rare
3. Occurs in patients 20 to 40 years of age
4. Males and females are affected equally (except subungual tumors, for which the male-to-female ratio = 1:3).

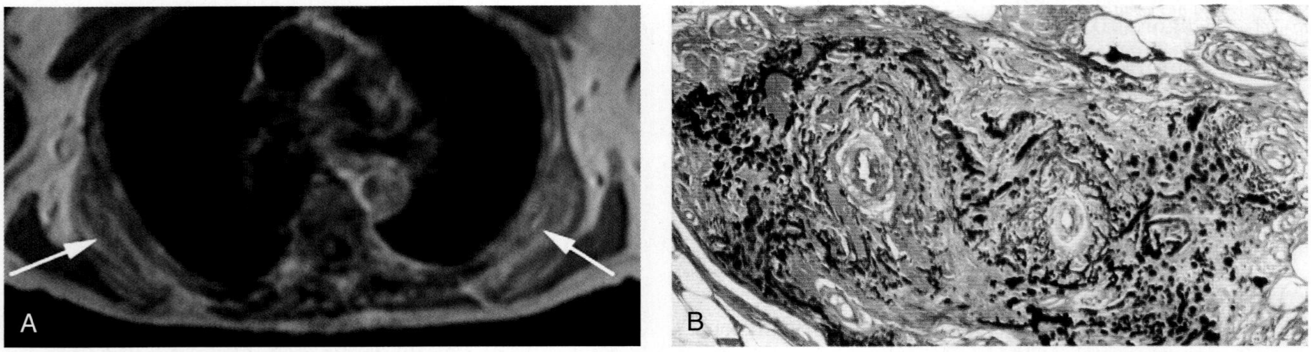

Figure 11 Elastofibroma. **A**, Axial MRI of the chest of a 73-year-old woman reveals bilateral soft-tissue masses (arrows) between the inferior tip of the scapula and the underlying chest wall consistent with elastofibromas. **B**, High-power histologic image reveals the beaded appearance of the elastic fibers admixed with the extensive collagen fibers. The elastin stain highlights the elastic fibers throughout the lesion (hematoxylin and eosin). Note the extensive vascularity.

B. Clinical presentation
   1. Small (<1 cm) red-blue nodule in the subungual region or other deep dermal layers in the extremities
   2. More difficult to see color in subungual region; may have ridging of the nail or discoloration of the nail bed
   3. Characteristic triad of symptoms: paroxysmal pain, cold insensitivity, localized tenderness
   4. Frequent delay in diagnosis
   5. Less common locations include the palm, wrist, forearm, and foot
   6. Multiple tumors in 10% of cases
C. Imaging appearance
   1. MRI
      a. Best imaging modality to identify glomus tumors
      b. Sensitivity: 90% to 100%; specificity: 50%
      c. Low signal intensity on T1-weighted sequences, high on T2-weighted sequences
   2. Plain radiographs
      a. Not very helpful in diagnosis
      b. Can show a scalloped osteolytic defect with a sclerotic border in the distal phalanx
D. Pathology
   1. Gross appearance—Small, red-blue nodule
   2. Histology
      a. Well-defined lesion of small vessels surrounded by glomus cells in a hyaline or myxoid stroma (**Figure 12**)
      b. Uniform, round cell with a prominent nucleus and eosinophilic cytoplasm
      c. Periodic acid-Schiff stain gives a chicken-wire appearance to the matrix between cells
E. Treatment/outcome
   1. Marginal excision is curative
   2. Extremely rare reports of malignant glomus tumors

X. SYNOVIAL CHONDROMATOSIS

A. Definition and demographics
   1. Synovial chondromatosis—A metaplastic proliferation of hyaline cartilage nodules in the synovial membrane.
   2. Occurs in patients 30 to 50 years of age
   3. Male-to-female ratio = 2:1
B. Genetics/etiology
   1. Generally thought to be a metaplastic condition
   2. Occasional chromosomal aberrations (hedgehog signaling) have been identified
C. Clinical presentation
   1. Joint pain, clicking, limited range of motion (ROM)
   2. Pain worse with activity
   3. Warmth, erythema, or tenderness may be present, depending on location
   4. Slow progression of symptoms over years
   5. Most common in the hip and knee, followed by shoulder and elbow
   6. Occasionally occurs in the bursa overlying an osteochondroma

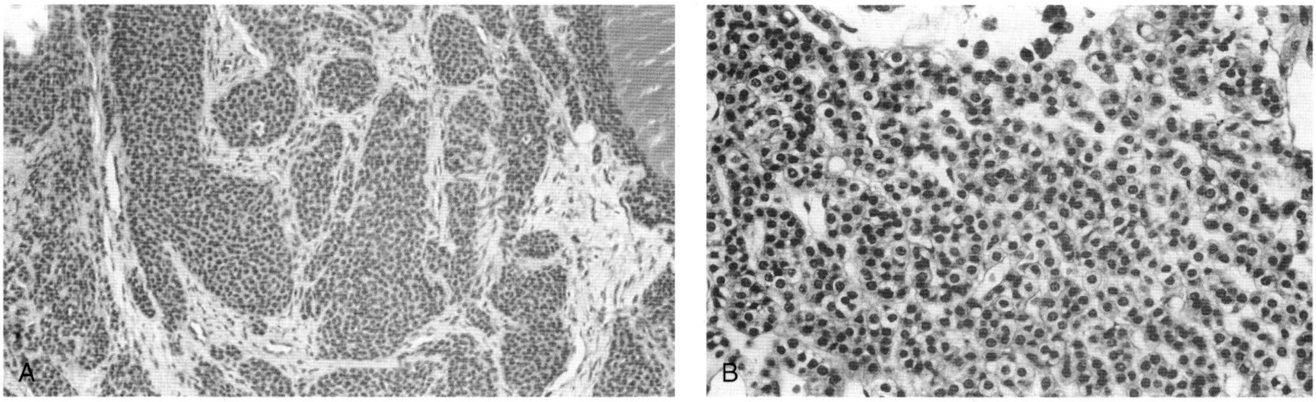

Figure 12 **A**, Low-power histologic image of a glomus tumor reveals small, rounded cells with dark nuclei in well-defined clumps. **B**, On higher power, the glomus cells and admixed capillaries are noted within a myxoid stroma (hematoxylin and eosin).

D. Imaging appearance
   1. Plain radiographs show variable appearance, depending on early or late disease.
   2. Cartilage nodules are not visible initially, except on MRI.
   3. Nodules calcify over time, then undergo endochondral ossification (**Figure 13**, A and B).
   4. Densities are smooth and well defined and remain within the confines of the synovial membrane.
   5. Erosion of cartilage and underlying bone may be seen.
   6. CT scan can define intra-articular loose bodies.
   7. MRI shows lobular appearance with signal dropout consistent with calcification.

E. Pathology
   1. Gross appearance—There may be hundreds of osteocartilaginous loose bodies within an affected joint.
   2. Histology
      a. Discrete hyaline cartilage nodules in various phases of calcification or ossification (**Figure 13**, C). Ossification starts on the periphery of the nodules.
      b. Cellular appearance of chondrocytes includes mild atypia, binucleate cells, and occasional mitoses (more cellular atypia than allowed in an intramedullary benign cartilage tumor) (**Figure 13**, D).

F. Treatment/outcome
   1. Treatment is open or arthroscopic synovectomy.
   2. Less than adequate removal of nodules increases risk for local recurrence.
   3. Natural history is self-limited, but the process can damage the joint.
   4. Differentiate between secondary synovial osteochondromatosis which can be associated with moderate/severe degenerative joint disease of a joint

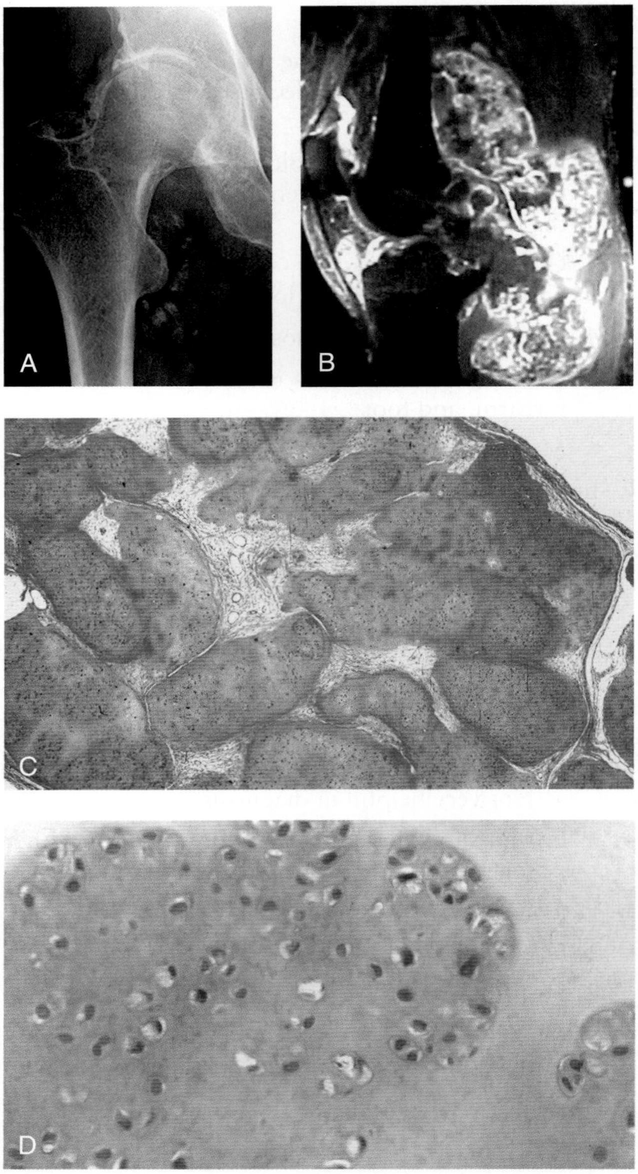

Figure 13 Synovial chondromatosis. **A**, AP radiograph of the right hip of a 46-year-old man with synovial chondromatosis demonstrates discrete calcifications superior and inferior to the femoral head, both within and external to the hip capsule. **B**, Sagittal T2-weighted MRI of the knee in a 33-year-old man with extensive synovial osteochondromatosis. Multiple ossified nodules within the joint required open synovectomies of the anterior and posterior compartments of the knee. **C**, Low-power histologic image of synovial osteochondromatosis reveals discrete hyaline cartilage nodules (hematoxylin and eosin). **D**, Higher power reveals increased cellularity with occasional binucleate cells (hematoxylin and eosin).

XI. TENOSYNOVIAL GIANT CELL TUMOR

A. Definition and demographics
   1. Tenosynovial giant cell tumor (TSGCT) or giant cell tumor of tendon sheath is a family of soft-tissue lesions involving tendon sheaths or synovium of joints
   2. Can be intra- or extra-articular
   3. Can be localized (nodular) or diffuse (latter was previously referred to as PVNS)
   4. Localized form most commonly affects patients 40 to 60 years of age. Diffuse form affects slightly younger patients. Localized/nodular form more common in females (2:1); only slight female predominance in diffuse form

B. Genetics/etiology
 1. An earlier traumatic incident is reported by 50% of patients.
 2. Minor population of intratumoral cells harbor a recurrent translocation (1p 13), and these cells overexpress colony-stimulating factor-1 (CSF1).
 3. Tumor cells recruit macrophages expressing the CSF-1 receptor (CSF-1R)

C. Clinical presentation
 1. Localized form: found in digits (85%), wrist, foot/ankle, knee (extra-articular) and knee (intra-articular)
 2. Diffuse form: mostly intra-articular in the knee (75%), hip, ankle, shoulder
 3. Localized form symptoms: slowly progressive, painless mass along tendon sheaths, or mechanical joint symptoms with focal involvement
 4. Diffuse form symptoms: pain, swelling, decreased joint ROM, recurrent effusions
 5. Natural history of extra-articular or intra-articular disease is very slow progression
 6. Joint deterioration with intraosseous extension over time

D. Imaging appearance
 1. Plain radiographs—Well-defined erosions on both sides of a joint signify advanced, diffuse intra-articular disease (**Figure 14**, A).
 2. MRI
  a. Localized forms are well-demarcated eccentric along tendon sheath or completely encasing the tendon.
  b. Diffuse intra-articular process and joint effusion with low/intermediate signal intensity (due to hemosiderin deposits) on T1- and spin echo T2-weighted images (**Figure 14**, B and C).
  c. Signal enhanced with gadolinium.
  d. Gradient echo sequences reveal hemosiderin deposits (blooming appearance).
 3. Differential diagnosis includes reactive or inflammatory synovitis, hemophilia, and synovial chondromatosis.

E. Pathology
 1. Gross appearance (diffuse intra-articular form)—Reddish-brown stained synovium with extensive papillary projections (**Figure 14**, D).
 2. Histology (diffuse type)
  a. Diagnostic mononuclear stromal cell infiltrate within the synovium (**Figure 14**, E).
  b. Cells are round with a large nucleus and eosinophilic cytoplasm.
  c. Hemosiderin-laden macrophages, multinucleated giant cells, and foam cells present; not required for diagnosis.
  d. Mitotic figures are relatively common.

F. Treatment/outcome
 1. Localized form
  a. Marginal excision of extra-articular disease along tendon sheaths
  b. Arthroscopic or open removal of a focal intra-articular lesion
  c. Local recurrence rate 0% to 15%
 2. Diffuse intra-articular form
  a. Arthroscopic total synovectomy of major joints
  b. Can combine anterior arthroscopic synovectomy with open excision of posterior disease around the knee
  c. High local recurrence rate 21% to 50% (27% in knee)
 3. Progression is highly variable, and there can be disease stabilization without treatment or after incomplete synovectomy.
 4. Total joint arthroplasty is indicated for advanced intra-articular disease with secondary degenerative changes.
 5. External beam radiation (30 to 50 Gy) is used occasionally following multiple local recurrences.
 6. The tyrosine kinase inhibitor, imatinib, has been used with variable success
 7. Inhibition of CSF1 receptor (CSF1R) using small-molecule inhibitors or a monoclonal antibody has shown some efficacy.
 8. Malignant progression of disease has been exceptionally rare.

XII. MYOSITIS OSSIFICANS

A. Definition and demographics
 1. Myositis ossificans—A reactive process characterized by a well-circumscribed proliferation of fibroblasts, cartilage, and bone within a muscle (or, rarely, within a nerve, tendon, or fat).
 2. Occurs in young, active individuals (most common in individuals 15 to 35 years of age).
 3. More common in males than in females.

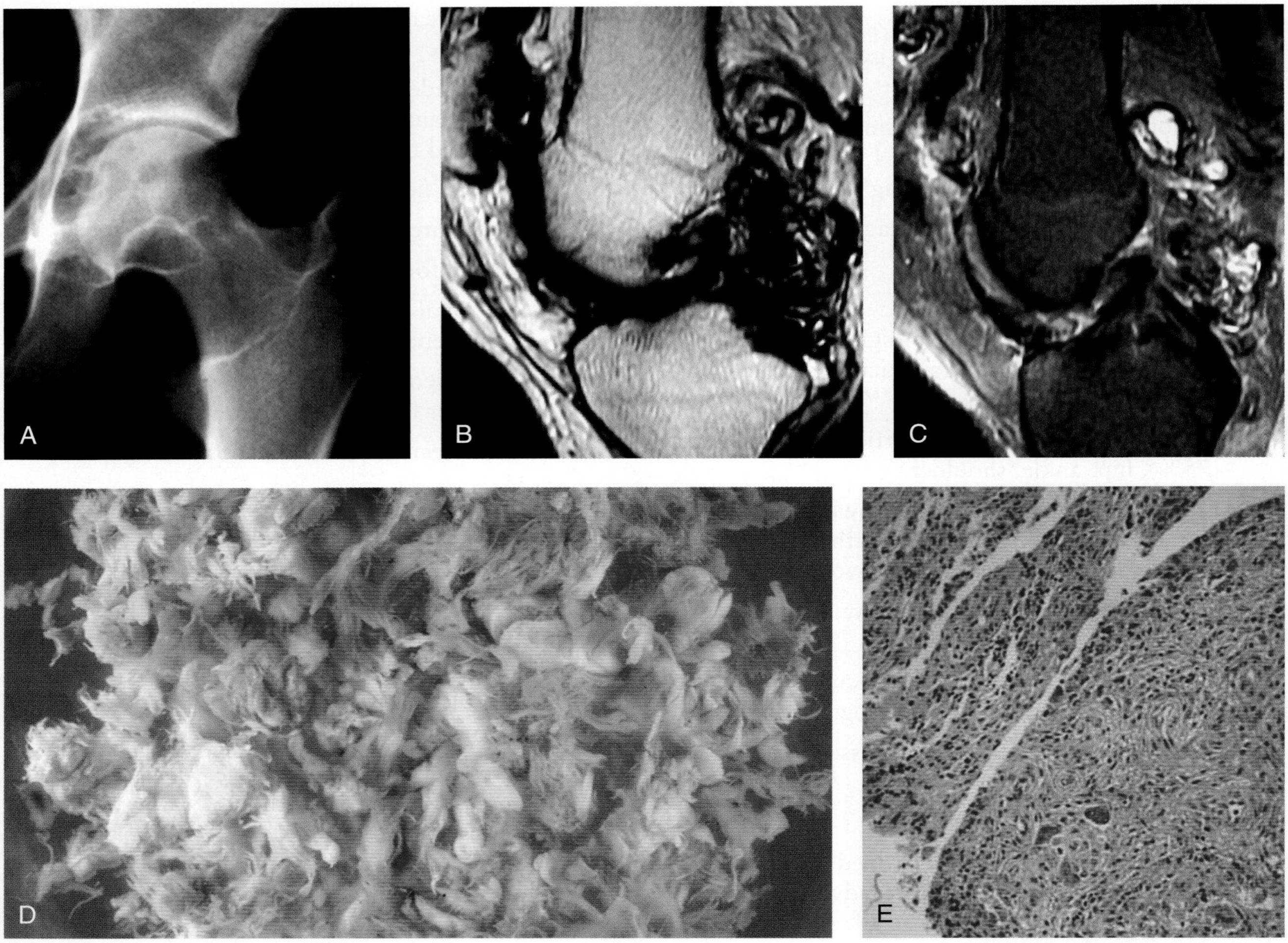

Figure 14 Examples of diffuse, intra-articular tenosynovial giant cell tumor. **A**, AP radiograph of the left hip of a patient with diffuse disease reveals osteolytic lesions with sclerotic rims on both sides of the joint. Sagittal T1-weighted (**B**) and T2-weighted (**C**) MRIs of a knee show extensive disease in the posterior aspect of the knee. The lesion is both intra-articular and extra-articular. Dark signal is seen on both of the images as a result of the hemosiderin deposits within the synovium. **D**, Gross appearance of the reddish-brown synovial fronds. **E**, Histologic image reveals a cellular infiltrate within the synovium with multinucleated giant cells and faint hemosiderin (hematoxylin and eosin). The round, mononuclear stromal cells are the key to the diagnosis.

B. Genetics/etiology—Almost always a posttraumatic condition.

C. Clinical presentation

1. Pain, tenderness, swelling, and decreased ROM, usually within days of an injury.
2. Mass that increases in size over several months (usually 3 to 6 cm); then growth stops and mass becomes firm.
3. Commonly occurs in the quadriceps, brachialis, and gluteal muscles.

D. Imaging appearance

1. Mineralization begins 3 weeks after injury.
2. Initially, irregular, fluffy densities in the soft tissues are noted on plain radiographs (**Figure 15**, A).
3. Adjacent periosteal reaction in the bone may be seen.
4. Rim enhancement is seen on MRI with gadolinium within the first 3 weeks.
5. With time and maturation, a zoning pattern occurs, with increased peripheral mineralization and a radiolucent center.
6. CT defines the ossified lesion, which looks like an eggshell (**Figure 15**, B).

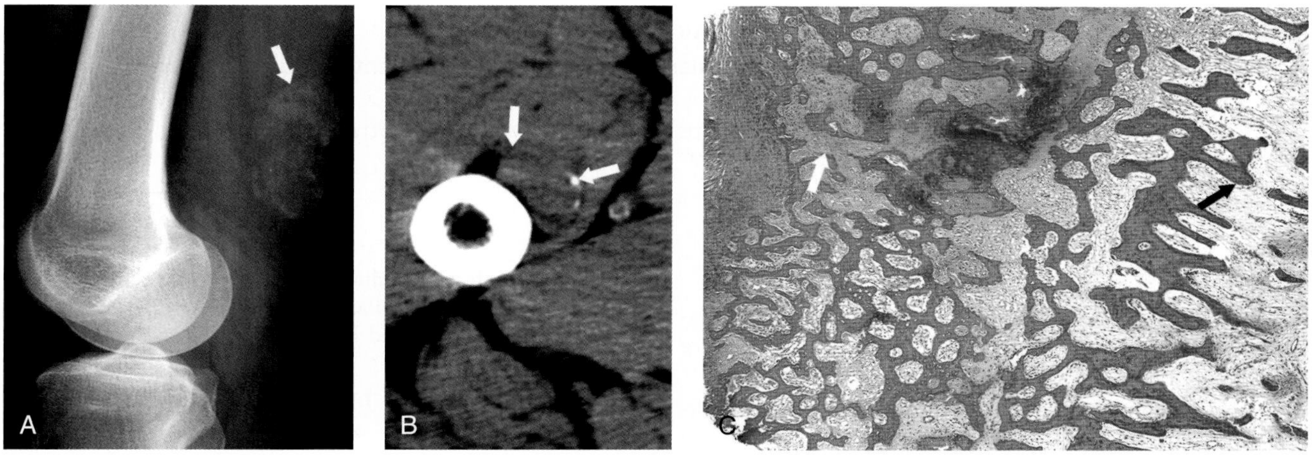

Figure 15 Examples of myositis ossificans. **A**, Lateral radiograph of a knee obtained 4 weeks after a football injury to the posterior thigh in a 19-year-old man reveals fluffy calcifications (arrow) in the posterior thigh musculature consistent with early myositis ossificans. **B**, CT scan of the thigh of a patient with traumatic myositis ossificans reveals the calcified outline of the lesion (arrows) with more mature tissue on the periphery. **C**, Histologic image of a myositis ossificans lesion reveals a zonal pattern (hematoxylin and eosin), with more mature bone toward the periphery (white arrow) and looser fibrous tissue toward the center (black arrow).

7. Differential diagnosis includes extraskeletal and parosteal osteosarcoma (more ossified in the center with peripheral lucencies).

E. Pathology
1. Gross appearance—Immature tissue in center of lesion with mature bone around outer edge.
2. Histology
   a. Zonal pattern (**Figure 15**, C)
      - Periphery: mature lamellar bone
      - Intermediate: poorly defined trabeculae with osteoblasts, fibroblasts, and large ectatic blood vessels
      - Center: immature, loose, fibrous tissue with moderate pleomorphism and mitoses
   b. Skeletal muscle can be entrapped in the periphery of the lesion
   c. No cytologic atypia
3. Differential diagnosis includes extraskeletal osteosarcoma (periphery is least ossified and cells show extreme pleomorphism).

F. Treatment/outcome
1. Myositis ossificans is a self-limited process, so observation and physical therapy to maintain motion are indicated.
2. Repeat radiographs should be obtained to confirm maturation and stability of the lesion.
3. Excision is indicated only when the lesion is mature (approximately 6 to 12 months) and if symptomatic; excision at initial stages predisposes to local recurrence.
4. The size of the mass often decreases after 1 year.

TOP TESTING FACTS

1. Lipomas should image the same as fat on all MRI sequences.
2. Vascular malformations are either low- or high-flow lesions and best treated nonsurgically (sclerotherapy or embolization).
3. Neurilemomas have Antoni A (cellular) and Antoni B (myxoid) areas on histology.
4. NF1 involves an abnormal chromosome 17; malignant transformation of a lesion will occur in 8% to 13% of patients.
5. Treatment of desmoid tumors requires a multidisciplinary team with consideration of initial medical management for most tumors.
6. Surgical resection for small, operable lesions requires a wide margin.
7. Elastofibromas commonly occur between the scapula and chest wall; they stain positive for elastin.

8. Glomus tumors usually occur in a subungual location.
9. Synovial chondromatosis and diffuse, intra-articular forms of tenosynovial giant cell tumor require a complete synovectomy to achieve local control.
10. The imaging and histologic appearance of myositis ossificans show a zonal pattern with increased peripheral mineralization and immature tissue in the center.

Bibliography

Feldman DS, Jordan C, Fonseca L: Orthopaedic manifestations of neurofibromatosis type 1. *J Am Acad Orthop Surg* 2010;18(6):346-357.

Flors L, Leiva-Salinas C, Maged IM, et al: MR imaging of soft-tissue vascular malformations: Diagnosis, classification, and therapy follow-up. *Radiographics* 2011;31(5):1321-1341.

Fouin F: Noailles: Localized and diffuse forms of tenosynovial giant cell tumor (formally giant cell tumor of the tendon sheath and pigmented villonodular synovitis). *Orthop Traumatol Surg Res* 2017;103:S91-S97.

Furlong MA, Fanburg-Smith JC, Miettinen M: The morphologic spectrum of hibernoma: A clinicopathologic study of 170 cases. *Am J Surg Pathol* 2001;25(6):809-814.

Goldblum JR, Weiss SW, Folpe AL eds: *Enzinger and Weiss's Soft Tissue Tumors*, ed 6. Saunders, 2014.

Gounder MM, Mahoney MR, Van Tine VA, et al: Sorafenib for advanced and refractory desmoid tumors. *N Engl J Med* 2018;379:2417-2428.

Jee WH, Oh SN, McCauley T, et al: Extraaxial neurofibromas versus neurilemmomas: Discrimination with MRI. *AJR Am J Roentgenol* 2004;183(3):629-633.

Kollipara R, Dinneen L, Rentas KE, et al: Current classification and terminology of pediatric vascular anomalies. *Am J Roentgenol* 2013;201:1124-1135.

Kransdorf MJ, Meis JM, Jelinek JS: Myositis ossificans: MR appearance with radiologic-pathologic correlation. *AJR Am J Roentgenol* 1991;157(6):1243-1248.

Lim SJ, Chung HW, Choi YL, Moon YW, Seo JG, Park YS: Operative treatment of primary synovial osteochondromatosis of the hip. *J Bone Joint Surg Am* 2006;88(11):2456-2464.

Martinez Trufero J, Pajares Bernad I, Torres Ramon I, Hernando Cubero J, Pazo Cid R: Desmoid-type fibromatosis: Who, when, and how to treat. *Curr Treat Options Oncol* 2017;18:29.

Murphey MD, Vidal JA, Fanburg-Smith JC, Gajewski DA: Imaging of synovial chondromatosis with radiologic-pathologic correlation. *Radiographics* 2007;27(5):1465-1488.

Oliveira AM, Chou MM: USP6-induced neoplasms: The biologic spectrum of aneurysmal bone cyst and nodular fasciitis. *Hum Pathol* 2014;45:1-11.

Parratt MT, Donaldson JR, Flanagan AM, et al: Elastofibroma dorsi: Management, outcome and review of the literature. *J Bone Joint Surg Br* 2010;92(2):262-266.

Peyraud F, Cousin S, Italiano A: CSF-1R inhibitor development: Current clinical status. *Curr Oncol Rep* 2017; 19:70.

Shin C, Low I, Ng D, Oei P, Miles C, Symmans P: USP6 gene rearrangement in nodular fasciitis and histological mimics. *Histopathology* 2016;69:784-791.

Smith K, Desai J, Lazarakis S, Gyorki D: Systematic review of clinical outcomes following various treatment options for patients with extraabdominal desmoid tumors. *Ann Surg Oncol* 2018;25:1544-1554.

Walker EA, Fenton ME, Salesky JS, Murphey MD: Magnetic resonance imaging of benign soft tissue neoplasms in adults. *Radiol Clin North Am* 2011;49(6):1197-1217, vi.

Chapter 146
Malignant Soft-Tissue Tumors

KRISTY L. WEBER, MD

I. SOFT-TISSUE SARCOMAS

A. Overview

1. Ratio of benign to malignant soft-tissue masses is 100:1 (sarcomas rare).
2. Males are affected more commonly than females.
3. Sixty percent of sarcomas affect the extremities (lower > upper).
4. Eighty-five percent occur in individuals older than 15 years.
5. Diagnostic appearance of most sarcomas on MRI is indeterminate; a biopsy is required.
6. Staging—The most common staging system is the American Joint Committee on Cancer system, which relies on tumor size, tumor grade, lymph node status, and whether distant metastases are present.

B. Surgery

1. The goal of surgery is to achieve an acceptable margin to minimize local recurrence and maintain reasonable function; limb salvage procedures are performed in approximately 90% of patients.
2. Sarcomas have a centripetal growth pattern.
3. A reactive zone around the tumor includes edema, fibrous tissue (capsule), inflammatory cells, and tumor cells.
4. "Shelling out" a sarcoma usually means excising it through the reactive zone, which leaves tumor cells behind in most cases.
5. Definition of surgical margins (Enneking)
   a. Intralesional: resection through the tumor mass for gross total resection
   b. Marginal: resection through the reactive zone
   c. Wide: resection with a cuff of normal tissue
   d. Radical: resection of the entire compartment (eg, quadriceps)
6. Indications for amputation
   a. When necessary to resect the entire tumor
   b. When major nerves cannot be saved
   c. In some locally recurrent sarcomas
   d. When the patient has significant comorbidities that preclude limb-sparing surgery
7. Standard oncologic techniques are used to resect soft-tissue sarcomas, including use of a tourniquet without exsanguination, excision of any open biopsy tract, and use of drains distal, close, and in line with the incision.
8. Surgical resection alone of large, deep, or high-grade tumors has an unacceptably high rate of local recurrence and requires adjuvant treatment (radiation with or without chemotherapy).
9. Soft-tissue reconstruction by free or rotational tissue transfer is often necessary; it minimizes wound complications after major resection, especially when preoperative radiation is used (**Figure 1**).

C. Radiation

1. Radiation is used routinely as an adjuvant to surgery in the treatment of soft-tissue sarcoma.
2. Noted exceptions to the use of radiation are when an amputation is performed or when the sarcoma is small, superficial, low grade, or amenable to a wide surgical resection.
3. Radiation is most often administered by external beam techniques (photons or protons). Some centers have options for intraoperative radiation to boost the total dose at a particular area of concern.
4. Early radiation effects: desquamation, delayed wound healing (**Figure 2**), infection. Late effects: fibrosis, fractures (**Figure 3**), joint stiffness, secondary sarcoma (depending on treatment dose, volume, and length of follow-up).

Dr. Weber or an immediate family member serves as a board member, owner, officer, or committee member of the American Academy of Orthopaedic Surgeons.

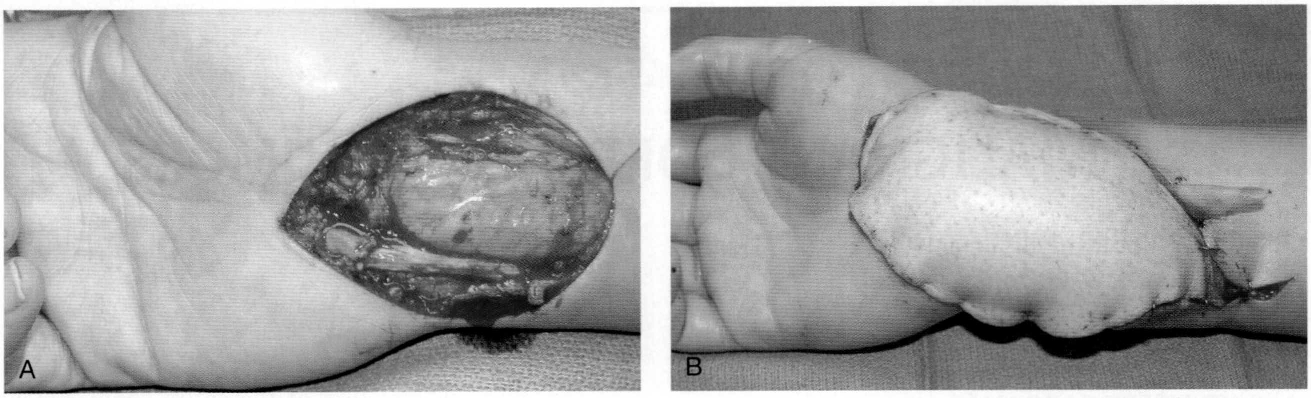

Figure 1 Clinical photographs show the wrist of a patient after soft-tissue sarcoma resection. **A**, Soft-tissue defect after wide resection of a clear cell sarcoma of the volar wrist. **B**, Soft-tissue reconstruction using free tissue transfer. This procedure is commonly performed to minimize wound breakdown and infection, especially when the patient has undergone preoperative radiation.

5. Preoperative radiation requires a lower dose (~50 Gy) than postoperative radiation (~66 Gy), decreases the surrounding edema, and helps form a fibrous capsule around the tumor. Surgery is delayed 3 to 4 weeks after completion of radiation.
6. Preoperative radiation incurs a higher wound complication rate (35%) than postoperative radiation (17%) (**Figure 2**).
7. No difference in overall survival related to timing of radiation.
8. External beam radiation (dose related) combined with extensive periosteal stripping during tumor resection increases the risk of postradiation fracture. In these cases, immediate or delayed prophylactic intramedullary or plate stabilization should be considered.
9. In the case of positive microscopic margins after surgical resection, there is no evidence for a radiation boost.

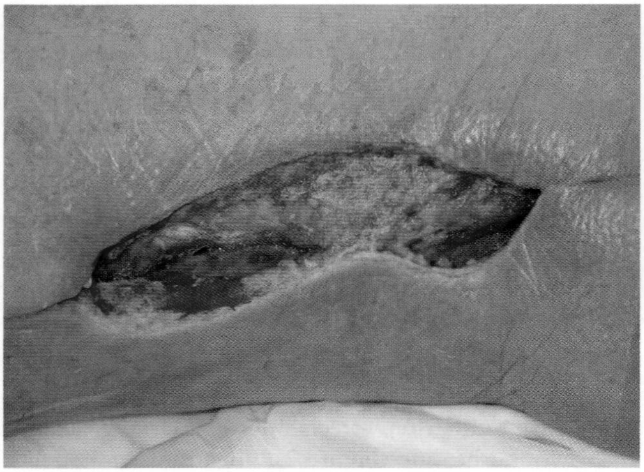

Figure 2 Clinical photograph shows wound breakdown in a patient who underwent preoperative radiation and surgical resection of a high-grade liposarcoma of the medial thigh.

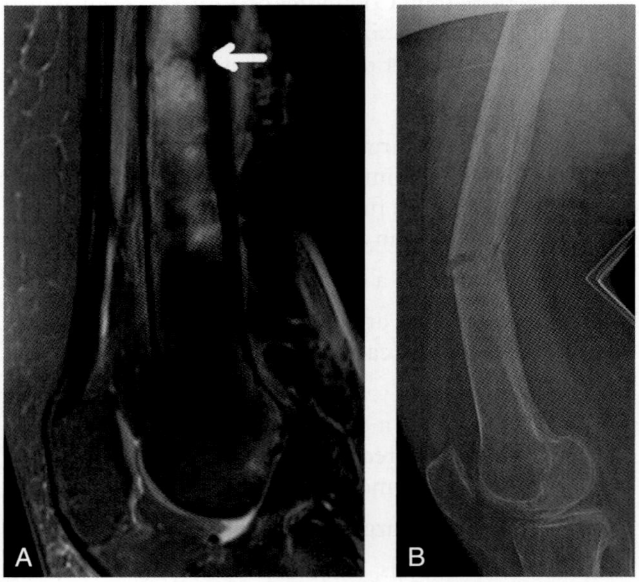

Figure 3 A 64-year-old woman who had 50 Gy of preoperative radiation for a large high-grade posterior thigh sarcoma 5 years earlier with periosteal stripping of 70% of the femur. **A**, Sagittal T2-weighted MRI of the right distal femur reveals marrow changes and a nondisplaced fracture (arrow) along the posterior cortex in the distal diaphysis. **B**, Lateral radiograph 1 week later showing an angulated postradiation femur fracture. The patient had femoral stabilization with an intramedullary nail.

D. Chemotherapy

1. Chemotherapy is considered the standard of care in the treatment of rhabdomyosarcoma and soft-tissue Ewing sarcoma/primitive neuroectodermal tumor.
2. Objective evidence of chemotherapy benefit for many other types of localized soft-tissue sarcoma is lacking. Studies show some effect on local or systemic disease recurrence but no difference in survival.
3. Given the high risk of metastasis in high-grade, large soft-tissue sarcomas, chemotherapy is frequently offered, often in a clinical trial setting. Patients with metastatic disease often receive systemic therapy to try and prolong lifespan.
4. Common agents include ifosfamide and doxorubicin, which have considerable toxicity in high doses. Taxanes can be used for angiosarcoma. Gemcitabine and docetaxel are used for leiomyosarcoma.
5. Patients with soft-tissue sarcoma who are older and have more comorbidities often cannot tolerate high-dose systemic treatment.
6. Recent clinical trials using targeted therapies, immunotherapy, and chimeric antigen receptor (CAR) T cell therapies show incremental progress in the treatment of various sarcoma subtypes.

E. Outcomes

1. The use of radiation and surgery minimizes the risk of local recurrence to less than 10%.
2. Tumor stage is the most important factor in determining overall prognosis/outcome.
3. Specific prognostic factors include presence of metastasis, grade, size, and depth of tumor.
4. Tumor grade is related to risk of metastasis (low grade, <10%; intermediate grade, 10% to 25%; high grade, >50%).
5. The most common site of metastasis is the lungs.
6. Lymph node metastasis (normally <5%) occurs more frequently in rhabdomyosarcoma, synovial sarcoma, epithelioid sarcoma, clear cell sarcoma, and angiosarcoma.
7. The outcome of individual soft-tissue sarcoma subtypes is rarely reported; approximately 50% of patients with high-grade soft-tissue sarcomas die of the disease.
8. Resection of pulmonary metastasis can cure up to 25% of patients.
9. Stereotactic body radiation therapy (SBRT) allows 86% local control of sarcoma lung metastasis at 24 months.
10. Patients require follow-up imaging of primary site of resection (MRI with/without contrast, or ultrasonography) and chest (radiography or CT) every 3 to 4 months for 2 years and then every 6 months for 3 years. Thereafter, annual chest studies are suggested for high-grade sarcomas.

II. UNDIFFERENTIATED PLEOMORPHIC SARCOMA

A. Definition and demographics

1. Undifferentiated pleomorphic sarcoma is pleomorphic in histologic appearance.
2. It is the most common soft-tissue sarcoma in adults 55 to 80 years of age.
3. Male-to-female ratio = 2:1
4. More common in Caucasian than in African American or Asian populations.

B. Genetics/etiology—Expression of PD-1 in 30% of undifferentiated pleomorphic sarcoma in small series

C. Clinical presentation

1. Usually a deep, slow-growing, painless mass.
2. More common in the extremities (lower more common than upper) than retroperitoneum.
3. Patients occasionally present with fever, elevated white blood cell count, and hypoglycemia.

D. Imaging appearance (indeterminate)—Low signal intensity on T1-weighted MRI; high signal intensity on T2-weighted MRI (**Figure 4, A** and **B**).

E. Pathology

1. Gross: a gray-white multinodular mass
2. Histologic subtypes include pleomorphic (80% to 85%), giant cell (10%), and inflammatory (<10%).
3. Storiform or cartwheel growth pattern is seen on low-power histologic images (**Figure 4, C**).
4. Cells are plump, spindled, and arranged around narrow vessels.
5. Haphazard histiocytic cells
6. Multinucleate eosinophilic giant cells (**Figure 4, D**)
7. Marked atypia, mitotic activity, and pleomorphism

F. Treatment/outcome

1. Radiation and wide surgical resection

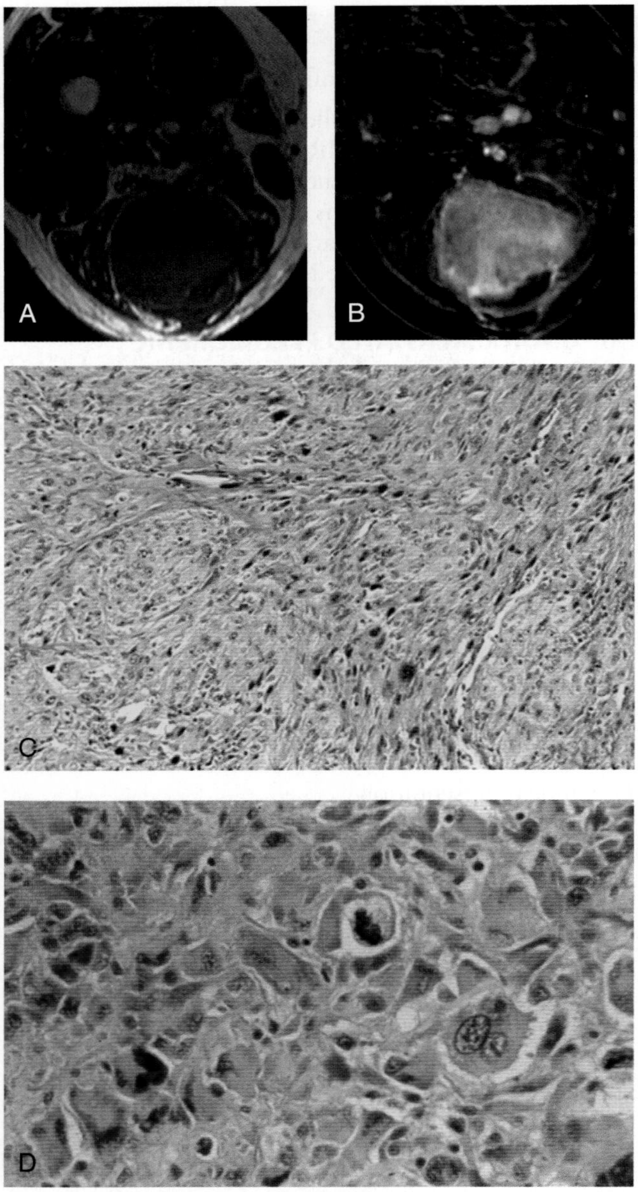

Figure 4 Undifferentiated pleomorphic sarcoma in a 68-year-old man who presented with a painless soft-tissue mass in the right posterior thigh. Axial T1-weighted MRI (**A**) and T2-weighted postcontrast MRI (**B**) show a mass indeterminate in appearance; a biopsy is required. **C**, Low-power histologic image reveals a storiform pattern with bizarre pleomorphic tumor cells and hyalinized collagen bundles consistent with undifferentiated pleomorphic sarcoma. **D**, Higher power histologic image reveals anaplastic tumor cells, multinucleated cells, and mitotic figures.

2. Chemotherapy in selected cases (ongoing clinical trial with pembrolizumab and neoadjuvant radiation)
3. Overall 5-year survival of 50% to 60% (depending on size, grade, depth, presence of metastasis)

III. LIPOSARCOMA

A. Definition and demographics

1. Composed of a variety of histologic forms related to the developmental stages of lipoblasts
2. Second most common soft-tissue sarcoma in adults
3. Occurs most commonly in patients 50 to 80 years of age
4. Affects males more commonly than females

B. Genetics/etiology

1. Liposarcoma originates from primitive mesenchymal cells; diagnosis does not require adipose cells.
2. Simple lipomas do not predispose a patient to liposarcomas.
3. Histologic types include well-differentiated, myxoid (most common, 50%), round cell, pleomorphic, and dedifferentiated.
4. Well-differentiated variants have giant marker and ring chromosomes and overexpression of *MDM2* (**Table 1**).
5. Well-differentiated and dedifferentiated liposarcoma are both characterized by chromosome 12q13-15 amplification.
6. Myxoid liposarcoma is associated with a translocation between chromosomes 12 and 16.

C. Clinical presentation

1. Wide spectrum of disease, depending on histologic type.
2. Slow growing; may become extremely large (10 to 20 cm), painless masses.
3. Pain may occur in larger lesions.
4. Occur in extremities (lower [thigh] more common than upper) and retroperitoneum (15% to 20%) (present at later age).
5. Well-differentiated liposarcoma is essentially the same histologic entity as atypical lipoma/atypical lipomatous tumor; however, the former term is used for retroperitoneal lesions and the latter term for extremity lesions.
6. The retroperitoneal lesions are more locally aggressive and likely to dedifferentiate than the extremity lesions.
7. Well-differentiated liposarcomas and atypical lipomas can transform into a dedifferentiated liposarcoma (also MDM2 positive). Rapid growth of a long-standing (usually > 5 years) painless mass is suspicious.

TABLE 1

Characteristic Cytogenetic and Molecular Events of Soft Tissue Sarcomas

Histologic Type	Cytogenetic Events	Molecular Events
Alveolar soft part sarcoma	t(X;17)(p11;q25)	*TFE3-ASPL* fusion
Clear cell sarcoma	t(12;22)(q13;q12) t(2;22)(q33;q12)	*EWSR1-ATF1* fusion *EWSR1-CREB1* fusion
Dermatofibrosarcoma protuberans	Ring form of chromosomes 17, 22 t(17;22)(q21;13)	*COL1A1-PDGFB* fusion *COL1A1-PDGFB* fusion
Desmoplastic small round cell tumor	t(11;22)(p13;q12)	*EWSR1-WT1* fusion
Extraskeletal myxoid chondrosarcoma	t(9;22)(q22;q12) t(9;17)(q22;q11) t(9;15)(q22;q21)	*EWS-NR4A3* fusion *TAF2N-NR4A3* fusion *TCF12-NR4A3* fusion
Fibrosarcoma, infantile	t(12;15)(p13;q26)	*ETV6-NTRK3* fusion
Inflammatory myofibroblastic tumor	t(1;2)(q22;p23) t(2;19)(p23;p13) t(2;17)(p23;q23) t(2;2)(p23;q13)	*TPM3-ALK* fusion *TPM4-ALK* fusion *CLTC-ALK* fusion *RANB2-ALK* fusion
Leiomyosarcoma	Complex with frequent deletions of 1p	
Liposarcoma		
Well-differentiated	Ring form of chromosome 12	Amplification of *MDM2, CDK4,* and others
Myxoid/Round cell	t(12;16)(q13;p11) t(12;22)(q13;q12)	*FUS-DDIT3* (*TLS-CHOP*) fusion
Pleomorphic	Complex	*EWSR1-DDIT3* (*EWSR1-CHOP*) fusion
Low-grade fibromyxoid sarcoma	t(7;16)(q33;p11)	*FUS-CREB3L2* fusion
Malignant peripheral nerve sheath tumor	Complex	
Malignant rhabdoid tumor	Deletion of 22q	*SMARCB1/INI1* inactivation
Myxofibrosarcoma	Ring form chromosome 12	
Rhabdomyosarcoma		
Alveolar	t(2;13)(q35;q14) t(1;13)(p36;q14), double minutes	*PAX3-FOO1A* fusion *PAX7-FOXO1A* fusion
Embryonal	t(2;2)(q35;p23) Trisomies 2q, 8 and 20	*PAX3-NCOA1* fusion *PAX3-AFX* fusion Loss of heterozygosity at 11p15
Solitary fibrous tumor	Inversion chromosome 12	*NAB2-STAT6*
Synovial sarcoma		
Monophasic	t(X;18)(p11;q11)	*SS18-SSX1, SS18-SSX2* or *SS18-SSX4* fusion
Biphasic	t(X;18)(P11;q11)	Predominantly *SS18-SSX1* fusion
Undifferentiated small round blue cell tumor	t(4;19)(q35;q13) t(10;19)(q26;q13) Xp11 (intrachromosomal inversion)	*CIC-DUX4* fusion *BCOR-CCNB3* fusion

Reproduced with permission from Wustrack R, Cooper K, Weber K: Molecular markers in bone and soft tissue tumors. *JBJS Rev* 2016;4:1-11.

D. Imaging appearance

1. Plain radiographs occasionally show foci of calcification or ossification in well-differentiated variants.
2. MRI appearance of well-differentiated variant is the same as a lipoma (**Figure 5**, A and B). Rare areas of dedifferentiation should be watched for (appear completely different than fat on imaging).

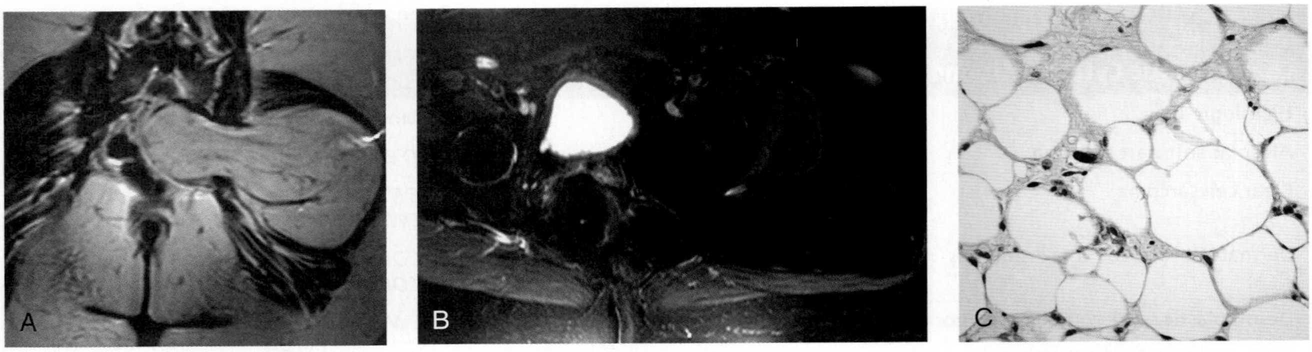

Figure 5 Well-differentiated liposarcoma. **A**, Coronal T1-weighted MRI reveals a large left retroperitoneal lipomatous lesion extending through the sciatic notch into the gluteal muscles. **B**, Axial T2-weighted fat-suppressed MRI reveals that the lesion completely suppresses with no concern for high-grade areas. **C**, Histologic image of the resected specimen reveals slight variation in the size and shape of the fat cells with hyperchromatic nuclei, consistent with a well-differentiated liposarcoma. The tissue had overexpression of MDM2, differentiating this from a benign lipoma.

3. MRI appearance of high-grade liposarcoma is indeterminate and similar to all sarcomas (low signal intensity on T1-weighted images; high signal intensity on T2-weighted images) (**Figure 6, A** and **B**).
4. Myxoid liposarcomas can metastasize to sites other than the lungs (such as the abdomen and spine), so staging for this tumor should include a CT scan of the abdomen and pelvis with contrast as well as a chest CT scan and an MRI scan of the spine.

E. Pathology
   1. Gross: large, well-circumscribed, lobular
   2. Well-differentiated liposarcoma
      a. Low-grade tumor
      b. Lobulated appearance of mature adipose tissue (**Figure 5, C**)
   3. Myxoid liposarcoma
      a. Low- to intermediate-grade tumor with lobulated appearance
      b. Composed of proliferating lipoblasts, a plexiform capillary network, and a myxoid matrix (**Figure 6, C**)
      c. Signet ring (univacuolar) lipoblasts occur at the edge of the tumor lobules
      d. Few mitotic figures
   4. Round cell liposarcoma
      a. Also considered a poorly differentiated myxoid liposarcoma

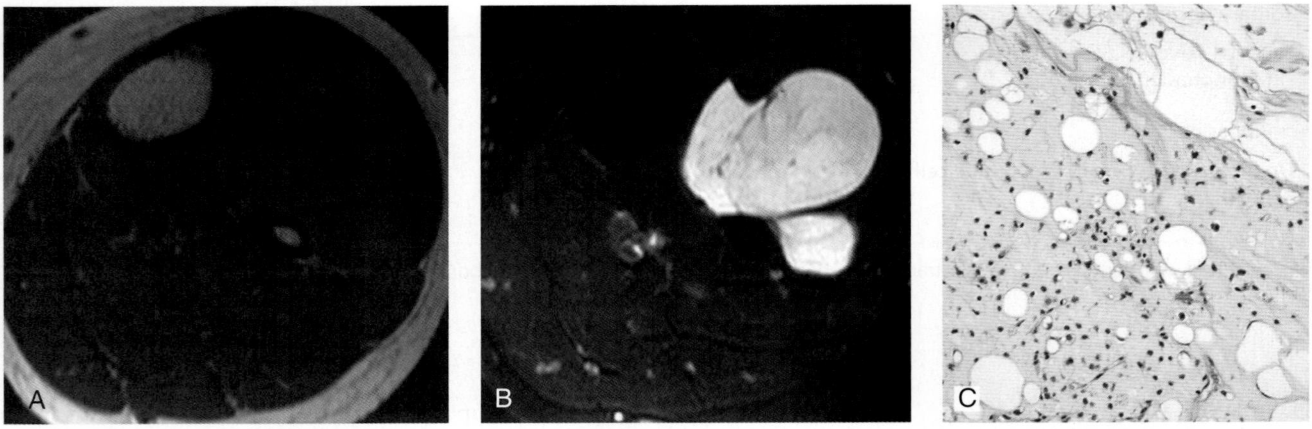

Figure 6 Myxoid liposarcoma in the left calf of a 27-year-old woman. Axial T1-weighted MRI (**A**) and T2-weighted short tau inversion recovery MRI (**B**) sequences reveal an indeterminate lesion that has low signal intensity on T1-weighted images and high signal intensity on T2-weighted images. No bony involvement is seen, but the mass is adjacent to the proximal fibula. **C**, Histologic image reveals lipoblasts (some with signet ring appearance), numerous capillaries, and a myxoid stroma between the tumor cells. No significant round cell component is noted.

b. Characteristic small round blue cells

c. Rare intracellular lipid formation and minimal myxoid matrix

5. Pleomorphic liposarcoma

a. High-grade tumor with marked pleomorphic appearance

b. Giant lipoblasts with hyperchromatic bizarre nuclei

c. Deeply eosinophilic giant cells

6. Dedifferentiated liposarcoma

a. High-grade sarcoma (undifferentiated pleomorphic sarcoma, fibrosarcoma, leiomyosarcoma)

b. Juxtaposed to well-differentiated lipomatous lesion

F. Treatment/outcome

1. Well-differentiated liposarcoma

a. Marginal resection without radiation or chemotherapy.

b. Metastasis extremely rare.

c. Risk of local recurrence is 25% to 50% at 10 years.

d. Dedifferentiation risk is 2% for extremity lesions and 20% for retroperitoneal lesions.

2. Intermediate- and high-grade variants

a. Radiation and wide surgical resection

b. Chemotherapy in selected patients

c. Incidence of pulmonary metastasis increases with grade.

d. Myxoid liposarcomas with more than 10% round cells have a higher likelihood of metastasis and are generally treated with chemotherapy.

e. Local recurrence is higher in retroperitoneal lesions.

IV. FIBROSARCOMA

A. Definition and demographics

1. Fibrosarcoma is a rare soft-tissue sarcoma of fibroblastic origin that shows no tendency to other cellular differentiation.

2. Occurs in adults 30 to 55 years of age.

3. Affects males more commonly than females.

B. Genetics/etiology—No data yet.

C. Clinical presentation

1. Slow-growing, painless mass (4 to 8 cm) most commonly noted around the thigh or knee

2. Ulceration of the skin in superficial lesions

D. Imaging appearance (indeterminate)—Low signal intensity on T1-weighted MRI; high signal intensity on T2-weighted MRI.

E. Pathology

1. Gross: shown in **Figure 7, A**

2. Histology

a. Uniform fasciculated growth pattern (herringbone) (**Figure 7, B**)

b. Spindle cells with minimal cytoplasm

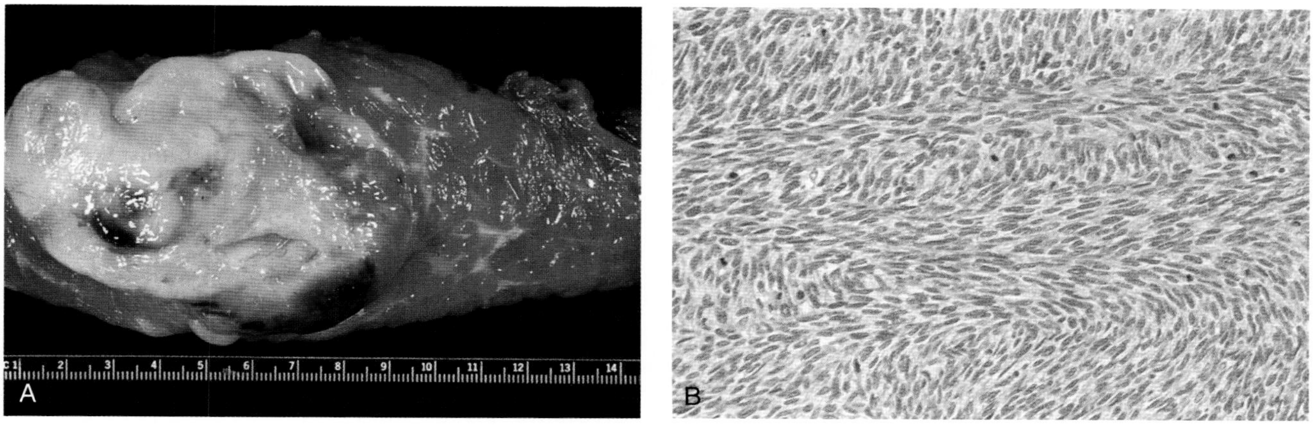

Figure 7 Fibrosarcomas. **A**, Photograph of gross appearance of a fibrosarcoma within the muscles of the anterior thigh. Areas of hemorrhage and cyst formation are present. **B**, High-power view of a fibrosarcoma reveals the distinct fascicular appearance of cells with little variation in size or shape. When the cells are cut in cross section, they appear round. The overall appearance is that of a herringbone pattern of spindle cells.

c. Collagen fibers commonly aligned in parallel throughout tumor
d. Mitotic activity varies

F. Treatment/outcome
1. Wide surgical resection and radiation
2. Chemotherapy for selected patients
3. Metastasis in approximately 50% of high-grade lesions

V. DERMATOFIBROSARCOMA PROTUBERANS

A. Definition
1. Rare, low-grade malignancy affecting dermal layers of skin
2. Occur in subcutaneous locations; 1 to 5 cm
3. Ninety percent have chromosomal translocation: t(17:22)(q22;q13) (**Table 1**)
4. Ten percent have fibrosarcomatous areas
5. Two percent to 5% can metastasize to lungs

B. Treatment
1. Treatment is surgical resection with wide margins because of propensity for local recurrence.
2. Tyrosine kinase inhibitors (imatinib) can be used.

VI. SYNOVIAL SARCOMA

A. Definition and demographics
1. Distinct lesion occurring in para-articular regions
2. Most common soft-tissue sarcoma in young adults
3. Occurs most commonly in patients 15 to 40 years of age
4. Affects males more commonly than females

B. Genetics/etiology
1. Characteristic translocation (X;18)
2. Represents the fusion of *SYT* with either *SSX1* or *SSX2*

C. Clinical presentation
1. Slow-growing soft-tissue mass; 3 to 5 cm
2. In some patients, 2 to 4 years can elapse before a correct diagnosis
3. Pain in 50% of patients; some have a history of trauma
4. Most commonly occur in para-articular regions around the knee, shoulder, arm, elbow, and foot (lower extremity in 60%)
5. Can arise from tendon sheath, bursa, fascia, and joint capsule, but only rarely involve a joint (**Figure 8**, A and B)

D. Imaging appearance
1. Calcification noted on plain radiographs in 15% to 20% of synovial sarcomas
2. MRI appearance indeterminate: low signal intensity on T1-weighted images; high signal intensity on T2-weighted images (**Figure 8**, A and B)

E. Pathology
1. Classically occurs as biphasic type, with epithelial cells forming glandlike structures alternating with elongated spindle cells (**Figure 8**, C).
2. Epithelial cells are large and round with distinct cell borders and pale cytoplasm.
3. Epithelial cells are arranged in nests or chords and stain positive with keratin.
4. Fibrous component involves plump, malignant spindle cells with minimal cytoplasm and dark nuclei; mast cells are common in fibrous sections.
5. Calcification more common at periphery.
6. Variable vascularity.
7. Less commonly, a purely monophasic histology is seen (either fibrous or epithelial) (**Figure 8**, D).

F. Treatment/outcome
1. Wide resection and radiation.
2. Chemotherapy effectiveness is variable; younger patients tolerate it better.
3. Lymph node metastasis occurs in 10% to 12% of patients.
4. Five-year survival = 50%, 10-year survival = 25%; better in heavily calcified lesions.

VII. EPITHELIOID SARCOMA

A. Definition and demographics
1. Distinct soft-tissue sarcoma often mistaken for a benign granulomatous process
2. Occurs in adolescents and young adults (10 to 35 years)
3. Male-to-female ratio = 2:1

B. Genetics/etiology-CA125 is highly expressed in the tumor.

C. Clinical presentation
1. Small, slow-growing soft-tissue tumor that can be superficial or deep

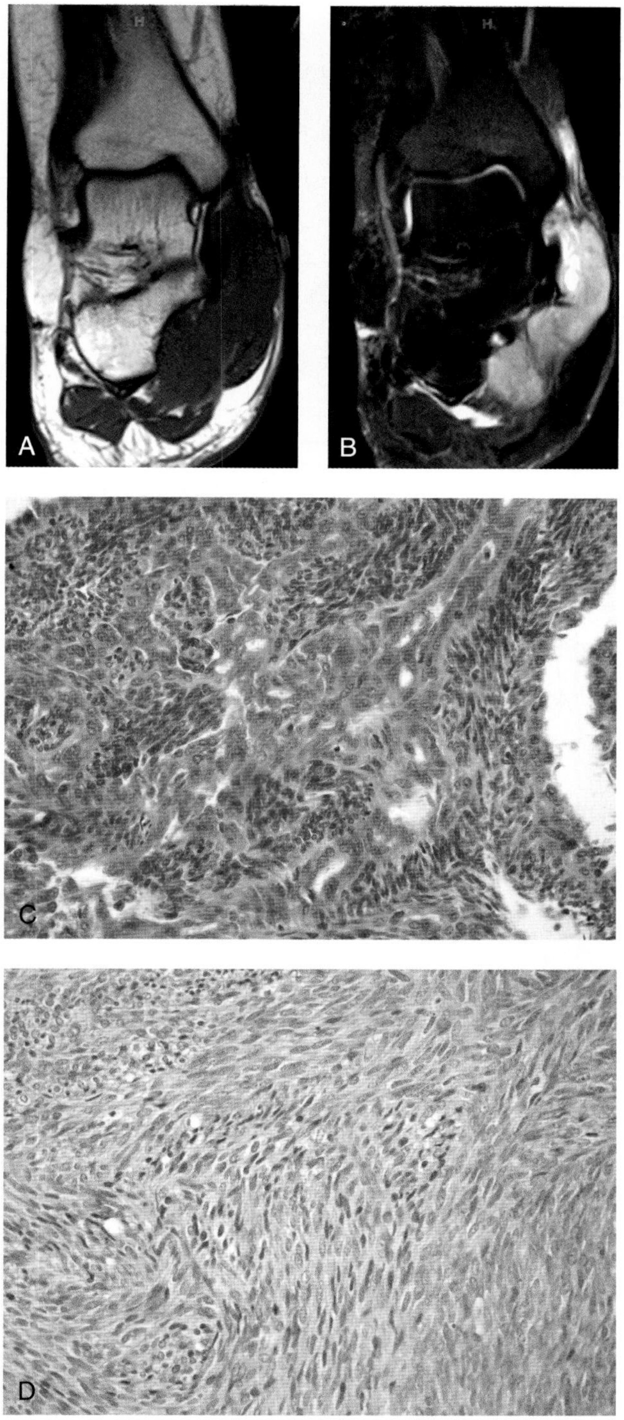

Figure 8 Synovial sarcoma around the foot. Coronal T1-weighted (**A**) and T2-weighted (**B**) MRIs of the ankle reveal a soft-tissue mass associated with the medial neurovascular bundle. The mass is indeterminate in appearance; a biopsy revealed it to be a synovial sarcoma. **C**, Histologic evaluation reveals the typical pattern of epithelial cells and fibrosarcoma-like spindle cells noted in a biphasic synovial sarcoma. **D**, An example of histologic evaluation of a monophasic synovial sarcoma variant shows only spindle cells (would be keratin positive).

2. Frequently involves hand, forearm, fingers; 3 to 6 cm (**Figure 9, A**)
3. Most common soft-tissue sarcoma in the hand/wrist
4. Occurs as firm, painless nodule(s); may ulcerate when superficial
5. When deep, attached to tendons, tendon sheaths, or fascia
6. Confused with granuloma, rheumatoid nodule, or skin cancer, often resulting in delay in diagnosis or inappropriate treatment

D. Imaging appearance

1. Occasional calcification within lesion
2. Can erode adjacent bone
3. MRI reveals nodule along tendon sheaths of upper or lower extremity
    a. Low signal intensity on T1-weighted images; high signal intensity on T2-weighted images
    b. Indeterminate in appearance; requires biopsy

E. Pathology

1. A nodular pattern with central necrosis within granulomatous areas is seen on low-power histologic images (**Figure 9, B**).
2. Higher power reveals an epithelial appearance with eosinophilic cytoplasm.
3. Minimal cellular pleomorphism.
4. Intercellular deposition of dense hyalinized collagen.
5. Calcification/ossification in 10% to 20% of patients.
6. Cells are keratin positive.

F. Treatment/outcome

1. Wide surgical resection and radiation (if limb-sparing).
2. Regional lymph node metastasis is common. Sentinel node biopsy may be indicated.
3. Often mistaken for a benign lesion and inadequately excised, leading to a high rate of multiple recurrences.
4. Amputation is frequently necessary to halt spread of disease.
5. Late regional or systemic metastasis to lungs is common.
6. Overall, extremely poor prognosis and chemotherapy is not effective.

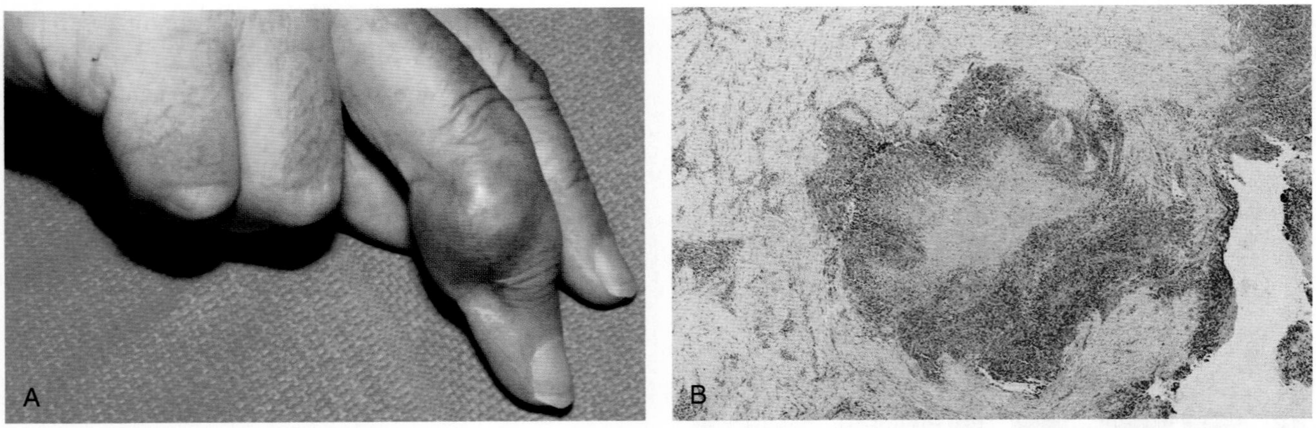

Figure 9 Epithelioid sarcoma. **A**, Clinical photograph shows an epithelioid sarcoma in the dorsal aspect of the distal long finger. Note the nodule in the superficial tissues. **B**, Low-power histologic image reveals a nodule with central necrosis consistent with an epithelioid sarcoma; these are often mistaken for a benign granulomatous process. (Reproduced from Scarborough MT, ed: *Musculoskeletal Tumors and Diseases Self-Assessment Examination*. Rosemont, IL, American Academy of Orthopaedic Surgeons, 2008.)

VIII. CLEAR CELL SARCOMA

A. Definition and demographics
   1. Rare soft-tissue sarcoma that has the ability to produce melanin
   2. Occurs in young adults (age range, 20 to 40 years)
   3. Affects females more commonly than males
   4. Also called "malignant melanoma of soft parts"

B. Genetics/etiology
   1. Frequent translocation of chromosomes 12 and 22 (not seen in malignant melanoma) (**Table 1**)
   2. Etiology thought to be neuroectodermal

C. Clinical presentation
   1. Occurs in deep tissues associated with tendons, aponeuroses
   2. Most common soft-tissue sarcoma of the foot; also occurs in ankle, knee, and hand
   3. Two to six centimeters
   4. Slow-growing mass; pain in 50% of patients; present for many years before diagnosis
   5. Often mistaken for a benign lesion and inadequately excised

D. Imaging appearance
   1. Nonspecific appearance; may be nodular in foot
   2. MRI: indeterminate; requires a biopsy; low signal intensity on T1-weighted images; high signal intensity on T2-weighted images (**Figure 10, A**)

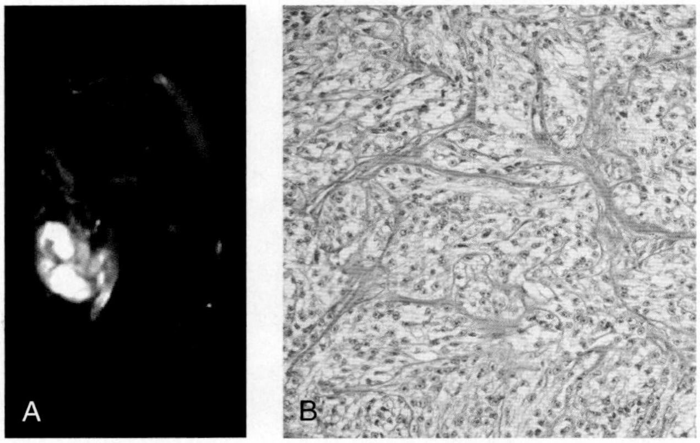

Figure 10 Clear cell sarcoma. **A**, Short tau inversion recovery MRI sequence of the left foot reveals a soft-tissue lesion abutting the medial calcaneus. Additional views revealed involvement of the neurovascular bundle. **B**, Histologic image shows fibrous septa separating the tumor into well-defined fascicles of cells with clear cytoplasm, consistent with a clear cell sarcoma.

E. Pathology
   1. Gross: no connection to overlying skin but may be attached to tendons
   2. Nests of round cells with clear cytoplasm are seen on histologic images (**Figure 10, B**)
   3. Uniform pattern of cells with a defined fibrous border that might be continuous with surrounding tendons or aponeuroses
   4. Occasional multinucleate giant cells but rare mitotic figures

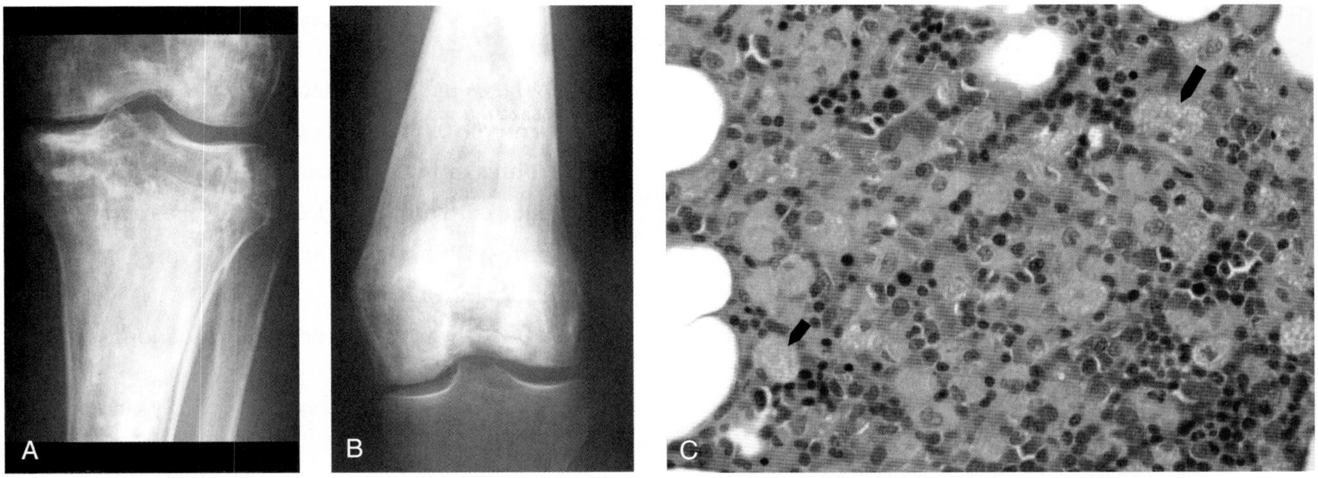

Figure 2 Gaucher disease. **A**, AP radiograph of the tibia shows sclerosis in the medullary cavity. **B**, AP radiograph of the distal femur shows the Erlenmeyer flask deformity, typical of Gaucher disease. Note the widened metaphyses. **C**, Hematoxylin/eosin preparation of high power view of Gauchers disease.

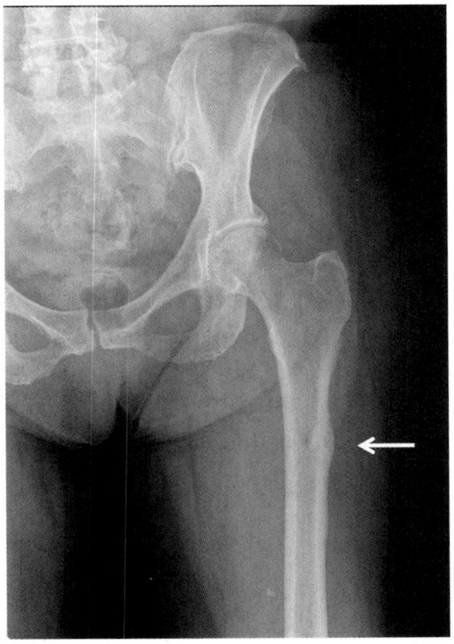

Figure 3 Anteroposerior view of the proximal right femur showing a characteristic "beaking" of the lateral cortex.

C. Imaging appearance
   1. Radiographs/CT
      a. Diaphysis
         - Linear cortical radiolucency
         - Endosteal thickening
         - Periosteal reaction and cortical thickening
         - Beaking in the lateral cortex of the subtrochanteric region of the femur
      b. Metaphysis: focal linear increased mineralization (condensation of the trabecular bone)
      c. Endosteal and periosteal new bone formation (**Figure 4**)
   2. Technetium Tc-99m bone scan—Area of focal uptake in the cortical and/or trabecular region.
   3. MRI (**Figure 5**)
      a. Periosteal high signal intensity on T2-weighted images (earliest finding).
      b. Linear zone of low signal intensity on T1-weighted images.
      c. Broad area of increased signal intensity on T2-weighted images.
      d. When a stress fracture is advanced in clinical course, low signal intensity lines representing the fracture may be seen.

D. Pathology
   1. Callus formation
   2. Woven new bone
   3. Enchondral bone formation

E. Treatment
   1. Rest
   2. Protected weight bearing until symptoms resolve and fracture heals
   3. Prophylactic fixation in selected cases
      a. Tension-side femoral neck fractures in athletes
      b. Anterior tibial diaphysis in athletes (dreaded black line)

c. Patients with low bone mass, especially patients older than 60 years and those with lesions on the tension side of the subtrochanteric region of the femur

V. NEUROPATHIC ARTHROPATHY

A. Definition and demographics

1. Neuropathic arthropathy is the destruction of a joint following loss of protective sensation.
2. Common locations include the foot, ankle, elbow, and shoulder.

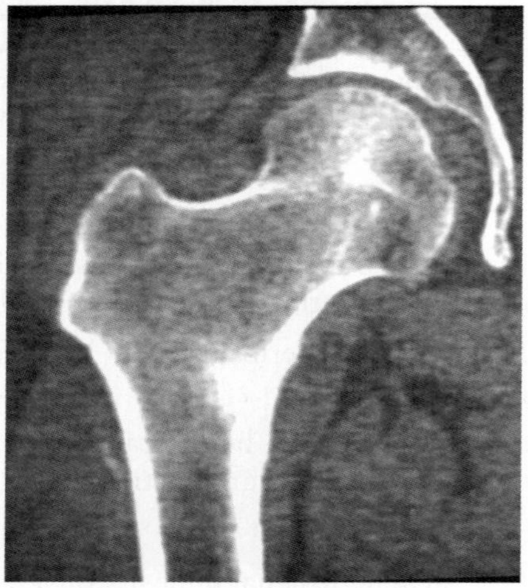

Figure 4 Coronal CT reconstruction shows a stress fracture of the proximal femur. Note the focal endosteal new bone formation and the periosteal new bone formation on the medial femoral cortex.

B. Etiology—Disease processes that damage sensory nerves.

1. Diabetes mellitus: affects the foot and ankle
2. Syringomyelia: affects the shoulder and elbow
3. Syphilis: affects the knee
4. Spinal cord tumors: affect the lower extremity joints
5. Leprosy: can affect any joint

C. Clinical presentation

1. Swollen, warm, and erythematous joint with little or no pain
2. Often mimics infection, especially in patients with diabetes
3. In the lower extremity, diabetes is the most common cause (**Figure 6, A**) while in the upper extremity, syringomyelia is the most common cause (**Figure 6, B**)

D. Radiographic appearance

1. Characteristic feature: destruction of the joint
2. Initial changes may simulate osteoarthritis
3. Late changes
   a. Fragmentation of the joint
   b. Subluxation/dislocation
   c. Fracture
   d. Collapse

E. Pathology

1. Productive/hypertrophic changes secondary to conditions involving the spinal cord (generally do not involve the sympathetic nervous system)
   a. Spinal cord traumatic injury

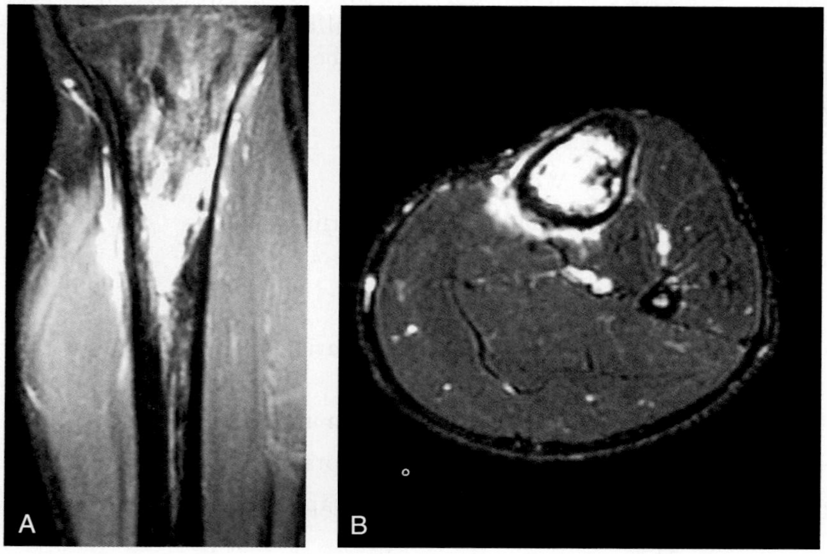

Figure 5 Stress fracture of the tibia. **A**, Coronal T2-weighted MRI shows high signal intensity in the medullary cavity and on the periosteal surface. **B**, Axial T2-weighted MRI shows high signal intensity in the medullary cavity and over the posteromedial cortical surface of the tibia.

b. Neoplasms

c. Spinal cord malformations

d. Syphilis

e. Syringomyelia

2. Destructive/atrophic changes usually secondary to peripheral nerve damage. Conditions that cause atrophic changes include

a. Diabetes

b. Alcoholism

3. Histologic changes

a. Synovial hypertrophy

b. Fragments of bone and cartilage in the synovium (detritic synovitis)

F. Treatment

1. Rest, elevation, protected weight bearing

2. Total contact casting when ulcers are present in the foot and ankle

VI. HEMOPHILIC ARTHROPATHY

A. Definition and demographics

1. Hemophilic arthropathy is the destruction of a joint secondary to repetitive bleeding into the synovial cavity

2. Classic hemophilia or hemophilia A (deficiency of factor VIII); Christmas disease or hemophilia B (deficiency of factor IX)

3. Locations: knee, ankle, elbow

B. Genetics/etiology—X-linked recessive (it is always helpful to draw the Punnet square).

1. Father does not have hemophilia; the mother is a heterozygous carrier

a. 50% of the daughters are heterozygous carriers

b. 50% of the sons have hemophilia

2. Father does have hemophilia; the mother is not a carrier

a. 100% of the daughters are heterozygous carriers

b. 0% of the sons have hemophilia

C. Clinical presentation

1. Hemarthrosis: often seen in young males, 3 to 15 years of age

2. Severity

a. Severe hemophilia—<1% normal clotting factor

b. Moderate hemophilia—1% to 5% normal clotting factor

c. Mild hemophilia—5% to 40% normal clotting factor

3. Target joint

a. > 3 bleeds into the same joint within a six month period

4. Temporal changes

a. Acute hemarthrosis: tense, painful effusion

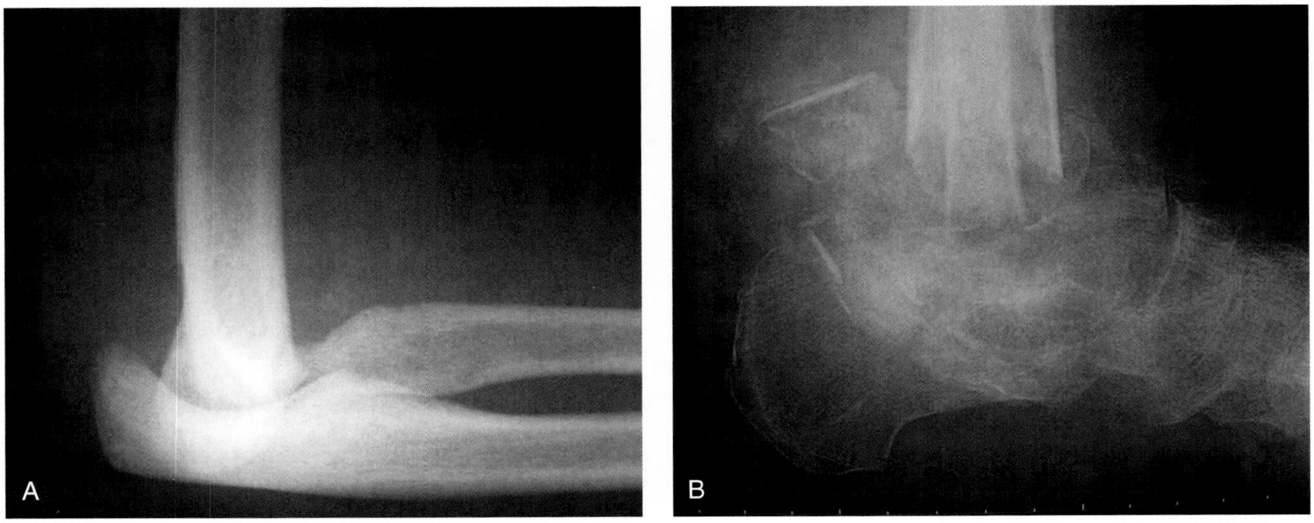

Figure 6 Neuropathic arthropathy. **A**, Lateral radiograph of the elbow of a patient with syringomyelia. Note the prominent neuropathic changes with complete destruction of the articular surfaces. **B**, Lateral radiograph of the ankle of a patient with diabetes mellitus. Note the complete destruction of the articular surfaces with dissolution and fragmentation.

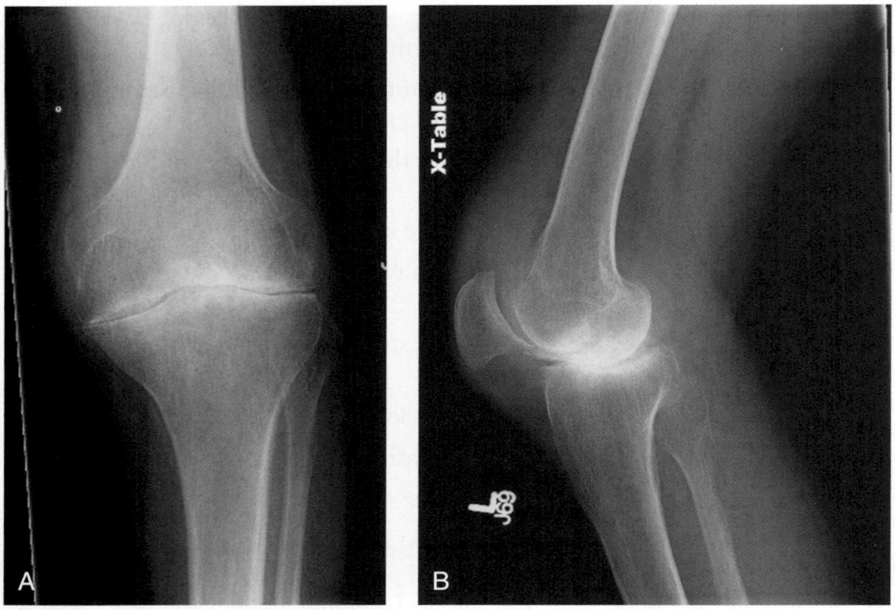

Figure 7 **A**, AP radiograph of the knee. This antero-posterior of the knee in a patient with severe hemophilia shows flattening of the joint surfaces. **B**, Lateral radiograph of the knee shows overgrowth of the patella and squaring of the inferior border.

b. Subacute hemarthrosis: occurs after two previous bleeds

c. Chronic hemarthrosis: arthritis, contractures

D. Radiographic appearance

1. Arnold/Hilgartner stages

a. Stage I: soft-tissue swelling

b. Stage II: osteoporosis

c. Stage III: bone changes (subchondral cysts) with intact joint

d. Stage IV: cartilage loss

e. Stage V: severe arthritic changes

2. Radiographic changes (**Figures** 7 and 8)

a. Knee

- Overgrowth of distal femur and proximal tibia
- Distal condylar surface appears flattened
- Squaring of the inferior portion of the patella

b. Ankle: arthritic changes of the tibiotalar joint

c. Elbow: arthritic changes and contractures

E. Pathology

1. Synovial hypertrophy and hyperplasia

2. Synovium covers and destroys the cartilage

F. Treatment

1. Factor replacement

a. Prophylactic treatment is one has a target joint

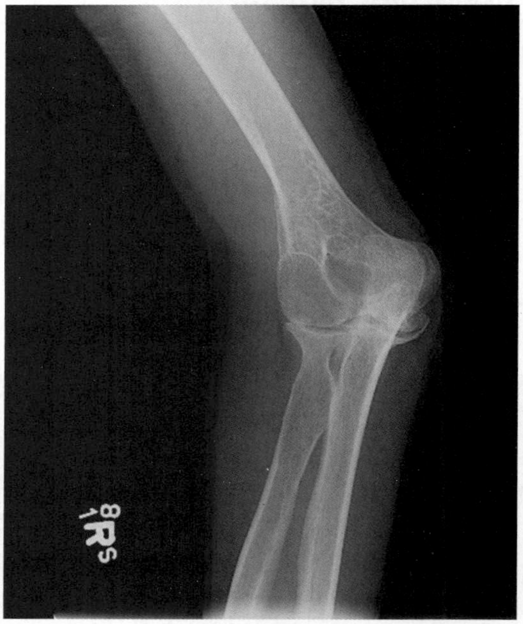

Figure 8 Antero-posterior view of the elbow in a patient with severe hemophilia demonstrating arthritis of the joint surfaces and overgrowth of the patella.

b. 100% factor replacement for 4 weeks if the patient has an arthroplasty

2. Prophylaxis against recurrent hemarthroses (factor replacement twice week)

3. Arthroplasty if the joint surfaces are destroyed

VII. BENIGN VASCULAR LESIONS (HEMANGIOMA AND LYMPHANGIOMA)

A. Definition and demographics

1. Hemangiomas of bone are collections of blood vessels and fat in the intramedullary cavity or the cortex. Long bone hemangiomas are very rare while vertebral hemangiomas are very common.
2. Most hemangiomas are solitary when they occur in long bones while they are often multiple when they involve the vertebra.
3. Bone involvement can also occur with soft-tissue hemangiomas.

B. Genetics/etiology—there is no genetic or inheritary predilections with bone hemangiomas.

C. Clinical presentation

1. Virtually all hemangiomas in bone are asymptomatic.
2. Occasionally vertebral hemangiomas will have soft-tissue extension and impinge on the spinal cord, or they may fracture and cause instability.

D. Imaging appearance

1. Long bone hemangiomas can have a very variable appearance with areas of lucency and sclerosis.
2. Vertebral hemangiomas can have a striated appearance which is quite characteristic (**Figure 9**).
3. On CT scanning, the clinician can detect "polka dots" in some vertebral hemangiomas (not all of them; **Figure 10**).
4. On magnetic resonance scanning, T1-weighted sequences will often show areas of high signal (most likely fat) and on T2-weighted sequences; there are high signal areas (most likely blood products) [high on T1 and T2] (**Figure 11, A** and **B**).

E. Pathology

1. Most bone hemangiomas are composed of large (cavernous) and small (capillary) vessels in variable proportions.

F. Treatment

1. Virtually all bone hemangiomas are asymptomatic. Occasionally, a long bone hemangioma requires biopsy to determine the correct diagnosis and curettage to prevent fracture and control progression.
2. Almost all vertebral hemangiomas are asymptomatic and are incidental to a patient's back pain.

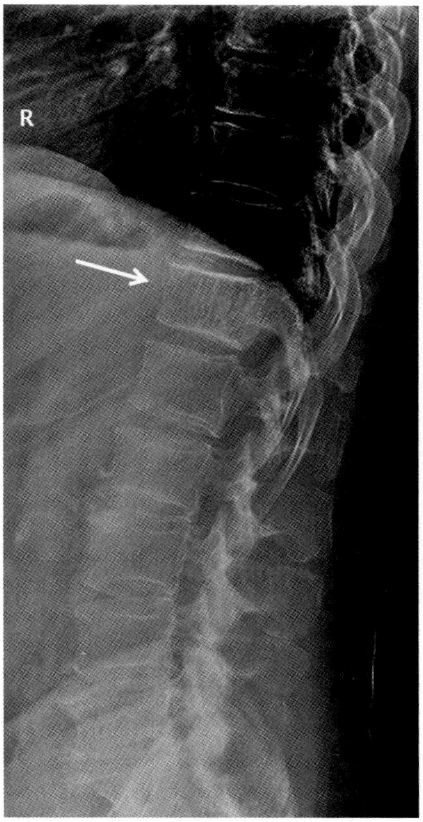

Figure 9 Lateral radiograph of the spine demonstrating the striations in the vertebra characteristic of vertebral hemangiomas.

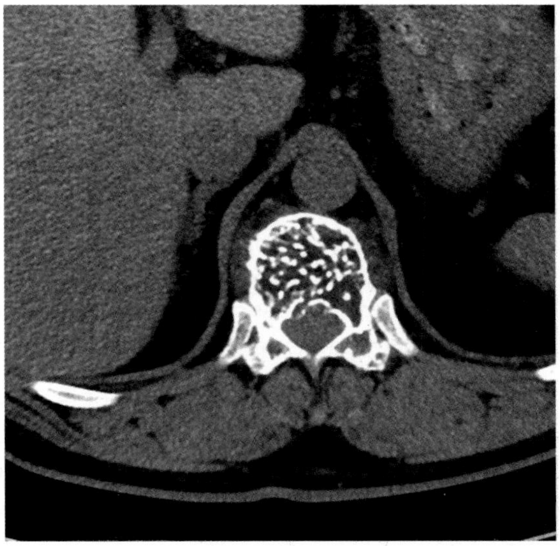

Figure 10 CT scan of T12 demonstrating the "polka dot" appearance of vertebral hemangiomas.

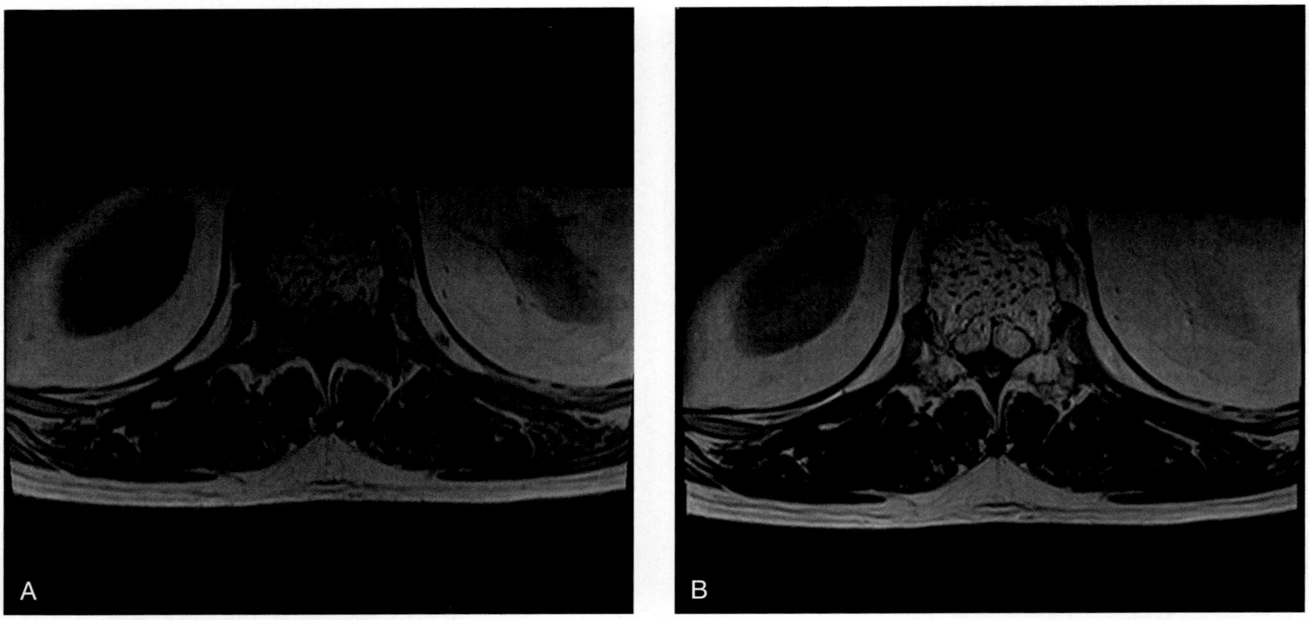

Figure 11 **A,** T1-weighted axial image of T12 showing the high signal, which probably represents fat and epidural extension and compression. **B,** T2-weighted axial image of T12 showing the high signal, which probably represents blood and epidural extension and compression.

3. Occasional vertebral hemangiomas with epidural extension require treatment. Patients can be treated with external beam irradiation or surgical decompression with or without external beam irradiation.
4. Vertebral hemangiomas which result in fracture and instability often require surgical treatment (rare occurrence).

VIII. BONE LYMPHANGIOMA

Lymphangiomas of bone is a very controversial topic. Separating bone lymphangioma from bone hemangioma is difficult and not easily done.

TOP TESTING FACTS

1. Melorheostosis is characterized by nodular, heavily mineralized bone on the surface of bones and in the soft tissues, which gives a dripping candle wax appearance on radiographs.
2. Massive osteolysis (Gorham-Stout disease) is purely lytic resorption of large segments of bone.
3. Radiographic findings for Gaucher disease include Erlenmeyer flask deformity (widened metaphyses).
4. Gaucher disease is caused by a deficiency of the enzyme glucocerebrosidase (acid β-glucosidase, lysosomal enzyme); treatment consists of enzyme replacement.
5. Imaging findings for stress fractures: radiographs show periosteal new bone formation; T1-weighted MRIs show normal marrow except for linear areas of low signal intensity; T2-weighted MRIs show high signal intensity in the medullary cavity and on the periosteal surface.
6. Stress fractures from prolonged diphosphonate therapy often occur on the lateral diaphyseal area of the subtrochanteric region and have a beaked appearance on radiographs.
7. The area affected by neuropathic arthropathy varies with the condition: syringomyelia, shoulder and elbow; syphilis, knee; diabetes mellitus, foot and ankle; spinal cord tumors, lower extremity joints; leprosy, any joint.
8. Radiographic findings for neuropathic arthropathy include fragmentation, subluxation, and dissolution of the joint.

9. Hemophilic arthropathy is characterized by factor deficiencies, including factor VIII (hemophilia A) and factor IX (hemophilia B).
10. Key radiographic findings for hemophilic arthropathy include squaring of the inferior patellar pole and femoral condyles.
11. Vertebral hemangiomas have a very characteristic appearance on radiographs or magnetic resonance imaging such that treatment does not require a biopsy.

Bibliography

Chisholm KA, Gilchrist JM: The Charcot joint: A modern neurologic perspective. *J Clin Neuromuscul Dis* 2011;13(1):1-13.

Engl W, Patrone L, Abbuehl BE: Target joint status in patients with hemophilia a during 18 consecutive months of prophylaxis with a pegylated full-length recombinant factor VIII with extended half-life *Blood* 2016;128:2592.

Ihde LL, Forrester DM, Gottsegen CJ, et al: Sclerosing bone dysplasias: Review and differentiation from other causes of osteosclerosis. *Radiographics* 2011;31(7):1865-1882.

Jain VK, Arya RK, Bharadwaj M, Kumar S: Melorheostosis: Clinicopathological features, diagnosis, and management. *Orthopedics* 2009;32(7):512.

Katz R, Booth T, Hargunani R, Wylie P, Holloway B: Radiological aspects of Gaucher disease. *Skeletal Radiol* 2011;40(12):1505-1513.

McCarthy EF, Frassica FJ: *Genetic diseases of bones and joints*, in *Pathology of Bone and Joint Disorders With Clinical and Radiographic Correlation*. Philadelphia, PA, Saunders, 1998, pp 54-55.

O'Hara J, Walsh S, Camp C, Mazza G, Carroll L, Hoxer C, Wilkinson L: The relationship between target joints and direct resource use in severe haemophilia. *Health Econ Rev* 2018;8:1.

Resnick D: Neuropathic osteoarthropathy, in Resnik D, ed: *Diagnosis of Bone and Joint Disorders With Clinical and Radiographic Correlation*, ed 3. Philadelphia, PA, Saunders, 1995, pp 3413-3442.

Ruggieri P, Montalti M, Angelini A, Alberghini M, Mercuri M: Gorham-Stout disease: The experience of the Rizzoli Institute and review of the literature. *Skeletal Radiol* 2011;40(11):1391-1397.

Vigorita VJ: *Osteonecrosis, Gaucher's disease*, in *Orthopaedic Pathology*. Philadelphia, PA, Lippincott Williams & Wilkins, 1999, pp 503-505.

Chapter 148
METASTATIC BONE DISEASE

KRISTY L. WEBER, MD

I. EVALUATION/DIAGNOSIS

A. Overview

1. Demographics

a. Metastatic bone disease occurs in patients older than 40 years.

b. Most common reason for destructive bone lesion in adults.

c. More than 1.73 million cases of cancer per year in the United States; bone metastasis develops in about 50% of patients.

d. Bone is the third most common site of metastasis (after lung and liver).

e. Most common primary cancer sites that metastasize to bone are breast, prostate, lung, kidney, and thyroid.

2. Genetics/etiology

a. Two main hypotheses

- 1889: Paget's "seed and soil" hypothesis (ability of tumor cells to survive and grow in addition to the compatible end-organ environment)
- 1928: Ewing's circulation theory
  - Tumors colonize particular organs because of the routes of blood flow from the primary site.
  - Organs are passive receptacles.
  - Batson plexus—Valveless plexus of veins around the spine allows tumor cells to travel to the vertebral bodies, pelvis, ribs, skull, and proximal limb girdle (eg, prostate metastases).

Dr. Weber or an immediate family member serves as a board member, owner, officer, or committee member of the American Academy of Orthopedic Surgeons.

b. Mediators of bone destruction include tumor necrosis factors; transforming growth factors (TGFs); 1,25 dihydroxyvitamin D3; and parathyroid hormone–related protein (PTHrP).

B. Clinical presentation (**Table 1**)

1. History

a. Progressive pain that occurs at rest and with weight bearing

b. Constitutional symptoms (weight loss, fatigue, loss of appetite)

c. Personal or family history of cancer

d. History of symptoms related to possible primary sites (hematuria, shortness of breath, hot/cold intolerance)

e. Primary tumors may metastasize quickly or take 10 to 15 years or longer (breast, renal, prostate)

2. Physical examination findings

a. Occasional swelling, limp, decreased joint range of motion, and neurologic deficits (10% to 20%) at metastatic bone sites

b. Possible breast, prostate, thyroid, or abdominal mass

c. Stool guaiac

d. Regional adenopathy

3. Laboratory studies

a. Complete blood cell count (anemia suggests myeloma)

b. Serum protein electrophoresis/urine protein electrophoresis (abnormal in myeloma)

c. Thyroid function tests (may be abnormal in thyroid cancer)

d. Urinalysis (microscopic hematuria in renal cancer)

TABLE 1

Workup of Patients Older Than 40 Years With a Destructive Bone Lesion[a]

Thorough history (history of cancer, weight loss, malaise, gastrointestinal bleeding, pain, etc)
Physical examination (focus on breast, lung, prostate, thyroid, lymph nodes)
Laboratory studies (electrolyte panel [calcium], alkaline phosphatase, complete blood cell count, tumor-specific markers as appropriate (eg, PSA, CA 125), serum protein electrophoresis/urine protein electrophoresis)
Plain radiographs of the bone lesion (two planes, include entire bone)
CT scan of chest, abdomen, pelvis
Total body bone scan

[a]Identifies primary site in 85% of patients.
CA 125 = cancer antigen 125, PSA = prostate-specific antigen

e. Basic chemistry panel: calcium, phosphorus, alkaline phosphatase, lactate dehydrogenase (LDH)

f. Specific tumor markers: prostate-specific antigen (PSA) (prostate); carcinoembryonic antigen (CEA) (colon, pancreas); cancer antigen 125 (CA 125) (ovarian)

4. Common scenarios

a. Known cancer patient with multiple bone lesions—Does not usually require confirmatory biopsy.

b. Known cancer patient with bone pain and normal radiographs—May be symptomatic from chemotherapy/osteoclast inhibitors or may require bone scan or MRI to define an early destructive lesion.

c. Patient without history of cancer with a destructive bone lesion—Must differentiate between metastatic disease and primary malignant bone tumor.

C. Radiographic appearance/workup

1. Appearance

a. Osteolytic (most bone metastases): lung, thyroid, kidney, gastrointestinal (**Figure 1, A**).

b. Osteoblastic: prostate, bladder (**Figure 1, B**).

c. Mixed osteolytic/osteoblastic: breast.

d. Most common locations include spine (40%), pelvis, proximal long bones, and ribs.

e. The thoracic spine is the most common vertebral location of metastasis.

f. Metastatic carcinoma to the spine spares the intervertebral disk.

g. Lesions distal to the elbow/knee are most commonly from the lung as a primary site.

h. Pathologic fracture is a common presentation (25%) and occurs more commonly in osteolytic versus osteoblastic lesions.

i. An avulsion of the lesser trochanter implies a pathologic process in the femoral neck with impending fracture.

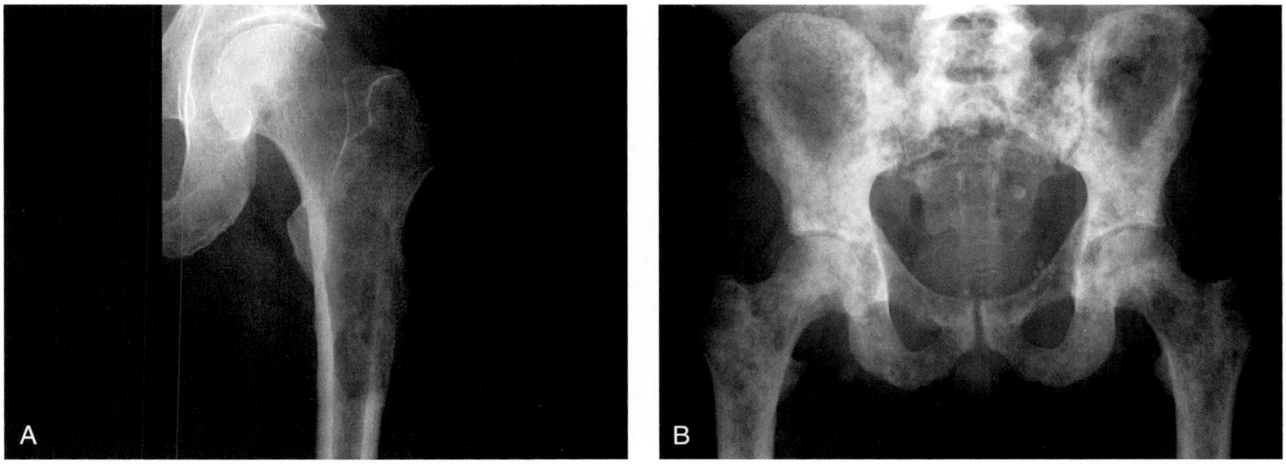

Figure 1 Osteolytic and osteoblastic metastases. **A**, Lung cancer metastases are generally purely osteolytic, as demonstrated in this AP radiograph of a left hip. Note the lesion in the left proximal femur that is destroying the lateral cortex. **B**, Prostate cancer metastases are osteoblastic, as noted throughout the pelvis, spine, and proximal femurs in this AP pelvic radiograph.

2. Workup (**Table 1**)
   a. Plain radiographs—Images in two planes and of the entire bone should be obtained (consider referred pain).
   b. Differential diagnosis of lytic bone lesion in patient older than 40 years includes metastatic disease, multiple myeloma, lymphoma, and, less likely, primary bone tumors, Paget sarcoma, and hyperparathyroidism (**Table 2**).
   c. Bone scan
      - Detects osteoblastic activity (may be negative in myeloma, metastatic renal cancer).
      - Identifies multiple lesions, which are common in metastatic disease (**Figure 2, A**).
   d. CT scan of chest, abdomen, and pelvis to identify primary lesion.
   e. Staging evaluation of lytic bone lesion will identify primary site in 85% of patients (**Table 1**).
   f. Bone marrow biopsy when considering myeloma as a diagnosis.
   g. MRI scan of the primary lesion is generally not necessary unless defining disease in the spine (**Figure 2, B**).
   h. Difficult to differentiate osteoporosis from metastatic disease with a single vertebral compression fracture; tumor is suggested by soft-tissue mass and pedicle destruction.

D. Biopsy/pathology
   1. A biopsy of a destructive bone lesion must be performed unless the diagnosis is certain.

TABLE 2

Differential Diagnosis of Destructive Bone Lesion in Patients Older Than 40 Years

Metastatic bone disease[a]
Multiple myeloma[a]
Lymphoma[a]
Primary bone tumors (chondrosarcoma, osteosarcoma, undifferentiated pleomorphic sarcoma, chordoma)
Pelvic/sacral insufficiency fractures
Postradiation/Paget sarcoma
Giant cell tumor
Hyperparathyroidism
Infection

[a]Most common diagnoses.

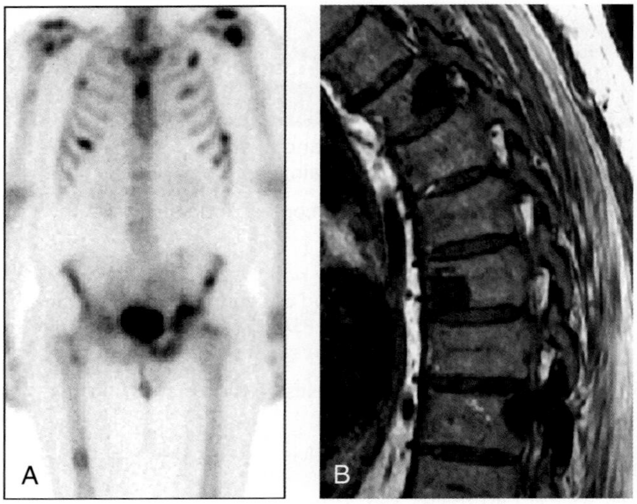

Figure 2 Metastases seen on a total body bone scan and MRI. **A**, Total body bone scan shows increased uptake in the sacroiliac region and metastases in the anterior pelvis, ribs, and shoulder girdle. **B**, Sagittal MRI of the thoracic spine shows vertebral lesions.

   2. Placing an intramedullary device in a 65-year-old patient with a lytic lesion in the femur without appropriate workup is risky (could be a primary malignant bone tumor).
   3. An open incisional biopsy or closed needle biopsy (fine-needle aspiration/core) can be performed.
   4. Histologic appearance of metastatic carcinoma is islands of epithelial cells with glandular or squamous differentiation (**Figure 3, A** and **B**).
   5. The carcinoma cells have tight junctions and reside within a fibrous stroma.
   6. Thyroid (follicular): follicles filled with colloid material (**Figure 3, C**).
   7. Renal cancer often has a clear appearance to the cytoplasm within the epithelial cells (**Figure 3, D**); in some cases, it may be poorly differentiated or have a sarcomatoid pattern.
   8. Epithelial cells are keratin positive.
   9. Special immunohistochemistry stains can sometimes determine the primary site of disease.
      a. Lung: Thyroid transcription factor-1 (TTF-1), NAPSIN-A
      b. Thyroid: TTF-1, thyroglobulin, PAX-8
      c. Breast: Estrogen and progesterone receptors, GATA-3, mammaglobin
      d. Prostate: PSA, NKX3.1
      e. Kidney: CDE10, vimentin, PAX-8

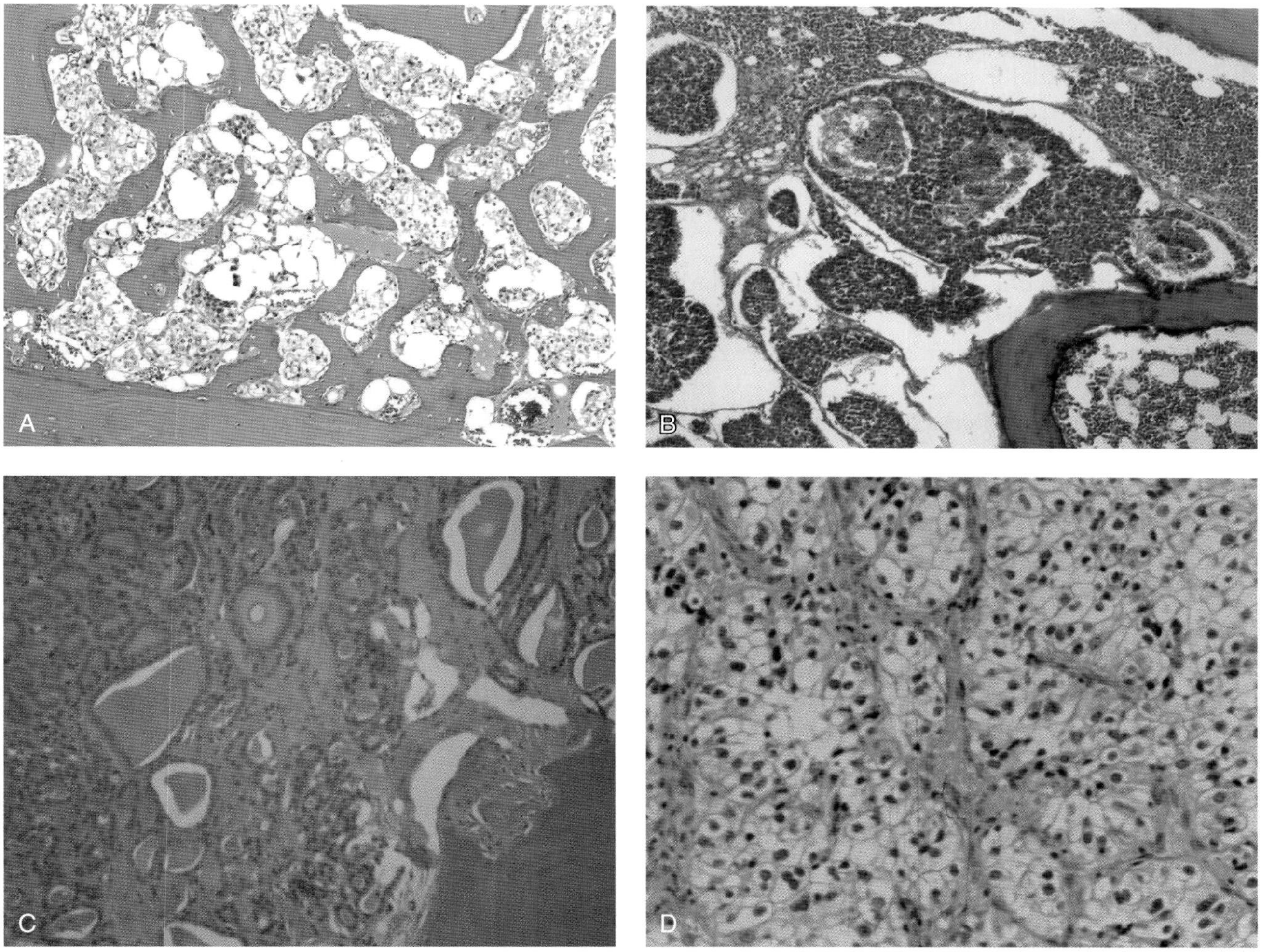

Figure 3 Histologic specimens show bone metastasis from the most common primary lesions. **A**, Prostate—note the new bone formation by the osteoblasts that are stimulated by factors secreted by the tumor cells. **B**, Lung—note the clumps of epithelial cells characterized by tight cell-cell junctions. **C**, Thyroid (follicular)—the epithelial cells are forming follicles surrounding a central colloid substance. **D**, Renal—the epithelial tumor cells are characterized by clear cytoplasm.

II. PATHOPHYSIOLOGY/MOLECULAR MECHANISMS

A. Metastatic cascade

1. Primary tumor cells proliferate and stimulate angiogenesis.
2. Tumor cells cross the basement membrane into capillaries and must avoid host defenses.
3. Tumor cells disseminate to distant sites.
4. Cells arrest in distant capillary bed, adhere to vascular endothelium, and extravasate into end-organ environment (integrins, cadherins, matrix metalloproteinases).
5. Tumor cells interact with local host cells and growth factors (TGF-β, insulinlike growth factor, fibroblast growth factor, bone morphogenetic protein).
6. Tumor cells proliferate to become a site of metastasis.

B. RANKL/osteoprotegerin

1. Tumor cells do not destroy bone; cytokines from the tumor stimulate osteoclasts or osteoblasts to destroy or generate new bone, respectively.
2. Osteoblasts/stromal cells secrete receptor activator of nuclear factor κ B ligand (RANKL).
3. Osteoclast precursors have receptors for RANKL (RANK).

4. Increased secretion of RANKL by osteoblasts causes an increase in osteoclast precursors, which eventually results in increased bone destruction.
5. Osteoprotegerin (OPG) is a decoy receptor that binds to RANKL and inhibits an increase in osteoclasts.

C. Vicious cycle in breast cancer
1. TGF-β is stored in the bone and released during normal bone turnover.
2. TGF-β stimulates metastatic breast cancer cells to secrete PTHrP.
3. PTHrP from cancer cells stimulates osteoblasts to secrete RANKL.
4. RANKL from osteoblasts stimulates osteoclast precursors and increases osteoclasts.
5. Osteoclasts destroy bone and release TGF-β, and the cycle of destruction repeats.

D. Other disease-specific factors
1. Breast cancer cells also secrete osteoclastic stimulants (interleukin [IL]-6, IL-8).
2. Prostate cancer—Endothelin-1 stimulates osteoblasts to produce bone.
3. Overexpression of growth factors and their receptors is common in renal cell carcinoma (epidermal growth factor receptor [EGFR], vascular endothelial growth factor receptor [VEGFR], platelet-derived growth factor receptor [PDGFR]).

E. Fracture healing in pathologic bone
1. Likelihood of pathologic fracture healing: multiple myeloma > renal carcinoma > breast carcinoma > lung carcinoma (ie, pathologic fracture healing is most likely in patients with myeloma and least likely in patients with metastatic lung cancer).
2. Most important factor in determining healing potential is the length of patient survival.

F. Other physiologic disruptions
1. Calcium metabolism—Hypercalcemia is present in 10% to 30% of cases.
   a. Common with lung and breast cancer metastasis
   b. Does not correlate with number of bone metastases or osteolytic nature
   c. Early symptoms: polyuria/polydipsia, anorexia, weakness, easy fatigability
   d. Late symptoms: irritability, depression, coma, profound weakness, nausea/vomiting, pruritus, vision abnormalities
   e. Treatment requires aggressive hydration and intravenous diphosphonate therapy
2. Hematopoiesis—Normocytic/normochromic anemia is common with breast, prostate, lung, and thyroid cancer metastasis.
3. Thromboembolic disease
   a. Patients with malignancy have increased thromboembolic risk
   b. Requires prophylaxis, especially after lower extremity/pelvic surgery
4. Pain control/bowel abnormalities
   a. Use narcotics for pain control
   b. Requires laxatives/stool softener to avoid severe constipation

III. BIOMECHANICS

A. Stress riser in bone occurs whenever there is cortical destruction.

B. Defects
1. Open section defect—When the length of a longitudinal defect in a bone exceeds 75% of diameter, there is a 90% reduction in torsional strength.
2. Fifty percent cortical defect (centered) = 60% bending strength reduction.
3. Fifty percent cortical defect (eccentric) = >90% bending strength reduction.

IV. IMPENDING FRACTURES/PROPHYLACTIC FIXATION

A. Indications for fixation
1. Snell/Beals criteria
   a. A 2.5-cm lytic bone lesion
   b. Fifty percent cortical involvement
   c. Pain persisting after radiation
   d. Peritrochanteric lesion
2. Mirels scoring system (**Table 3**)
   a. Four factors are scored: radiographic appearance, size (proportion of bone diameter occupied by the lesion), site, and pain.
   b. Prophylactic fixation is recommended for a score ≥9 (33% fracture risk).

TABLE 3

Mirels Scoring System for Prediction of Pathologic Fracture in Patients With Metastatic Bone Lesions

Factor	Points		
	1	2	3
Radiographic appearance	Blastic	Mixed	Lytic
Size (as a proportion of shaft diameter)	<1/3	1/3 to 2/3	>2/3
Site	UE	LE	Peritrochanteric
Pain	Mild	Moderate	Mechanical

UE = upper extremity; LE = lower extremity
Adapted with permission from Mirels H: Metastatic disease in long bones: A proposed scoring system for diagnosing impending pathologic fractures. *Clin Orthop* 1989;249:256-265.

3. Spinal lesions—impending fracture/collapse
   a. Thoracic
      - Risk of fracture/collapse exists when 50% to 60% of the vertebral body is involved (without other abnormalities).
      - Risk of fracture/collapse exists when only 20% to 30% of the vertebral body is involved if there is also costovertebral joint involvement.

   b. Lumbar
      - Risk of fracture/collapse exists when 35% to 40% of the vertebral body is involved (without other abnormalities).
      - Risk of fracture/collapse exists when 25% of vertebral body is involved if there is also pedicle/posterior element involvement.

B. Other factors to consider
1. Scoring systems are not exact and cannot predict all human factors
2. Histology of primary lesion
3. Expected lifespan, comorbid conditions, and activity level
4. Most surgical decisions can be based on plain radiographs (MRI not needed for extremity lesions)
5. Prophylactic fixation compared with fixation of actual pathologic fracture
   a. Decreased perioperative morbidity/pain
   b. Shorter operating room time
   c. Faster recovery/shorter hospital stay
   d. Ability to coordinate care with medical oncology

V. NONSURGICAL TREATMENT

A. Indications
1. Nondisplaced fractures (depending on location)
2. Non–weight-bearing bones (**Figure 4**)
3. Poor medical health/shortened lifespan

B. Observation/pain management/bracing treatment
1. Observation or activity modifications are used for patients with very small lesions or advanced disease.
2. Functional bracing treatment can be used in the upper and lower extremities and spine.
3. Pain management is important in all symptomatic patients.
   a. Opioids
   b. Nonopioids: NSAIDs, tricyclic antidepressants, muscle relaxants, steroids
   c. A bowel program is necessary to prevent severe constipation

C. Medical
1. Cytotoxic chemotherapy
2. Hormonal treatment (prostate, breast metastasis)
3. Growth factor receptor inhibitors (lung, renal cell metastasis)
4. Bisphosphonates
   a. Inhibit osteoclast activity by inducing apoptosis
   b. Inhibit protein prenylation and act on the mevalonate pathway
   c. Significant decrease in skeletal events (breast, prostate, lung)

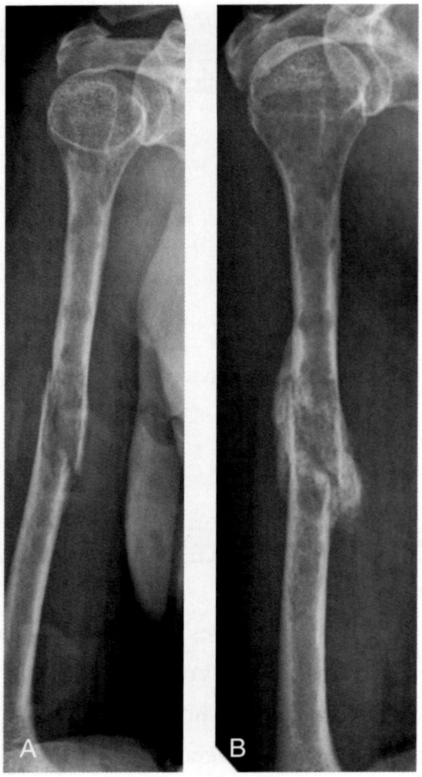

Figure 4 **A**, AP radiograph of the right humerus of a 68-year-old woman with metastatic breast cancer and a pathologic fracture. She was treated nonsurgically due to multiple comorbidities. **B**, In this radiograph, note the callus formation about the healed fracture site 2 months later.

d. Reduced pain

e. Used commonly in metastatic bone disease (intravenous zoledronic acid)

f. Complications: Osteonecrosis of the jaw and occasional nephrotoxicity

5. Denosumab—Human monoclonal antibody to RANKL

a. Subcutaneous injection

b. Does not require monitoring of renal function

c. Superior to zoledronic acid in delaying time to first skeletal-related event (in metastatic breast cancer patients)

d. Noninferior to zoledronic acid in delaying time to first skeletal event in multiple myeloma and tumors other than breast/prostate cancer

e. Greater reduction of bone turnover markers compared with zoledronic acid (metastatic breast cancer)

f. No difference between denosumab and zoledronic acid in terms of survival or disease progression (metastatic breast cancer)

g. Complications: Hypocalcemia and osteonecrosis of the jaw (<0.5%)

D. Radiation

1. External beam radiation

a. Indications: pain, impending fracture, neurologic symptoms

b. Dose: usually 30 Gy in 10 fractions to bone lesion (but can use higher dose/less fractions)

c. One dose of 8 Gy is effective for palliative pain relief although retreatment rates are higher

d. Pain relief in 70% of patients

e. Postoperatively, the entire implant should be irradiated after wound healing (~2 weeks) to decrease fixation failure and improve local control

f. Should be used for patients with radiosensitive tumors of the spine who have pain or tumor progression without instability or myelopathy

2. Radiopharmaceuticals

a. Samarium Sm-153 or strontium chloride 89 for refractory pain

b. Delivery of radiation to the entire skeleton (bone scan concept)

c. Palliation of pain—may delay progression of lesions

d. Use requires normal renal function and blood counts (radium-223 less toxicity)

e. Iodine-131 is used to treat metastatic thyroid cancer

E. Minimally invasive techniques

1. Radiofrequency ablation or cryoablation—Used for palliative pain control (commonly used in pelvis/acetabulum)

2. Kyphoplasty/vertebroplasty (**Figure 5**)

a. Pain relief in patients with vertebral compression fractures from metastasis.

b. The risk of cement leakage in vertebroplasty (35% to 65%) is usually not clinically relevant.

c. Vertebroplasty is not indicated for osteoporotic spinal compression fractures, but it is still used for metastatic disease and multiple myeloma affecting the spine.

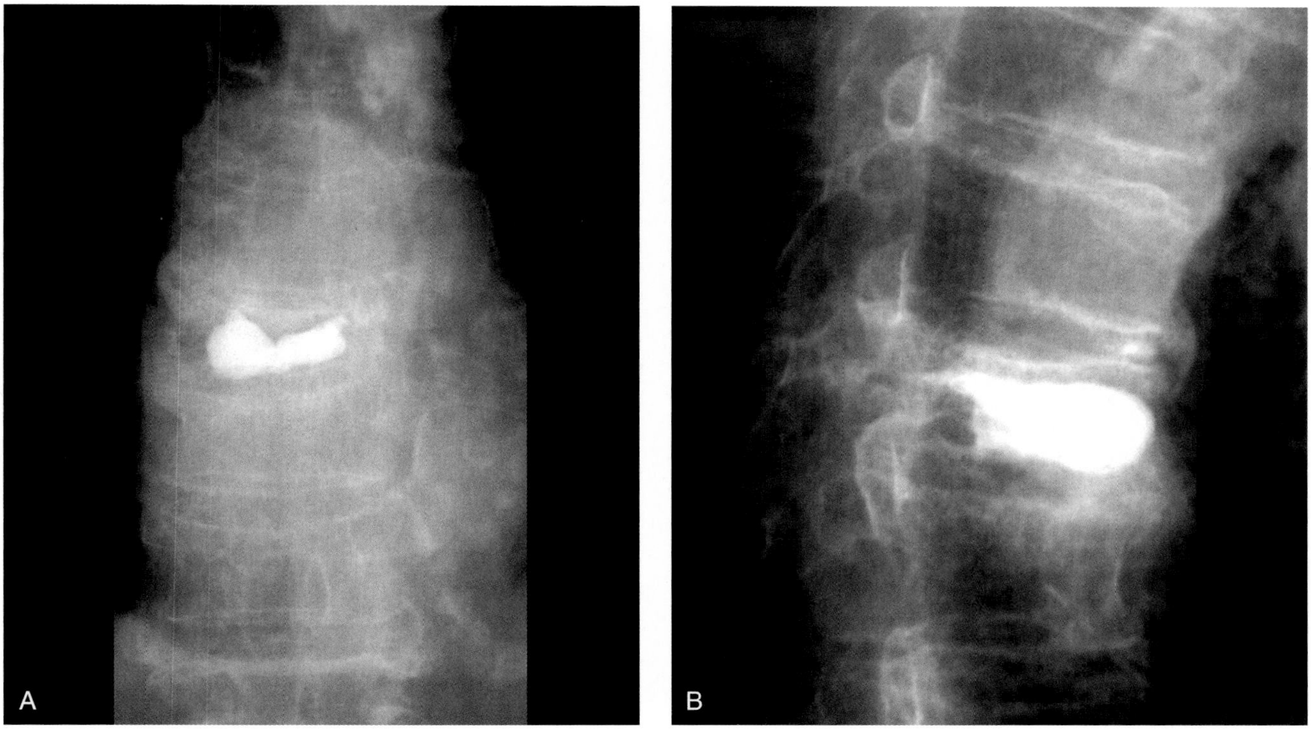

Figure 5 AP (**A**) and lateral (**B**) radiographs of the spine of a woman with metastatic lung cancer to the thoracic vertebra, causing painful collapse. The patient was treated with vertebroplasty and experienced marked pain relief.

VI. SURGICAL TREATMENT/OUTCOME

A. Overview

1. Goals of surgical treatment
    a. Relieve pain
    b. Improve function
    c. Restore skeletal stability
2. Considerations before surgery
    a. Patient selection (functional status, activity level, comorbidities)
    b. Stability/durability of planned construct (withstand force of six times body weight around hip)
    c. Address all areas of weakened bone
    d. Preoperative embolization for highly vascular lesions (renal, thyroid metastasis)
    e. Extensive use of methyl methacrylate (cement) to improve stability of construct
    f. Cemented (rather than noncemented) joint prostheses are more widely used in patients with bone metastasis

B. Upper extremity

1. Overview
    a. Upper extremity metastases affect activities of daily living, use of external aids, bed-to-chair transfers
    b. Much less common (20%) than lower extremity metastases
2. Scapula/clavicle—Usually nonsurgical treatment/radiation
3. Proximal humerus
    a. Resection and proximal humeral replacement (megaprosthesis); excellent pain relief but poor shoulder function
    b. Intramedullary locked device (closed versus open with curettage/cement) if bone quality allows (**Figure 6**)
4. Humeral diaphysis
    a. Intramedullary fixation: closed versus open with curettage/cement
    b. Intercalary metal spacer: selected indications for extensive diaphyseal destruction or failed prior implant

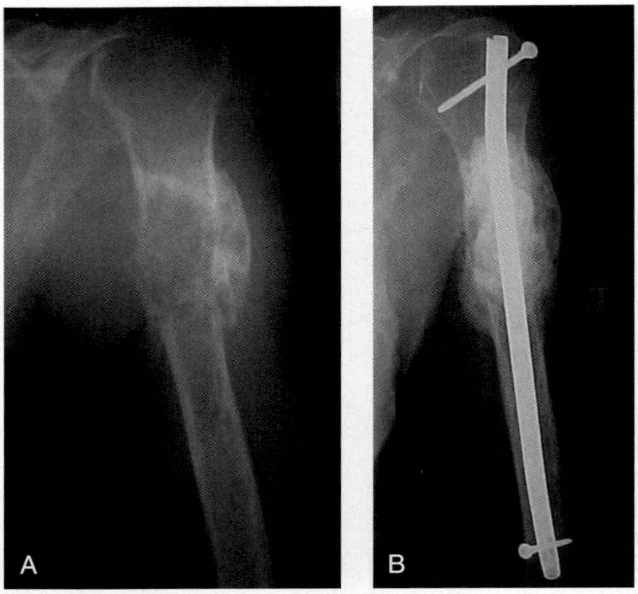

Figure 6 Radiographs of the left humerus of a 52-year-old right-handed man with metastatic renal carcinoma and a pathologic fracture. **A**, AP radiograph shows a fracture through the osteolytic lesion in the left proximal humerus. **B**, Postoperative radiograph obtained after placement of a locked left humeral intramedullary rod. This lesion was curetted and cemented during the surgery and received radiation after 2 weeks.

5. Distal humerus
   a. Flexible crossed nails can be supplemented with cement and extend the entire length of bone (insert at elbow).
   b. Orthogonal plating—Combine with curettage/cement (**Figure 7**).
   c. Resection and modular distal humeral prosthetic reconstruction.
6. Distal to elbow—Individualize treatment with plates or intramedullary devices versus nonsurgical treatment.

C. Lower extremity
1. Overview
   a. Common location for bone metastasis
   b. Surgical treatment if patient has ≥3 months to live (but displaced femoral diaphyseal fractures may be fixed in patients with less time to live)
2. Pelvis (**Figure 8**)
   a. Treat non–weight-bearing areas with radiation or minimally invasive techniques.
   b. Resection or curettage in selected cases

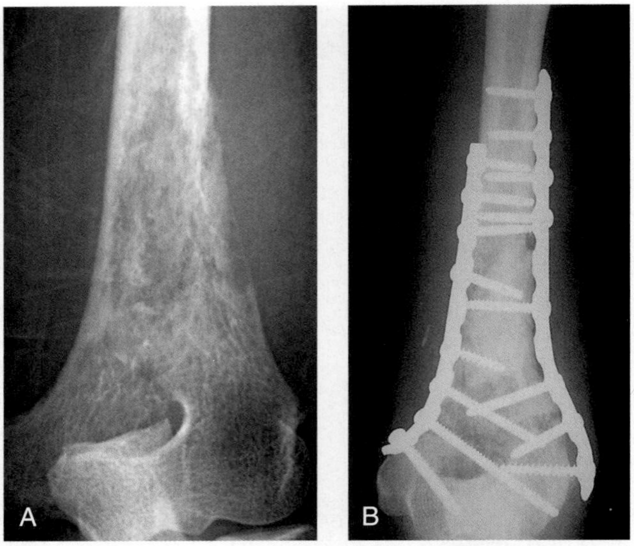

Figure 7 Radiographs of the distal humerus of a 56-year-old woman with metastatic endometrial cancer. **A**, AP view demonstrates the permeative appearance of the lesion. The patient had persistent pain after radiation of the metastasis. **B**, Postoperative AP view obtained after curettage, cementation, and double plating of the lesion.

3. Acetabulum (**Figure 9, A** and **B**)
   a. Surgical treatment requires extensive preoperative planning (cross-sectional imaging, embolization for vascular lesions).
   b. Extent of bone destruction delineates treatment options (standard total hip arthroplasty, acetabular mesh/cage, rebar reconstruction to transmit stresses from acetabulum to unaffected ilium/sacrum).
   c. Girdlestone procedure is appropriate in patients with end-stage disease, severe pain, and substantial periacetabular bone loss (**Figure 9, C**).

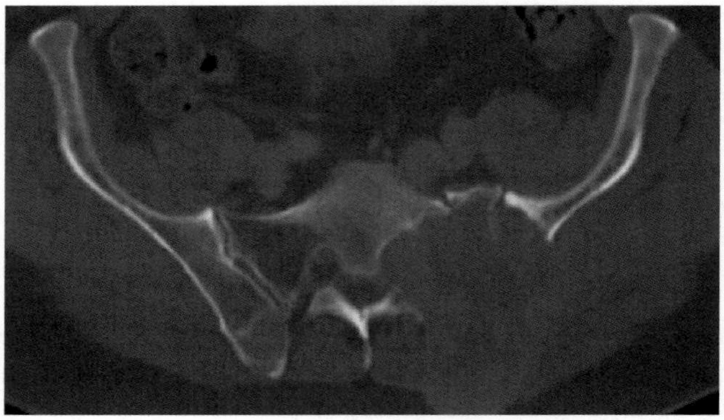

Figure 8 Axial CT scan of the pelvis of a 47-year-old man with metastatic thyroid cancer defines a large, destructive lesion in the left sacroiliac region.

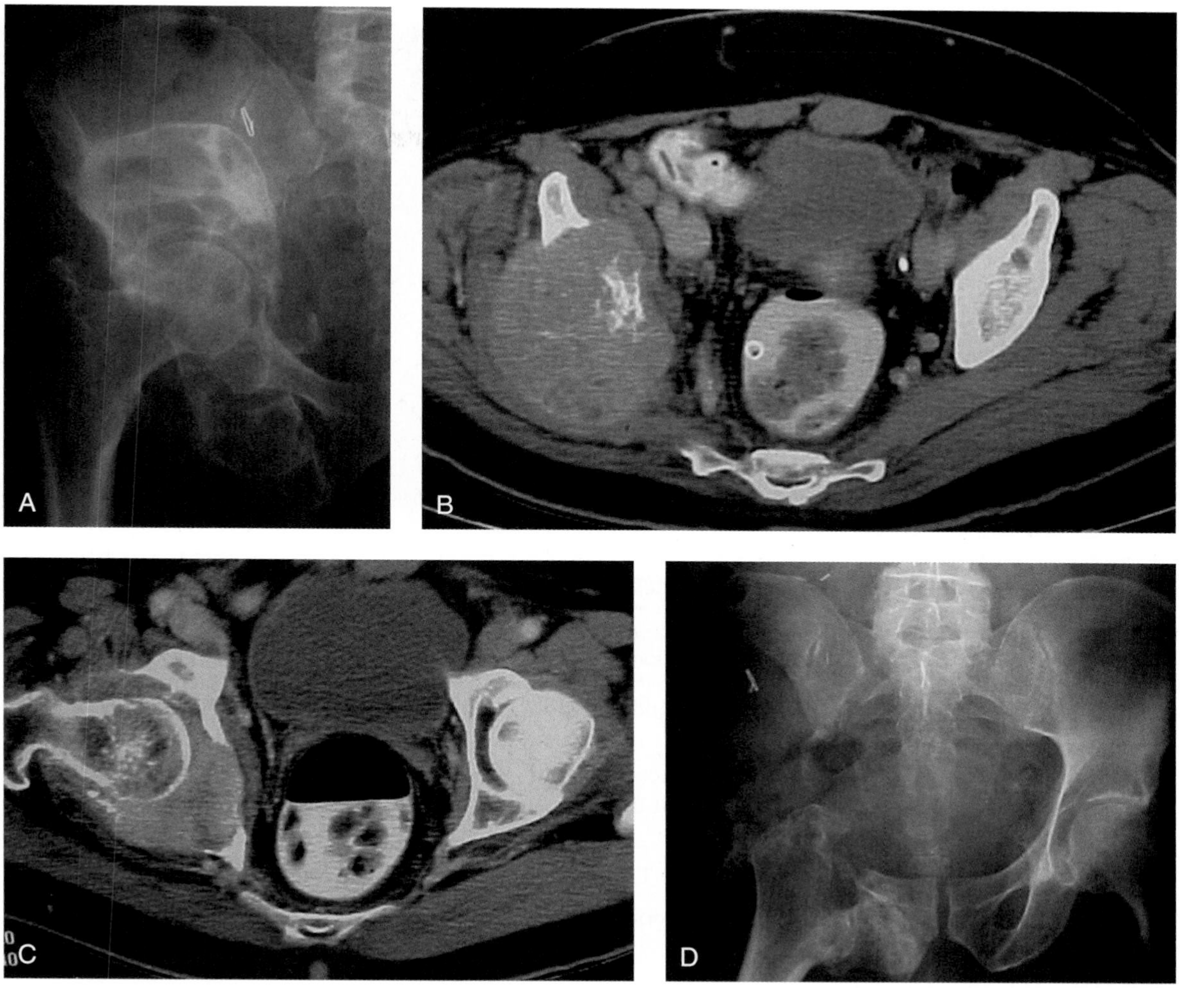

Figure 9 Imaging studies in patients with metastatic disease to the right hemipelvis. **A**, AP radiograph of the right pelvis in a 78-year-old woman with metastatic renal cell carcinoma to the right acetabulum, ischium, and ilium after prior radiation. **B** and **C**, CT scans of the pelvis defines the destruction of the ilium and acetabulum with a large associated soft-tissue mass. **D**, AP radiograph of the pelvis after a Girdlestone procedure which was deemed the safest procedure given the extent of disease, patient comorbidities, and potential for marked blood loss.

4. Femoral neck (**Figure 10**)
   a. Pathologic fractures or impending fractures require prosthetic reconstruction.
   b. Internal fixation with cement has an unacceptably high failure rate because of the likelihood of disease progression.
   c. Usually a bipolar cup is satisfactory; a total hip arthroplasty should be performed only if the acetabulum is involved with metastatic disease or the patient has extensive degenerative joint disease.
5. Intertrochanteric (**Figure 11**)
   a. Intramedullary reconstruction nail (open versus closed) protects the entire femur (**Figure 11**)
   b. Calcar replacement prosthesis for lesions with extensive bone destruction
6. Subtrochanteric
   a. Intramedullary locked reconstruction nail (**Figures 12 and 14**)
   b. Resection and prosthetic replacement (megaprosthesis)
      - Patients with periarticular bone destruction that does not allow rigid fixation
      - Displaced pathologic fracture through large osteolytic lesion
      - Radioresistant lesion (large renal cell metastasis)

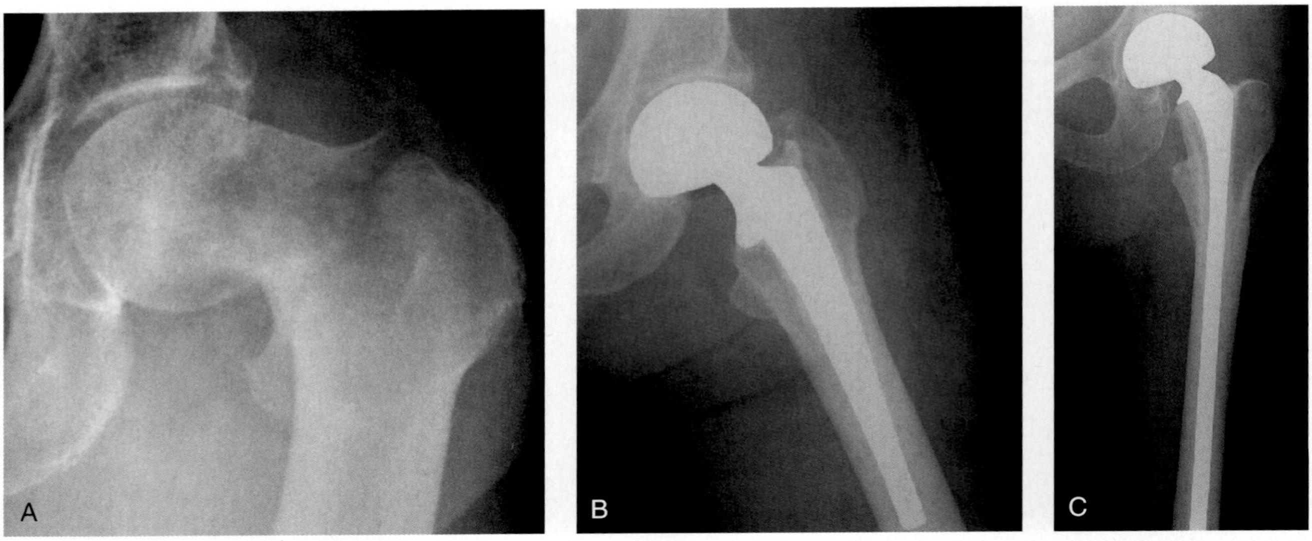

Figure 10 Metastases to the femoral neck. **A**, AP radiograph of the left hip in a 70-year-old woman with metastatic breast cancer reveals a pathologic femoral neck fracture. No other lesions were noted throughout the femur. **B**, AP radiograph obtained after a cemented bipolar hip reconstruction. Most patients with femoral neck disease do not require acetabular components. Internal fixation of a pathologic hip fracture is not indicated. **C**, AP radiograph of a hip obtained after implantation of a long-stemmed femoral implant, which can be used to prevent pathologic fractures in the femoral diaphysis. Patients with long-stemmed prostheses have a higher risk of cardiopulmonary complications due to intraoperative/postoperative thromboembolic events.

- Solitary lesion (some series indicate improved survival for resection of solitary metastasis from renal carcinoma)
- Salvage of failed fixation devices (**Figure 13**)

7. Femoral diaphysis: intramedullary locked reconstruction nail
8. Distal femur
   a. Locking plate/screws/cement

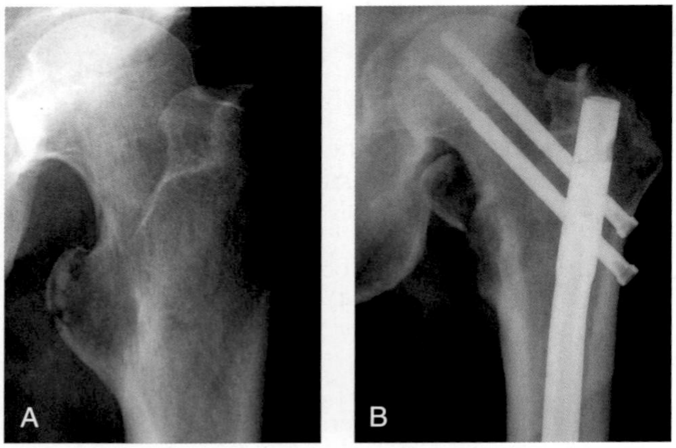

Figure 11 Intertrochanteric lesions. **A**, AP radiograph of the hip of a patient with metastatic thyroid cancer. A lesser trochanter avulsion or osteolytic lesion indicates a pathologic process in the older patient. **B**, AP radiograph obtained after the patient was treated prophylactically with a locked femoral reconstruction nail.

   b. Retrograde intramedullary device (less ideal because of tumor reaming in knee joint and stress riser at tip of rod in proximal femur)
   c. Resection and distal femoral replacement
9. Distal to knee
   a. Individualize treatment with prostheses, intramedullary devices, plates/screws/cement (**Figure 15**).
   b. Avoid amputation if possible.

D. Spine
1. Risk factors for progressive neurologic deficit
   a. Osteolytic lesions
   b. Pedicle involvement ("winking owl" sign on AP radiograph)
   c. Posterior column involvement
2. Indications for surgical treatment
   a. Significant or progressive neurologic deficit
   b. Intractable pain
   c. Progression of deformity
3. Surgical options
   a. Anterior vertebrectomy
   b. Posterior decompression/instrumentation
   c. Anterior/posterior combination approach (**Figure 16**)

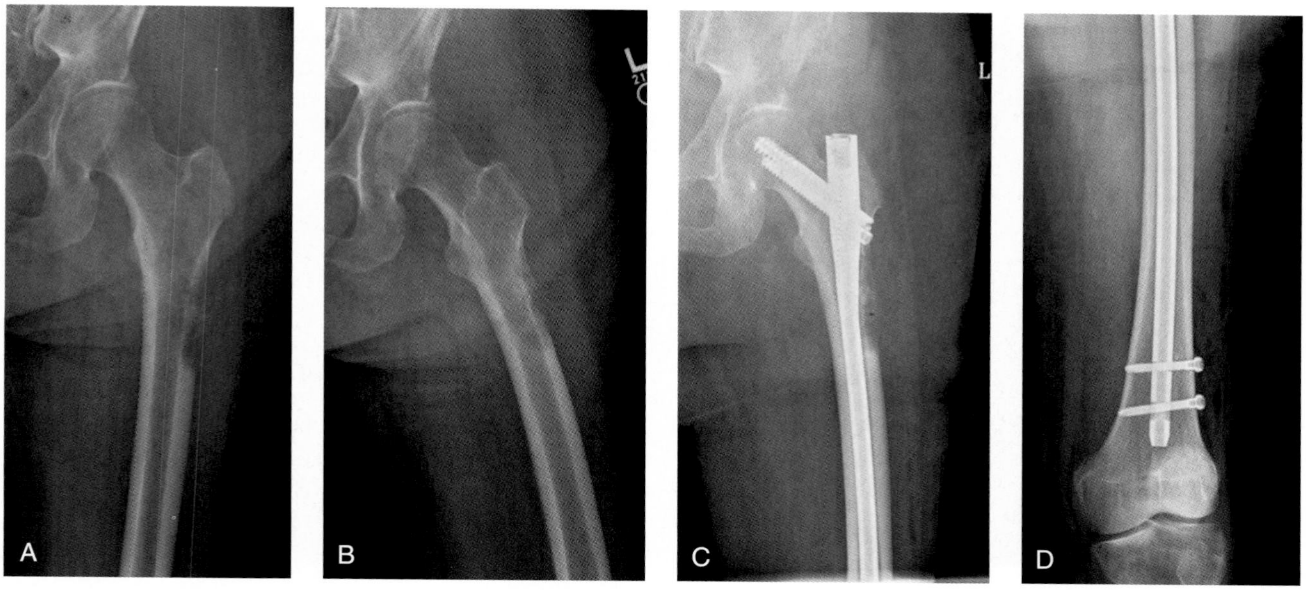

Figure 12 Radiographs of the left femur of a 62-year-old woman with metastatic lung cancer. **A**, AP and **B**, lateral radiographs of the left proximal femur reveal a large subtrochanteric lytic lesion at high risk for pathologic fracture. **C** and **D**, Postoperative radiographs of the left femur show stabilization of the entire femur with an intramedullary reconstruction nail.

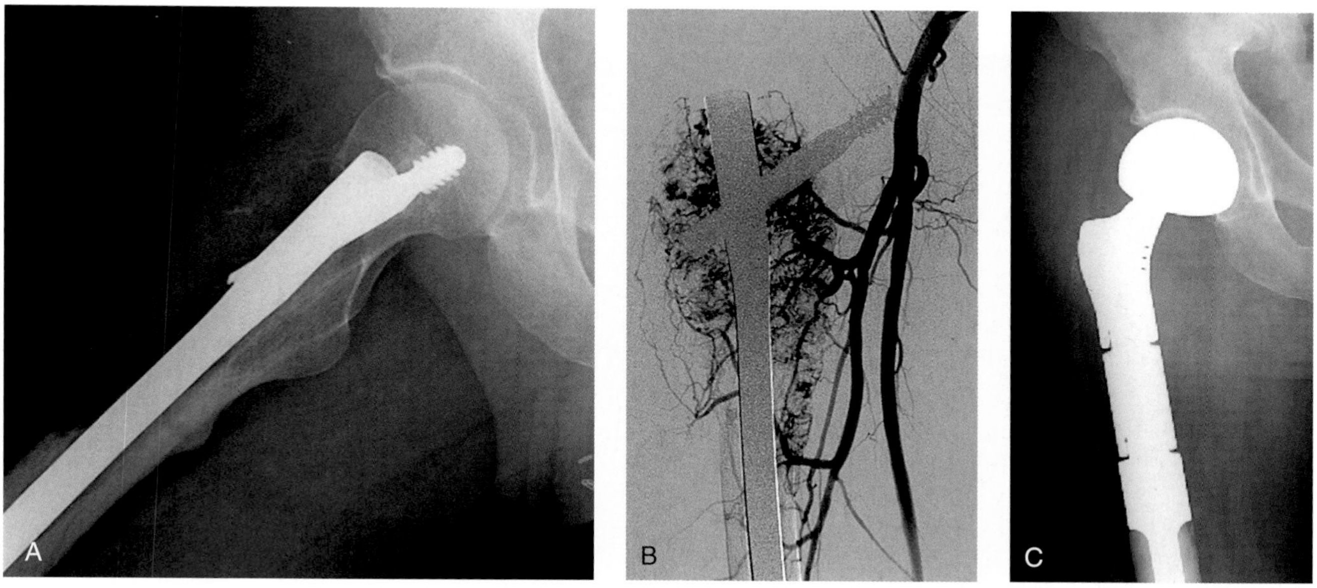

Figure 13 Imaging studies of a 49-year-old man with metastatic renal cell carcinoma and painful progression of disease after placement of an intramedullary reconstruction nail in the right femur. **A**, Lateral radiograph demonstrates the loss of anterior cortex proximally. **B**, Prior to salvage of the impending hardware failure, embolization of the feeding vessels is performed, as shown in this angiogram. This should be done routinely for patients with metastatic renal carcinoma unless a tourniquet can be used for surgery. **C**, AP radiograph obtained after the proximal femur was resected shows the defect reconstructed with a cemented megaprosthesis using a bipolar acetabular implant.

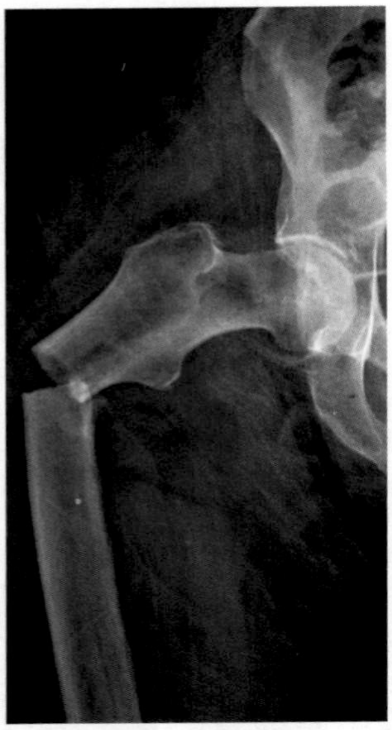

Figure 14 Radiograph of the right femur of a 77-year-old woman demonstrates a pathologic subtrochanteric fracture. A staging workup did not reveal a primary site of disease, but an intraoperative biopsy of the femoral lesion showed carcinoma on frozen section. The patient should be treated with a femoral reconstruction nail.

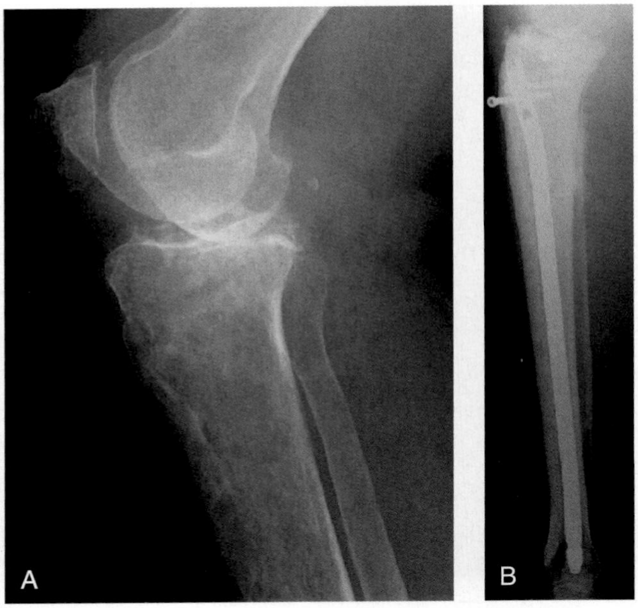

Figure 15 Radiographs of the right knee of a 67-year-old woman with metastatic breast cancer to the tibia. **A**, Lateral radiograph demonstrates the destruction of the tibia with concomitant severe osteopenia. This extends throughout the length of the bone. **B**, Lateral radiograph obtained after 18 months reveals a locked intramedullary tibial rod in good position. With postoperative radiation, bisphosphonates, and hormonal treatment, the bone quality greatly improved.

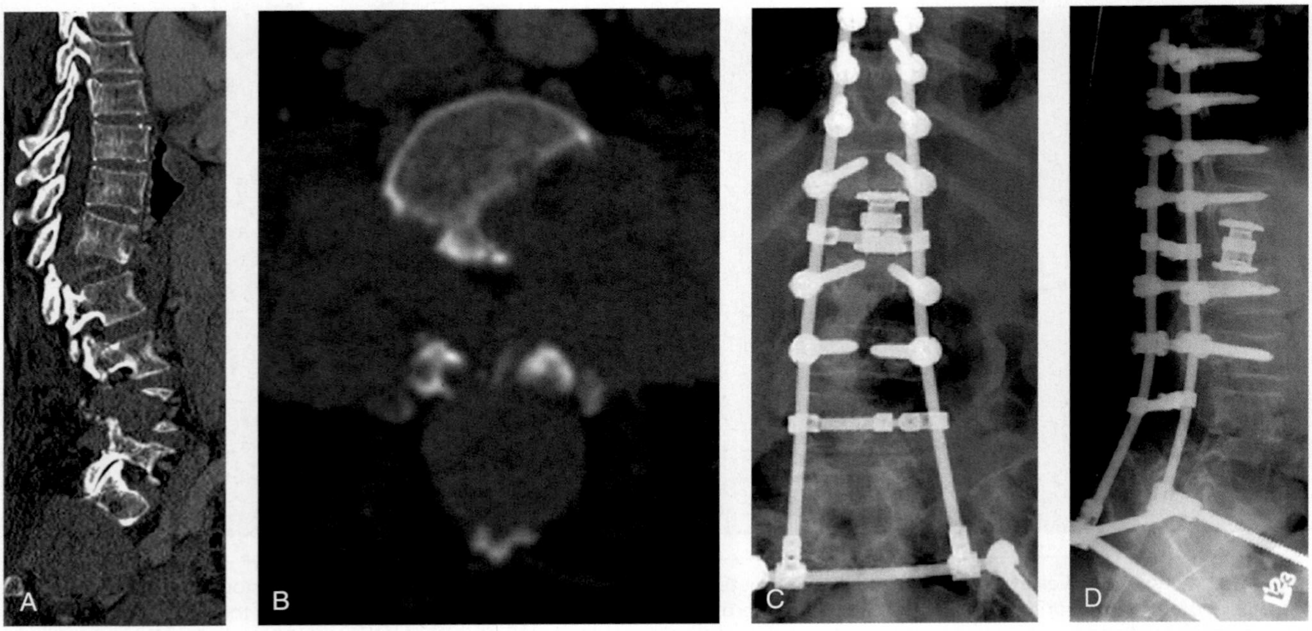

Figure 16 Images of the spine of a 57-year-old woman with metastatic thyroid cancer. **A**, A CT sagittal reconstruction of the thoracolumbar spine demonstrates complete destruction and collapse of L1, with severe central canal obstruction at this level. Note also the extensive disease at L4 and S2. **B**, Axial CT image at L4 demonstrates the canal compromise at this level and the extent of the soft-tissue mass. AP (**C**) and lateral (**D**) radiographs obtained after L1 corpectomy, partial L4 corpectomy, and posterior thoracic-lumbar-pelvic fixation with pedicle screws, rods, and a transiliac bar. A distractible cage is shown at L1.

TOP TESTING FACTS

1. The most common diagnosis of a lytic, destructive lesion in a patient older than 40 years is bone metastasis.
2. The most common primary sites that metastasize to bone are breast, prostate, lung, kidney, and thyroid.
3. Careful history, physical examination, and radiographic staging will identify 85% of primary lesions; biopsy is needed when the primary lesion has not been identified.
4. The histologic features of metastatic carcinoma include epithelial cells in a fibrous stroma.
5. Breast carcinoma cells secrete PTHrP, which signals osteoblasts to release RANKL, which causes osteoclast activation and further bone resorption.
6. Osteolytic lesions have a greater likelihood of pathologic fracture than osteoblastic lesions.
7. Bisphosphonates cause osteoclast apoptosis by inhibiting protein prenylation and act via the mevalonate pathway.
8. RANKL inhibitors (denosumab) work as a human monoclonal antibody to block RANKL binding to the RANK receptor on osteoclast precursors.
9. External beam radiation is helpful for pain control and is important in maintaining local tumor control postoperatively.
10. Pathologic femoral neck lesions require prosthetic replacement, not in situ fixation.
11. Locked intramedullary fixation is used for impending or actual diaphyseal fractures. (Femoral rods usually have proximal screws to protect the femoral neck.)

Bibliography

Chow R, Hoskin P, Hollenberg D et al: Efficacy of single fraction conventional radiation therapy for painful uncomplicated bone metastases: A systematic review and meta-analysis. *Ann Palliat Med* 2017;6:125-142.

Damron TA, Morgan H, Prakash D, Grant W, Aronowitz J, Heiner J: Critical evaluation of Mirels' rating system for impending pathologic fractures. *Clin Orthop Relat Res* 2003;415(415, suppl):S201-S207.

Expert panel on radiation oncology-Bone metastasis; Lo SS, Lutz ST, Chang EL, et al: ACR appropriateness criteria spinal bone metastases. *J Palliat Med* 2013;16:9-19.

Harrington KD: The management of acetabular insufficiency secondary to metastatic malignant disease. *J Bone Joint Surg Am* 1981;63(4):653-664.

Henry DH, Costa L, Goldwasser F, et al: Randomized, double-blind study of denosamab versus zoledronic acid in the treatment of bone metastases in patients with advanced cancer (excluding breast and prostate cancer) or multiple myeloma. *J Clin Oncol* 2011;29:1125-1132.

Kirkinis MN, Lyne CJ, Wilson MD, Choong PF: Metastatic bone disease: A review of survival, prognostic factors and outcomes following surgical treatment of the appendicular skeleton. *Eur J Surg Oncol* 2016;42:1787-1797.

Lutz ST, Lo SS, Chang EL, et al: ACR Appropriateness Criteria® non-spine bone metastases. *J Palliat Med* 2012;15(5):521-526.

O'Carrigan B, Wong MH, Wilson ML, Stockler MR, Pavlakis N, Goodwin A: Bisphosphonates and other bone agents for breast cancer. *Cochrane Database Syst Rev* 2017;10:CD003474.

Patchell RA, Tibbs PA, Regine WF, et al: Direct decompressive surgical resection in the treatment of spinal cord compression caused by metastatic cancer: A randomised trial. *Lancet* 2005;366(9486):643-648.

Roodman GD: Mechanisms of bone metastasis. *N Engl J Med* 2004;350(16):1655-1664.

Rosenthal D, Callstrom MR: Critical review and state of the art in interventional oncology: Benign and metastatic disease involving bone. *Radiology* 2012;262(3):765-780.

Scolaro JA, Lackman RD: Surgical management of metastatic long bone fractures: Principles and techniques. *J Am Acad Orthop Surg* 2014;22:90-100.

Shiloh R, Krishnan M: Radiation for treatment of painful bone metastases. *Hematol Oncol Clin North Am* 2018;32:459-468.

Siegel RL, Miller KD, Jemal A: Cancer statistics, 2018. *CA Cancer J Clin* 2018;68:7-30.

Stopeck AT, Lipton A, Body J-J, et al: Denosumab compared with zoledronic acid for the treatment of bone metastases in patients with advanced breast cancer: A randomized, double-blind study. *J Clin Oncol* 2010;28(35):5132-5139.

Weber KL: Evaluation of the adult patient (aged >40 years) with a destructive bone lesion. *J Am Acad Orthop Surg* 2010;18:169-179.

Chapter 149
METABOLIC BONE AND INFLAMMATORY JOINT DISEASE

FRANK J. FRASSICA, MD

I. OSTEOPETROSIS (ALBERS-SCHONBERG DISEASE) (MARBLE BONE DISEASE)

A. Definition and demographics

1. Osteopetrosis is a rare disorder characterized by deficient formation or function of osteoclasts with resultant dense bone and no medullary cavity.
2. Autosomal recessive forms are diagnosed in children; the delayed type is more common and often is not diagnosed until adulthood.

B. Genetics/etiology

1. The lethal form is autosomal recessive.
2. The delayed type is autosomal dominant (the patients usually present with fractures).
3. If in a mouse model one deletes or knockouts the RANKL, the mouse gets osteopetrosis (this is not seen in humans).
4. When osteopetrosis occurs with renal tubular acidosis and cerebral calcification, an associated carbonic anhydrase II deficiency is present.
5. Deactivating mutations in multiple genes have been found. Major sites of the defects include:
   a. IKBKG gene—most cases of X-linked recessive
   b. *TCIRG1 ATPase* (*ATP6i*) gene mutation most common autosomal recessive form
   c. CNCL7 (chloride channel 7)—most of the autosomal dominant forms

C. Clinical presentation

1. Fracture (long bones, ribs, acromion)
2. Complications following tooth extraction due to poor tooth quality
3. Pancytopenia
4. Central nervous system and eye problems (lack of bone remodeling results in cranial nerve compression)
5. Short stature (in childhood form)
6. Hypocalcemia
7. Respiratory compromise

D. Radiographic appearance (**Figure 1**) (quite simply there is obliteration of the medullary cavity)

1. Symmetric increase in bone mass
2. Thickened cortical and trabecular bone
3. Often alternating sclerotic and lucent bands
4. Widened metaphyses (Erlenmeyer flask deformity)

E. Pathology

1. Islands or bars of calcified cartilage within mature trabeculae
2. Osteoclasts without ruffled borders

F. Treatment

1. Bone marrow transplantation for infantile form
2. Interferon gamma-1β for delayed type

II. ONCOGENIC OSTEOMALACIA (TUMOR-INDUCED OSTEOMALACIA)

A. Definition and demographics

1. **Oncogenic** c osteomalacia is a rare paraneoplastic syndrome of renal phosphate wasting caused by a bone or soft-tissue tumor that secretes a substance that leads to osteomalacia.
2. Tumor-overexpressed fibroblast growth factor-23 (FGF23), a phosphatonin, is responsible for hypophosphatemia and osteomalacia.

Neither Dr. Frassica nor any immediate family member has received anything of value from or has stock or stock options held in a commercial company or institution related directly or indirectly to the subject of this chapter.

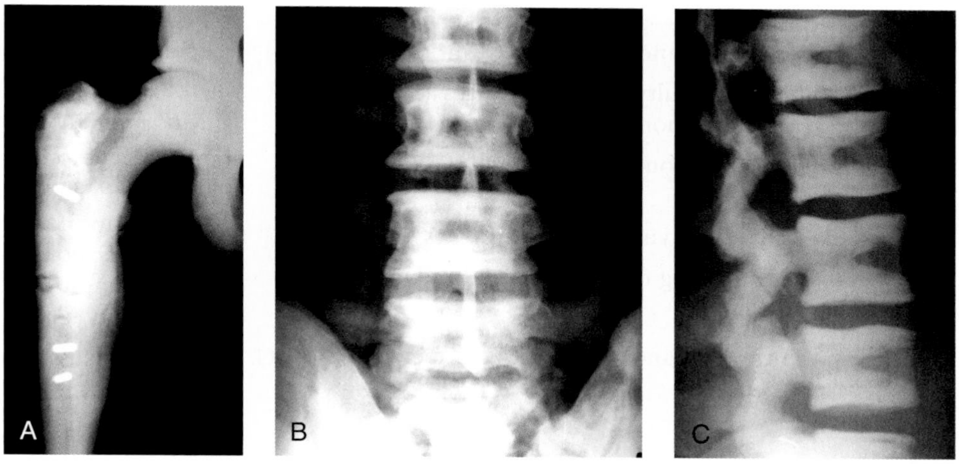

Figure 1 Osteopetrosis. **A**, AP radiograph of the hip in a patient with osteopetrosis. The medullary cavity is intensely sclerotic and is absent in the periacetabular region. **B**, AP view of the spine of a patient with osteopetrosis demonstrates the dense sclerosis at the superior and inferior end plates of the vertebral bodies. **C**, Lateral view of the lumbosacral spine showing the "rugger jersey" appearance. Note the complete obliteration of the medullary cavity.

3. A long delay in detecting the tumor, which may be very small, is common.

B. Genetics/etiology—Common bone and soft-tissue tumors that cause **oncogenic** osteomalacia:
   1. Phosphaturic mesenchymal tumor, mixed connective tissue type (majority)
   2. Hemangioma
   3. Hemangiopericytoma
   4. Giant cell tumor
   5. Osteoblastoma
   6. Nonossifying fibroma
   7. Sarcomas
   8. Nasal sinuses

C. Clinical presentation
   1. Progressive bone and muscle pain
   2. Weakness and fatigue
   3. Fractures of the long bones, ribs, and vertebrae

D. Imaging appearance
   1. Radiographs: diffuse osteopenia, pseudofractures
   2. Octreotide scan (indium-111-pentetreotide scintigraphy, radiolabeled somatostatin analogue): tumors can be detected

E. Laboratory features
   1. Hypophosphatemia
   2. Phosphaturia due to low proximal tubular reabsorption
   3. Low or normal serum 1,25-dihydroxyvitamin D level
   4. Elevated serum alkaline phosphatase level

F. Treatment
   1. Removal of the tumor
   2. Phosphate supplementation with 1,25-dihydroxyvitamin D

III. HYPERCALCEMIA OF MALIGNANCY

A. Definition and demographics
   1. Hypercalcemia may develop in 10% to 30% of patients with cancer and is a poor prognostic sign.
      a. Hypercalcemia with diffuse lytic metastases (20% of cases) is commonly associated with the following:
         - Breast cancer
         - Hematologic malignancies (eg, multiple myeloma, lymphoma, leukemia)
      b. Hypercalcemia without diffuse lytic metastases (80% of cases) is commonly associated with the following:
         - Squamous cell carcinoma
         - Renal or bladder carcinoma
         - Ovarian or endometrial cancer
         - Breast cancer

B. Genetics/etiology
   1. Humoral hypercalcemia due to secreted factors such as parathyroid-related hormone (most common cause is squamous cell tumor of the lung)
   2. Local osteolysis due to tumor invasion of bone
   3. Absorptive hypercalcemia due to excessive vitamin D produced by malignancies

C. Clinical presentation—proportional to the severity of calcium elevation and the rate of elevation
   1. Neurologic: difficulty concentrating, sleepiness, depression, confusion, coma
   2. Gastrointestinal: constipation, anorexia, nausea, vomiting
   3. Genitourinary: polyuria, dehydration
   4. Cardiac: shortening of QT interval, bradycardia, first-degree block

D. Radiographic appearance—Diffuse lytic metastases may be present.

E. Laboratory features
   1. Hypercalcemia
      a. Mild—10.5 to 11.9 mg/dL
      b. Moderate—12.0 to 13.9 mg/dL
      c. Severe—Greater than or equal to 14.0 mg/dL
   2. Normal or high serum phosphorus level
   3. Low parathyroid hormone level

F. Pathology—Osteoclastic bone resorption

G. Treatment
   1. Aggressive volume expansion with intravenous saline solution
   2. Diphosphonate therapy to halt osteoclastic bone resorption (usually intravenous pamidronate or zoledronic acid)
   3. Discontinuing all medications that increase serum calcium levels such as calcium, vitamin D, thiazide diuretics, lithium)
   4. Loop diuretics cautiously
   5. Combination therapy (chemotherapy and radiation) to kill the cancer cells

IV. PAGET DISEASE

A. Definition and demographics
   1. Paget disease is a remodeling disease characterized initially by increased osteoclast-mediated bone resorption and then disordered bone turnover.
   2. Usually occurs in patients older than 50 years

B. Genetics/etiology
   1. Caused by dysregulation of osteoclast differentiation and function
   2. Possibly caused by a slow viral infection (paramyxovirus, respiratory syncytial virus, canine distemper virus)
   3. Most common in Caucasians of Anglo-Saxon descent
   4. Strong genetic tendency (autosomal dominant)—Most important predisposing gene is *SQSTM1*, which harbors mutations that cause osteoclast activation in 5% to 20% of patients with a positive family history.

C. Clinical presentation
   1. No sex predilection
   2. May be monostotic or polyostotic; the number of sites remains constant.
   3. Common sites: femur, pelvis, tibia, skull, spine (often axial skeleton) (**Figure 2**)
   4. Often asymptomatic and found incidentally on a bone scan, chest radiograph, or in patients with elevated alkaline phosphatase levels
   5. Progresses through three phases
      a. Lytic phase
         - Profound resorption of the bone
         - Purely lucent on radiographs, with expansion and thinned but intact cortices
      b. Mixed phase: combination of osteolysis and bone formation with coarsened trabeculae
      c. Sclerotic phase: enlargement of the bone with thickened cortices and both sclerotic and lucent areas
   6. Bone pain may be present, possibly caused by increased vascularity and warmth or by stress fractures.
   7. Bowing of the femur or tibia
   8. Fractures, most commonly femoral neck
   9. Arthritis of the hip and knee
   10. Lumbar spinal stenosis
   11. Deafness
   12. Malignant degeneration
      a. Occurs in 1% of patients
      b. Most common locations: pelvis, femur, humerus
      c. Patients often note a marked increase in pain and may note a soft-tissue mass.

D. Laboratory features
   1. Increased alkaline phosphatase level (95%) of patients

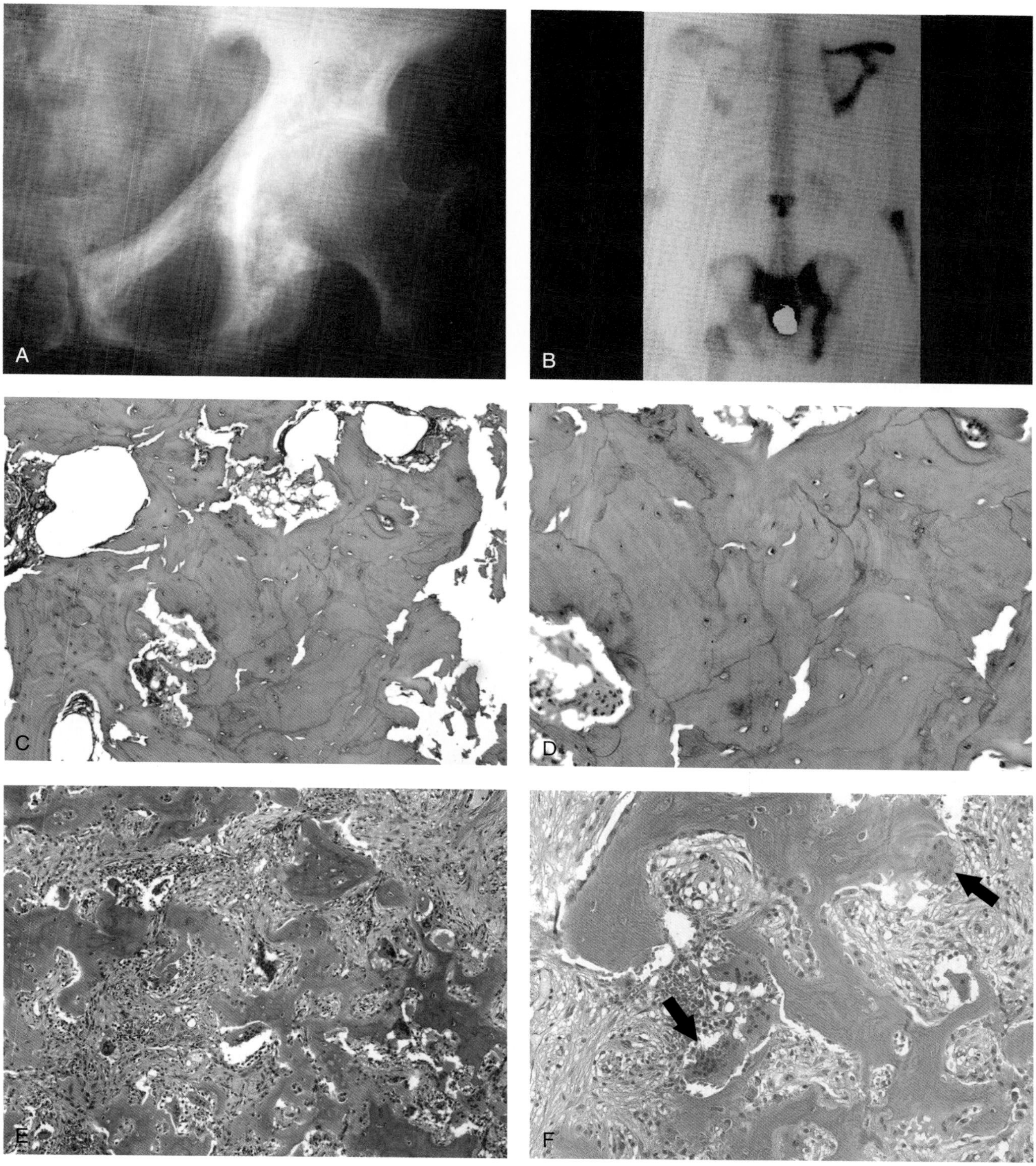

Figure 2 Paget disease. **A**, AP view of the pelvis in a patient with Paget disease. Note the coarsened trabeculae from the pubis to the supra-acetabular area and marked thickening of the iliopectineal line. **B**, Technetium Tc-99m bone scan of a patient with Paget disease. Note the intense uptake in the scapula, lumbar vertebral body, right ilium, and right ulna. **C** and **D**, Hematoxylin and eosin stain of pagetic bone. Note the disordered appearance of the bone and the multiple cement lines (curved blue lines). **E**, Low power hematoxylin/eosin stain demonstrating numerous giant cells and woven bone indicative of the lytic phase of Paget disease. **F**, High power hematoxylin/eosin stain demonstrating numerous giant cells and woven bone indicative of the lytic phase of Paget disease (black arrows pointing to the giant cells).

2. Increased urinary markers of bone turnover
   a. Collagen cross-links
   b. N-telopeptide, hydroxyproline, deoxypyridinoline
3. Normal calcium level

E. Imaging
1. Appearance on plain radiographs (**Figure 2**, A)
   a. Coarsened trabeculae
   b. Cortical thickening
   c. Lucent advancing edge ("blade of grass" or "flame-shaped") in active disease
   d. Loss of distinction between the cortices and medullary cavity
   e. Enlargement of the bone
2. Technetium Tc-99m bone scans—Increased uptake accurately marks sites of disease (**Figure 2**, B).
   a. Intense activity, which often outlines the shape of the bone, during the active phase
   b. Mild to moderate activity in the sclerotic phases
3. Appearance on CT scans
   a. Cortical thickening
   b. Coarsened trabeculae

F. Pathology
1. Profound osteoclastic bone resorption
2. Abnormal bone formation: mosaic pattern
   a. Woven bone and irregular sections of thickened trabecular bone
   b. Numerous cement lines

G. Treatment
1. Therapy is aimed at stopping the osteoclasts from resorbing bone.
2. Diphosphonates
   a. Oral agents: alendronate and risedronate
   b. Intravenous agents: pamidronate and zoledronic acid

V. OSTEONECROSIS (BONE INFARCT)

A. Osteonecrosis is the death of bone cells and bone marrow secondary to a loss of blood supply.

B. Genetics/etiology
1. Four mechanisms have been proposed.
   a. Mechanical disruption of the blood vessels (trauma, such as a hip dislocation)
   b. Arterial vessel occlusion: nitrogen bubbles (bends), sickle cell disease, fat emboli
   c. Injury or pressure on the blood vessel wall: marrow diseases (such as Gaucher), vasculitis, radiation injury
   d. Venous outflow obstruction
2. Associated with hypercoagulable states
   a. Decreased anticoagulants—proteins C, S
   b. Increased procoagulants

C. Clinical presentation—The patient may present with a dull pain in the joint or severe arthritic pain with collapse of the joint, or may be asymptomatic.

D. Imaging
1. Appearance on radiographs
   a. Initially normal
   b. Sclerosis and cyst formation
   c. Subchondral fracture (crescent sign), subchondral collapse
   d. Arthritic changes: osteophytes, loss of joint space
2. Appearance on MRI: characteristic marrow changes in the metaphyseal marrow and subchondral locations (**Figure 3**)

E. Pathology
1. Osteocyte death (no cells in the bone lacunae)
2. Marrow necrosis
3. Loss of the vascular supply

F. Treatment
1. Core decompression or vascularized bone graft if the joint surfaces remain intact (no collapse)
2. Arthroplasty or osteotomy for joint collapse

VI. RHEUMATOID ARTHRITIS

A. Definition and demographics
1. Rheumatoid arthritis is a systemic inflammatory disease of the synovium.
2. Twice as common in females as in males
3. According to the American College of Rheumatology revised criteria (2010), the patient must score at least 6 points based on joint distribution, serology, symptom duration, and presence of acute-phase reactants (**Table 1**). Radiographs are no longer required for diagnosis.

B. Genetics/etiology
1. Genetic marker HLA-DR4 (in patients of northern European descent)

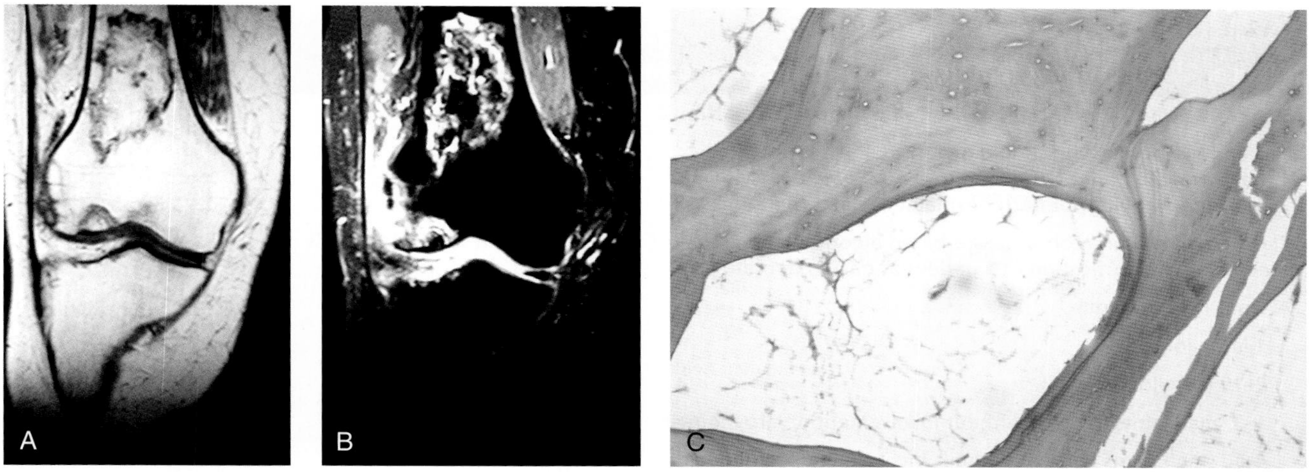

Figure 3 Osteonecrosis. **A**, T1-weighted coronal MRI of the knee of a patient with osteonecrosis shows a large metaphyseal lesion and a wedge-shaped area of necrosis at the subchondral region of the lateral femoral condyle. **B**, T2-weighted coronal MRI of the knee of a patient with osteonecrosis demonstrates a large metaphyseal lesion with a large subchondral wedge-shaped lesion in the lateral femur. **C**, Hematoxylin and eosin stain demonstrates the complete loss of the bone marrow and an absence of osteocytes in the trabecular lacunae.

2. Monozygotic twins have a concordance rate of 15% to 30% while dizygotic twins have a concordance rate of only 5%
3. HLA-DRB1 (self versus nonself)

C. Clinical presentation
1. Morning stiffness, pain
2. Joint swelling (most prominent in small joints of the hands and feet)
    a. Effusions
    b. Synovial proliferation
3. Hand deformities: metacarpophalangeal joint, subluxation, ulnar drift of the fingers, swan-neck deformity, boutonniere deformity

D. Imaging appearance (**Figure 4**)
1. Periarticular osteopenia
2. Juxta-articular erosions
3. Joint space narrowing

E. Laboratory features
1. Approximately 90% of patients are positive for rheumatoid factor.
2. Elevation of acute-phase reactants: erythrocyte sedimentation rate (ESR), C-reactive protein (CRP) level

F. Pathology—Inflammatory infiltrate destroys cartilage, ligaments, and bone.

G. Treatment
1. Nonsteroidal anti-inflammatory drugs
2. Aspirin
3. Disease-modifying antirheumatic drugs (DMARDs)
    a. Methotrexate (current treatment of choice)
    b. Others (D-penicillamine, sulfasalazine, gold, antimalarials)
4. Cytokine-neutralizing
    a. Etanercept (soluble p75 tumor necrosis factor [TNF] receptor immunoglobulin G–fusion protein)
    b. Infliximab (chimeric monoclonal antibody to TNF-α)
    c. Rituximab (monoclonal antibody to CD20 antigen; inhibits B-cells)
5. Physical therapy—To maintain joint motion and muscle strength.

VII. ANKYLOSING SPONDYLITIS (MARIE-STRUMPELL DISEASE)

A. Definition and demographics
1. Inflammatory disorder that affects the spine, sacroiliac joints, and large joints (hip) in young adults
2. Male-to-female ratio = 3:1

B. Genetics/etiology
1. Ninety percent of patients have HLA-B27.
2. Autoimmune disorder

TABLE 1

Clinical Classification of Rheumatoid Arthritis: A Scoring System

2010 ACR-EULAR Classification Criteria for Rheumatoid Arthritis	Score
Target population (Who should be tested?): Patients who 1. have at least 1 joint with definite clinical synovitis (swelling)[a] 2. with the synovitis not better explained by another disease[b]	
Classification criteria for RA (score-based algorithm: add score of categories A-D; a score of ≥ 6/10 is needed for classification of a patient as having definite RA)[c]	
A. Joint involvement[d]	
1 large joint[e]	0
2–10 large joints	1
1–3 small joints (with or without involvement of large joints)[f]	2
4–10 small joints (with or without involvement of large joints)	3
>10 joints (at least one small joint)[g]	5
B. Serology (at least one test result is needed for classification)[h]	
Negative RF *and* negative ACPA	0
Low-positive RF *or* low-positive ACPA	2
High-positive RF or high-positive ACPA	3
C. Acute-phase reactants (at least one test result is needed for classification)[i]	
Normal CRP *and* normal ESR	0
Abnormal CRP *or* abnormal ESR	1
D. Duration of symptoms[j]	
< 6 wk	0
≥ 6 wk	1

Reproduced with permission from Aletaha D, Neogi T, Silman AJ, et al: 2010 Rheumatoid arthritis classification criteria: An American College of Rheumatology/European League Against Rheumatism collaborative initiative. *Arthritis Rheum* 2010;62(9):2569-2581.

[a]The criteria are aimed at classification of newly presenting patients. In addition, patients with erosive disease typical of RA with a history compatible with prior fulfillment of the 2010 criteria should be classified as having RA. Patients with long-standing disease, including those whose disease is inactive (with or without treatment) and who, based on retrospectively available data, have previously fulfilled the 2010 criteria should be classified as having RA.

[b]Differential diagnoses vary among patients with different presentations, but may include conditions such as systemic lupus erythematosus, psoriatic arthritis, and gout. If it is unclear about the relevant differential diagnoses to consider, an expert rheumatologist should be consulted.

[c]Although patients with a score of < 6/10 are not classifiable as having RA, their status can be reassessed and the criteria might be fulfilled cumulatively over time.

[d]Joint involvement refers to any swollen or tender joint on examination, which may be confirmed by imaging evidence of synovitis. Distal interphalangeal joints, first carpometacarpal joints, and first metatarsophalangeal joints are excluded from assessment. Categories of joint distribution are classified according to the location and number of involved joints, with placement into the highest category possible based on the pattern of joint involvement.

[e]"Large joints" refers to shoulders, elbows, hips, knees, and ankles.

[f]"Small joints" refers to the metacarpophalangeal joints, proximal interphalangeal joints, second through fifth metatarsophalangeal joints, thumb interphalangeal joints, and wrists.

[g]In this category, at least one of the involved joints must be a small joint; the other joints can include any combination of large and additional small joints, as well as other joints not specifically listed elsewhere (eg, temporomandibular, acromioclavicular, sternoclavicular).

[h]Negative refers to IU values that are less than or equal to the upper limit of normal (ULN) for the laboratory and assay; low-positive refers to IU values that are higher than the ULN but ≤ 3 times the ULN for the laboratory and assay; high-positive refers to IU values that are > 3 times the ULN for the laboratory and assay. Where RF information is only available as positive or negative, a positive result should be scored as low-positive for RF.

[i]Normal/abnormal is determined by local laboratory standards.

[j]Duration of symptoms refers to patient self-report of the duration of signs or symptoms of synovitis (eg, pain, swelling, tenderness) of joints that are clinically involved at the time of assessment, regardless of treatment status.

ACPA = anticitrullinated protein antibody, ACR-EULAR = American College of Rheumatology/European League Against Rheumatism, CRP = C-reactive protein, ESR = erythrocyte sedimentation rate, RA = rheumatoid arthritis, RF = rheumatoid factor

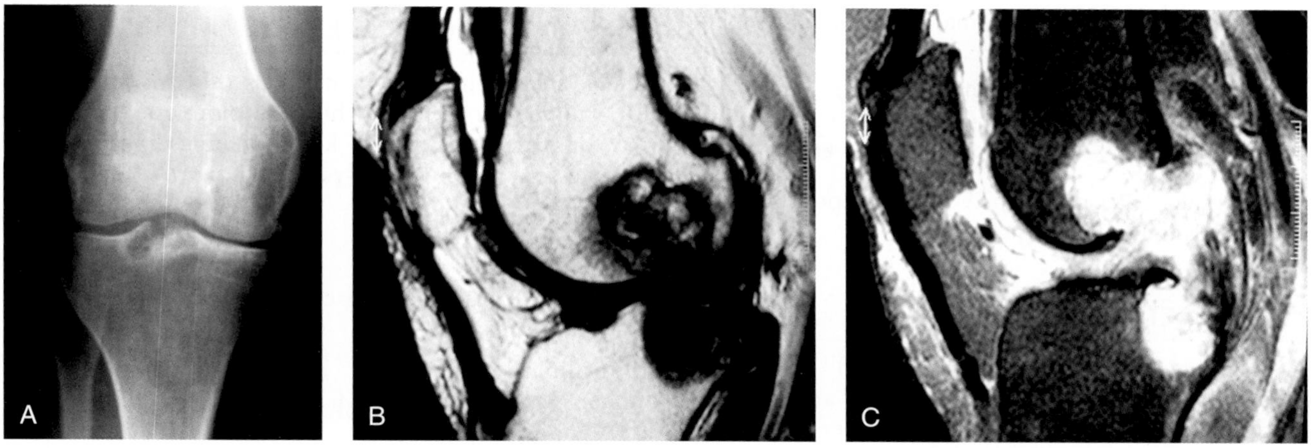

Figure 4 Rheumatoid arthritis. **A**, AP radiograph of the knee shows a subchondral cyst in the proximal tibia with narrowing of the medial compartment of the knee. **B**, T1-weighted sagittal MRI of the knee shows a large subchondral lesion in the distal femur and proximal tibia and an erosion on the tibial condylar surface. **C**, T2-weighted sagittal MRI of the knee demonstrates a large erosion on the distal femur and proximal tibia, an effusion, and diffuse synovial thickening.

a. High levels of TNF are found.

b. CD4+, CD8+ T cells are present

C. Clinical presentation

1. Young adults
2. Low back and pelvic pain
3. Morning stiffness
4. Hip arthritis in approximately one-third of patients
5. Uveitis: pain, light sensitivity
6. Heart involvement
   a. Aortic valve insufficiency
   b. Third-degree heart block

D. Radiographic appearance

1. Sacroiliac joint inflammation
   a. Blurring of subchondral margins
   b. Erosions
   c. Bony bridging
2. Cervical spine involvement
   a. Fracture may occur in the cervical spine and be unnoticed on plain radiographs
      - CT or MRI should be used to detect an occult fracture
3. Lumbar spine involvement (**Figure 5**)
   a. Loss of lumbar lordosis
   b. Squaring of the vertebrae
   c. Osteophytes bridging the vertebrae

E. Pathology

1. Laboratory findings
   a. HLA-B27 in 90% of patients
   b. Elevated ESR and CRP level
2. Inflammation of ligamentous attachment sites
   a. Erosions, subchondral inflammation
   b. Ossification of joints (sacroiliac joint)

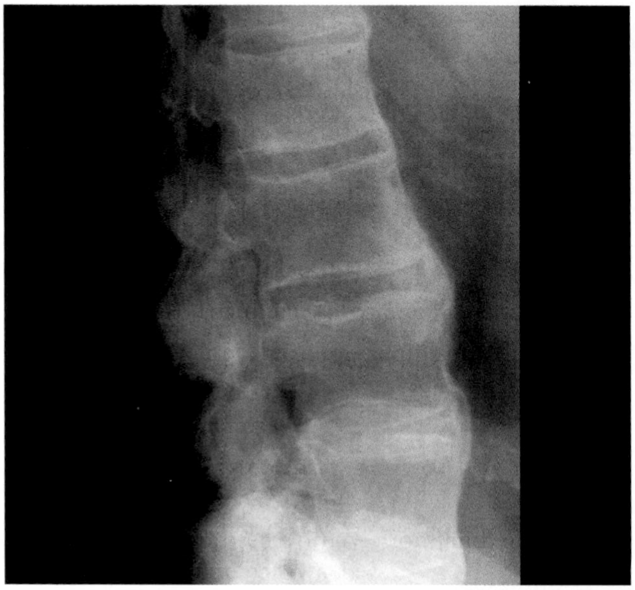

Figure 5 Lateral radiograph of the spine of a patient with ankylosing spondylitis. Note the anterior osteophytes bridging all the lumbar vertebrae.

3. Arthritis—Pannus formation with lymphoid infiltration

F. Treatment: anti-TNF therapy

1. Infliximab (chimeric monoclonal antibody to TNF-α)
2. Etanercept (soluble p75 TNF receptor immunoglobulin G–fusion protein)

VIII. REACTIVE ARTHRITIS

A. Reactive arthritis (formerly called Reiter syndrome) is a type of inflammatory arthritis that occurs after an infection at another site in the body.

B. Genetics/etiology—Affected individuals are genetically predisposed (high incidence of HLA-B27).

C. Clinical presentation

1. An infection will have occurred 1 to 8 weeks before the onset of the arthritis.
   a. Post venereal type—*Chlamydia trachomatis*
   b. Post enteric type—*Salmonella*, *Shigella*, *Campylobacter*, *Yersinia*
2. Common extraskeletal involvement
   a. Urethritis, prostatitis
   b. Uveitis
   c. Mucocutaneous involvement
3. Systemic symptoms: fatigue, malaise, fever, weight loss
4. Arthritis is asymmetric.
5. Common sites include the knee, ankle, subtalar joint, and metatarsophalangeal and interphalangeal joints.
6. Tendinitis/fasciitis (common)
   a. Achilles tendon insertion
   b. Plantar fascia
7. Recurrent joint symptoms and tendinitis are common even after treatment.

D. Radiographic appearance

1. Juxta-articular erosions
2. Joint destruction

E. Pathology

1. Synovial inflammation
2. Enthesitis

F. Treatment: indomethacin and referral to a rheumatologist

IX. SYSTEMIC LUPUS ERYTHEMATOSUS

A. Systemic lupus erythematosus (SLE) is an autoimmune disorder in which autoimmune complexes damage joints, skin, kidneys, lungs, heart, blood vessels, and nervous system.

B. Genetics/etiology

1. Multiple genes
2. HLA class II, HLA class III, HLA-DR, HLA-DQ are associated

C. Clinical presentation

1. Multiple joint involvement
2. Osteonecrosis of the hips (common, especially in patients taking glucocorticoids)

D. Radiographic appearance

1. Erosions or joint destruction (uncommon)
2. Osteonecrosis may be seen as a result of corticosteroid treatment.

E. Pathology—Antinuclear antibodies are present in 95% of patients.

1. Anti-ds DNA

F. Treatment

1. Analgesics
2. Glucocorticoids
3. Antimalarials
4. Immunosuppressive medications
   a. Cyclophosphamide
   b. Azathioprine
   c. Methotrexate

X. GOUT

A. Definition and demographics

1. Gout is a metabolic disorder manifested by uric acid crystals in the synovium.
2. Affects older men and postmenopausal women.
3. Prevalence is increasing.

B. Clinical presentation

1. Involvement of a single joint is common.
2. Gout is often polyarticular in men with hypertension and alcohol abuse.
3. Involved joints are intensely painful, swollen, and erythematous.

C. Radiographic appearance (**Figure 6**, A)

1. Periarticular erosions

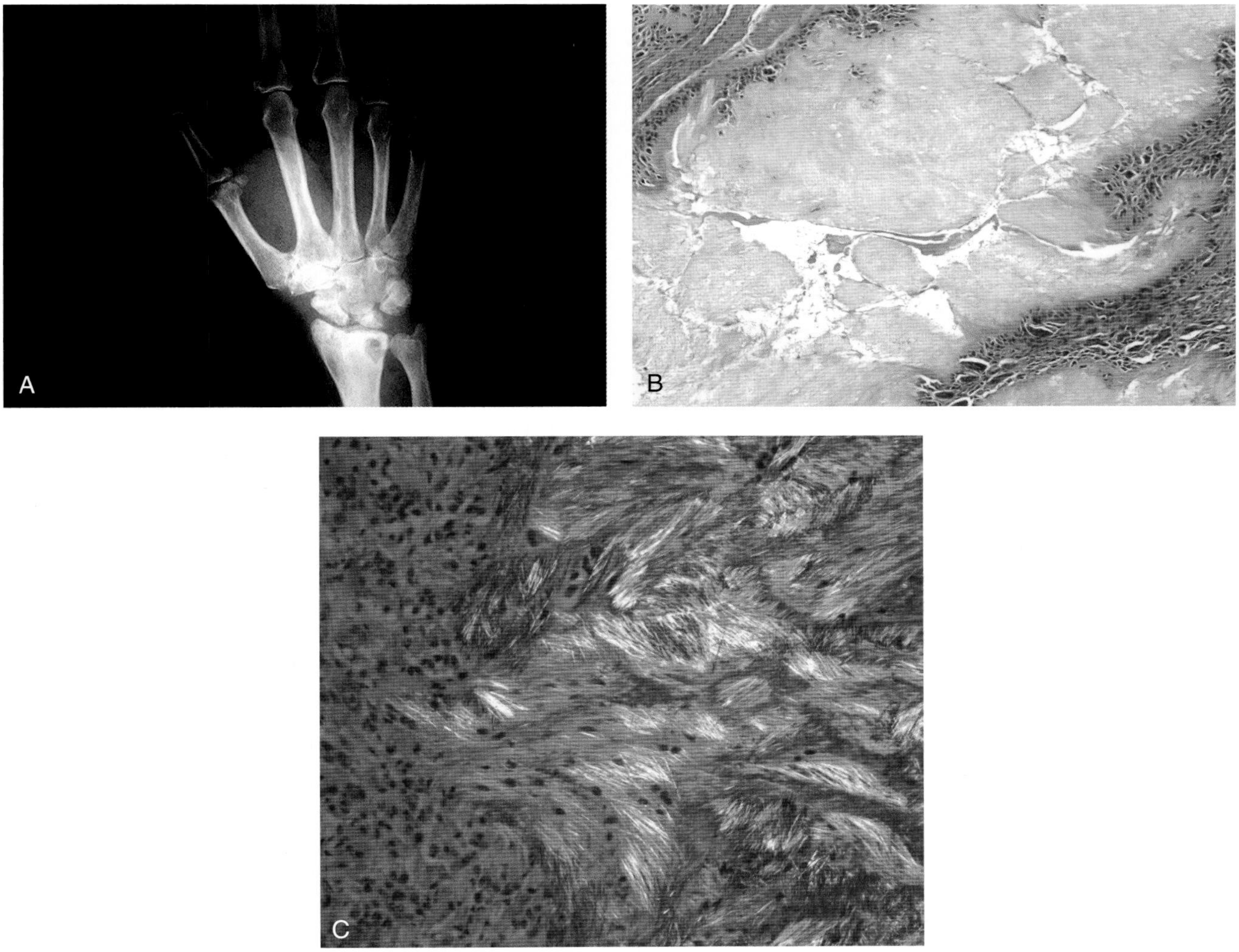

Figure 6 Gout. **A**, PA radiograph of the hand of a patient with gout shows a lucent lesion in the distal radius and erosive changes in the carpal bones. **B**, Hematoxylin and eosin stain of a lesion in a patient with gout. Note that the tophaceous areas are amorphous and white and are bordered by inflammatory cells. **C**, Birefringent crystals of gout (white needle-shaped objects). Note the reactive inflammatory cells on the left side of the figure.

2. The peripheral margin of the erosion often has a thin overlying rim of bone (cliff sign).

D. Pathology

1. Joint aspiration is the only definitive diagnostic procedure. Needle- and rod-shaped crystals with negative birefringence are seen.
2. Joint white blood cell count is usually less than 50,000 to 60,000/μL.
3. Serum uric acid level is often elevated (but not always).
4. Hematoxylin and eosin staining shows amorphous material and inflammatory cells (**Figure 6**, B).

E. Treatment

1. Nonsteroidal anti-inflammatory drugs
2. Colchicine
3. Hypouricemic therapy: allopurinol, probenecid

XI. OSTEOPOROSIS

A. Definition and demographics

1. Characteristics
   a. Low bone mass
   b. Microarchitectural deterioration
   c. Fractures

2. Bone mass is acquired between 2 and 30 years of age; failure to attain adequate bone mass during this period is one of the main determinants in the development of osteoporosis. Peak bone mass (PBM) is related to the development of osteoporosis.
3. World Health Organization definition (T-score is comparison to patients at PBM, whereas Z-score is a comparison to patients of a similar age)
   a. Normal: within 1 SD of PBM (T-score = 0 to −1.0)
   b. Low bone mass (osteopenia): 1.0 to 2.5 SDs below PBM (T-score = −1.0 to −2.5)
   c. Osteoporosis: more than 2.5 SDs below PBM (T-score < −2.5)

B. Genetics/etiology
1. Causes are multifactorial.
2. Withdrawal of estrogen is one of the main causes in women; this deficiency results in an increase in receptor activator of nuclear factor κB ligand expression.
3. Genetic predisposition is important.
4. Genes associated with the development of osteoporosis
   a. *COL1A1*
   b. Vitamin D receptor
   c. *LRP5* (codes for low-density lipoprotein receptor–related protein)

C. Clinical presentation
1. Patient usually presents with a fracture following minor trauma.
2. Low bone mineral density (found on routine screening)
3. Most important risk factors
   a. Increasing age (geriatric patient)
   b. Female sex
   c. Early menopause
   d. Fair-skinned
   e. Maternal/paternal history of hip fracture
   f. Low body weight
   g. Cigarette smoking
   h. Glucocorticoid use
   i. Excessive alcohol use
   j. Low protein intake
   k. Anticonvulsant or antidepressant use

D. Radiographic appearance
1. Osteopenia
2. Thinning of the cortices
3. Loss of trabecular bone

E. Pathology
1. Loss of trabecular bone
2. Loss of continuity of the trabecular bone

F. Treatment
1. Adequate calcium and vitamin D intake
2. Antiresorptive therapy for patients with osteoporosis
3. Diphosphonates (analogues of pyrophosphate). The potency of diphosphonates is related to their chemical structure.
   a. Actions: cause apoptosis of the osteoclast and withdrawing of the osteoclast from the bone surface (hence, bone resorption is halted).
   b. Mechanism
      - Inhibit protein prenylation
      - Act via the mevalonate pathway
      - Specifically inhibit farnesyl pyrophosphate
      - Disrupt the ruffled border of osteoclasts
   c. Side effects
      - Myalgias, bone pain, or weakness (up to one-third of patients) (when delivered in intravenously in up to 25% of patients)
      - Gastric irritation (when delivered orally)
      - Osteonecrosis of the jaw (occurs in patients on long-term therapy, most common in the myeloma patient on intravenous zoledronic acid)
         - Patient who are candidates for diphosphonate therapy should undergo a dental evaluation before starting treatment.
      - Atypical fractures of the subtrochanteric and diaphyseal areas of the femur (stress fractures)
      - Atrial fibrillation
4. Anabolic therapy with parathyroid hormone 1 to 34 (PTH [1-34]) (teriparatide).
   a. Indications: Intermittent PTH at a low dose is an anabolic factor in the treatment of osteoporosis. Teriparatide is approved for the treatment of osteoporosis in women and men at high risk for fracture (T-score less than −3.0 with or without

a history of previous fragility fracture). The maximum period of administration is 2 years.

b. Mechanism: The precise mechanism is unknown, although PTH most likely has direct and indirect effects positive for osteoblast differentiation, function, and survival.

c. Side effects: mild hypercalcemia

d. Contraindications: children, active Paget disease, hypercalcemia, previous history of irradiation (risk of development of osteosarcoma)

TOP TESTING FACTS

1. Osteopetrosis is a rare disorder characterized by a failure of osteoclastic resorption with resultant dense bone with no medullary cavity (prone to fracture).
2. Oncogenic osteomalacia is a paraneoplastic syndrome characterized by renal phosphate wasting. It is caused by a variety of bone and soft-tissue tumors (osteoblastoma, hemangiopericytoma, and phosphaturic mesenchymal tumor).
3. Hypercalcemia may occur as a complication of breast cancer, multiple myeloma, lymphoma, lung cancer, and leukemia.
4. Paget disease is a remodeling disease characterized by disordered bone formation; it is treated with diphosphonates.
5. Rheumatoid arthritis is a systemic inflammatory disorder characterized by morning stiffness and joint pain; approximately 90% of patients are positive for rheumatoid factor.
6. Ankylosing spondylitis is an inflammatory disorder of the spine and sacroiliac joints characterized by HLA-B27 positivity; it is treated with anti-TNF therapy.
7. Gout is a metabolic disorder caused by uric acid crystals in the synovium, resulting in periarticular erosions.
8. Osteoporosis is characterized by low bone mass (>2.5 SDs below the mean) and an increased risk of fracture.
9. The action of diphosphonates is through inhibition (apoptosis) of osteoclasts through protein prenylation. The specific enzyme inhibited is farnesyl pyrophosphate.
10. Possible side effects of diphosphonate therapy: atypical stress fractures of the subtrochanteric and diaphyseal region of the femur.
11. Intermittent PTH (teriparatide) is approved for patients at high risk for osteoporotic fractures.

Bibliography

Bukata SV, Tyler WK: Metabolic bone disease, in O'Keefe RJ, Jacobs JJ, Chu CR, Einhorn TA, eds: *Orthopaedic Basic Science: Foundations of Clinical Practice*, ed 4. Rosemont, IL, American Academy of Orthopaedic Surgeons, 2013, pp 331-333.

Canalis E, Giustina A, Bilezikian JP: Mechanisms of anabolic therapies for osteoporosis. *N Engl J Med* 2007;357(9):905-916.

Carter JD: Treating reactive arthritis: Insights for the clinician. *Ther Adv* 2(1):45-54, 2010.

Chong WH, Molinolo AA, Chen CC, Collins MT: Tumor-induced osteomalacia. *Endocr Relat Cancer* 2011;18(3):R53-R77.

Fauci AS, Langford CA, eds: *Harrison's Rheumatology*. New York, NY, McGraw-Hill, 2010.

Favus MJ: Bisphosphonates for osteoporosis. *N Engl J Med* 2010;363(21):2027-2035.

Goldner W. Cancer-related hyercalcemia. *J Oncol Pract* 2016;12(5):426-432.

Jiang Y, Xia WB, Xing XP, et al: Tumor-induced osteomalacia: An important cause of adult-onset hypophosphatemic osteomalacia in China. Report of 39 cases and review of the literature. *J Bone Miner Res* 2012;27(9):1967-1975.

Kuhn A, Bonsmann G, Anders HJ, Herzer P, Tenvrock K, Schneider M: The diagnosis and treatment of systemic lupus erythematosus. *Dtsch Arztebl* 2015;112(25):423-432.

Neogi T: Gout. *N Engl J Med* 2011;364:443-452.

Ralston SH, Layfield R: Pathogenesis of Paget disease of bone. *Calcif Tissue Int* 2012;91(2):97-113.

Ralston SH: Pagets disease of bone. *N Engl J Med* 2013;368:644-650.

Rosen CJ, ed: *Primer on the Metabolic Bone Diseases and Disorders of Mineral Metabolism*, ed 8. Washington, DC, American Society for Bone and Mineral Research, 2013.

Rosner MH, Dalkin AC: Onco-nephrology: The pathophysiology and treatment of malignancy-associated hypercalcemia. *Clin J Am Soc Nephrol* 2012;7(10):1722-1729.

Siris ES, Roodman GD: *Paget's Disease of Bone*, ed 6. Washington, DC, American Society for Bone and Mineral Research, 2006, pp 320-329.

Shekelle PG, Newberry SJ, Fitzgerald JD, et al: Management of gout: A systematic review in support of an American College of Physicians Clinical Practice Guideline. *Ann Intern Med* 2017;166(1):37-51.

Sozen T, Ozisik L, Basaran NC: An overview and management of osteoporosis. *Eur J Rheum* 2017;4(1):46-56.

Steward CG: Hematopoietic stem cell transplantation for osteopetrosis. *Pediatr Clin North Am* 2010;57(1):171-180.

Tolar J, Teitalabaum SL, Orchard PJ: Osteopetrosis. *N Engl J Med* 2004;351:2839-2849.

Tsokos T: The diagnosis and treatment of systemic lupus erythematosus. *N Engl J Med* 2011;365:2110-2121.

Werner BC, Samartzis D, Shen FS: Spinal fractrues in patients with ankylosing spondylitis. *J Am Acad Orthop Surg* 2016;24(4):241-249.

Index

Note: Page numbers followed by "f" indicate figures, "t" indicates tables.

D

E

F

G

J

K

P

Q

R

S

U

V

